PRINCIPLES AND PRACTICE OF
CARDIOPULMONARY PHYSICAL THERAPY

THIRD EDITION

PRINCIPLES AND PRACTICE OF
CARDIOPULMONARY PHYSICAL THERAPY
THIRD EDITION

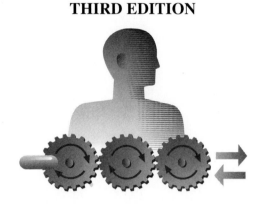

Edited by:

Donna Frownfelter, MA, PT, CCS, RRT
NovaCare, Inc.
Contract Services
Region 7
Northwestern University
Programs in Physical Therapy
Chicago, Illinois
Committed to Excellence
Glenview, Illinois

Elizabeth Dean, PhD, PT
Associate Professor
University of British Columbia
School of Rehabilition Sciences
Vancouver, British Columbia

With 22 contributors and 401 illustrations

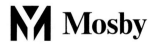 Mosby

St. Louis Baltimore Boston Carlsbad Chicago Naples New York Philadelphia Portland
London Madrid Mexico City Singapore Sydney Tokyo Toronto Wiesbaden

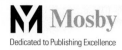

Dedicated to Publishing Excellence

A Times Mirror
Company

Vice President and Publisher: Don Ladig
Editor: Martha Sasser
Developmental Editors: Kellie White, Amy Dubin
Project Manager: Deborah L. Vogel
Production Editor: Mamata Reddy
Designer: Pati Pye
Manufacturing Supervisor: Linda Ierardi

THIRD EDITION

Printed in the United States of America
Composition by Times Mirror Higher Education Group, Inc. Print Group
Printing/binding by R.R. Donnelley & Sons Company

Mosby-Year Book, Inc.
11830 Westline Industrial Drive
St. Louis, Missouri 63146

**International Standard Book Number
0-8151-3340-5**

96 97 98 99 00 / 9 8 7 6 5 4 3 2 1

CONTRIBUTORS

Michael Wade Baskin, PT, RRT
Owner/Executive Director
GT Physical Therapy and Rehabilitation
West Point, Mississippi

Jean K. Berry, PhD, RN
Senior Research Specialist
Medical-Surgical Nursing
University of Illinois at Chicago
Chicago, Illinois

Gary Brooks, MS, PT, CCS
Associate Professor
Health and Rehabilitation Sciences
The Sage Colleges
Troy, New York

Susan M. Butler, MMSc, PT, CCS
Division of Physical Therapy
Department of Rehabilitation Medicine
Maine Medical Center
Portland, Maine

Margaret K. Covey, MS, RN
Senior Research Specialist and Doctoral Candidate
Medical-Surgical Nursing
University of Illinois at Chicago
Chicago, Illinois

Linda D. Crane, MMSc, PT, CCS
Instructor
Division of Physical Therapy
University of Miami School of Medicine
Miami, Florida

Anne Mejia Downs, PT, CCS
Department of Physical and Occupational Therapy
Instructor, Division of Physical Therapy
Department of Medical Allied Health Professions
School of Medicine
University of North Carolina
Chapel Hill, North Carolina

Willy E. Hammon, BSc, PT
Chief of Rehabilitative Services
The University Hospitals
Special Instructor in Physical Therapy
College of Health
Clinical Instructor, College of Nursing
University of Oklahoma Health Sciences Center
Oklahoma City, Oklahoma

Scott M. Hasson, EdD, PT
Director
Advanced Studies
School of Physical Therapy
Texas Woman's University
Houston, Texas

Lyn Hobson, PT, RRT
Rush-Presbyterian-St. Luke's Medical Center
Chicago, Illinois

Gail M. Huber, MHPE, PT
Instructor
Programs in Physical Therapy
Northwestern University
Chicago, Illinois

Thomas Johnson, MD
Associate Professor in Radiological Sciences
University of Oklahoma Health Sciences Center
Oklahoma City, Oklahoma

Phyllis G. Krug, MS, PT, CCS
President, Long Life, Inc.
Teaneck, New Jersey

Susan K. Ludwick, MS, PT
Supervisor, Rehabilitation Therapy Services
Henry Ford Hospital
Detroit, Michigan

Mary Massery, PT
President, Massery Physical Therapy
Glenview, Illinois
Adjunct Faculty
Programs in Physical Therapy
Northwestern University
Chicago, Illinois

Mary Mathews, BS, RN, CCRN, RRT
Neonatal and Pediatrics Chest Physical Therapist
Coordinator
Respiratory Care Services
Rush-Presbyterian-St. Luke's Medical Center
Chicago, Illinois

Lisa Sigg Mendelson, MS, RN, CPAN
Practitioner-Teacher, College of Nursing
Rush Presbyterian-St. Luke's Medical Center
Rush University
Chicago, Illinois

Victoria A. Moerchen, MS, PT
Doctoral Candidate in Motor Control
Department of Kinesiology
Staff Physical Therapist
Bridges-For-Families Early Intervention
Waisman Center
Pediatric Consultant and Lecturer
University of Wisconsin
Madison, Wisconsin

Claire Peel, PhD, PT
Department of Physical Therapy
School of Pharmacy and Allied Health Professions
Creighton University
Omaha, Nebraska

Arthur V. Prancan, PhD
Associate Professor
Department of Pharmacology
Rush Medical College
Chicago, Illinois

Elizabeth J. Protas, PhD, PT, FACSM
Assistant Dean and Professor
School of Physical Therapy
Texas Woman's University
Houston, Texas

Michael Ries, MD, FCCP
Assistant Professor of Medicine
Rush Medical College
Chicago, Illinois

Susan Scherer, MA, PT
Assistant Professor
Physical Therapy Program
University of Colorado Health Sciences Center
Denver, Colorado

Alexandra J. Sciaky, MS, PT, CCS
Education Coordinator
University of Michigan Medical Center
Physical Therapy Division
Physical Medicine and Rehabilitation Department
Ann Arbor, Michigan

Maureen Shekleton, DNSc, RN, FAAN
Satellite Site Coordinator
DuPage Community Clinic
Wheaton, Illinois
Adjunct Clinical Faculty
Rush University College of Nursing
University of Illinois College of Nursing
Chicago, Illinois

To our students
—Past, Present, and Future—
For Their Inspiration, Inquiry, and Enthusiasm

CONTEMPORARY DEFINITION OF
CARDIOPULMONARY PHYSICAL THERAPY

The purpose of cardiopulmonary physical therapy (CPPT) is to prevent, mitigate, or reverse cardiopulmonary dysfunction, and hence, the impairment of or threat to oxygen transport. Oxygen transport refers to the delivery, uptake, and extraction of oxygen at the tissue level, thus it reflects the adequacy of the structure and function of the airways, lungs, pulmonary circulation, blood, heart, peripheral circulation, microcirculation, and tissue. CPPT refers to the prescription for and delivery of noninvasive interventions in the comprehensive management (diagnosis, assessment, treatment, and follow-up) of patients with primary or secondary cardiopulmonary dysfunction resulting from acute, chronic, and acute-on-chronic conditions, and the cardiopulmonary/cardiovascular manifestations of systemic disease. CPPT interventions include mobilization, exercise, body positioning, breathing control, coughing and airway clearance maneuvers, and manual techniques. Wherever possible and appropriate, CPPT is applied to optimize oxygen transport and to thereby replace, augment, or reduce the need for invasive medical and surgical management including pharmacological agents. Patient education and patient-driven treatment planning are fundamental components of CPPT. In addition, CPPT has an essential role in the promotion of optimal cardiopulmonary and cardiovascular health and fitness in the general population.

FOREWORD

Donna Frownfelter and Elizabeth Dean have succeeded in creating a unique set of resources for students and clinicians. The importance of the oxygen transport mechanism is woven throughout this text and accompanying case study book, *Clinical Case Study Guide*. The disruption of the mechanism can create cardiopulmonary dysfunction and can result in reduced function, reduced functional work capacity, and death. A comprehensive understanding of oxygen transport and the factors that determine and influence it is therefore essential in order to assess the deficits of the mechanism and determine treatment interventions.

The third edition of *Principles and Practice of Cardiopulmonary Physical Therapy* is not simply a new edition of the former, *Chest Physical Therapy and Pulmonary Rehabilitation*. It is a totally new textbook, encompassing both the cardiac and pulmonary systems in health and dysfunction. The two previous editions have been praised for their clinical relevance. The new books go a long way to support the state of the art clinical practice with documented scientific literature.

The authors have many years of experience teaching undergraduate students as well as consulting and teaching in professional postgraduate courses. These books have been written in response to questions and concerns raised by students and clinicians. This is the only text in which Mary Massery has published her work on neuropulmonary rehabilitation. Several chapters emphasize positioning for respiratory success and ventilatory strategies to improve rehabilitation potential.

The books are very user-friendly. Each chapter of the text has key terms and questions for discussion to help the reader focus on the important concepts presented in the chapter. The combination of the text and case study guide will be an asset in teaching cardiopulmonary physical therapy. However, either book can be effectively used independently of the other. The case study guide can be of assistance to physical therapists in helping them focus on patient evaluation, cardiopulmonary dysfunction, and treatment approaches. I applaud the authors for these new books and would highly recommend them for students and clinicians.

Sally C. Edelsberg, MS, PT
Director and Associate Professor
Programs in Physical Therapy
Northwestern University Medical School

PREFACE

The work that has gone into this third edition has resulted in a completely new book! When we first discussed the possibilities of a new edition, we knew it would be a total change from *Chest Physical Therapy and Pulmonary Rehabilitation.* We wanted to present a new approach, not just a revision. Elizabeth's research and study of oxygen transport mechanisms in relation to patient treatment highlighted this concept as the primary thread that would pull the new book together. The cardiopulmonary system must be viewed as a whole, interacting with other body systems for optimal function. Therapy interventions must incorporate cardiopulmonary goals as well as neuromuscular and musculoskeletal goals for patients to reach maximal rehabilitation potential.

We have attempted to pull together physiological as well as clinical data to meet the changing needs of health care to provide objective documentation for our interventions. Yet we were diligent in maintaining a text aimed at the undergraduate student or practicing therapist with minimal background in cardiopulmonary physical therapy. To that end we have tried to keep the material readable and very user-friendly. Our hope is that virtually any question that may arise about treating a patient with cardiopulmonary dysfunction would have some answers in this book.

We both teach undergraduate physical therapy students and thank them for their input, questions, and concerns about patients with cardiopulmonary dysfunction who have helped us focus this text to meet students' needs. In addition, through our continuing education seminars with postgraduate physical therapists, we have been challenged to apply the concepts in light of the changing health care scene. How can we be most effective and scientifically correct in choosing treatment techniques that have demonstrated improvement in the oxygen transport mechanism and patient function? We always learn when we teach, and we hope to share that learning with others through this text.

We are excited about being able to present an accompanying text, *Clinical Case Study Guide.* We are attempting to show the physiological principles presented in our text, by identifying real-life case studies that physical therapists deal with every day in their practice. Our hope is that this will be used widely in teaching physical therapy students and will facilitate their understanding of how to effectively integrate cardiopulmonary concepts in each of their patients, not just in patients with a primary cardiopulmonary diagnosis.

To our knowledge, this is the first international book written dealing with cardiopulmonary physical therapy. It is a blend of physiology and international approaches to the patient with cardiopulmonary dysfunction. We have had the privilege of teaching and consulting internationally and have tried to make this text applicable to all therapists regardless of their situation and the degree of sophisticated equipment.

We realize that in some Third-World nations, hands-on therapy and positioning is the only mode of therapy available. We believe that this is often all that is needed when applied with the proper concepts and thought processes.

We are delighted with the way this edition has come together. We have many new chapter authors who have added depth and direction for both cardiac and pulmonary foci.

We are pleased this is finally completed and thank our families, friends, and colleagues for supporting us and encouraging us through the rough times to see this book to completion. Our hope is that this will be a welcome addition to your professional library, and we welcome your comments and suggestions for future work.

Donna Frownfelter
Elizabeth Dean

ACKNOWLEDGMENTS

There are so many people that I want to thank and acknowledge for their support and contributions to this book. First, my family, for their understanding and support during stressful deadlines and crunch spots. My husband David has been there for me since I went to physical therapy school and has always encouraged me to do what my vision led me to do. My three teenagers, Lauren, Daniel, and Kristin, have helped keep my life on track and grounded in the reality of daily life while taking time to "smell the roses." You are special gifts to me, and I love you.

To my students, I thank you for your questions, concerns, and wonderings about what this cardiopulmonary stuff really means to your patients. You wonder if you can really be a better therapist because you take these things into account in evaluation and treatment. Please remember the difference between ordinary and extraordinary is just that little "extra." I believe *that* is what incorporating cardiopulmonary attention does; it adds the little extra. Be an extraordinary therapist, no matter what the health care environment.

To the contributing authors, I thank you for your time and significant effort in bringing together the literature and clinical aspects of cardiopulmonary physical therapy. Your dedication to this project has made it much more than Elizabeth and I could have done alone. *You* know how important it is to convey the message of treating the whole patient and helping them reach his or her potential.

To my colleague and soul mate Mary Massery, who I have taught with, travelled with, given seminars with, laughed with, and cried with, I thank you for all you have taught me and how special it is to have someone you can always count on to discuss a difficult patient or a personal issue. We have become quite a team, and I value our professional and personal relationships. Your contributions to the clinical chapters we have done together this time have been significant. I look forward to many more projects and fun times together. There is no greater pleasure for a teacher than to see a former student travel in that teacher's tracks and surpass her. Thanks Spike!

My deepest thanks go to Elizabeth Dean. You have been an incredible colleague who has given new life to this book. You have, in a gentle way, helped to ensure that physiologic and scientific evidence be paired with our clinical experience and treatment techniques. You have truly brought about a book that I could never have completed alone. Words are not enough to thank you for your commitment to this project and the countless hours you have spent in a major revision of the former textbook. I am delighted at what you have done and the depth of knowledge you have brought in your content and organization of this book. I am honored that you chose this text in which to share your work, and I have enjoyed working with you and learning from you. We share a common bond in the relationships we have with our students and our desire to spread the word about the importance of including cardiopulmonary concerns in the patient's evaluation and plan of treatment. We have grown close in the last 10 years, and I value our friendship as well as our professional work together. Thank you hardly is enough, but "Thanks!"

To my friends, family, and fellow workers at NovaCare, Inc. Contract Services, I thank you for your patience and understanding of the demands on my time and your encouragement to continue and finish this project. Your support has meant a great deal and I hope you feel a part of this, for it is because of you this has really happened. I'm glad to have a work environment that supports personal and professional growth.

To our Mosby staff: Martha Sasser, thanks for your ideas and vision for going with this new book. You saw the possibilities and were there with other suggestions to make it even better (even if some of them came when we thought we were done!). To Kellie White, you kept us on track and helped catch up with chapter authors who needed a nudge and still had time to have Julia Isabelle—quite an accomplishment! You will now find what we have, that motherhood is often harder than your other job! Best wishes! To Mamata Reddy and Amy Dubin, you have pushed us through the editing process with the gentle and firm hand that we needed and with much support and help. Thank you for your cooperation and critical eye in making this an excellent outcome.

Finally, and most importantly, I thank God for the vision, strength, and energy to undertake this book and see it through to completion. My involvement in spreading the word about the need for optimizing the cardiopulmonary system has always felt like a mission. It has been amazing to me how many therapists don't see the need and how they can have an *"Aha!"* experience in a seminar or class, or even just reading this book. If I can have a small part in that experience, my "mission" has been fulfilled, and for that I am grateful.

Donna Frownfelter

To Donna, for having made this dream come true. Our working relationship and friendship began 10 years ago when I first approached Donna to review a manuscript entitled "The Pulmonary Effects of Body Positioning," published in *Physical Therapy* in 1985. This publication was the stepping stone to a prolonged and ever-growing interest in oxygen transport and how it is affected by cardiopulmonary interventions such as body positioning and mobilization. The enthusiasm, interest, and support of Donna and my former graduate student, Jocelyn Ross, have fueled my energies in the exciting dynamic area of cardiopulmonary physical therapy. My heartfelt gratitude to you both.

To Daniel Perlman, for your encouragement and support of my liaison with Donna at the outset and over the years. You knew a good thing when you saw it.

To Doug Frost, for your support in getting this project into the end zone. Thank you for your support and for being there as the book continued to evolve.

To our dedicated contributors, for your expertise, which has contributed to a volume on the principles and practice of cardiopulmonary physical therapy that is on the cutting edge with respect to the scientific and physiologic literature. Thank you for your contributions and team effort.

To my cardiopulmonary physical therapy colleagues and students for your inquisitiveness and enthusiasm. Thank you all for your inspiration.

And not to forget the Mosby crew—Martha Sasser, Kellie White, Mamata Reddy, and Amy Dubin—I thank each one of you for your commitment to making this book the best it can be.

Elizabeth Dean

CONTENTS

PART 1

Cardiopulmonary Function in Health and Disease

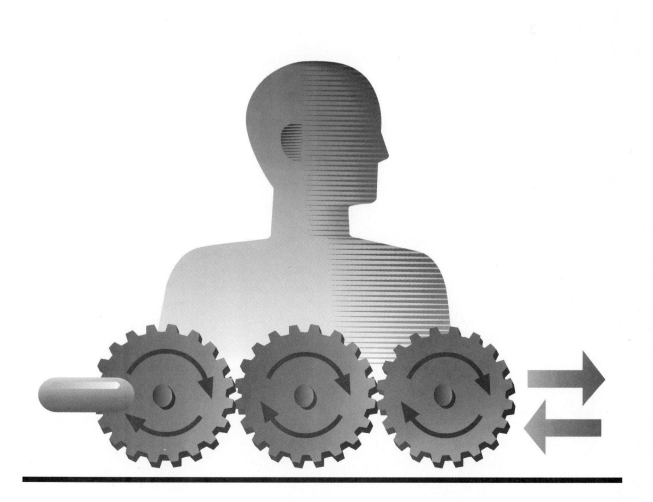

CHAPTER 1

Oxygen Transport: The Basis for Cardiopulmonary Physical Therapy

Elizabeth Dean

KEY TERMS   Cellular respiration   Gravitational stress
                Exercise stress   Oxygen transport pathway

INTRODUCTION

Cardiopulmonary physical therapy is an essential non-invasive medical intervention that can reverse or mitigate insults to oxygen transport. It can avoid, delay, or reduce the need for medical interventions, such as supplemental oxygen, intubation, mechanical ventilation, suctioning, bronchoscopy, chest tubes, surgery, and medications. A comprehensive understanding of oxygen transport and the factors that determine and influence it is therefore essential to the comprehensive assessment of oxygen transport and optimal treatment prescription to effect these outcomes.

This chapter details the oxygen transport system, the pathway, and the component steps that provide a con-ceptual basis for cardiopulmonary physical therapy practice. Oxygen transport is the basis for life. Impaired or threatened oxygen transport, hence, cardiopulmonary dysfunction, is a physical therapy priority.

In health, the oxygen transport system is normally perturbed by movement and activity, changes in body position, and emotional stress. In disease, disruption of or threat to this system is always a medical priority because of the threat to life or impairment of functional capacity.

The fundamental steps in the oxygen transport pathway, and their function and interdependence are described first. Special attention is given to cellular respiration and the utilization of oxygen during me-

3

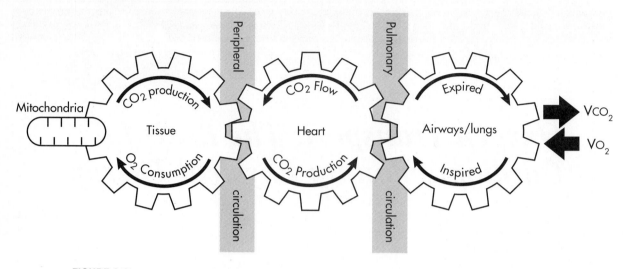

FIGURE 1-1
Scheme of components of ventilatory-cardiovascular-metabolic doupling underlying oxygen transport. (Modified from Wasserman K et al: Principles of exercise testing and interpretation, Philadelphia, 1987, Lea & Febiger.)

tabolism at the cellular level in muscle. Second, the factors that normally perturb oxygen transport in health are described, namely gravitational stress secondary to changes in body position, exercise stress secondary to increased oxygen demand of the working muscles, emotional stress, and arousal. A thorough understanding of the effects of those factors that normally perturb oxygen transport is essential to accurately assess and treat deficits in oxygen transport.

OXYGEN TRANSPORT

Oxygen transport refers to the delivery of fully oxygenated blood to peripheral tissues, the cellular uptake of oxygen, the utilization of oxygen from the blood, and the return of partially desaturated blood to the lungs. The oxygen transport pathway consists of multiple steps ranging from the ambient air to the perfusion of peripheral tissues with oxygenated arterial blood (Figure 1-1). Oxygen transport has become the basis for conceptualizing cardiopulmonary function, and diagnosing and managing cardiopulmonary dysfunction (Dantzker, 1983; Dantzker, Boresman, and Gutierrez, 1991; Dean, 1994a; Dean and Ross,

1992a; Goldring, 1984; Johnson, 1973; Ross, and Dean, 1989; Weber et al, 1983).

Oxygen transport variables include oxygen delivery (Do_2), oxygen consumption (Vo_2) and the oxygen enhancement ratio (OER) or the utilization coefficient. Oxygen demand is the amount of oxygen required by the cells for aerobic metabolism. Oxygen demand is usually reflected by Vo_2; however, in cases of severe cardiopulmonary dysfunction and compromise to oxygen transport, Vo_2 can fall short of the demand for oxygen. Oxygen transport variables, including the components of Do_2, Vo_2, and the OER, are shown in Figure 1-2. Do_2 is determined by arterial oxygen content and cardiac output, oxygen consumption by the arterial and venous oxygen content, difference and cardiac output, and oxygen extraction by the ratio of Do_2 to Vo_2.

Measures and indices of oxygen transport that reflect the function of the component steps of the oxygen transport pathway are shown in the box above.

Energy Transfer and Cellular Oxidation

Cellular metabolism and survival depend on the continuous synthesis and degradation of adenosine

Measures and Indices of the Function of the Steps in the Oxygen Transport Pathway

Control of Ventilation

PO.1 (central drive to breathe)
Ventilatory responses of hypoxia and hypercapnia
PaO_2 and SaO_2 responses to exercise

Inspired Gas

Alveolar oxygen pressure
Alveolar carbon dioxide pressure
Alveolar nitrogen pressure

Hematologic Variables

Hemoglobin
Plasma proteins and their concentrations
Red blood cells and count
White blood cells and count
Platelets
Clotting factors
Clotting times
Hematocrit
PaO_2
$PaCO_2$ (end tidal CO_2)
$P(A-a)O_2$
CaO_2
CvO_2
$C(a-v)O_2$ difference
HCO_3
SaO_2
pH
PaO_2/PAO_2
PaO_2/FIO_2
Serum lactate

Pulmonary Variables

Minute ventilation
Tidal volume
Respiratory rate
Dead space volume
Alveolar volume
Alveolar ventilation
Distribution of ventilation
Static and dynamic lung compliance
Airway resistance
Functional residual capacity
Closing volume
Vital capacity
Forced expiratory volumes and flows
Other pulmonary volumes, capacities, and flow rates
Inspiratory and expiratory pressures
Work of breathing
Respiratory muscle strength and endurance

Pulmonary Hemodynamic Variables

Cardiac output
Total perfusion
Distribution of perfusion
Anatomic shunt
Physiologic shunt
Systolic and diastolic pulmonary artery pressures
Pulmonary capillary blood flow
Pulmonary capillary wedge pressure
Pulmonary vascular resistance
Pulmonary vascular resistance index
Systemic hemodynamic variables
Heart rate
Electrocardiogram (ECG)

Systemic blood pressure

Mean arterial blood pressure
Systemic vascular resistance
Systemic vascular resistance index
Central venous pressure
Pulmonary artery pressures
Wedge pressure
Blood volume
Cardiac output
Cardiac index
Stroke volume
Stroke index
Shunt fraction
Ejection fraction
Left ventricular work
Right ventricular work
Fluid balance
Renal output
Creatinine clearance and blood urea nitrogen (BUN)

Diffusion

$D (A-a)O_2$
Diffusing capacity
Diffusing capacity/alveolar volume

Gas Exchange

Oxygen consumption (VO_2)
Carbon dioxide production (VCO_2)
Respiratory exchange ratio (VCO_2/VO_2)
Ventilation and perfusion matching
PaO_2/PAO_2
$P(A-a)O_2$

Oxygen Extraction and Utilization

Oxygen extraction ratio (VO_2/DO_2)
$C(a-v)O_2$ difference
$P(a-v)O_2$ difference
SvO_2
Metabolic enzymes at the cellular level
Oxyhemoglobin dissociation

Adequacy of Tissue Perfusion and Oxygen Transport

Tissue oxygenation
Tissue pH

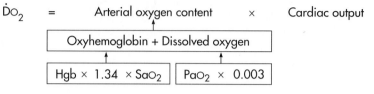

Oxygen delivery

$$\dot{D}o_2 \;=\; \underbrace{\text{Arterial oxygen content}}_{\boxed{\text{Oxyhemoglobin + Dissolved oxygen}}} \;\times\; \text{Cardiac output}$$

| Hgb × 1.34 × SaO₂ | PaO₂ × 0.003 |

Oxygen consumption

$$\dot{V}o_2 \;=\; (\text{Arterial oxygen content} - \text{Venous oxygen content}) \;\times\; \text{Cardiac output}$$

Oxyhemoglobin + Dissolved oxygen

| Hgb × 1.34 × SvO₂ | PaO₂ × 0.003 |

Oxygen enhancement ratio

$$\text{OER} \;=\; \frac{\text{Oxygen consumption}}{\text{Oxygen delivery}} \;=\; \frac{\dot{V}o_2}{\dot{D}o_2}$$

FIGURE 1-2

Formulas for determining oxygen delivery (Do₂), oxygen consumption (V̇o₂), and oxygen extraction ratio (OER). (Modified from Epstein C.D., Henning R.J.: Oxygen transport variables in the identification and treatment of tissue hypoxia, *Heart Lung* 22:328–348, 1993.)

triphosphate (ATP); the major source of energy for biological work. Work is performed in biological systems for contraction of skeletal, cardiac, and smooth muscle (e.g., exercise, digestion, glandular secretion and thermoregulation, and nerve impulse transmission) (see box below). These processes require a continuous supply of ATP, which is made available by aerobic (oxygen requiring) processes primarily. In the event

that oxygen delivery is inadequate, nonaerobic (anaerobic or non–oxygen-requiring) energy-transferring processes can also supply ATP. However, supplying energy anaerobically is more costly metabolically, that is, it is not efficient, is limited, and cannot be sustained because of the disruptive effects of lactate, a cellular byproduct of anaerobic metabolism, on physiological processes in general. Metabolic acidosis is a consequence of lactate accumulation. In critically ill patients, the presence of metabolic acidosis secondary to anaerobic metabolism can be life-threatening. Prolonged anaerobic metabolism is lethal in two respects. First, the patient is increasingly dependent on anaerobic metabolism because of inadequate oxygen delivery to peripheral tissues, and second, acidosis interferes with normal cellular processes and homeostasis, which require an optimal pH of 7.40.

The ATP molecule consists of an adenine and a ri-

> **Biological Work Requiring Continuous Oxygen Supply**
>
> Contraction of skeletal muscle
> Contraction of cardiac muscle
> Contraction of smooth muscle
> Nerve impulse transmission
> Active cellular metabolic processes
> Active pumping mechanisms

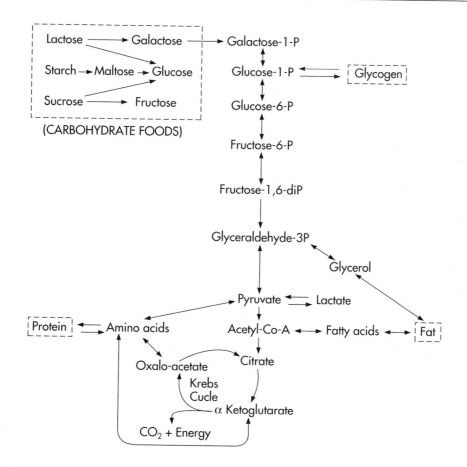

FIGURE 1-3

Interrelationships among carbohydrate, fat, and protein metabolism and their points of entry into the Krebs cycle. (Printed with permission from Shepard R.J.: *Physiology and biochemistry of exercise*, Philadelphia, 1985, Praeger Scientific.)

bose molecule with three phosphates attached. Splitting of the terminal phosphate bond or the two terminal phosphate bonds generates considerable amounts of energy. This energy is used to power various chemical reactions associated with metabolism. These metabolic processes take place in specialized organelles in the cells called mitochondria. The primary pathways that are responsible for the formation of ATP are the Krebs cycle and the electron transfer chain.

The complex, enzymatically controlled chemical reactions of metabolism are designed to form and conserve energy through the Krebs cycle and the electron transfer chain and then use this energy for biological work (Ganong, 1993; Shephard, 1985). Carbohydrates, fats, and proteins, ingested from foodstuffs in the diet, are oxidized to provide the energy for phosphorylation of adenosine diphosphate (ADP), that is, the formation of ATP by combining ADP with phosphate. These substances are broken down, and they access the Krebs cycle at the pyruvic acid or acetyl coenzyme A (CoA) levels (Figure 1-3). Some amino acids can enter the Krebs cycle directly.

The Krebs cycle degrades acetyl CoA to carbon dioxide (CO_2) and hydrogen atoms (H_2). The primary

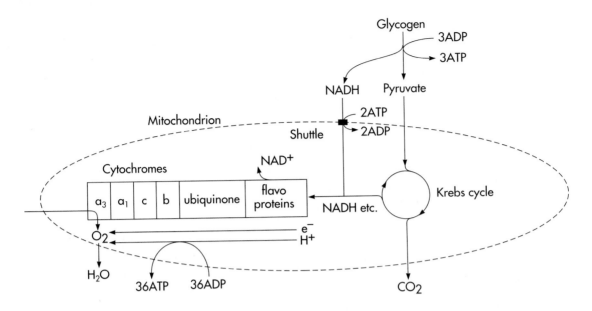

FIGURE 1-4

Electron transfer chain and its relationship with the Krebs cycle. (Printed with permission from Shepard R.J.: *Physiology and biochemistry of exercise,* Philadelphia, 1985, Praeger Scientific.)

purpose of this cycle is to generate hydrogen ions for the electron transfer chain by two principal electron acceptors, nicotinamide adenine dinucleotide (NAD) and flavin adenine dinucleotide (FAD). Many acids catalyze the numerous reactions of the Krebs cycle.

Cellular oxidation or respiration refers to the function of the electron transfer chain to release energy in small amounts and to conserve energy in the formation of high energy bonds. It is this process that ensures a continual energy supply to meet the needs of metabolism (Figure 1-4).

Three major systems of energy transfer exist to supply energy during all-out exercise over varying durations (McArdle, Katch, and Katch, 1994). Although these systems are discrete they overlap. Cellular ATP and creatine phosphate (CP) are immediate energy sources for the first 10 seconds of exercise. From 30 to 60 seconds, glycolysis provides a short-term energy source. The ATP-CP system and the glycolytic system are anaerobic processes. As exercise persists for several minutes, the long-term aerobic system predominates. Thus for sustained physical activity and exercise, energy is primarily provided by aerobic metabolism. Oxygen for this process is provided by the oxygen transport pathway. Carbon compounds that enter the body in the form of carbohydrate, fat, and protein undergo oxidative metabolism in the form of aerobic glycolysis in the mitochondria in the cytoplasm of the cells.

The Krebs cycle and the electron transfer chain are the biochemical pathways in the mitochondria of the cell responsible for harnessing the oxygen for aerobic metabolism and ensuring a continuous supply of oxygen for this process (Shephard, 1985). Initially, glucose is phosphorylated to produce two molecules of ATP (glycolysis). Glucose is oxidized to produce two molecules of pyruvic acid, yielding a net gain of two molecules of ATP per molecule of glucose. The two pyruvate molecules enter the Krebs cycle where they are oxidized to CO_2 and water. This process yields 30 ATP molecules. Hydrogen ions released in the process are transferred to the electron transfer chain yielding 4 ATP molecules for cellular metabolism. Electrons are removed from hydrogen and funnelled

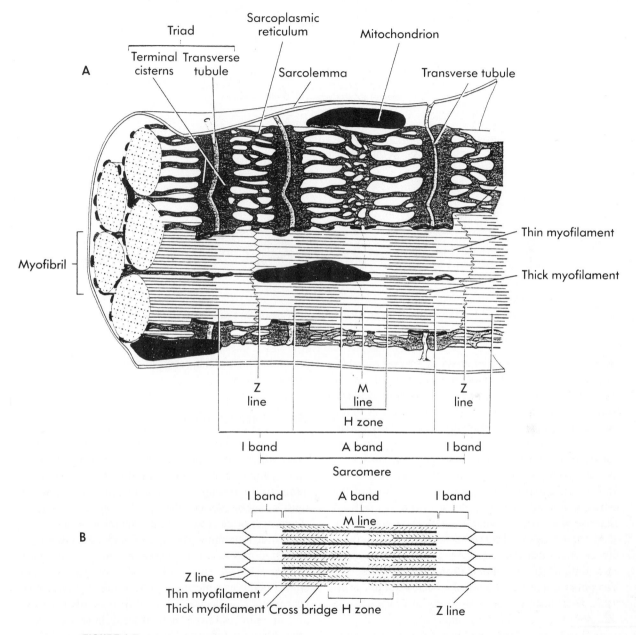

FIGURE 1-5
Schematic of the ultrastructure of a muscle fiber. **A,** View of muscle membrane structure and
myofibril arrangement. **B,** A single functional unit (sarcomere) of a myofibril showing the
interdigitation of the actin and myosin filaments. (Printed with permission from Tortora, G.J.,
Anagnostakos N.P.: *Principles of anatomy and physiology,* New York, 1990, Harper & Row.)

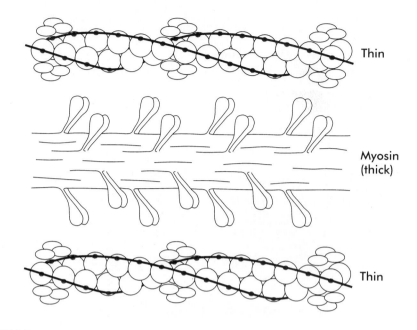

FIGURE 1-6
Arrangement of the thick and thin myofilaments. (From Hasson S.: *Clinical exercise physiology,*
St. Louis, 1994, Mosby.)

down the electron transport chain by specialized electron carrier molecules, cytochromes 1 to 5. It is only the last of these cytochromes, cytochrome oxidase, that can reduce molecular oxygen to water. This process is driven by a gradient of high-to-low potential energy. The energy transferred as electrons are passed from H_2 to O_2, and is trapped and conserved as high energy phosphate bonds. Oxygen is *only* involved in these metabolic pathways at the end of the electron transfer chain, where oxygen is the final electron acceptor and combines with H_2 to form H_2O. More than 90% of ATP synthesis takes place through the electron transfer chain by oxidative reactions combined with phosphorylation, that is, oxidative phosphorylation. An individual's peak aerobic capacity is determined by the availability of oxygen at the end of the electron transport chain.

For each molecule of glucose that is metabolized, 36 molecules of ATP are produced; four molecules from substrate phosphorylation (anaerobic), and 32 from oxidative phosphorylation (aerobic). The low ATP yield from anaerobic metabolism explains why

anaerobic metabolism can only serve as a short-term energy source.

Muscle Contraction and Metabolism

The basic mechanism for muscle contraction is excitation contraction coupling (Kirchberger, 1991; Tortora, and Anagnostakos, 1990). Action potentials mediated centrally or through the spinal cord depolarize the muscle cell membrane, the sarcolemma, and stimulate the release of calcium from the lateral sacs of the sarcoplasmic reticulum. The sarcoplasmic reticulum is an extensive network of invaginations and tubular channels encasing the muscle fibers or myofibrils. The calcium floods over the myofilaments of the myofibrils. Myofilaments consist of thin and thick fibers, actin, and myosin protein, which interdigitate with each other giving the typical striated appearance to skeletal muscle (Figures 1-5 and 1-6). Actin is a helical molecule with tropomyosin intertwined along its length. Tropomyosin normally inhibits the interaction of actin and myosin. Calcium causes a conformational change of the tropomyosin molecule that enables troponin, also distributed along the actin molecule, to combine with calcium. The combining of calcium and troponin triggers the movement of actin and myosin. Contraction involves the attaching and detaching of the myosin heads (cross bridges) to actin in a cyclical manner, which causes the actin and myosin filaments to slide past each other. In this way, the muscle is shortened without shortening of the myofilaments.

The energy for muscle contraction in the form of ATP is generated within the mitochondria of the myofibrils (Shephard, 1985). Myosin ATPase splits ATP so that the transfer of this energy can be used for muscle contraction. Specifically, the enzyme ATPase is activated when actin and myosin are joined. ATP is then available to bind with the cross bridge, causing it to detach from actin. Relaxation occurs with the cessation of electrical excitation and the rapid removal or sequestration of calcium into the lateral sacs of the sarcoplasmic reticulum.

The specific metabolic properties of muscle depend on the constituent muscle fiber types (Fox, Bowers, and Foss, 1993). The three primary muscle fiber groups are fast twitch fibers, slow twitch fibers, and intermediate fibers, which have properties of both. The fast twitch fibers (fast glycolytic fibers) are recruited during short-term sprint type exercise, which relies mainly on anaerobic metabolism. These fibers are well-adapted for rapid forceful contractions, because they have large amounts of myosin ATPase, rapid calcium release and uptake and high rate of cross bridge cycling. Slow twitch fibers (slow oxidative fibers) are recruited during prolonged aerobic exercise. These fibers have large amounts of myoglobin, mitochondria, and myochondrial enzymes. Compared with the fast twitch fibers, slow twitch fibers are fatigue-resistant. The intermediate fibers have both anaerobic and aerobic metabolic enzymes, which make these fibers capable of both types of muscle work. Although the characteristics of the fiber types are distinct, activity and exercise recruits both types of fibers. Depending on the particular activity or exercise, one fiber type may be preferentially recruited over the others.

Principles of Oxygen Transport

A continuous supply of oxygen is needed to meet moment-to-moment demands for oxygen commensurate with changing metabolic demands for energy at the cellular level in addition to basal metabolic demands (Cone, 1987; Dantzker, 1991; Samsel and Schumacker, 1991). Oxygen transport occurs either by convection or diffusion. Convection of oxygen refers to the movement of oxygen from the alveoli to the tissue capillaries. Convection is primarily determined by the hemoglobin concentration, oxygen saturation, and cardiac output. The diffusion of oxygen refers to the movement of oxygen from the capillaries to the mitochondria. Diffusion is determined by metabolic rate, vascular resistance, capillary recruitment, tissue oxygen consumption, and extraction.

Normally, D_{O_2} is regulated by tissue metabolism and the overall demand for oxygen. Typically, D_{O_2} is 3 to 4 times greater than oxygen demand, and V_{O_2} is not directly dependent on D_{O_2}. In health, the increased metabolic demands of exercise constitute the greatest challenge to the oxygen transport system. The V_{O_2} can increase 20 times. In response to increased muscle metabolism, blood flow increases to the peripheral muscles through vasodilatation and capillary recruitment, thereby increasing the availability of oxygen to the working tissues and its extraction from the arterial blood. As D_{O_2} and V_{O_2} increase, venous return, stroke volume, and heart rate also increase, thereby increasing cardiac output (CO). The CO can increase more than five times in strenuous exercise.

At rest, regional differences in the proportion of CO normally delivered to the body organs reflects differences in organ functions and is not necessarily matched to the metabolic rate (Guyton, 1987). For example, the distribution of CO to the kidneys is 20%, and to the mesenteric, splenic, and portal tissues is 20% to 30%. Comparatively, muscle at rest is 10% and the brain and myocardium are less than 5% each.

Oxygen Content of the Blood

Oxygen is transported in arterial blood to the tissues in combination with hemoglobin (98%) and dissolved in plasma (2%) The majority of oxygen is carried in the blood by hemoglobin, compared with a relatively minimal amount of oxygen that is dissolved in the blood. The oxyhemoglobin dissociation curve represents the relationship between the affinity of hemoglobin for oxygen and arterial oxygen tension. The affinity of hemoglobin for oxygen depends on the tissue oxygen demand. In health, exercising muscle increases the demand for oxygen. The heat of the working muscles and the acidic environment result in reduced oxyhemoglobin affinity, and increased oxygen release. This is reflected by a shift to the right of the oxyhemoglobin dissociation curve (see Chapter 9). The affinity of hemoglobin and oxygen is increased with the cessation of exercise, which is reflected by a leftward shift of the curve.

Oxygen Delivery to the Tissues

The final steps in oxygen transport involve the dissociation of oxygen from hemoglobin and the diffusion of oxygen from the capillaries to the cells (Schumacker, Samsel, 1989). Diffusion depends on the quantity and rate of blood flow, the difference in capillary and tissue oxygen pressures, the capillary surface area, capillary permeability, and diffusion distance (West, 1995). With increased metabolic demand of the tissues, capillary dilatation and recruitment increase capillary surface area and reduce vascular resistance to flow. Diffusion distance is decreased, the movement of oxygen into the cell is facilitated, and the tissue oxygen tension is increased.

The two diffusion gradients that determine effective oxygen transport are between the pulmonary capillaries and the alveoli, and between the peripheral capillaries and the tissue cells. Diffusion of oxygen occurs as the blood moves from the aorta to the arterioles. The mean oxygen tension in the aorta is about 95 mm Hg and in the arterioles is 70 to 80 mm Hg. The oxygen gradient between the arterioles and the cells is the most steep. The mean oxygen pressure is less than 50 mm Hg in the capillaries. The oxygen tension in the capillaries determines the rate of diffusion to the cells. An optimal diffusion gradient maintains the oxygen tension in the cell between 1 to 10 mm Hg; oxygen tension is less than 0.5 mm Hg in the

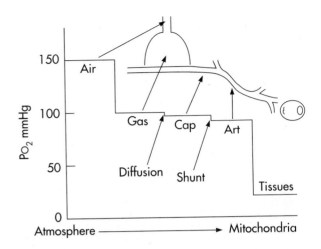

FIGURE 1-7
Scheme of oxygen partial pressures from air to tissue. The cascade reflects the removal of oxygen by the pulmonary capillary blood and the tissues. Depressions caused by the effects of diffusion and shunt are also illustrated. (Used with permission from West J.B.: *Respiratory physiology—the essentials,* ed 5, Baltimore, 1995, Williams & Wilkins.)

mitochondria (Guyton, 1991). This decremental Pa_{O_2} profile down the oxygen transport pathway, from the airways to the tissues, is termed the oxygen cascade (Figure 1-7).

Cardiac Output

In addition to arterial oxygen content, CO is a primary determinant of Do_2 (Dantzker, 1991). The transport of oxyhemoglobin to the tissues is dependent on convective blood flow by way of CO. The CO is the volume of blood pumped from the right or left ventricle per minute. The components of CO are stroke volume (SV) and heart rate (HR), that is, CO = SV × HR. Stroke volume is the amount of blood ejected from the left ventricle during each ventricular systole or heartbeat and is determined by the preload, myocardial distensibility, myocardial contractility, and afterload. The Do_2 is optimized in patients by increasing CO through the therapeutic manipulation of preload, myocardial contractility, afterload, and heart rate.

Preload

Preload is the end diastolic muscle fiber length of the ventricle before systolic ejection, and reflects the left ventricular end diastolic volume (LVEDV). The LVEDV is dependent on venous return, blood volume, and left atrial contraction. An increase in ventricular volume stretches the myocardial fibers and increases the force of myocardial contraction (Starling effect) and stroke volume. This effect is limited by the physiologic limits of distension of the myocardium. Excessive stretching such as in fluid overload of the heart leads to suboptimal overlap of the actin and myosin filaments, thus impairing rather than enhancing contractility.

Afterload

Afterload is the resistance to ejection during ventricular systole. Afterload of the left ventricle is primarily determined by four factors: the distensibility of the aorta, vascular resistance, patency of the aortic valve, and viscosity of the blood.

Myocardial Contractility

Myocardial contractility reflects actin-myosin coupling during contraction. Myocardial contractility is assessed by the ejection fraction, rate of circumferential muscle fiber shortening, pressure volume relationships, and the rate of change of ventricular pressure over time.

Oxygen Debt

Tissue oxygen debt or recovery oxygen consumption is the difference between oxygen demand and oxygen consumption. In health, oxygen debt can be sustained for short periods during intense exercise. Anaerobic metabolism is stimulated to produce ATP under these conditions. In patients, the degree of oxygen debt significantly correlates with survival (Fenwick et al, 1990).

Oxygen Extraction Ratio or Utilization Coefficient

The oxygen extraction ratio (OER), or utilization coefficient, reflects the proportion of oxygen delivered to that consumed. The OER is calculated by dividing Vo_2 by Do_2. Normally, the OER is 23%.

Supply-dependent Oxygen Consumption

Normally, a decrease in Do_2 does not reduce Vo_2 (Phang, Russell, 1993). With a decrement in Do_2, the tissues extract a proportionate amount of oxygen from the blood. In critically ill patients, the Do_2 may be significantly limited to the point where basic metabolic needs for oxygen (300 ml/min/M^2) are not being met (Fenwick et al, 1990; Lorente et al, 1991; Phang, Russell, 1993). The critical level at which Vo_2 falls is associated with tissue anaerobic metabolism and the development of lactic acidosis and decreased pH (Figure 1-8) (Mizock, Falk, 1992; Schumaker, Cain, 1987). Serum lactates correspondingly increase and provide a valid index of anaerobic metabolism in patients with multiorgan system failure.

The Oxygen Transport Pathway

Oxygen transport is dependent on several interconnecting steps ranging from oxygen-containing air being inhaled through the nares to oxygen extraction at the cellular level in response to metabolic demand (see Figure 1-1, p. 4). These steps provide the mechanism for ventilatory, cardiovascular, and metabolic coupling. In addition, blood is responsible for transporting oxygen within the body, thus its constituents and consistency directly affect this process.

The Quality and Quantity of Blood

Although not considered a discrete step in the oxygen transport pathway, blood is the essential medium for transporting oxygen. To fulfill this function, blood must be delivered in an adequate yet varying amount proportional to metabolic demands, and have the appropriate constituents and consistency. Thus consideration of the characteristics of the circulating blood volume is essential to any discussion of oxygen transport.

Blood volume is compartmentalized within the intravascular compartment such that 70% is contained within the venous compartment, 10% in the systemic arteries, 15% in the pulmonary circulation, and 5% in the capillaries (Sandler, 1986). The large volume of blood contained within the venous circulation permits adjustments to be made as cardiac output demand changes. The veins constrict, for example, when cardiac output needs to be increased. When blood volume is normal and body fluids are appropriately distributed between the intra- and extravascular compartments, fluid balance is considered normal. When these are disrupted, a fluid balance problem exists. In addition, fluid imbalance affects the concentration of electrolytes, and particularly sodium, which is in the highest concentration in the extracellular fluid. Four primary fluid problems that have implications for oxygen transport are water deficit, water excess, sodium deficit, and sodium excess (see Chapter 15). Other ions that are often affected in fluid and electrolyte imbalance deficits include potassium, chloride, calcium, and magnesium (Figure 1-8). These electrolyte disturbances also contribute to impaired oxygen transport by affecting the electrical and mechanical behavior of the heart and blood vessels, and hence cardiac output and the distribution of oxygenated arterial blood to the periphery.

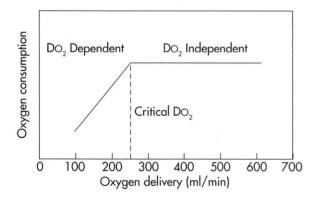

FIGURE 1-8

Relationship between oxygen consumption ($\dot{V}o_2$) and oxygen delivery (Do_2). The Do_2-independent phase represents the normal metabolic state. The Do_2-dependent phase represents the dependency of $\dot{V}o_2$ on Do_2 when Do_2 Falls below the critical Do_2. (Modified from Phang, P.T. and Russel, J.A.: When does $\dot{V}o_2$ depend on Do_2? *Resp Care 38:* 618-630, 1993.)

Blood is a viscous fluid composed of cells and plasma. Because 99% of the blood is red blood cells, the white blood cells play almost no role in determining the physical characteristics of blood.

Hematocrit refers to the proportion of blood that is cells. The normal hematocrit is 38% for women and 42% for men. Blood is several times as viscous as water, which increases the difficulty with which blood is pumped through the heart and flows through vessels; the greater the number of cells, the greater the friction between the layers of blood, which results in increased viscosity. Thus the viscosity of the blood increases significantly with increases in hematocrit. An increase in hematocrit such as in polycythemia increases blood viscosity several times over. The concentration and types of protein in the plasma can also affect viscosity but to a lesser extent.

In the adult, red blood cells are produced in the marrow of the membranous bones such as the vertebrae, sternum, ribs, and pelvis. The production of red blood cells from these sites diminishes with age. Tissue oxygenation is the basic regulator of red blood cell production. Hypoxia stimulates red blood cell production through erythropoietin production in bone (Guyton, 1991).

Viscosity of the blood has its greatest effect in the small vessels. Blood flow is considerably reduced in small vessels, resulting in aggregates of red blood cells adhering to the vessel walls. This effect is not offset by the tendency of the blood to become less viscous in small vessels as a result of the alignment of the blood cells flowing through, which minimizes the frictional forces between layers of flowing blood cells. In addition, in small capillaries, blood cells can become stuck particularly where the nuclei of endothelial cells protrude and momentarily block blood flow.

The major function of the red blood cells is to transport hemoglobin, which in turn carries oxygen from the lungs to the tissues. Red blood cells also contain a large quantity of carbonic anhydrase, which catalyzes the reaction between CO_2 and H_2O. The rapidity of this reaction makes it possible for blood to react with large quantities of CO_2 to transport it from the tissues to the lungs for elimination.

Hemoglobin is contained within red blood cells up to a concentration of 34 gm/100 ml of cells. Each gram of hemoglobin is capable of combining with 1.34 ml of oxygen (see Figure 1-2, p. 6). Therefore in healthy women, 19 ml of oxygen and in healthy men, 21 ml of oxygen can be carried in the blood, given that the whole blood of women contains an average of 14 gm/100 ml of blood and 16 gm/100 ml of blood in men.

Clotting factors of the blood are normally in a proportion that does not promote clotting. Factors that promote coagulation (procoagulants), and factors that inhibit coagulation (anticoagulants) circulate in the blood. In the event of a ruptured blood vessel, prothrombin is converted to thrombin, which catalyzes the transformation of fibrinogen to fibrin threads. This fibrin mesh captures platelets, blood cells, and plasma to form a blood clot.

The extreme example of abnormal clotting is disseminated intravascular coagulation, where both hemorrhage and coagulation occur simultaneously. The acute form of this syndrome occurs in critically ill patients with multiorgan system failure. The mechanism appears to involve tissue factors, factors that damage the blood vessel wall, and factors that increase platelet aggregation (Green and Esparaz, 1990). The chronic form of the syndrome occurs in chronic conditions such as neoplastic disease.

Plasma is the extracellular fluid of the blood and contains 7% proteins, namely albumin, globulin, and fibrinogen. The primary function of the albumin and to a lesser extent, globulin and fibrinogen, is to create osmotic pressure at the capillary membrane and to prevent fluid leaking into the interstitial spaces. The globulins serve as carriers for transporting substances in the blood and provide immunity as the antibodies that fight infection and toxicity. Fibrinogen is fundamental to blood clotting. The majority of blood proteins, including hemoglobin, are also excellent acid-base buffers and are responsible for 70% of all buffering power of whole blood.

Blood flow (Q) depends on a pressure gradient (P) and vascular resistance (R), that is, $Q = P/R$. Hence blood flow equals the pressure gradient divided by resistance. The length of a given blood vessel and the viscosity of the blood are also determinants of blood flow.

The average blood volume is 5,000 ml. Approximately 3,000 ml of this is plasma and 2,000 ml is red blood cells. These values vary according to gender, weight, and other factors. Normally, changes in blood volume reflect deficits and excesses of fluid through imbalances created by losses through the skin and respiratory tract, and through urinary, sweat, and fecal losses. Exercise and hot weather are major challenges to fluid balance in health.

The plasma contains large quantities of sodium and chloride ions, and small amounts of potassium, calcium, magnesium, phosphate, sulfate, and organic acid ions. In addition, plasma contains a large amount of protein. The large ionic constituents of the plasma are responsible for regulating intracellular and extracellular fluid volumes and the osmotic factors that cause shifts of fluid between the intracellular and extracellular compartments.

Oxyhemoglobin Dissociation

The demand for oxygen at the cellular level changes from moment to moment. The properties of oxyhemoglobin dissociation ensure that there is a continuous supply of oxygen at the cellular level. Oxygen combines with the hemoglobin molecules in the pulmonary circulation and then is released in the tissue capillaries in response to a reduced arterial oxygen tension. The S-shaped oxyhemoglobin dissociation curve (see Chapter 9) shifts to the right in response to reduced tissue pH, increased CO_2, increased temperature and increased diphosphoglycerate (DPG), a constituent of normal blood cells.

The delivery of blood and its ability to effectively transport oxygen is central to all steps in the oxygen transport pathway and must be considered at each step in clinical problem solving and decision making.

Steps in the Oxygen Transport Pathway

Step One: inspired oxygen and quality of the ambient air

In health, the concentration of inspired oxygen is relatively constant at 21% unless the individual is at altitude. In which case, the fraction of inspired oxygen is reduced the higher the elevation.

Atmospheric air consists of 79% nitrogen, 20.97%

oxygen and 0.03% CO_2. Because nitrogen is not absorbed in the lungs, it has a crucial role in maintaining the lung tissue patent. The constituents of the air have become an increasingly important social, environmental, and health issue because of environmental hazards, pollution, and thinning of the ozone layer resulting in deterioration of air quality, an increase in toxic oxygen free radicals and a reduction in atmospheric oxygen pressure.

Many factors influence air quality, (e.g., geographical area, season, urban vs. rural area, high vs. low elevation, home environment, work environment, indoor vs. outdoor, level of ventilation, air conditioning, enclosed buildings, areas with high particulate matter, areas with gaseous vapors and toxic-inhaled materials, and smoke-filled vs. smoke-free environments). Poor air quality contributes to changes in the filtering ability of the upper respiratory tract, airway sensitivity, and lung damage, acutely and over time. Chronic irritation of the lungs from poor air quality can lead to allergies, chronic inflammatory reactions, fibrosis, and alveolar capillary membrane thickening. At the alveolar level, the inspired air is saturated with water vapor. In dry environments, however, the upper respiratory tract may become dehydrated, lose its protective mucous covering, become eroded, and provide a portal of infection even though the air is adequately humidified by the time it reaches the lower airways and alveoli.

Step Two: airways

The structure of the airways down the respiratory tract change according to their function. The main airway, the trachea, consists of cartilagenous rings, connective tissue, and small amounts of smooth muscle. This structure is essential to provide a firm and relatively inflexible conduit for air to pass from the nares through the head and neck to the lungs, and avoid airway collapse. As the airways become smaller and branch throughout the lung tissue, they consist primarily of smooth muscle. Airway narrowing, or, obstruction and increased resistance to airflow, is caused by multiple factors, including edema, mucus, foreign objects, calcification, particulate matter and space-occupying lesions, as well as hyperreactivity of bronchial smooth muscle. The airways are lined with cilia, fine microscopic hair-like projections, which are responsible for wafting debris, cells, and microorganisms away from the lungs into larger airways to be removed and evacuated. The airways are also lined with mucus, which consists of two layers, the upper gel layer and the lower sol layer with which the cilia communicate.

Step Three: lungs and chest wall

Air entry to the lungs depends on the integrity of the respiratory muscles, in particular, the diaphragm, the lung parenchyma, and the chest wall. Contraction and descent of the diaphragm inflates the lungs. The distribution of ventilation is primarily determined by the negative intrapleural pressure gradient down the lungs. The negative intrapleural pressure gradient results in uneven ventilation down the lung, and interregional differences (see Chapter 3). However, there are other factors, intraregional differences, that contribute to uneven ventilation within regions of the lung. These intraregional differences reflect regional differences in lung compliance and airway resistance (Ross, Dean, 1992). In patients with partially obstructed airways, reduced lung compliance, and increased airway resistance increase the time for alveolar filling. Gas exchange is compromised if there is inadequate time for alveolar filling or emptying, that is, increased time constants (West, 1995). Different time constants across lung units contribute to uneven patterns of ventilation during inspiration. A lung unit with a long time constant is slow to fill and to empty, and may continue to fill when surrounding units are emptying. A second factor is altered diffusion distance. In diseases where diffusion distance is increased, ventilation along lung units is uneven.

The lungs and the parietal pleura are richly supplied with thin-walled lymphatic vessels (Guyton, 1991). Lymphatic vessels have some smooth muscle and thus can actively contract to propel lymph fluid forward. This forward motion is augmented by valves along the lymphatic channels. The rise and fall of the pleural pressure during respiration compresses lymphatic vessels with each breath, which promotes a continuous flow of lymph. During expiration and increased intrapleural pressure, fluid is forced into the lymphatic vessels. The visceral pleura continuously drains fluid from the lungs. This creates a negative pressure in the pleural space, keeping the lungs expanded. This pressure exceeds the elastic recoil pressure of the lung parenchyma, which collapses the lungs.

The peritoneal cavity of the abdomen consists of a visceral peritoneum containing the viscera and a parietal peritoneum lining the abdominal cavity. Numerous lymphatic channels interconnect the peritoneal cavity and the thoracic duct; some arise from the diaphragm. With cycles of inspiration and expiration, large amounts of lymph are moved from the peritoneal cavity to the thoracic duct. High venous pressures and vascular resistance through the liver can interfere with normal fluid balance in the peritoneal cavity. This leads to the transudation of fluid with a high protein content into the abdominal cavity. This accumulation of fluid is referred to as ascites. Large volumes of fluid can accumulate in the abdominal cavity and significantly compromise cardiopulmonary function secondary to increased intraabdominal pressure on the underside of the diaphragm.

Optimal diaphragmatic excursion requires a balance between thoracic and intraabdominal pressures. Increases in abdominal pressure secondary to factors other than fluid accumulation can impair diaphragmatic descent and chest wall expansion, for example, gas entrapment, gastrointestinal (GI) obstruction, space-occupying lesions, and paralytic ileus.

Step Four: diffusion

Diffusion of oxygen from the alveolar sacs to the pulmonary arterial circulation depends on five factors: the area of the alveolar capillary membrane, diffusing capacity of the alveolar capillary membrane, pulmonary capillary blood volume, and ventilation and perfusion ratio (Ganong, 1993). The transit time of blood at the alveolar capillary membrane is also an important factor determining diffusion. The blood remains in the pulmonary capillaries for 0.75 seconds at rest. The blood is completely saturated within one third of this time. This provides a safety margin during exercise or other conditions in which cardiac output is increased and the pulmonary capillary transit time is reduced. The blood can normally be fully oxygenated even with reduced transit time.

Step Five: perfusion

The distribution of blood perfusing the lungs is primarily gravity dependent, thus the dependent lung fields are perfused to a greater extent than the nondependent lung fields. In the upright lung, the bases are better perfused than the apices (see Chapter 3). Ventilation and perfusion matching is optimal in the midzones of the upright lungs (West, 1985). In health, the ventilation to perfusion ratio is a primary determinant of arterial oxygenation. In the upright lung this ratio is 0.8 in the mid-zone.

Step Six: myocardial function

Optimal myocardial function and cardiac output depends on the synchronized coupling of electrical excitation of the heart and mechanical contraction. The sinoatrial node located in the right atrium is the normal pacemaker for the heart and elicits the normal sinus rhythm with its component P-QRS-T configuration. This wave of electrical excitation spreads throughout the specialized neural conduction system of the atria, interventricular septum, and the ventricles, and is followed by contraction of the atria and then the ventricles. Contraction of the right and left ventricles ejects blood into the pulmonary and systemic circulations respectively.

Cardiac output depends on several factors in addition to the integrity of the conduction system and the adequacy of myocardial depolarization (dromotropic effect). The amount of blood returned to the heart (preload), determines the amount ejected (Starling effect). The distensibility of the ventricles to accommodate this blood volume needs to be optimal, neither too restrictive nor compliant. The contractility of the myocardial muscle must be sufficient to eject the blood (inotropic effect). And finally, cardiac output is determined by the aortic pressure needed to overcome peripheral vascular resistance and eject blood into the systemic circulation (afterload).

The pericardial cavity, like the pleural and peritoneal cavities, is a potential space containing a thin film of fluid. The space normally has a negative pressure. During each expiration, pericardial pressure is increased, and fluid is forced out of the space into the mediastinal lymphatic channels. This process is normally facilitated with increased volumes of blood in the heart and each ventricular systole.

Step Seven: peripheral circulation

Once oxygenated blood is ejected from the heart, the peripheral circulation provides a conduit for supplying this blood to metabolically active tissue. Blood vessels throughout the body are arranged both in series and in parallel. The arteries and capillaries are designed to advance blood to perfuse the tissues with oxygenated blood. The vasculature is architected so that the proximal large arteries have a higher proportion of connective tissue and elastic elements than distal medium and small arteries, which have a progressively higher proportion of smooth muscle. This structure enables the large proximal arteries to withstand high pressure when blood is ejected during ventricular systole. Considerable potential energy is stored within the elastic walls of these blood vessels as the heart contracts. During diastole, the forward propulsion of blood is facilitated with the elastic recoil of these large vessels. The thin-walled muscular arterioles serve as the stopcocks of the circulation and regulate blood flow through regional vascular beds and maintain peripheral vascular resistance to regulate systemic blood pressure. Blood flow through these regional vascular beds is determined by neural and humoral stimulation, and by local tissue factors. Blood pressure control is primarily regulated by neural stimulation of the peripheral circulation and these vascular beds.

The microcirculation consists of the precapillary arteriole, the capillary, and the venule. The Starling effect governs the balance of hydrostatic and oncotic pressures within the capillary and the surrounding tissue. The balance of these pressures is 0.3 mm Hg; its net effect is a small outward filtration of fluid from the microvasculature into the interstitial space (see Chapter 3). Any excess fluid or loss of plasma protein is drained into the surrounding lymphatic vessels, which usually has a small negative pressure as does the interstitium. The integrity of the microcirculation is essential to regulate the diffusion of oxygen across the tissue capillary membrane, and to remove CO_2 and waste products.

The greater the muscular component of blood vessels, the greater their sensitivity to both exogenous neural stimulation and endogenous stimulation by circulating humoral neurotransmitters such as catecholamines and local tissue factors. This sensitivity is essential for the moment-to-moment regulation of the peripheral circulation with respect to tissue perfusion and oxygenation, commensurate with tissue metabolic demands, and control of total peripheral resistance and systemic blood pressure.

Step Eight: tissue extraction and utilization of oxygen

Perfusion of the tissues with oxygenated blood is the principal goal of the oxygen transport system (Dantzker, 1993). Oxygen is continually being used by all cells in the body, thus it diffuses out of the circulation and through cell membranes very rapidly to meet metabolic needs. Diffusion occurs down a gradient from areas of high to low oxygen pressure. The distance between the capillaries and the cells is variable, thus a significant safety factor is required to ensure adequate arterial oxygen tensions. Intracellular PO_2 ranges from 5 to 60 mm Hg, with an average of 23 mm Hg (Guyton, 1991). Given that only 3 mm Hg of oxygen pressure are needed to support metabolism, 23 mm Hg of oxygen pressure provide an adequate safety margin. These mechanisms ensure an optimal oxygen supply over a wide range of varying oxygen demands in health and in the event of impaired oxygen delivery because of illness. Normally, the rate of oxygen extraction by the cells is regulated by oxygen demand by the cells, that is, the rate at which ADP is formed from ATP and not by the availability of oxygen.

The adequacy of the quality and quantity of the mitochondrial enzymes, required to support the Krebs cycle and electron transfer chain, and the availability of myoglobin may be limiting factors in the oxygen transport pathway secondary to nutritional deficits and muscle enzyme deficiencies. Myoglobin is a comparable protein to hemoglobin that is localized within muscle mitochondria. Myoglobin combines reversibly with oxygen to provide an immediate source of oxygen with increased metabolic demands and facilitate oxygen transfer within the mitochondria.

Normally, the amount of oxygen extracted by the tissues is 23%, that is, the ratio of oxygen consumed to oxygen delivered. Thus this ratio ensures that considerably greater amounts of oxygen can be extracted during periods of increased metabolic demand.

Step Nine: return of partially desaturated blood and CO_2 to the lungs

Partially desaturated blood and CO_2 are removed from the cells via the venous circulation to the right side of the heart and lungs. CO_2 diffuses across the alveolar capillary membrane and is eliminated from the body through the respiratory system, and the deoxygenated venous blood is reoxygenated. The oxygen transport cycle repeats itself and is sensitively tuned to adjust to changes in the metabolic demand of the various organ systems, such as digestion in the GI system, and cardiac and muscle work during exercise.

Factors that interfere with tissue oxygenation and the capacity of the tissue to use oxygen include abnormal oxygen demands, reduced hemoglobin and myoglobin levels, edema, and poisoning of the cellular enzymes (Kariman, Burns, 1985).

FACTORS THAT NORMALLY PERTURB OXYGEN TRANSPORT

Basal metabolic rate (BMR) reflects the rate of metabolism when the individual is in a completely rested state, that is, no food intake within several hours, after a good night's sleep, no arousing or distressing emotional stimulation, and at a comfortable ambient temperature. Normally, the BMR is constant within and between individuals if measured under standardized conditions. This rate reflects resting energy expenditure of the body's cells to maintain resting function, including the work of breathing; heart, renal, and brain function; and thermoregulation.

Normally, over the course of the day, the human body is exposed to fluctuations in ambient temperature and humidity, ingestion states, activity and exercise levels (exercise stress), body positions and body position changes (gravitational stress), emotional states (emotional stress) and states of arousal. These factors significantly influence oxygen consumption and energy expenditure, and thus increase rate of metabolism.

Several factors related to disease can significantly increase oxygen consumption and metabolic rate over and above BMR. Such factors include fever, the disease process itself, the process of healing and recovery from injury or disease, thermoregulatory disturbance, reduced arousal, increased arousal resulting from anxiety and pain, sleep loss, medical and surgical interventions, fluid imbalance, and medications Dean, 1994b). These factors may contribute to a systemic increase in BMR or may reflect local changes in tissue metabolism. Autoregulation of the regional vascular beds promotes increased regional blood flow in accordance with their local tissue metabolic demand.

Because gravitational stress and exercise stress are fundamental to normal cardiopulmonary function and oxygen transport, the effects of gravity and exercise are highlighted. It should be emphasized that the effects of gravity on fluid shifts and the systemic effects of exercise are physiologically distinct, that is, exposing an individual to a gravitational stress does not adapt that individual to an exercise stress and vice versa. These two factors also augment arousal, through stimulation of the reticular activating system in the brain stem and the autonomic nervous system (ANS), which when depressed, significantly compromises oxygen transport in patient populations. The impact of emotional stress on oxygen transport is discussed briefly. These concepts are described further in Chapters 17 and 18.

Gravitational Stress

Humans are designed to function in a 1 G gravitational field. Given that 60% of the body weight is fluid contained within the intra- and extravascular compartments, and that this fluid has considerable mass, changes in body position result in significant fluid shifts instantaneously and threaten hemodynamic stability (Dean, Ross, 1992a; Dean, Ross, 1992b). To maintain consciousness and normal body function during changes in body position, the heart and peripheral vasculature are designed to detect these fluid shifts and accommodate quickly to avoid deleterious functional consequences (e.g., reduced stroke volume, CO, circulating blood volume, and cerebral perfusion). The preservation of the fluid-regulating mechanisms is essential to counter the hemodynamic effects of changing body position. This capacity is quickly lost with recumbency and is the primary cause of bed rest deconditioning in patient and older populations (Chase, Grave, Rowell, 1966; Winslow, 1985). Restoration of gravitational stress with upright positioning is the *only* means by which these fluid-regulating mechanisms can be maintained and orthostatic intolerance and its short- and long-term sequelae averted.

Exercise Stress

Exercise constitutes the greatest perturbation to homeostasis and oxygen transport in humans. Cardiac output can increase five times to adjust to the metabolic demands of exercise stress. All steps in the oxygen transport pathway are affected by exercise stress. Ventilation is increased, and ventilation and perfusion matching is optimized to maximize oxygenation of blood. Heart rate and stroke volume are increased to effect greater cardiac output of oxygenated blood to the tissues. At the tissue level, oxygen extraction is enhanced.

Emotional Stress

The body responds to emotional stress similar to exercise stress with the sympathetic stress reaction. Perceived threat, the basis of emotional stress, triggers the fight, flight, or fright mechanism and a series of sympathetically mediated physiological responses. This reaction that prepares the body for flight includes an increase in heart rate, blood pressure, CO, blood glucose, muscle strength, mental alertness, cellular metabolism, and increased local blood flow to specific muscle groups, as well as inhibition of involuntary function.

SUMMARY

This chapter described the oxygen transport system, its component steps, and their interdependence. This framework provides a conceptual basis for the practice of cardiopulmonary physical therapy.

The oxygen transport system is designed to deliver oxygen from the ambient air to every cell in the body to support cellular respiration, that is, the metabolic utilization of oxygen at the cellular level. Blood is the essential medium in which cellular and noncellular components transport oxygen from the cardiopulmonary unit to the peripheral tissues. The fundamental steps in the oxygen transport pathway were described. These steps included the quality of the ambient air, the airways, lungs, chest wall, pulmonary circulation, lymphatics, heart, peripheral circulation, and the peripheral tissues of the organs of the body.

In health, the most significant factors that perturb oxygen transport are changes in gravitational stress secondary to changes in body position, exercise stress secondary to increased oxygen demand of working muscles, arousal, and emotional stress. A thorough understanding of the normal effects of gravitational and exercise stress and arousal is essential to understand deficits in oxygen transport. In disease, numerous factors impair and threaten oxygen transport, that is, underlying pathophysiology, restricted mobility, recumbency, factors related to the patient's care, and factors related to the individual (see Chapter 16). Thus the physical therapist needs a detailed understanding of these concepts to diagnose these deficits and prescribe efficacious treatments.

REVIEW QUESTIONS

1. Describe the oxygen transport pathway, its steps and their interdependence.
2. Describe the physiological processes of energy transfer and cellular oxidation.
3. Explain oxygen transport with respect to oxygen delivery, uptake and utilization and the interrelationship among these processes.
4. Outline the factors that perturb oxygen transport in health.

References

Chase, G.A., Grave, C., & Rowell, L.B. (1966). Independence of changes in functional and performance capacities attending prolonged bed rest, *Aerospace Medicine 37:*1232–1237.

Cone, J.B. (1987). Oxygen transport from capillary to cell. In Snyder, J.V., Pinsky, M.R. (eds). *Oxygen transport in the critically ill,* Chicago: Year Book.

Dantzker, D.R. (1993). Adequacy of tissue oxygenation. *Critical Care Medicine 21:*S40–S43.

Dantzker, D.R. (1991). *Cardiopulmonary Critical Care,* ed 2. Philadelphia: WB Saunders.

Dantzker, D.R. (1985). The influence of cardiovascular function on gas exchange. *Clinical Chest Medicine* 4:149–159.

Dantzker, D.R., Boresman, B., & Gutierrez, G. (1991). Oxygen supply and utilization relationships. *American Review of Respiratory Disorders* 143:675–679.

Dean, E. (1994a). Oxygen transport: a physiologically-based conceptual framework for the practice of cardiopulmonary physiotherapy, *Physiotherapy 80:*347–355.

Dean, E. (1994b). Physiotherapy skills: positioning and mobilization of the patient. In Webber, B.A., Pryor, J.A., editors. (1994b). *Physiotherapy for respiratory and cardiac problems,* Edinburgh: Churchill Livingstone.

Dean, E., & Ross, J. (1992a). Discordance between cardiopulmonary physiology and physical therapy. *Chest 101:*1694–1698, 1992a.

Dean, E., & Ross, J. (1992b). Oxygen transport. The basis for contemporary cardiopulmonary physical therapy and its optimization with body positioning and mobilization, *Physical Therapy Practice* 1:34–44.

Epstein, C.D. & Henning, R.J. (1993). Oxygen transport variables in the identification and treatment of tissue hypoxia, *Heart Lung, 22:*328–348.

Fenwick, J.C., et al: Increased concentrations of plasma lactate predict pathologic dependence of oxygen consumption on oxygen delivery in patients with adult respiratory distress syndrome, *Journal of Critical Care* 5:81–86, 1990.

Fox, E., Bowers R., & Foss M. (1993). *The physiological basis for exercise and sport,* ed 5, Madison: Wis. 1993, Brown & Benchmark.

Ganong, W.F.: *Review of medical physiology,* ed 16, Los Altos, Calif: Lange Medical Publications.

Goldring, R.M.: Specific defects in cardiopulmonary gas exchange, *American Review Respiratory Disorders 129:*S57–S59, 1984.

Green, D., & Esparaz, B. (1990). Coagulopathies in the critically-ill patient. In Cane, R.D., Shapiro, B.A., & Davison, R. (Ed.). (1990). *Case studies in critical care medicine,* ed 2, Chicago: Year Book.

Guyton, A.C. (1991). *Textbook of medical physiology,* ed 8, Philadelphia, 1991, WB Saunders.

Guyton, A.C. (1987). *Human physiology and mechanisms of disease,* ed 4, Philadelphia: WB Saunders.

Johnson, R.L. (1973). The lung as an organ of oxygen transport, *Basic Respiratory Diseases 2:*1–6, 1973.

Kariman, K., & Burns, S.R. (1985). Regulation of tissue oxygen extraction in disturbed in adult respiratory distress syndrome, *American Review Respiratory Diseases* 132:109–114, 1985.

Kirchberger, M.A. (1991). Excitation and contraction of skeletal muscle. In West J.B., editor (1991). *Best and Taylor's physiological basis of medical practice.* Baltimore: Williams & Wilkins.

Lorente, J.A., et al (1991). Oxygen delivery-dependent oxygen consumption in acute respiratory failure, *Critical Care Medicine 19:*770–775, 1991.

McArdle, W.D., Katch, F.I., & Katch, V.L. (1994). *Essentials of exercise physiology,* Philadelphia: Lea & Febiger.

Mizock, B.A., & Falk, J.L. (1992). Lactic acidosis in critical illness, *Critical Care Medicine* 20:80–93, 1992.

Phang, P.T., Russell, J.A. (1993). When does V_{O_2} depend on D_{O_2}? *Respiratory Care* 38:618–630.

Ross, J., & Dean, E. (1989). Integrating physiological principles into the comprehensive management of cardiopulmonary dysfunction. *Physical Therapy* 69:255–259, 1989.

Ross, J., & Dean, E. (1992). Body positioning. In C.C. Zadai (Ed.). *Clinics in physical therapy. Pulmonary management in physical therapy.* New York: Churchill Livingstone.

Samsel, R.W., & Schumacker, P.T. (1991). Oxygen delivery to tissues, *European Respiratory Journal* 4:1258–1267.

Sandler, H. (1986). Cardiovascular effects of inactivity. In Sandler, H., Vernikos, J., (Eds.). *Inactivity physiological effects.* Orlando, Fla: Academic Press.

Schumacker, P.T., & Cain, S.M.: The concept of critical oxygen delivery, *Intensive Care Medicine 13:*223–229.

Schumaker, P.T., & Samsel, R.W. (1989). Oxygen delivery and uptake by peripheral tissues: physiology and pathophysiology, *Critical Care Clinics* 5:255–269.

Shephard, R.J. (1985). *Physiology and biochemistry of exercise,* Philadelphia: Praeger Scientific.

Tortora, G.J., & Anagnostakos N.P. (1990). *Principles of anatomy and physiology,* New York: Harper & Row.

Wasserman, K., et al (1987). *Principles of exercise testing and interpretation,* Philadelphia: Lea & Febiger.

Weber, K.T., et al (1983). The cardiopulmonary unit: The body's gas exchange system, *Clinics Chest Medicine 4:*101–110.

West, J.B. (1985). *Respiratory physiology—the essentials,* ed 5, Baltimore: Williams & Wilkins.

West, J.B.: *Ventilation, blood flow and gas exchange,* (ed 4). Oxford: Blackwell Scientific.

Winslow, E.H. (1985). *Cardiovascular consequences of bed rest, Heart Lung* 14:236–246.

CHAPTER 2

Cardiopulmonary Anatomy

Elizabeth Dean
Lyn Hobson

KEY TERMS

Cardiopulmonary unit
Heart
Heart-lung interdependence
Lymphatic circulation
Parenchyma

Peripheral circulation
Pulmonary circulation
Respiratory muscles
Thoracic cavity
Tracheobronchial tree

INTRODUCTION

The heart lies in series with the lungs, constituting the cardiopulmonary unit, the central component of the oxygen transport pathway (Scharf and Cassidy, 1989; Weber et al, 1983). Virtually all the blood returned to the right side of the heart passes through the lungs and is delivered to the left side of the heart for ejection to the systemic, coronary, and bronchopulmonary circulations. Because of this interrelationship, changes in either lung or heart function can exert changes in the function of the other organ. A detailed understanding of the anatomy of the heart and lungs, and how these organs work synergistically is essential to the practice of cardiopulmonary physical therapy.

This chapter presents the anatomy of the cardiopulmonary system, including the skeletal features of the thoracic cavity; muscles of respiration; anatomy of the tracheobronchial tree; lung parenchyma; basic anatomy of the heart; and peripheral, pulmonary, and lymphatic circulations (Berne and Levy, 1992; Burton and Hodgkin, 1984; Ganong, 1993; Guyton, 1991; Katz, 1992; Murray, 1986; Murray and Nadel, 1988; Nunn, 1993; West, 1991; West, 1995; and Williams et al, 1989).

THORAX

The bony thorax covers and protects the principal organs of respiration and circulation, as well as the

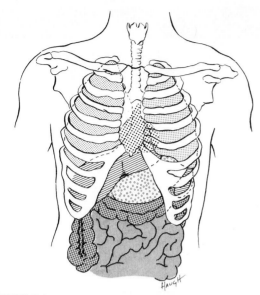

FIGURE 2-1
The relationship of the bony thorax and lungs to the abdominal contents (anterior view).

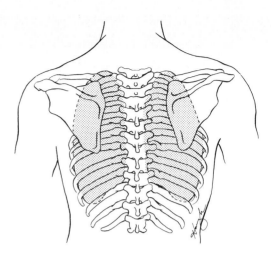

FIGURE 2-2
The relationship of the lungs to the bony thorax (posterior view).

liver and the stomach (Figures 2-1 and 2-2). The posterior surface is formed by the 12 thoracic vertebrae and the posterior part of the 12 ribs. The anterior surface is formed by the sternum and the costal cartilage. The lateral surfaces are formed by the ribs. At birth, the thorax is nearly circular, but during childhood and adolescence, it becomes more elliptical until adulthood. It is wider from side to side than it is from front to back.

Sternum

The sternum, or breastbone, is a flat bone with three parts: the manubrium, body, and xiphoid process. The manubrium is the widest and thickest bone of the sternum. Its upper border is scalloped by a central jugular notch, which can be palpated, and two clavicular notches that house the clavicles. Its lower border articulates with the upper border of the body at a slight angle, the sternal angle or angle of Louis. This angle can be easily palpated, is a landmark located between thoracic vertebrae T4 and T5, and is on a

level with the second costal cartilages. The bifurcation of the trachea into the right and left mainstem bronchi also occurs at the sternal angle. The manubrium and body are joined by fibrocartilage, which may ossify in later life.

The body of the sternum is twice as long as the manubrium. It is a relatively thin bone and can be easily pierced by needles for bone marrow aspirations. The heart is located beneath and to the left of the lower one third of the body of the sternum. Although it is attached by cartilage to the ribs, this portion of the sternum is flexible and can be depressed without breaking. This maneuver is used, with care, in closed cardiac massage to artificially circulate blood to the brain and extremities. The lower margin of the body is attached to the xiphoid process by fibrocartilage. This bone is the smallest of the three parts of the sternum and usually fuses with the body of the sternum in later life.

Ribs

A large portion of the bony thoracic cage is formed by 12 ribs located on either side of the sternum. The first seven ribs connect posteriorly with the vertebral

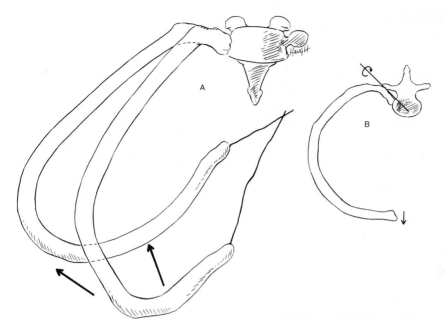

FIGURE 2-3
The movements of the ribs. **A,** "Bucket handle," lower rib. **B,** "Pump handle," first rib.

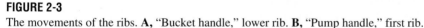

column and anteriorly through costal cartilages with the sternum. These are known as the true ribs. The remaining five ribs are known as the false ribs. The first three have their cartilage attached to the cartilage of the rib above. The last two are free or floating ribs. The ribs increase in length from the first to the seventh rib, and then decrease to the twelfth rib. They also increase in obliquity until the ninth rib and then decrease in obliquity to the twelfth rib.

Each rib has a small head and a short neck that articulate with two thoracic vertebrae. The shaft of the rib curves gently from the neck to a sudden sharp bend, the angle of the rib. Fractures often occur at this site. A costal groove is located on the lower border of the shaft of the ribs. This groove houses the intercostal nerves and vessels. Chest tubes and needles are inserted above the ribs to avoid these vessels and nerves. The ribs are separated from each other by the intercostal spaces that contain the intercostal muscles.

MOVEMENTS OF THE THORAX

The frequency of movement of the bony thorax joints is greater than that of almost any other combination of joints in the body. Two types of movements have been described—the pump-handle movement and the bucket-handle movement (Figure 2-3) (Cherniack and Cherniack, 1983). The upper ribs are limited in their ability to move. Each pair swings like a pump handle, with elevation thrusting the sternum forward. This forward movement increases the anteroposterior diameter and the depth of the thorax and is called the pump-handle movement. In the lower ribs, there is little antero-posterior movement. During inspiration, the ribs swing outward and upward, each pushing against the rib above during elevation. This bucket-handle movement increases the transverse diameter of the thoracic cage. Thus during inspiration, the thorax increases its volume by increasing its anteroposterior and transverse diameters.

MUSCLES OF RESPIRATION

Inspiration

Inspiration is an active movement involving the contraction of the diaphragm and intercostals. Additional muscles may come into play during exertion in health. In disease, the role of these accessory muscles of inspiration may have an important role even at rest. The accessory muscles include the sternocleidomastoids, scalenes, serratus anterior, pectoralis major and minor, trapezius, and erector spinae. The degree to which these accessory muscles are used by the patient is dependent on the severity of cardiopulmonary distress (Clemente, 1985; Murray and Nadel, 1988; and Williams et al, 1989).

Diaphragm

The diaphragm is the principal muscle of respiration. During quiet breathing, the diaphragm contributes approximately two thirds of the tidal volume in the sitting or standing positions, and approximately three fourths of the tidal volume in the supine position. It is also estimated that two thirds of the vital capacity in all positions is contributed by the diaphragm.

The diaphragm is a large, dome-shaped muscle that separates the thoracic and abdominal cavities. Its upper surface supports the pericardium (with which it is partially blended), heart, pleurae, and lungs. Its lower surface is almost completely covered by the peritoneum and overlies the liver, kidneys, suprarenal glands, stomach, and spleen (Figure 2-4). This large muscle can be divided into right and left halves. Each half is made up of three parts—sternal, lumbar, and costal. These three parts are inserted into the central tendon, which lies just below the heart. The sternal part arises from the back of the xiphoid process and descends to the central tendon. On each side is a small gap, the sternocostal triangle, which is located between the sternal and costal parts. It transmits the superior epigastric vessels and is often the site of diaphragmatic hernias. The costal parts form the right and left domes. They arise from the inner surfaces of the lower four ribs and the lower six costal cartilages. They interdigitate and transverse the abdomen to insert into the anterolateral part of the central tendon. The lumbar part arises from the bodies of the upper

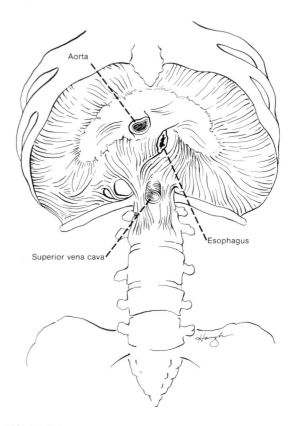

FIGURE 2-4
The diaphragm from below.

lumbar vertebrae and extends upward to the central tendon. The central tendon is a thin, strong aponeurosis situated near the center of the muscle, somewhat closer to the front of the body. It resembles a trefoil leaf with three divisions or leaflets. The right leaflet is the largest, the middle is the next largest, and the left leaflet is the smallest.

Major vessels traverse the diaphragm through one of three openings (see Figure 2-4). The vena caval opening is located to the right of the midline in the central tendon and contains branches of the right phrenic nerve and the inferior vena cava. The esophageal opening is located to the left of the midline and contains the esophagus, the vagal nerve trunks and branches of the gastric vessels. The aortic opening is located in the midline and contains the

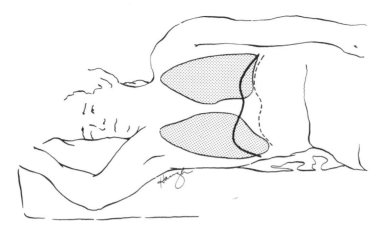

FIGURE 2-5
When the patient is lying on side, the dome of the diaphragm on the lower side rises further in the thorax than the dome on the upper side.

aorta, thoracic duct, and sometimes the azygos vein. The diaphragm is also pierced by branches of the left phrenic nerve, small veins, and lymph vessels.

The position of the diaphragm and its range of movement vary with posture, the degree of distention of the stomach, size of the intestines, size of the liver, and obesity. The average movement of the diaphragm in quiet respiration is 12.5 mm on the right and 12 mm on the left. This can increase to a maximum of 30 mm on the right and 28 mm on the left during increased ventilation. The posture of the individual determines the position of the diaphragm. In the supine position, the resting level of the diaphragm rises. The greatest respiratory excursions during normal breathing occur in this position. However, the lung volumes are decreased because of the elevated position of the abdominal organs. In a sitting or upright position, the dome of the diaphragm is pulled down by the abdominal organs, allowing a larger lung volume. For this reason, individuals who are short of breath are more comfortable sitting than reclining. In a side-lying position, the dome of the diaphragm on the lower side rises farther into the thorax than the dome on the upper side (Figure 2-5). The abdominal organs have a tendency to fall forward out of the way, allowing greater excursion of the dome on the lower side. In contrast, the upper side moves little with respiration

in this position. On x-ray, the position of the diaphragm can indicate whether the film was taken during inspiration or expiration, and may also indicate pathology in the lungs, pleurae, or abdomen.

Each half of the diaphragm is innervated by a separate nerve—the phrenic nerve on that side. Although the halves contract simultaneously, it is possible for half of the muscle to be paralyzed without affecting the other half. Generally, the paralyzed half remains at the normal level during rest. However, with deep inspiration, the paralyzed half is pulled up by the negative pressure in the thorax. A special x-ray, moving fluoroscopy, is used to determine paralysis of the diaphragm.

Contraction of the diaphragm increases the thoracic volume vertically and transversely. The central tendon is drawn down by the diaphragm as it contracts. As the dome descends, abdominal organs are pushed forward, as far as the abdominal walls will allow. When the dome can descend no farther, the costal fibers of the diaphragm contract to increase the thoracic diameter of the thorax. This occurs because the fibers of the costal part of the diaphragm run vertically from their attachment at the costal margin. Thus contraction of these fibers elevates and everts the ribs (Figure 2-6). If the diaphragm is in a low position, it will change the angle of pull of the muscle's

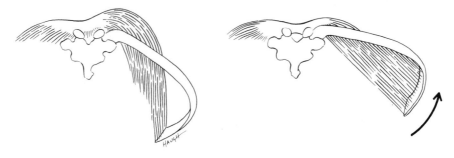

FIGURE 2-6
Contraction of the costal fibers of the diaphragm causes rib eversion and elevation.

costal fibers. Contraction of these fibers creates a horizontal pull, which causes the lateral diameter to become smaller as the ribs are pulled in toward the central tendon.

As the diaphragm descends, it compresses the abdominal organs, increasing intraabdominal pressure. At the same time, the intrathoracic pressure decreases as the lung volume is increased by the descending diaphragm. Inspiratory airflow occurs as a result of this decrease in intrathoracic pressure (see Chapter 3). The pressure gradient between the abdominal and thoracic cavities also facilitates the return of blood to the right side of the heart.

Movement of the diaphragm can be controlled to some extent voluntarily. Vocalists spend years learning to manipulate their diaphragms to produce the controlled sounds during singing. The diaphragm momentarily ceases movement when a person holds his or her breath. The diaphragm is involuntarily involved in parturition, bearing down in bowel movements, laughing, crying, and vomiting. Hiccups are spasmodic, sharp contractions of the diaphragm that may indicate disease (e.g., a subphrenic abscess) if they persist.

Intercostals

The external intercostals extend from the tubercles of the ribs, above, down, and forward to the costochondral junction of the ribs below, where they become continuous with the anterior intercostal membrane (Figure 2-7). This membrane extends the

muscle forward to the sternum. There are 11 external intercostal muscles on each side of the sternum. They are thicker posteriorly than anteriorly, and thicker than the internal intercostal muscles. They are innervated by the intercostal nerves, and contraction draws the lower rib up and out toward the upper rib. This action increases the volume of the thoracic cavity.

There are also 11 internal intercostals per side. These are considered primarily expiratory in function. Studies have shown that the intercartilaginous or parasternal portion of the internal intercostals contracts with the external intercostals during inspiration to help elevate the ribs. Besides their respiratory functions, the intercostal muscles contract to prevent the intercostal spaces from being drawn in or bulged out during respiratory activity.

Sternocleidomastoid

The sternocleidomastoids (SCMs) are strong neck muscles arising from two heads, one from the manubrium and one from the medial part of the clavicle (see Figure 2-7, p. 29). These two heads fuse into one muscle mass that is inserted behind the ear into the mastoid process. It is innervated by the accessory nerve and the second cervical nerve. There are two of these muscles, one on each side of the neck. When one SCM contracts, it tilts the head toward the shoulder of the same side and rotates the face toward the opposite shoulder. If the two SCM muscles contract together, they pull the head forward into flexion. When the head is fixed, they assist in elevating the sternum, increasing

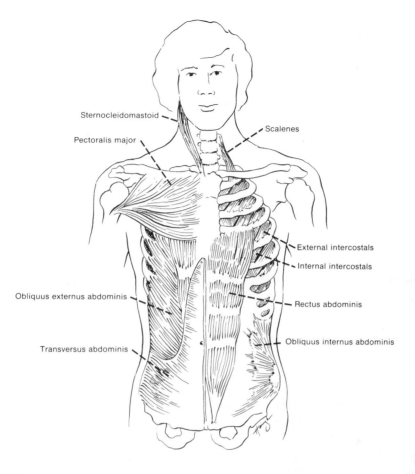

FIGURE 2-7
Respiratory muscles (anterior view).

the anteroposterior (AP) diameter of the thorax.

The SCMs are the most important accessory muscles of inspiration. Their contractions can be observed in all patients during forced inspiration and in all patients who are dyspneic. These muscles become visually predominant in patients who are chronically dyspneic (see Chapter 4).

Scalenes

The anterior, medial, and posterior scalenes are three separate muscles that are considered as a functional unit. They are attached superiorly to the transverse processes of the lower five cervical vertebrae

and inferiorly to the upper surface of the first two ribs (see Figure 2-7). They are innervated by related cervical spinal nerves. These muscles are primarily supportive neck muscles, but they can assist in respiration through reverse action. When their superior attachment is fixed, the scalenes act as accessory respiratory muscles and elevate the first two ribs during inspiration.

Serratus Anterior

The serratus anterior arises from the outer surfaces of the first eight or nine ribs. It curves backward, forming a sheet of muscle that inserts into the medial border of the scapula. It is innervated by the long thoracic nerve (cervical nerves C5, C6, and C7). There are two of these muscles, one on each side of the body. Normally, they assist in forward pushing of the arm (as in boxing or punching). When the scapulae are fixed, they act as accessory respiratory muscles and elevate the ribs to which they are attached.

Pectoralis Major

The pectoralis major is a large muscle arising from the clavicle, the sternum, and the cartilages of all the true ribs (see Figure 2-7, p. 29). This muscle sweeps across the anterior chest to insert into the intertubercular sulcus of the humerus. It is innervated by the lateral and medial pectoral nerves and cervical nerves C5, C6, C7, C8, and T1. There are two of these muscles, one on each side of the body. This muscle acts to rotate the humerus medially and to draw the arm across the chest. In climbing and pull-ups, it draws the trunk toward the arms. In forced inspiration when the arms are fixed, it draws the ribs toward the arms, thereby increasing thoracic diameter.

Pectoralis Minor

The pectoralis minor is a thin muscle originating from the outer surfaces of the third, fourth, and fifth ribs near their cartilages. It inserts into the coracoid process of the scapula. It is innervated by the pectoral nerves (cervical nerves C6, C7, and C8). There are two of these muscles, one on each side of the body. They contract with the serratus anterior to draw the scapulae toward the chest. During deep inspiration, they contract to elevate the ribs to which they are attached.

Trapezius

The trapezius consists of two muscles that form a huge diamond-shaped sheet extending from the head down the back and out to both shoulders (Figure 2-8). Its upper belly originates from the external occipital protuberance and curves around the side of the neck to insert into the posterior border of the clavicle. The middle part of the muscle arises from a thin diamond-shaped tendinous sheet, the supraspinous ligaments and the spines of the upper thoracic region, and runs horizontally to insert into

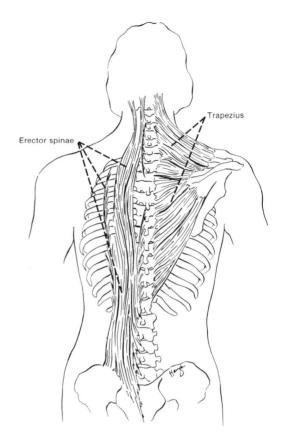

FIGURE 2-8
Respiratory muscles (posterior view).

the spine of the scapula. Its lower belly arises from the supraspinous ligaments and the spines of the lower thoracic region, and runs upward to be inserted into the lower border of the spine of the scapula. This large muscle is innervated by the external or spinal part of the accessory nerve and cervical nerves C3 and C4. Its main function is to rotate the scapulae in elevating the arms and to control their gravitational descent. It also braces the scapulae and raises them, as in shrugging the shoulders. Its ability to stabilize the scapulae makes it an important accessory muscle in respiration. This stabilization enables the serratus anterior and pectoralis minor to elevate the ribs.

Erector Spinae

The erector spinae is a large muscle extending from the sacrum to the skull (see Figure 2-8, p. 30). It originates from the sacrum, iliac crest, and the spines of the lower thoracic and lumbar vertebrae. It separates into a lateral iliocostalis, an intermediate longissimus, and a medial spinalis column. This muscle mass inserts into various ribs and vertebral processes all the way up to the skull. It is innervated by the related spinal nerves. These muscles extend, laterally flex, and rotate the vertebral column. They are considered accessory respiratory muscles through their extension of the vertebral column. In deep inspiration, these muscles extend the vertebral column, allowing further elevation of the ribs.

Expiration

Expiration is a passive process, occurring when the intercostals and diaphragm relax. Their relaxation allows the ribs to drop to their preinspiratory position and the diaphragm to rise. These activities compress the lungs, raising intrathoracic pressure above atmospheric pressure, and thereby contributing to air flow out of the lungs.

Rectus Abdominis

The rectus abdominis rises from the pubic crest and extends upward to insert into the xiphoid process and the costal margin of the fifth, sixth, and seventh costal cartilages (see Figure 2-7, p. 29). It is innervated by related spinal nerves, and its action is considered within the context of the other abdominal muscles.

Obliquus Externus Abdominis

This muscle arises in an oblique line from the fifth costal cartilage to the twelfth rib (see Figure 2-7, p. 29). Its posterior fibers attach in an almost vertical line with the iliac crest. The other fibers extend down and forward to attach to the front of the xiphoid process, the linea alba, and below with the pubic symphysis. It is innervated by the lower six thoracic spinal nerves.

Obliquus Internus Abdominis

This muscle originates from the lumbar fascia, the anterior two thirds of the iliac crest, and the lateral two thirds of the inguinal ligament (see Figure 2-7, p. 29). Its posterior fibers run almost vertically upward to insert into the lower borders of the last three ribs. The other fibers join an aponeurosis attached to the costal margin above, the linea alba in the midline and the pubic crest below. It is innervated by the lower six thoracic nerves and the first lumbar spinal nerves.

Transversus Abdominis

The transversus abdominis arises from the inner surface of the lower six costal cartilages, the lumbar fascia, the anterior two thirds of the iliac crest, and the lateral one third of the inguinal ligament (see Figure 2-7, p. 29). It runs across the abdomen horizontally to insert into the aponeurosis, extending to the linea alba. It is innervated by the lower six thoracic nerves and the first lumbar spinal nerves.

Action of the Abdominal Muscles

These four muscles work together to provide a firm but flexible wall to keep the abdominal viscera in position. The abdominal muscles exert a compressing force on the abdomen when the thorax and pelvis are fixed. This force can be used in defecation, urination, parturition, and vomiting. In forced expiration, the abdominal muscles help force the diaphragm back to its resting position and thus force air from the lungs. If the pelvis and vertebral column are fixed, the obliquus externus abdominis aids expiration further by depressing and compressing the lower part of the thorax. Patients with chronic obstructive pulmonary disease (COPD) have difficulty in exhalation, which causes them to trap air in their lungs. The continued contraction of the abdominal muscles throughout exhalation helps them force this air from the lungs. The abdominal muscles also play an important role in coughing. First, a large volume of air is inhaled, and the glottis is closed. Then the abdominal muscles contract, raising intrathoracic pressure. When the glottis opens, the large difference in intrathoracic and atmospheric pressure causes the air to be expelled forcefully at tremendous flow rates (tussive blast).

Patients with weak abdominal muscles (from neuromuscular diseases, paraplegia, quadriplegia or extensive abdominal surgery) often have ineffective coughs (see Chapters 28 and 33).

The four abdominal muscles have many other nonrespiratory functions both individually and as a group; these are not discussed here.

Internal Intercostals

There are 11 internal intercostal muscles on each side of the thorax. Each muscle arises from the floor of the costal groove and cartilage, and passes inferiorly and posteriorly to insert on the upper border of the rib below. These internal intercostals extend from the sternum anteriorly, around the thorax to the posterior costal angle. They are generally divided into two parts—the interosseous portion located between the sloping parts of the ribs, and the intercartilaginous portions located between costal cartilages. As discussed previously, the intercartilaginous portions are considered inspiratory in function. Contraction of the interosseous portions of the intercostals depresses the ribs and may aid in forceful exhalation. This muscle is innervated by the adjacent intercostal nerves.

SUMMARY OF RESPIRATORY MOVEMENTS

In quiet inspiration, the diaphragm, external intercostals, and intercartilaginous portions of the internal intercostals are the primary muscles that contract. The diaphragm contracts first and then descends, enlarging the thoracic cage vertically. When abdominal contents prevent its further descent, the costal fibers of the diaphragm contract, causing the lower ribs to swing up and out to the side (bucket-handle movement). This lateral rib movement is assisted by the external intercostals and the intercartilaginous portion of the internal intercostals. The transverse diameter of the thorax is increased by this bucket-handle movement. Finally, the upper ribs move forward and upward (pump-handle movement) also through contraction of their external intercostals and the intercartilaginous portions of the internal intercostals. This increases the AP diameter of the thorax. During quiet inspiration, the epigastric area protrudes, then the ribs swing up and out laterally, and finally the upper ribs move forward and upward (Cherniack and Cherniack, 1983).

Quiet expiration is passive and involves no muscular contraction although some electrical activity can be detected. The inspiratory muscles relax, causing intrathoracic pressure to be raised as the ribs and diaphragm compress the lungs by returning to their preinspiratory positions. This increased pressure allows air flow from the lungs.

In forced inspiration, a large number of accessory muscles may contract in addition to the normal inspiratory muscles mentioned. The erector spinae contract to extend the vertebral column. This extension permits greater elevation of the ribs during inspiration. Various back muscles (e.g., erector spinae, trapezius, and rhomboids) contract to stabilize the vertebral column, head, neck, and scapulae. This enables accessory respiratory muscles to assist inspiration through reverse action. The SCM raises the sternum. The scalenes elevate the first two ribs. The serratus anterior, pectoralis major, and pectoralis minor assist in elevating the ribs bilaterally. All these accessory muscles tend to elevate the ribs, thus increasing the AP diameter but not the transverse diameter of the thorax. (In fact, the transverse diameter does increase slightly as a result of the increased strength of the contraction of the normal inspiratory muscles.) The marked increase in AP diameter in relation to transverse diameter creates an impression of *en bloc* breathing in the patient using accessory muscles.

In forced expiration, the interosseous portion of the internal intercostals and the abdominal muscles contract to force air out of the lungs. Forced expiration can be slow and prolonged (as in patients with COPD) or rapid and expulsive (as in a cough). If the abdominal contractions are strong enough, the trunk flexes during exhalation. This flexion further compresses the lungs, forcing more air from them.

UPPER AIRWAYS

Nose

Noses vary in size and shape with individuals and nationalities. Its framework is comprised of bony and cartilaginous parts. The upper one third is primarily bony and contains the nasal bones, the frontal processes of the maxillae and the nasal part of the frontal bone. Its lower two thirds are cartilaginous and contain the septal, lateral, and major and minor alar nasal cartilages. The nasal cavity is divided into right and left halves by the nasal septum. This cavity extends from the nostrils to the posterior apertures of the nose in the nasopharynx. The lateral walls of the cavity are irregular as a result of projecting superior, middle, and inferior nasal chonchae. There is a meatus located beneath or lateral to each choncha through which the sinuses drain. The chonchae increase the surface area of the nose for maximum contact with inspired air. The superior chonchae and adjacent septal wall are referred to as the olfactory region. They

are covered with a thin, yellow olfactory mucous membrane that consists of bipolar nerve cells that are olfactory in function. Only a portion of inspired air reaches the olfactory region to provide a sense of smell. When people smell something specific, they *sniff*. This action lifts the inspired air so that more of it comes in contact with the olfactory region.

The anterior portion (vestibule) of the nasal cavity (Figure 2-9) is lined with skin and coarse hairs (vibrissae) that entrap inhaled particles. The rest of the cavity and sinuses (with the exception of the olfactory region) are lined with respiratory mucous membrane. This membrane is composed of pseudostratified columnar ciliated epithelium (Figure 2-10). It contains goblet cells, as well as mucous and serous glands that produce secrete mucus and serous secretions. These secretions

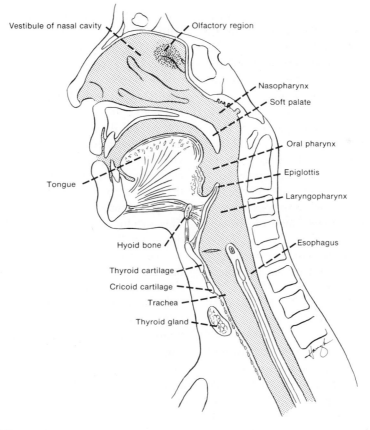

FIGURE 2-9
Sagittal section of the head and neck.

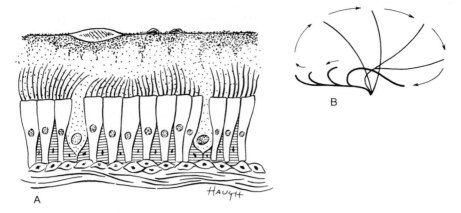

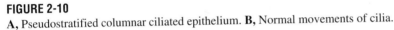

FIGURE 2-10
A, Pseudostratified columnar ciliated epithelium. **B,** Normal movements of cilia.

entrap foreign particles and bacteria. This mucus is then swept to the nasopharynx by the cilia at a rate of 5 to 15 mm/min, where it is swallowed or expectorated. The mucous membrane is vascular, with arterial blood supplied by branches of the internal and external carotid arteries. Venous drainage occurs through the anterior facial veins. The mucous membrane is thickest over the chonchae. As air is inhaled, it passes around and over the chonchae, whose vascular moist surfaces heat, humidify, and filter the inspired air. The mucous membrane may become swollen and irritated in upper respiratory infections and may secrete copious amounts of mucus. Because this membrane is continuous with sinuses, auditory tubes and lacrimal canaliculi, people suffering from colds often complain of sinus headaches, watery eyes, earaches, and other symptoms. Secretions are often so copious that the nasal passages become completely blocked.

Pharynx

The pharynx is an oval fibromuscular sac located behind the nasal cavity, mouth, and larynx. It is approximately 12 to 14 cm long and extends from the base of the skull to the esophagus below, at the level of the cricoid cartilage opposite the sixth cervical vertebra. Anteriorly, it opens into the nasal cavity (nasopharynx), mouth (oral pharynx) and larynx (laryngopharynx). The pharyngeal walls are lined with ciliated respiratory mucous membrane in the nasal portion, and stratified squamous in the oral and laryngeal parts.

The nasopharynx is a continuation of the nasal cavities (see Figure 2-9, p. 33). It lies behind the nose and above the soft palate. With the exception of the soft palate, its walls are immovable, so its cavity is never obliterated, as is the oral and laryngeal pharynx. The nasopharynx communicates with the nasal cavity anteriorly through the posterior apertures of the nose. It communicates with the laryngeal and oral pharynx through an opening, the pharyngeal isthmus. This opening is closed by elevations of the soft palate during swallowing.

The oral pharynx extends from the soft palate to the epiglottis (see Figure 2-9, p. 33). It opens into the mouth anteriorly through the oropharyngeal isthmus. Its posterior walls lie on the bodies of the second and third cervical vertebrae. Laterally, two masses of lymphoid tissue—the palatine tonsils—may be seen. These tonsils form part of a circular band of lymphoid tissue surrounding the opening into the digestive and respiratory tracts.

The laryngopharynx lies behind the larynx and extends from the epiglottis above to the inlet of the esophagus below (see Figure 2-9, p. 33). The fourth to sixth cervical vertebrae lie behind the laryngeal

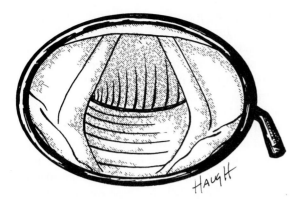

FIGURE 2-11
Visualization of the larynx via a laryngoscope.

pharynx. In front of the laryngopharynx are the epiglottis, the inlet of the larynx and the posterior surfaces of the arytenoid and cricoid cartilages.

Larynx

The larynx is a complex structure composed of cartilages and cords moved by sensitive muscles (Figure 2-11), and is located between the trachea and laryngopharynx, for which it forms an anterior wall. It acts as a sphincteric valve with its rapid closure, preventing food, liquids, and foreign objects from entering the airway. It controls airflow, and at times closes so that thoracic pressure may be raised and the upper airways cleared by a propulsive cough when the larynx opens. Expiratory airflow vibrates as it passes over the contracting vocal chords, producing the sounds used for speech. (The larynx is not essential for speech. Humans can speak by learning to dilate the upper part of the esophagus so that air vibrates as it passes over; this is called esophageal speech).

In adult men, the larynx is situated opposite the third, fourth and fifth cervical vertebrae; it is situated somewhat higher in women and children. In children, the larynx is essentially the same in girls and boys. At puberty, the male larynx increases in size considerably until its AP diameter is almost doubled. All the cartilages enlarge, with the thyroid cartilage becoming prominent anteriorly.

The laryngeal skeleton contains the hyoid bone

and the cartilages of the larynx (e.g., thyroid, cricoid, epiglottic, right and left arytenoids, corniculates, and cuneiforms). The thyroid cartilage is the largest. It has a V-shaped notch in its upper one third, which projects forward, forming the "Adam's apple." The entire cartilage is pulled up in swallowing, with the upper part of the cartilage passing beneath the hyoid bone. The cricoid cartilage is shaped like a signet ring, with the signet part facing the posterior. The anterior part of the cartilage is easily palpated just below the thyroid cartilage. It is thicker and more prominent than the tracheal rings, which lie below. It is the only cartilage that completely circles the airway. The cricoid cartilage is connected to the thyroid cartilage by the cricothyroid membrane. (This membrane is often punctured to establish an airway in an emergency when the upper airway is obstructed.) The epiglottic cartilage is the elastic skeleton of the epiglottis. It is a leaflike structure attached by ligaments to the hyoid bone anteriorly and the thyroid cartilage below. It is considered a vestigial structure, and its removal causes little effect. Finally, the arytenoid cartilages are two small pyramid-shaped cartilages that articulate with the posterior part of the cricoid cartilage. The vocal cords attach from these cartilages to the thyroid cartilage.

The true vocal cords (or vocal folds) are two pearly white folds of mucous membrane that stretch from the arytenoid cartilage to the thyroid cartilage. The space between the true vocal cords is called the *rima glottidis.* It changes shape with movement of the cords but is generally triangular when the cords are open. The rima glottidis and the true vocal cords are grouped together under the term *glottis.* The glottis is the narrowest part of the adult airway.

Just above the true vocal cords are two shallow grooves in the mucous membrane lining of the larynx. These grooves (ventricles of the larynx) contain numerous glands that secrete the mucus that covers the larynx. The false vocal cords (vestibular or ventricular folds) lie just above the ventricles of the larynx. They are two soft, pink masses of mucous membrane raised slightly from the laryngeal wall. They extend from the thyroid cartilage to the arytenoids. The false cords are not as well developed as the true cords and do not approximate completely during phonation. However, their closure can help protect the airway from aspiration of foreign material.

There are two main groups of muscles that control the opening and closing of the glottis—the abductors and adductors. The posterior cricoarytenoid muscle is the most important muscle in the larynx, since it is the only abductor of the vocal folds. It is vital for respiration. Contraction of this muscle separates the vocal folds and widens the lumen of the glottis. There are eight adductors of the vocal folds: (1) aryepiglottic, (2) thyroepiglottic, (3) thyroarytenoid, (4) vocalis, (5) cricothyroid, (6) lateral cricoarytenoid, (7) transverse arytenoid and (8) oblique arytenoid muscles. Contraction of these muscles results in approximation of the vocal cords and narrowing of the glottis. The adductors of the cords are important in protecting the lower airways. Their contraction prevents fluids, food, and other substances from being aspirated. All the intrinsic laryngeal muscles are innervated by the recurrent laryngeal nerve (a branch of the vagus nerve) with the exception of the cricothyroid muscle, which is supplied by the external branch of the superior laryngeal nerve (also a branch of the vagus nerve).

The mucous membrane of the larynx is continuous with that of the laryngopharynx above and the trachea below. It lines the cavity of the larynx and the structures found within. On the anterior surface and upper half of the posterior surface of the epiglottis, and the vocal folds, the mucous membrane is stratified squamous epithelium. The rest of the laryngeal mucosa is ciliated columnar epithelium. The mucous membrane of the larynx has many mucous glands. They are especially numerous in the epiglottis, in front of the arytenoid cartilages and in the ventricles of the larynx. Some taste buds are also located on the epiglottis and irregularly throughout the rest of the larynx.

LOWER AIRWAYS

Trachea

The trachea is a semi-rigid, cartilaginous tube approximately 10 to 11 cm long and 2.5 cm wide. It lies in front of the esophagus, descending with a slight incli-

nation to the right from the level of the cricoid cartilage (see Figure 2-11, p. 35, and Figure 2-12). It travels behind the sternum into the thorax to the sternal angle (opposite the fifth thoracic vertebra), where it divides to form the right and left main-stem bronchi. The tracheal wall is strengthened by 16 to 20 horseshoe-shaped cartilaginous rings. The open parts of the tracheal rings are completed by fibrous and elastic tissue and unstriated transverse muscle. This part of the ring faces the posterior and is very flexible. It indents or curves inward during coughing, which increases the velocity of expelled air. These cartilages lie horizontally one above the other, separated by narrow bands of connective tissue. The trachea is lengthened during hyperextension of the head; swallowing, which raises the trachea; and inspiration, when the lungs expand and pull the trachea downward. Its cross-sectional area becomes smaller with contraction of the unstriated transverse muscle fibers that complete the tracheal rings.

The mucous membrane of the trachea also contains columnar ciliated epithelium and goblet cells. Each ciliated epithelial cell contains approximately 275 cilia. These structures beat rapidly in a coordinated and unidirectional manner, propelling a sheet of mucus cephalad from the lower respiratory tract to the pharynx, where it is swallowed or expectorated. The cilia beat in this layer of mucus with a strong, forceful forward stroke, followed by a slow ineffective backward stroke that returns the cilia to their starting position. This propelling of mucus by the cilia (mucociliary escalator) is essential. When cilia are paralyzed by smoke, alcohol, dehydration, anesthesia, starvation, or hypoxia, mucus begins to accumulate in distal, gravity-dependent airways, causing infiltrates and eventually localized areas of collapse referred to as atelectasis.

The number of mucus-containing goblet cells is approximately equal to the number of ciliated epithelial cells. Reserve cells lie beneath the ciliated and goblet cells. These reserve cells can differentiate into either goblet cells or ciliated cells. Beneath the reserve cells lie the gland cells. There are approximately 40 times more gland cells than goblet cells. Mucus is composed of 95% water, 2% glycoprotein, 1% carbohydrate, trace amounts of lipid, deoxyri-

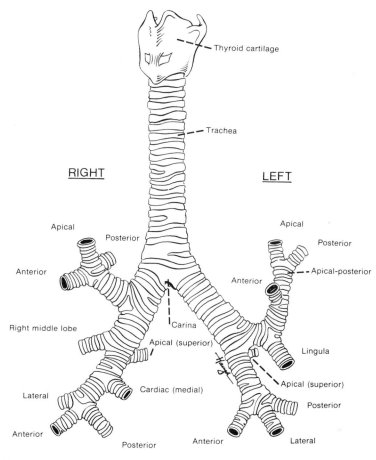

Thyroid cartilage

Trachea

RIGHT

LEFT

Apical

Apical

Posterior

Posterior

Apical-posterior

Anterior

Anterior

Right middle lobe

Carina

Lingula

Apical (superior)

Cardiac (medial)

Apical (superior)

Lateral

Posterior

Anterior

Posterior

Anterior

Lateral

FIGURE 2-12

Tracheobronchial tree (a three-quarter view, rotated toward the right side).

bonucleic acid (DNA), dead tissue cells, phagocytes, leukocytes, erythrocytes, and entrapped foreign particles. Mucus lines the airways from the trachea to the alveoli. Two separate layers have been observed—the sol layer, which lies on the mucosal surface and contains high concentrations of water, and the gel layer, which is more superficial and more viscous because of its lower concentration of water.

The right main-stem bronchus appears to be an extension of the trachea, being wider, shorter, and more vertical than the left main-stem bronchus. Its greater width and more vertical course cause a majority of aspirated foreign material to pass through the right

main-stem bronchus. The azygos vein arches over the right main-stem bronchus, the right pulmonary artery lies beneath. The right main-stem bronchus divides to form the right upper lobe bronchus, the right middle lobe bronchus and the right lower lobe bronchus. The right upper lobe divides into three segmental bronchi—apical, posterior, and anterior. The apical bronchus runs almost vertically toward the apex of the lung. The posterior bronchus is directed posteriorly in a horizontal direction, while the anterior bronchus is directed anteriorly in an almost horizontal direction. The right middle lobe bronchus divides about 10 mm below the right upper lobe bronchus and descends downward anterolaterally. The right lower lobe bronchus divides into five segmental bronchi. The apical or superior bronchus runs almost horizontally, posteriorly. The medial or cardiac bronchus descends downward medially toward the heart. The anterior basal bronchus descends anteriorly. The lateral basal bronchus descends laterally and the posterior bronchus descends posteriorly. Note that each segment describes its position.

The left main-stem bronchus is narrower and runs more horizontally than the right main-stem bronchus. The aortic arch passes over it, while the esophagus, descending aorta, and thoracic duct lie behind it. The left pulmonary artery lies anteriorly and above the left main-stem bronchus. The left main-stem bronchus has two major divisions—the left upper lobe bronchus and the left lower lobe bronchus. The left upper lobe bronchus has three major segmental bronchi. The anterior bronchus ascends at approximately a 45-degree angle. The apical-posterior bronchus has two branches; one runs vertically and the other posteriorly toward the apex of the left lung. The lingular bronchus descends anterolaterally, much like the right middle lobe bronchus of the right lung. The right lower lobe bronchus divides into four segmental bronchi. The superior or apical bronchus runs posteriorly in a horizontal direction. The anterior bronchus descends anteriorly. The lateral bronchus descends laterally, while the posterior bronchus descends posteriorly. Again the segments describe their anatomical position.

The bronchi of the airways continue to divide until there are approximately 23 generations (Table 2-1). The main, lobar, and segmental bronchi are made up of the first four generations. The walls contain U-shaped cartilage in the main bronchi. This cartilage becomes less well-defined and more irregularly shaped as the bronchi continue to divide. In the segmental bronchi the walls are formed by irregularly shaped helical plates with bands of bronchial muscle. The mucous membrane of these airways is essentially the same as in the trachea, but the cells become more cuboidal in the lower divisions.

The subsegmental bronchi extend from the fifth to the seventh generation. The diameter of these airways becomes progressively smaller, although the total cross-sectional area increases because of the increased number of divisions of the airways. The mucous membrane is essentially the same, with helical cartilaginous plates and cilia becoming more sparse. These changes continue throughout the eighth to eleventh generations, which are referred to as bronchioles.

The terminal bronchioles extend from the twelfth to the sixteenth generation. The diameter of these airways is approximately 1 mm. Cartilage is no longer present to provide structural rigidity. The airways are embedded directly in the lung parenchyma, and it is the elastic properties of this parenchyma that keep these lower airways open. Strong helical muscle bands are present, and their contraction forms longitudinal folds in the mucosa that sharply decrease the diameter of these airways. The epithelium of the terminal bronchioles is cuboidal and no longer ciliated. The cross-sectional area of the airways increases sharply at this level, as the diameter of the terminal bronchioles ceases to decrease as markedly with each generation. All the airways to this level (1 to 16 generations) are considered conducting airways, because their purpose is to transport gas to the respiratory bronchioles and alveoli, where gas exchange occurs. The conducting airways receive their arterial blood from the bronchial circulation (branches of the descending aorta). Airways from below this point receive their arterial blood from the pulmonary arteries.

The respiratory bronchioles extend from the seventeenth to the nineteenth generation. They are considered a transitional zone between bronchioles and alveoli. Their walls contain cuboidal epithelium interspersed with some alveoli. The number of alveoli increases with each generation. The walls of the bronchioles are also buried in the lung parenchyma. The airways depend on traction of this parenchyma to maintain their lumen. Muscle bands are also present between alveoli.

Alveolar ducts extend from the twentieth to the twenty-second generation. Their walls are composed entirely of alveoli, which are separated from one another by their septae. Septae contain smooth muscle, elastic and collagen fibers, nerves, and capillaries.

The twenty-third generation of air passages is called alveolar sacs. They are essentially the same as alveolar ducts, except that they end as blind pouches.

TABLE 2-1

Structural Characteristics of the Air Passages

	GENERATION (MEAN)	NUMBER	MEAN DIAMETER (MM)	AREA SUPPLIED	CARTILAGE	MUSCLE	NUTRITION	EMPLACEMENT	EPITHELIUM
Trachea	0	1	18	Both lungs	U-shaped		Links open end of cartilage		
Main bronchi	1	2	13	Individual lungs				Within connective tissue sheath alongside arterial vessels	
Lobar bronchi	2 → 3	4 → 8	7 → 5	Lobes	Irregular shaped and helical plates	Helical bands	From the bronchial circulation		Columnar ciliated
Segmental bronchi	4 → 5	16 → 32	4 → 3	Segments Secondary lobules					
Small bronchi	11	2,000	1						
Bronchioles and terminal bronchioles	12 → 16	4,000 → 65,000	1 → 0.5			Strong helical muscle bands		Embedded directly in the lung parenchyma	Cubiodal
Respiratory bronchioles	17 → 19	130,000 → 500,000	0.5	Primary lobes	Absent	Muscle band between alveolar			
Alveolar ducts	20 → 22	1,000,000 → 4,000,000	0.3	Alveoli		Thin bands in alveolar septa	From the pulmonary circulation	Forms the lung parenchyma	Cubiodal to flat between the alveoli
Alveolar sacs	23	8,000,000	0.3	Alveoli					Alveolar epithelium

From Weibel *Morphometry of the human lung*, New York, 1963, Springer. Used with permission.

(Actually, communication occurs between "blind pouches" in the form of the pores of Kohn's, which are channels in alveolar walls, and Lambert's canals, which are communications between bronchioles and alveoli. These communications are thought to be responsible for the rapid spread of lung infection. They also provide collateral ventilation to alveoli, whose bronchi are obstructed. Although this ventilation does little to arterialize blood, it does help prevent collapse of these alveoli.) Each alveolar sac contains approximately 17 alveoli. There are about 300 million alveoli in an adult man, 85% to 95% of which are covered with pulmonary capillaries. Alveolar epithelium is composed of two cell types. Type I cells, squamous pneumocytes, have broad thin extensions that cover about 95% of the alveolar surface. Type II cells, the granular pneumocytes, are more numerous than type I cells but occupy less than 5% of the alveolar surface. This is because of their small, cuboidal shape. These cells are responsible for the production of surfactant, a phospholipid that lines the alveoli. Surfactant keeps alveoli expanded by lowering their surface tension. Type II cells have been shown to be the primary cells involved in repair of the alveolar epithelium. (This has been shown in experiments where O_2 toxicity was induced in monkeys and in numerous other conditions where type I cells were destroyed.) Type III cells, alveolar brush cells, are rare and are found only occasionally in humans.

An additional type of cell, the alveolar macrophage, is found within the alveolus. These cells are thought to originate from stem cell precursors in the bone marrow and reach the lung through the blood stream. They are large, mononuclear, ameboid cells that roam in the alveoli, alveolar ducts, and alveolar sacs. They contain lysosomes, which are capable of killing engulfed bacteria. (Studies show them to be most effective in neutralizing inhaled gram-positive organisms.) They also engulf foreign matter and are either transported to the lymphatic system or migrate to the terminal bronchioles where they attach themselves to the mucus. They are then carried by the mucus to larger airways and eventually to the pharynx. Since cilia are not present below the eleventh generation of air passages, clearance of matter and bacteria from these areas is largely dependent on the macrophages.

Other cells located in the distal airways that are important in the defense of the lung are the lymphocytes and polymorphonuclear leukocytes. Immunoglobulins (IgA, IgG, and IgM) in the blood serum appear to enhance the engulfing activity of the macrophages. There are two types of lymphocytes found in the lung—the B-lymphocyte and the T-lymphocyte. The B-lymphocytes produce gamma globulin antibodies to fight lung infections, whereas the T-lymphocytes release a substance that attracts macrophages to the site of the infection. The polymorphonuclear leukocytes are important in engulfing and killing blood-borne gram-negative organisms.

LUNGS

Two lungs, each covered with its pleurae—the visceral pleura and the parietal pleura—lie within the thoracic cavity. Each lung is attached to the heart and the trachea by its root and the pulmonary ligament. It is otherwise free in the thoracic cavity. The lungs are light, soft spongy organs, whose color darkens with age as they become impregnated with inhaled dust. They are covered with the visceral pleura, a thin, glistening serous membrane that covers all surfaces of the lung. The visceral pleura reflects and continues on the mediastinum and inner thoracic wall, where it becomes known as the parietal pleura. The space between the two pleurae is minuscule and contains a negative pressure at all times, which helps keep the lungs inflated. A small amount of pleural fluid lubricates the two pleurae as they slide over each other during breathing. In disease, fluid, tumor cells, or air may invade the pleural space and collapse the underlying lung. Each lung has an apex, base, and three surfaces (costal, medial, and diaphragmatic). There are also three borders (anterior, inferior, and posterior). Each lung is divided by fissures into separate lobes. In the right lung the oblique fissure separates the lower lobe from the middle, whereas the horizontal fissure separates the upper lobe from the middle. The right lung is heavier and wider than the left lung. It is also shorter because of the location of the right lobe of the liver. The left lung is divided into upper and lower lobes by the oblique fissure. It is longer and thinner than the right lung, because the heart and pericardium are located in the left thorax. Numerous structures enter the lung at the hilus, or root of the lung, including the main-stem bronchus, the pulmonary artery, pulmonary veins, bronchial arteries and veins, nerves, and lymph vessels. The root, or hilus, of the lungs lies opposite the bodies of the fifth, sixth, and seventh thoracic vertebrae. The lungs are connected to the upper airways by the trachea and main-stem bronchi.

Surface markings

Surface markings of the lungs can be outlined over the chest with a basic knowledge of bony landmarks and gross anatomy of each lung (Table 2-2, and Figures 2-13, 2-14, and 2-15). The apices of both lungs extend 1 in above the clavicles at the medial ends. The anterior medial border of the right lung runs from the sternoclavicular joint, to the sternal angle downward to the xiphisternum. The inferior border runs from the xiphisternum laterally to the sixth rib in the midclavicular line, the eighth rib in the midaxillary line, and the tenth rib in the midscapular line. The midscapular line runs downward from the infe-

rior angle of the scapula with the arm at rest. The inferior border joins the posterior medial border of the lung 2 cm lateral to the tenth thoracic vertebra. The posterior medial border runs 2 cm lateral to the vertebral column from the seventh cervical vertebra to the tenth thoracic vertebra.

The left lung is generally smaller than the right and accommodates the position of the heart. The medial border on the anterior aspect runs from the sternoclavicular joint to the middle of the sternal angle, down the midline of the sternum to the fourth costal cartilage. A lateral indentation of about 1½ in forms the cardiac notch at the level of the fifth and sixth costal cartilages. The courses of the inferior and medial borders on the posterior aspect are similar in the left and right lungs. In the left lung, however, the inferior border crosses at the level of the tenth thoracic vertebra, not the twelfth observed in the right lung.

The position of the fissures of the lungs can be outlined over the chest wall. In both lungs, the oblique fissure begins between the second to fourth thoracic vertebrae. This can be roughly estimated by

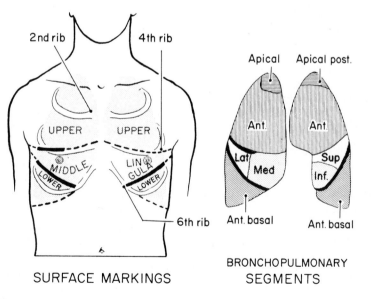

SURFACE MARKINGS

BRONCHOPULMONARY SEGMENTS

FIGURE 2-13
Surface markings of the lungs (anterior aspect). The underlying bronchopulmonary segments are also shown. (Printed with permission from Cherniak RM, Cherniack L: *Respiration in health and disease,* ed 3, Philadelphia, 1983, WB Saunders.)

TABLE 2-2

Anatomical Arrangement of the Bronchopulmonary Segments

LOBE	RIGHT LUNG: BRONCHOPULMONARY SEGMENTS	LOBE	LEFT LUNG: BRONCHOPULMONARY SEGMENTS
Upper	Apical—extends above the clavicle anteriorly; smaller area posteriorly Anterior—occupies area between the clavicle and horizontal fissure Posterior—remainder of upper lobe on the posterior aspect down to the oblique fissure	Upper	Apical posterior—extends above the clavicle anteriorly; occupies comparable area as the apical and posterior segments of the right lung Anterior—occupies area between the clavicle and theborder of the lingula (comparable line to the horizontal fissure of the right lung)
Middle	Lateral—extends medially from junction of the two fissures at the third intercostal space to occupy one third of the anterior surface of the lobe Medial—occupies the remaining anterior surface of the lobe	(Lingula)‡	Superior—occupies upper half of the lingula Inferior—occupies lower half of the lingula
Lower (Base)	Anterior—occupies basal area beneath the oblique fissure anteriorly Superior—occupies half the area from the oblique fissure downward* on the posterior aspect Lateral—extends from the junction of the middle lobe over the midaxillary area to occupy one third the area inferior to the superior segment on the posterior aspect Posterior—occupies two thirds of the area posteriorly beneath the superior segment Medial—occupies a space on the inner aspect of the right base†	Lower (Base)	Anterior—occupies area inferior to the oblique fissure anteriorly Superior—occupies one third of the basal area posteriorly from the oblique fissure downward Lateral—occupies the lateral half of the remaining two thirds of the left lower lobe beneath the superior segment on the posterior aspect Posterior—occupies the medial portion of the remaining two thirds of the left ower lobe beneath the superior segment on the posterior aspect

* This segment can be drained preferentially when the patient lies prone. Superior segments also called apical.

† Medial basal segent has no direct exposure to the chest wall, therefore, cannot be directly auscultated. This segment preferentially drains when the patient is positioned for the left lateral basal segment because of the comparable angle of its bronchus.

‡ Lingula is not an anatomically distinct area compared with the right middle lobe; rather, it is anatomically part of the left upper lobe.

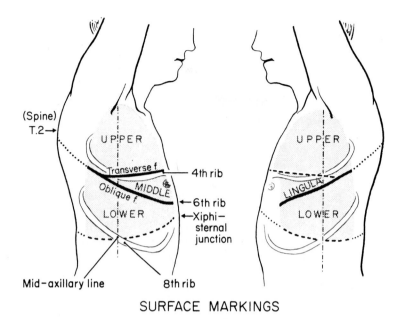

SURFACE MARKINGS

FIGURE 2-14

Surface markings of the lungs (lateral aspect). (Printed with permission from Cherniak RM, Cherniack L: *Respiration in health and disease,* ed 3, Philadelphia, 1983, WB Saunders.)

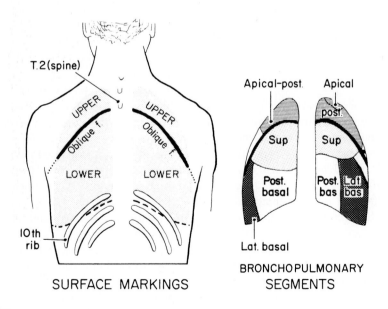

SURFACE MARKINGS

BRONCHOPULMONARY SEGMENTS

FIGURE 2-15

Surface markings of the lungs (posterior aspect). The underlying bronchopulmonary segments are also shown. (Printed with permission from Cherniak RM, Cherniack L: *Respiration in health and disease,* ed 3, Philadelphia, 1983, WB Saunders.)

following a line continuous with the medial border of the abducted scapula, around the midaxillary line at the fifth rib, and terminating at the sixth costal cartilage anteriorly. The horizontal fissure of the right lung originates from the oblique fissure at the level of about the fourth intercostal space in the midaxillary line, and courses medially and slightly upward over the fourth rib anteriorly. The left lung has no horizontal fissure.

Bronchopulmonary Segments

The bronchopulmonary segments lie within the three lobes of the right lung and the two lobes of the left lung. There are 10 bronchopulmonary segments on the right and eight on the left. Brief anatomic descriptions of the position of each lobe are provided in Table 2-2, p. 42. Figure 2-13, p. 41, illustrates the surface markings on the anterior view of the lungs and the position of the various bronchopulmonary segments within the major anatomic divisions provided by the fissures. Figure 2-14, p. 43, shows some of these features from the lateral views. Figure 2-15, p.43 illustrates the surface markings and bronchopulmonary segments of the posterior aspect of the lungs.

HEART

The heart is a conical, hollow muscular pump enclosed in a fibroserous sac, the pericardium. Its size is closely related to body size and corresponds remarkably to the size of an individual's clenched fist. It is positioned in the center of the chest behind the lower half of the sternum. The largest portion of the heart lies to the left of the midsternal line; the apex is found approximately 9 cm to the left in the fifth intercostal space.

The surface markings of the heart can be traced by joining four points over the anterior chest wall. On the right, the heart extends from the third to the sixth costal cartilages at a distance of about 10 to 15 mm from the sternum. On the left, the heart extends from the second costal cartilage to the fifth intercostal space 12 to 15 mm, and 9 cm from the left sternal border, respectively. Joining the two points on the left side outlines the left atrium and ventricle. The

heart is rotated to the left in the chest, resulting in the right side of the heart being foremost. Thus joining the two uppermost points outlines the level of the atria and joining the two lower points represents the margin of the right ventricle.

The heart as a whole is freely movable within the pericardial cavity, changing position during both contraction and respiration. During contraction, the apex moves forward, strikes the chest and imparts the chest and apex beat, which may be felt and seen. Abnormal position of the apex beat can indicate cardiac enlargement or displacement. During breathing, the movements of the diaphragm determine the position of the heart. This is because of the attachment of the central tendon of the diaphragm to the pericardium. Changes in position during quiet breathing are hardly noticeable, but with deep inspirations, the downward excursion of the diaphragm causes the heart to descend and rotate to the right. The opposite occurs during expiration. Pathology of the lungs can also change the position of the heart. Atelectasis shifts the heart to the same side. In tension pneumothorax, where air enters the chest usually through an opening in the chest wall and cannot escape, the positive pressure shifts the heart away from the side of the pathology.

The heart is enclosed by the pericardium, whose two surfaces can be visualized by considering the heart as a fist that is plunged into a large balloon. The outer surface, a tough fibrous membrane, is called the fibrous pericardium. It encases the heart and the organs and terminations of the great vessels. This membrane is so unyielding that when fluid accumulates rapidly in the pericardial cavity, it can compress the heart and impede venous return. When this occurs often, a window is cut in the pericardium, allowing the fluid to escape. The inner surface, the serous pericardium, is a serous membrane that lines the fibrous pericardium. Ten to 20 ml of clear pericardial fluid separates and moistens the two pericardial surfaces. The pericardium with its fluid minimizes friction during contraction. It also holds the heart in position and prevents dilation. The serous pericardium consists of an outer layer, the parietal layer, and an inner layer—the visceral layer, or epicardium.

The heart is divided into right and left halves by an obliquely placed longitudinal septum (Figure 2-16).

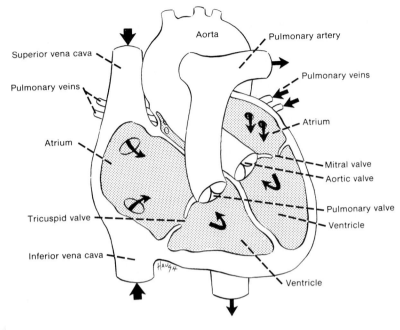

FIGURE 2-16
Blood flow of the heart.

Each half has two chambers—the atrium, which receives blood from veins, and the ventricles, which eject blood into the arteries. The superior vena cava, inferior vena cava, and intrinsic veins of the heart deposit venous blood into the right atrium. Blood then passes through the tricuspid valve to the right ventricle. The right ventricle projects the blood through the pulmonary valve into the pulmonary arteries, which are the only arteries in the body containing deoxygenated blood. Pulmonary veins return the blood to the left atrium and from there, it passes through the mitral valve to the left ventricle. From the left ventricle it is ejected through the aortic valve into the main artery of the body—the aorta.

The heart is divided into three layers—the epicardium, myocardium, and endocardium. The outermost layer, the epicardium, is visceral pericardium and is often infiltrated with fat. The coronary blood vessels that nourish the heart run in this layer before entering the myocardium. The myocardium consists of cardiac muscle fibers. The thickness of the layers of cardiac muscle fibers is directly proportional to the amount of work they perform. The ventricles do more work than the atria, and their walls are thicker. The pressure in the aorta is higher than that in the pulmonary trunk. This requires greater work from the left ventricle, so its walls are twice as thick as those of the right ventricle. The innermost layer, the endocardium, is the smooth endothelial lining of the interior of the heart.*

Heart Valves

The four valves of the heart, although delicate in appearance, are designed to withstand repetitive closures against high pressures (see Figure 2-16) (French, Criley, 1983). Normally, they operate for more than 80 years without need of repair or replacement. The tricuspid and mitral valves function differently from the other valves of the heart. Being

*For additional information of the clinical aspects of heart anatomy, refer to Andreoli et al, 1991; Goldberger, 1990; Sokolow, McIlroy, Cheitlin, 1990; and Gray's Anatomy.

located between the atria and ventricles, they must effect a precise closure within a contracting cavity.

During diastole, the two leaflets or cusps of the mitral valve and the three cusps of the tricuspid valve relax into the cavities of the ventricles, allowing blood to flow between the two chambers. As the ventricular chambers fill with blood, the cusps of the valves are forced up into a closed position. Fibrous cords, the chordae tendinae, are located on the ventricular surfaces of these cusps. These cords connect the cusps of the valve with the papillary muscles of the ventricular walls. As pressure builds in the ventricular chambers, contraction of these muscles prevents the cusps from being forced up into the atria. Dysfunction or rupture of the chordae tendinae or the papillary muscles may undermine the support of one or more valve cusps, producing regurgitation from the ventricles to the atria.

The pulmonic and aortic valves are similar in appearance but the aortic cusps are slightly thicker than the pulmonic cusps. Each valve has three fibrous cusps, the bases of which are firmly attached to the root of the aorta or the pulmonary artery. The free edges of these valves project into the lumen of the vessels. At the end of systole, blood in the aorta and pulmonary artery forces the cusps of the valves shut. These valves are attached in such a manner that they cannot be everted into the ventricles by increased pressure in the vessels. During diastole, the cusps support the column of blood filling the ventricles. Contraction of the ventricles during systole increases pressure within the ventricular chambers, forcing the cusps to open and allow blood flow into the vessels.

The arterial supply of the heart muscle is derived from the right and left coronary arteries, which arise from the aortic sinuses (Figure 2-17). The left coronary artery (LCA) divides into the anterior descending artery and the left circumflex artery. These arteries supply most of the left ventricle, the left atrium, most of the ventricular septum and, in 45% of people, the sinoatrial (SA) node. The right coronary artery (RCA) supplies most of the right ventricle, the atrioventricular (AV) node and, in 55% of people, the SA node. Infarction of these arteries or their branches can thus cause interruption

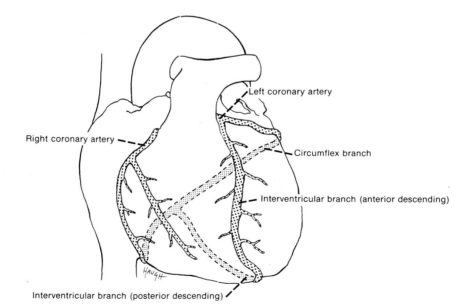

FIGURE 2-17
Blood supply of the heart.

or cessation of the conduction system and death of the myocardial muscle in the area supplied by the artery. The severity of the infarction is dependent on the size of the artery and the importance of the area it supplies.

The heart is drained by a number of veins. Most of the veins of the heart enter the coronary sinus, which then empties into the right atrium. A small portion of veins, the thebesian veins, empty directly into the right and left ventricles.

Innervation

Innervation of the heart involves a complex balance between its intrinsic automaticity and extrinsic nerves (Figure 2-18). The SA and AV nodes provide the heart with an inherent ability for spontaneous rhythmic initiation of the cardiac impulse. The rate of this impulse formation is regulated by the autonomic nervous system (ANS), which also influences other phases of the cardiac cycle. It controls the rate of spread of the excitation impulse and the contractility of both atria and ventricles.

The ANS extends its influence to the heart via the vagus nerve (parasympathetic) and upper thoracic nerves (sympathetic). These nerves mingle together around the root and arch of the aorta near the tracheal bifurcation, forming the cardiac plexus. Extensions from the cardiac plexus richly supply the SA and AV nodes. They are so well-mingled that scientists are unable to determine which nerves supply which parts of the heart. Stimulation of the sympathetic nervous system causes acceleration of the discharge rate in the SA node, increase in AV nodal conduction, and increase in the contractile force of both atrial and ventricular muscles. Stimulation of the vagus nerve causes cardiac slowing and decreased AV nodal conduction. Thus the parasympathetic system decelerates heart rate and the sympathetic system accelerates heart rate.

Intrinsic innervation of the heart centers around the SA node, which lies near the junction of the superior vena cava and the right atrium. It is the normal pacemaker of the heart, sending concentric waves of excitation throughout the atrium. Without neural influence, impulse formation from this node would be greater than 100 beats/minute. However, vagal influence decreases the impulse formation to 60–90 beats/minute. The SA

node retains its position as pacer of the heart as long as it generates impulses at a faster rate than any other part of the myocardium and as long as these impulses are rapidly conducted from the atria to the ventricles. Normal impulse formation may be interrupted by vascular lesions (occlusion of the coronary arteries) or by cardiac disease (pericarditis). The SA node is especially susceptible to pericarditis and all other surface cardiac diseases because of its superficial position immediately beneath the epicardium.

The muscle fibers of the heart are self-excitatory, which enables the heart to rhythmically and automatically contract. The normal pacemaker of the heart is the sinoatrial node located in the posterior wall of the right atrium. The concentric waves of excitation sent out by the SA node must travel through the AV node to reach the ventricles. This node is located in the floor of the right atrium, just above the insertion of the tricuspid valve. Its main function is to cause a 0.04 second delay in the atrioventricular transmissions. This has two advantages. It postpones ventricular excitation until the atria have had time to eject their contents into the ventricles. It also limits the number of signals that

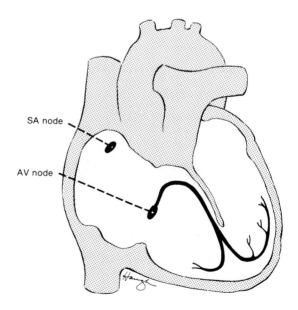

FIGURE 2-18
Electrical conduction of the heart.

can be transmitted by the AV node. The AV node also has its own inherent rhythmicity, firing at a much slower rate than the SA node (40–60 beats/minute). Its main pathology is a result of occlusion of the right coronary artery, which supplies the AV node in 90% of the cases. From the AV node arises a triangular group of fibers known as the AV bundle or bundle of His. This bundle divides in the ventricular septum into two branches—the left bundle branch and the right bundle branch. Each of these bundles continues to divide into many fine strands that spread across the ventricles. At the end of the bundle's ramifications are Purkinje's fibers, which are continuous with the cardiac muscle. The waves of excitation pass through the bundle of His, down the bundle branches, and through the Purkinje fibers, which permeate the ventricles and cause them to contract. This wave of depolarization gives rise to the normal P-QRS-T configuration of the electrocardiogram (ECG) tracing (Figure 2-19) (see Chapter 11). The P-wave indicates atrial depolariza-

tion, the QRS complex indicates ventricular depolarization and the T-wave indicates ventricular repolarization. There is no wave indicating atrial repolarization, since this is embedded in the QRS complex (Andreoli et al, 1991; Wagner, 1994). See Physiology of the Electrical Excitation of the Heart and ECG Interpretation, Chapter 11; Dubin, 1989; Marriott, Conover, 1989; and Wagner, 1994.

SYSTEMIC CIRCULATION

The systemic vascular system is a complex series of blood vessels throughout the entire body. It conveys nutrition and oxygen to all tissues of the body and carries away their waste products. The driving force for this system is the heart. The vascular system can be considered to have two major components—the peripheral and pulmonary circulations (Schlant et al, 1994).

Blood vessels are designed to forward oxygenated blood from the heart during systolic ejection of the

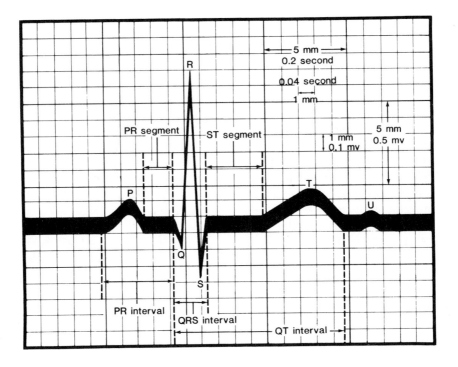

FIGURE 2-19
A normal ECG showing characteristic waves, intervals, and segments.

left ventricle, perfuse the vascular beds commensurate with their metabolic needs and remove metabolic excreta. Anatomically, the proximal vessels have a higher proportion of connective tissue and elastin to withstand high pulse pressures (e.g., the aorta, which carries blood to the head, viscera, and limbs). In addition, potential energy is stored in the walls of the larger vessels during systole. During diastole, the elastic recoil of these vessels maintains the forward motion of the blood between ventricular systoles. The medium-size blood vessels have comparable proportions of connective tissue and elastin to smooth muscle. As the blood vessels become smaller, smooth muscle predominates. The arterioles are primarily smooth muscle and their diameter can alter significantly. They regulate the blood flow to regional tissue beds and are also responsible for regulating total peripheral resistance and systemic blood pressure. They are called the stopcocks of the circulation. Many factors (e.g., nervous impulses, hormonal stimulation, drugs, oxygen, and carbon dioxide concentrations) determine the degree of contraction of vascular smooth muscle and whether contraction occurs locally or throughout the entire body.

Arterioles branch to form the smallest vessels, the capillaries, which consist of a single layer of endothelial cells forming lumen just large enough for the red blood cells to roll along. The capillary bed is enormous; its capacity far exceeding 5 L. Its network is finer and denser in active tissue like muscle and brain, and less dense in less active tissue such as tendon. Gas exchange occurs in the capillary bed, where the red blood cells give up their oxygen, and blood plasma transudes capillary walls, carrying nutrition to tissue.

The microcirculation specifically consists of the metarterioles, the capillary bed, and the venules. The capillary wall is a semipermeable membrane that is responsible for the transfer of oxygen, nutrients, and waste between the circulation and the interstitial fluid (see Chapters 1 and 3). The capillary pores selectively allow different-size molecules to pass through them. This is an essential feature that regulates the movement of fluid in and out of the intra- and extravascular compartments. This process is fundamental to maintaining and regulating normal hemodynamics.

Capillaries form venules, which are the smallest

veins. These veins branch and become increasingly larger. Blood flow through the veins is largely dependent on muscular or visceral action or pressures. These pressures are intermittent and, were it not for double-cusp valves located within the veins, blood would flow backward when the pressure ceases. In the extremities, muscular contractions move blood into the trunk. In the pelvic and abdominal region, blood flow is dependent on intraabdominal pressure exceeding intrathoracic pressure. Blood flows through the trunk in veins that become increasingly larger until they finally enter the superior and inferior vena cavae.

PULMONARY CIRCULATION

The vena cavae empty directly into the right atrium. Blood flow from the right side of the heart through the lungs is known as the pulmonary circulation. The quantity of blood flowing through the pulmonary circulation is approximately equal to that flowing through systemic circulation. Blood flows from the right ventricle into the pulmonary artery, which divides into right and left branches 4 cm from the ventricle. These branches then separate, one going to each lung, where they continue to divide into smaller arteries. The pulmonary arteries and arterioles are much shorter, have thinner walls and larger diameters, and are more distensible than their systemic counterparts. This gives the pulmonary system a compliance as great as that of the systemic arterial system, thereby allowing the pulmonary arteries to accommodate the stroke volume output of the right ventricle. Pulmonary vascular resistance and arterial pressure are one sixth that of the systemic system (pulmonary arterial pressure is 20/10 mm Hg compared with 120/80 mm Hg systemically).

Pulmonary capillaries are short and arise abruptly from much larger arterioles. They form a dense network over the walls of the alveoli, making a minimum distance over which gas exchange occurs. The pulmonary veins are also very short but have distensibility characteristics similar to those of the systemic system. Unlike systemic veins, these veins have no valves. Pulmonary veins act as a capacitance vessel, or a blood reservoir for the left atrium. Contraction of smooth muscle in the veins makes the reservoir constrict. This increases blood volume in relation to the internal volume of the vessels. The pulmonary veins become larger until they converge into two veins from each lung, which then carry oxygenated blood to the left atrium.

LYMPHATIC CIRCULATION

The lymphatic circulation provides an additional route for fluid to be returned from the interstitium to the systemic circulation, and thus has a central role in the regulation of interstitial fluid dynamics. Lymph, the fluid that flows in the lymphatic channels, is interstitial fluid with similar composition to tissue fluid. The lymphatics remove excess fluid, large proteins, and other large molecules away from the interstitial spaces. Although relatively little protein leaks from the capillaries into the surrounding tissue, the absence of its immediate removal is life-threatening.

Virtually all areas of the body drain into a network of lymphatic channels. From the lower portion of the body, and left head and neck, excess tissue fluid and protein drain into the thoracic duct, which empties into the venous circulation at the junction of the left internal jugular vein and subclavian vein. Lymph from the right side of the head, neck, arm, and parts of the right thorax drain into the right lymph duct, which empties into the venous circulation at the junction of the right internal jugular vein and subclavian vein. Lymph from the lower part of the body drains into the inguinal and abdominal lymphatic channels. The pressure in the lymphatic system is usually slightly negative which helps to keep the interstitium "dry." The lymph vessels are thin-walled with some smooth muscle and thus can contract to propel their contents. In addition, lymph vessels have valves to facilitate the forward motion and to minimize retrograde movement of lymph.

SUMMARY

This chapter reviewed the anatomy of the cardiopulmonary system. The anatomical features of the respiratory pump were described with respect to the structure of the bony thorax, the muscles of respiration associated with the chest wall and of the diaphragm. The upper and lower respiratory tracts were described, as well as the relationship of the tracheobronchial tree to the lung parenchyma. The lung parenchyma is defined anatomically in terms of discrete bronchopulmonary segments contained within three major divisions of each lung. The specific surface markings defined by the lung fissures and the landmarks for the bronchopulmonary segments were emphasized. The basic anatomy of the heart was described. The structure of the peripheral and pulmonary circulations was also presented. Special reference was made to the lymphatic circulation and its central role in the regulation of capillary fluid dynamics. A detailed understanding of cardiopulmonary anatomy is fundamental to the knowledge base underlying the assessment and management of cardiopulmonary dysfunction and impaired oxygen transport, by physical therapists.

REVIEW QUESTIONS

1. Describe the thorax and its movements.
2. Describe the respiratory muscles and their function.
3. Explain the pathway of oxygen from the atmosphere to the alveolar capillary membrane.
4. Describe the movement of oxygenated blood from the periphery through the heart to the pulmonary and peripheral circulations.
5. Describe the movement of deoxygenated blood from the periphery back to the heart.
6. Explain the role of the lymphatic circulation and its physiological significance.

References

Andreoli, K.G., Fowkes, V.K., Zipes, D.P., & Wallace, A.G. (Eds). (1991). *Comprehensive cardiac care* (7th ed.). St. Louis: Mosby.

Berne, R.M., & Levy, M.N. (1992). *Cardiovascular physiology* (6th ed.). St Louis: CV Mosby.

Burton, G.G., & Hodgkin, J.E. (1984). *Respiratory care: A guide to clinical practice* (2nd ed.). Philadelphia: JB Lippincott.

Cherniack, R.M., & Cherniack, L. (1983). *Respiration in Health and Disease* (3rd ed.). Philadelphia: WB Saunders.

Clemente, C.D. (Ed.). (1985). *Anatomy of the human body* (30th ed.). Philadelphia: Lea & Febiger.

Dubin, D. (1989) *Rapid interpretation of EKGs* (4th ed.). Tampa, Florida: Cover Publishing.

French, W.G., & Criley, J.M. (Eds.). (1983). *Practical cardiology: Ischemic and valvular heart disease.* New York: John Wiley & Sons.

Ganong, W.F. (1993). *Review of medical physiology* (16th ed.). Los Altos, Calif.: Lange Medical Publications.

Goldberger, E. (1990). *Essentials of clinical cardiology.* Philadelphia: JB Lippincott.

Guyton, A.C. (1991). *Textbook of medical physiology* (8th ed.). Philadelphia: WB Saunders.

Katz, A.M. (1992). *Physiology of the heart* (2nd ed.). New York: Raven Press.

Marriott, H.J.L., & Conover, M.B. (1989). *Advanced concepts in arrhythmias* (2nd ed.). St. Louis: Mosby.

Murray, J.F. (1986). *The normal lung.* Philadelphia: WB Saunders.

Murray, J.F., & Nadel, J.A. (1988). *Textbook of respiratory medicine.* Philadelphia: WB Saunders.

Nunn, J.F. (1993). *Applied respiratory physiology* (4th ed.). London: Butterworths.

Scharf, S.M. & Cassidy, S.S. (Eds.). (1989). *Heart-lung interactions in health and disease.* New York: Marcel Dekker.

Sokolow, M., McIlroy, M.B., & Cheitlin, M.D. (1990). *Clinical cardiology* (5th ed.). Norwalk, Conn.: Appleton & Lange.

Schlant, R.C., Alexander, R.W., O'Rourke, R.A., Roberts, R., & Sonnenblick, E.H. (Eds.). (1994). *Hurst's the heart: arteries and veins* (8th ed.). New York: McGraw-Hill.

Wagner, G.S. (1994). *Marriott's practical electrocardiography* (9th ed.). Baltimore: Williams & Wilkins.

Weber, K.T., Janicki, J.S., Shroff, S.G., & Likoff, M.J. (1983). The cardiopulmonary unit. The body's gas transport system, *Clinics in chest medicine, 4,* 101-110.

Weibel, E.R. (1963). *Morphometry of the human lung.* New York: Springer-Verlag.

West, J.B. (Ed.). (1991). *Best and Taylor's physiological basis of medical practice* (12th ed.). Baltimore: Williams & Wilkins.

West, J.B. (1995). *Respiratory physiology—the essentials* (5th ed.). Baltimore: Williams & Wilkins.

Williams, P.L., Warwick, R., Dyson, M., & Bannister, L.H. (Eds.). (1989). *Gray's anatomy* (37th ed.). Edinburgh: Churchill Livingstone.

CHAPTER 3

Cardiopulmonary Physiology

Elizabeth Dean
Lyn Hobson

KEY TERMS

Control of breathing
Control of the heart
Diffusion
Electromechanical coupling
Gas exchange

Oxyhemoglobin dissociation
Respiratory mechanics
Ventilation and perfusion matching
Ventilation perfusion

INTRODUCTION

This chapter reviews the basics of cardiopulmonary physiology. A thorough understanding of normal physiology provides a basis for understanding the deficits of cardiopulmonary dysfunction and adaptation to it, and conducting a thorough assessment and prescribing treatment (Bates, 1989; Berne and Levy, 1992; Clemente, 1985; Goldberger, 1990; Guyton, 1991; Katz, 1992; Murray and Nadel, 1988; Nunn, 1993, Scharf and Cassidy, 1989; Schlant, Alexander, O'Rourke, Roberts, and Sonnenblick, 1994; Sokolow, McIlroy, and Cheitlin, 1990; and West, 1995.

CONTROL OF BREATHING

The act of breathing is a natural process to which most of us give little thought. Unconsciously, it adjusts to various degrees of activity, maintaining optimum arterial levels of P_{O_2} and P_{CO_2}, whether we are resting or physically active. Sighing, yawning, hiccuping, laughing, and vomiting are all involuntary acts using respiratory muscles. Breathing is also under our voluntary control. A person can stop it temporarily by holding his or her breath or can increase it by rapidly panting until he or she faints (from cerebral vascular constriction as a result of a decrease in arterial P_{CO_2}).

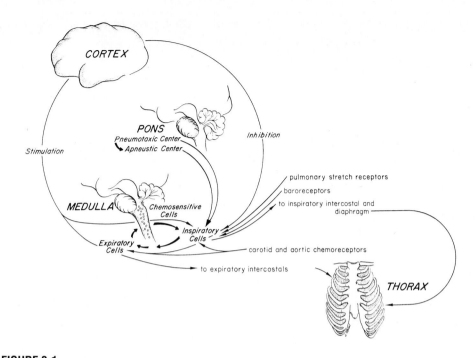

FIGURE 3-1
Control of breathing.

Exhalation is used in singing, speaking, coughing, and blowing, whereas inspiration is used for sniffing and sucking. Parturition, defecation, and the Valsalva maneuver are all performed while voluntarily holding our breath. These activities are directed by control centers located in the brain. The centers integrate a multitude of chemical, reflex, and physical stimuli before transmitting impulses to the respiratory muscles. The cerebral hemispheres control voluntary respiratory activity, whereas involuntary respiratory activity is controlled by centers located in the pons and medulla (Figure 3-1).

Medullary and Pontine Respiratory Centers

The respiratory center in the medulla is in the reticular formation. It contains the minimum number of neurons necessary for the basic sequence of inspiration and expiration. Although this center is capable of maintaining some degree of respiratory activity, these respirations are not normal in character.

The apneustic center is in the middle and lower pons. If uncontrolled by the pneumotaxic center, prolonged inspiratory gasps (apneustic breathing) occur.

The pneumotaxic center is in the upper one third of the pons. It maintains the normal pattern of respiration, balancing inspiration, and expiration by inhibiting either the apneustic center or the inspiratory component of the medullary center.

Central Chemoreceptors

These receptors are located on the ventral lateral surfaces of the upper medulla. They are bathed in the cerebrospinal fluid (CSF), which is separated from blood by the blood-brain barrier. Although this barrier is relatively impermeable to hydrogen (H) and bicarbonate (Hco_3) ions. Carbon dioxide (CO_2) diffuses through the barrier easily. Increased stimulation of central chemoreceptors by a rising arterial Pco_2 results in increased rate and depth of ventilation.

Peripheral Chemoreceptors

These receptors are located in the carotid bodies, which lie in the bifurcations of the common carotid artery and in the aortic bodies located above and below the aortic arch. These bodies receive blood from small branches of the vessels on which they are located. The receptors respond to an increase in arterial Pco_2 by increasing ventilation but are much less important in their response to Pco_2 than are the central chemoreceptors.

The main role of the peripheral chemoreceptors is to respond to hypoxemia by increasing ventilation. If arterial Pco_2 is normal, the Po_2 must drop to 50 mm Hg before ventilation increases. A rising Pco_2 causes the peripheral chemoreceptors to respond more quickly to a decreasing Po_2. In some patients with severe lung disease, this response to hypoxemia (the hypoxic drive) becomes very important. These patients often have a permanently elevated Pco_2 (CO_2 retention). The CSF in these patients compensates for a chronically elevated arterial Pco_2, by returning the pH of the CSF to near normal values. When these patients have lost the ability to stimulate ventilation in response to an elevated Pco_2, arterial hypoxemia becomes the major stimulus to ventilation (hypoxic drive).

REFLEXES

Hering-Breuer Reflex

Hering and Breuer noted in 1868 that distention of anesthetized animal lungs caused a decrease in the frequency of inspiration and an increase in expiratory time. Receptors for this reflex are thought to lie in the smooth muscle of airways from the trachea to the bronchioles. In humans, it takes a lung inflation of more than 800 ml above functional residual capacity to activate the reflex and delay the next breath.

Cough Reflex

Mechanical or chemical stimuli to the larynx, trachea, carina, and lower bronchi result in a reflex cough and bronchoconstriction. The high velocity created by the cough sweeps mucus and other irritants up toward the pharynx (see Chapter 21).

Stretch Reflex

The intercostal muscles and the diaphragm contain sensory muscle spindles that respond to elongation. A signal is sent to the spinal cord and anterior horn motor neurons. These neurons signal more muscle fibers to contract (recruitment) and thus increase the strength of the contraction. Theoretically, such a stretch reflex may be useful when there is an increase in airway resistance or a decrease in lung compliance. Stretching the ribs and the diaphragm may activate the stretch reflex and help the patient take a deep breath. The fundamental pathways of the stretch reflex are shown in Figure 3-2. Research is needed, however, to establish the therapeutic role of proprioceptive

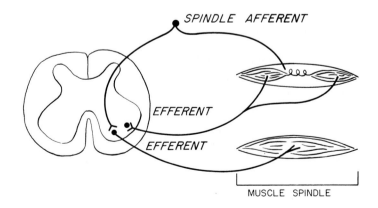

FIGURE 3-2
Stretch reflex.

neurofacilitation techniques based on stretch reflex theory in altering pulmonary function.

Joint and Muscle Receptors

Peripheral joints and muscles of the limbs are believed to have receptors that respond to movement and enhance ventilation in preparation for activity. Ventilation has also been shown to be stimulated by a similar reflex in humans and anesthetized animals in response to passive movement of the limbs. The precise pathways for these reflexes have not been well-established.

Mechanoreceptors

Changes in systemic blood pressure cause corresponding changes in pressure receptors in the carotid and aortic sinuses. Increase in blood pressure causes mechanical distortion of the receptors in these sinuses, producing reflex hypoventilation. Conversely, a reduction in blood pressure can result in hyperventilation.

MECHANICAL FACTORS IN BREATHING

The flow of air into the lungs is a result of pressure differences between the lungs and the atmosphere. In normal breathing, for inspiration to occur, alveolar pressure must be less than atmospheric pressure. Muscular contraction of the respiratory muscles lowers alveolar pressure and enlarges the thorax (Goldman, 1979). The decreased pressure causes air to flow from the atmosphere into the lungs. Patients who are unable to create adequate negative pressure may have to be mechanically ventilated. The ventilators create a positive pressure (greater than atmospheric pressure) that forces air into the lungs where there is atmospheric pressure. The iron lung used during the poliomyelitis epidemic of the 1950s assisted ventilation using cycles of negative pressure to inflate the lungs.

Exhalation occurs when alveolar pressure is greater than atmospheric pressure. At the cessation of inspiration, the respiratory muscles return to their resting positions. The diaphragm rises, compressing the lungs and increasing alveolar pressure. As the intercostals relax, the ribs drop back to their preinspiratory position, further compressing the lungs and in-

creasing alveolar pressure. The increased alveolar pressure contributes to air flowing from the lungs. Normally, expiration is a passive process reflecting elastic recoil of the lung parenchyma.

Resistance to Breathing

Compliance

The inner walls of the thorax, lined with parietal pleura, and the parenchyma of the lung, enclosed in visceral pleura, lie in close proximity to one another. The pleurae are separated by a potential space containing a small amount of pleural fluid. Muscular contraction of the intercostals and the diaphragm mechanically enlarges the thorax. The lungs are enlarged at this time because of their close proximity to the thorax. The healthy lung resists this enlargement and tries to pull away from the chest wall. The ease with which the lungs are inflated during inspiration is known as compliance and is defined as the volume change per unit of pressure change. The normal lung is very distensible or compliant. It can become more rigid and less compliant in diseases that cause alveolar, interstitial or pleural fibrosis, and alveolar edema. Compliance increases with age and in emphysema.

The elastic recoil or compliance of the lung is also dependent on a special surface fluid called surfactant, which lines the alveoli. This fluid increases compliance by lowering the surface tension of the alveoli, thereby reducing the muscular effort necessary to ventilate the lungs and keep them expanded. It is a complex lipoprotein that is thought to be produced in the type II alveolar cells (see Chapter 2). A decrease in surfactant causes the alveoli to collapse. Reexpanding these alveoli requires a tremendous amount of work on the part of the patient. The patient may become fatigued and need mechanical ventilation. This occurs in respiratory distress syndrome of the premature infant (previously called hyaline membrane disease) and in adult respiratory distress syndrome. In another disease, alveolar proteinosis, there is excessive accumulation of protein in the alveolar spaces. This may be because of excessive production of surfactant or deficient removal of surfactant by alveolar macrophages.

The elastic properties of the lung tend to collapse the lung if not counterbalanced by external forces.

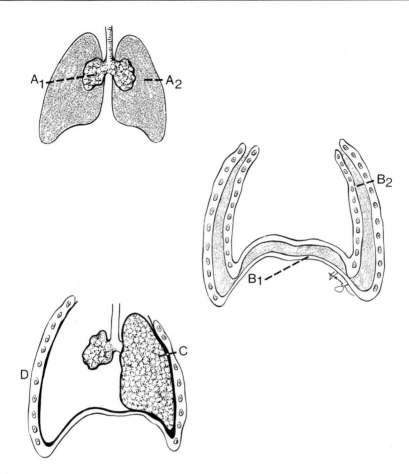

FIGURE 3-3

Various relationships between the lungs and the thorax. A_1, The size the lungs would assume if they were not acted on by the elastic recoil of the thoracic wall. A_2, normal size of lungs within the thorax B_1, The size the thorax would assume if it were not acted on by elastic recoil of the lungs. B_2, Normal position of the chest wall when acted on by elastic recoil of the lungs C, The normal relationship of lung to thorax. D, The positions assumed by the lung and thorax in a tension pneumothorax.

The tissues of the thoracic wall also have elastic recoil, which cause it to expand considerably if unopposed. These two forces oppose each other, keeping the lungs expanded and the thoracic cage in a neutral position. If these forces are interrupted (as in pneumothorax), the lung collapses and the thoracic wall expands (Figure 3-3). Similarly, the overinflated, barrel-shaped chest of the patient with chronic obstructive pulmonary disease (COPD) is explained in part by the elastic tension of the chest wall being unopposed by the usual elastic forces of the lungs, which have been damaged by disease.

Pressure Volume Relationships

Pressure volume curves help to define the elastic properties of the chest wall and lungs (Cherniack, Cherniack, 1983; Comroe, Forster, Dubois, Briscoe, and Carlsen, 1986). The elasticity of the respiratory system as a whole is the sum of its two

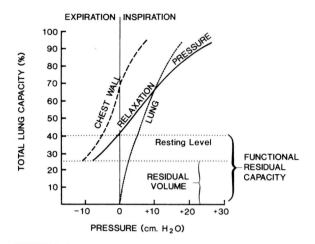

FIGURE 3-4

The relaxation pressure curve. The pressure in the lung at any volume reflects elastic forces of the lung and chest wall.

major components, the lungs and the chest wall. The so-called relaxation pressure curve is shown in Figure 3-4. The curve illustrates the static pressure of the lungs, chest wall, and the combination of the two measured at given lung volumes. Functional residual capacity reflects the balance of elastic forces exerted by the chest wall and the lungs. This is an important point with significant implications for the clinical presentation and management of patients with cardiopulmonary dysfunction.

The relaxation pressure curve represents static pressure measurements. This means that the respiratory muscles are inactive, and the volume in the lungs at a given point in the respiratory cycle is determined by the balance of forces between the chest wall and the lungs. The chest wall and lungs exert elastic forces that oppose each other. The chest wall attempts to pull the lung out and the lungs attempt to recoil and pull in the chest wall. The curves labeled lung and chest wall are theoretical and illustrate the elastic force exerted by each when permitted to act unopposed by the other. Normally, these two forces are exerted together and give the pressure volume relaxation curve. It can be seen that at functional residual capacity (FRC), these forces are in equilibrium,

and therefore functional residual capacity is the resting volume of the respiratory system. Active muscular work is required to effect inspiration. Expiration is normally a passive process. The pressure volume curve also shows the range of lung volumes, specifically tidal volume, over which the energy expenditure for breathing is most economical. In other words, large volume changes result from relatively small changes in pressure as noted from the slope of the curve over tidal volume.

In lung disease, this balance of forces is disrupted (West, 1992). More work and more energy are required to sustain the respiratory effort. The patient is less able to rely on normal elastic recoil of either the chest wall, lungs, or both. Therefore, the patient must put more energy into the system to produce the same respiratory function. The limits of respiratory excursion are determined by both elastic and muscular forces. At total lung capacity, the elastic forces of the respiratory system are balanced by the inspiratory muscle force. At residual volume, the elastic forces of the chest wall are balanced by the maximum expiratory muscle force. This volume excursion from total lung capacity to residual volume reflects vital capacity.

Although the curves representing the elastic forces of the lungs and chest wall are theoretical, they are helpful in understanding the effect of lung dysfunction on pulmonary function and on the clinical presentation of the patient (Burrows, Knudson, Quan, and Kettel, 1983). For example, in COPD, the characteristic barrel chest reflects the unopposed elastic forces of the chest wall, succeeding in increasing the excursion of the chest as a result of reduced elastic recoil of the lungs. At the other extreme is the effect of a puncture wound to the chest wall, which disrupts the intrapleural pressure gradient that normally keeps the lung expanded and the chest wall contained. The result of such a puncture is to produce a pneumothorax where the lung collapses down to the hilum and the chest wall springs outward (see Figure 3-3, p. 57).

Airway Resistance

The flow of air into the lungs depends on pressure differences and on the resistance to flow by the airways. Resistance is defined as the pressure difference required for one unit flow change. The air passages in

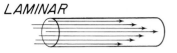

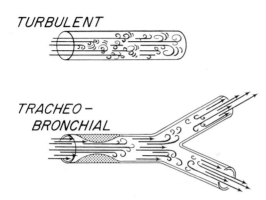

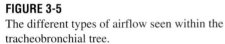

FIGURE 3-5
The different types of airflow seen within the tracheobronchial tree.

humans are divided into upper and lower airways (see Chapter 2). The upper airways are responsible for 45% of airway resistance. The resistance to airflow by the lower airways depends on many factors and is therefore difficult to predict. The branching of the lower airways is irregular, and the diameter of the lumen may vary because of external pressures, and contraction or relaxation of bronchial or bronchiolar smooth muscle. The lumen diameter may also decrease as a result of mucosal congestion, edema, or mucus. Any of these changes in the airway diameter may cause an increase in airway resistance. Flow of air through these airways can be either laminar or turbulent (Figure 3-5). Laminar flow is a streamlined flow where resistance occurs mainly between the sides of the tubes and the air molecules. It tends to be cone-shaped, with the molecules in contact with the walls of the tubes moving more slowly than the molecules in the middle of the tube. Turbulent flow occurs when there are frequent molecular collisions in addition to the resistance of the sides of the tubes seen in laminar flow. This type of flow occurs at high flow rates and in airways where there are irregularities caused by mucus, exudate, tumor, and other obstructions. In normal lungs, airflow is a combination of laminar and turbulent flow and is known as tracheobronchial flow.

The airways are distensible and compressible, and thus are susceptible to outside pressures. As these pressures compress the airways, they alter the airway resistance. Transmural pressure is the difference between the pressures in the airways and the pressures surrounding the airways. In erect humans, there is a higher transmural pressure at the apices of the lungs than at the bases. This expands the alveoli at the apices relative to those at the bases. Although the alveoli in the apices have a greater volume at end expiration, the alveoli in the bases are better ventilated. This is because the alveoli in the bases operate at lower transmural pressures and thus accommodate a greater volume during inspiration than those at higher pressures.

Airway resistance decreases during inspiration as a result of widening of the airways. During expiration, airways narrow, thus increasing resistance. The positive alveolar pressure that occurs during expiration partially compresses the airways. If these airways have lost their structural support as a result of disease, they may collapse and trap air distally (as in emphysema).

VENTILATION

Ventilation is the process by which air moves into the lungs. The volume of air inhaled can be measured with a spirometer. The various lung capacities and volumes are defined in chapter 8.

Regional differences in ventilation exist throughout the lung. Studies using radioactive inert gas have shown that when the gas is inhaled by an individual in the seated position, and measurements are taken with a radiation counter over the chest wall, radiation counts are greatest in the lower lung fields, intermediate in the midlung fields, and lowest in the upper lung fields. This effect is position or gravity dependent. In the supine position, the apices and bases are ventilated comparably, and the lowermost lung fields are better ventilated than the uppermost lung fields. Similarly, in the lateral or sidelying position, the lower lung fields are preferentially ventilated compared with the upper lung fields (see Chapter 18).

The causes of regional differences in ventilation

can be explained in terms of the anatomy of the lung and mechanics of breathing. An intrapleural pressure gradient exists down the lung. In the upright position, the intrapleural pressure tends to be more negative at the top of the lung, and becomes progressively less negative toward the bottom of the lung. This pressure gradient is thought to reflect the weight of the suspended lung. The more negative intrapleural pressure at the top of the lung results in relatively greater expansion of that area and a larger resting alveolar volume. The expanding pressure in the bottom of the lung, however, is relatively small and hence has a smaller resting alveolar volume. This distinction between the upper and lower lung fields is fundamental to understanding differences in regional ventilation. The regional differences in resting alveolar volume should not be confused with regional differences in ventilation volume. Ventilation refers to volume change as a function of resting volume. The relatively higher resting volume in the upper lung fields renders it stiffer or less compliant compared with the low lung volumes and greater compliance in the lower lung fields. The lower lung fields therefore exhibit a

greater volume change in relation to resting volume which effects greater overall ventilation compared with the upper lung fields. In summary, ventilation is favored in the lowermost lung fields regardless of the position of the body.

DIFFUSION

Once air has reached the alveoli, it must cross the alveolar-capillary (A-C) membrane (Figure 3-6). The gases must cross through the surfactant lining, the alveolar epithelial membrane and the capillary endothelial membrane. Oxygen has to travel further through a layer of plasma, the erythrocyte membrane and intracellular fluid in the erythrocyte, until it encounters a hemoglobin molecule. This distance is actually small in normal lungs, but in disease states, it may increase. The alveolar wall and the capillary membrane often become thickened. Fluid, edema, or exudate may separate the two membranes. These conditions are often first detected when arterial P_{O_2} becomes chronically lower than normal. Oxygen diffuses slowly through the A-C membrane in compari-

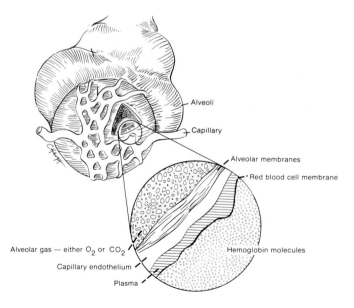

FIGURE 3-6
The components of the alveolar-capillary membrane.

son to CO_2 diffusion. As a result, patients with diffusion problems frequently have hypoxemia with a normal P_{CO_2}. Sarcoidosis, berylliosis, asbestosis, scleroderma, and pulmonary edema are some diseases that decrease the diffusing capacity of the gases. The capacity may also decrease in emphysema because of a decrease in surface area for gas exchange.

PERFUSION

Perfusion of the lung refers to the blood flow of the pulmonary circulation available for gas exchange. The pulmonary circulation operates at relatively low pressures compared with the systemic circulation. For this reason, the walls of the blood vessels in the pulmonary circulation are significantly thinner than comparable vessels in the systemic circulation. Pulmonary arterial pressure is low, because perfusion of the top of the lung is the most distal area. Compared with the systemic circulation, there is little requirement for significant regional differences in perfusion.

Hydrostatic pressure has a significant effect on perfusion of the lower lobes. The hydrostatic pressure reflects the effect of gravity on the blood, tending to favor perfusion of the lower lung fields. This fact has been substantiated using radioactive tracers in the pulmonary circulation and measuring radiation counts over the lung fields. The nonuniformity of perfusion reflects the interaction of alveolar, arterial, and venous pressures down the lung. Normally, blood flow is determined by the arterial venous pressure gradient. In the lungs, there are regional differences in alveolar pressure that can exert an effect on the arterial venous pressure gradient. For example, in the upper lung fields, alveolar pressure approximates atmospheric pressure, which overrides the arterial pressure and effectively closes the pulmonary capillaries. In the lower lung fields, the opposite occurs. The relatively low volume of air in the alveoli is overridden by the greater capillary hydrostatic pressure. Thus the capillary pressure effectively overcomes the alveolar pressure.

Pulmonary blood vessels constrict in response to low arterial pressures of oxygen. This is termed hypoxic vasoconstriction. Hypoxic vasoconstriction in the lung is believed to serve as an adaptive mechanism for diverting blood away from underventilated or poorly oxygenated lung areas. Although hypoxic vasoconstriction may have an important role to improve the efficiency of the lungs as a gas exchanger, this mechanism may be potentially deleterious to a patient who has reduced arterial oxygen pressure secondary to pulmonary pathology.

The acid base balance of the blood also affects pulmonary blood flow. A low blood pH or acidemia, for example, potentiates pulmonary vasoconstriction. Thus impaired ventilatory function can disturb blood gas composition and in turn, acid base balance. This effect can be amplified because of the cyclic reaction of pH on pulmonary vasoconstriction. Consideration of these basic physiologic mechanisms are tantamount to optimizing physical therapy intervention.

Ventilation and Perfusion Matching

It is essential that ventilated areas of the lung are in contact with perfused areas of the lung to effect normal gas exchange. Conditions that alter the ventilation or perfusion of part of the lung also affect the gas exchange in that portion of the lung. Uneven ventilation occurs where there is uneven compliance or uneven airway resistance in different parts of the lung. The lung is more compliant, that is, easier to inflate at low lung volumes. In the upright position, the apices have a higher resting volume because of a more negative intrapleural pressure than the bases, which renders the apices less compliant than the bases with relatively low resting volumes. Ventilation as previously described is favored in the lower lung regions rather than the apices. Uneven airway resistance may result from airway narrowing (bronchoconstriction in asthma, mucous plugs, edema, tumor,) or collapse from external pressures as with tumors or emphysema). Uneven compliance may also result from fibrosis, emphysema, pleural thickening, effusions, or pulmonary edema.

Nonuniform perfusion or blood flow can be a result of gravity, regional differences in intrapleural pressure, regional changes in alveolar pressure, and obstruction or blockage of part of the pulmonary circulation. Gravity increases blood flow in the dependent portions of the lung and decreases it in the nondependent portions of the lung. Regional differences

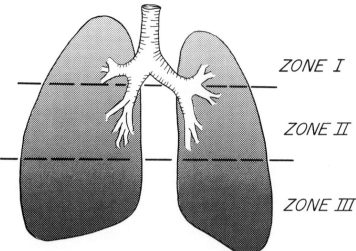

FIGURE 3-7

The perfusion of the lung is dependent on posture. In the upright position three areas can be seen. Zone III has perfusion in excess of ventilation, in Zone II perfusion and ventilation are fairly equal and in Zone I ventilation occurs in excess of perfusion.

in intrapleural pressure change the transmural pressure of blood vessels and thereby the amount of blood flowing through those vessels. Changes in alveolar pressure also affect the amount of blood flowing through the vessels. Overexpanded alveoli can compress blood vessels, while underexpanded alveoli may allow more blood to flow through those vessels. Blood clots, fat, parasites, or tumor cells may constrict or block part of the pulmonary circulation.

As discussed previously, gravity tends to pull blood into the dependent positions of the lung (Figure 3-7). In erect humans, therefore, there is greater blood flow at the bases of the lung. In places, the arterial blood pressure exceeds the alveolar pressure and causes compression or collapse of the airways (Figure 3-8). Blood flow to the apices is decreased because of gravity. Alveoli in this region are more fully expanded as a result of high transmural pressures and may further decrease blood flow by compressing blood vessels. It follows that the areas of optimal gas exchange occur where there is the greatest

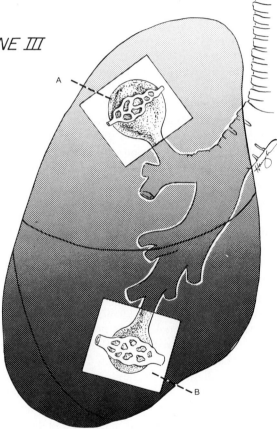

FIGURE 3-8

Relationship between the size of the airways and the amount of perfusion in the area in the upright position. **A,** Perfusion is decreased in the apices due to gravity. This enables the alveoli to fully expand. This expansion may compress blood vessels and thereby further decrease blood flow. **B,** Perfusion is increased in the bases of the lungs due to gravity. The enlarged vessels prevent full expansion of alveoli and may in fact compress them to a smaller size.

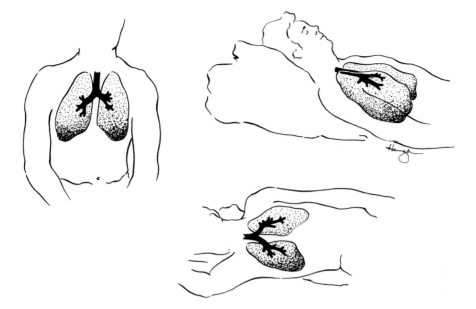

FIGURE 3-9
The effect of positioning on perfusion of the lung. Note that gravity-dependent segments have the greatest amount of perfusion.

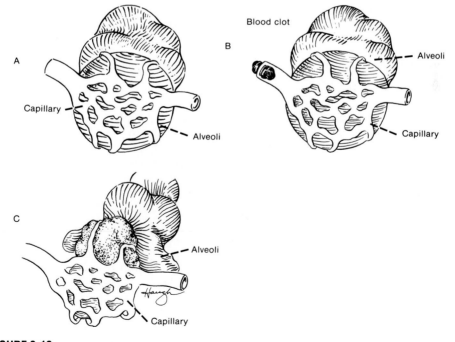

FIGURE 3-10
A, Normal alveolus. **B,** Dead space. **C,** Shunt.

amount of perfusion and ventilation. This occurs toward the base of the lungs in erect humans. Changes in posture cause changes in perfusion and ventilation. Generally, greater air exchange occurs toward the gravity-dependent areas. In side lying, there is greater gas exchange in the dependent lung (Figure 3-9).

In normal lungs, there is an optimal ratio or matching of gas and blood. This ratio of ventilation to perfusion is 0.8 to maintain normal blood gas values of P_{O_2} and P_{CO_2}. Therefore the lungs must be able to supply four parts ventilation to about five parts perfusion. When the ratio is not uniform throughout the lung, the arterial blood cannot contain normal blood gas values. Regions with low ratios (perfusion in excess of ventilation) act as a shunt, while regions with high ratios (ventilation in excess of perfusion) act as dead space (Figure 3-10). Hypoxemia results if regions of abnormal V:Q ratio predominate. An

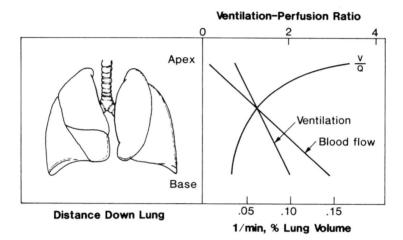

FIGURE 3-11
The effect of gravity on ventilation, perfusion and ventilation-perfusion matching (V/Q ratio).

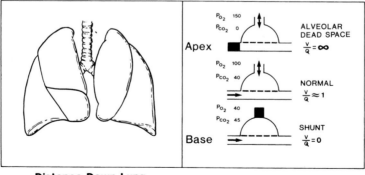

FIGURE 3-12
Schemata showing the effect of gravity on ventilation and perfusion down the upright lung.

elevation in arterial P_{CO_2} may also occur unless the patient increases ventilation. Therapists who are positioning patients with cardiopulmonary pathology may find that their patients experience greater distress when placed in certain positions. Such position-dependent distress can be explained by ventilation-perfusion inequalities that cause poor gas exchange in the dependent lung.

The relationship of ventilation and perfusion in the lung is summarized in the following figures. Figure 3-11 shows increases in ventilation and perfusion down the upright lung. Optimal ventilation and perfusion matching, V:Q occurs in the mid-lung zones. In the upright position, ventilation is in excess of perfusion in the apices, and perfusion is in excess of ventilation in the bases. Figures 3-12 illustrate the effects of shunt and physiologic dead space on V:Q matching in the upright lung, and their effect on alveolar gas. Specifically, Figure 3-12 shows a schematic representation of regional differences in ventilation and perfusion in the upper, middle, and lower zones of the upright lung. These gradients are reflected in the alveolar P_{O_2} and P_{CO_2} levels associated with alveolar dead space of the apices, appropriate ventilation-perfusion matching in the mid-lung, and shunt in the bases.

CARDIAC REFLEXES

The heart behaves automatically, thus is termed a functional syncytium. Three primary reflexes enable the heart to increase stroke volume and cardiac output with moment-to-moment changes in myocardial demand (French and Criley, 1983).

The first reflex is the Starling effect which refers to the increased force of contraction that occurs with increased venous return (preload). The second reflex, the Anrep effect, refers to the increase in ventricular contractile force as a result of an increase in aortic pressure (afterload). And third, the Bowdich effect refers to the corresponding increase in heart rate when myocardial contractile force increases. The integrated function of these three reflexes ensures that cardiac output adjusts as demands on the heart change, that is in health, primarily in response to exercise, body position and emotional stress.

COORDINATION OF CARDIAC EVENTS

The mechanical activity of the heart is precisely regulated with the electrical activity of the heart to effect optimal cardiac output to the organs of the body (Andreoli, Fowkes, Zipes, and Wallace, 1991; Dubin, 1989; Wagner, 1994). The electrical and mechanical events of the cardiac cycle are summarized in Figure 3-13. These events include the spread of the wave of electrical excitation throughout the myocardium, the resulting sequence of contraction of the atria and ventricles followed by dynamic changes in pressure and blood volume in the heart chambers, the heart sounds

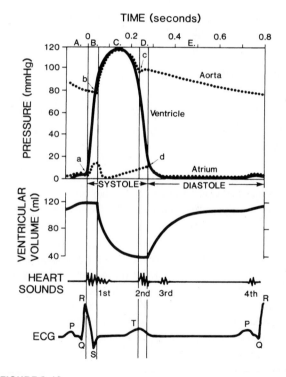

FIGURE 3-13
Summary of electrical and mechanical events of the heart. **A,** Atrial systole. **B,** Isovolumetric contraction. **C,** Ejection. **D,** Isovolumetric relaxation. **E,** Rapid inflow, diastasis, and active rapid filling. Note relationship of ventricular pressure and volume. *(a)* closure of the atrioventricular valves; *(b)* opening of the semilunar valves; *(c)* closure of the semilunar valves; *(d)* opening of the atrioventricular valves.

and the timing of these events. The cardiac cycle takes 0.8 second in a heart beating at 75 beats/min. Ventricular systole or ejection takes about one-third of this time. Its onset and termination are marked respectively by closure and opening of the atrioventricular valves (mitral and tricuspid). Diastole, or the period between successive ventricular systoles in which the ventricles fill with blood, takes two thirds of the 0.8 second of each cardiac cycle.

Phases of Systole and Diastole

Ventricular systole normally has three phases: isovolumetric contraction period, rapid ejection period, and a slower ejection period. Ventricular diastole also has three phases: passive rapid-filling phase, diastasis (a slower filling phase), and active rapid-filling phase.

Heart Sounds

The heart sounds are described as a low-pitched long duration sound (S_1) followed by a higher-pitched slower duration sound (S_2) that resembles the phonic sounds of LUB-dub. S_1 is associated with closure of the atrioventricular valves. S_2 is associated with closure of the semilunar valves. In inspiration, the aortic valve closes several milliseconds before the pulmonic valve, resulting in a splitting of the second heart sound, S_2. During inspiration, intrathoracic pressure becomes more negative, venous return and right heart volume increase, hence pulmonary ejection is prolonged in this situation, and closure of the pulmonary valve is delayed. Other variations in splitting of S_2 occur with pathology. The presence of a third (S_3) or fourth (S_4) heart sound is usually considered abnormal. S_3 is usually associated with the passive rapid-filling phase, and S_4 with the active rapid-filling phase.

Volume and Pressure Changes

Changes in the ventricular volume curve and aortic pressure wave reflect changes in atrial and ventricular pressure during systole and diastole (Ganong, 1993; Guyton, 1991). The sequence of events appears in a flow chart in Figure 3-14. Pressure gradients within the

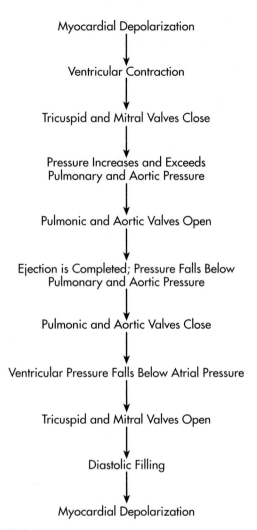

FIGURE 3-14
The sequence of pressure changes in the heart during the cardiac cycle.

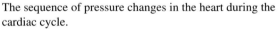

heart are responsible for the opening and closing of the valves. Coordinated valve opening and closure are important in promoting the forward movement of blood and preventing mechanical inefficiency of the heart pump resulting from valvular regurgitation of blood during ventricular contraction. Regurgitation of blood in the retrograde direction gives rise to heart murmurs audible on auscultation of the heart (Goldberger, 1990).

TABLE 3-1

**Balance of Forces Moving Fluid
In and Out of the Capillary**

	mm Hg
Mean forces moving fluid out of capillary	
Mean capillary pressure	17.0
Negative interstitial pressure	6.3
Oncotic interstitial pressure	5.0
TOTAL OUTWARD PRESSURE	28.3
Mean forces moving fluid into capillary	
Plasma oncotic pressure	28.0
TOTAL INWARD PRESSURE	28.0
OUTWARD PRESSURE – INWARD PRESSURE = NET OUTWARD PRESSURE	0.3

Peripheral Circulation

The purpose of the peripheral circulation including the microcirculation at the tissue level is to provide saturated oxygenated blood and remove partially de-saturated blood. The microcirculation within each organ regulated the blood flow both exogenously via the neurological system and endogenously via the humoral system commensurate with the metabolic needs of that tissue bed (see Chapter 2). The four principal factors that determine the movement of fluid in the microcirculation include the following:

1. The capillary hydrostatic pressure from the blood pressure, which tends to move blood across the capillary membrane out of the circulation into the interstitium
2. The capillary oncotic pressure from the proteins within the blood vessels, which tends to retain fluid in the circulation
3. The interstitial hydrostatic pressure, which tends to move fluid back into the circulation
4. The interstitial oncotic pressure, which tends to draw fluid out of the circulation into the interstitium

The net forces acting on the capillary fluid are nearly in equilibrium with a slight tendency for fluid to be filtered out of the systemic circulation into the interstitium. Table 3-1 illustrates the mean pressures determining normal fluid dynamics across capillary membranes.

TRANSPORT OF OXYGEN BY THE BLOOD

Once oxygen reaches the blood, it rapidly combines with hemoglobin to form oxyhemoglobin (West, 1995). A small proportion of oxygen is dissolved in the plasma. The use of the hemoglobin molecule as an oxygen carrier allows for greater availability and efficiency of oxygen delivery to the tissues in response to changes in metabolism. Saturation of the oxygen-carrying sites on the hemoglobin molecule is curvilinearly related to the partial pressure of oxygen in the tissues. This relationship is called the oxyhemoglobin dissociation curve and is a sigmoid or S-shaped curve (Figure 3-15). The hemoglobin of arterial blood is 98% or almost completely saturated with oxygen. Under normal circumstances, arterial blood is mixed with a small proportion of venous blood from the coronary and pulmonary circulation, resulting in arterial saturation of less than 100%. The graph shows a range of partial pressures of oxygen that may exist in the tissues. At relatively high arterial oxygen pressures, the oxygen saturation is high. This reflects high association or low dissociation between oxygen and hemoglobin. Saturation does not fall significantly until the partial pressure of oxygen falls below 80 mm Hg. Even at Po_2 levels of 40 to 50 mm Hg, arterial saturation is still 75%. This suggests an enormous capacity of the oxyhemoglobin dissociation system to meet the varying needs of different tissues without severely compromising arterial saturation. A Po_2 of less than 50%, for example, has a profound effect on arterial saturation. This demonstrates an adaptive response of hemoglobin dissociation to respond to low oxygen tissue pressures by greater dissociation of oxygen from hemoglobin as the need arises. As the Po_2 improves as a result of increased supply of oxygen or decreased demand, the affinity between oxygen and hemoglobin increases, and arterial saturation increases. Thus oxygen is not released unless there is a need for greater oxygen delivery to the tissues.

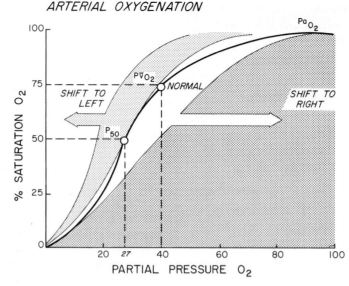

FIGURE 3-15
The oxyhemoglobin dissociation curve.

Different conditions can increase or decrease hemoglobin affinity for oxygen and thereby cause a shift in the oxyhemoglobin dissociation curve (West, 1995) (Figure 3-15). A shift to the right results in decreased oxygen affinity and greater dissociation of oxygen and hemoglobin. In this instance, for any given partial pressure of oxygen, there is a lower saturation than normal. This means that there is more oxygen available to the tissues. Shifts in the curve to the right occur with increasing concentration of hydrogen ions (i.e., decreasing pH), increasing P_{CO_2}, increasing temperatures, and increasing levels of 2,3-DPG (diphosphoglycerate), a byproduct of red blood cell metabolism. West (1995) suggests, "A simple way to remember these shifts is that an exercising muscle (increased metabolic demand), is acid, hypercarbic, (hypercapnic) and hot, and it benefits from increased unloading of oxygen from its capillaries."

A shift of the curve to the left results in increased oxygen affinity. Thus for any given partial pressure of oxygen, there is a higher saturation than normal. This means that there is less oxygen available to the tissues. This occurs in alkalemia, hypothermia, and decreased 2,3-DPG.

Anemia (reduced red blood cell count and hemoglobin) and polycythemia (excess red blood cells and hemoglobin) produce changes in oxygen content of the blood as well as saturation. Anemia shifts the curve to the right and lowers the maximal saturation achievable. Polycythemia has the opposite effect. The curve is shifted to the left and maximal saturation approaches 100%.

TRANSPORT OF CARBON DIOXIDE

CO_2 is an acid produced by cells as a result of cell metabolism. It is carried in various forms by venous blood to the lungs, where it is eliminated. Most of the CO_2 added to plasma diffuses into the red blood cells, where it is buffered and returned to the plasma to be carried to the lungs. The buffering mechanism is so effective that large changes in dissolved CO_2 can occur with small changes in blood pH.

The transport of CO_2 has an important role in the acid-base status of the blood and maintenance of normal homeostasis (Comroe, Forster, Dubois, Briscoe, and Carlsen, 1986). The lung excretes 10,000 mEq of carbonic acid per day. (Carbonic acid is broken down into water and CO_2. The CO_2 is buffered and eliminated through the lungs.) The kidney can excrete only 100 mEq per day of acids. Therefore alterations in alveolar ventilation can have profound effects on the body's acid-base status. A decrease in the lung's ability to ventilate causes a sharp rise in P_{CO_2} and a drop in pH. This causes an acute respiratory acidosis. If this change occurs gradually, the pH will remain within normal limits while the P_{CO_2} is elevated. This is known as a compensated respiratory acidosis. Hyperventilation or excessive ventilation causes rapid elimination of CO_2 from the blood. This results in a decreased P_{CO_2} and an increased pH and is known as an acute respiratory alkalosis. Again, if the change occurs gradually, the pH remains within normal limits even though the P_{CO_2} is decreased. This is a compensated respiratory alkalosis.

SUMMARY

This chapter presented an overview of cardiopulmonary physiology with respect to breathing control, both central and peripheral mechanisms such as muscle, joint, and lung and chest wall stretch receptors, involved with the regulation of respiration. Mechanical factors of breathing, chest wall and lung compliance, and airway resistance are described. The elastic properties of the respiratory system, that is, chest wall and lungs, are reflected in the pressure volume relaxation curve. This curve has important implications for the clinical presentation of the patient with cardiopulmonary dysfunction, and in particular, the efficiency and energy requirement of the respiratory system. Ventilation and perfusion matching is the basis of gas exchange and the adequacy of lung function. Many factors in addition to disease, however, can affect ventilation and perfusion matching, including age, body position, breathing at low lung volumes and smoking history. The relationship of such factors are discussed. The purpose of the heart is to provide an adequate cardiac output, hence, adequate oxygen delivery to the vital organs and peripheral tissues. The optimal coupling of electrical and mechanical events in the heart to effect cardiac output are described.

Arterial P_{O_2} and P_{CO_2} are normally maintained within certain prescribed limits. In health, oxyhemo-globin dissociation ensures adequate oxygen delivery to the tissues once oxygen has diffused through the alveolar capillary membrane into the circulation. Transport of CO_2 and its buffering mechanisms are central to acid base balance and normal homeostasis.

REVIEW QUESTIONS

1. Describe the control of breathing.
2. Explain respiratory mechanics with respect to airway resistance and lung compliance.
3. Describe the distributions of ventilation, perfusion and diffusion.
4. Explain the determinants of ventilation and perfusion matching.
5. Describe electromechanical coupling in the heart.
6. Describe oxyhemoglobin dissociation and the oxyhemoglobin dissociation curve.

REFERENCES

Andreoli, K.G., Fowkes, V.K., Zipes, D.P., & Wallace, A.G. (Eds.). (1991). *Comprehensive cardiac care* (7th ed.). St Louis: Mosby.

Bates, D.V. (1989). *Respiratory function in disease.* (3rd ed.). Philadelphia: WB Saunders.

Berne, R.M., & Levy, M.N. (1992). *Cardiovascular physiology* (6th ed.). St Louis: CV Mosby.

Burrows, B., Knudson, R.J., Quan, S.F., & Kettel, L.J. (1983). *Respiratory disorders: A pathophysiologic approach* (2nd ed.). Chicago: Year Book Medical.

Cherniack, R.M., & Cherniack, L. (1983). *Respiration in health and disease* (3rd ed.). Philadelphia: WB Saunders.

Clemente, C.D. (Ed.). (1985). *Anatomy of the human body* (30th ed.). Philadelphia: Lea and Febiger.

Comroe, J.H., Jr., Forster, R.E., II, Dubois, A.B., Briscoe, W.A., & Carlsen, E. (1986). *The lung; Clinical physiology and pulmonary function tests* (3rd ed.). Chicago: Year Book Medical.

Dubin, D. (1989). *Rapid interpretation of EKGs* (4th ed.). Tampa, FL: Cover.

French, W.G., & Criley, J.M. (Eds.). (1983). *Practical cardiology: Ischemic and valvular heart disease.* New York: John Wiley and Sons.

Ganong, W. F. (1993). *Review of medical physiology* (16th ed.). Los Altos: Lange Medical Publications.

Goldberger, E. (1990). *Essentials of clinical cardiology.* Philadelphia: JB Lippincott.

Goldman, M. (1979). Mechanical interaction between diaphragm and rib cage. *American Review of Respiratory Disease, 119*(Part 2), 23-26.

Guyton, A.C. (1991). *Textbook of medical physiology.* (8th ed.). Philadelphia: WB Saunders.

Katz, A.M. (1992). *Physiology of the heart* (2nd ed.). New York: Raven Press.

Murray, J.F., & Nadel, J.A. (1988). *Textbook of respiratory medicine.* Philadelphia: W.B. Saunders.

Nunn, J.F. (1993). *Applied respiratory physiology* (4th ed.). London: Butterworths.

Scharf, S.M., & Cassidy S.S. (Eds.). (1989). *Heart-lung interactions in health and disease.* New York: Marcel-Dekker, Inc.

Schlant, R.C., Alexander, R.W., O'Rourke, R.A., Roberts, R., & Sonnenblick, E. H. (Eds.). (1994). *Hurst's the heart: Arteries and veins* (8th ed.). New York: McGraw-Hill.

Sokolow, M., McIlroy, M.B., & Cheitlin, M.D. (1990). *Clinical cardiology* (5th ed.). Norwalk: Appleton & Lange.

Wagner, G.S. (1994). *Marriott's practical electrocardiography* (9th ed.). Baltimore: Williams and Wilkins.

West, J.B. (1995). *Respiratory physiology—The essentials* (5th ed.). Baltimore: Williams and Wilkins.

West, J.B. (1992). *Pulmonary pathophysiology: The essentials* (4th ed.). Baltimore: Williams and Wilkins.

West, J.B. (1991). *Best and Taylor's physiological basis of medical practice* (12th ed.). Baltimore: Williams and Wilkins.

CHAPTER 4

Cardiopulmonary Pathophysiology

Willy E. Hammon
Scott Hasson

KEY TERMS

Angina
Bronchiectasis
Coronary artery disease
Emphysema

Fibrosis
Myocardial infarction
Obstructive lung disease
Restrictive lung disease

INTRODUCTION

The first part of this chapter, beginning with obstructive lung disease, describes the pathophysiology of chronic pulmonary disease. Chronic pulmonary disease can be categorized broadly into obstructive and restrictive disorders.

Obstructive disorders are characterized by a decreased rate of airflow during expiration (as a result of increased airway resistance). Restrictive disorders are conditions in which the inspiratory capacity of the lungs is restricted to less than the predicted normal. Overlap between the two categories does exist.

The second part of this chapter, beginning with coronary artery disease (CAD), describes the pathophysiology of cardiovascular disease. Cardiovascular disease is also known primarily as CAD, and is manifested in various clinical syndromes. CAD is an atherosclerotic process that occurs in the right and left coronary arteries, which ultimately affects heart per-

formance. The parameters affected by CAD can be the volume of blood pumped and the heart rate. The major purposes of this portion of the chapter are to describe the etiologic factors of clinical syndromes associated with CAD, briefly describe medical treatment, and discuss issues of prognosis.

OBSTRUCTIVE LUNG DISEASE

Several abbreviations can be found in the literature for a pulmonary disorder characterized by increased airway resistance, particularly noticeable by a prolonged forced expiration. Some of these are chronic obstructive pulmonary disease (COPD), chronic obstructive airway disease (COAD), chronic airway obstruction (CAO), and chronic obstructive lung disease (COLD) (Fishman, 1988).

The first part of this chapter describes chronic bronchitis, emphysema, asthma, and bronchiectasis

71

individually. With the possible exception of asthma and bronchiectasis, however, it is unusual in the clinical setting to find a patient with only one of these conditions. Most patients have some combination of chronic bronchitis, emphysema, and asthma, and in this chapter, these individuals are referred to as having COPD. These patients have intermittent episodes of wheezing, along with a variable degree of chronic bronchitis and emphysema (Hodgkin, 1975). Radiologically, they may have hyperinflated lungs, flattened diaphragms, and an enlarged right ventricle as a result of increased pulmonary artery pressure. Other findings vary from patient to patient, depending on the predominant disease process contributing to their COPD.

COPD is very common. In 1994 the American Lung Association (ALA) estimated that 14.2 million Americans have COPD. In the United States alone, health care costs for COPD exceed $7.6 billion annually. Deaths from COPD numbered more than 85,000 in 1991; it is the fourth leading cause of death in the United States.

Chronic Bronchitis

Chronic bronchitis is a disease characterized by a cough producing sputum for at least 3 months and for 2 consecutive years (American Thoracic Society, 1962).

Pathologically, there is an increase in the size of the tracheobronchial mucous glands (increased Reid index) and goblet cell hyperplasia (Mitchell, 1968; Reid, 1960; Stoller and Wiedemann, 1990). Mucous cell metaplasia of bronchial epithelium results in a decreased number of cilia. Ciliary dysfunction and disruption of the continuity of the mucous blanket are common. In the peripheral airways, bronchiolitis, bronchiolar narrowing, and increased amounts of mucus are observed (Cosio, 1978; Wright, 1992).

The cause of chronic bronchitis is believed to be related to long-term irritation of the tracheobronchial tree. The most common cause of irritation is cigarette smoking (*US Surgeon General,* 1984). Inhaled cigarette smoke stimulates the goblet cells and mucous glands to secrete more mucus. This smoke also inhibits ciliary action. The hypersecretion of mucus and impaired cilia lead to a chronic productive cough. The fact that smokers secrete an abnormal amount of mucus makes them susceptible to respiratory infections, and it takes them longer to recover from these infections. In addition, the irritation of smoke in the tracheobronchial tree causes bronchoconstriction. Although smoking is the most common cause of chronic bronchitis, other agents that have been implicated are air pollution, bronchial infections, and certain occupations.

These patients are referred to as "blue bloaters," because they usually have stocky body build and are "blue" as a result of hypoxemia (Dornhorst, 1955; Filley et al, 1968; Fishman, 1988; Nash, Briscoe, and Cournand, 1965. Although many of these patients have a high arterial partial pressure of carbon dioxide ($Paco_2$), the pH is normalized by renal retention of bicarbonate (Hco_3). In the patient with chronic bronchitis, bone marrow tries to compensate for chronic hypoxemia by increased production of red blood cells, leading to polycythemia (Snider, Faling, and Rennard, 1994). Polycythemia, in turn, makes the blood more viscous, forcing the heart to work even harder to pump it. Long-term hypoxemia leads to increased pulmonary artery pressure and right ventricular hypertrophy.

Individuals with bronchitis often expectorate mucoid brownish-colored sputum. In an exacerbation, usually from infection, they have an even greater amount of purulent sputum. Ventilation-perfusion abnormalities are common, which increase hypoxemia and $Paco_2$ retention (Rochester and Brown, 1976). The respiratory rate increases, as does the use of accessory muscles. The resultant increased work of breathing requires greater oxygen consumption by these muscles, with a greater production of carbon dioxide (CO_2) than the respiratory system can adequately meet. This contributes to a further drop in the arterial partial pressure of oxygen (Pao_2) and a rise in $Paco_2$. The hypoxemia and acidemia increase pulmonary vessel constriction, which raises pulmonary artery pressure and ultimately leads to right heart failure (cor pulmonale).

In the following example, a patient is admitted to the hospital with an exacerbation of chronic bronchitis and presents the following picture: he is of stocky body build, his color is dusky, and he breathes with moderate-to-marked use of the respiratory accessory muscles, depending on the degree of respiratory distress. Wheezing may be audible or noted by auscultation. Intercostal (or sternal) retractions may be present, also depending on the degree of respiratory distress. Edema in the extremities (especially in the ankle area) and neck vein distention reflect decompensated cor pulmonale. The patient may report that this breathing difficulty began with increased amounts of secretions (showing a change in normal color) or decreased amounts of sputum (reflecting increased retention of secretions). Arterial blood gases show the individual with bronchitis to have a lowered Pao_2, a raised $Paco_2$ and a lowered pH.

Pulmonary function tests indicate a reduced vital capacity, forced expiratory volume in 1 second (FEV_1), maximum voluntary ventilation and diffusing capacity, as well as an increased functional residual capacity and residual volume.

During an exacerbation, these patients are usually treated with intravenous (IV) fluids, antibiotics, bronchodilator and low-flow oxygen. Cortiocosteroids may be administered. Some patients with increased secretions respond to chest physical therapy and bronchial

hygiene methods (Snider, Faling, and Rennard, 1994, Sutton et al, 1988; Sutton et al, 1983). Diuretics and digitalis are often given to treat cor pulmonale.

Emphysema

There are two main types of emphysema—centrilobular and panlobular (Reid, 1976; Thurlbeck, 1974). It has been suggested that centrilobular emphysema is 20 times more common than panlobular emphysema, although both types are often found in the same pair of lungs.

As its name implies, centrilobular emphysema is characterized by destruction of the respiratory bronchiole, edema, inflammation, and thickened bronchiolar walls. These changes are more common and more marked in the upper lobes and superior segments of the lower lobes (Thurlbeck, 1963). This form of emphysema is found more often in men than in women, is rare among nonsmokers, and is common among patients with chronic bronchitis.

Panlobular emphysema, on the other hand, is

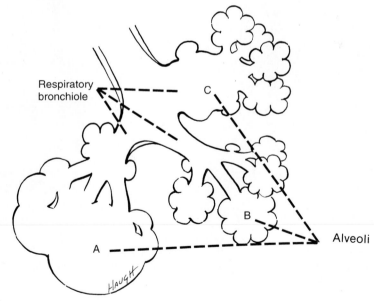

FIGURE 4-1
A, Panlobular emphysema is characterized by a destructive enlargement of the alveoli, **B,** A normal respiratory bronchiole and alveoli. **C,** Centrilobular emphysema is characterized by a selective enlargement and destruction of the respiratory bronchiole.

characterized by destructive enlargement of the alveoli, distal to the terminal bronchiole (Figure 4-1). It most often involves the lower lobes. This type of emphysema is also found in subjects that have alpha$_1$-antitripsin deficiency. Airway obstruction in these individuals is caused by loss of lung elastic recoil or radial traction on the bronchioles. When individuals with normal lungs inhale, the airways are stretched open by the enlarging elastic lung, and during exhalation the airways are narrowed as a result of the decreasing stretch of the lung. However, the lungs of patients with panlobular emphysema have decreased elasticity because of disruption and destruction of surrounding alveolar walls. This in turn leaves the bronchiole unsupported and vulnerable to collapse during exhalation.

Bullae, emphysematous spaces larger than 1 cm in diameter, may be found in patients with emphysema (Figure 4-2) (Reid, 1967; Thurlbeck, 1991; Thurlbeck, 1976). It is thought that bullae develop from a coalescence of adjacent areas of emphysema or an obstruction of the conducting airways that permits the flow of air into the alveoli during inspiration but does not allow air to flow out again during expiration. This causes the alveoli to become hyperinflated and eventually leads to destruction of the alveolar walls with a resultant enlarged air space in the lung parenchyma. These bullae can be more than 10 cm in diameter, and by compression, can compromise the function of the remaining lung tissue (Figure 4-3). If this happens, surgical intervention to remove the bulla is often necessary. Pneumothorax, a serious complication, can result from the rupture of one of these bullae.

The emphysema patient's most common complaint is dyspnea. Physically, these patients appear thin and have an increased anteroposterior chest di-

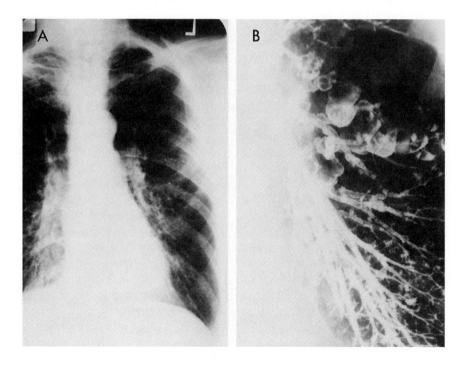

FIGURE 4-2
A, AP chest film reveals bullous emphysema with multiple, thin, rounded fibrotic lucencies. **B,** The spot film bronchogram of the left midlung field shows intact bronchi and distal emphysematous blebs. (Courtesy of T. H. Johnson, M.D.)

ameter. Typically, they breathe using the accessory muscles of inspiration. These patients are often seen leaning forward, resting their forearms on their knees or sitting with their arms extended at their sides and pushing down against the bed or chair to elevate their shoulders and improve the effectiveness of the accessory muscles of inspiration. They may breathe through pursed lips during the expiratory phase of breathing. These patients have been referred to as "pink puffers" because of the increased respiratory work they must do to maintain relatively normal blood gases (Dornhorst, 1955; Filley et al, 1968; Fishman, 1988; Nash, Briscoe, and Cournand, 1965). On auscultation, decreased breath sounds can be noted throughout most or all of the lung fields. Radiologically, the emphysema patient has overinflated lungs, a flattened diaphragm, and a small, elongated

heart (Figure 4-4). Pulmonary function tests show a decreased vital capacity, FEV_1, maximum voluntary ventilation and a greatly reduced diffusing capacity. The total lung capacity is increased, while the residual volume and functional residual capacity are even more increased. Arterial blood gases reflect a mildly or moderately lowered Pao_2, a normal or slightly raised $Paco_2$ and a normal pH. These patients, unlike patients with chronic bronchitis, normally will develop heart failure in the end stage of the disease (Figure 4-5).

Treatment of progressive emphysema that requires hospitalization often includes IV fluids, antibiotics, and low-flow oxygen (Snider, Faling, and Rennard, 1994). Some of these patients also receive bronchodilators, corticosteroids, diuretics, and digitalis. Pursed-lip breathing can relieve dyspnea and improve

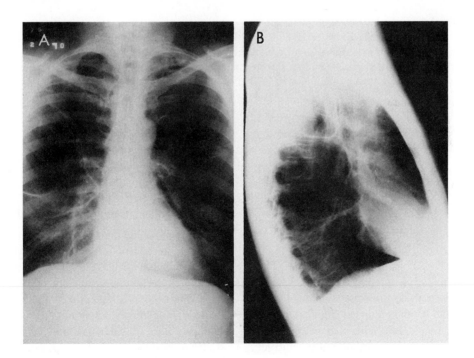

FIGURE 4-3
A, AP and **B,** lateral views of the chest of a patient with advanced bullous emphysematous changes. Note the bullae in the upper lung fields. The lateral film reveals an increased A-P diameter of the thorax, flattening of the diaphragms and in increased anterior clear space. (Courtesy of T. H. Johnson, M.D.)

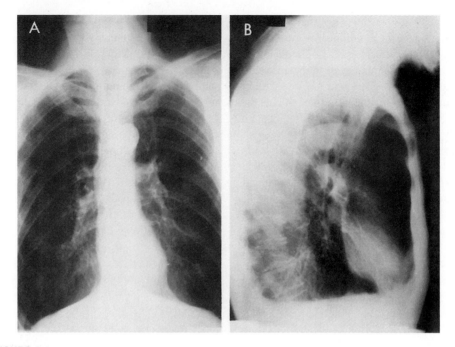

FIGURE 4-4

A, AP chest film reveals the increased lucency of lung fields and flattening of the diaphragm of emphysema. The vascular structures are crowded medially. **B,** Lateral chest film reveals an increased AP diameter and flattening of the diaphragms. There is an increase in the anterior clear space. These are all findings of emphysema. (Courtesy of T. H. Johnson, M.D.)

arterial blood gasses (Muller, Petty, and Filley, 1970; Petty and Guthrie, 1974).

The cause of emphysema is uncertain. It is known that the incidence of emphysema increases with age. It is most often found in chronic bronchitics, and there is no question that emphysema is more prevalent in cigarette smokers than in nonsmokers (*US Surgeon General,* 1984). The risk of developing COPD is 30 times greater in smokers than nonsmokers (Fielding, 1985). There also seems to be an hereditary factor, evident in the severe panlobular emphysema that patients with an alpha$_1$-antitrypsin deficiency develop relatively early in life, even though they may never have smoked (Eriksson, 1965; Tobin, Cook, and Hutchinson, 1983). Repeated lower respiratory tract infections may also play a role. However, the interrelationship of

these and other factors in producing emphysema is still not well understood.

Prognosis of chronic bronchitis and emphysema

Chronic bronchitis and emphysema are marked by a progressive loss of lung function. At the end of 5 years, patients with COPD have a death rate four to five times greater than the normal expected value. Death rates reported by various studies depend on the method of selection of patients, types of diagnostic tests and other criteria (Anthonisen, 1989; Bousky et al, 1964; Kanner et al, 1983; Kanner and Renzetti, 1984). One study reported a 3-year overall mortality rate of 23%, with patient age and the initial FEV$_1$ value being the most accurate predictors of death (Anthonisen, Wright, and Hodgkin, 1986). In general,

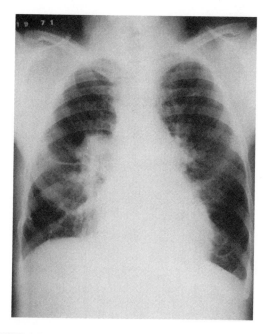

FIGURE 4-5

The chest film reveals peripheral emphysematous lucency. The hilar areas are tremendously enlarged by the pulmonary arteries in a typical cor pulmonale configuration. Cardiomegaly is also present. (Courtesy of T. H. Johnson, M.D.)

the death rates 5 years after diagnosis are 20% to 55%. Other investigators reported an overall mortality of 47 percent at the end of 5 years (Burrows, and Earle, 1969). They believed a 5-year survival rate can be estimated as follows: 80% in patients with an FEV_1 close to 1.0 L; and 40% for patients with an FEV_1 less than 0.75 L. However, if the above flow rates are found in patients with complications of resting tachycardia, chronic hypercapnia and a severely impaired diffusing capacity, the survival rates should be reduced by 25%. Other factors that have been associated with a poor prognosis are cor pulmonale, weight loss, radiologic evidence of emphysema, a dyspneic onset, polycythemia, and Hoover's sign (an inward movement of the ribs on inspiration) (Mitchell, Webb, and Filley, 1964; Renzetti, 1967).

The most common cause of death in patients with COPD (in descending order of frequency) are con-

gestive heart failure (CHF), which is secondary to cor pulmonale; respiratory failure; pneumonia; bronchiolitis; and pulmonary embolism.

Asthma

Asthma is a disease characterized by an increased responsiveness of the trachea and bronchi to various stimuli, and is manifested by widespread narrowing of the airways that changes in severity either spontaneously or as a result of treatment. During an asthma attack, the lumen of the airways is narrowed or is occluded by a combination of bronchial smooth muscle spasm, inflammation of the mucosa, and an overproduction of a viscous, tenacious mucus.

Asthma is certainly a widespread disease in the world today. Its incidence is about 3% to 7% in adults (Barnes, 1993; National Asthma Education Program, 1991). It is found more often in individuals under age 25, where estimates of prevalence vary from 5% to 15% (Williams and McNicol, 1969). About 80% of children with asthma do not have asthma after the age of 10.

Asthma that begins in patients under the age of 35 is usually allergic or extrinsic. These asthma attacks are precipitated when an individual comes in contact with a specific substance to which that person is sensitive, such as pollens or household dust (see box 4-1 below). Often people with asthma are allergic to a number of substances, not only one or two.

If a patient's first asthma attack occurs after the age of 35, usually there is evidence of chronic airway obstruction with intermittent episodes of acute bronchospasm. These individuals, whose attacks are not triggered by specific substances, are referred to as having nonallergic or intrinsic asthma (see box below). Chronic bronchitis is commonly found in this group, and this is the type of individual often seen in the hospital setting.

The individual with an acute asthma attack usually has been awakened at night or early in the morning with one or more of the following symptoms: cough, dyspnea, wheezing, or chest tightness (McFadden, 1988). In fact, nocturnal awakenings are such a common occurrence with asthma, that their absence from the history causes even experienced clinicians to doubt the diagno-

Factors That May Precipitate an Asthma Attack
Allergic or extrinsic asthma
Pollen (especially ragweed)
Animals
Feathers
Molds
Household dust
Food
Nonallergic or intrinsic asthma
Inhaled irritants
Cigarette smoke
Dust
Pollution
Chemicals
Weather
High humidity
Cold air
Respiratory infections
Common cold
Bacterial bronchitis
Drugs
Aspirin
Emotions
Stress
Exercise

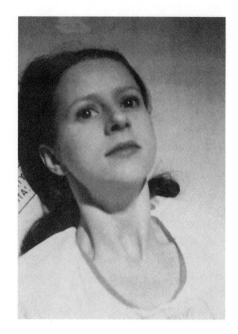

FIGURE 4-6
A patient in respiratory distress during an acute asthma attack. Note the marked use of the sternocleidomastoids and other accessory muscles during inspiration.

sis (Turner-Warwick, 1988). The patient has a rapid rate of breathing and is using the accessory respiratory muscle (Figure 4-6). The expiratory phase of breathing is prolonged with audible wheezing and rhonchi. However, when severe obstruction is present, the chest becomes silent (Gold, 1976). The patient may cough often, though unproductively, and may complain of tightness in his chest. Radiologically, the lungs may appear hyperinflated or show small atelectatic areas from retained secretions. The degree of tachypnea, hyperinflation, accessory muscle use, and pulsus paradoxus (difference in systolic blood pressure during inspiration and expiration) are useful guides for determining the degree of airway obstruction present (Woolcock, 1994). Early in the attack, arterial blood gases reflect slight hypoxemia and a low Pa_{CO_2} (from hyperventilation). If the attack progresses, the Pa_{O_2} continues to fall as the Pa_{CO_2} climbs above the normal range. As obstruction becomes severe, deterioration of the patient occurs, evident by a

high Pa_{CO_2}, a low Pa_{O_2}, and a pH of less than 7.30 (McFadden and Lyons, 1968).

Medical management of acute asthma has three goals: (1) relief of bronchospasm, (2) mobilization of secretions, and (3) maintenance of alveolar ventilation. Therefore most hospitalized patients with asthma are treated with IV fluids, bronchodilators, supplemental oxygen, and corticosteroids.

An asthma attack that persists for hours and is unresponsive to medical management is referred to as status asthmaticus. The patient may appear dehydrated, cyanotic, and near exhaustion from labored breathing. In contrast to the audible wheezing and rhonchi heard early in the attack, the chest now has greatly diminished or absent breath sounds. Status asthmaticus results in a significant death rate and is regarded as a medical emergency. Bilateral manual lower chest compression assists expiration and has value as an emergency treatment of asthma (Fisher, Bowery, and Ladd-

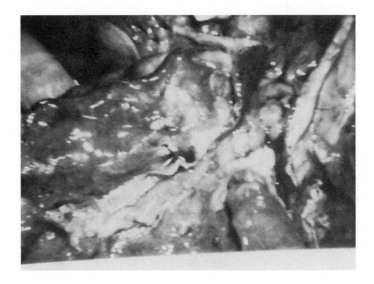

FIGURE 4-7
Gross specimen of lung showing large mucus plug within the bronchial tree of a patient who died from status asthmaticus. (Courtesy of J. J. Coalson, Ph.D.)

Hudson, 1989; Watts, 1989). Patients in respiratory failure may require mechanical ventilation.

Studies that examine the lungs of patients who die from status asthmaticus find lungs that are significantly hyperinflated and do not deflate even when the thorax is opened (Huber and Koessler, 1922; Dunnill, 1960; Saetta et al, 1991). Examination of the airways reveals a mucosa that is edematous and inflamed. Characteristic of asthma, the basement membrane is thickened. The mucous glands are enlarged, and there is an increase in the number of goblet cells. Evidence of bronchospasm is seen by the hypertrophied and thickened smooth muscle. The lumens of most bronchioles, down to the terminal bronchioles, are filled with viscous, sticky mucus (Figure 4-7). It is evident that the occluded bronchioles have caused death by asphyxiation. Secretions in the tracheobronchial tree of the patient with asthma are a combination of mucus, secreted by the mucous glands, and an exudate from the dilated capillaries just below the basement membranae. It has been shown that cilia do not sweep the mucoserous fluid nearly as effectively as pure mucus. In addition, sheets of ciliated epithelium have been shed into the

bronchial lumen, further contributing to the stasis of secretions. Although the alveoli are overinflated, the permanent destructive changes found in emphysema are not present.

Prognosis of asthma

Most studies following children with asthma for a number of years report a death rate of about 1% (Ogilvie, 1962). One large study of 1,000 people with asthma of all ages in England reported a mortality of 7% as a result of asthma or its complications. This study reported that 2% of the patients with intermittent asthma died, compared with 9% of those with continuous asthma. During the 1960s, there was a sharp increase in the number of deaths among people with asthma reported by countries around the world. At the peak of this increase, England and Wales reported that 7% of the deaths in children between 10 and 14 years of age were attributable to asthma. This reflected a 700% increase in only 7 years. Some medical authorities feel this increase in deaths was related to widespread use or abuse of certain pressurized aerosol nebulizers containing isoproterenol, but this has been disputed (Gandevia, 1973). In 1987 there were more than 4,300 deaths from asthma in the Untied States, 31% more than in 1980 (McFadden and Gilbert, 1992).

Bronchiectasis

Bronchiectasis is defined as an abnormal dilation of medium-size bronchi and bronchioles (about the fourth to ninth generations), generally associated with a previous, chronic necrotizing infection within these passages. Ordinarily, there is sufficient cartilage within the walls of the larger bronchi to protect them from dilation.

The airway deformities can be classified into three types (Reid, 1950; Luce, 1994). Cylindrical (or longitudinal) bronchiectasis is the most common type, with a uniform dilation of the airways. Varicose bronchiectasis refers to a greater dilation than in cylindrical bronchiectasis, causing the walls of the bronchi to resemble varicose veins (Figure 4-8). Saccular (or cystic) bronchiectasis refers to airways that have intermittent spherical ballooning (Figure 4-9).

Bronchiectasis is usually localized in a few segments or in an entire lobe of the lung. Most commonly, it is unilateral (although 40% to 50% of the cases are bilateral) and affects the basal segments of the lower lobes. When the left lower lobe is involved, it is not unusual to find bronchiectasis in the lingula of the left upper lobe as well. Interestingly, bronchiectasis of the right middle lobe is relatively common in older adults and can contribute to both hemoptysis and repeated infections of this lobe. Upper lobe bronchiectasis generally involves the apical and posterior segments and is usually caused by tuberculosis or bronchopulmonary aspergillosis.

Pathologically, the mucosa appears edematous and ulcerated. Destruction of the elastic and muscular structures of the airway walls is evident with resultant

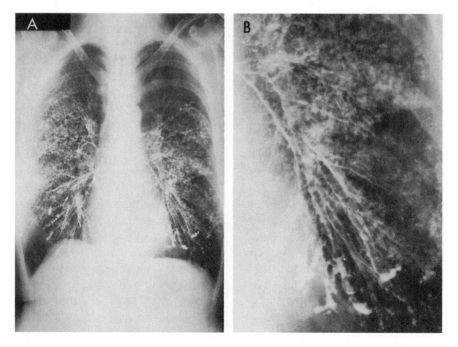

FIGURE 4-8
A, AP chest film of a bronchogram with cylindrical and varicose bronchiectasis in the lower lung fields. **B,** Close-up view of cylindrical and varicose bronchiectatic changes in the left lower lobe. (Courtesy of T. H. Johnson, M.D.)

dilation and fibrosis. The walls are lined with hyperplastic, nonciliated, mucus-secreting cells that have replaced the normal ciliated epithelium. This change is significant, because it interrupts the mucociliary blanket and causes pooling of infected secretions, which further damage and irritate the bronchial wall (Barker and Bardana, 1988; Currie et al, 1987).

The etiology of bronchiectasis is related to obstruction of the airways and respiratory infections (Luce, 1994; Simpson, 1975). Some 60% of the cases of bronchiectasis are preceded by an acute respiratory infection. The infection involves the bronchial walls. Portions of the mucosa are destroyed and are replaced by fibrous tissue. The radial traction of the lung parenchyma on the damaged bronchi causes the involved airways to become permanently dilated and distorted (Barker and Bardana, 1988). These areas, devoid of normal ciliated cells, contain secretions that eventually become chronically infected.

Obstruction can cause bronchiectasis by collapsing lung tissue (atelectasis) distal to the obstruction (Barker and Bardana, 1988). The increased negative pressure in the chest (from the collapsed lung) exerts a greater traction on the airways, causing them to expand and to become distorted. Secretions are retained, and if the obstruction is prolonged, an infection occurs that begins to destroy the walls of the bronchi, as described above. There has been a significant reduction in the number of patients with bronchiectasis since the introduction of antibiotics to treat respiratory infections.

Twenty-four–hour sputum volume has been used as an indicator of severity of disease to categorize patients with bronchiectasis (Ellis et al, 1981). Those producing less than 10 ml per day have been categorized as having mild bronchiectasis, 10 to 150 ml as moderate bronchiectasis and greater than 150 ml as having severe bronchiectasis.

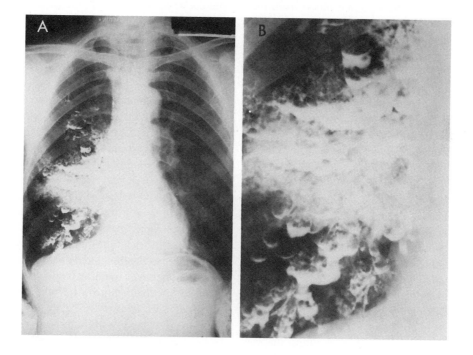

FIGURE 4-9

A, AP chest film of a bronchogram shows saccular bronchiectasis. **B,** Close-up view of bronchiectatic areas with grapelike saccular bronchiectasis. (Courtesy of T. H. Johnson, M.D.)

Patients with severe, diffuse, long-standing bronchiectasis are rare today. Physically, they are emaciated, and as many as 25% of them may have clubbed fingers. A chronic cough, with expectoration of unpleasant-tasting, purulent sputum is typical in these patients. When this sputum is collected and allowed to stand, it may separate into three distinct layers: the uppermost layer is frothy, the middle layer is serous or mucopurulent, and the lowest layer is purulent and may contain small grayish or yellowish plugs (Dittrich's plugs). Changes of body position, while sleeping or on arising, often stimulate coughing as the pooled secretions again spill onto the mucosa of normal, larger airways. These individuals may have cor pulmonale from fibrosis that has extended to involve the pulmonary capillary bed. Patients with widespread bronchiectasis appear dyspneic and have increased work of breathing as a result of hypoxemia and hypercapnia from ventilation-perfusion mismatching. Anastomosis of the bronchial and pulmonary vascular systems causes shunting of the systemic blood from the hypertrophied bronchial arteries. It also may contribute to a decreased capability to take oxygen into the involved segments of the lung (Liebow, Hales, and Lindskog, 1949; Luce, 1994).

Most patients complain of relatively few symptoms, except during a respiratory infection when they have an increased cough and sputum production. The amount of sputum expectorated and the severity of the cough vary from patient to patient, according to the amount of involvement. Hemoptysis does occur in about half of the older patients, evidently because of erosion of enlarged bronchial arteries that accompany the dilated bronchi.

Effective postural drainage, percussion, vibration, and the forced expiratory technique (FET) are important in the management of bronchiectasis (Gallon, 1991; van Hengstum et al, 1988; Sutton, 1983; Verboom, Bakker, and Sterk, 1986) (see Chapter 20). It should be done as frequently as indicated in patients with a productive cough. Postural drainage should be done 1 hour before retiring at night to facilitate the expectoration of secretions that would interfere with rest by stimulating violent coughing when the patient changes positions. It should also be done on arising in the morning to clear the lungs of secretions that have accumulated overnight. Therapists teaching the patient postural drainage positions devised to drain the involved segments should keep in mind that this disease causes distortion and dilation of the bronchi; hence the traditional positions found in books may be of limited value in determining the precise segment of the lung that is the source of the secretions. If the involvement is in the lower lobes, the patient should be placed in the Trendelenburg position and should be gradually rotated from lying on one side, to supine, to lying on the opposite side, and prone, if tolerated, while doing the FET and/or receiving percussion and vibration 5 to 10 minutes per segment over all surfaces of the lower lobe being treated. A similar procedure may be followed while sitting if the upper lobes require drainage, but these segments rarely require drainage, since they usually drain during the course of the day while the individual is in a more or less erect position. Positions that are especially productive should be emphasized and drained longer. The patient should be instructed to do the postural drainage even if the treatment seems unproductive. Secretions may be mobilized during treatment and it can take several minutes for the remaining cilia to sweep the mucus far enough up the tracheobronchial tree to be expectorated or swallowed.

Pulmonary function tests of patients with localized bronchiectasis show few or no abnormalities. However, in more widespread disease, there is a reduction in the FEV_1, maximum midexpiratory flow rate, maximal voluntary ventilation (MVV), diffusing capacity, and an increase in the residual volume (Luce, 1994).

Hospitalized patients with bronchiectasis may be treated with postural drainage, percussion, vibration, and/or the forced expiratory technique, intravenous fluids, antibiotics, supplemental oxygen and other medications (Stoller and Wiedemann, 1990; Luce, 1994). Long-term medical management may include a broad-spectrum antibiotic taken orally 10 to 14 days per month, low-flow oxygen for hypoxemia, postural drainage, avoidance of bronchial irritants (e.g., cigarette smoke and air pollution) and other measurers. Some patients may have surgical resection if their area of involvement is quite limited or to control hemoptysis. It is most important that these patients drink large volumes of water each day (2 to

3 L) to keep their secretions thin so they can be expectorated more easily (unless fluid intake is limited for cardiac reasons).

Prognosis of bronchiectasis

Before the antibiotic era, the prognosis for individuals with bronchiectasis was poor. As might be expected, infection was usually the precipitating cause of death. However, at the present time, the prognosis of patients with proper medical management is much improved (Sanderson et al, 1974; Ellis et al, 1981). Most studies show that about 75% of the patients have an improved symptom complex since diagnosis and lead relatively normal lives. Cor pulmonale, a complication of diffuse, long-standing bronchiectasis, accounts for about 50% of the deaths (Konietzki, Carton, and Leroy, 1969). Pneumonia and hemorrhage are less common causes of death. With modern therapy, only a few patients succumb to respiratory infections or their complications. Few children who develop bronchiectasis live beyond their 40s. Repeated bronchopulmonary infections can contribute to worsening pulmonary function and an earlier death. Before the antimicrobial era, most patients with untreated, widespread, severe bronchiectasis died within 25 years. Today prognosis for each individual depends on the extent of the disease process at the time of diagnosis and on proper medical management. Patients with moderate, localized disease, if treated properly, may have a relatively normal life expectancy.

RESTRICTIVE LUNG DISEASE

A restrictive disease is characterized by lungs that are prevented from expanding fully. Normally during inspiration, the diaphragm descends, the dimension of the chest increases laterally and anteriorly, and the lung tissue expands as it fills with air. Hence an abnormality in any of these areas can produce a restrictive pattern. For example, a decrease in compliance or elasticity of the lung parenchyma, such as interstitial fibrosis, sarcoidosis, pneumoconiosis, and scleroderma, can produce this defect. Pleural abnormalities such as pleural effusion (by direct compression) can prevent the lungs from expanding fully. Thoracic changes such as kyphoscoliosis and ankylosing

spondylitis can cause lung restriction. Obesity and ascites, by limiting diaphragmatic movement, can also produce a restrictive defect.

Pulmonary function tests generally show a decreased vital capacity, inspiratory capacity, and total lung capacity, whereas the residual volume can be normal or reduced. If the restriction is pulmonary in origin, there is a reduction in the lung compliance and the diffusing capacity.

Many of these restrictive disorders are discussed in Chapter 5. Since obstructive lung diseases are encountered much more often than restrictive disorders, they have been discussed in greater detail. The following is a brief examination of some of the restrictive lung diseases.

Diffuse Interstitial Pulmonary Fibrosis

This disease is known as diffuse interstitial pulmonary fibrosis (IPF) in the United States and cryptogenic fibrosing alveolitis in Europe (Reynolds, and Matthay, 1990). IPF represents a common histologic response to a wide variety of insults (Weg, 1982). Initially, some type of injury to the pulmonary parenchyma causes an influx of inflammatory and immune cells, resulting in a diffuse inflammatory process distal to the terminal bronchiole (alveolitis). This can progress to subacute interstitial disease with the presence of acute and chronic inflammatory cells. Chronic disease is manifest by thickened alveolar walls and progression to fibrosis.

The etiologic factors of this condition are uncertain. Similar conditions can be produced by certain drugs or poisons and are found in patients with rheumatoid arthritis and systemic sclerosis. There appears to be a genetic factor, since twins, siblings, and other members of the same family have been reported with diffuse interstitial pulmonary fibrosis. This condition has also been reported in a few individuals with Raynaud's phenomenon, ulcerative colitis, and other diseases, but their exact relationship remains unclear.

The most common early symptoms are fatigue, dyspnea on exertion, and a chronic unproductive cough. As the disease progresses, the patient becomes steadily more dyspneic and cyanotic. On auscultation, one notes sharply crackling rales. Chest expansion is reduced and clubbing of the digits is often present.

The chest x-ray usually indicates diffuse reticular markings, most prominent in the lower lung fields. Sometimes, a gallium citrate Ga 67 isotope scan of the lungs is conducted to assess the overall inflammation of the lung parenchyma (Line et al, 1978; Turner-Warwick and Haslam, 1987).

Pulmonary function tests show a reduced vital capacity and total lung capacity with no impaired flow rates (Keogh and Crystal, 1980; Reynolds and Matthay, 1990). Compliance is markedly reduced to less than half of the predicted value. A reduced diffusing capacity is the earliest and most consistent change. At first, the arterial PaO_2 may be normal at rest but may drop significantly with exercise. The $PaCO_2$ is reduced as a result of hyperventilation, and the pH is kept normal by renal compensation. Later the PaO_2 is markedly reduced because of the thickened alveolar membrane and ventilation-perfusion mismatching.

Bronchoalveolar lavage (BAL) is often used to assess the amount of inflammation and the accumulation of immune effector cells and proteins in the alveoli (Crystal, et al, 1981; Rudd, Halslam, and Turner-Warwick, 1981). The technique consists of wedging a fiberoptic bronchoscope in a sublobar airway, then infusing 20 to 50 ml aliquots of saline into the peripheral airway, which are immediately aspirated by syringe. A total of 150 to 300 ml is instilled and recovered. The fluid and cells are analyzed (Reynolds, 1987). High-intensity alveolitis is defined by 10% or more polymorphonuclear granulocytes (PMNs) in BAL cell differential counts; low-intensity alveolitis consists of 10% PMNs or less (Reynolds, 1986).

Lung biopsies that demonstrate an abundance of inflammatory cells suggest early disease, whereas a prevalence of fibrosis is indicative of advanced disease. A distinct category of IPF has been described and may be clinically useful (Liebow, Steer, and Billingsley, 1965). Desquamative interstitial pneumonitis (DIP) is characterized by an intraalveolar accumulation of mononuclear cells, relatively intact alveolar walls without destruction or fibrinous exudates (numerous inflammatory cells with little or no fibrosis). This pattern has correlated with a more benign course and a better response to corticosteroids.

Since a pattern of DIP is commonly seen along with usual interstitial fibrosis (UIP) or IPF, some believe that DIP likely represents an earlier and more reversible stage of IPF.

Corticosteroids are the mainstay of treatment for IPF (Reynolds and Matthay, 1990). A trial of immunosuppressive therapy is almost always prescribed for a period of time. Objective measures such as blood counts, erythrocyte sedimentation rate, pulmonary function testing, particularly exercise tests with measurement of arterial oxygen desaturation and diffusing capacity BAL fluid analysis and the patient's symptoms must demonstrate improvement or the medication should be discontinued. A composite clinical roentgenographic, physiological score (CRP score) of eight variables has been developed that allows quantification of the clinical course and the response to therapy in individual patients (Watters et al, 1986). If effective, medications are usually continued for a year and then a decision is made about continuing or tapering the dosage.

Individuals who are not responsive to corticosteroids may be placed on other immunosuppressive drugs such as cyclophosphamide, azathioprine, or penicillamine (Turner-Warwick, 1987; Reynolds and Matthay, 1990). Penicillamine is more effective in patients with connective tissue diseases and interstitial fibrosis other than those with IPF.

Patients should stop smoking at once. Supplemental oxygen is important with exercise as there is a characteristic significant fall in arterial oxygen tension (PaO_2) (Hammon and McCaffree, 1985; Reynolds and Matthay, 1990). Individuals that require more than 4 L flow/min by nasal prongs may prefer direct administration of oxygen into the trachea. In addition to supplying higher concentrations of oxygen to the lungs, many patients prefer the cosmetic effective of not wearing obvious nasal prongs.

Patients that have refractory disease limited to the lungs may be candidates for single or double lung transplantation. There have been significant advances in the success of lung transplantation in recent years (Toronto Lung Transplant Group, 1988) (see Chapter 38).

Individuals with the subacute form described by Hamman and Rich usually die within 6 months (Hamman, 1944). Patients with the chronic form, treated with steroids, may survive for as long as 15 years. Untreated, these patients most often die within 1 to 4 years. Cause of death is usually related to respiratory or heart failure, although an unexpected number have died from adenocarcinoma and undifferentiated or alveolar cell carcinoma of the lung.

Pulmonary Infiltrates With Eosinophilia

Eosinophils are commonly present in lung tissue as part of the body's cellular response to a variety of agents and systemic immunologic diseases (Butterworth and David, 1981). They are present in the airways and lung tissue of patients with idiopathic pulmonary fibrosis. In interstitial lung disease that appears to have an allergic component (e.g., hypersensitivity pneumonitis, drug-induced lung syndromes, sarcoidosis) eosinophils are a minor component of tissue reaction. However, in certain primary or systemic diseases, eosinophils can be the most conspicuous inflammatory cell present in the lung. These conditions can be grouped together and referred to as eosinophilic syndromes (Crofton et al, 1952). Considerable overlapping exists among these syndromes as their etiologic factors and pathogenesis remains poorly understood (Reynolds and Matthay, 1990).

Simple pulmonary eosinophilia

This is a self-limiting disease with chest x-ray demonstrating migratory, fleeting areas of pulmonary infiltrates located in the periphery of the lungs along with minimal respiratory symptoms and blood eosinophilia (Crofton et al, 1952). Certain drugs such as sulfonamides have been implicated as a cause (Reynolds and Matthay, 1990). This disease is also referred to as Loeffler's pneumonia and the PIE syndrome (peripheral infiltrates with blood eosinophilia) (Crofton et al, 1952). If the disease is related to an allergic response to microfilaria, human parasites (e.g., *Ascaris lumbriocoides, Strongyloides stercoralis*), or cat and dog parasites (ascarids) that produce visceral larva migrans, it is termed tropical eosinophilia.

Prolonged pulmonary eosinophilia

As implied by the name, this disease is more chronic than the simple form, with a more severe symptom complex. Over time, it can eventually result in a form of interstitial pulmonary fibrosis with honeycombed lung changes on chest x-ray and a restrictive pattern on pulmonary function tests.

This disease is more common in women (Sederlinic, Sicilian, and Gaensler, 1988). Their symptoms include an acute respiratory illness with fever, night sweats, weight loss, and dyspnea. It can be confused with tuberculosis, but these patients deteriorate when treated with antituberculosis drugs. This disease must also be differentiated from eosinophilic granuloma and the desquamative form of idiopathic interstitial pneumonitis. Dense infiltrates located in the periphery of the lung on chest x-ray provide an important clue. Often, a lung biopsy is necessary to confirm the diagnosis. Treatment with corticosteroids produces a striking improvement in the patient's symptoms and chest x-ray in just a few weeks.

Eosinophilic granuloma

Eosinophilic granuloma (or histiocytosis X) can either be a unifocal disease effecting only the lungs or a multifocal disease involving the bones of the skull, mandible, vertebra, pelvis, ribs, and extremities (Groopman and Golde, 1981; Marcy and Reynolds, 1985). Lung involvement is characterized by an interstitial granuloma composed of moderately large, pale histiocytes and eosinophils, and arteriolitis with eosinophils. The histiocytic process with eosinophils then involves bronchioles, alveolar ducts, and alveolar septa, which results in their destruction. The proliferative endarteritis causes necrosis.

This disease most commonly effects men in their 30s or 40s. They usually have symptoms of fatigue, malaise, weight loss, a nonproductive cough, dyspnea on exertion, and chest pain, sometimes related to a pneumothorax or rib lesions. The chest radiograph often indicates a diffuse micronodular and interstitial infiltrate initially involving the middle and lower lung fields. In more advanced disease, small cystic areas develop in the infiltrate, producing a honeycomb pattern. Spontaneous pneumothorax is a complication in approximately 25% of cases.

The course of the disease varies (Reynolds and Matthay, 1990). Spontaneous regression with residual symptoms may occur in 10% to 25% of cases. In many patients, the disease stabilizes or "burns out," leaving them with a moderate pulmonary impairment as a result of fibrosis, cystic lung changes and a restrictive defect on pulmonary function tests. Dyspnea on exertion is common. Some patients have persistent bronchitis. Cortiocosteroids are not particularly effective. Treatment is mainly symptomatic, with judicious use of antibiotics and bronchodilators. Occasionally, progressive pulmonary disease leads to cor pulmonale and respiratory failure.

Pulmonary Alveolar Proteinosis

Pulmonary alveolar proteinosis is a rare disease of unknown origin, characterized by alveoli filled with lipid-rich "proteinaceous" material and no abnormality of the alveolar wall, interstitial spaces, conducting airways or pleural surfaces. Most often it is found in men between the ages of 30 and 50, although it has been reported in patients of all ages and both sexes.

The most common symptoms are progressive dyspnea and weight loss, with cough, hemoptysis and chest pain reported less frequently (Claypool, Rogers, and Matuschak, 1984). Chest x-ray reveals diffuse bilateral (commonly perihilar) opacities (Figure 4-10). Physical findings may include fine inspiratory rales, dullness to percussion and, in the later stages, cyanosis and clubbing. Pulmonary function studies usually show a decreased vital capacity, functional residual capacity and diffusing capacity. Arterial blood gases indicate a low Pa_{O_2}, especially during exercise, with normal Pa_{CO_2}, and pH (Rogers et al, 1978).

The treatment of choice for patients with moderate to severe dyspnea on exertion from alveolar proteinosis is bronchial alveolar lavage (Rogers and Tatum, 1970; Rogers, Graunstein, and Shuman 1972). The patient is taken to the operating room where, after general anesthesia and placement of a double-lumen tube (which isolates each lung), the patient is turned in the lateral decubitus position with the lung to be lavaged downward. The double-lumen tube enables the patient to be ventilated by the uppermost lung while the lower lung is carefully filled with saline to the functional residual capacity. Then an additional 300 to 500 ml saline are alternately allowed

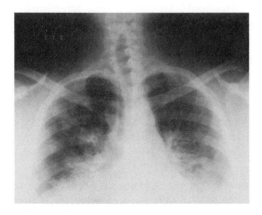

FIGURE 4-10
Pulmonary alveolar proteinosis. PA chest film demonstrates an irregular, patchy, poorly defined confluence of acinar shadows which are symmetrical in both lower lung fields. The appearance is very similar to pulmonary edema. (Courtesy of T. H. Johnson, M.D.)

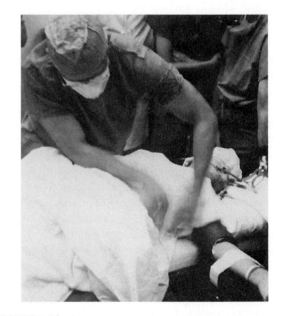

FIGURE 4-11
A patient with pulmonary alveolar proteinosis in the operating room undergoing bronchial alveolar lavage of her left lung. Percussion is done over the left lung as the saline runs out, increasing the amount of proteinaceous material removed during this procedure.

to run into and out of the lung by gravitational flow. As the saline flows out, percussion is done over the lung being lavaged, and this greatly increases the amount of proteinaceous material washed from the lung (Figure 4-11). The effectiveness of mechanical percussion, manual vibration, and manual percussion in removing the material from involved lungs has been compared and manual percussion has been found to be superior (Hammon, 1983; Hammon, Freeman, and McCaffree, 1986; Hammon, McCaffree, and Cucchiara, 1993). In this procedure, a patient is usually lavaged with 20 to 30 L saline and is then taken to the recovery room and later back to his or her own room. After 2 or 3 days, the procedure is repeated on the opposite lung.

Most patients have significant clinical improvement following bronchial alveolar lavage, and many have an improvement in their chest x-rays (Claypool, Rogers, and Matuschak, 1984). After lavage, for reasons that are unclear, the material may reaccumulate slowly or not at all. Some patients do have spontaneous remissions without undergoing lavage.

Before bronchial alveolar lavage was done on these patients, almost all children with alveolar proteinosis died, and 20% to 25% of the adults died within 5 years, usually because of respiratory failure or cor pulmonale. Some 60% to 70% improved greatly or recovered. The effect that bronchial alveolar lavage has on the long-term outcome remains to be seen, but present results are encouraging (Claypool, Rogers, and Matuschak, 1984).

Idiopathic Pulmonary Hemosiderosis

Idiopathic pulmonary hemosiderosis (IPH) is a disease of unknown origin and is characterized by repeated episodes of pulmonary hemorrhage, iron-deficiency anemia, and in long-term patients, pulmonary insufficiency (Soergel and Sommers, 1962). IPH is most commonly found in children under the age of 10. In children, it is found with equal frequency in both genders, but in adults, it is twice as common in men as it is women.

This disease has an insidious onset. The patient has symptoms of weakness, anemia, pallor, lethargy, and occasionally, a nonproductive cough (Reynolds

and Matthay, 1990). If the patient is assessed during an acute episode of pulmonary hemorrhage, fine rales and dullness to percussion are present on physical examination. An enlarged liver, spleen, and lymph nodes may be noted on palpation in 20% to 25% of cases. The chest x-ray during acute episodes show acinar consolidation for 2 to 3 days, then a reticular pattern identical to other interstitial diseases. The chest x-ray usually returns to normal in 10 to 12 days. However, after recurrent episodes with hemosiderin deposited in the interstitial spaces, there is progressive interstitial fibrosis. Pulmonary function tests indicate a decreased diffusing capacity, with or without a fall in the patient's resting Pao_2.

The hemorrhage is ordinarily confined to the peripheral airspaces. Interestingly, massive blood loss into lung tissue can occur without hemoptysis or noticeable blood in the trachea or major bronchi (Reynolds and Matthay, 1990). Sputum samples of BAL fluid may contain hemosiderin-laden macrophages. After recurrent episodes of hemoptysis, interstitial fibrosis is present in most cases.

The prognosis of IPH is variable with death occurring somewhere between 2½ to 20 years after the onset of symptoms. Permanent remissions may occur with or without corticosteroid administration. No treatment has been shown to effectively alter the outcome of this disease.

Sarcoidosis

Sarcoidosis is a granulomatous disorder of unknown origin that can effect multiple body systems (Mitchell and Scadding, 1974). Typically, initial findings can include bilateral hilar adenopathy, pulmonary infiltration and skin or eye lesions (Sharma, 1977). The lungs are the organs most often involved and some 20% to 50% of these patients first seek medical attention because of respiratory symptoms. It affects blacks 10 to 20 times more often than whites and women twice as often as men. It usually occurs in the third or fourth decade of life.

The intrathoracic changes can be classified into four stages (Siltzbach et al, 1974; Weg, 1982). In the first stage, the patient is asymptomatic, with the chest x-ray showing bilateral hilar adenopathy and right

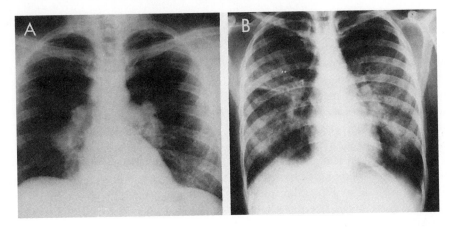

FIGURE 4-12

A, Sarcoidosis in its first stage is manifested by bilateral hilar adenopathy. Usually there are no significant physical symptoms. **B,** Disseminated sarcoidosis (third stage) reveals widespread parenchymal changes with scarring. The hilar adenopathy is usually decreased. (Courtesy of T. H. Johnson, M.D.)

paratracheal adenopathy (Figure 4-12, *A*). In the second stage a diffuse pulmonary infiltration is found along with the bilateral hilar adenopathy. Interstitial infiltration or fibrosis, without hilar adenopathy, characterizes the third stage (Figure 4-12, *B*). In the fourth stage, emphysematous changes, cysts, and bullae are found.

In 60% to 90% of these patients with hilar adenopathy, the disease spontaneously regresses over a period of 1 to 2 years. About one third of the patients with sarcoidosis involving the lungs also have a spontaneous regression, usually leaving some residual fibrosis. The remaining two thirds that have chronic sarcoidosis have progressive pulmonary impairment, along with a variable degree of involvement of the heart, liver, spleen, lymph nodes, muscles, bones, and central nervous system (CNS).

Most patients with sarcoidosis need no treatment. Corticosteroids, although controversial, are the most effective forms of therapy for patients with sarcoidosis that requires treatment (DeRemee, 1977; Turner-Warwick et al, 1986).

Rheumatoid Arthritis

Rheumatoid arthritis (RA) is a systemic disease that principally involves the joints but also often affects

the lungs and pleurae. The most common thoracic complication of RA is pleurisy, with or without pleural effusions. Although RA occurs twice as often in women, pleuritis has a striking predilection for men (Reynolds and Matthay, 1990). Pleural disease is one manifestation of RA, occasionally causing fibrothorax and restrictive lung disease that requires decortication.

Interstitial lung disease, indicated by abnormal pulmonary function tests demonstrating a restrictive ventilatory impairment and a reduced ventilatory capacity, is evident in about 40% of RA patients (Frank et al, 1973). It is also more prevalent in men. The chest x-ray demonstrates diffuse interstitial infiltrates, especially in the lung bases. Pulmonary nodules, which are pathologically identical to the subcutaneous nodules found in RA, may also occur and cavitate (Weg, 1982).

Coal miners with RA may have chest x-rays demonstrating rounded densities that evolve rapidly and undergo cavitation (Caplan's syndrome) in contrast to the massive fibrosis found in coal miners' pneumoconiosis (Caplan, 1953).

Systemic Lupus Erythematosus (SLE)

Although systemic lupus erythematosus (SLE) is a systemic collagen vascular disease, some 50% to

90% of these patients have pleural or pulmonary involvement (Hunninghake and Fauci, 1979). Pleuritic chest pain often signals polyserositis associated with SLE. Pleural effusions are a manifestation of polyserositis and are present in 40% to 60% of individuals with SLE. Most often they are bilateral.

Patients with pulmonary involvement present with dyspnea on exertion and cough productive of mucoid sputum (Weg, 1982). Rarely do SLE patients complain of supine dyspnea, which suggests diaphragmatic paralysis or a diffuse myopathy of the diaphragm (Gibson, Edmonds, and Hughes, 1977).

The chest x-ray usually indicates patchy, nonspecific densities and/or basilar linear or platelike atelectasis. Pleural effusions and pulmonary infiltrates are common, whereas diffuse interstitial fibrosis is rarely seen (Hunninghake and Fauci, 1979).

Pulmonary function tests often indicate a restrictive pattern with a decreased diffusing capacity and a reduced arterial oxygen saturation.

Progressive Systemic Sclerosis (Scleroderma)

Progressive systemic sclerosis (scleroderma) is a rare disease that causes thickening and fibrosis of the connective tissue of multiple parts of the body with replacement of many elements of the connective tissue by colloidal collagen. The skin is most often involved, although the lungs, heart, kidney, bones, and other parts of the body can also be affected.

Approximately one half to two thirds of the patients with progressive systemic sclerosis have pulmonary involvement (Reynolds and Matthay, 1990).

Many of these patients with pulmonary involvement are asymptomatic, although symptoms can include weight loss, progressive dyspnea, low-grade fever, and cough (sometimes producing mucoid sputum). Chest x-ray shows a characteristic fibrosis of the mid and lower lung fields. Auscultation often reveals bibasilar rales. Pulmonary function tests reveal a restrictive defect with impaired diffusion.

D-penicillamine is the best treatment for pulmonary involvement in patients with progressive systemic sclerosis (DeClerk et al, 1987).

Prognosis of patients with only skin and joint involvement is much better than for those that have involvement of the heart, lungs and kidneys. In the latter group, progression results in death after several years. Women seem to have a poorer prognosis than men.

CORONARY ARTERY DISEASE

Atherosclerosis

Pathophysiology

To discuss CAD the process of atherosclerosis must first be described. Although the specific pathogenesis of atherosclerosis is not known, it is hypothesized that the process is initiated by trauma to the intima of the arterial wall. The trauma may be related to various primary risk factors such as: high blood pressure and cigarette smoking.

High blood pressure has been indicated as a potential trauma inducer, since increased pressure and turbulence may damage the endothelial cells of the intima, thus exposing the media to the circulation. The media, which is composed primarily of smooth muscle is thought to be the origin of the atherosclerotic lesion.

Cigarette smoking has also been indicated as a potential trauma inducer. However, the hypothesized mode of injury is different than that observed with increased blood pressure. Cigarette smoke is high in carbon monoxide and hydrocarbons that are carried by the red blood cells and the plasma. It is thought that the hydrocarbons or carbon monoxide bind to the endothelial cells, causing damage and possibly death to these cells.

Once the media is sufficiently exposed to the circulation the process of atherosclerosis is initiated. Platelets aggregate at the injury site and release substances that induce endothelial and smooth muscle cell replication. It is at this site that fatty streaks and fibrous plaques are developed. The cause of fatty streak development is that low-density lipoproteins (LDLs) deposit fat into the smooth muscle of the media. Why this occurs is unknown, but apparently is related to the smooth muscle cell proliferation and perhaps increased need for energy. The initial fatty streaks are generally only slightly raised and do not imperil circulation. However, when a fibrous plaque develops, the characteristic impingement of the vessel lumen occurs. The plaque is somewhat hard and consists of connective "scar-like" tissue, smooth muscle and fat. Finally, the plaque may undergo calcification or lead to hemorrhaging if the vessel wall necroses. The result is decreased blood flow (ischemia) and oxygenation (hypoxia), or complete lack of blood flow and oxygen (anoxia) to the target organ.

Risk factors

As described above high blood pressure, cigarette smoking and hyperlipidemia are direct or primary risk factors for causing atherosclerosis. Secondary risk factors are age, gender, race, obesity, stress, and activity level. Several risk factors are modifiable and include: (1) hypertension, (2) hyperlipidemia, (3) smoking, (4) obesity, (5) stress level, and activity level. It is interesting to note that the "big three" primary risk factors are all modifiable by the individual. Reducing risk factors can reduce the probability of CAD by five- to ten-fold (Ornish et al, 1990).

CLINICAL SYNDROMES ASSOCIATED WITH CAD

Angina Pectoris

Angina pectoris is defined as chest pain that is related to ischemia of the myocardium. However, the pain referred from ischemia may be in the left shoulder, jaw, or between the shoulder blades. Angina can be classified as stable, unstable, or variant.

Stable angina

Stable angina generally occurs during physical effort but may be related to stress. The individual is able to describe what type and intensity of activity causes the angina. Stable angina is characterized by substernal, usually nonradiating pain that lasts between 5 to 15 minutes after the offending incident. Care would involve sublingual nitrates and cessation of the activity causing the angina. Usually the angina subsides completely with treatment. However, angina brought about by emotional stress is more difficult to treat, since the stress cannot be stopped as easily as cessation of exercise.

Unstable angina

Unstable angina also occurs during physical exertion or psychological stress. The major difference between stable and unstable angina is the frequency, duration and intensity of the pain. In unstable angina, the episodes are more frequent and the duration of each event is usually greater than 15 minutes. In addition the intensity of the pain may be more severe. Unstable angina is usually an indicator of CAD progression. Individuals with unstable angina are at greater risk to have a myocardial infarction (MI). Unstable angina is less responsive to treatment using rest and sublingual nitrates. Often times, the individual must be hospitalized and treated with IV nitrates.

Variant angina

Variant angina occurs while the individual is at rest, usually during waking and often at the same time period. Exertion does not influence variant angina. However, the angina may benefit from rest and sublingual nitrates. Like unstable angina the pain is intense and of longer duration and likely to lead to an MI. In addition, arrhythmias are more likely to occur with an individual who has variant angina, as compared with exertion related angina (i.e., stable and unstable). Stable and unstable angina are believed to be caused primarily by progressive arterial occlusion and ischemia. It is believed that variant angina is caused by a combination of occlusion and coronary artery spasm. Therefore variant angina has been successfully treated with calcium channel blockers.

Prognosis of angina

Individuals do not die from angina. The progression of atherosclerosis of coronary arteries is a change from the clinical signs of angina to MI, which is discussed on p. 91. However, even though there is no risk for mortality from angina, an individual's lifestyle can change drastically. People with angina may be fearful of being active and may deny that they are having exertion-related chest pain. Denial of CAD, depression and anger are common manifestation for individuals with angina, though it has rarely been studied (Beckham et al, 1994). The result of angina (diagnosed or undiagnosed and denied) can be depression and potentially further decline in physical activity. Although rest is an important aspect of treatment, it is well-documented that even low levels of activity can modify several risk factors and arrest the progression of the disease process (Niebauer et al, 1995). Research is still underway to determine if

CAD is reversible when lifestyle adjustments are initiated (Ornish et al, 1990; Schuler et al, 1992).

Myocardial Infarction

MI is defined as necrosis of a portion of the myocardium. The death of the myocardium occurs as a result of ischemia and anoxia. The vessels affected are the right and left coronary arteries. The right coronary artery supplies portions of the inferior section of the left ventricle and the posterior section. The left coronary artery branches and forms the circumflex and anterior descending arteries. The circumflex supplies the lateral portion of the left ventricle, while the anterior descending artery supplies the anterior portion. In addition, the right coronary artery supplies the right atrium atrial-ventricular (AV) bundle and the right ventricle. The left coronary artery supplies the left atrium and the primary portion of the conduction pathway. Generally, the clinical symptoms are similar to that of angina, with emphasis on extreme pressure as well as tightness over the sternum region. In addition, pain can radiate to the jaw, upper back, and shoulders (with left more frequent than right).

MIs can be classified into categories by size, location, and degree of myocardial wall involvement. The terms small and large are often used to describe MIs. However, degrees of complication are also used in conjunction with size. MIs can be described as uncomplicated and complicated based on size of the MI and recovery of the patient. Location indicates the portion of the heart involved and also what coronary artery or branch that is at fault. As described above, the general regions of the heart are anterior, posterior, lateral, and inferior. Finally, MIs are classified by the extent of the wall damage. A transmural infarct (or full wall) extends from the endocardium to the epicardium. There is the potential that only a small portion of the ventricle wall is affected, such as just below the epicardium (subepicardial) and just below the endocardium (subendocardial).

Uncomplicated myocardial infarction

An uncomplicated MI is described as a small infarction with no complications during recovery. Usually the result is full recovery without a significant de-

crease in cardiac performance at rest and during minimal to moderate activity (Cahalin, 1994). However the location and the extent of the MI is also critical. MIs located in the inferior portion of the heart are the least significant, and partial wall thickness is less significant than a transmural MI.

Treatment. The treatment for an uncomplicated MI is initially like the complicated MI, where the patient is cared for in the coronary care unit. The medical treatment is designed to decrease myocardial work and oxygen demand. Therefore patients are on oxygen and administered vasodilators (nitroglycerin) to increase myocardial blood flow and analgesics to help further reduce ischemic pain. In addition, to reduce contractility of the myocardium, calcium channel blockers or beta-blockers are administered. Finally, antiarrhythmia medication may be prescribed if an aberrant cardiac rhythm is present or is highly probable to occur.

Since the course is uncomplicated, this means that a patient's stay in the coronary care unit may be only 2 to 3 days, with a total hospital stay of 7 to 10 days. Treatment following ICU discharge is oriented toward increasing physical activity and in educating the patient and family in risk factor reduction. This process is described as cardiac rehabilitation Phase I.

Complicated myocardial infarction

A complicated MI is different from an uncomplicated case since the patient may have one, a combination, or all four of the following conditions/complications: (1) arrhythmia, (2) heart failure, (3) thrombosis, and (4) damage to heart structures.

Arrhythmias. Arrhythmias occur in 95% of all patients with MIs. The type and severity of the arrhythmia is dependent on the extent of myocardial damage and the location of the damage. As described earlier, the uncomplicated MI patient usually has a small area of the myocardium involved; thus the potential arrhythmias are less dangerous and occurrence is less common. Arrythmias that are life-threatening include (1) complete AV heart block, (2) ventricular paced arrhythmia, and (3) ventricular tachycardia, including ventricular flutter and fibrillation. In these conditions, either the heart rate is too slow and thus cardiac output is impaired, or the heart rate is too rapid with poor stroke volume and ejection fraction, and again impaired cardiac output. Treatment of the above conditions is immediate and requires drugs and potentially, electrical shock (for flutter/fibrillation). Usually, an artificial pacemaker is implanted once the patient is stabilized.

Heart failure. Another complication following MI is heart failure. Heart failure is a condition where the heart is weakened and is unable to produce a significant cardiac output to meet the bodies need for oxygen, nutrition, and removal of waste products. When the heart experiences ischemia the myocardium contracts with less force, and conduction abnormalities may alter the mechanics of the contraction. If an area of the heart is infarcted, the affected myocardium does not contract, thus affecting overall cardiac output. Another type of heart failure not directly related to ischemia and infarction is congestive heart failure (CHF) (see Congestive Heart Failure, p. 000).

Immediately post-MI, cardiac output is reduced significantly. However, the compensatory response is to increase sympathetic innervation, resulting in increased heart rate and myocardial contractility. The result of this compensation is a cardiac output that may approach normal resting values. However, if the damage has been great, the kidneys compensate by retaining sodium and water in an attempt to improve circulatory volume and venous return. Depending on the amount of myocardial tissue death, the individual may survive with resulting chronic congestive heart failure through persistent fluid retention and hypotension. If greater than 40% of the left ventricle is infarcted, the result is usually cardiogenic shock followed by death of the individual.

Thrombosis. Another complication is increased incidence of thrombosis from deep leg veins and from the damaged heart itself. Thrombosis from deep leg veins occurs from lower limb inactivity and circulatory stasis. This is a complication that can be observed for all surgical patients. Emboli from deep leg vein thrombus usually result in pulmonary complications. If the emboli are large or numerous the result can be pulmonary tissue infarction and potentially death. The incidence of pulmonary emboli has grown less since early ambulation is now the rule rather than the exception. However, a pulmonary emboli must be considered a distinct possibility in all surgical, MI, and gunshot patients.

Heart wall or mural wall thrombosis can lead to an emboli lodging in the brain, intestine, kidney, artery to the extremities, or any location in the systemic arterial circulation. Usually mural thrombosis do not affect the pulmonary system, since even the smallest fragments are caught in capillary beds and do not enter into the venous system.

Structural damage. The last complication is structural damage to critical myocardial tissue that affects heart function. If conductant pathway (bundle branch) tissue located primarily at the septum is damaged, arrhythmias result. In addition, papillary muscles that assist in closing valves can be infarcted. The result of improper valve function is decreased cardiac output. Besides these two critical tissues, if significant full thickness damage occurs to the myocardial wall cardiac function is compromised. Heart wall damage can result in ventricular aneurysms or ventricular wall rupture. Ventricular aneurysm or bulging of the weakened ventricular wall occurs in transmural (full wall thickness) infarcts. Ventricular wall rupture, which can occur acutely following transmural infarction, but more often occurs in the first to second week post-MI following an aneurysm is usually fatal. Therefore following an MI, it is critical to determine if an aneurysm has occurred in the myocardium so that appropriate surgical intervention can be performed.

Treatment. The treatment for a complicated MI is initially like the uncomplicated MI, where the patient is cared for in the coronary care unit. The medical treatment once again is designed to decrease myocardial work and oxygen demand. Patients are on oxygen and administered vasodilators (nitroglycerin) to increase myocardial blood flow and analgesics to help further reduce ischemic pain. Myocardium calcium channel blockers or beta-blockers are administered to reduce contractility. Finally, antiarrhythmia medication are prescribed if an aberrant cardiac rhythm is present.

Individuals with a complicated MI have a much longer stay in the coronary care unit, and their total hospital stay time is greatly increased when compared with the uncomplicated MI patient (Topol, 1988). The time in coronary care and total hospital stay are dependent on the complications that occur following the MI. Individuals with heart failure, thrombolytic events, or structural damage requiring surgery may be in the coronary care unit for more than 2 weeks. Total hospital stay time for complicated MI patients may exceed 2 to 3 weeks (Topol, 1988). However, treatment following ICU discharge is similar to that of the uncomplicated MI patient with the goal of increasing physical activity and in educating the patient and family in risk factor reduction. The major difference in Phase I cardiac rehabilitation for the complicated versus the uncomplicated MI patient is the initial workload intensity, duration, and frequency (i.e., much lower workload for complicated MI patient) (Rowe, 1989). Progression is also usually a bit more conservative, since the probability for a recurrent MI event is much greater in the complicated MI patient (Rowe, 1989).

Prognosis post-myocardial infarction

Prognosis following MI is dependent on many factors. Usually cardiovascular performance is reduced, unless the structural damage to the ventricle is minor (as in the case of many uncomplicated MI patients). The most important factor is extent of ventricular damage. However, with early detection of transmural infarction and improvement in surgical intervention and coronary care, acute post-MI deaths have been reduced (Wenger, 1984). Other critical factors include remaining cardiac capacity and status of CAD. Even though CAD mortality has declined in the United States, the disease remains the top cause of sudden death in adults.

Congestive Heart Failure

CHF is characterized by the inability of the heart to maintain adequate cardiac output. The etiologic factors of heart failure is usually from ischemia and MI secondary to CAD. For the heart to maintain an appropriate amount of blood flow to the pulmonary and systemic circulation, heart rate and stroke volume must be adequate. Usually, stroke volume is the critical factor to maintain adequate cardiac output. Stroke volume is a function of the amount of blood in the left ventricle at the end of diastole (preload); the amount

of pressure and resistance the heart must overcome to eject blood into the systemic circulation (afterload); and myocardial contractility, which is the amount of force the left ventricle can apply to the blood within the chamber. If any of these three variables are negatively affected then cardiac output is reduced. The cause of heart failure is often decreased contractility.

Acute heart failure

If an individual has a significant myocardial infarction, the contractility and pumping ability of the heart is immediately reduced. The initial result is decreased cardiac output and damming of blood in the veins. The result is increased systemic venous pressure. This acute phase, which may reduce cardiac output to 40% of normal resting values is short-lived lasting only a few seconds before the sympathetic nervous system is stimulated, and the parasympathetics become reciprocally inhibited. Sympathetic innervation causes an increase in contractility of viable myocardial tissue, and the increase in cardiac output may be 100%. In addition, sympathetic innervation also increases venous return, since the tone of blood vessels is increased. The result is increased systemic filling pressure, and thus increased preload. The sympathetic reflex following MI becomes maximally operational within 30 seconds; therefore, besides some pain and fainting, an individual with a mild MI may not know they just suffered a heart attack! The sympathetic response can continue with cardiac output maintained at an adequate level for quiet rest. However, the individual may still have persistent ischemic pain that should be assessed as quickly as possible.

Chronic heart failure

Following a MI several physiological responses occur besides sympathetic reflex compensation. The kidney begins to retain fluid almost immediately following an MI. The reasons appear to be related to decreased glomerular pressure secondary to decreased cardiac output. In addition, there is an increase in renin output and therefore an increase in angiotensin production. Angiotensin promotes reabsorption of water and salt from the renal tubules. The effect of moderate fluid retention is an increase in blood volume and an increase in venous return. This once again increases preload and thus cardiac output. However, if the MI was severe, the result can be excess fluid retention. This results in detrimental effects of edema and overstretching of the heart, since blood volume and venous return is too great.

In addition to increased kidney retention of fluid, a second process that is activated immediately following an MI is recovery of the myocardium. New collateral arteries are formed to supply the peripheral portions of the infarcted region. This revascularization can assist cells that were marginally active to become fully functional again. In addition, the unaffected myocardial cells hypertrophy. The result in a mild to moderate MI is a great improvement in cardiac function that takes 6 weeks to several months, depending on extent of injury.

Compensated and decompensated heart failure

The final state following acute and chronic physiological changes is called compensated heart failure. In this state, the heart is able to pump blood effectively, but at a reduced cardiac output compared with the pre-MI condition. The individuals cardiac reserve has been greatly reduced. The cardiac reserve can be defined as the difference between the maximum cardiac output attainable minus the resting cardiac output. When an individual exercises or is active at a heavy load, they experience the same symptoms of acute heart failure, because the heart is unable to supply the cardiac output required of the activity. The symptoms include rapid heart rate, pallor, and diaphoresis. Decompensated failure occurs when the heart is so severely damaged or weakened that normal cardiac output can not be attained. The result is that cardiac output is not high enough to allow for normal renal function. Fluid continues to be accumulated and the heart is stretched more and weakened further so that only moderate-to-low quantities of blood can be pumped. With unilateral left ventricle heart failure the left ventricle fails, while the right ventricle continues to pump vigorously. The result can be increased blood volume and pulmonary capillary pressure in the lungs. If this occurs, fluid begins to filter into the interstitial spaces of the alveoli resulting in pulmonary edema and suffocation. Even if the heart does not have a unilateral dysfunction the result can be deterioration of the myocardium. As the heart weakens, not only is systemic blood flow compromised, but so is the coronary system. The area most affected is the subendocardial region. As these cells become infarcted, the heart weakens further until other regions of the heart also become ischemic and infarcted. The entire process described from the acute to chronic stages is congestive heart failure.

Prognosis

The result without pharmaceutical or surgical intervention (heart transplantation) is death. Pharmaceutical intervention to halt or to delay heart failure is with diuretics to reduce fluid levels and cardiac glycosides such as digitalis to improve myocardial contractility. This pharmacological treatment is combined with modification of salt and fluid intake. Finally, in cases when the heart has not compensated well and the myocardium has sufficiently weakened so that cardiac output is minimal, then heart transplant is the only recourse. Since organ donors are not readily available, the number of individuals who need new hearts far outnumber the donor organs. As described previously, once the heart has had enough tissue damage to greatly reduce the cardiac reserve, the prognosis is poor.

SUMMARY

The first portion of the chapter has described the essential pathophysiological features of obstructive and restrictive lung diseases. Obstructive disorders are characterized by a decreased rate of airflow during expiration (as a result of increased airway resistance). Restrictive disorders are conditions in which the inspiratory capacity of the lungs is restricted to less than the predicted normal.

A knowledge of the pathophysiology of pulmonary dysfunction assists the practitioner in relating the pathophysiology to the clinical signs and symptoms, and the appropriate treatment goals and interventions.

The second portion of this chapter has described the essential pathophysiological features of CAD. CAD results from atherosclerosis. The clinical syndromes associated with CAD are angina, MI, and heart failure.

A knowledge of the pathophysiology of CAD enables the clinical practitioner to relate the etiologic factors and pathophysiology to the clinical signs and symptoms exhibited by this patient population, and prescribes treatment.

REVIEW QUESTIONS

1. What are the two broad categories of lung disease?
2. What is the major characteristic of obstructive lung disease?
3. How does emphysema differ from chronic bronchitis?
4. How does asthma differ from emphysema?
5. What is the major characteristic of restrictive lung disease?
6. How is diffuse interstitial fibrosis diagnosed and managed?

References

American Thoracic Society (statement by the Committee on Diagnostic Standards for Non-Tuberculous Respiratory Diseases) (1962). Definitions and classification of chronic bronchitis, asthma, and pulmonary emphysema. *American Review of Respiratory Diseases 85*, 762.

Anthonisen, N. (1989). Prognosis in chronic obstructive pulmonary disease: results from multicenter clinical trials. *American Review of Respiratory Diseases 140*, 595-599.

Anthonisen, N., Wright, E., & Hodgkin, J., (1986). Prognosis in chronic obstructive pulmonary disease. *American Review of Respiratory Diseases 133*, 14-20.

Barker, A., & Bardana, E. (1988). Bronchiectasis: update of an orphan disease, *American Review of Respiratory Diseases 137*, 969–978.

Barnes, P. (1993). Asthma. In Bone, R. (Ed.). *Pulmonary and critical care medicine.* Vol. 1. St. Louis: Mosby.

Beckham, J.C., et al (1995). Pain coping strategies in patients referred for evaluation of angina pectoris. *Journal of Cardiopulmonary Rehabilitation 15*, 173-180.

Bousky S., et al (1964). Factors affecting prognosis in emphysema, *Diseases of the Chest 45*, 402.

Burrows, B., & Earle, R. (1969). Predictability of survival in patients with chronic airway obstruction. *American Review of Respiratory Diseases 99*, 865.

Butterworth, A., & David, J., (1981). Eosinophil function. New England Journal of Medicine *304*, 154-156.

Cahalin, L.P., (1994). Exercise tolerance and training for healthy persons and patients with cardiovascular disease. In Hasson, S. (Ed.). *Clinical exercise physiology.* St. Louis: Mosby.

Caplan, A. (1953). Certain unusual radiological appearances in chest of coal miners suffering from rheumatoid arthritis. *Thorax 8*, 29-37.

Claypool, W., Rogers, R., & Matuschak, G. (1984). Update on the clinical diagnosis, management and pathogenesis of pulmonary alveolar proteinosis (Phospholipidosis). *Chest 85*, 550-558.

Cosio, M. (1978). The relations between structural changes in small airways and pulmonary function tests. *New England Journal of Medicine 298:*1277-1281.

Crofton, J., et al (1952). Pulmonary eosinophilia. *Thorax 7*, 1-35.

Crystal, R., et al (1981). Interstitial lung disease: current concepts of pathogenesis, staging and therapy. *American Journal of Medicine 70*, 542-558.

Currie, D., et al (1987). Impaired tracheobronchial clearance in bronchiectasis. *Thorax 42*, 126-130.

DeClerk, C., et al (1987). D-penicillamine therapy and interstitial lung disease in scleroderma. A long-term follow-up study. *Arthritis Rheumatism 30:* 643-650.

DeRemee, R. (1977). The present status of treatment of sarcoidosis: a house divided. *Chest 71*, 388-393.

Dornhorst, A. (1955). Respiratory insufficiency. *Lancet 1*, 1185-1187.

Dunnill, M. (1960). The pathology of asthma, with special reference to changes in the bronchial mucosa. *Journal of Clinical Pathology 13*, 27-33.

Ellis, D., et al (1981). Present outlook in bronchiectasis: clinical and social study and review of factors influencing prognosis. *Thorax 36*, 659-664.

Eriksson, S. (1965). Studies in alpha$_1$-antitrypsin deficiency. *ACTA Medica Scandinavica 177*, 1-85.

Fielding, J., (1985). Smoking: health effect and control. *New England Journal of Medicine 313*, 491-498.

Filley, G., et al (1968). Chronic obstructive bronchopulmonary disease II. Oxygen transport in two clinical types. *American Journal of Medicine 44*, 26-38.

Fisher, M., Bowery, C., & Ladd-Hudson, K. (1989). External chest compression in acute asthma: a preliminary study. *Critical Care Medicine 17*, 686-687.

Fishman, A. (1988). The spectrum of chronic obstructive disease of the airway. In Fishman, A. (Ed.). Pulmonary Diseases and Disorders (2nd ed.). New York: McGraw-Hill.

Frank, S., et al (1973). Pulmonary dysfunction in rheumatoid disease. *Chest 63*, 27-34.

Gallon, A. (1991). Evaluation of chest percussion in the treatment of patients with copious sputum production. *Respiratory Medicine 85*, 45-51.

Gandevia, B. (1973). Pressurized sympathomimetic aerosol and their lack of relationship to asthma mortality in Australia. *Medical Journal of Australia 1*, 273.

Gibson, G., Edmonds, J., & Hughes, G. (1977). Diaphragm function and lung involvement in systemic lupus erythematosus. *American Journal of Medicine 63:*926-930.

Gold, W. (1976). Asthma. *Basic Respiratory Diseases 4:*1-4.

Groopman, J., & Golde, D. (1981). The histiocytic disorders: a pathophysiologic analysis. *Annals of Internal Medicine 94*, 95-107.

Hamman, L. Rich AR. (1994). Acute diffuse interstitial fibrosis of the lungs. *Bull Johns Hopkins Hospital 74*, 177.

Hammon, W. (1983). Chest physical therapy in the operating room: A six year experience. *Physical Therapy 63*, 786.

Hammon, W., Freeman, P., & McCaffree, D. (1986). Manual percussion versus manual vibration for alveolar clearance. Physical Therapy *66*, 754

Hammon, W., & McCaffree, D. (1985). Improving exercise tolerance in diffuse interstitial lung disease. *Cardiopulmonary Quarterly, Winter V* (4), 6-7.

Hammon, W., McCaffree, D., & Cucchiara, A. (1993). A comparison of manual to mechanical chest percussion for clearance of alveolar material in patients with pulmonary alveolar proteinosis (Phospholipidosis). *Chest 103*, 1409-1412.

Hodgkin JE, et al (1975). Chronic obstructive airway diseases—current concepts in diagnosis and comprehensive care. *Journal of the American Medical Association 232*, 1243.

Huber, H., & Koessler, K. (1922). The pathology of bronchial asthma. *Archives of Internal Medicine 30*, 689-760.

Hunninghake, G., & Fauci, A. (1979). Pulmonary involvement in the collagen vascular diseases (state of the art). *American Review of Respiratory Diseases 119*, 471-480.

Kanner, R., et al (1983). Predictions of survival in subjects with chronic airflow limitations. *American Journal of Medicine 74*, 249-255.

Kanner, R., & Renzetti, A. (1984). Predictions of spirometric changes and mortality in the obstructive airway disorders. *Chest 85*, 155-175.

Kao, D., et al (1975). Advances in the treatment of pulmonary alveolar proteinosis. *American Review of Respiratory Diseases 111*, 361-363.

Keogh, B., & Crystal, R. (1980). Pulmonary function testing in interstitial pulmonary disease. *Chest 78*, 856-865.

Konietzki, N., Carton, R., & Leroy, E. (1969). Causes of death in patients with bronchiectasis. *American Review of Respiratory Diseases 100*, 852.

Liebow, A., Hales, M., & Lindskog, G. (1949). Enlargement of the bronchial arteries and their anastomoses with the pulmonary arteries in bronchiectasis. *American Journal of Pathology 25*, 211-231.

Liebow, A., Steer, A., & Billingsley, J. (1965). Desquamative interstitial pneumonia. *American Journal of Medicine 39*, 369-404.

Line, B., et al (1978). Gallium-67 citrate scanning in the staging of idiopathic pulmonary fibrosis: correlation with physiologic and morphologic features and bronchoalveolar lavage. *American Review of Respiratory Diseases 118*, 355-365.

Luce, J. (1994). Bronchiectasis. In Murray, J., Nadel, J. (Eds.). *Textbook of respiratory medicine* (2nd ed.). (pp 1398-1417). Philadelphia: WB Saunders.

Marcy, T., & Reynolds, H. (1985). Pulmonary histiocytosis. *Lung 163*, 129-150.

McFadden, E. (1988). Asthma: acute and chronic therapy. In Fishman, A. (Ed.). *Pulmonary diseases and disorders* (2nd ed.) New York: McGraw-Hill.

McFadden, E., & Gilbert, I. (1992). Asthma. *New England Journal of Medicine 327* (27), 1928-1937.

McFadden, E., & Lyons, H. (1968). Arterial blood gas tensions in asthma. New England Journal of Medicine *278*, 1027-1032.

Mitchell, R., et al (1968). Clinical and morphologic correlations in chronic airway obstruction. *American Review of Respiratory Diseases 97*, 54-61.

Mitchell, D., Scadding, J. (1974). Sarcoidosis (state of the art). *American Review of Respiratory Diseases 110*, 774-802.

Mitchell, R., Webb, W., & Filley, G. (1964). Chronic obstructive bronchopulmonary disease. III. Factors influencing prognosis. *American Review of Respiratory Diseases 89*, 878.

Muller, R., Petty, T., & Filley, G. (1970). Ventilation and arterial blood gas changes induced by pursed-lip breathing. *Journal of Applied Physiology 28*, 784.

Nash, E., Briscoe, W., & Cournand, A. (1965). The relationship between clinical and physiological findings in chronic obstructive disease of the lungs. *Medicina Thoracalis 22*, 305-327.

National Asthma Education Program (1991). Expert Panel Report. Guidelines for the diagnosis and management of asthma. DHHS Pub. No. 91-3042. Bethesda, MD: Department of Health and Human Services.

Niebauer, J., et al. (1995). Five years of physical exercise and low fat diet: Effects on progression of coronary artery disease. *Journal of Cardiopulmonary Rehabilitation 15*, 47-64, 1995.

Ogilvie, A.G. (1962). Asthma: A study on prognosis of 1,000 patients. *Thorax 17*, 183.

Ornish D., et al. (1990). Can lifestyle changes reverse coronary heart disease? Lancet 336: 129-133.

Oxman, A., et al (1993). Occupational dust exposure and chronic obstructive pulmonary disease: a systematic overview of the evidence. *American Review of Respiratory Diseases 148*(1), 38-41.

Petty, T., & Guthrie, A. (1974). The effects of augmented breathing maneuvers on ventilation in severe chronic airway obstruction. *Respiratory Care 16*, 104.

Reid, L. (1967). *The pathology of emphysema.* Chicago: Year-Book Medical Publishers.

Reid, L. (1976). Anatomy of the lung and patterns of structural change in disease. *Physiotherapy 62*, 44.

Reid, L. (1960). Measurement of bronchial mucus gland layer. A diagnostic yardstick in chronic bronchitis. *Thorax 15*, 132-141.

Reid, L. (1950). Reduction in bronchial subdivision in bronchiectasis. *Thorax 5*, 233-247.

Renzetti, A. (1967). Prognosis in chronic obstructive pulmonary disease. *Medical Clinics of North America, 51*, 363.

Reynolds, H. (1987). Bronchoalveolar lavage. *American Review of Respiratory Diseases 135*, 250-263.

Reynolds, H. (1986). Idiopathic interstitial pulmonary fibrosis: contribution of bronchoalveolar lavage analysis. *Chest 89*, 139-144.

Reynolds, H., & Matthay, R. (1990). Diffuse interstitial and alveolar inflammatory disease. In George, R. et al. (Eds). *Chest medicine: Essentials of pulmonary and critical care medicine* (2nd ed.).

Rochester, D., & Brown, N. (1976). Chronic obstructive pulmonary diseases. *Resident and Staff Physician 22*, 44.

Rogers, R., et al (1978). Physiologic effects of bronchial alveolar lavage in alveolar proteinosis. *American Review of Respiratory Diseases 118*, 255-264.

Rogers, R., Graunstein, M., & Shuman, J. (1972). Role of bronchial alveolar lavage in the treatment of respiratory failure: a review. *Chest (Supplement) 62,* 95.

Rogers, R., & Tatum, K. (1970). bronchial alveolar lavage: a new approach to old problems. *Medical Clinic of North America 54,* 755.

Rowe MH: Effect of rapid mobilization on ejection fractions and ventricular volumes after myocardial infarction. *American Journal of Cardiology 63,* 1037-1041, 1989.

Rudd, R., Halslam, P, & Turner-Warwick, M. (1981). Cryptogenic fibrosing alveolitis: relationship of pulmonary physiology and bronchoalveolar lavage to response to treatment and prognosis. *American Review of Respiratory Diseases 124,* 1-8.

Saetta, M., et al (1991). Quantitative structural analysis of peripheral airways and arteries in sudden fatal asthma. *American Review of Respiratory Diseases 143,* 138-143.

Sanderson, J., et al (1974). Bronchiectasis: results of surgical and conservative management: A review of 393 cases. *Thorax 29,* 407-416.

Schuler et al: Myocardial perfusion and regression of coronary artery disease in patients on a regimen of intensive physical exercise and low fat diet. J Am Coll Cardiol 19:34-42, 1992.

Sederlinic, P., Sicilian, L., & Gaensler, E. (1988). Chronic eosinophilic pneumonia: A report of 19 cases and a review of the literature. *Medicine 67,* 154–162.

Sharma, O. (1977). A clinical picture sarcoidosis: Treatment and Prognosis. *Resident and Staff Physician 23,* 123.

Siltzbach, L., et al (1974). Course and prognosis of sarcoidosis around the world. *American Journal of Medicine 57,* 847-852.

Simpson, D. (1975). Bronchiectasis. *Hosp Med 11,* 94.

Snider, G., Faling, C., & Rennard, S. (1994). Chronic bronchitis and emphysema. In Murray, J., Nadel, J. (Eds.). *Textbook of respiratory medicine.* Philadelphia: WB Saunders.

Soergel, K., & Sommers, S. (1962). Idiopathic pulmonary hemosiderosis and related syndromes. *American Journal of Medicine 32,* 499-511.

Stoller, J., & Wiedemann, H. (1990). Chronic obstructive lung diseases: asthma, emphysema, chronic bronchitis, bronchiectasis, and related disorders. In George, R., et al. (Eds.). Chest medicine: Essentials of pulmonary and critical care medicine (2nd ed.). Baltimore: Williams and Wilkins.

Sutton, P., et al (1988) Use of nebulized saline and nebulized terbutaline as an adjunct of chest physiotherapy. *Thorax 43,* 57-60.

Sutton, P., et al (1983). Assessment of the forced expiratory technique, postural drainage and directed coughing in chest physiotherapy. *European Journal of Respiratory Diseases 64,* 62-68.

Thurlbeck, W. (1991). Pathology of chronic airflow obstruction. In Cherniack, N. (Ed.), *Chronic obstructive pulmonary disease.* Philadelphia: WB Saunders.

Thurlbeck, W. (1976). *Chronic airflow obstruction in lung disease.* Philadelphia: WB Saunders.

Thurlbeck, W. (1974) Chronic bronchitis and emphysema—the pathophysiology of chronic obstructive lung disease. *Basic Respiratory Diseases 3,* 1.

Thurlbeck, W. (1963). The incidence of pulmonary emphysema: with observations on the incidence and spatial distribution of various types of emphysema. *American Review of Respiratory Diseases, 87,* 206-215.

Tobin, M., Cook, P., & Hutchinson, D., (1983). Alpha$_1$-antitrypsin deficiency: the clinical and physiological features of pulmonary emphysema is subjects homozygous for Pi type Z. A survey by the British Thoracic Association. *British Journal of Diseases of the Chest 77,* 14-27.

Topol EJ: A randomized controlled trial of hospital discharge after myocardial infarction in the era of reperfusion. *New England Journal of Medicine* 318:1083-1088, 1988.

Toronto Lung Transplant Group (1988). Experience with single lung transplantation for pulmonary fibrosis. *Journal of American Medical Association 259,* 2258-2262.

Turner-Warwick, M. (1988). Epidemiology of nocturnal asthma. *American Journal of Medicine 85,* Suppl 1B:6-8.

Turner-Warwick, M., et al (1986). Corticosteroid treatment in pulmonary sarcoidosis: do serial lavage lymphocyte counts, serum angiotensin converting enzyme measurements, and gallium-67 scans help management: *Thorax 41,* 903-913.

Turner-Warwick, M., & Haslam, P. (1987). The value of serial bronchoalveolar lavages in assessing the clinical progress of patients with cryptogenic fibrosing alveolitis. *American Review of Respiratory Diseases 135,* 26-34.

US Surgeon General. (1984). The Health Consequences of Smoking: Chronic Obstructive Lung Disease. Pub. No. 84-50205. Washington, DC: US Department of Health and Human Resources.

van Hengstum M., et al (1988). Conventional physiotherapy and forced expiratory manoeuvres have similar effects on tracheobronchial clearance. *European Journal of Respiratory Diseases 1,* 758-761.

Verboom J., Bakker, W., & Sterk, P. (1986). The value of the forced expiratory technique with and without postural drainage in adults with cystic fibrosis. *European Journal of Respiratory Diseases 69,* 169-174.

Watters, H. et al (1986). A clinical, radiological and physiological scoring system for the longitudinal assessment of patients with idiopathic pulmonary fibrosis. *American Review of Respiratory Diseases 133,* 97-103.

Watts, J. (1989). Thoracic compression for asthma. *Chest 86,* 505.

Weg, J. (1982). Chronic noninfectious parenchymal diseases. In Guenter, C., & Welch, M. (Eds.). *Pulmonary medicine* (2nd ed.). Philadelphia: JB Lippincott.

Wenger N: Early ambulation physical activity: Myocardial infarction and coronary artery bypass surgery. Heart Lung 1: 14-17, 1984.

Williams, H., & McNicol, R. (1969). Prevalence, natural history, and relationship of wheezy bronchitis and asthma in children: An epidemiological study. *British Medical Journal 4,* 321.

Woolcock. A. (1994). Asthma. In Murray, J., Nadel, J. (Eds.). Textbook of Respiratory Medicine (2nd ed.). Philadelphia: WB Saunders.

Wright, J., et al (1992). Diseases of the small airways. *American Review of Respiratory Diseases 146,* 240-262.

CHAPTER 5

Cardiopulmonary Manifestations of Systemic Conditions

Elizabeth Dean

KEY TERMS

Connective tissue dysfunction
Endocrine dysfunction
Gastrointestinal dysfunction
Hematologic dysfunction
Hepatic dysfunction
Immunological dysfunction

Malnutrition
Musculoskeletal dysfunction
Neurological dysfunction
Obesity
Renal dysfunction
Systemic disease

INTRODUCTION

This chapter describes the cardiopulmonary consequences of systemic diseases. Systemic diseases can
significantly affect oxygen transport either directly or
in combination with primary cardiopulmonary dysfunction. Although these effects can be as cata-
strophic as those resulting from primary cardiopulmonary dysfunction, their presentation is often subtle
and may elude detection until significant impairment
is apparent. The pulmonary and pleural complications
of cardiac disease and the cardiac complications of
pulmonary disease are described first. Then the cardiopulmonary complications of conditions involving
the following systems are described including the fol-

lowing: musculoskeletal, connective tissue, neurological, gastrointestinal (GI), hepatic, renal, hematological, endocrine, and immunological systems. Finally,
the cardiopulmonary manifestations of nutritional
disorders, specifically obesity and starvation
(anorexia nervosa) are presented.

Physical therapists (PTs) need to be able to predict
the impact of systemic disease on oxygen transport
for a given patient to maximize the efficacy of their
treatment prescriptions. Complications of systemic
disease appear to be increasingly prevalent. This may
reflect both the aging of the population and improved
survival and prognosis of patients with multisystem
disease. Furthermore, PTs are treating an increasing

number of patients without referral, and thus may not be alerted by a referring practitioner to the presence and significance of underlying systemic disease. Lastly, physical therapy by definition physiologically stresses the patient, therefore, the PTs must be able to identify all factors that compromise or threaten oxygen transport so that treatment can be prescribed most effectively with minimal risk.

A comprehensive understanding of all factors that affect or threaten oxygen transport is essential particularly in those patients who are not obviously at risk, that is, those without overt cardiopulmonary disease. The PT must be able to "red flag" a patient with an underlying problem for which physical therapy may be contraindicated or an untoward treatment response anticipated. Alternatively, treatment may need to be modified or treatment responses monitored more often.

Specific diagnosis of those factors that contribute to or threaten cardiopulmonary and cardiovascular dysfunction is, therefore, tantamount to efficacious treatment across all physical therapy specialties. The capacity of the oxygen transport system needs to be established to ensure that it can adequately respond to changes in metabolic demand, including those imposed by physical therapy treatment. Even though cardiopulmonary dysfunction may not be the primary problem, identifying whether cardiopulmonary dysfunction can limit a patient's response to treatment,

whether treatment should be modified to avert an incident, or whether treatment is contraindicated all together, is essential.

Oxygen transport can be significantly affected by dysfunction in the major organ systems of the body (see box below). The pulmonary and pleural complications of heart disease and the cardiac complications of pulmonary disease are usually predictable and therefore most readily detected clinically. The cardiopulmonary complications of conditions affecting other organ systems, however, can be more subtle, if not more devastating.

CARDIAC CONDITIONS

The pulmonary complications of heart disease and the cardiac complications of pulmonary disease are well known (Scharf and Cassidy, 1989). The mechanically inefficient heart disrupts the normal forward propulsion of deoxygenated and oxygenated blood to and from the lungs. Because the right and left sides of the heart are in series, a problem on one side inevitably has some effect, that can lead to a problem on the other side, thus the heart and lung should be thought of as a single functioning unit. Disruption of the cardiopulmonary circuit leads to backlogging of blood and an increased volume of blood in the capacitance vessels, or the veins. Right heart failure contributes to increased central venous pressure (i.e., right atrial pressure) and if sufficiently severe, leads to peripheral edema in the dependent body parts. Because blood is not being forwarded to the lungs adequately, hypoxemia can result. In turn, hypoxic vasoconstriction of the pulmonary circulation leads to increased pulmonary vascular resistance, and hence, increased right ventricular afterload and work. Left heart failure can result in inadequate forward movement of blood through the left heart, resulting in backlogging in the pulmonary circulation and cardiogenic pulmonary edema. Pulmonary edema alters lung mechanics and lymphatic drainage, and in turn, these effects contribute to an increased risk of infection secondary to impaired macrophage function and bacterial growth. Excess pulmonary fluid around the alveolar capillary membrane creates a diffusion defect. If fluid accumulation is extreme, backlogging may be transmitted to

---

Systems and Systemic Conditions That Affect the Cardiopulmonary System and Oxygen Transport

Cardiopulmonary system
Musculoskeletal system
Connective tissue conditions
Collagen vascular conditions
Neurological system
Gastrointestinal system
Hepatic system
Renal system
Hematological system
Endocrine system
Immunological system
Nutritional disorders

the right side of the heart and to the periphery. Comparable to excess fluid in the lungs, backup of fluid in the peripheral circulation can impair tissue perfusion. Other cardiovascular conditions such as systemic hypertension increases systemic afterload, which in turn increases the work of the heart thereby reducing its mechanical efficiency.

Pulmonary function can be significantly altered in cardiac disease (Bates, 1989). Left heart failure, for example, is associated with accumulation of fluid in the pulmonary interstitium. This leads to reduced caliber of the airways and early airway closure, air trapping and increased residual volume. The fluid can produce reflex constriction of bronchial smooth muscle leading to the syndrome of cardiac asthma. The combination of airway collapse and bronchoconstriction decreases total lung capacity, flow rates and forced expiratory volumes. Ventilation and perfusion abnormalities are also associated with cardiac disease. Ventilation of underperfused lung zones contributes to increased ventilatory dead space, and perfusion of underventilated lung zones leads to a right to left shunt. In left heart failure, airway resistance contributes to inhomogeneous ventilation and perfusion. The normal pattern of increased ventilation to the bases is reversed in left heart failure, that is, the apices of the lungs are better ventilated (James, Cooper, White, and Wagner, 1971).

With progression of the pulmonary edema, the alveoli become flooded resulting in reduced ventilation, and significant ventilation and perfusion mismatching. The alveolar-arterial gradient ($A-a_{O_2}$ gradient) is then increased, diffusing capacity decreased, and arterial partial pressure of oxygen (Pa_{O_2}) decreased. Lung compliance is inversely related to pulmonary artery pressures and interstitial fluid accumulation (Saxton, Rabinowitz, Dexter, and Haynes, 1956). The net effect of these abnormalities is both obstructive and restrictive pathophysiologic patterns of lung dysfunction, that is, reduced forced expiratory volumes and vital capacity, and an overall increase in the work of breathing.

Pleural effusions can result from heart disease, in particular, congestive heart failure (CHF). Changes in intravascular pressures lead to transudative pleural effusions and cardiac injury leads to exudative effusions. Comparable to fluid balance in other parts of the circulation, fluid balance in the lung is dependent on Starling's forces, that is, hydrostatic and oncotic pressures. In health, several liters of fluid are absorbed from the pleural space, thus when the balance of these forces is disrupted in disease, considerable fluid can accumulate in the pleural space. Impaired alveolar expansion from pleural effusions is of clinical concern. There is some evidence, however, to support that small effusions displace rather than compress the lung (Anthonisen and Martin, 1977).

PULMONARY CONDITIONS

Lung disease can contribute to cardiac dysfunction in several ways. First, lung disease invariably threatens oxygen transport by its effects on respiratory mechanics, and ventilation and perfusion matching. To compensate, the heart attempts to increase cardiac output which produces a corresponding increase in cardiac work. Overall, ventilation and oxygen transport is less efficient. Hypoxemia secondary to inadequate ventilation and perfusion matching may predispose the patient to cardiac dysrhythmias.

Pleural complications can arise from either heart or lung disease. Both heart and lung function can be compromised by altered fluid balance of the pleurae. Fluid balance in the pleural space is comparable in terms of its regulation to that in the alveolar space. Both are determined by Starling forces. Specifically, hydrostatic pressure pushes fluid into these space while oncotic pressure counters the effect of the hydrostatic forces. The net effect of these filtration and absorption forces is a minimal net filtration pressure. When the balance of these forces is disrupted, heart and lung function can be threatened. Excessive fluid floods the space usually reflecting both excessive hydrostatic pressure and diminished oncotic pressure. The lymphatic vessels become overwhelmed and are unable to keep the pleural space dry. Pleural fluid accumulates and either displaces lung tissue (small-to-moderate effusions) or restricts opening of adjacent alveolar sacs, causing atelectasis (severe effusions) (Brown, Zamel, and Aberman, 1978), and if sufficiently severe, may restrict cardiac filling. Pleural fluid accumulation poses a unique threat to oxygen transport as a result of its direct physical effect on the lungs, heart, or both, thus it warrants special attention by PTs.

Pulmonary lymphatics control fluid balance within the lung parenchyma. Lymphatic vessels arise within the pleurae and not within the alveolar capillary space. They drain fluid from the interlobular septae and subpleural areas, to the hilar vessels and the primary tracheobronchial lymph nodes. Problems arising within the heart or lungs can contribute to imbalances in the major lymphatic inflow and outflow channels. This contributes to fluid accumulation, stagnation, and physical compression of the myocardium and lungs (Guyton, 1991).

Both heart and lung disease can produce deleterious hematologic changes to compensate for hypoxemia. Increases in the number of red blood cells raise the hematocrit and the viscosity of the blood. This phenomenon increases the work of the heart further. In addition, viscous blood increases the probability of thromboemboli. This risk is superimposed on the existing risk of thromboemboli in hypoeffective hearts.

A thorough understanding of the interrelationship of the heart and lungs is essential for diagnosis and optimal management. In addition, the cardiopulmonary and cardiovascular manifestations of other primary organ systems must be recognized and anticipated particularly in patients with multisystem disease.

MUSCULOSKELETAL CONDITIONS

Musculoskeletal conditions impact on cardiopulmonary function secondary to their effects on muscle, in particular, the diaphragm, muscles of the chest wall, oropharynx, larynx and abdomen, and on bones and joints (e.g., arthritis, ankylosing spondylitis, kyphoscoliosis, and the deformity secondary to neuromuscular diseases and chronic lung diseases). Additional effects are imposed by inactivity, (i.e., muscle wasting and increased joint rigidity). Increased joint rigidity limits the amount of physical activity a patient may perform, which contributes to cardiopulmonary compromise, in addition to the local effect of increased chest wall rigidity and compromised bucket-handle and pump-handle motions. The normal three-dimensional movement of the chest wall and normal pulmonary circulation and lymphatic function is compromised (Chapter

---

Cardiopulmonary Manifestations of Musculoskeletal Conditions

General Manifestations
Reduced alveolar ventilation

Altered respiratory mechanics
Chest wall rigidity
Reduced chest wall excursion

Impaired mucocilary transport

Airflow obstruction
Pulmonary restriction
Atelectasis
Inspissated secretions

Increased work of breathing

Inefficient breathing pattern

Increased work of the heart

Inefficient breathing pattern
Constrictive pericarditis

Reduced aerobic capacity

Manifestations in Specific Conditions
Rheumatoid arthritis

Pleuritis with or without effusion
Diffuse interstitial pneumonitis and fibrosis
Pulmonary arteritis
Bronchiolitis
Pleural effusions

Ankylosing spondylitis

Upper lobe fibrobullous disease
Chest wall restriction

---

22). The cardiopulmonary manifestation of musculoskeletal conditions are summarized in the box above.

The cardiopulmonary deficits associated with musculoskeletal disorders of the chest wall include reduced lung volumes consistent with pulmonary restriction, reduced flow rates, reduced inspiratory and expiratory pressures, increased atelectasis, increased dynamic airway compression, ventilation and perfusion mismatching, inefficient breathing pattern, impaired cough and gag reflexes, increased risk of aspiration, increased risk of obstruction secondary to impaired mucociliary clearance, restricted mobility, compression of mediastinal structures and heart, and impaired lymphatic drainage which depends on normal expiratory and inspiratory cycles (Bates, 1989).

CONNECTIVE TISSUE CONDITIONS

Connective tissue/virgule collagen vascular disorders (e.g., scleroderma and systemic lupus erythematosus [SLE]), invariably affect the cardiopulmonary system (Bagg and Hughes, 1979). Inflammation and tissue injury can affect the airway, lung parenchyma, pulmonary vasculature, pleurae, respiratory muscles, heart and pericardium. Shrinking lung syndrome associated with chronic connective tissue changes is a feature of advanced disease and is characterized by a significant loss of alveolar surface area, diffusion capacity, and lung volumes. Fibrotic changes increase the elasticity of the lung parenchyma and reduce lung compliance, thereby increasing work of breathing. These changes are comparable to those in idiopathic pulmonary fibrosis. Both the electrical conduction system of the heart and its mechanical behavior are adversely affected by systemic connective tissue changes (Goldman and Kotler, 1985). Furthermore,

---

Cardiopulmonary Manifestations of Connective Tissue/Collagen Vascular Conditions

General Manifestations

Acute injury to the alveolar-capillary unit
Alveolar hemorrhage
Interstitial pneumonitis
Interstitial pulmonary fibrosis
Pulmonary hypertension
Respiratory muscle dysfunction
Pulmonary edema
Pulmonary infection
Abnormal diffusing capacity
Chest wall restriction

Manifestations in Scleroderma

Restrictive ventilatory impairment
Decreased diffusing capacity
Diaphragmatic dysfunction
Gastroesophageal reflux and aspiration

---

connective-tissue changes in the skin can lead to chest wall restriction. The cardiopulmonary manifestations of connective tissue conditions are summarized in the box below.

NEUROLOGICAL CONDITIONS

Cardiopulmonary consequences of neurological disease reflects the specific pathophysiologic mechanisms involved (Griggs and Donohoe, 1982). There are three basic patterns of pathology: (1) involvement of the central nervous system (CNS), (2) the peripheral nervous system, and (3) the autonomic nervous system. The cardiopulmonary manifestations of neurological conditions are summarized in the box on p. 104.

Involvement of the CNS

The primary centers for breathing control and control of the heart emanate from the midbrain. The generator for breathing control produces a regular respiratory rate through modulation of inspiratory and expiratory inhibitory and excitatory neurons.

Activity of the central generator is affected by arousal and the general alerting reaction of the reticular activating system. In addition, breathing control is influenced by the hypothalamus, the orbital cortex, forebrain, and amygdala (Hitchcock and Leece, 1967).

Insult to the CNS can result in cardiovascular responses that precipitate neurogenic pulmonary edema. Such responses include systemic hypertension, pulmonary hypertension, intracranial hypertension and bradycardia. The medulla is believed to mediate the cardiovascular responses associated with neurogenic pulmonary edema. Marked sympathetic stimulation, catecholamine release, and vagotonia appear to precipitate neurogenic pulmonary edema and the resulting leaking of the alveolar capillary membrane and alveolar flooding (Colice, 1985). However, the possibility of a primary pulmonary endothelial permeability abnormality has been suggested (Peterson, Ross, and Brigham, 1983).

Cortical disturbances may have a direct effect on cardiopulmonary function. Among the most common disturbances seen clinically are cortical infarction and seizures. Hemispheric infarction can lead to

General Manifestations
Impaired mucociliary transport

Reduced mobility
Cilia dyskinesia
Increased mucus accumulation
Reduced cough and gag reflexes
Impaired airway protection
Increased airway resistance
Increased risk of airway obstruction
Impaired glottic closure
Increased risk of aspiration

Impaired alveolar ventilation

Reduced lung volumes and capacities, as well as flow rates
Weakness of pharyngeal and laryngeal structures
Respiratory muscle weakness
Reduced respiratory muscle endurance

Increased work of breathing

Reduced aerobic capacity and deconditioning

Manifestations in Specific Conditions
Multiple sclerosis

Respiratory muscle weakness
Impaired ventilation secondary to spasm
Increased oxygen consumption secondary to spasm
Increased oxygen consumption secondary to impaired posture and gait
Impaired gag and cough reflexes
Ineffective cough

Cerebral palsy

Increased oxygen consumption secondary to increased muscle tone
Significantly reduced mobility and activity
Impaired movement economy
Impaired swallowing
Impaired saliva control
Reduced gag and cough reflexes
Impaired coordination of thoracic and abdominal motion during respiration
Ineffective cough and airway clearance mechanisms

Stroke

Reduced movement economy
Spasticity and increased oxygen demands
Flaccidity of respiratory muscles
Impaired respiratory muscle strength
Impaired pulmonary function
Asymmetric chest wall
Weak and ineffective cough

Parkinson's disease

Increased oxygen consumption secondary to increased muscle tone
Reduced movement economy
Chest wall restriction and impaired pulmonary function
Ineffective cough

contralateral weakness of the diaphragm and other respiratory muscles. Epileptic seizures disrupt breathing, which causes hypoxemia, respiratory acidosis, and a metabolic acidosis secondary to extreme muscle contraction and lactate accumulation. The associated increase in sympathetic stimulation can precipitate cardiac dysrhythmias and pulmonary edema.

Demyelinating diseases such as multiple sclerosis result in progressive deterioration of neuromuscular function. The muscles of respiration become increasingly involved, resulting in respiratory insufficiency (Cooper, Trend, and Wiles, 1985). In addition, with increasing debility cardiopulmonary conditioning is reduced. Weakness of the pharyngeal musculature contributes to loss of airway protection in addition to the loss of cough and gag reflexes. Aspiration is problematic for these patients as the disease advances.

Stroke patients may have central involvement that affects cardiopulmonary regulation and function, including reduced electrical activity of the respiratory muscles, or peripheral involvement such that weakness, spasticity, impaired biomechanics, and gait directly affect respiratory muscle function and chest wall excursion (DeTroyer, De Beyl, and Thirion, 1981). Abdominal muscle weakness contributes to impaired cough effectiveness. Pharyngeal weakness contributes to sleep apnea in these patients. The common clinical presentation of unilateral involvement leads to a posture listing to the affected side when recumbent, sitting and during ambulation. This posture impairs ventilation and chest wall expansion on the affected side. Abdominal muscle involvement directly affects intraabdominal pressure and the efficiency of diaphragmatic descent during contraction, that is, should the abdominal muscles become flaccid the efficiency of diaphragmatic contraction is significantly reduced. Lung volumes and flow rates are reduced proportionately giving a restrictive pattern of lung function. Reduced activity and exercise around the time of the stroke contributes to reduced cardiopulmonary conditioning and capacity of the oxygen transport system. Finally, a high proportion of patients with strokes are hypertensive and older, a population with a higher prevalence of heart disease and atherosclerosis (Chimowitz and Mancini, 1991).

Cerebral palsy is associated with significantly increased muscle tone, which correspondingly increases basal and exercise oxygen consumption, resulting in increased oxygen demands. Even though the demands are increased in this condition, oxygen delivery is compromised. For example, thoracic deformity and spasm of the muscles of the chest wall and abdomen impair breathing pattern and its efficiency (Fullford and Brown, 1976). The airways of patients with cerebral palsy are vulnerable because of poor gag, cough, and swallowing reflexes. In addition, these patients often have poor saliva control, which increases the risk of aspiration further. Mental retardation (Bates, 1989) often complicates the presentation of cerebral palsy and prevents these patients from responding adequately to their hydration needs or being able to cooperate with life-preserving treatments. These patients harbor numerous microorganisms, which adds further to their general risk of infection.

Patients with Parkinson's disease also exhibit significant cardiopulmonary deficits (Mehta, Wright, and Kirby, 1978). Oxygen demand is increased commensurate with increased muscle tone. Comparable to the patients described above, patients with Parkinson's also have reduced cardiopulmonary conditioning levels as a result of compromised agility and ability to be independently mobile in many cases. These patients also have a restrictive pattern of lung disease with most lung volumes and capacities being reduced. Chest wall rigidity impairs the normal pump-handle and bucket-handle movements, thus it reduces breathing efficiency. The energy cost of breathing is correspondingly increased. Respiratory insufficiency of Parkinson's disease likely reflects an increase in tone of the respiratory muscles, chest wall rigidity, as well as increased parasympathetic tone and resulting airway obstruction.

Patients with a history of poliomyelitis with or without cardiopulmonary complications at onset, may exhibit pulmonary limitation several decades later (Dean, Ross, Road, Courtenay, and Madill, 1991; Steljes, Kryger, Kirk, and Millar, 1990). These individuals are at risk for developing respiratory insufficiency as a result of respiratory muscle weakness, chest wall deformity, minor infection and periods of relative immobility, or secondary to medical interventions, (e.g., anesthesia, sedation).

Diseases and lesions involving the brainstem can lead to various abnormal breathing patterns. Some common breathing aberrations are Cheyne-Stokes respiration, central neurogenic hyperventilation, apneustic breathing, and ataxic breathing. Cerebellar and basal ganglia lesions may produce respiratory muscle discoordination and dyspnea (Hormia, 1957; Neu, Connolly, Schwertley, Ladwig, and Brody, 1967).

Spinal cord lesions have a variable effect on cardiopulmonary function depending on the level of the lesion. Cervical lesions result in a high mortality rate as a result of cardiopulmonary complications. All lung volumes are diminished with the exception of total lung capacity (TLC), which over time returns to normal; tidal volume (TV), which is usually preserved (10% of TLC); and residual volume (RV), which is significantly increased (Estenne and DeTroyer, 1987; Fugl-Meyer, 1971). Quadriplegic patients tend to have a greater diaphragmatic contribution to tidal ventilation compared with healthy people (Estenne and DeTroyer, 1985). In addition, these patients have impaired cough as a result of loss of innervation and paresis of the diaphragm in some cases, and abdominal and intercostal muscles. The contribution of accessory muscle activity to ventilation varies considerably (McKinley, Auchincloss, Gilbert, and Nicholas, 1969). In quadriplegia, with only the accessory muscles and diaphragm spared, platypnea (increased dyspnea when upright) may occur (Dantzker, 1991). In the upright position, the diaphragm is flattened and less efficient when moved downward by reduced abdominal pressures.

Thoracic lesions tend to have less effect on pulmonary function (vital capacity and forced expiratory volumes in particular) than cervical lesions, and the significance of this effect is reduced as the level of the lesion is reduced. Lumbar lesions may have minimal or no effect on pulmonary function; however, involvement of the abdominal muscles may limit cough effectiveness.

Involvement of the Peripheral Nervous System

Disorders of the peripheral nervous system include those of the motor neuron, peripheral nerve, neuromuscular junction and muscle. Neuromuscular disorders of the larynx, pharynx, and tongue can lead to upper airway obstruction and increased airway resistance, and interfere with maintaining a clear airway. Aspiration is a common and serious problem associated with impaired motor control of the larynx, pharynx, and tongue.

Involvement of the Autonomic Nervous System

Cardiopulmonary consequences of disorders of the autonomic nervous system have been documented. Of those diseases with an autonomic component, autonomic neuropathies, diabetes, and alcoholism have been the most studied. Multiple system atrophy accompanies autonomic failure affecting multiple systems. Because of the anatomic proximity of the autonomic, respiratory and hypnogenic neurons and the degeneration of these structures in this condition, dysfunction of the respiratory control mechanisms parallels autonomic and somatic dysfunction. The respiratory dysrhythmias that are seen in multiple system atrophy include central, upper airway obstruction, irregular rate, rhythm, and amplitude of respiration with or without oxygen desaturation, transient uncoupling of the intercostal and diaphragmatic muscle activity, prolonged periods of apnea, Cheyne-Stokes respiration, inspiratory gasps, and transient sudden respiratory arrest (Bannister, 1989).

Patients with diabetes and autonomic neuropathies exhibit variable effects on cardiopulmonary status. Postural hypotension is a complication of diabetic autonomic neuropathy and efferent sympathetic vasomotor denervation. Norepinephrine levels are generally reduced in these patients. The splanchnic and peripheral circulations fail to constrict in response to standing, thus cardiac output falls. The postural effect is exacerbated by reduced cardiac acceleration in patients with diabetes. Insulin has been associated with cardiovascular effects, including reduced plasma volume, increased peripheral blood flow secondary to vasodilatation, and increased heart rate. In the presence of autonomic neuropathies, insulin can induce postural hypotension. Diabetic diarrhea secondary to abnormal gut motility can contribute to fluid loss and its sequelae. Cardiopulmonary changes associated with autonomic neuropathy secondary to diabetes include altered ventilatory responses to hypoxia and hypercapnia, altered respiratory pattern and apneic episodes during sleep, altered bronchial reactivity and impaired cough (Bannister, 1989; Montserrat et al., 1985).

GASTROINTESTINAL CONDITIONS

The cardiopulmonary manifestations of GI dysfunction are summarized in the box below. Inflammatory bowel disease and pancreatitis are principal examples of GI dysfunction that affects on cardiopulmonary function. Aspiration is a significant cause of morbidity and mortality in patients with GI dysfunction, thus it should be prevented or detected early. The pathophysiology, management, and outcome depend on the nature of the aspirate. Several predisposing factors produce aspiration pneumonia including a decreased level of consciousness, disorders of pharyngeal and esophageal motility, altered anatomy, disorders of gastric and intestinal motility, and iatrogenic factors such as surgery, nasogastric (NG) intubation, and general anesthesia.

Inflammatory bowel disease can lead to the following cardiopulmonary pathologies: vasculitis, fibrosis, granulomatous disease, and pulmonary thromboembolism. Bronchitis and bronchiectasis have also been associated with inflammatory bowel disease; however, their occurrence is not related to the activity or therapy. Biopsy specimens have shown basement membrane thickening, thickening of the epithelium, and infiltration of the underlying connective tissue with inflammatory cells (Higenbottom, et al., 1980).

The pulmonary manifestations of pancreatitis are among the most important sequelae of this disease. Of the deaths that occur in the first week of hospitalization, 60% are associated with respiratory failure (Renner, Savage, Pantoja, and Renner, 1985). Problems include elevated hemidiaphragms particularly on the right side, basal atelectasis, diffuse pulmonary infiltrates appearing more often on the right side than the left side, pleural effusions on the left side more than the right side, and pneumonitis. These findings are not specific for pancreatitis and are probably secondary to localized peritonitis, subphrenic collections, ascitis, pain, and abdominal distension. In chronic pancreatitis, abdominal symptoms may be reduced and thoracic symptoms such as dyspnea, chest pain, and cough may predominate. Chronic effusions may result in pleural thickening.

LIVER CONDITIONS

Both acute and chronic liver conditions can predispose a patient to cardiopulmonary and cardiovascular complications (see the box, on p. 108, at left). Hepatic failure can lead to hypoxemia secondary to intrapulmonary vascular dilatation and noncardiogenic pulmonary edema. Hepatopulmonary syndrome, hallmarked by intrapulmonary vascular dilatation, produces both diffusion and perfusion defects in the lungs and is the principal reason for severe hypoxemia (Sherlock, 1988). The origin of pulmonary edema is secondary to hepatic encephalopathy and cerebral edema (Trewby, et al., 1978).

With respect to chronic liver conditions, cardiopulmonary manifestations have been associated with cirrhosis of the liver and hepatitis. The most common pulmonary abnormalities associated with these conditions are intrapulmonary vascular dilatation with and without shunt, pulmonary hypertension, airflow obstruction, chest wall deformity, pleural effusions, pancinar emphysema, pleuritis, bronchitis,

---

Cardiopulmonary Manifestations of GI Conditions

Risk of aspiration
Gastroesophageal reflux

Increased airway resistance
Bronchospasm

Reduced lung volumes
Elevated hemidiaphragms
Compression atelectasis

Arterial hypoxemia
Alveolar capillary leak and V/Q mismatch
Alveolar hemorrhage and consolidation worsen shunt
Increased pulmonary vascular resistance

Cardiopulmonary Manifestations of Liver Conditions

Intrapulmonary vascular dilatation
Pulmonary hypertension
Expiratory airflow obstruction
Chest wall deformity
Pleural effusions
Panacinar emphysema
Pleuritis
Bronchitis
Bronchiectasis
Impaired hypoxic vasoconstriction
Interstitial pneumonitis
Pulmonary fibrosis

Cardiopulmonary Manifestations of Renal Conditions

Alveolar hemorrhage
Airway obstruction
Reduced lung volumes
Reduced diffusing capacity

---

bronchiectasis, hypoxic vasoconstriction, and interstitial pneumonitis, fibrosis. Hypoxemia results from shunting, ventilation and perfusion mismatching and diffusion abnormalities.

Pleural effusions and ascites interfere with diaphragm function and present unique problems in the patient with liver disease. Rich lymphatic connections exist between the abdominal and thoracic cavities. Because of the rich lymphatic supply of the pleural space, ascitic fluid can flow into the pleural space. This effect is enhanced during inspiration when the intraabdominal pressure is relatively positive and the intrapleural space is negative (Crofts, 1954).

RENAL CONDITIONS

Cardiopulmonary complications can result from renal disease and the category of disorders referred to as pulmonary-renal syndromes (see the box above, at right). (Rankin and Matthay, 1982; Matthay, Bromberg, and Putman, 1980). The pathophysiologic characteristics of these disorders include alveolar hemorrhage, interstitial and alveolar inflammation, and involvement of the pulmonary vasculature. Pulmonary function testing may detect both obstructive and restrictive abnormalities as a result of bronchial complications, and inflammation and hemorrhage respectively.

In systemic illness, pathology of the lungs and kidneys often coexist. Like the medical management of these patients, physical therapy warrants being especially aggressive given the course of the pulmonary-renal syndromes and the potential for relapses and irreversible organ damage.

HEMATOLOGIC CONDITIONS

Hematologic disorders that can manifest cardiopulmonary symptoms include abnormalities of the fluid and cellular components of the blood, and coagulopathies (Bromberg and Ross, 1988). Cardiopulmonary manifestations of hematologic conditions are summarized in (the box on p. 109). The primary underlying mechanisms by which these conditions disrupt gas exchange include hemorrhage, infection, edema, anemia, fibrosis, and malignancies.

Abnormalities related to red blood cells and their ability to transport hemoglobin and oxygen may produce signs resembling pulmonary pathology, (e.g., tachypnea, dyspnea, and cyanosis). Abnormalities of the deformability of red blood cells alter blood viscosity and pulmonary blood flow. The interstitium can be disrupted by such factors as hemorrhage and malignancies. Coagulopathies disrupt the normal hemostasis and clotting mechanisms of the blood. Pulmonary hemorrhage and hemoptysis are common sequelae. The most common causes of pulmonary hemorrhage include vitamin-K deficiency, hemophilia, hepatic failure, and disseminated intravascular coagulation. Pharmacologic agents such as platelet inhibitors and anticoagulants can also result in pulmonary hemorrhage. Pulmonary thromboemboli are common events with symptoms including pleuritic chest pain, dyspnea, and hemoptysis.

Of the erythrocyte disorders sickle cell anemia is probably the most common. Acute chest infection and thrombosis leading to pulmonary infarction may

Cardiopulmonary Manifestations of Hematologic Conditions
General Cardiopulmonary Manifestations Hemorrhage Edema Polycythemia Anemia Infection **Abnormalities of the Fluid Portion of the Blood** Abnormal blood volume Abnormal fluid balance (water excesses and deficits) Abnormal electrolytes Abnormal plasma proteins Abnormal procoagulants and anticoagulants Abnormal clotting times **Abnormalities of the Cellular Portion of the Blood** Abnormal red blood cell count Abnormal red blood cells Abnormal deformability of the red blood cells Abnormal hemoglobin Abnormal oxyhemoglobin dissociation (e.g., carbon monoxide poisoning) Abnormal white blood cells and antibodies Blood dyscrasias

occur with clinical symptoms such as fever, pleuritic chest pain, cough, and pulmonary infiltrates. The pulmonary function of patients with sickle cell anemia is abnormal with reduced TLC, vital capacity, diffusing capacity, arterial oxygen tensions, and reduced exercise capacity (Femi-Pearse, Gazioglu, and Yu, 1970).

The hematologic malignancy disorders that can affect pulmonary function include the leukemias and Hodgkin's disease. The three primary mechanisms by which these disorders can affect pulmonary function include direct infiltration, increased risk of opportunistic infection and secondary effects of treatment, such as interstitial pneumonitis and fibrosis.

Disorders of plasma proteins can have significant effects on the Starling's forces maintaining normal fluid balance within the tissue vascular beds. De-

pending on the amount of plasma protein, particularly albumin, fluid is retained or lost from the circulation. With reduced protein and oncotic pressure within the vasculature, more fluid is filtered out of the circulation into the interstitium. In catabolic states in which protein is broken down in the body, more protein leaks through the capillaries taking water with it, thus leading to edema.

ENDOCRINE CONDITIONS

Endocrine and metabolic disorders can be associated with cardiopulmonary complications (see the box on p. 110). (Civetta, Taylor, and Kirby, 1989; Guyton, 1991). Disorders of the thyroid gland, pancreas (diabetes mellitus [DM]) and adrenal glands are such disorders that are often seen clinically. Thyroid hormone influences the central drive to breathe and surfactant synthesis. Hypothyroidism can lead to sleep apnea, pleural effusions secondary to altered capillary permeability, and pericardial effusions. Decreases in vital capacity have also been reported secondary to muscle weakness. Hyperthyroidism increases cellular oxidative metabolism (the metabolic rate) leading to an increase in oxygen consumption and CO_2 production, and an overall increase in minute ventilation. Vital capacity, lung compliance, and diffusion capacity can be reduced. In addition, maximal inspiratory and expiratory pressures can be reduced secondary to muscle weakness.

Patients with diabetes are prone to aspiration and respiratory infections. Late complications of diabetic neuropathy include renal failure, which may be accompanied by pleural effusions and pulmonary edema. Autonomic neuropathy may affect vagal activity and airway tone. Ischemic heart disease and cardiomyopathies are common in patients with diabetes and may cause CHF and cardiogenic pulmonary edema. Patients with diabetes have been reported to have reduced sensitivity to inspiratory loading (O'Donnell, Friedman, Russomanno, and Rose, 1988), which may impair their subjective responses to exercise.

Adrenal insufficiency can also compromise oxygen transport (Civetta, Taylor, and Kirby, 1989). Reduced aerobic capacity results from symptoms of weakness, fatigue, and associated muscle and joint complaints. Orthostatic intolerance primarily reflects

---

Cardiopulmonary Manifestations of Endocrine Conditions

Thyroid Disorders
Hypothyroidism

Hypometabolic
Fatigue and excessive sleep
Reduced conditioning
Decreased vital capacity secondary to muscle
  weakness
Sleep apnea
Decreased heart rate
Decreased cardiac output
Decreased blood volume
Pleural effusions
Pericardial effusions

Hyperthyroidism

Hypermetabolic
Decreased vital capacity and diffusing capacity
Fluid loss (diarrhea)
Respiratory muscle weakness
Fatigue and inability to sleep
Reduced conditioning

Pancreatic Disorders (Diabetes)

Pulmonary endothelial thickening
Reduced TLC
Reduced vital capacity and forced expiratory
  volumes
Reduced airway vagal tone
Increased risk of aspiration
Possible reduced elastic recoil
Impaired hypoxic and hypercapnic responses
Impaired ventilatory response to exercise
Defective neutrophil production
Colonization with gram-negative bacilli
Pleural effusions and pulmonary edema with
  diabetic nephropathy
Reduced sensitivity to increases in inspiratory
  resistive loading
Accelerated atherosclerotic vascular and cardiac
  changes
Increased ischemic heart disease
Cardiomyopathy
Increased risk of infection

Adrenal Insufficiency

Orthostatic symptoms
Reduced aerobic capacity secondary to anorexia,
  weakness and fatigue
Impaired breathing mechanics secondary to GI
  symptoms
Tendency to retain fluid

---

reduced inotrophic capacity of the heart and reduced systemic vascular resistance.

IMMUNOLOGICAL CONDITIONS

Congenital and acquired defects in the immunological status of the lung lead to cardiopulmonary dysfunction, including infection and inflammation. In addition, patients who are immunodeficient have an increased risk of pulmonary malignancies (Shackleford and McAlister, 1975).

Acquired immunodeficiency syndrome (AIDS), an example of a primary disorder of cell-mediated immunity, has reached epidemic proportions over the past 20 years. This syndrome leads to lymphocyte death. The most serious pulmonary infections associated with AIDS is *Pneumocystis carinii* pneumonia (Murray, Felton, and Garay, 1984). The fact that the patient with the human immunodeficiency virus (HIV) is more likely to have recurrent pneumonia suggests that the infecting organisms persist in the lung despite treatment (Shelhamer, et al., 1984). The clinical presentation includes diffuse pulmonary infiltrates, cough, dyspnea, and hemoptysis. These patients can also have symptoms of upper airway obstruction.

NUTRITIONAL DISORDERS

The two most common nutritional disorders seen in Western countries are obesity, and anorexia nervosa, which is akin to starvation. Obesity contributes in several ways to impaired oxygen transport (Alexander, 1985; Bates, 1989). These include alveolar hypoventilation and impaired Pao_2 and gas exchange as a result of the increased weight of adipose tissue over the thoracic cavity. Systemic and pulmonary blood pressures are increased. In addition, large abdomens, and abdominal contents impinge on diaphragmatic motion, and can restrict diaphragmatic descent. This can lead to compression of the dependent lung fields. Recumbency can induce respiratory insufficiency, that is positional respiratory failure. Obese individuals have a higher incidence of snoring and obstructive sleep apnea secondary to weakness, and increased compliance of the postpharyngeal structures. In addition, these patients often have weak ineffectual coughs resulting from expiratory muscle weakness and mechanical inefficiency of these muscles. Work of breathing is markedly increased. Furthermore, in chronic cases, reactive pulmonary vasoconstriction in response to chronic hypoxemia contributes to right ventricular insufficiency and increased work of the heart and cardiomegaly.

The major cardiopulmonary manifestations of anorexia nervosa relate to generalized weakness and reduced endurance of all muscles, including the respiratory muscles. Cough effectively is correspondingly compromised. Oxygen transport reserve is minimal. Because of poor nutrition and fluid intake, the patient is at significant risk of anemia, fluid and electrolyte imbalances, and cardiac dysrhythmias (Wilson, et al, 1991). Common manifestations of nutritional disorders are summarized in the box below.

Cardiopulmonary Manifestations of Nutritional Disorders

Obesity

Alveolar hypoventilation
Obstructive sleep apnea
Reduced outward recoil of the chest wall
Increased abdominal contents
Increased mass of the abdominal wall
Reduced functional residual capacity
Reduced expiratory reserve volume
Marked reductions lung volumes, arterial oxygen tension (Pao_2) and saturation (Sao_2) in recumbency
Basal airway closure and resulting decrease in Pao_2
Marked pulmonary abnormalities during sleep
Reduced ventilatory responses to CO_2
Cardiomegaly
Rotation and horizontal position of the heart
Axis deviation
Reduced myocardial pumping efficiency
Reduced aerobic conditioning and oxygen transport reserve capacity

Starvation or Anorexia Nervosa

Generalized weakness, debility, and loss of cardiopulmonary conditioning
Impaired mucociliary transport
Ineffective cough
Fluid and electrolyte disturbances
Cardiac dysrhythmias
Respiratory muscle weakness

SUMMARY

This chapter described the cardiopulmonary consequences of systemic diseases. Oxygen transport, the purpose of the cardiopulmonary system, can be significantly affected by dysfunction in virtually all organ systems of the body. The pathophysiological consequences of diseases of the following systems on oxygen transport were presented: cardiac, pulmonary, musculoskeletal, connective tissue/collagen vascular, neurological, gastrointestinal, hepatic, renal, hematologic, endocrine, and immunological systems. In addition, the cardiopulmonary manifestations of nutritional disorders, including obesity and anorexia nervosa, were described.

A knowledge of these effects is essential to the practice of physical therapy across all specialties in that the prevalence of systemic disease appears to be increasing. The presentation of cardiopulmonary consequences of systemic disease is often subtle or obscured, and is associated with a poor prognosis, thus early detection and appropriate management is essential.

PTs need to be able to distinguish diagnostically cardiopulmonary manifestations of systemic diseases to appropriately identify indications for physical therapy, contraindications, side effects, and unusual treatment responses. In addition, detailed assessment of the patient's problems ensures that problems amenable to physical therapy are appropriately treated, and those that are not are referred back to a physician.

REVIEW QUESTION

- Describe the cardiopulmonary manifestions of:
1. Musculoskeletal dysfunction
2. Connective tissue dysfunction
3. Neurological dysfunction
4. Hepatic dysfunction
5. Renal dysfunction
6. Hematologic dysfunction
7. Endocrine dysfunction
8. Obesity
9. Malnutrition (e.g. anorexia nervosa)

References

Alexander, J.K. (1985). The cardiomyopathy of obesity. *Progress in Cardiovascular Disease, 27,* 325-334.

Anthonisen, N.R., & Martin, R.R. (1977). Regional lung function in pleural effusions. *American Review of Respiratory Diseases, 116,* 201-206.

Bagg, L.R., & Hughes, D.T. (1979). Serial pulmonary function tests in progressive systemic sclerosis. *Thorax, 34,* 224-228.

Bannister, R. (1989). *Autonomic Failure.* (2nd ed.). Oxford Medical Publications: Oxford.

Bates, D.V. (1989). *Respiratory Function in Disease* (3rd ed.). Philadelphia: W.B. Saunders.

Bromberg, P.A., & Ross, D.W. (1988). The lungs and hematologic disease. In: Murray, J.F., & Nadel, J. (Eds.). *Textbook of Respiratory Medicine.* Philadelphia, W.B. Saunders, pp. 1906-1920.

Brown, N.E., Zamel, N., & Aberman, A. (1978). Changes in pulmonary mechanics and gas exchange following thoracentesis. *Chest, 74,* 540-542.

Chimowitz, M.I., & Mancini, G.B.J. (1991). Asymptomatic coronary artery disease in patients with stroke. *Current Concepts of Cerebrovascular Diseases and Stroke, 26,* 23-27.

Civetta, J.M., Taylor, R.W., & Kirby, R.R. (1989). *Critical Care.* Philadelphia: Lippincott.

Colice, G.L. (1985). Neurogenic pulmonary edema. *Clinics in Chest Medicine, 6,* 473-489.

Cooper, C.B., Trend, P.S., & Wiles, C.M. (1985). Severe diaphragm weakness in multiple sclerosis. *Thorax, 40,* 631-632.

Crofts, N.F. (1954). Pneumothorax complicating therapeutic pneumoperitineum. *Thorax, 9,* 226-228.

Dantzker, D.R. (1991). *Cardiopulmonary Critical Care.* (2nd ed.). Philadelphia: W.B. Saunders.

Dean, E., Ross, J., Road, J.D., Courtenay, L. & Madill, K. (1991). Pulmonary function in individuals with a history of poliomyelitis. *Chest, 100,* 118-123.

DeTroyer, A., De Beyl, D.Z., & Thirion, M. (1981). Function of the respiratory muscles in acute hemiplegia. *American Review of Respiratory Diseases, 123,* 631-632.

Estenne, M., & DeTroyer, A. (1985). Relationship between respiratory muscle electromyogram and rib cage motion in tetraplegia. *American Review of Respiratory Diseases, 132,* 53-59.

Estenne, M., & DeTroyer, A. (1987). Mechanism of the postural dependence of vital capacity in tetraplegic subjects. *American Review of Respiratory Diseases, 135,* 367-371.

Femi-Pearse, D., Gazioglu, K.M., & Yu, P.N. (1970) Pulmonary function and infection in sickle cell disease. *Journal of Applied Physiology, 28,* 574-577.

Fugi-Meyer, A.R. (1971). A model for treatment of impaired ventilatory function in tetraplegic patients. *Scandinavian Journal of Rehabilitation Medicine, 3,* 168-177.

Fullford, F.E., & Brown, J.K. (1976). Position as a cause of deformity in children with cerebral palsy. *Developmental Medicine in Child Neurology, 18,* 305-314.

Goldman, A.P., & Kotler, M.N. (1985). Heart disease in scleroderma. *American Heart Journal, 110,* 1043-1046.

Griggs, R.C., & Donohoe, K.M. (1982). Recognition and management of respiratory insufficiency in neuromuscular disease. *Journal of Chronic Diseases, 35,* 497-500.

Guyton, A.C. (1991). *Textbook of Medical Physiology.* (8th ed.). Philadelphia: W.B. Saunders.

Higenbottom, T., Cochrane, G.M., Clark, T.J.H., Turner, D., Millis, R., & Seymour, W. (1980). Bronchial disease in ulcerative colitis. *Thorax, 35,* 581-585.

Hitchcock, E., & Leece, B. (1967). Somatotopic representation of the respiratory pathways in the cervical cord of man. *Journal of Neurosurgery, 27,* 320-329.

Hormia, A.L. (1957). Respiratory insufficiency as a symptom of cerebellar ataxia. *American Journal of Medical Science, 233,* 635-640.

James, A.E., Cooper, M., White, R.I., & Wagner, H.N. (1971). Perfusion changes on lung scans in patients with congestive heart failure. *Radiology, 100,* 99-106.

Matthay, R.A., Bromberg, S.I., & Putman, C.E. (1980). Pulmonary renal syndromes--a review. *Yale Journal of Biology and Medicine, 53,* 497-523.

Mehta, A D., Wright, W.B., & Kirby, B. (1978). Ventilatory function in Parkinson's disease. *British Medical Journal, 1,* 1456-1457.

McKinley, C.A., Auchincloss, J.H., Gilbert, R., & Nicholas, J. (1969). Pulmonary function, ventilatory control, and respiratory complications in quadriplegic subjects. *American Review of Respiratory Diseases, 100,* 526-532.

Montserrat, J.M., Cochrane, G.M., Wolf, C., Picado, C., Roca, J., & Agustidval, A. (1985). Ventilatory control in diabetes mellitus. *European Journal of Respiratory Disease, 67,* 112-117.

Murray, J.F., Felton, C.P., Garay, S.M., et al. (1984). Pulmonary complications of the acquired immunodeficiency syndrome. *New England Journal of Medicine, 310,* 1682-1688.

Neu, H.C., Connolly, J.J., Schwertley, F.W., Ladwig, H.A., & Brody, A.W. (1967). Obstructive respiratory dysfunction in Parkinsonian patients. *American Review Respiratory Diseases, 95,* 33-47.

O'Donnell, C.R., Friedman, L.S., Russomanno, J.H., & Rose, R.M. (1988). Diminished perception of inspiratory-resistive loads in insulin-dependent diabetics. *New England Journal of Medicine, 319,* 1369-1373.

Peterson, B.T., Ross, J.C., & Brigham, K.L. (1983). Effect of naloxone on the pulmonary vascular responses to graded levels of intracranial hypertension in anesthetized sheep. *American Review of Respiratory Diseases, 128,* 1024-1029.

Rankin, J.A., & Matthay, R.A. (1982). Pulmonary renal syndromes. II. Etiology and pathogenesis. *Yale Journal of Biology and Medicine, 55,* 11-26.

Renner, I.G., Savage, W.T., Pantoja, J.L., & Renner, V.J. (1985). Death due to acute pancreatitis: a retrospective analysis of 405 autopsy cases. *Digestive Diseases and Sciences, 30,* 1005-1008.

Saxton, G.A., Rabinowitz, W., Dexter, L., & Haynes, F. (1956). The relationship of pulmonary compliance to pulmonary vascular pressures in patients with heart disease. *Journal of Clinical Investigation, 35,* 611-618.

Shackleford, M.D., & McAlister, W.H. (1975). Primary immunodeficiency diseases and malignancy. *American Journal of Roentgenology, Radium Therapy & Nuclear Medicine, 123,* 144-153.

Scharf, S.M. & Cassidy, S.S. (1989). *Heart-Lung Interactions in Health and Disease.* New York: Marcel Dekker, Inc.

Shelhamer, J.H., Ognibene, F.P., Macher, A.M., Tuacon, C, Steiss, R., Longo, D., Kovacs, J.A., Parker, M.M., Natanson, C., & Lane H.C. (1984). Persistence of Pneumocystis carinii in lung tissue of acquired immunodeficiency syndrome patients treated for pneumocystis pneumonia. *American Review of Respiratory Diseases, 130,* 1161-1165.

Sherlock S. (1988). The liver lung interface. *Seminars in Respiratory Medicine, 9,* 247-253.

Steljes, D.G., Kryger, M.H., Kirk, B.W., & Millar, T.W. (1990). Sleep in postpolio syndrome. *Chest, 98,* 133-140.

Trewby, P.N., Warren, R., Contini, S, Crosbie, W.A., Wilkinson, S.P., Laws, J.W., & Williams, R. (1978). Incidence and pathophysiology of pulmonary edema in fulminant hepatic failure. *Gastroenterology, 74,* 859-865.

Wilson, J.D., Braunwald, E., Isselbacher, J.K., Petersdorf, R.G., Martin, J.B., Fauci, A.S., & Root, R.K. (eds). (1991). Harrison's Principles of Internal Medicine. (12th ed.). New York: McGraw Hill.

PART II

Cardiopulmonary Assessment

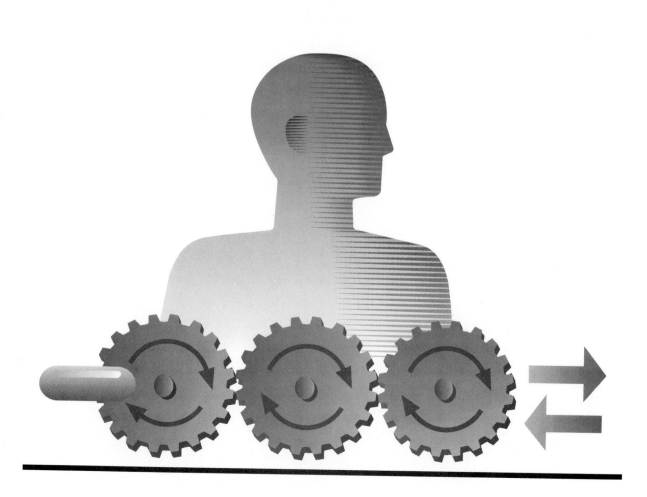

CHAPTER 6

Measurement and Documentation

Claire Peel

KEY TERMS

Documentation
Measurement
Objective assessment

Reliability
Subjective assessment
Validity

INTRODUCTION

Measurement and documentation are critical components of the process of providing patient care. Measurements form the basis for deciding treatment strategies and therefore influence patients' responses to therapeutic interventions. Measurements are also used during treatment sessions to determine rate of progression and appropriateness of exercise prescriptions. Typically, therapists make a series of measurements and in combination with the results of measurements made by other health care professionals, form an impression of the client. The impression includes both physical and psychosocial aspects. If parts of the impression are incorrect because of inaccurate measurements, then the course of treatment may be misdirected. The result could be treatment that is either not effective or unsafe. Consequently, knowledge of the qualities of mea-

surements that relate to the cardiovascular and pulmonary systems is essential for quality patient care.

Documentation of the results of measurements, the interpretation of the results and the patient care plan is important not only for reimbursement but also to assure communication among health care team members. Timely and appropriate sharing of information on physiological responses to activity is often critical for optimal medical management. Documentation needs to be written clearly and concisely, and to include objective findings that will facilitate efficient and continuous care from all members of the health care team.

This chapter provides a discussion of types and characteristics of measurements that are common to cardiopulmonary physical therapy, followed by a discussion of the process of selecting, performing, and interpreting measurements. A discussion of the purposes and types of documentation follows, including suggestions for providing objective and outcome-oriented information.

CHARACTERISTICS OF MEASUREMENTS

The purpose of performing a measurement is to assess or evaluate a characteristic or attribute of an individual. The characteristic to be measured first must be defined, and the purpose of performing each measurement must be clear. Therapists then can select the most appropriate method of measurement given the available resources and their clinical skills.

Levels or Types of Measurements

Measurements can be described according to their type or level of measurement. There are four levels of measurements which are nominal, ordinal, interval and ratio (Rothstein, Echternach, 1993). Recognizing the level of measurement aids in the understanding and interpretation of the result.

Nominal

Objects or people are often placed in categories according to specific characteristics. If the categories have no rank or order, then the measurement is considered nominal. An example of a nominal measurement is the classification of patients with pulmonary dys-

function into those with obstructive lung disease, restrictive lung disease, or a combination of both types of dysfunction. The categories are mutually exclusive, that is, all patients fit into one and only one category.

The categories of a nominal measurement scale are defined using objective indicators that are universally understood. For example, the classification of patients with heart failure could be based on the primary cause for the development of the condition (see the box below, at left). In each case, the cause could be determined by diagnostic testing such as angiography or echocardiography. Clear descriptions of the criteria for inclusion in each category facilitate clinicians' agreement on the assignment of patients to categories. A high percentage of agreement indicates high interrater reliability.

Ordinal

Ordinal measurements are similar to nominal measurements with the exception that the categories are ordered or ranked. The categories in an ordinal scale indicate more or less of an attribute. The scale for rating angina is an example of an ordinal scale (Pollock, Willmore, and Fox, 1978) (see the box below, at right). Each category is defined and a rating of grade 1 angina is less than a rating of grade 4. In an ordinal scale, the differences between consecutive ratings are not neces-

---

> **Common Causes for the Development of Heart Failure**
>
> Myocardial infarction (MI) or ischemia
> Cardiac arrhythmias
> Renal insufficiency
> Cardiomyopathy
> Heart valve abnormalities
> Pericardial effusion or myocarditis
> Pulmonary embolism or pulmonary hypertension
> Spinal cord injury
> Congenital abnormalities
> Aging

From Cahalin, L. P. (1994). Cardiac muscle dysfunction. In Hillegass, E. A., & Sadowsky, H. S. (Eds.). *Essentials of cardiopulmonary pulmonary physical therapy.* Philadelphia: WB Saunders.

> **Angina Scale**
>
> Grade 1: **Light**—The discomfort that is established, but just established
>
> Grade 2: **Light-moderate**—Discomfort from which one can be distracted by a noncataclysmic event; it can be "pain" but usually is not
>
> Grade 3: **Moderate-severe**—Discomfort or pain that prevents distraction by a beautiful woman, handsome man, television show, or other consuming interest; only a tornado, earthquake or explosion can distract one from a grade 3 discomfort or pain
>
> Grade 4: **Severe**—Discomfort that is the most excruciating pain experienced or imaginable

sarily equal. The difference between grade 1 angina and grade 2 is not necessarily the same as between grade 3 and grade 4 angina. Consequently, if numbers are assigned to categories, they can be used to represent rank, but cannot be subjected to mathematical operations. Averaging angina scores is incorrect because by averaging, it is assumed that there are equal intervals between categories.

Categorical measurements are considered ordinal if being assigned to a specific category is considered "better than" or "worse than" another category. For example, patients with angina could be classified as having either stable or unstable angina. This measurement would be considered ordinal, because stable angina usually is considered a better condition to have compared with unstable angina (Hurst, 1990).

Ratio

Ratio measurements have scales with units that are equal in size, and have a zero point that indicates absence of the attribute that is being measured. Examples of ratio measurements that are used in cardiopulmonary physical therapy include vital capacity, cardiac output, and oxygen consumption. Ratio measurements are always positive values, and can be subjected to all arithmetic operations. For example, an aerobic capacity of 4 L/min is twice as great as an aerobic capacity of 2 L/min.

When deciding if a measurement is ratio level or not, the attribute that is being measured is defined. If the zero point indicates absence of the attribute, then the scale would be considered ratio. For example, cardiac output can be defined as the amount of blood in liters ejected from the left ventricle over a 1-minute period. A measurement of zero cardiac output would be absence of the characteristic, or no blood ejected from the left ventricle.

Interval

Measurements that are at interval level have units on a scale with equal distance between consecutive measurements. Interval measurements are differentiated from ratio measurements, because the zero point is arbitrary rather than absolute. An arbitrary zero point is one that does not mean an absence of the characteristic that is being measured. Temperature can be mea-

sured using either an interval or a ratio scale. The Fahrenheit temperature scale assigns the zero point to the temperature at which water freezes, whereas the Kelvin scale assigns the zero point to an absence of heat. The Fahrenheit scale is an example of an interval level of measurement, and the Kelvin scale is a ratio level of measurement.

Measuring force production using an isokinetic dynamometer is an example of an interval measurement commonly used in physical therapy. Patients may be able to generate muscle tension and move an extremity, but register a score of zero because they cannot move as fast as the dynamometer. Interval measurements can have negative values, and can be subjected to some arithmetic operations. Adding and subtracting values is logical. A patient who generates 10 ft-lbs at one session and 20 ft-lbs at the following session increased their torque production by 10 ft-lbs. Interval values cannot be subjected to division or multiplication. It cannot be stated that the patient generated twice as much torque on the second session compared with the first session because it cannot be assumed that a reading of zero indicated no torque production.

Reliability

Reliability is defined as the consistency or reproducibility of a measurement. Ideally, if attempting to measure a specific attribute, the value of the measurement should change only when the attribute changes. However, all measurements have some element of error that contributes to the variability of the measurement. When the error is relatively high, the value of the measurement can change, even though the attribute has not changed. Believing that a change occurred when it did not could result in an inaccurate clinical decision related to treatment planning or progression.

Many factors contribute to variability in the results of measurements. The characteristic being measured may demonstrate a certain degree of variability. Both blood pressure and heart rate vary depending on both mental and physical factors such as body position, hydration level, anxiety and time of day. For these attributes, multiple measurements often are used to provide the best estimate of the patient's true heart rate and blood pressure.

Another factor that contributes to the variability of a measurement is changes in the testing instrument. Testing instruments may vary in their readings because of changes in environmental conditions or malfunction of parts of the instrument. Instruments should be calibrated, that is, compared with a known standard, on a regular basis to assure accuracy of the readings. Some instruments are relatively easy to calibrate. For example, values obtained using aneroid blood pressure devices can easily be compared with values obtained using mercury manometers. Values obtained using either palpation or a heart rate monitor can be compared with values obtained from ECG recordings. The mercury manometer and the electrocardiograph (ECG) would be considered the standard method of measurement. Other devices, such as cycle ergometers, are more difficult to calibrate, and the usual approach is to rely on the manufacturer's specifications as to the accuracy of the work rate readings.

A third factor contributing to measurement variability is differences in the methods that therapists use to make measurements. If a result is consistent when one therapist repeats a measurement, then the measurement is said to have high intrarater reliability. Measurements that are consistent when multiple therapists perform the measurement under the same conditions are said to have high interrater reliability. Often, measurements have high interrater reliability, but lower intrarater reliability because therapists vary in the specific methods of making the measurement. For example, a slight variation in the anatomical site used for measuring skinfold thickness can produce relatively large differences in percent fat estimates (Ruiz, Colley, and Hamilton, 1971). Interrater reliability is important in clinical settings where a patient may be evaluated and treated by more than one therapist. If the interrater reliability of a measurement is low, then changes in the patient over time may not be accurately reflected.

Validity

Valid measurements are those that provide meaningful information and that accurately reflect the characteristic for which the measurement is intended. For a measurement to be useful in a clinical setting, the measurement must possess a certain degree of validity. Measurements can be reliable but not valid. For example, measurements made using bioelectrical impedance analyses have been shown to be valid for the estimation of total body water, but uncertainty exists as to the validity of estimates of percent body fat made with this device (Kusher and Schoeller, 1986).

There are various types of validity. Of importance in clinical practice are concurrent, predictive, and prescriptive validity. Concurrent validity is when a measurement accurately reflects measurements made with an accepted standard. Comparing bioelectrical impedance measurements for estimating percent body fat with estimates made from hydrostatic weighing is an example of determining concurrent validity. In this example, hydrostatic weighing would be considered the "gold" or accepted standard. Measurements with predictive validity can be used to estimate the probability of occurrence of a future event. Screening tests often involve measurements that are used to predict future events. For example, by identifying people with risk factors for coronary artery disease (CAD), a prediction is made that the likelihood of developing CAD is higher than normal. Measurements with prescriptive validity provide a guide to the direction of treatment. The categorical measurement of determining a person's risk for a future coronary event is a measurement that would need to have predictive validity. By classifying patients into high vs. low risk categories based on the results of a diagnostic exercise test, the intensity, and rate of progression of treatment is determined.

The accuracy of various types of exercise tests often is described by reporting sensitivity and specificity. Sensitivity is the ability of a test to identify individuals who are "positive," or who have the characteristic that is being measured. Specificity is the ability of a test to identify individuals who are "negative," or who do not have the characteristic. If a test produces a high number of "false positive" results, then the sensitivity will be low. A false positive result means that the test result was positive but the characteristic was absent. Young women often have positive stress test results but do not have CAD. The consequence of a false positive test result could be unnecessary treatment. A high number of "false negative" results would produce a low specificity. A false negative result would be a negative test result, even though the disease or characteristic is present. The consequence of a false negative test result is not receiving treatment when it is indicated.

Objective and Subjective Measurements

Measurements vary in degree of subjectivity vs. objectivity. Subjective measurements are those that are affected in some way by the person taking the measurement, that is, the measurer must make a judgment as to the value assigned. The assessment of a patient's breath sounds is influenced by many factors including the therapist's choice of terminology for describing the findings, their perception of normal breath sounds, and their hearing acuity. The grading of functional skills may be influenced by the therapist's interpretation of what constitutes minimal vs. moderate assistance. Because of the influence of the person performing the measurement, subjective measurements usually have lower interrater reliability compared to objective measurements (Rothstein and Echternach, 1993).

Objective measurements are not affected by the person performing the measurement, that is, these measurements do not involve judgement of the measurer. Heart rate measured by a computerized ECG system is an example of an objective measurement. Other examples include measurement of blood pressure using an intraarterial catheter or oxygen consumption using a metabolic system. Objective measurements are not necessarily accurate, but usually have high interrater reliability (Rothstein, and Echternach, 1993).

Most measurements cannot be classified as either objective or subjective. The quality of a measurement can be placed on a continuum based on the degree of reliability, as shown in Figure 6-1. The attribute or characteristic that is being measured also can be viewed as a subjective or objective phenomena

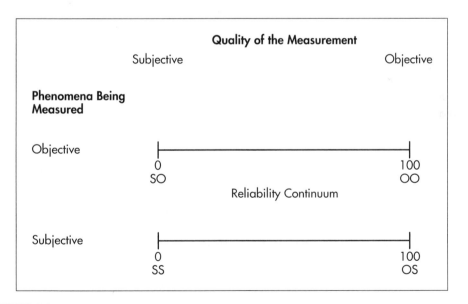

FIGURE 6-1

Illustration of the relationship between the quality of a measurement as being subjective or objective, and the phenomenon being measured. The scales indicate that the objectivity of a measurement, or reliability, lies along a continuum. For example, a subjective phenomenon may be measured subjectively (subjective sign [SS]) or objectively (objective sign [OS]). (From Rothstein JM: On defining subjective and objective measurements, *Phys Ther* 69:577-579, 1989.)

(Rothstein, 1989). A subjective attribute such as pain can be measured in either a subjective manner with a low degree of reliability, or in an objective manner with a high degree of reliability.

SELECTING MEASUREMENTS

At the initial session with a client, how do therapists decide on the measurements to be performed? And what additional measurements need to be performed during the course of treatment and at follow-up evaluations? Many factors influence the choice of the therapist, including information obtained from the medical record and the patient interview, and knowledge of available treatment options. Therapists also must strive for efficiency and not repeat tests that have been performed by other health care professionals. Characteristics or qualities of measurements, such as reliability and validity also influence the therapist's decision.

Medical and personal information about the client will be a primary factor guiding the selection of measurements. For example, appropriate measurements differ for a patient with an acute MI vs. a patient who is 3 weeks post-MI. Other factors to consider include the size of the infarction and associated complications such as arrhythmias, heart failure, or angina. Information collected during the patient interview also may guide the selection. For example, for patients who display anxiety when walking on a treadmill is discussed, another mode of exercise may be more appropriate. Measurements need to be selected that are appropriate to the specific pathology, the severity of the condition, and other characteristics unique to the patient.

Another important factor to consider in selecting measurements is the application of the information. Every measurement should contribute to the decisions made by the therapist on the course and progression of treatment. Measurements that do not contribute to the assessment of the patient result in an inefficient use of the therapist's time and add unnecessary costs to medical care.

Another factor that influences the selection of measurements is the risk-benefit ratio. How do risks of conducting a test or measurement relate to the value of the information gained? Subjecting a patient to a symptom-limited exercise test during the acute stage post-MI could provide information to formulate an exercise prescription. However, the risks of performing this procedure at this time in the recovery period may outweigh the benefits.

PERFORMING MEASUREMENTS

When performing measurements, care must be taken to use procedures that can be replicated for future comparisons. Time must be taken to ensure that conditions are optimal and that the patient is informed of his or her part in the activity. For example, measuring blood pressure in a noisy treatment area immediately when the patient arrives for an appointment may not provide an accurate measurement of resting or baseline blood pressure. Documenting the conditions in which a measurement was made also is important. Conditions may include, but are not limited to, time of day, room temperature, recent activities performed by the patient, and type of measuring device.

Measurements should be made with an objective and open mind, that is, without anticipating the result of the measurement. A measurement that is approached with a preconceived idea of the outcome may be affected by the therapist's expectations. Having confidence in the results of one's measurements is important, and is developed as clinical skills are developed.

In clinics where more than one therapist is likely to evaluate or treat a patient, written procedures for performing measurements are needed. Therapists also need to review the written procedures on a regular basis and practice performing the measurements as a group. Practicing together is especially important for therapists who are new to the clinic. The interrater reliability for commonly used measurements then can be determined. If the reliability is low, the written procedures may need to be revised to assure optimal consistency of measurement.

INTERPRETING MEASUREMENTS

Interpreting the results of measurements often is a difficult task. Usually patients' problems are understood not by reviewing the results of a single measurement, but by viewing the relationships between the results of several measurements. For example, the finding that blood pressure does not increase with activity by itself may not be considered abnormal, if the activity level is low and the patient is taking a beta receptor antagonist medication. The finding of no increase in blood pressure with signs and symptoms of exercise intolerance during moderate level activity in another patient may be indicative of inadequate cardiac output.

A knowledge of what is "normal" is important to be able to interpret the results of tests. For some measurements, normal values are well-defined. Measurements of resting blood pressure, cholesterol, and blood glucose have defined categories of normal, borderline, and elevated. For other measurements, population normative standards are not well-defined. For example, what is the normal increase in heart rate when walking at 3.5 mph on a level surface? Values for individuals differ, depending on age, medications, fitness level, and walking efficiency. Results need to be interpreted by considering these factors and pathological conditions if present. Each individual has their own "normal" or usual response, and variations from this value could be considered abnormal.

Interpreting the results of tests is similar to putting the pieces of a puzzle together to create a picture of the patient and their limitations. Information is collected from several sources, including the medical record, patient interview and physical therapy evaluation. Measurements performed and interpreted by other health care professionals can be obtained from the medical record and include chest x-ray, blood analyses, and echocardiography. During an interview, the patient reports information about his current and past medical problems. It is important to be sensitive to the patient's feelings about his condition, noting his stage of emotional recovery. Detecting attitudes related to changing lifestyle habits also is important. After the interview, the therapist should have a sense of the patient as a person and begin to plan a strategy for optimizing his or her physical function.

Measurements made during the physical examination may include physiological responses to activity, breathing patterns, ventilatory capacity, and breath sounds. The results of these measurements are integrated with results collected during the chart review and viewed in the context of the patient's personal goals. Therapists develop a picture of the severity of the cardiopulmonary condition, the stage of recovery, and the presence of coexisting conditions. A treatment plan is developed based on the composite of findings. The plan is implemented and is continuously checked for appropriate direction by measurements made during treatment sessions. Because of the progressive nature of many of the conditions that affect the cardiovascular and pulmonary systems, each treatment session can be viewed as a reassessment.

PURPOSES OF DOCUMENTATION

To be useful, measurements need to be recorded or documented in a concise and organized manner. Measurements that remain in the mind of the evaluator often are forgotten or not remembered accurately. Documentation is becoming more important to assist and to maximize reimbursement, as well as to facilitate efficiency of care through communication between health care professionals.

Documentation includes information about evaluative findings, the assessment of the patient's condition, and the plan for future care. Reasons for documentation include the following:

1. To provide information for other therapists, assistants, or aides who may evaluate and/or treat the client.
2. To provide data for comparison for follow-up visits.
3. To provide data to determine treatment effectiveness and efficiency through collection of information on the results or outcomes of various types of care.
4. To assist therapists in organizing findings to facilitate logical decisions on the treatment approach and overall care plan.

TYPES OF DOCUMENTATION

Systems for documenting information vary between facilities. In acute care hospitals, physical therapy notes may be included as a part of the patient's comprehensive medical record. In other facilities such as private practice clinics the patient's record may consist of physical therapy notes and medical information that is relative to the physical therapy care plan. Whatever the system, notes can be classified according to the timing and purpose of the documentation, using the following categories:

1. Initial evaluation, assessment, and plan
2. Interim or progress notes
3. Discharge notes
4. Follow-up or reevaluation notes

The initial note usually is the longest, containing information on the reason for referral, other medical conditions and information that could affect physical therapy management, data collected during the patient interview and physical examination, an assessment or interpretation of the findings and the care plan. Interim or progress notes record short-term changes in the patient's status, and typically are written on a daily or weekly basis. The discharge note records the specific outcomes of treatment, the plan for discharge, including home program, and the plan for follow-up. At follow-up visits, a note is written to assess changes since the time of discharge and plans for additional treatment.

GENERAL GUIDELINES FOR CONTENT AND ORGANIZATION

Writing notes in a clear and concise format is important so that information is conveyed accurately. Examples of unclear notes are ones in which the handwriting is illegible, or that contain vague statements that could be interpreted in more than one way. Concise notes are more likely to be read by other health care professionals. In most clinicians' schedules, time is not available to read through extensive information about a patient that may not be relevant. A concise note only includes essential information in a writing style that is clear and does not include unnecessary phrases. Another important rule is to use only standard or accepted abbreviations. Facilities have lists of approved abbreviations for that facility. The list should be available to those who write, read, and review records. Within a physical therapy department, common terms need to be clearly defined and used in a consistent manner by all staff. Terms that often generate confusion and carry multiple meanings include "minimally assisted," "functional

ambulation," and "abnormal tone." Written definitions of commonly used terms that include examples of characteristics that illustrate the definition can help to decrease confusion.

Notes also need to clearly demonstrate the need for professional skills if a physical therapist is performing the evaluation and/or treatment. Activities that can be performed by physical therapists assistants, aides, nursing personnel or family members need to be delegated to the appropriate individual. In addition, patients can be instructed in those activities in which they can perform independently.

Another time in which documentation is essential is when an unusual or adverse event occurs. For example, abnormal responses to activity that may appear relatively benign are important to record. Abnormal responses may include dizziness, anginal or musculoskeletal pain, or arrhythmias. An unusually high or low heart rate or blood pressure response also should be noted. Combined with findings noted by the patient or other health care professionals, these results may indicate significant changes in the patient's cardiopulmonary status.

The organization of documentation varies between facilities. Many facilities use the SOAP (subjective, objective, assessment, plan) format (Kettenbach, 1990). Other facilities have modified this format, with the same information organized in a different way. The following section presents an overview of relevant subjective and objective information, and a description of items to include in the assessment and plan.

Subjective Information

Subjective information contains a degree of judgement or interpretation by the person reporting the information. The patient and family's perceptions of their cardiac or pulmonary condition are considered subjective information. In the initial note, descriptions of pain or discomfort that may be associated with either a cardiac event or a pulmonary complication are important to include. Some of the information reported by the patient may be objective, such as blood cholesterol levels, resting blood pressure values or number of cigarettes smoked per day.

In the interim note, it is important to record the patient's responses to treatment including feelings of angina, dyspnea, or fatigue. Whether a prescribed home or ward activity program is performed and the patient's subjective responses to the program also are important to note. Any reported changes in the ability to function either at home or in the community are important to record. The most important subjective finding to report in the discharge note is whether the patient believes personal treatment goals were achieved.

Objective Information

Measurable or observable information that is collected during the interview, evaluation, and treatment is considered objective. Information from the medical record may be included if it is relevant to the patient's current condition. To be relevant, the information should have potential impact on the direction of the evaluation and treatment of the patient, such as current medications and results of diagnostic tests. Results of tests and measurements conducted as a part of the initial evaluation are objective information. A description of the treatment that is provided, and the patient's physiological responses to treatment also are considered objective information.

When recording information collected during the evaluation, the results of various tests can be categorized as impairments or as functional limitations. An impairment is an abnormality of physiological function or anatomical structure at the tissue, organ or body system level (Jette, 1994). Examples of impairments include decreases in muscle strength or range of motion, or abnormal heart rate and blood pressure values. A functional limitation is a restriction in performance at the level of the whole person (Jette, 1994). Functional limitations can be attributed to physical, social, cognitive, or emotional factors. Examples of functional limitations include the inability to dress, transfer, ambulate, or climb stairs. Improvements in functional status usually are of primary interest to patients and families and to those who reimburse for health care. Measurements of impairments are important, because they assist therapists in deciphering the causes or reasons for limitations in function.

The description of the evaluation and treatment results needs to include specific information on the activity, or exercise stress, and on the physiological responses. Components of the activity description include the following:

1. Mode of activity (corridor or track walking, lower extremity cycling)
2. Work level or rate (mph, percent grade, estimated resting metabolic rate level)
3. Duration of activity at each work level

The description of the activities should be written clearly so that the workload can be reproduced. The responses to activity include changes in heart rate and rhythm, blood pressure, respiratory rate, oxygen saturation levels, and heart and breath sounds as compared with from preactivity to either during or immediately after activity. Signs of exercise intolerance, such as changes in skin color, incoordination, and sweating, also need to be documented. Whether the patient used oxygen during treatment, or required physical assistance also should be noted. By objectively recording the activity prescription and the physiological responses, therapists can estimate the patient's activity tolerance.

Assessment

The purpose of the assessment part of a note is to list the client's major problem(s), identify treatment goals or outcomes, and provide an interpretation of the subjective and objective findings. The problem list is limited to problems that can be addressed by physical therapy. Problems can be listed in order of priority and stated in functional terms. For example, stating "patient unable to climb stairs because of abnormal ECG responses and dizziness," rather than stating "abnormal ECG response during activity."

Goals are the outcomes to be achieved by participating in a physical therapy program and are generated by the therapist and patient in consultation. Goals are stated in functional terms as to what the patient will be able to do at discharge. The following is an example:

Patient will be able to carry one 25-lb. bag a distance of 50 feet with appropriate heart rate and rhythm responses, within 2 weeks.

To be able to determine if a goal has been met, the therapist must be able to observe or to measure the activity. Therapists also estimate the time that it will take to achieve the outcome. In the discharge note, whether each goal has been met is stated. If a goal has not been achieved, then a reason or explanation is provided.

The assessment also includes a brief interpretation of the subjective and objective findings. Therapists can use this section to state their "clinical hypothesis," or explanation of the primary problem that produces the objective and subjective findings. The initial note may include statements about the individual's potential to succeed in a rehabilitation program, or reasons for not performing tests that would typically be performed with individuals with similar diagnoses. Whether the patient needs to be referred to other health care professionals or to community services also can be included.

Plan

The plan provides a description of the approach that will be taken to assist the patient in achieving the stated goals. The plan may include a description of treatment that can be provided, education for the patient and/or family, and referrals to other services. Descriptions of home or ward programs should be included in the plan. At discharge from an inpatient unit, the plan includes where the patient will be residing and plans for follow-up. At discharge from an outpatient facility, the plan contains recommendations for follow-up care.

SUMMARY

Measurement and documentation are important components of the process of providing patient care. Therapists select measurements because they reveal information about patient characteristics that is needed to determine appropriate directions for treatment. Performing measurements in a consistent way allows comparison of patient characteristics at varied points in time. The recording, or documentation, of the results of measurements and other information about the patient serves as a legal record. Although documentation formats vary between facilities, information from records can be organized into sections describing subjective and objective information, assessment or interpretation of the findings, and the care plan. Subjective and objective information is collected during an interview, medical record review, and evaluation and/or treatment session. The assessment provides an interpretation of the subjective and objective findings, and states the desired treatment outcomes. A specific plan to achieve the outcomes then is described. Documentation can be viewed as a way to assist therapists to organize their findings, reflect on the significance of the findings, and generate an efficient and comprehensive care plan.

REVIEW QUESTIONS

1. Describe and give examples of nominal, ordinal, ratio and interval measurements.
2. Identify three factors that contribute to the variability of measurements.
3. Define sensitivity and specificity of tests.
4. Differentiate between objective and subjective measurements.
5. Identify four purposes for documenting the results of evaluation and treatment sessions.

References

Hurst, J.W. (1990). The recognition and treatment of four types of angina pectoris and angina equivalents. In Hurst, J.W., Schlant, R.C., Rackley, C.E., Sonnonblick, E.H., & Wenger, N.K. (Eds.). The heart (7th ed.). New York: McGraw-Hill.

Jette, A.M. (1994). Physical disablement concepts for physical therapy research and practice. *Physical Therapy 74*, 380-386.

Kettenbach, G. (1990). *Writing S.O.A.P. notes.* Philadelphia: FA Davis.

Kusher, R.F. & Schoeller, D.A. (1986). Estimation of total body water by bioelectrical impedance analysis. *American Journal of Clinical Nutrition. 44*, 417-424.

Pollock, M.L., Wilmore, J.H., & Fox, S.M. (1978). *Health and fitness through physical activity.* New York: John Wiley and Sons.

Rothstein, J.M. (1989). On defining subjective and objective measurements. *Physical Therapy 69*, 577-579.

Rothstein, J.M., & Echternach, J.L. (1993). *Primer on measurement: An introductory guide to measurement issues.* Alexandria, VA: American Physical Therapy Association.

Ruiz, L., & Colley, J.R.T. & Hamilton, P.J.S. (1971). Measurement of triceps skinfold thickness: An investigation of sources of variation. *British Journal of Preventive and Social Medicine 25*, 165-167.

CHAPTER 7

History

Willy E. Hammon

INTRODUCTION

The value of the history depends in large part on the skill of the interviewer. When eliciting the history from a patient, therapists must be alert to recognize the symptoms that are indicative of cardiac and pulmonary disease. This information is then used in the decision-making process to select the most appropriate intervention for the individual.

THE INTERVIEW

Obtaining a thorough and accurate patient history is truly an art. One important goal of history taking is to establish a good patient-therapist rapport. The patient must be allowed to explain the history in his or her own words and pace (Hurst, et al, 1990). If the therapist appears hurried, distracted, preoccupied, irritated, or uncaring; is often interrupted; or fails to be an attentive listener, the patient-therapist relationship will likely suffer.

The interviewer must be careful not to allow personal feelings about the patient's grooming, appearance, demeanor, and behavior during the interview to unduly question the validity of the chief complaints (Birdwell, 1993). By the time the patient is referred for physical therapy, he or she may have seen one or more physicians, have been subjected to a number of noninvasive or invasive studies, or have been prescribed oral or inhaled medications with variable or unsatisfactory alleviation of symptoms. The patient is likely to manifest a degree of anxiety and frustration.

Therefore the therapist's approach, history-taking and interviewing style is important for gaining the patient's confidence and cooperation.

The patient history interview can be divided into the data-gathering and interpretative sections (Snider, 1994). The data-gathering segment begins with asking why the patient has sought medical attention and has been referred for physical therapy services. In other words, what is the patient's chief complaint—the symptom that caused the patient to seek help?

Each chief complaint should be carefully explored. Supplementary questions should be nonleading, using words the patient can easily understand. This allows the interviewer to determine the significance of the complaint. An in-depth knowledge of cardiopulmonary pathophysiology allows the therapist to almost simultaneously gather data about the patient's symptoms and to interpret the likely type of cardiopulmonary dysfunction that exists. This in turn serves as a basis for the therapist to begin to select the appropriate assessment and treatment modalities for the individual.

It is important to remember that patient satisfaction is greatest if the patient is allowed to fully express major concerns without interrupting. In addition, the risk of missing what is really of greatest concern to the patient is reduced if the patient is allowed sufficient time to describe it in his or her own words. Studies have shown this usually only takes from 1 to 3 minutes.

The patient's view of what is the problem and his or her suggestions for addressing the problem should be included in the interview. Patient satisfaction is improved by his or her involvement in the interview as well as later in the establishment of short- and long-term goals.

The depth of the history taken by the physical therapist (PT) can vary according to the following factors:

1. **Whether the individual is an inpatient or an outpatient.** Many inpatients have detailed medical records available for the therapist to review. This significantly reduces the amount of information the therapist needs to obtain from the patient during an interview. If the information in the chart is scant, or if the individual is an outpatient with only a treatment referral and little or no medical records available, the therapist should obtain a more detailed history.

2. **Whether the treatment order is narrow or broad in scope.**
3. **The acuteness of the patient's illness, level of consciousness, and his ability to provide accurate information.**

This chapter presents a comprehensive approach to history taking. Therapists may find part or all of this information applicable, depending on their particular circumstances.

QUESTIONNAIRES

Printed symptom or medical questionnaires can be beneficial or detrimental to the patient-therapist relationship, depending on how they are used. Questionnaires can expedite the data-gathering portion of the initial visit by allowing the patient to note in advance, all symptoms, medical conditions, surgeries, occupations, medications, and other factors that may influence physical therapy intervention. They can reduce the amount of nontreatment time therapists may otherwise spend inquiring about irrelevant symptoms and conditions. Printed questionnaires also allow patients sufficient time to recall relevant information and respond more accurately than they often do in an interview setting (Miller, 1980). Used in this way, a printed questionnaire can be a valuable tool for expediting a comprehensive evaluation of cardiopulmonary patients.

However, if questionnaires are used improperly, they can depersonalize the history-taking portion of the initial visit (Hurst, et al, 1990). If the therapist allows the printed form to become a substitute for interaction with the patient, patient satisfaction will be low and the patient-therapist relationship will suffer.

DYSPNEA

Dyspnea, breathlessness or shortness of breath, can be defined as the sensation of difficulty in breathing (George, 1990). It is one of the most common reasons that patients seek medical attention. Dyspnea is difficult to quantitate, because it is subjective and at times is normal (i.e., at high altitudes, and during or following vigorous exercise). Dyspnea is a symptom of cardiac and pulmonary diseases, as well as other conditions.

When a patient complains of shortness of breath or

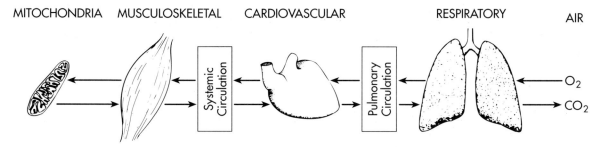

MITOCHONDRIA   MUSCULOSKELETAL   CARDIOVASCULAR   RESPIRATORY   AIR

Systemic Circulation

Pulmonary Circulation

O_2

CO_2

FIGURE 7-1

Schematic illustration of the oxygen transport system, which involves the interaction between the respiratory, cardiovascular, and musculoskeletal systems. (Reprinted with permission from Mahler D: Dyspnea: diagnosis and management. *Clin Chest Med* 8 [2], 215–230, 1987.)

breathlessness, it should be noted that this complaint is often unrelated to the patient's arterial oxygen level (Pao_2). Many times, it appears that altered mechanical factors during breathing contribute to the sensation of breathlessness (Mahler, 1987). Numerous receptors that have a role in sensing dyspnea have been identified and include vagal receptors (e.g., irritant, stretch, and J-receptors), chemoreceptors, proprioceptive receptors (tendon organs, muscle spindles, joint and/or skin receptors), and upper airway receptors (Snider, 1994).

Analyzing the oxygen transport system (Figure 7-1) can help the therapist determine the likely cause of each patient's dyspnea and the most appropriate physical therapy intervention. The delivery of oxygen from ambient air to the mitochondrion within the cell depends on the intact interaction of the respiratory, cardiovascular, and muscular systems. Also, carbon dioxide (CO_2) is eliminated in the opposite direction. Dyspnea can be caused by dysfunction in any of the systems.

Dyspnea commonly occurs when the body's requirement for breathing (ventilation) exceeds the body's capacity to provide (Snider, 1994). In other words, the symptom varies directly with the body's demand for ventilation and inversely with ventilatory capacity.

There are three basic causes of dyspnea: (1) an increased awareness of normal breathing, (2) an increase

in the work of breathing, and (3) an abnormality in the ventilatory system itself (George, 1990).

An increased awareness of normal breathing is usually related to anxiety (Miller, 1980). The patient commonly complains of "not getting a deep enough breath," a feeling of "smothering," or "not getting air down in the right places" (Szidan and Fishman, 1988). These sensations have been designated as psychogenic dyspnea. The patient's breathing pattern is irregular, with frequent sighs. When severe, it is associated with tingling of the hands and feet, circumoral numbness, and lightheadedness. Coaching the patient to hyperventilate and to reproduce the symptoms may help the patient better understand the cause of these symptoms and how to control them (Miller, 1980). The hyperventilation syndrome is properly diagnosed only after organic causes have been excluded and pulmonary function tests indicate normal respiratory mechanics and Pao_2.

The second cause of dyspnea is an increase in the work of breathing. Greater inspiratory pressures must be generated by the respiratory muscles to move air in and out of the lungs when the mechanical properties of the lungs have changed. This may be related to an increase in lung water resulting from cardiac disease or the high cardiac output of anemia. A loss of compliance (increased lung stiffness) because of diffuse inflammatory or fibrotic lung disease often causes shortness of breath. Small or large airways obstruction as a result of bronchoconstriction, sputum, inflammation, and other effects commonly produces dyspnea.

The third cause of dyspnea is an abnormality in the ventilatory apparatus or pump. The ventilatory apparatus consists of the thoracic cage, respiratory muscles, and nerves. Any of these may become dysfunctional. Thoracic cage abnormalities include kyphoscoliosis, extreme obesity, and large pleural effusions. Diseases of the respiratory muscles include polymyositis and muscular dystrophy. Neurologic abnormalities include spinal cord injuries, phrenic nerve injuries, brachial plexus neuropathy, ascending polyneuritis (Guillain-Barre syndrome), myasthenia gravis, amyotrophic lateral sclerosis, poliomyelitis, neurotoxins, and exposure to paralytic agents.

The time course of the appearance and progression of dyspnea should be identified (Sharf, 1989). Acute dyspnea is common in pulmonary embolism, pneumothorax, acute asthma, pulmonary congestion related to congestive heart failure (CHF), pneumonia, and upper airways obstruction. Most of these conditions require immediate physician evaluation of the acute problem before physical therapy intervention. Subacute or chronic progression of dyspnea generally presents as increasingly severe dyspnea with exertion over time. It occurs with emphysema, restrictive lung disorders such as pulmonary fibrosis, chest wall deformities, respiratory muscle dysfunction, occupational lung diseases, chronic CHF, or large pleural effusions.

Dyspnea may also be related to body position. Therefore when evaluating dyspnea, the patient should be asked if he or she has difficulty breathing when reclining horizontally. Is it necessary to be propped up on several pillows to sleep at night (orthopnea)? Does she have more difficulty breathing when reclining on one side (trepopnea)? Does he ever wake up at night short of breath, and need to sit up or walk around the room to "catch his breath" (paroxysmal nocturnal dyspnea)?

Acute Dyspnea

The patient that has acute dyspnea requires a rapid and thorough history and physical assessment. The therapist should ask several important questions to address the possible causes of acute dyspnea (Mahler, 1987):

1. **Are you short of breath at rest?** If the answer is yes, it suggests a severe physiological dysfunction. The patient likely needs prompt evaluation by a physician if this is of recent onset and has not had a medical workup.
2. **Do you have chest pain?** If so what part of your chest? Unilateral localized chest pain raises the possibility of spontaneous pneumothorax, pulmonary embolism, or chest trauma.
3. **What were you doing immediately before or at the time of onset of shortness of breath?** Approximately 75% of spontaneous pneumothoraces occur during sedentary activity, 20% during some strenuous activity, and 5% are related to coughing or sneezing. A history of immobilization of a lower extremity, recent surgery, bed rest, travel requiring prolonged sitting, obesity, CHF, venous disease of the lower extremities, are all risk factors for pulmonary embolism. If the patient's symptoms are related to chest trauma, the fact that a fall, a blow, or an accident occurred can usually be quickly established.
4. **Do you have any major medical or surgical conditions?** Cystic fibrosis, chronic obstructive pulmonary disease (COPD), interstitial lung disease, and malignancies are important causes of secondary spontaneous pneumothorax.

If the therapist strongly suspects pneumothorax or pulmonary emboli because of the history and physical assessment, the patient should be referred for immediate medical evaluation.

Dyspnea on Exertion

Dyspnea on exertion is a common complaint of patients with cardiopulmonary dysfunction. Dyspnea during exercise or exertion usually precedes dyspnea at rest (Wasserman, 1982). It most often is a result of chronic pulmonary disease or CHF. Some causes of dyspnea during exertion or exercise are listed in Table 7-1.

It is important to establish the amount of activity required to produce dyspnea. Various scales (Borg, 1982; Mahler and Harver, 1990) have been developed to categorize the level of dyspnea and impairment present in patients (Figures 7-2, 7-3 and Table 7-2). The patient should be asked about daily activity, and what activities

TABLE 7-1

Disorders Limiting Exercise Performance, Pathophysiology, and Discriminating Measurements*

DISORDERS	PATHOPHYSIOLOGY	MEASUREMENTS THAT DEVIATE FROM NORMAL
Pulmonary		
Airflow limitation	Mechanical limitation to ventilation mismatching of V_A/Q, hypoxic stimulation to breathing	V_E max/MVV, expiratory flow pattern, V_D/V_T; Vo_2 max, V_E/Vo_2 V_E response to hyperoxia, (A-a)Po_2
Restrictive	Mismatching V_A/Q, hypoxic stimulation to breathing	
Chest wall	Mechanical limitation to ventilation	V_E max/MVV, $Paco_2$ VO_2 max
Pulmonary circulation	Rise in physiological dead space as fraction of V_T, exercise hypoxemia	V_D/V_T, work-rate-related hypoxemia Vo_2 max, V_E/Vo_2, (a-ET)Pco_2, O_2–pulse
Cardiac		
Coronary	Coronary insufficiency	Electrocardiogram (ECG), Vo_2 max, anaerobic threshold O_2, V_E/Vo_2 O_2-pulse, blood pressure (BP) (systolic, diastolic, pulse)
Valvular	Cardiac output limitation (decreased effective stroke volume)	
Myocardial	Cardiac output limitation (decreased ejection fraction and stroke volume)	
Anemia	Reduced O_2 carrying capacity	O_2-pulse, anaerobic threshold Vo_2, Vo_2 max, V_E/Vo_2
Peripheral circulation	Inadequate O_2 flow to metabolically active muscle	Anaerobic threshold Vo_2, Vo_2 max
Obesity	Increased work to move body; if severe, respiratory restriction and pulmonary insufficiency	Vo_2-work rate relationship, Pao_2, $Paco_2$, Vo_2 max
Psychogenic	Hyperventilation with precisely regular respiratory rate	Breathing pattern, Pco_2
Malingering	Hyperventilation and hypoventilation with irregular respiratory rate	Breathing pattern, Pco_2
Deconditioning	Inactivity or prolonged bedrest; loss of capability for effective redistribution of systemic blood flow	O_2-pulse, anaerobic threshold Vo_2, Vo_2 max

*V_A—alveolar ventilation; Q—pulmonary blood flow; MVV—maximum voluntary ventilation; V_D/V_T—physiologic dead space/tidal volume ratio; O_2—oxygen; Vo_2—O_2 consumption; (A-a)Po_2—alveolar-arterial Po_2 difference; (a-ET)Pco_2—arterial-end tidal Pco_2 difference. (Reprinted with permission from Wasserman K: Dyspnea on exertion: Is it the heart or lungs? *JAMA* 248: 2039–2043, 1982. © 1982 American Medical Association.)

produce breathlessness (Constant, 1993). Does the patient become short of breath climbing a flight of stairs or walking uphill? Is the patient able to walk and talk simultaneously? Does walking slower affect the individual's dyspnea?

In addition, when the patient began to notice an increase in shortness of breath should be noted. A recent onset of dyspnea is more characteristic of heart failure than chronic lung disease, which has a longer, insidious onset. Acute pulmonary problems such as pneumothorax, atelectasis, pneumonia, and other conditions superimposed on chronic lung disease can also explain a recent increase in symptoms.

Is wheezing present with the dyspnea on exertion?

TABLE 7-2

American Thoracic Society Dyspnea Scale

GRADE	DEGREE	
0	None	Not troubled with breathlessness except with strenuous exercise
1	Slight	Troubled by shortness of breath when hurrying on the level or walking up a slight hill
2	Moderate	Walks slower than people of the same age on the level because of breathlessness or has to stop for breath when walking at own pace on the level
3	Severe	Stops for breath after walking about 100 yards or after a few minutes on the level
4	Very severe	Too breathless to leave the house or breathless when dressing or undressing

Reprinted with permission from Brooks SM (Chairman): Task group on surveillance for respiratory hazards in the occupational setting. Surveillance for respiratory hazards, *ATS News* 12–16, 1982.

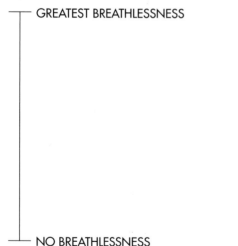

0	Nothing at all
0.5	Very, very slight (just noticeable)
1	Very slight
2	Slight
3	Moderate
4	Somewhat severe
5	Severe
6	
7	Very severe
8	
9	Very, very severe (almost maximal)
10	Maximal

FIGURE 7-2

The visual analogue scale is a vertical line of 100 mm in length. The patient is asked to make a mark along this line that represents his level of breathlessness. The distance of the patient's mark above zero represents the measurement of dyspnea. (Reprinted with permission from Mahler D: Dyspnea: diagnosis and management, *Clin Chest Med* 8 [2], 215–230, 1987.)

FIGURE 7-3

The Borg category scale for rating breathlessness. (Reprinted with permission from Borg G: Psychophysical bases of perceived exertion, *Med Sci Sports Exerc* 14, 377–381, 1982.)

Has there been an associated weight gain? Does the patient have a positive smoking history and sputum production? If a positive response is received, these suggest that COPD is the primary cause of symptoms (Constant, 1993).

The basic defect that cardiac diseases produce during exertion is a limited cardiac output, primarily caused by a reduced stroke volume (Wasserman, 1982). To compensate for the relatively low stroke volume, the patient develops a rapid heart rate and a wide arteriovenous O_2 difference (decreased capillary PO_2) at an inappropriately low work rate. Therefore the exercising muscles (both skeletal and myocardial) have increased difficulty getting an adequate oxygen supply to perform the necessary work, which results in dyspnea, fatigue or pain. The lactic acidosis that results from the low oxygen delivery to the muscles can be measured by either invasive or noninvasive

---

Functional and Therapeutic Classification of Patients with Heart Disease

Functional Classification
Class I

Patients with cardiac disease but without resulting limitations of physical activity; ordinary physical activity does not cause undue fatigue, palpitation, dyspnea, or anginal pain.

Class II

Patients with cardiac disease resulting in slight limitation of physical activity; they are comfortable at rest. Ordinary physical activity results in fatigue, palpitation, dyspnea, or anginal pain.

Class III

Patients with cardiac disease resulting in marked limitation of physical activity; they are comfortable at rest. Less than ordinary physical activity causes fatigue, palpitation, dyspnea, or anginal pain.

Class IV

Patients with cardiac disease resulting in inability to carry on any physical activity without discomfort; symptoms of cardiac insufficiency or of the anginal syndrome may be present even at rest. If any physical activity is undertaken, discomfort increases.

Therapeutic Classification
Class A

Patients with cardiac disease whose physical activity need not be restricted in any way.

Class B

Patients with cardiac disease whose ordinary physical activity need not be restricted but who should be advised against severe or competitive efforts.

Class C

Patients with cardiac disease whose ordinary activities should be moderately restricted and whose more strenuous efforts should be discontinued.

Class D

Patients with cardiac disease whose ordinary activity should be markedly restricted.

Class E

Patients with cardiac disease who should be at complete rest, confined to bed or chair.

Reprinted with permission from the New York Heart Association (1964). *Diseases of the heart and blood vessels; Nomenclature and criteria for diagnosis.* (6th ed.). Boston: Little, Brown.

gas-exchange methods during exercise testing. The functional and therapeutic capacity of the patient with heart disease can be estimated based on the history and symptoms (see box on p. 133).

Dyspnea in cardiac patients is usually related to metabolic acidosis-induced hydrogen ion stimulus. Also, increased pressure in the right side of the heart and pulmonary circulation during exertion may stimulate mechanoreceptors that increase ventilation and induce dyspnea.

Diseases that involve the lungs or thoracic cage generally prevent external respiration (ventilation) from keeping pace with internal respiration (in the cells) (Wasserman, 1982). In other words, patients outwalk or outrun their lungs during activities or exertion. The primary symptom that limits exercise in pulmonary patients is dyspnea because of the difficulty they have eliminating CO_2 produced by metabolism. Some individuals such as those with pulmonary fibrosis and some with COPD do experience a decrease in PO_2 with exercise. Hence, dyspnea on exertion in pulmonary patients is usually related to hypoxic or hypercapnic stimuli.

Dyspnea in Cardiac Patients

The cause of dyspnea in cardiac patients depends on whether an associated stiffness of the lungs (fall in compliance) is also present (Szidan and Fishman, 1988). Dyspnea is the primary symptom of a decompensating left ventricle (Marriott, 1993). As the ventricle fails to eject the normal volume of blood, it produces chronic pulmonary venous hypertension, congestion, and pulmonary edema, resulting in stiff or less compliant lungs. This, along with modest hypoxemia that augments the respiratory drive, increases ventilation and the work of breathing. Tachypnea is often seen at rest. Exercise exaggerates the pulmonary congestion and edema, promotes arterial and mixed venous hypoxemia, which also increases the amount of dyspnea and tachypnea manifested. Fatigue, resulting from low cardiac output, also affects the respiratory muscles, further increasing the sensation of breathlessness.

Dyspnea in cardiac patients without stiff lungs is primarily seen during exertion or exercise (Szidan, and Fishman, 1988). In uncomplicated pulmonic stenosis, it is probably related to an inadequate cardiac output during exercise. Patients with tetralogy of Fallot and other forms of cyanotic heart disease, experience both dyspnea and fatigue during exercise when the arterial oxyhemoglobin saturation has fallen appreciatively below the resting level.

Orthopnea

Orthopnea is dyspnea brought on in the recumbent position (Hurst, 1990). The patient may state the need for two or three pillows under the head to rest at night. This symptom is commonly associated with CHF but may also be associated with severe chronic pulmonary disease.

Paroxysmal Nocturnal Dyspnea

Paroxysmal nocturnal dyspnea (PND) is an important type of shortness of breath. This symptom has strong predictive value as a sign of CHF (Hurst, et al, 1990). The patient usually falls asleep in the recumbent position, and 1 or 2 hours later, awakens from sleep with acute shortness of breath. The patient sits upright on the side of the bed or goes to an open window to breathe "fresh air" to get relief from shortness of breath.

The mechanism of PND is the transfer of fluid from extravascular tissues into the bloodstream (or intravascularly) during sleep (Constant, 1993). The intravascular volume of fluid gradually increases until the compromised left ventricle can no longer manage it. The left atrial pressure rises when the rate of lymphatic drainage from the lungs is unable to keep up with the increased volume of fluid. The increased atrial pressure leads to a sufficiently elevated pulmonary capillary pressure to produce interstitial edema. Patients who are light sleepers awaken early with dyspnea. Deep sleepers may not awaken until they develop alveolar edema.

Classic PND cannot usually be eliminated by only elevating the trunk without lowering the legs. The patient must pool blood in the extravascular tissues of the legs to get adequate relief, which usually takes at least 30 minutes. This is why the patient must sit up or stand up, and ambulate.

The patient should be asked about the amount of

exercise or work performed during the day before an attack on PND. A true left ventricular failure episode of PND is more likely to occur after a day of unusual exertion, which has caused an increased amount of extravascular fluid to accumulate in the legs. If the patient is participating in an exercise or rehabilitation program, the level of exercise may need to be reduced to prevent PND.

Platypnea

Platypnea is the onset of dyspnea when assuming the sitting position from the supine position (Sharf, 1989). This unusual phenomenon is often found in patients with basilar pulmonary fibrosis or basilar arteriovenous malformation. It can be related to the redistribution of blood flow to the lung bases in the sitting position with resultant ventilation-perfusion mismatching and hypoxemia.

Trepopnea

Trepopnea refers to dyspnea in one lateral position but not the other (Snider, 1994). It is often produced by unilateral respiratory system pathology such as lung disease, pleural effusion, or airway obstruction. It also is commonly seen in patients with mitral stenosis (Constant, 1993). Occasionally it may be the result of a fall in blood pressure in the left lateral decubitus position. If the patient has ischemic heart disease, the reduction in coronary perfusion can cause either angina or dyspnea.

Functional Dyspnea

Functional dyspnea is defined as shortness of breath at rest but not during exertion (Sharf, 1989). It is most commonly seen in young women who complain of the need to take a deep breath or to sigh and interpret this sensation as shortness of breath. The physical examination and pulmonary function tests are negative. Reassurance is usually all that is necessary.

WHEEZING

Patients that complain of wheezing associated with dyspnea may have pulmonary or cardiac disease. This symptom, if first reported in patients over age 40, is often related to heart failure (Hurst, et al, 1990). When confirmed that the wheezing is because of heart disease, the patient is said to have cardiac asthma. Wheezing in cardiac patients is a manifestation of narrowed airways and thickened bronchial walls as a result of pulmonary edema (Szidan, and Fishman, 1988). However, if patients have a history of episodes of wheezing and dyspnea since childhood, COPD, or asthma is the likely cause. Other pulmonary conditions such as eosinophilic pneumonia, bronchopulmonary aspergillosis, allergic granulomatosis, etc., can cause wheezing (Miller, 1980). Wheezing must be differentiated from stridor, which is commonly caused by laryngotracheal narrowing due to tracheostomy scar, trauma of intubation, laryngeal paralysis, epiglottitis, or tumors. Chronic pulmonary patients may also develop heart conditions, so it is good to remember patients that complain of wheezing may have both cardiac and pulmonary disease.

COUGH

Cough is a common symptom of pulmonary disease. The cough mechanism consists of three phases: (1) an inspiratory phase, (2) a compressive phase, and (3) an expiratory phase (Irwin, 1977).

There are numerous cough irritant receptors located on the mucosa of the larynx, trachea, bronchi, pleura, and external auditory canal. These receptors are most sensitive at the glottis and carina, and diminish rapidly beyond the fourth generation bronchi. A cough follows stimulation of these mucosal receptors by any of a number of factors including inflammation, sputum, foreign bodies, noxious gases or odors, chemical substances, endobronchial tumors, and extrabronchial pressure on the trachea or bronchi (Sharf, 1989).

A productive cough is beneficial for clearing the airways of sputum and foreign material, and generally should not be inhibited. However, a dry, hacking cough is usually of no value and can have a self-perpetuating irritant effect on the respiratory mucosa. A dry cough may be the initial symptom of certain interstitial lung diseases such as allergic alveolitis, sarcoidosis, and pulmonary fibrosis. Some causes and characteristics of coughs are listed in Table 7-3.

TABLE 7-3

Some Causes and Characteristics of Coughs

CAUSE	CHARACTERISTICS
Acute infection of lungs	
Tracheobronchitis	Cough associated with sore throat, running nose, and eyes
Lobar pneumonia	Cough often preceded by symptoms of upper respiratory infection; cough dry, painful at first; later becomes productive
Bronchopneumonia	Usually begins as acute bronchitis; dry or productive cough
Mycoplasma and viral pneumonia	Paroxysmal cough, productive of mucoid or blood-stained sputum associated with influenza-like syndrome
Exacerbation of chronic bronchitis	Cough productive of mucoid sputum becomes purulent
Chronic infections of lungs	
Bronchitis	Cough productive of sputum on most days for more than 3 consecutive months and for more than 2 successive years; sputum mucoid until acute exacerbation, when it becomes mucopurulent
Bronchiectasis	Cough copious, foul, purulent, often since childhood; forms layer on standing
Tuberculosis or fungus	Persistent cough for weeks to months often with blood-tingling of sputum
Parenchymal inflammatory processes	
Interstitial fibrosis and infiltrations	Cough nonproductive, persistent, depends on etiologic factors
Smoking	Cough usually associated with injected pharynx; persistent, most marked in morning, usually only slightly productive unless succeeded by chronic bronchitis
Tumors	
Bronchogenic carcinoma	Nonproductive to productive cough for weeks to months; recurrent small hemoptysis common
Alveolar cell carcinoma	Cough similar to bronchogenic carcinoma, except in occasional instance when large quantities of watery, mucoid sputum are produced
Benign tumors in airways	Cough nonproductive, occasionally hemoptysis
Mediastinal tumors	Cough, often with breathlessness, caused by compression of trachea and bronchi
Aortic aneurysm	Brassy cough
Foreign body	
Immediate, while still in upper airway	Cough associated with progressive evidence of asphyxiation
Later, when lodged in lower airway	Nonproductive cough, persistent, associated with localizing wheeze
Cardiovascular	
Left ventricular failure	Cough intensifies while supine along with aggravation of dyspnea
Pulmonary infarction	Cough associated with hemoptysis, usually with pleural effusion

Reprinted with permission from Szidon J, Fishman A: Approach to the pulmonary patient with respiratory signs and symptoms. In Fishman A, editor: *Pulmonary diseases and disorders.* New York, 1988, McGraw-Hill.

Cough may be the only presenting symptom of asthma. In asthmatics, cough is precipitated by inhaling cold air or exercise, and is dry. Cough can precipitate an asthma attack in sensitive patients and is known as cough-induced bronchospasm.

It is important to determine the length of time cough has been present (Sharf, 1989). The most common cause of an acute cough is a viral respiratory infection, which generally resolves within a few days or 2 to 3 weeks. Exposure to noxious gases also precipitates acute coughing.

A cough that has persisted for more than 3 weeks can be termed chronic (Snider, 1994). The most common cause of chronic cough is chronic bronchitis, and is present in up to 30% of cigarette smokers. The next most common cause is the postnasal discharge syndrome. Patients describe a sensation of secretions dripping from the back of the nose into the throat, prompting throat clearing or coughing.

Various cardiac conditions may stimulate receptors in the bronchi and provoke coughing (Goldberger, 1990). Because the bronchial veins empty into the pulmonary veins (leading to the left side of the heart), systemic veins, and the superior vena cava (leading to the right side of the heart), venous congestion and coughing may occur with either right- or left-side CHF. It is more common, however, with left-sided CHF. The onset of a cough in a patient with paroxysmal tachycardia or acute myocardial infarction (MI) is often an early symptom of acute left-side heart failure.

Coughing may be caused by other cardiovascular conditions such as a large left atrium displacing the left main-stem bronchus upward, aortic aneurysms placing pressure on the bronchi, or a double aortic arch compressing the trachea.

A specific diagnosis can be made in 80% of cases of chronic cough by an appropriate history alone (Stulberg, 1985). Determining the precipitating causes or the time of onset points the clinician to a probable diagnosis. For example, does the patient cough primarily at night? If so, it points to heart failure, esophageal problems, bronchiectasis or asthma as the potential cause. An early morning cough is more common in bronchitis and individuals with postnasal drip. Cough following meals suggests esophageal disease. Cough precipitated by exertion or deep breathing suggests asthma or interstitial lung disease. Allergens or irritant fumes at home or at work may be a cause of cough. Postviral cough may be present for weeks following a viral illness.

Some medications can elicit coughing. Beta-blockers prescribed to treat hypertension, migraine headaches, cardiovascular disease (CVD), or glaucoma may precipitate asthma. Many drugs, including chemotherapeutic agents, can cause interstitial lung disease and coughing.

Cough and wheezing may result from COPD, asthma, or early left heart failure. Early left heart failure predisposes the patient to respiratory infections and may be responsible for chronic bronchitis.

Cough Complications

One of the more common complications of cough is syncope. Tussive or cough-induced syncope, which is more common in men than women, can be recognized through accurate history taking (Miller, 1980). It is typically reported by middle-age men who "smoke hard, eat hard, drink hard, and cough hard." They experience fainting or near-fainting following cough paroxysms. The cause is obscure but may be related to vagal-induced cardiac slowing or vasodilatation, or high intrathoracic pressures that impair venous return, decrease cardiac output, increase intracranial pressure, and result in a reduced cerebral blood flow. Cough syncope is often resolved by smoking cessation.

Complications of cough include headache, back pain, muscular tears, hematomas, rib fractures (along the posterior axillary line), occasionally vertebral compression fractures (in osteopenic patients), urinary incontinence (UI) (in women), and inguinal hernias (in men) may occur (Braman and Corrao, 1987).

CHEST PAIN

Taking an accurate history is crucial to the proper evaluation of chest pain (Snider, 1994). Although the definitive cause of chest pain cannot be fully established without diagnostic medical tests, it is usually possible to determine whether the pain originates in the pleura, chest wall, or thoracic organs by means of careful history taking.

Chest pain can be divided into two basic types: chest wall pain and visceral pain (George, 1990). The first arises from involved thoracic cage structures and tends to be superficial and well-localized. The latter arises from the heart, pericardium, aorta, mediastinum, bronchi, or esophagus. It is described as deep and difficult to localize.

Pleuritic

Pleuritic chest pain originates from the parietal pleura or endothoracic fascia, but not the visceral pleura, which has no pain receptors. The patient can usually identify it as being close to the thoracic cage (Szidan, Fishman, 1988). Pleuritic chest pain worsens sharply with inspiration as the inflamed parietal pleura is stretched with chest wall motion. Deep breathing, coughing, or laughing are extremely painful, requiring the patient to apply pressure over the involved area to control the pain.

Pleuritic chest pain is ordinarily found in patients that have other signs of respiratory illness, such as cough, fever, chills, malaise. Inflammation of the diaphragmatic pleura produces ipsilateral shoulder pain by way of the phrenic nerve (Miller, 1980).

The onset of pleuritic chest pain varies according to its cause (Snider, 1994). Sudden severe pleuritic chest pain suggest a spontaneous pneumothorax, pulmonary embolism, or infarct. Pulmonary embolism is usually accompanied by sudden dyspnea, hemoptysis, tachycardia, cyanosis, hypotension, anxiety, and agitation (Marriott, 1993).

Cardiac

There are three cardinal features that are characteristic of cardiac chest pain. The patient should be asked the following questions (Marriott, 1993):

1. **Does the pain have maximal intensity from the onset or does it build up for several seconds?** Ischemic cardiac pain or angina is caused by the myocardium contracting in the absence of an adequate oxygen supply. The same type of pain can be produced by placing a blood pressure cuff around the upper arm and inflating it until the brachial pulse is no longer palpated at the wrist. If a patient opens and closes a fist, pain will gradually appear and escalate in the forearm. The causal mechanism of this pain is the same as that of myocardial pain: continuing muscular contraction in the absence of an adequate oxygen supply. This type of pain requires several contractions of the myocardium to reach its maximal intensity. In other words, there is a characteristic buildup or escalation of angina pain.

2. **Can you point to the area of pain with one finger?** Anginal pain is characteristically demonstrated by patients using their entire hand or closed fist against the anterior chest wall. It is described as a sign of angina, because it is so typical (Marriott, 1993). By contrast, any pain that can be localized by pointing with a fingertip is unlikely to be angina.

3. **Is the pain deep inside your chest or does it seem as though it is close to the surface?** Anginal pain is visceral pain that may be referred superficially but always has a deep internal component to it.

Myocardial ischemia may be completely painless (silent ischemia). Angina may in fact not be painful but rather described as discomfort, pressure, squeezing, a tight band, heaviness, burning, indigestion. It usually is located substernally and radiates into one or both arms, neck, jaw, or back.

Angina is not limited only to patients with CAD (Marriott, 1993). Individuals that have normal coronary arteries but an insufficient oxygen supply for a given cardiac workload can also experience angina. These include individuals with anemia, hypertension, tachycardia, and thyrotoxicosis. Hypertrophic and dilated cardiomyopathy can produce typical angina pain, although the latter tends to be intermittent, usually occurring with episodes of CHF. Aortic valve disease can cause angina as a result of impairment of adequate coronary artery blood flow.

Angina is usually precipitated by exertion such as walking uphill, against the wind, or in cold weather (Marriott, 1993). It also is more likely to be brought on after a meal or by emotional stress. The rapid resolution of chest pain by rest or sublingual nitroglycerin strongly suggests a cardiac origin. The pain produced by MI is longer, persisting more than 20 minutes; occurs at rest; and is accompanied by nausea, diaphoresis, hypotension, and dyspnea.

Pulmonary Hypertension

Chest pain related to pulmonary hypertension may mimic angina pectoris. It is usually found in patients with mitral stenosis or Eisenmenger's syndrome (pulmonary hypertension related to an interventricular septal defect, patent ductus arteriosus, or atrial septal defect). This type of chest pain is usually absent at rest, occurs during exertion, and is invariably associated with dyspnea (Hurst, et al, 1990). It is believed to be because of dilation of the pulmonary artery or right ventricular ischemia. The pain is not relieved by nitrates. Primary pulmonary hypertension may be accompanied by syncope and Raynaud's phenomenon (Sharf, 1989).

Pericardial

Pericardial chest pain is also midline, but because of its anatomical relationship with the mediastinal pleura, it has features that suggest pleural involvement (Snider, 1994). Deep breathing, coughing, swallowing, movement and lying down may make it worse. If the central tendon of the diaphragm is involved, the pain may be referred to the left shoulder or scapular area (Marriott, 1993). The patient may report that each heartbeat affects the pain. Sitting up and leaning forward, or lying on the right side often relieves the pain.

Esophageal

Diffuse esophageal spasm or esophageal colic is a common cause of chest pain. It is often confused with cardiac pain because it is located substernally, has a squeezing or aching quality, and may radiate into one or both arms (George, 1990). Furthermore, diffuse esophageal spasm may be relieved by sublingual nitroglycerin as a result of its generalized function as a smooth muscle relaxant.

Pain that radiates through the chest to the back, pain that decreases by a change in position from supine to upright, or relief by ingesting antacids, all suggest an esophageal origin (Snider, 1994). Also, diffuse esophageal spasm is often associated with pain on swallowing (odynophagia), dysphagia, and regurgitation of stomach contents. Swallowing hot or cold liquids, or emotional stress tend to precipitate this type of chest pain.

Chest Wall

Chest wall pain is the most common type of chest pain. Clues in the patient's history to this type of pain include intermittent occurrence, variable intensity, and local tenderness (Miller, 1980). Because it is often located on the anterior chest wall, many patients believe it is heart pain. However, an important differentiation from cardiac pain is that it does not occur during but rather following exertion. It may worsen with inspiration, but its association with trunk motions (flexion, extension, rotation) distinguish it from pleuritic chest pain.

Localized anterior chest pain as a result of costochondritis of the second to fourth costosternal articulations (Tietze's syndrome) is described as tender to touch (George, 1990). A complaint of rib tenderness, together with a history of trauma, fall, long-term steroid use, coughing, or upper extremity exertion, suggests rib fracture.

Degenerative disk disease and arthritis of the cervical or thoracic spine, thoracic outlet syndrome, spondylitis, fibromyalgia, kyphoscoliosis, and herpes zoster can all produce chest wall pain (Epstein, Gerber, and Borer, 1979; Miller, 1980; Pellegrino, 1990; Snider, 1994; Wise, Semble, and Dalton, 1992). Primary lung cancer that invades the adjoining chest wall, ribs, or spine produces severe persistent localized pain (Snider, 1994). Pancoast's syndrome (superior sulcus tumor), in which a primary lung tumor located in the extreme apex of the lung invades the brachial plexus and produces pain in the shoulder, scapular region, or medial aspect of the arm and hand.

Chest wall pain may rarely be caused by thrombosis of a superficial vein on the chest wall (Mondor's disease). It is a self-limiting condition of unknown origin and can last several weeks (Snider, 1994). The only physical finding is a subcutaneous cord that can be palpated along the lateral chest wall.

HEMOPTYSIS

Hemoptysis is defined as coughing up blood. It can vary in amount from blood-streaked sputum to containing virtually all blood. The bleeding site may be anywhere in the upper or lower respiratory tract.

The timing and frequency of hemoptysis, as determined in the history, can offer clues about its cause. A history of nosebleeds is significant since blood may be aspirated during sleep at night and expectorated the following morning. Intermittent bouts of hemoptysis is more characteristic of respiratory infections such as bronchiectasis, tuberculosis, fungus infections, or broncholithiasis (Miller, 1980). Persistently expectorating blood-streaked sputum on a daily basis is highly suggestive of bronchogenic neoplasm.

The lung receives its blood supply in two ways: the pulmonary arteries (a low pressure system) and the bronchial arteries (a high pressure system) off of the aorta (Sharf, 1989). The appearance of hemoptysis may vary according to which blood supply is involved. If the bronchial vessels are the source, there tends to be large or massive amounts of bright red blood. This is often the site of bleeding in bronchiectasis, since bronchial arteries undergo enlargement and extensive anastomosis with the pulmonary artery system. Or, in mitral stenosis, where there is increased pulmonary vascular resistance, hemoptysis arises from passively engorged submucosal bronchial veins (Szidan and Fishman, 1988).

Hemoptysis from the low-pressure pulmonary artery system tends to occur in small amounts and is composed of dark or clotted venous blood (Snider, 1994). It may arise from the pulmonary parenchyma, as in the case of the highly vascular granulation tissue found in the walls of lung abscesses. These abscesses may be caused by infections such as tuberculosis, anaerobic bacteria, staphylococci, or chronic irritation from a fungus ball in an abscess cavity. If a blood vessel ruptures in an abscess cavity, hemorrhage tends to be massive, even exsanguinating.

Cardiovascular conditions such as mitral stenosis, pulmonary infarction, Eisenmenger physiology, and aortic aneurysm are also associated with hemoptysis (Hurst, et al, 1990). Pink frothy sputum is often found with acute pulmonary edema. Therapists should carefully evaluate complaints of hemoptysis and be certain of its cause before cautiously conducting treatment.

FATIGUE AND WEAKNESS

There are multiple causes of fatigue and weakness (Hurst, et al, 1990). Therapists should not conclude too quickly that they are related to physical inactivity and decreased muscular strength in sedentary cardiopulmonary patients. The most common causes of fatigue and weakness complaints are depression, anxiety, and emotional stress. They often accompany anemia, hypothyroidism, and chronic disease states.

Fatigue is often associated with CHF. In this condition, it probably is related to an insufficient cardiac output to adequately perfuse the entire body, including the skeletal muscles. Generally, fatigue caused by cardiac disease is related to exertion, but fatigue related to anxiety tends to be continuous (Hurst, et al, 1990).

Diuretics used to treat CHF can cause potassium depletion and hypokalemia with resultant weakness. Antihypertensive medications can produce weakness by postural hypotension.

PEDAL EDEMA

CHF is a common cause of bilateral pedal edema (Marriott, 1993). However, several pounds of fluid (10 to 20 lbs.) generally accumulate in the body before foot and ankle swelling is evident. Therefore weight gain is an even earlier indication of fluid retention due to CHF. Occasionally, patients may only complain about an increase in abdominal girth resulting from ascites. When caused by CHF, the onset of ascites virtually always occurs after pedal edema is present. If the amount of ascites is disproportionate to that of pedal edema, restrictive cardiomyopathy or constrictive pericarditis should be a consideration.

It is important to determine whether the patient had dyspnea on exertion before the onset of lower-extremity edema. If the edema is a result of a poorly functioning left ventricle, mitral stenosis, or cor pulmonale, it usually follows dyspnea on exertion.

Patients with CHF and altered renal function commonly report edema of the ankle and lower legs while upright during the day, but indicate a decrease during the night (Hurst, et al, 1990). This is a result of local hydrostatic factors related to the upright position.

Edema may be present in nephrosis or starvation

when the total blood protein falls below 5 gm/100 ml (hypoproteinemia). Other causes of pedal edema include liver disease, kidney disease, and anemia. Edema of one leg is ordinarily because of local factors such as thrombophlebitis or varicose veins.

HOARSENESS

Hoarseness, abnormal vocal cord motion during phonation, is a symptom of laryngeal dysfunction (Miller, 1980). It is usually associated with upper respiratory tract infections or allergies, and resolves in 1 to 2 weeks (Sharf, 1989). Trauma following intubation, laryngeal polyps, or tumors are other common causes of hoarseness. However, this symptom is also related to cardiopulmonary conditions. Because the recurrent laryngeal nerves pass through the upper thorax, intrathoracic pathology that involves one of these nerves can cause unilateral vocal cord paralysis, resulting in hoarseness (Sharf, 1989). These include lung or mediastinal tumors, granulomatous disease, enlarged mediastinal lymph nodes, and pericardial or mediastinal adhesions.

Several cardiovascular conditions can produce hoarseness, because the left recurrent laryngeal nerve loops under the arch of the aorta and above the pulmonary artery as it returns to the neck (Hurst, et al, 1990). Therefore an aneurysm of the arch of the aorta, a dilated pulmonary artery or atrium resulting from an atrial septal defect, or mitral stenosis can cause hoarseness (Goldberger, 1990).

Hence, if patients manifest hoarseness, it is necessary to inquire about the length of time it has been present, the patient's smoking history, and any history of cardiac or pulmonary diseases.

OCCUPATIONAL HISTORY

Taking an occupational history is particularly important for pulmonary patients who arrive for physical therapy with little or no accompanying medical information. The internal surface of the lung measures 50 to 100 m^3 and is in constant contact with the environment (Miller, 1980). Jobs that involve exposure to silica or silicates (e.g., miners, sandblasters, foundry workers, stone cutters, brick layers, or quarry workers) or other inorganic substances place workers at risk for combinations of obstructive and restrictive lung disease (e.g., silicosis). Construction workers, shipyard workers, pipefitters, and other industrial workers exposed to asbestos are at increased risk for developing a restrictive lung disease such as asbestosis (Varkey, 1983). Benign pleural plaques may be found on the diaphragmatic pleura and bilaterally between the sixth and tenth ribs on the anterolateral or posterolateral chest wall. Progressive pleural thickening rarely occurs. These individuals have an increased incidence of malignant neoplastic diseases such as bronchogenic carcinoma and malignant mesothelioma.

Coal workers are exposed to coal mine dust. About 10% have simple pneumoconiosis, whereas a smaller proportion develop the complicated form—progressive massive pulmonary fibrosis (Brandstetter and Sprince, 1982).

A history of paroxysmal coughing, chest tightness, or dyspnea that is worse during the week but remits on weekends strongly suggests occupational asthma (Brandstetter, and Sprince, 1982). This condition is difficult to diagnose because symptoms often occur several hours after exposure to the provoking agent. Causal agents include grain dusts, wood dusts, formalin, enzyme detergents, ethanolamines (in spray paints and soldering flux), nickel and hard metals (tungsten carbide). Workers exposed to cotton flax and hemp dusts may develop byssinosis, an obstructive lung disease. In the early stages, it is reversible, but long-term exposure over a number of years causes chronic irreversible obstructive lung disease.

A history of fever, cough, shortness of breath, and recurrent pneumonias in farmers in the northern United States suggests farmer's lung (Brandstetter, and Sprince, 1982). This is the most common hypersensitive pneumonitis, caused by inhaling fungal agents such as thermophilic actinomycetes. Long-term exposure can lead to pulmonary fibrosis. There are numerous occupations that expose workers to etiologic factors that cause hypersensitive pneumonitis.

SMOKING HISTORY

The patient should be asked their tobacco-smoking history (Snider, 1994). The number of pack-years of cigarettes smoked may be calculated (average number of packs/day × number of years smoked) as a relative risk of lung cancer and COPD. Regular smoking of marijuana is more damaging to the lungs than cigarette smoking.

FAMILY HISTORY

The family history is useful in evaluating the possibility of hereditary pulmonary diseases such as alpha$_1$-antitrypsin deficiency, cystic fibrosis, allergic asthma, hereditary hemorrhagic telangiectasia, and others (Miller, 1980; Szidan, and Fishman, 1988). A family history of diabetes, hypertension, CAD, or rheumatic fever raises the possibility of these conditions existing in the patient as well (Marriott, 1993).

PRIOR TREATMENT

It is important to determine what treatment(s) the patient has received for his or her condition. Specifically, has the patient ever received physical therapy for this or any other condition? What type of treatments were done? Were they helpful in improving or resolving the condition? In this way we determine what treatment modalities have been used, which of these the patient believes may have merit, and those with which the patient finds objectionable or lacks confidence, thus avoiding alienating the patient by not repeating what he or she believes to be ineffective therapy is avoided.

SUMMARY

Obtaining an accurate and thorough history is the cornerstone of the physical therapy evaluation process. The probable cause and severity of many cardiopulmonary symptoms can be determined by careful history taking. This information enables therapists to select the most appropriate evaluation and treatment techniques. When properly performed, accurate history taking gains the patient's confidence and cooperation, and provides the basis for a good patient-therapist relationship.

REVIEW QUESTIONS

1. What are the basic causes of dyspnea?
2. What questions can be asked of a patient with dyspnea to determine the likely cause?
3. What scales have been developed to quantitate dyspnea?
4. What are the principal features of chest pain that originate from the pleurae? The chest wall? The thoracic organs?
5. What are the cardinal features of cardiac chest pain?
6. What occupations can place workers at rish for respiratory disease?

References

Birdwell, B., Herbers, J., & Kroenke, K. (1993). Evaluating chest pain: the patient's presentation style alters the physician's diagnostic approach. *Archives of Internal Medicine, 153,* 1991–1995.

Borg, G. (1982). Psychophysical bases of perceived exertion. *Medicine and Science in Sports and Exercise, 14,* 377–381.

Braman, S., Corrao, W. (1987). *Cough: differential diagnosis and treatment. Clinical Chest Medicine 8(2),* 177–188.

Brandstetter, R., Sprince, N. (1982). Occupational lung disease. *Medical Times,* June, 56–63.

Constant, J. (1993). The evolving checklist in history-taking. In Constant J. *Bedside cardiology.* Boston: Little, Brown.

Epstein, S., Gerber, L., & Borer, J. (1979). Chest wall syndrome: a common cause of unexplained cardiac pain. *Journal of the American Medical Association, 241,* 2793–2797.

George, R. (1990). History and physical examination. In George, R., et al (Eds.), *Chest medicine: Essentials of pulmonary and critical care medicine.* Baltimore: Williams and Wilkins.

Goldberger, E. (1990). Symptoms referable to the cardiovascular system. In Goldberger, E. *Essentials of clinical cardiology.* Philadelphia: JB Lippincott.

Irwin, R., Rosen, M., & Braman, S. (1977). Cough: a comprehensive review. *Arch Intern Medicine 137,* 1186–1191.

Hurst, J., et al. (1990). The history: past events and symptoms related to cardiovascular disease. In Hurst, J. (Ed.). *The heart.* New York: McGraw-Hill.

Mahler, D. (1987). Dyspnea: diagnosis and management. *Clinics in Chest Medicine, 8(2),* 215–230.

Mahler, D., & Harver, A. (1990). Clinical measurements of dyspnea. In Mahler, D. (Ed.). *Dyspnea.* Mount Kisco, NY: Futura.

Marriott, H. (1993). Taking the history. In Marriott, H. *Bedside cardiac diagnosis.* Philadelphia: JB Lippincott.

Miller, D. (1980). The medical history. In Sackner, M. (Ed.). Diagnostic techniques in pulmonary disease. New York: Marcel Dekker.

Pellegrino, M. (1990). Atypical chest pain as an initial presentation of primary fibromyalgia. *Archives of Physical Medicine and Rehabilitation 71,* 526–528.

Sharf, S. (1989). History and physical examination. In Baum, G., & Wolinski, E. (Eds.). Textbook of pulmonary diseases. (4th ed.). Boston: Little, Brown.

Snider, G. (1994). History and physical examination. In Baum, G., & Wolinski, E. (Eds.), Textbook of pulmonary diseases. (5th ed.). Little, Brown.

Stulberg, M. (1985). Evaluating and treating intractable cough—Medical Staff Conference, University of California, San Francisco. *West J Med, 143,* 223–228.

Szidan, P., & Fishman, A. (1988). Approach to the pulmonary patient with respiratory signs and symptoms. In Fishman, A. (Ed.). Pulmonary diseases and disorders. (2nd ed.). New York: McGraw-Hill.

Varkey, B., (1983). Asbestos exposure: An update on pleuropulmonary hazards. *Postgraduate Medicine, 74(4),* 93–103.

Wasserman, K., (1982). Dyspnea on exertion: is it the heart or the lungs? *Journal of the American Medical Association, 248,* 2039–2043.

Wise, C., Semble, E., & Dalton, C. (1992). Musculoskeletal chest wall syndromes in patients with noncardiac chest pain: A study of 100 patients. *Archives of Physical Medicine and Rehabilitation, 73,* 147–149.

CHAPTER 8

Pulmonary Function Tests

Donna Frownfelter

KEY TERMS

Dead space
Lung capacities
    Functional residual capacity
    Inspiratory capacity
    Total lung capacity
    Vital capacity
Lung volume

Expiratory reserve volume
Inspiratory reserve volume
Residual volume
Tidal volume
Obstructive component
Predicted values
Restrictive component

INTRODUCTION

Pulmonary function tests (PFTs) help in the evaluation of the mechanical function of the lungs. (Cherniak, Crapo, and Youtsey, 1992). They are based on researched norms taking into account sex, height, and age. For example, there are predicted values for a male, age 65 who is 6 feet tall. (Morris, Koski, and Johnson, 1971). When the patient performs the test actual results (observed) will be compared with the predicted value expected of a person of gender, height, and age to see if he falls within the "normal" range, or has a restrictive or obstructive component based on the tests. If the patient is not within the normal range, a bronchodilator is given, and the test will be repeated to see if there is significant improvement with medication. Basically, the pulmonary function tests are categorized as volume, flow, or diffusion studies. Diagno-sis of pulmonary disease or dysfunction and improvement with treatment will be evaluated as a result of interpreting a patient's pulmonary function tests.

DEAD SPACE

The most important function of the lungs is to supply the body with oxygen and to remove carbon dioxide (CO_2) produced as a waste product of metabolism. As this continuous gas exchange takes place sufficient ventilation is needed to move the gases to the alveoli. There is a series of conducting airways in the lungs from the trachea down to the terminal bronchi, which do not participate in respiration but only move the gases to the alveoli. This is the volume known as anatomic dead space. Generally, the anatomic dead space is appropriately equal to the adult body weight. For example, in a 150-lb. person, there is an approximately 150 mL anatomic dead space. A normal tidal volume (TV), the breath normally taken, needs to be large enough to reach the alveoli well past the anatomic dead space. In a normal adult, the TV is generally 450 to 600 mL. The anatomic dead space would thus represent about one third TV volume. The rest of the breath would reach the alveoli and be considered "alveolar ventilation." With many neurologically impaired patients who have a limited TV, it is important to note that little alveolar ventilation may be taking place when the patient is breathing in a rapid and shallow pattern. For example, if a patient's TV was 200 mL, 150 mL would be anatomic dead space and only 50 mL of each breath would be alveolar ventilation.

There are many diseases or conditions that can alter the volume of dead space that needs to be ventilated. In some cases the dead space decreases, such as in a pneumonectomy, where it is physically removed, or in asthma, where bronchospasm may narrow the airways. In other conditions such as pulmonary embolus, dead space increases when ventilated areas of lung cease to be perfused. The alveoli continue to receive fresh gas, but there is no blood available for gas exchange. This type of dead space is known as physiologic dead space.

When dead space is increased, a larger percentage of the tidal volume is ventilating the dead space, leaving a smaller percentage for alveolar ventilation. The patient must work harder to get enough air to the

functioning alveoli. This causes increased work of breathing and may result in patient fatigue. Neurological and neuromuscular weakness may result in an inability to take a normal TV. Similarly, surgical procedures or pain from fractured ribs can also compromise a patient's ability to take a breath. As the TV drops a large percentage of the breath is anatomic dead space. This results in increased work of breathing for the patient and may ultimately result in respiratory failure if the patient is unable to provide alveolar ventilation.

LUNG VOLUMES

The lung has four volumes, TV, inspiratory reserve volume (IRV), expiratory reserve volume (ERV), and residual volume (RV) (Figure 8-1).

- TV is the normal breath.
- IRV is the maximal amount of air that can be inhaled from the end of a normal inspiration.
- ERV is the maximal amount of air that can be expired after a normal exhalation.
- RV is the volume of gas that remains in the lungs at the end of a maximum expiration.

Changes in RV can help in the diagnosis of certain medical conditions. An increase in RV means that even with maximum effort, the patient cannot exhale excess air from the lungs. This results in hyperinflated lungs and indicates that certain changes have

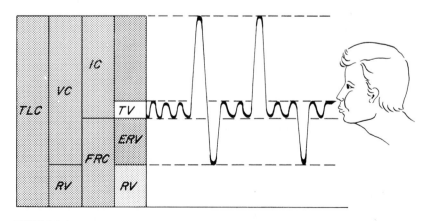

FIGURE 8-1
A spirogram (pulmonary function testing).

occurred in the pulmonary tissue, which in time may cause mechanical changes in the chest wall (e.g., increased AP diameter, flattened diaphragms). These changes may be reversible in patients with partial bronchial obstruction, such as young asthmatics, or irreversible, as in patients with advanced emphysema. Restrictive lung disease can cause a decrease in residual volume, as can cancer of the lung, microatelectasis, or musculoskeletal impairment. (Smith and Dickson, 1994).

LUNG CAPACITIES

A lung capacity is two or more volumes added together (Figure 8-1). The capacities include total lung capacity (TLC), vital capacity (VC), inspiratory capacity (IC) and functional residual capacity (FRC).

TLC is the amount of gas the lung contains at the end of a maximum inspiration. It is made up of all four lung volumes. An increased TLC is seen with hyperinflation such as emphysema. A decrease in TLC may be seen in restrictive lung disease such as pulmonary fibrosis, atelectasis, neoplasms, pleural effusions, and hemothorax, as well as in restrictive musculoskeletal problems such as spinal cord injury, kyphoscoliosis, or as secondary to morbid obesity or pregnancy.

VC is the maximum amount of gas that can be expelled from the lungs by forceful effort following a maximum inspiration. It contains the IRV, TV, ERV. A decrease in VC can occur as a result of absolute reduction in distensible lung tissue. This is seen in pneumonectomy, atelectasis, pneumonia, pulmonary congestion, occlusion of a major bronchus by a tumor or foreign object, or restrictive lung disease.

A decrease in VC may also be seen without primary lung disease or airway obstruction. In neuromuscular or musculoskeletal dysfunction, VC can be compromised (Guillain-Barré, spinal cord injury, drug overdose, motor vehicle accident with fractured ribs, severe scoliosis, and kyphoscoliosis). Restrictive contributing factors such as morbid obesity, pregnancy, enlarged heart, and pulmonary effusion may involve the limitation of expansion of the lungs.

IC is the maximal amount of air that can be inspired from the resting expiratory level. It contains the IRV and the TV.

FRC is the volume of air remaining in the lungs at the resting expiratory level. It contains the ERV and the RV.

The FRC prevents large fluctuations in PaO_2 with each breath. An increase in FRC represents hyperinflation of the lungs. It causes the thorax to be larger than normal, which results in muscular inefficiency and some mechanical disadvantage. Patients on mechanical ventilators may increase their FRC with positive pressure and by additional modes such as positive end expiratory (PEEP), or BiPap. Spontaneously breathing patients can also be on continuous positive airway pressure (CPAP), which keeps the lungs at a positive airway pressure to improve oxygenation.

AIR FLOW MEASUREMENTS
Forced Expiration

When patients perform a VC maneuver, it can either be slow or fast. During exhalation, the amount of air exhaled over time can be measured. In a slow VC a patient with emphysema can take a great deal of time to empty his lungs. In a forced VC a normal individual can exhale 75% of the VC in the first second of exhalation (FEV_1). Patients with emphysema often have greatly decreased VCs, only 40% of which are predicted.

Flow Volume Curve

The flow volume curve is helpful in diagnosing lung disease, since it is independent of effort. The curve in Figure 8-2 demonstrates that flow rises to a high value and then declines over most of expiration (Rahn, et al, 1946). In restrictive lung disease, the maximum flow rate is reduced, as is the total volume exhaled. In obstructive lung disease, the flow rate is low in relation to lung volume, and a scooped-out appearance is often seen (see Figure 8-2).

Another diagnostic test that uses forced expiration is the flow volume loop. It is a graphic analysis of the flow generated during a forced expiratory volume maneuver followed by a forced inspiratory volume maneuver (Figure 8-3). This graph offers a pictorial representation of data from many individual tests (e.g., peak inspiratory and expiratory flow rates,

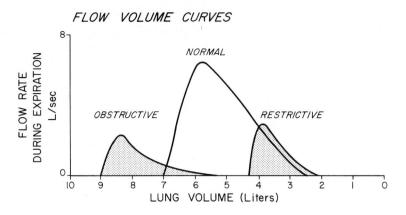

FIGURE 8-2

Comparison of flow volume curves in the normal patient and in the patient with obstructive and restrictive lung disease.

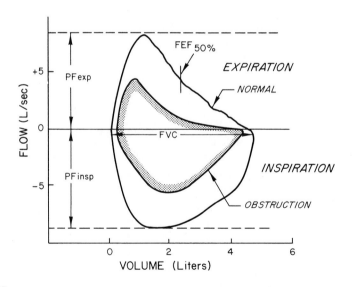

FIGURE 8-3

Comparison of flow volume loops in the normal patient and in the patient with obstructive lung disease.

FVC, and FEV). The shape of the graph may also be helpful in diagnosing disease, again seeing a more scooped-out appearance with obstructive disease.

CLOSING VOLUME AND AIRWAY CLOSURE

The assessment of closing volume is used to help diagnose small airway disease. A test called the single breath nitrogen (N_2) washout is used for assessing closing volume and closing capacity of the small airways. In this test, the patient takes a single VC breath of 100% oxygen. During complete exhalation, the N_2 concentration can be measured. The characteristic tracing of N_2 concentration can be measured. The characteristic tracing of N_2 concentration vs. lung volume reflects sequential emptying of differentially ventilated lung units, resulting in different expiratory N_2 concentrations. Four phases can be identified (Figure 8-4). Phase I contains pure dead space and virtually none of the potential N_2 from the RV. Phase II is associated with an increasing N_2 concentration of a mixture of gas from the dead space and alveoli. The plateau in N_2 concentration observed in Phase III reflects pure alveolar gas emanating from the bases and middle lung zones. Phase IV occurs toward the end of expiration and is characterized by an abrupt increase

in N_2 concentration. This high N_2 concentration reflects closure of airways at the base of the lungs and expiration of gas from the upper lung zones, because in the single breath of 100% oxygen, less oxygen was initially directed to this area.

Closing volume is the lung volume at which the inflection of Phase IV, the marked increase in N_2 concentration after the plateau, is observed. Closing capacity refers to closing volume and RV. The same characteristic tracing of the single breath nitrogen washout test can be obtained with an inhalation of a bolus of tracer gas (e.g., argon, helium, xenon-133).

The closing volume is 10% of the vital capacity in young, healthy individuals. It increases with age and is 40% of the vital capacity at age 65. Closing volume is used as an aid in the diagnosis of small airway disease and as a means of evaluating treatment or drug response.

MAXIMAL VOLUNTARY VENTILATION

Maximal voluntary ventilation measures the maximal breathing capacity of the patient. It reflects strengths and endurance of the respiratory muscles. The patient is asked to pant for 15 seconds into the spirometer tubing. This is often examined preoperatively with the

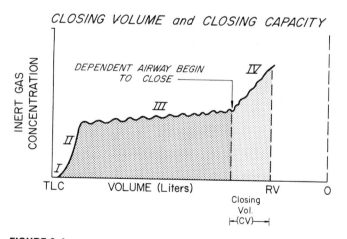

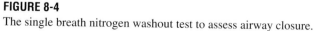

FIGURE 8-4

The single breath nitrogen washout test to assess airway closure.

other results to determine a patient's prognosis for success after surgery, such as his or her ability to cough, to take deep breaths, and to enhance airway clearance.

DIAGNOSIS OF RESTRICTIVE AND OBSTRUCTIVE LUNG DISEASE

Physicians use the results of pulmonary function tests to diagnose lung disease or characteristic components of lung disease, such as bronchospasm. A restrictive component describes conditions that limit the amount of volume coming into the lungs (restriction to inspi-

ration). An obstructive component generally relates to problems in exhalation air flows and characteristic patterns of obstruction, such as in the first second of expiration FEV_1 measurement). Patients do not often have only one primary disease process but many times have overlapping lung conditions (Clausen, 1984). A diagnosis may read: PFTs consistent with moderate emphysema with bronchospastic component; good response to bronchodilators. A patient with an abnormal PFT is given a bronchodilator and retested. If there is a 15% to 20% increase in the PFT after bronchodilators are administered, they will be a recommended

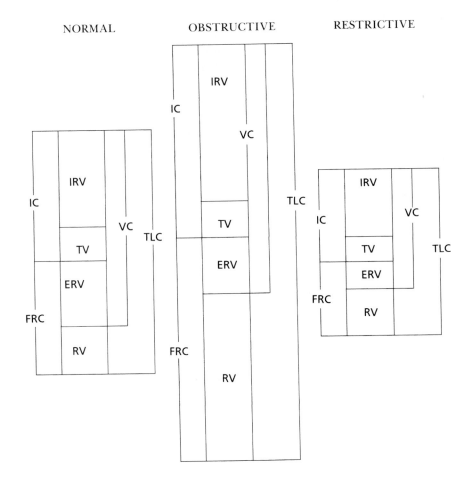

FIGURE 8-5
Examples of proportional changes of lung volumes and capacities characteristic of obstructive and restrictive lung diseases.

part of the patients' medications. However, some patients are given a trial of bronchodilators, even if there is not such a dramatic response on PFTs).

A pictorial demonstration of the differences in obstructive and restrictive lung disease is shown in Figure 8-5. Disease has a marked effect on pulmonary function, yet TV usually remains 10% of total lung capacity until the disease is relatively severe. Physiologic pulmonary reserves in both disease processes are limited and generally affect a patient's response to exercise. Exercise will be limited by the ventilatory status rather than by a cardiac end point. As obstructive lung disease progresses, TLC, FRC, and RV are markedly increased. In severe COPD, the increased FRC can compromise the VC. More energy is expended to breathe compared with that expended by a normal individual. This effect can be disproportionally increased with minimal amounts of activity. In restrictive lung disease, restriction of the chest wall or lung tissue can produce a decrease in TLC. A VC of 80% or less of predicted values for a patient is considered a diagnostic feature. A residual decline in FRC potentiates airway closure.

The phenomenon of closing volume in the lungs is particularly significant to physical therapists (PTs) who prescribe breathing exercises and body positioning, and can thereby alter pulmonary mechanics and gas exchange. These treatment interventions may have a pronounced effect on the lung volumes and airway closure (Dean, 1985). At low lung volumes (e.g., breathing at FRC, Trendelenberg position, and in lung disease) intrapleural pressures are generally less negative and the pressure of dependent lung regions may equal or exceed atmospheric pressure. Intrapleural pressure is less negative because the lungs are less expanded and elastic recoil is decreased. As a result, airway closure is potentiated. In young individuals, closure is evident at RV; however, in older individuals, closure is observed at higher lung volumes, such as at FRC. Premature closure of the small airways results in uneven ventilation and impaired gas exchange with a given lung unit. Airway closure occurs more readily in chronic smokers and in patients with lung disease.

Aging has a significant effect on airway closure. With aging, a loss of pulmonary elastic recoil results in a loss of intrapleural negative pressure. In older individuals, therefore, airway closure occurs at higher lung volumes. For example, closure has been reported to occur at the age of 65 in the upright lung during normal breathing. In the supine position, where FRC is reduced, closure occurs at a significantly younger age (about age 44). In addition to the often compounding effect of age, the lung volume at which airway closure occurs increases with chronic smoking and lung disease, and is changed with the alterations in body position (Berry, Pai, and Fairshter, 1990; Zadai, 1985).

SUMMARY

Pulmonary functions change as a patient's condition gets better or worse (Emery et al, 1991; Emerson, Lukens, Effron, 1994). There are normal declines in volumes and flows with aging as well as disease processes. Basic bedside spirometry is often done to assess the patient's breathing mechanical ability. For example, in a patient with Guillain Barré, as breathing becomes labored, the VC is monitored to determine whether a ventilator is needed. On the other hand, a patient with obstructed airways, such as the patient with cystic fibrosis, the pulmonary function tests will improve (Versteegh, et al, 1986). In patients with spinal cord injury or neuromuscular weakness, as their strength improves, their vital capacity increases. However, because of the lack of abdominal muscles, the flows may be reduced.

REVIEW QUESTIONS

1. What effect will an obstructive component have on exercise performance? What effect will a restrictive component have on excercise performance?
2. Why is it important to compare the patient's predicted values with the actual observed values in a pulmonary function test?
3. What response should you see to determine if bronchodilators have a positive effect on pulmonary function?
4. How can pulmonary function tests be used to assess patient improvement or decline?
5. How valuable are pulmonary function tests if patients do not give maximal effort?

References

Berry, R., Pai, U. & Fairshter, R. (1990). Effect of age on changes in flow rates and airway conductance after a deep breath. *Journal of Applied Physiology, 68,* 635–643.

Cherniak, R.M. (1992). Evaluation of respiratory function in health and disease. *Dis Mon, 38 (7),* 505–76.

Clausen, J.L. (1984). Pulmonary function testing guidelines and controversies. London: Grune and Stratton.

Crapo, R.O. (1994). Pulmonary function testing, *New England Journal of Medicine, 331(1),* 25–30.

Dean, E. (1985). The effect of body position on pulmonary function, *Physical Therapy 65,* 613–618.

Emerson, C.L., Lukens, T.W., Effron, D. (1994). Physician estimation of FEV1 in acute exacerbation of COPD. *Chest, 105(6),* 1709–1712.

Emery, C.E., et al. (1991). Psychological outcome of a pulmonary rehab program. *Chest, 100 (3),* 613–617.

Morris, J., Koski, A., & Johnson, L. (1971). Prediction nomograms (BTPS) spirometric values in normal males and females. *American Review of Respiratory Diseases, 163,* 57–67.

Rahn, H., et al. (1946). The pressure-volume diagram of the thorax and lung. *American Journal of Physiology, 146,* 161.

Smith, R.M., & Dickson, R.A. (1994). Changes in residual volume relative to vital capacity and total lung capacity after arthrodesis of the spine in patients who have idiopathic scoliosis. *Bone and Joint Surgery of America, 76 (1),* 153.

Versteegh, F.G.A., et al. (1986). Relationship between pulmonary function, O_2 saturation during sleep and exercise with cystic fibrosis. *Advanced Cardiology, 35,* 151–155, 1986.

Williams-Russe, P., et al. (1992). Predicting postoperative complications. Is it a real problem? *Archives of Internal Medicine, 152 (6),* 1209–1213.

Youtsey, J.W. (1990). Basic pulmonary function measurement. In Scanlon, C.L., Spearman, C.B., & Sheldan, R.L. (Eds.). Egan's fundamentals of respiratory care. (5th ed.). St. Louis: Mosby.

Zadai, C. (1985). Pulmonary physiology of aging: The role of rehabilitation. *Topics in Geriatric Rehabilitation, 1,* 49–56.

CHAPTER 9

Arterial Blood Gases

Donna Frownfelter

KEY TERMS   Acid/base balance   Hypoxemia
                 Alveolar ventilation   Oxygen saturation
                 Arterial blood gas   Partial pressure of gases

INTRODUCTION

Arterial blood gases are assessment tools to help the physical therapist (PT) understand the patient's acid/base balance, alveolar ventilation and oxygenation status (Cherniak, 1992). They are valuable resources of information, from respiratory monitoring in the intensive care unit to following outpatients to evaluate the therapy and progress of their diseases.

The purpose of this chapter is to help the clinician evaluate and interpret arterial blood gases more effectively and to integrate the information into treatment planning and progression of the patient.

ACID/BASE BALANCE

Normal body metabolism consists of consumption of nutrients and excretion of acid metabolites. Acid metabolites must be kept from accumulating in high amounts, because the body's cardiovascular and nervous systems operate in a relatively narrow free H^+ ion range (narrow pH). Free H^+ ion concentration is discussed as pH ($-\log [H^+]$). Maintenance of body systems requires an appropriate acid/base balance (Shapiro, 1994).

Approximately 98% of normal metabolites are in the form of carbon dioxide (CO_2). Carbon dioxide reacts readily with water to form carbonic acid:

$$CO_2 + H_2O \rightleftarrows H_2CO_3$$

Carbonic acid can exist either as a liquid or a gas. Because carbonic acid can change to CO_2, much of the acid content can be excreted through the lungs during respiration.

The Henderson-Hasselbach equation demonstrates

how the H^+ ion concentration results from the dissociation of carbonic acid and the interrelationship of the blood acids, bases, and buffers:

$$H_2O + CO_2 \rightleftarrows H_2CO_3 \; H+ + HCO_3^-$$

Renal Buffering Mechanisms

The kidneys are the main route of excretion for the normal metabolic acids. Hydrogen ions are excreted in the urine and also resorbed by bicarbonate into the blood. In this manner, the kidneys can respond when there is an acid/base imbalance to return to normal homeostasis.

Normal Blood Gas Values

Acid/base is denoted by the pH. The pH values are normally 7.35 to 7.45. If the pH is below 7.35, the patient is considered to be in an acidotic state (more acid). If the pH is above 7.45, the patient is considered to be in an alkalotic state (more basic).

Alveolar ventilation is reflected in the partial pressure of carbon dioxide (Pco_2). Normal Pco_2 values are 35 mmHg to 45 mmHg. If the PCO_2 is below 35 mmHg the patient is said to be hyperventilating (increased ventilation, blowing off more CO_2 than normal). If the Pco_2 is above 45 mmHg the patient is hypoventilating, or not having enough alveolar ventilation or not blowing off enough CO_2 to maintain normal alveolar ventilation.

Arterial oxygen is measured as Po_2, the partial pressure of oxygen. Normal values are 80 to 100 mm Hg. If the Po_2 is below 80 mmHg in someone less than 60 years old, the patient is hypoxemic. A value of 60 to 80 mmHg is considered mild hypoxemia, 40 to 60 mmHg would be considered moderate hypoxemia, and less than 40 mmHg is severe hypoxemia (Cherniak, 1992).

Base Excess/Base Deficit

The blood normally has a capacity to buffer acid metabolites. The normal level of base Hco_3 in the blood is 22 to 26 milimoles per liter (mmol/L). This buffering capacity diminishes in the presence of acidemia or alkalemia. Acidosis is an abnormal acid/base balance where the acids dominate. Alkalemia is an abnormal acid/base balance where the bases dominate. When there is a decrease in the Hco_3^-, it is seen in a negative base excess and referred to as a base deficit, which is usually seen as a negative number on the blood gas report, that is, –3.

When interpreting a blood gas, it is helpful to determine whether the patient's condition is acute or chronic. Another method is to examine whether the situation is uncompensated, partially compensated or completely compensated. The pH is the key to making this determination. If the pH is not in the normal 7.35 to 7.45 range, then the patient will be in an acute state. As it progresses back toward normal, it may be partially compensated. When a normal pH exists, it is compensated or chronic.

For example, in a patient who is retaining a CO_2 of 55 mm Hg, the pH may read 7.25; this would be considered acute. As the body retains base, the pH will rise back toward the normal numbers. If the pH was 7.32 with a Pco_2 of 55 and + 3 base excess, the reading would be partially compensated. When the pH is within normal limits with the Pco_2 of 55 and a pH of 7.35, the reading would be compensated or chronic.

PARTIAL PRESSURE OF GASES

To better understand blood gases, it is important to remember the properties of gases. The earth's surface consists of gas molecules that have mass and are attracted to the earth's center of gravity. At the surface, this atmospheric weight exerts a pressure that can support a column of mercury 760 mm high.

Dalton's law states that in a mixture of gases, the total pressure is equal to the sum of the partial pressures of the separate gases. Oxygen is 20.9% of the atmosphere, so it has a partial pressure of 159 (760 × 20.9% = 159). Nitrogen is 79% of the atmosphere, so it has a partial pressure of 600 (760 × 79% = 600). Other gases make up 0.1% of the atmosphere.

Diffusion of gases across semipermeable membranes show gradients from higher concentrations to lower concentrations. Each gas moves independently from the others.

During respiration, oxygen and CO_2 exchange across the alveolar capillary membrane. Special situations may affect the normal progress of respiration and gas exchange.

Normally, alveolar units ventilate and capillary units bring oxygenated blood to the tissues, excreting CO_2 back into the alveoli to be removed through the lungs. However, some abnormal situations may occur, such as shunts and dead space units. In a shunt unit, the alveoli has collapsed, but blood flow continues and is unable to pick up oxygen. An example of this is atelectasis, where a lung segment or part of a segment has retained secretions and lung tissue distal to the mucous plug collapses. Circulation continues but oxygenation does not occur and the Po_2 decreases. On the other hand, a dead space unit can have ventilation but not perfusion. This occurs with pulmonary embolism, where a blood clot obstructs the circulation. The oxygen is available in the ventilated alveoli, but

with no circulation, a dead unit is credited. Figure 9-1 demonstrates the regional differences seen in respiratory units.

Hemoglobin

Hemoglobin (Hgb) is the main component of the red blood cell. It is crucial for oxygen transport. The normal Hgb is 12 to 16 gm/100 mL blood. In patients that have lost blood through surgical procedures or disease, the decreased hemoglobin can account for their extreme weakness as a result of decreased oxygen transport capacity. In addition, patients with advanced chronic obstructive pulmonary disease (COPD) can at times desaturate with exercise when their Po_2s are low; during exercise, they use increased oxygen.

Cyanosis, a bluish color to the skin, mucous membranes, and nailbeds, is indicative of an abnormal amount of reduced Hgb concentration, usually greater than 5 gm of reduced Hgb. The presence of cyanosis

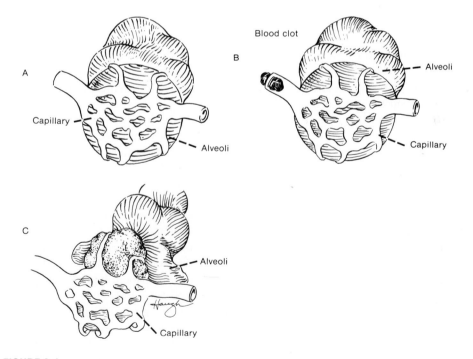

FIGURE 9-1
A, Normal alveolus. **B,** Dead space. **C,** Shunt.

suggests a high probability of hypoxemia; however, it can occur without cyanosis. Two examples may be cited, one in which an anemic patient with hypoxemia can have little cyanosis, and the other in which a patient with polycythemia can have cyanosis with minimal hypoxemia.

There is a predictable relationship between the arterial oxygen saturation of the Hgb and the P_{O_2}. It is represented in the oxyhemoglobin dissociation curve as follows. When oxygen saturation is monitored during exercise, saturation is kept at or above 90%. As the curve denotes at a level of approximately 60 mm Hg, the saturation is about 90%. As the P_{O_2} drops at the sharp part of the curve, for every mm Hg P_{O_2}, there is a marked decrease in oxygen saturation (Guyton, 1986).

Chemoreceptor Response to Hypoxemia

The peripheral chemoreceptors, the carotid, and the aortic bodies, are located at the bifurcation of the internal and external carotid arteries and the arch of the aorta. These receptors are nervous tissue that have a high metabolic rate and an abundant oxygen supply. When tissue P_{O_2} decreases, their response to the brain is to increase ventilation and cardiac output. When this is not sufficient to effect a normal P_{O_2}, supplemental oxygen or increased mechanical assistance such as continuous positive airway pressure (CPAP) is given (Tarpy, 1994).

BLOOD GAS INTERPRETATION

The norms for the pH, P_{CO_2}, P_{O_2}, and base have previously been given and should first be considered. Is the value normal or not? Is the patient acute, that is, uncompensated, partially compensated, or fully compensated (chronic)? There are also "acceptable" ranges to consider, as in the following:
- pH 7.30 to 7.50
- P_{CO_2} 30 to 50 mm Hg
- pH 7.45 alkalemia
- pH 7.35 acidemia
- Pa_{CO_2} 45 respiratory acidosis (hypercapnia)
- Pa_{CO_2} 35 respiratory alkalosis (hypocapnea)

A relationship between the pH and the PCO_2 also exists. There is a predictable change caused by variation in carbonic acid:

- For every 20 mm Hg increase in P_{CO_2}, the pH decreases by 0.10.
- For every 10 mm Hg decrease in P_{CO_2}, the pH increases by 0.10.

There is also a relationship between the P_{CO_2} and the plasma bicarbonate:
- For every increase of 10 mm Hg in the P_{CO_2}, there is a decrease of 1 mmol/L plasma bicarbonate
- For every 10 mm Hg P_{CO_2}, there is a decrease in plasma bicarbonate of 2 mmol/L.

Knowing these guidelines, it can be determined if the changes in the arterial blood gases are in line with respiratory problems vs. metabolic problems such as acidosis from diabetic ketoacidosis, where the base deficit can be very low, the pH can be low (acidemic), but the P_{CO_2} can be within normal limits (Shapiro, 1994; Shapiro, Peruzzi, and Templin, 1994).

RESPIRATORY FAILURE

Respiratory failure is defined as the failure of the pulmonary system to meet the metabolic demands of the body, that is, ventilation and oxygenation (Shapiro, Peruzzi, and Templin, 1994). The blood gases usually have a pH below 7.30 and a P_{CO_2} above 50. Generally the patient is also hypoxemic.

During the acute phase, the kidneys have not started to compensate and the base HCO_3^- is within normal limits. Later, a base excess can be noted as the kidneys try to compensate for the acidotic pH. Chronic respiratory failure can be noted by an increased P_{CO_2} with a pH within normal limits.

In assessing the P_{O_2}, the following ranges are used: mild hypoxemia less than 80 mm Hg, moderate hypoxemia 60 to 80 mm Hg, and severe hypoxemia below 40 mm Hg.

Positional changes can affect the oxygenation status. For example, unilateral right lower lobe atelectasis with the patient lying on the right side causes increased blood flow to the right lung, which is collapsed. This causes increased shunting and a decrease in oxygenation lying on the right side (differential shunting). If the patient lies on the left side, the oxygenation will improve. Lying supine, a mixed P_{O_2} can be observed.

When hypoxemia is noted, treatment consists of oxygen therapy and alleviation of the cause of hypoxemia, if possible. This may be airway clearance techniques or medication, in addition to the oxygen therapy. Oxygen therapy treats the hypoxemia, decreases the patient's work of breathing, and decreases myocardial work.

FACTORS AFFECTING ARTERIAL BLOOD GASES

There are many normal causes that have an affect on arterial blood gases, such as extremes of age-neonatal to geriatrics. The neonate has many changes going on in the initial life process; fetal circulation changes dramatically in the first hours and days of life. In the geriatric patient, decreases in cardiac output (CO), residual volume (RV) of the lungs, and maximal breathing capacity gradually decrease Po_2 over the life cycle. It is estimated that after 60 years of age, the Po_2 decreases by 1 mm Hg per year of age from 60 to 90 years.

Exercise or any increase in activity from rest may result in increased oxygen consumption for patients with cardiopulmonary dysfunction. In the normal population, the human body compensate by increasing oxygen consumption to meet the workload. Usually, a plateau is reached and a constant oxygen consumption for that activity is achieved. In patients with cardiopulmonary dysfunction, oxygen consumption continues to increase even at the same workload in untrained patients. It is important to monitor oxygen saturation to prevent desaturation of these patients (Guyton, 1986). During pregnancy, hormonal and mechanical factors have a negative effect on cardiopulmonary function. During the last trimester, women often observe shortness of breath and difficulty taking a deep breath secondary to diaphragmatic encroachment.

During sleep, there is a decrease in minute ventilation and a decreased responsiveness to CO_2 and hypoxemia. Many patients with spinal cord injury and COPD have been noted to have hypoxemia during sleep studies. This should be considered in any tired or groggy patient.

Low barometric pressure associated with high altitude significantly decreases the amount of oxygen available to the individual. As noted before, the partial pressure 20% of oxygen is dependent on the total atmospheric pressure. When the total pressure is reduced less O_2 is available. This is particularly important if a patient already has a decreased Po_2 and is traveling to an area with lower barometric pressure. Patients on oxygen will need an oxygen prescription based on the area in which they are living.

Barometric pressure increases, such as a hyperbaric oxygen chamber with higher barometric pressure, can be helpful in delivering increased oxygen for many patients. Wound-healing needs and carbon monoxide poisoning are two such indications.

Increased temperatures (febrile state) can increase metabolism and therefore increase oxygen consumption. Decreased temperatures can decrease the oxygen consumption, as seen in patients involved in cold water near drowning, where they survived several minutes under the water, and were resuscitated and resumed normal lives.

It is important to note on the arterial blood gas report the status of the patient when the blood gas was drawn. Usually patients are at rest when the blood gas is drawn. If the Po_2 is low at rest (60 mm Hg) it is close to the sharp part of the oxyhemoglobin dissociation curve and the patient may desaturate with exercise.

If the patient was on supplemental oxygen and the Po_2 was only 55 mm Hg, the Po_2 is still inadequate with additional O_2 (Carpenter, 1991). Similarly, if a patient is on mechanical ventilation, the blood gases should be within or near normal limits.

SUMMARY

This chapter discussed the normal arterial blood gases and what their values mean to the therapist. Relationships between pH and Pco_2, Pco_2 and Hco_3^-, and O_2 saturation and Po_2 have been examined. We saw predictable changes that are caused by respiratory changes were described. In addition we noted that metabolic changes can have marked effects on blood gases. Oxygen therapy and airway clearance techniques can improve hypoxemia, and position changes can be detrimental, causing differential shunting or improving the Po_2 by better ventilation/perfusion matching.

As PTs, it is necessary to be acutely aware of the respiratory monitors that can assess and progress patients safely to their optimal rehabilitation potential.

REVIEW QUESTIONS

1. Which factors affect arterial blood gases?
2. How can exercise have a deleterious effect on blood gases?
3. What predictable changes occur between pH and P_{CO_2} and P_{O_2} and oxygen saturation?
4. What two therapeutic techniques can improve hypoxemia?
5. What affect can body position have on blood gases?

References

Carpenter, K.D. (1991). Oxygen transport in the blood. *Critical Care Nurse, 11 (9),* 20-33.

Cherniak, R.M. (1992). Evaluation of respiratory function in health and disease. *Dis Mon, 38 (7),* 505-576.

Guyton, A. (1986). *Textbook of medical physiology* (7th ed.). Philadelphia: WB Saunders.

Shapiro, B.A. (1994). Evaluation of blood gas monitors: performance criteria, clinical impact, and cost/benefit (editorial comment). *Critical Care Medicine, 22 (4),* 546-548.

Shapiro, B.A., Peruzzi, W., & Templin, R. *Clinical application of blood gases,* (5th ed.). St. Louis: Mosby.

Tarpy, S.P., & Farber, H.W. (1994). Chronic lung disease: when to prescribe home oxygen. *Geriatrics, 49 (2),* 27-28, 31-33.

CHAPTER 10

Principles of Chest X-Ray Interpretation

Michael Ries
Thomas Johnson

KEY TERMS

Air bronchogram
Air fluid levels
Atelectasis
Densities
Diffuse patterns

Hyperlucency
Mass formations
Pneumonia
Radiograph
Silouette sign

There are three general categories of radiographic studies of the chest—fixed-position studies, suspended motion studies, and motion studies. The routine posteroanterior (PA) and lateral chest film is a fixed-position, suspended motion study. The patient is positioned with chest against the x-ray film holder and is asked to hold his breath in deep inspiration.

The radiograph (x-ray) is named from the source of the x-rays to the film. Thus a PA chest film is positioned so that the source of the x-rays is 72 in. behind the patient and the film is in front. An anteroposterior (AP) chest film is the reverse, with the back of the patient against the film. During interpretation, the conventional position of the film on the view box is as if the physical therapist (PT) were facing the patient.

One of the first things to check before interpreting the film is the quality of the film. An optimal PA chest film is one in which the dim outline of the vertebral bodies is seen through the mediastinum. Films may be overpenetrated (of increased density) or underpenetrated (of decreased density) and still be adequate for interpretation. Suboptimal films may also hide pathology and cause misinterpretation.

The purpose of a radiograph is to see inside the otherwise opaque body by shifting the spectrum of light to above the high ranges of the visible spectrum, thus converting the body structures into densities rather than colors. The densities recorded on the x-ray film range in shades of gray to black depending on the amount of x-ray energy the structures of the body absorb as the x-ray passes through them.

159

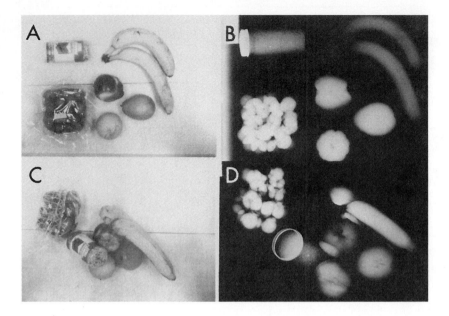

FIGURE 10-1

Familiar fruits such as an apple, orange, pear and banana (**A** and **C**) transform into two-dimensional objects when x-rayed (**B** and **D**). The pictures (**A** and **C**) also show a box of cherry tomatoes and a jar of bird seed (millet seed) and their x-rays. **B**, is the radiograph of **A**, and **D**, is the radiograph of **C**. Changes in position of the same objects from **A** to **C** illustrate the changes of shape in the corresponding x-rays. **B** to **D**, and emphasize the need for PA and lateral x-rays for evaluating three-dimensional structures.

There are five basic densities, varying from very radiolucent to very radiopaque. The darkest or most radiolucent density is gas or air. Fat is moderately radiolucent. An intermediate or water density is seen reflecting the connective tissues, blood, muscle, skin, and other structures. Bone and deposited calcium are moderately radiopaque. Metal is the most opaque (white or clear). The structures of the body absorb most of the x-rays as they pass through the body, and the remainder of the rays expose the film.

An example of an x-ray is the familiar fruits or objects that have been converted into a two-dimensional reproduction of densities in Figure 10-1. These three-dimensional structures are reduced to two dimensions and only the edges or structures tangential to the beam of the x-rays are recorded. Thus two views, taken at 90° from each other (PA and lateral), are required for a mental reconstruction of the third dimension, which is used to interpret the internal problems of a patient.

The routine examination of the chest should include a PA and lateral chest film on maximum inspiration at least for the first examination. Without the lateral film, disease processes behind the heart and posterior in the thorax may be missed. Very ill patients who cannot be transported to the radiology department must often be evaluated at the bedside from a single PA or AP view (taken with the portable x-ray unit). The size of the patient introduces mechanical limitations to the performance of a lateral chest film. Portable x-ray units are not as powerful as the stationary departmental machines.

Additional radiographic views may be ordered to verify or elucidate findings. These include (1) oblique views, (2) apical lordotic views, (3) decubitus views, (4) laminograms, (5) inspiration and

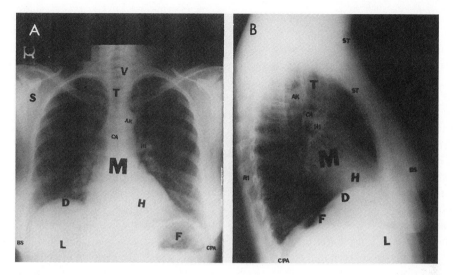

FIGURE 10-2

These **A,** PA and **B,** lateral x-rays anatomically localize the basic structures that must be reviewed during chest x-ray evaluation. Some of the structures are seen in both views and others are seen in only one view. During evaluation, one should identify and see the following basic anatomical structures.

Soft tissues and *extrathoracic structures:* soft tissues *(ST)*, breast shadows *(BS)*, diaphragm *(D)*, liver *(L)*, and fundus of stomach *(F)*.

Bony thorax: ribs *(RI)*, vertebrae *(V)*, scapulae *(S, seen best on PA)*, clavicles *(CL, seen best on PA)* and sternum *(SN, seen best on lateral)*.

Mediastinal structures: mediastinum *(M)*, trachea *(T)*, carina *(CA)*, aortic knob *(AK)*, heart *(H)*, anterior clear space *(ACS, seen on lateral)* and hilus of lungs *(HI)*.

Lung fields: hilus of lungs *(HI)*, pulmonary vessels (arise from hilus and branch outward), costophrenic angles *(CPA)* and lung apices *(LA, seen best on PA)*.

There are many other structures that must be evaluated in addition to these basic ones, and pathologies must be identified.

expiration films, (6) special studies requiring contrast materials, (7) physiologic motion evaluation with the fluoroscope, (8) computed tomography (CT scan), and (9) magnetic resonance imaging (MRI).

Film interpretation requires a solid knowledge of gross anatomy and gross pathology. The PT is literally examining the internal structures of the body without an autopsy or surgical intervention. The structures of the body are thus converted into the densities of air, fat, water, calcium, and metal. The PT should examine the entire film, not just one area, and should not get "tunnel vision." Once an abnormality is found, the PT should continue to evaluate the remainder of the film and should not stop at that point,

since other pathologies may be present. All the anatomical structures on the film should be examined. A body system approach is recommended: bones and soft tissues (including the abdomen), the mediastinum from larynx to abdomen, the cardiovascular system, the hila, and finally, the lungs (Figure 10-2).

The tools of radiographic interpretation include the following:

1. The principle of bilateral symmetry (when structures are paired, then in general one should look like the other).
2. The presence or absence of air fluid levels (there are almost no straight lines in the chest).

If a line appears to be straight, then it must be explained.

3. The silhouette sign. When densities are next to each other, they obliterate normal margins and show no separation (normal silhouette of a structure is obliterated). When densities or structures are in front or in back of other densities or structures, then a margin is seen.

4. An air bronchogram is seen when the air around a bronchus is pathologically filled with fluid or other material.

5. Lobar and segmental collapse follows the anatomy of the lung.

6. Pleural changes may be manifested by gas in a pneumothorax, fluid in a pleural effusion, calcium or soft tissue from scarring or mesothehome. A hydropneumothorax demonstrates an air fluid level.

7. The presence or absence of mass formation as in tumors, nodular changes or miliary changes. The conventional terminology depends on the size of the abnormality.

8. Air-containing spaces such as bullae or cysts.

Bronchi are not usually seen unless they are surrounded by fluid or have a disease causing thickening of the walls. The vascular pattern may be distorted, blurred, increased, or decreased by pulmonary disease. Air space or alveolar disease is manifested by opacification (white appearance) of air-filled structures of the lung. Thus pneumonia may appear as patchy coalescent areas of acini, or segmental and/or lobar consolidation. An air bronchogram is seen when the air-filled lung tissue about the bronchus is filled with fluid or other material and the bronchus is filled with air (Figure 10-3).

Certain lung diseases cause a decrease (increase in translucency), such as emphysema (generalized) or bullae (localized). Interstitial pulmonary disease is manifested by distortion or increase in volume of tissues surrounding the air spaces. An enormous number of diseases can produce interstitial roentgenographic changes. Sometimes a diagnosis is strongly suggested by the roentgenographic appearance, but in most, a histologic evaluation is required for diagnosis. Enlargement of the bronchi may result in bronchiectasis (Figure 10-4). Bronchiectasis is characterized by tubular

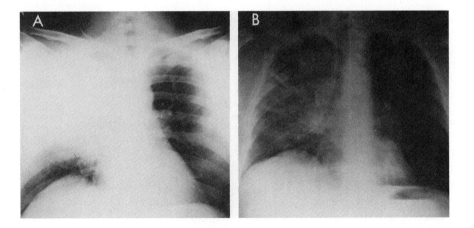

FIGURE 10-3
A, There is total pneumonic consolidation of right upper lobe with complete alveolar and bronchial filling. **B,** Approximately 24 to 36 hours later, the consolidation has cleared markedly with patchy coalescent residual. A few air bronchograms are seen in the perihilar region.

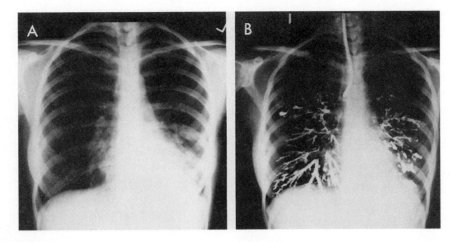

FIGURE 10-4
A, Fibrosis and saccular bronchiectatic changes are present in the left lower lobe. A few cystic "circular" changes are present in the right upper lobe but are best seen on the bronchogram. **B,** The bronchogram demonstrates the dilated abnormal bronchi of cystic and saccular bronchiectasis in the left lower lobe with fibrosis around them. The right upper lobe reveals a few cystic changes.

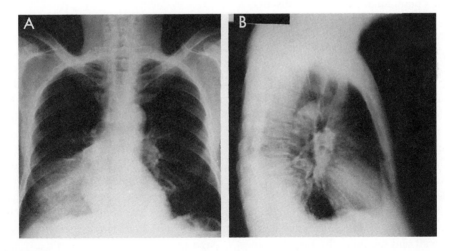

FIGURE 10-5
A, The PA chest film demonstrates the water density of a pneumonic consolidation in the right lower lobe. The diaphragm is blurred. **B,** The lateral film shows obliteration of the posterior right diaphragm and the costophrenic angle by the pneumonic consolidation.

shadows that are double-line parallel shadows following the bronchovascular distribution. The shadows may branch similar to the bronchial tree.

Pneumonias are usually classified by their causative agents of anatomical distribution. A lobar pneumonia is one that involves the entire lobe, and a segmental pneumonia involves the anatomical segment of a lobe. Generalized pneumonic processes occur with aspiration of vascular spread of an infectious agent (Figure 10-5). The roentgenographic findings of bronchopneumonia are varied. The earliest manifestation may consist only of peribronchial cuffing. The disease, however, spreads rapidly to the alveoli. More often, however, bronchopneumonia is manifested by multiple, ill-defined nodular densities (acinar nodules) that are patchy. As these acinar nodules become confluent, airspace consolidation develops. As the disease progresses, segmental and lobar pneumonias can be seen.

Pulmonary abscesses and cavities may occur secondary to pneumonia. An abscess occurs when there is a breakdown of the tissues of the lung, with the area replaced by infectious materials (of water density). When the infectious materials empty into the bronchus and air communicates with the abscess, a cavity develops in that area of the lung. Lung abscesses often result from aspiration and they are often found in the areas dependent at the time of the aspiration. Thus abscesses occur in the area that is downward by gravity, depending on the upright or reclining position of the individual (Figure 10-6). If the pleura is penetrated by the abscess, an empyema develops; and if a cavity communicates with the pleura, a pneumothorax develops with a bronchopleural fistula.

A pneumothorax or gas in the pleural space develops when the pleural space communicates air through either a defect in the chest wall or a defect in the pleural surface of the lung. As the air accumulates between the chest wall and the lung, the lung becomes compressed and moves away from the chest wall (separated by air) (Figure 10-7). Chronic interstitial disease and emphysema are often complicated by a spontaneous pneumothorax. Traumatic causes such as automobile accidents or insertion of central venous

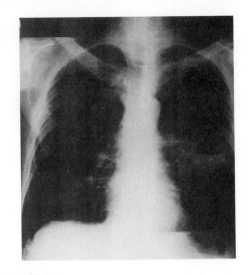

FIGURE 10-6
A 5-cm cavitary abscess is seen on the left with an air fluid level and a relatively smooth wall. This patient was probably recumbent and lying slightly on the left side to aspirate materials to this area, which was first a pneumonic process in the superior segment of the left lower lobe and progressed to an abscess cavity.

catheters may result in a traumatic pneumothorax. The appearance is fairly characteristic, and there may be an associated air fluid level with a hydropneumothorax (secondary to minor bleeding from the punctured lung). Pleural effusions, or the accumulation of fluid between the lung and chest wall, can be seen in increased hydrostatic pressure (congestive heart failure [CHF]), diseases of the pleurae (malignancies) or diseases of the lung (emphysema secondary to pneumonia).

Atelectasis is the term used for incomplete expansion of a portion or all of the lung. A loss of air in the alveoli in the atelectatic area occurs. Atelectasis is a sign of disease, since it is always secondary to another lesion, such as (1) obstruction of a bronchus; (2) loss of ability for pulmonary expansion as a result of pleural disease, diaphragmatic disease, and masses in the thorax; or (3) volume loss from local or generalized pulmonary fibrosis. Atelectasis is a loss of vol-

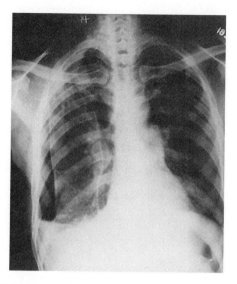

FIGURE 10-7

The chest x-ray reveals separation of the visceral from the parietal pleural line and absence of vessels laterally. A "straight line" is seen at the right base, indicating a gas fluid level in a hydropneumothorax. Fibrotic and irregular pulmonary changes in the lungs indicate underlying interstitial disease, which was a pneumoconiosis (silicosis).

ume in the area involved and results in a decrease in size or a change in position of the surrounding structures (Figure 10-8).

Congestive heart failure, uremia and pulmonary edema may be manifested by a "diffuse" pattern on the chest film (Figure 10-9). In CHF, there is a progression of roentgenographic changes as the disease evolves into pulmonary edema. The first manifestation is an increase in the antigravity vasculature of the lungs (redistribution of blood flow to the upper lobe vessels). The next stage is manifested by a loss of the distinct margins of the vessels. This is followed by accumulation of fluid in the interstitial spaces (around the alveoli). Pulmonary edema is present when the fluid seeps from the interstitium and makes the alveoli opaque. Pulmonary edema is radiographically indistinguishable from diffuse pneumonia. CHF usually is associated with cardiomegaly (enlargement of cardiac silhouette) and may be associated with pleural effusions and/or pericardial effusions (Figure 10-10).

Pulmonary malignancies may be both primary and metastatic. Mass formation is characteristic, and there may be atelectasis when the mass obstructs a

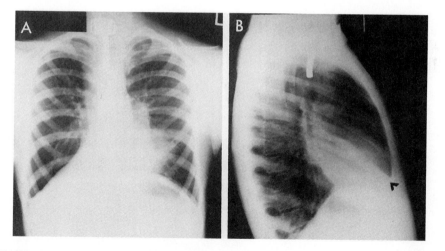

FIGURE 10-8

A, The PA film demonstrates loss of the right heart border and the downward shift of the minor fissure, with atelectasis of the right middle lobe secondary to a radiolucent foreign body in the right middle lobe bronchus. No air remains in the middle lobe, thus it is dense. **B,** The *arrow* on the lateral view points to the residual tissue density of the right middle lobe, which is atelectatic.

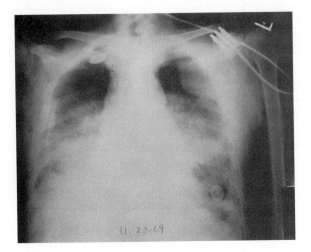

FIGURE 10-9
The central lung fields reveal increased density and there is sparing of the peripheral areas in "butterfly" pulmonary edema. The patient has had a thoracotomy, and chest tubes are in place.

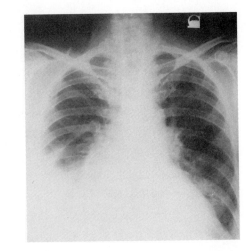

FIGURE 10-10
The chest film reveals cardiomegaly (enlargement of the cardiopericardial silhouette) and bilateral pleural effusions are more marked on the right than on the left. Vascular structures are blurred with interstitial edema.

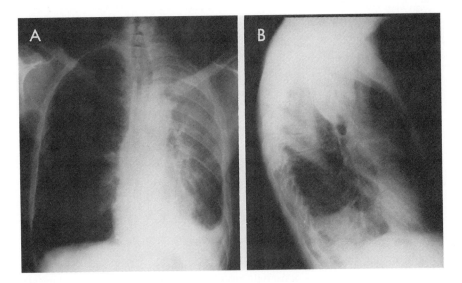

FIGURE 10-11
A, A mass is present in the left hilar area obstructing the left upper lobe bronchus. There is atelectasis of the left upper lobe and lingula secondary to the malignancy. **B,** The lateral view reveals an S-shaped curve of tumor mass and atelectasis.

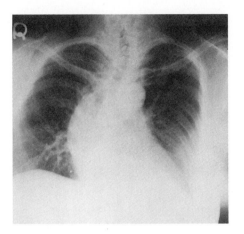

FIGURE 10-12
This chest x-ray of a kyphoscoliotic patient reveals a
markedly abnormal, reverse S-shaped curve of the thoracic
spine deforming the mediastinal structures and ribs. This
patient is breathing primarily with the diaphragms.

bronchus (Figure 10-11). Secondary findings such as
widening of the mediastinum, rib metastasis, pleural
masses or pleural fluid, and encasement of vasculature with hyperlucency beyond the tumor may be
seen. Alveolar cell carcinoma may appear like a
pneumonia. Involvement of the phrenic nerve may
result in paralysis of the diaphragm with elevation.

Thoracic deformities such as kyphoscoliosis may
severely impair the respiration of an individual (Figure 10-12). The abnormal shape and direction of the
spine interfere with the leverage necessary for movement of the ribs with respiration. Severe impairment
of respiration may occur when there is fusion of the

articulating facets in rheumatoid arthritis of the spine.
An obese individual may have severe difficulty with
respiration, not only because of the excess fat and
added weight on the thorax, but also because of the
increased load on the cardiovasculature system. This
increased load and hypoxemia may result in CHF.

REVIEW QUESTIONS

1. What are the three categories of radiographic
   studies of the chest?
2. How may the quality of the film impact interpretation?
3. What are the five basic densities seen on a radiograph?
4. What principles are used consistently to interpret
   radiographs?
5. How can lung disease cause a change in translucency of the Xray?
6. How can mediastinal deviation diagnose pneumothorax or atelectasis?

Bibliography

Felson, B. (1973). *Fundamentals of chest roentgenology* (2nd ed.).
    Philadelphia: WB Saunders.
Fraser, R.G. & Pare, J.A. (1988). *Diagnosis of diseases of the chest*
    (3rd ed.). Philadelphia: WB Saunders.
Freundlich, I.M. & Bragg, D.G. (1992). *A radiographic approach
    to diseases of the chest* Baltimore: Williams and Wilkins.
Meschan, I. (1976). *Synopsis of analysis of roentgen signs in gen-
    eral radiology* Philadelphia: WB Saunders.
Murray, J.F. & Jade, J.A. (1994). *Textbook of respiratory medicine*
    Philadelphia: WB Saunders.
Paul, L.W. & Juhl, J.H. *The essentials of roentgen interpretation*
    (3rd ed.). New York: Paul B Hober, 1972.

CHAPTER 11

Electrocardiogram Identification

Gary Brooks

KEY TERMS	Arrhythmia	Electrocardiogram (ECG)
	Artifact	Syncytium
	Bradycardia	Supraventricular
	Depolarization	Tachycardia

INTRODUCTION

The heart is a vital link in the oxygen transport system, pumping blood to the pulmonary and peripheral circulation systems to supply oxygen and other nutrients required for metabolism in all tissues. The beating heart generates rhythmic, electrical impulses that cause mechanical contraction, or the pumping action, of cardiac muscle. Some of the electrical current produced by these rhythmic impulses is detectable by electrodes that may be placed on the surface of the skin. Current flow during the cardiac cycle is then recorded as the characteristic waveforms of the electrocardiogram (ECG). Mechanical events such as contraction and relaxation of the myocardium are inferred from the waveforms produced by the ECG.

The ECG is an essential tool in the physician's diagnosis and medical treatment of cardiac disease. Information provided by the ECG may also assist the physical therapist (PT) in the assessment of a patient's readiness for and response to physical activity. PTs in many different practice environments have access to information afforded by the ECG. For example, in an acute care or rehabilitation setting, a patient's baseline ECG, with an interpretation, may be available within the medical record. Documentation accompanying a referral for outpatient physical therapy may include a reference to the patient's ECG. In other settings such as an intensive care unit or cardiac rehabilitation program, ongoing monitoring of a patient's ECG may be performed during evaluation and treatment procedures. It is therefore crucial that all PTs have a basic understanding of the uses and limitations of the ECG in their practices.

This chapter briefly reviews the basic anatomy and physiology of the myocardial conduction system as it relates to the ECG. The configuration of the normal ECG is presented and discussed along with several methods of quickly determining heart rate and rhythm from an electrocardiographic record or "strip." Some of the more common dysrhythmias are examined, as are some other pathologic features. Throughout the chapter, the uses and limitations of the ECG in physical therapy practice are highlighted.

PHYSIOLOGY AND ANATOMY OF THE CONDUCTION SYSTEM
Generation of the Action Potential

The action potential, or cardiac impulse, is generated by ionic flow across myocardial cell membranes. In the cell's resting state, a negative membrane potential exists, based on the relative concentrations of sodium (Na^+), Calcium (Ca^{++}), and Potassium (K^+) in the internal and external cellular environments. Membrane potential changes rapidly at the onset of depolarization, with the opening of Na^+ and Ca^{++} channels, allowing these ions to cross the membrane and enter the cell. Calcium then becomes available for contraction of cardiac muscle myofibrils. During depolarization, the membrane's potential becomes positive and the cell contracts. As in skeletal muscle, the Na^+ channels are fast-opening and fast-closing mechanisms, allowing Na^+ to rapidly enter the myocardial cell on depolarization. Unlike skeletal muscle, however, cardiac muscle has a prolonged depolarization phase as a result of the slower and extended opening of the Ca^{++} channels. During depolarization, there is also a decrease in membrane permeability to K^+, for which there is an outward gradient. A plateau phase of the action potential exists, during which outward flow of K^+ ions is inhibited. This prolongs depolarization and delays return to the resting membrane potential.

Each cell has an absolute refractory period during depolarization, meaning that an additional stimulus will not cause an additional depolarization. A brief, but significant, relative refractory period follows depolarization, during which a stimulus of greater than normal intensity is necessary to depolarize the cell again. The refractory period of atrial cells is significantly shorter than that of ventricular cells allowing a more rapid intrinsic atrial rhythm than intrinsic ventricular rhythm. Therefore atrial rhythms pace the heart, including the ventricles, given intact atrioventricular (AV) conduction.

Closure of the slow Ca^{++} channels at onset of repolarization is accompanied by opening of K^+ channels, causing a rapid outflow of K^+, which restores resting negative membrane potential. During the cell's resting phase, Na^+ and Ca^{++} are actively pumped out of the cell, and K^+ is pumped into the cell, restoring ionic gradients needed for repolarization (Shih, 1994; Guyton, 1991; Smith and Kampine, 1990).

It is the electrical current produced by ionic flow that is transmitted through the conductive tissues surrounding the heart. This current is detectable by surface electrodes, enabling the recording of the ECG.

The Conduction System

Because myocardial cells are arranged as a syncytium, an impulse propagates, or spreads to adjacent cells, causing them to make contact also. This arrangement alone does not permit the heart to function as an effective pump. It is the conduction system that initiates and rapidly transmits impulses to other locations within the myocardium, allowing for effective, coordinated myocardial contraction and pumping. The conduction system is comprised of specialized cardiac muscle that contracts minimally, because it contains few contractile myofibrils.

Any portion of the conduction system is capable of self-excitation and may act as a pacemaker, generating action potentials. However, because of the intrinsically more rapid rate of spontaneous depolarization of the sinoatrial (SA) node, it normally acts as the heart's pacemaker. The rate of depolarization of the SA node determines the heart rate. In the absence of an impulse from the SA node, the atrioventricular (AV) node depolarizes spontaneously, taking over as pacemaker, with the important difference that the rate of depolarization is lower than that of the SA node.

The pathway of a normal cardiac impulse may be

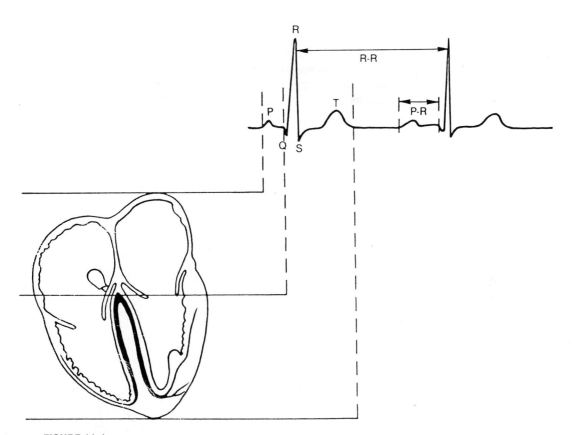

FIGURE 11-1
Relationship of ECG complex to conduction pathway. (From Brown, K.R., & Jacobson. (1988). *Mastering dysrhythmias: A problem-solving guide.* Philadelphia: FA Davis.)

followed, highlighting its relationship to the cardiac cycle. Figure 11-1 displays the association of the conduction system and its components with the ECG. Atrial depolarization is initiated by a spontaneously generated impulse that originates in the SA node. The impulse is then transmitted throughout the atrial muscle resulting in atrial contraction. This event is recorded as the P-wave of the ECG. The impulse is also transmitted, via rapidly conducting internodal pathways, to the AV node. Atrial repolarization is not recorded by the ECG, because it occurs during and is hidden by ventricular depolarization.

Impulse conduction within the AV node and the AV bundle (bundle of His) slows considerably, re-

sulting in a delaying of the impulse before it reaches the ventricular conduction system. This pause in impulse propagation allows the atria to contract and fill the ventricles with blood. The P-R interval of the ECG represents this period between onset of atrial depolarization and the onset of ventricular depolarization. Normally the P-R interval lasts between 0.12 and 0.20 seconds (Brown and Jacobson, 1988).

Following passage through the AV node, the impulse continues to the Purkinje's fibers, which transmit the impulse rapidly to the ventricular endocardium. This initiates ventricular depolarization, which is represented in the ECG by the QRS complex.

The depolarization wave propagates relatively slowly throughout the ventricular myocardium. The span of time elapsing during ventricular depolarization is reflected by the QRS interval, which normally ranges between 0.06 and 0.11 seconds (Brown and Jacobson, 1988; Smith and Kampine, 1990). Ventricular depolarization originates in the interventricular septum, creating the Q-wave, which is normally small or absent. The depolarization wave next spreads to the apex and then to the right and left ventricles, causing the R- and S-waves. Depolarization also propagates in an endocardial to epicardial direction within the ventricles (Lilly, 1993; Guyton, 1991).

The T-wave of the ECG represents ventricular repolarization. It is preceded by the S-T segment, during which depolarization has been completed and repolarization is yet to begin. The configuration of the S-T segment is an important marker of myocardial ischemia or infarction. Following the T-wave, a U-wave may be seen. The U-wave was considered to have little physiologic or pathologic significance (Smith and Kampine, 1990). However, U-wave inversion may now be considered to correlate with myocardial ischemia (American College of Sports Medicine, 1991). Note that the ventricles remain in a state of contraction until slightly after repolarization. This period of contraction corresponds to the Q-T interval on the ECG. Diastole, therefore, begins subsequent to the end of the T-wave and continues until the next ventricular depolarization. Note also that atrial depolarization and contraction occur during diastole.

THE ELECTROCARDIOGRAM
Recording the Electrocardiogram

Before examining the timing of the wave forms and the rhythms of the ECG, a basic understanding of the

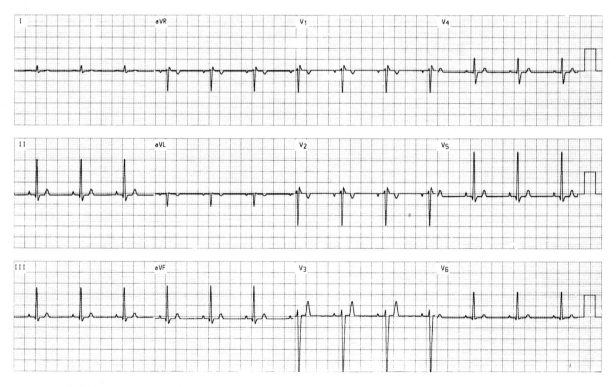

FIGURE 11-2
A normal 12-lead ECG tracing.

principles of electrocardiography is needed. A standard, 12-lead configuration is used for diagnosis and medical management of cardiac conditions. An example of a normal 12-lead ECG is seen in Figure 11-2. Six leads record the electrical signals in the frontal plane, and six leads record signals in the transverse plane.

The frontal plane leads include three standard limb leads—I, II, and III. Three augmented limb leads,

AVR, AVL, and AVF are derived from the electrical sum of the three standard limb leads. The transverse plane leads are referred to as the precordial leads. Imagine that each of the 12 leads "views" the heart from a different angle, therefore recording events in different locations of the heart (Figure 11-3). By convention, the waveform on the ECG is positive (upward) as current travels toward a lead and negative (downward) when current travels away from a lead.

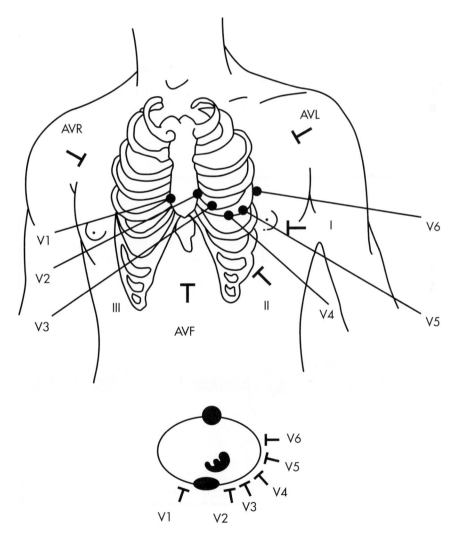

FIGURE 11-3
Electrocardiogram leads.

Other lead configurations may be used for exercise testing (American College of Sports Medicine, 1991). Single-lead monitoring is commonly used during exercise training or in acute care settings.

Evaluating the ECG Strip

The evaluation of an ECG should be approached in a systematic fashion. The following questions are useful to appreciate the information that is relevant to current clinical practice (Cummins, 1994).

• What is the rate and pattern (regularity) of the rhythm? If the R-R interval, that is, the distance between successive R-waves, is inconsistent, is the pattern irregular?
• Does a P-wave precede every QRS complex? This indicates appropriate atrial activity.
• Is there a QRS complex after every P-wave? This indicates appropriate conduction of impulses from atria to ventricles.
• What is the P-R interval? A P-R interval of greater than 0.20 seconds indicates delay in conduction from atria to ventricles.
• Is the QRS complex of normal duration and morphology (shape)? A QRS complex greater than 0.12 seconds indicates either that an impulse arose within a ventricle or was conducted abnormally through the ventricular conduction system.

By answering each of these questions, the tendency to "eyeball" the rhythm and make a quick but inaccurate assessment is avoided.

Determination of Heart Rate

Several quick methods estimate heart rate. Most printed and displayed ECG recordings indicate a heart

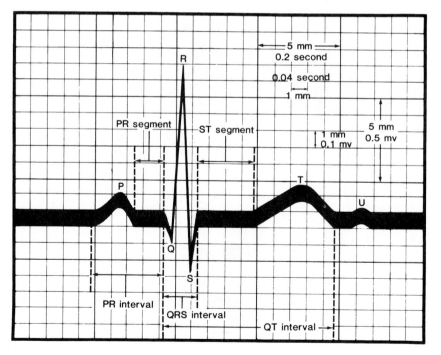

FIGURE 11-4

A normal ECG showing characteristic waves, intervals, and segments, and some of the features of the tracing paper.

rate. This must be interpreted with caution, however. The presence of artifact (extraneous deflections of the waveform caused by movement or electrical interference) may render inaccurate the displayed or printed heart rate. This is a common problem during activity or exercise, the circumstances during which many PTs monitor patients. It is possible to calculate or to estimate a heart rate from a printed ECG strip because, by convention, the recording paper is divided into 1 mm squares and larger 5 mm squares, which are defined by heavier lines (Figure 11-4). Also by convention, the standard paper speed for an ECG recording is a rate of 25 mm/second. Each millimeter of length then represents 1/25th, or 0.04 seconds, and each 5 mm block represents one fifth, or 0.20 seconds. Some monitor systems place a mark on the recording paper at 25 mm, or 1-second intervals.

There are several methods of estimating heart rate from a printed ECG strip. On a printed ECG strip, find an R-wave located on or near a heavy vertical line. Proceeding to the left of that R wave, for each subsequent heavy vertical line, assign the following numbers: 300 for the first heavy line encountered, 150 for the next followed by 100, 75, 60, 50, and 42 (Figure 11-5). Stop at the first heavy vertical line following the next R wave that is encountered. The heart rate may be estimated as falling between the two most recently assigned values. In Figure 11-5,

the rate would be estimated as falling between 100 and 75, or close to 80 beats per minute (BPM).

In many clinics, rulers are available that are calibrated so that heart rate may be estimated quickly by aligning markings on the ruler with features of the ECG strip. For example, after the arrow on the ruler is placed on an R-wave, count two R-waves to the left and read the number at that position on the ruler. In Figure 11-6, this method approximates the heart rate as 74 BPM.

It is important to note that the preceding two methods are useful *only* if the rhythm of the ECG strip is regular, that is the R-waves are equally spaced, occurring at consistent intervals. Should the rhythm be irregular, with R-waves appearing at varying intervals, another method must be employed to estimate the heart rate.

Recall that the ECG graph paper is divided into boxes, with the horizontal spacing representing time intervals of 0.04 seconds for each small (1 mm) box and 0.20 seconds for each larger (5 mm) box. It follows that 1 second in time is represented by five larger boxes. A mark may be placed at 1- or 3-second intervals, enabling quicker appraisal of heart rate based on a 6-second strip. The procedure is as follows. Obtain a printed strip of sufficient length, covering more than 6 seconds. If 1-second marks are not present, it may be convenient to place a mark at every

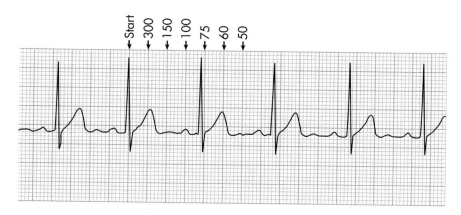

FIGURE 11-5
"Count-off" method of estimating heart rate.

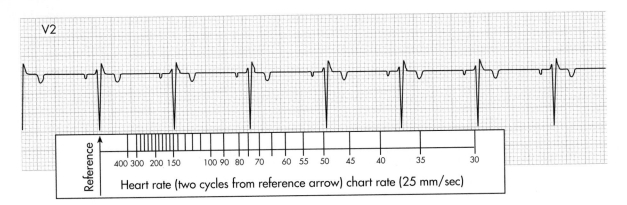

FIGURE 11-6
Using a rate-ruler to confirm heart rate.

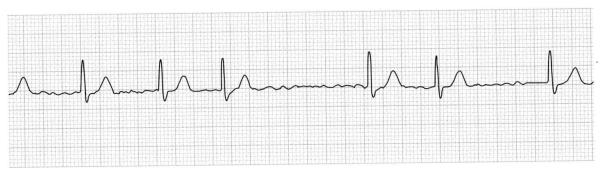

FIGURE 11-7
Heart rate estimation in an irregular rhythm (atrial fibrillation).

fifth large block. Next, select a 1-second mark or a heavy vertical line on the left side of the strip, and proceed to the right for a length corresponding to 6 seconds. If 1-second marks are counted, do not count the starting mark or there will be only a 5-second strip. Count the number of R-waves within the 6-second recording, and multiply by 10. That is estimated heart rate. Several 6-second strips may be analyzed to document a heart rate range of an irregular rhythm (Figure 11-7). The rate of this irregular rhythm is estimated at 70 BPM.

Evaluation of Rhythms

Electrocardiographic monitoring is an important evaluation tool during the treatment of individuals with history of or potential for acute myocardial infarction (MI) or myocardial ischemia. Most cardiac deaths are a result of lethal arrhythmias, for which there is increased risk in the presence of infarction or ischemia. Rapid recognition of lethal arrhythmias, or arrhythmias that may deteriorate into lethal arrhythmias, is essential for all health professionals involved in the care of individuals with cardiac disease. The arrhythmias described in

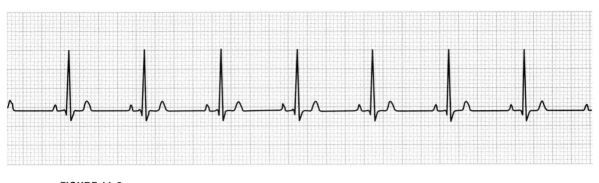

FIGURE 11-8
Normal sinus rhythm.

this chapter are those that must be recognized by providers of Advanced Cardiac Life Support as determined by the American Heart Association (Emergency Cardiac Care Committee and Subcommittees, 1992).

Normally, a cardiac impulse is generated by the SA node, causing atrial depolarization. This is followed by a slight delay in the AV node, after which the impulse is conducted to the ventricles causing ventricular depolarization. These events are seen in their normal spatial and temporal sequence in normal sinus rhythm (Figure 11-8). A P-wave precedes every QRS complex and every P-wave is, in turn, succeeded by a QRS complex. This occurs within an interval of 0.20 seconds (one large box), as determined by the P-R interval. The QRS complexes occur within a range of 0.04 to 0.11 seconds, indicating that ventricular impulse conduction and depolarization is occurring in a normal interval. The positively deflected T-wave indicates normal ventricular repolarization. Because the SA node spontaneously depolarizes at a rate of between 60 and 100 BPM, the rate of normal sinus rhythm must fall within these limits.

The identification of arrhythmias affects clinical decision making, particularly with regards to a patient's readiness for and/or response to activity. Clinical significance of arrhythmias range from benign to lethal. The clinical significance of a given arrhythmia is determined by a number of considerations. Some of these considerations include the following: Is there evidence of hemodynamic compromise? Is the arrhythmia a new or unusual finding? Might the arrhythmia be a precursor to a more serious or perhaps lethal arrhythmia? Is this an acute occurrence or a chronic arrhythmia pattern? The clinical response to a patient with an arrhythmia depends on the answers to these questions and the treatment setting.

ARRHYTHMIA IDENTIFICATION
Supraventricular Arrhythmias

Supraventricular arrhythmias arise from an abnormality of impulse generation or conduction "above" the level of the ventricles. The abnormality may occur in the atria or at the level of the AV junction. Supraventricular arrhythmias may be categorized as sinus, atrial, or junctional arrhythmias.

A cardiac rhythm may be a sinus rhythm, but with an irregular or abnormally rapid or slow rate. Sinus arrhythmia is an irregular sinus rhythm with varying R-R intervals (Figure 11-9). This is a normal variant that is associated with the individual's respiratory pattern. *Sinus bradycardia* is a sinus rhythm occurring at a rate of less than 60 BPM (Figure 11-10). This rhythm may significantly reduce cardiac output, causing hemodynamic compromise, manifested by hypotension or symptoms such as dizziness, lightheadedness, or syncope. On the other hand, individuals taking beta-blockers, medication that slows the heart, may exhibit this as their normal rhythm, as may individuals who achieve a high level of physical conditioning. *Sinus tachycardia* is a sinus rhythm occurring at a rate of greater than 100 BPM (Figure 11-11). Sinus tachycardia, or any other

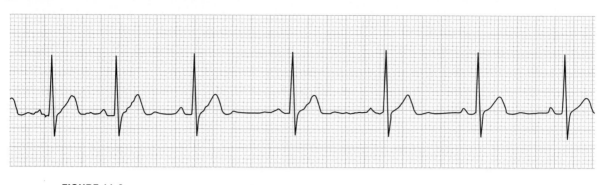

FIGURE 11-9
Sinus arrhythmia.

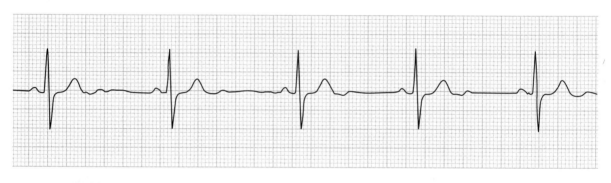

FIGURE 11-10
Sinus bradycardia.

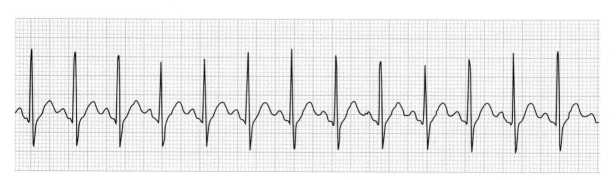

FIGURE 11-11
Sinus tachycardia.

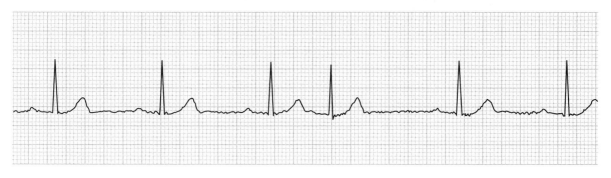

FIGURE 11-12
Premature atrial complex.

form of tachycardia, increases myocardial oxygen demand, or the workload on the heart. This may initiate or exacerbate ischemia in the presence of coronary artery disease (CAD).

A common form of arrhythmia is a "premature" complex, that is, a beat that occurs sooner than expected given the established rhythm. A premature atrial complex, or PAC, is an early beat of atrial origin (Figure 11-12). An R-wave appears closer to its preceding R-wave than the other R-waves in the established rhythm. Closer inspection reveals the presence of a P-wave associated with the QRS complex, meaning that the impulse first depolarized the atria before being conducted to the ventricles. Sometimes the AV junction may initiate an early beat, causing a premature junctional complex or PJC. When this occurs, the R-wave appears earlier; however, there may be no associated P-wave, or there may be an unusual P-wave, one that is inverted or following the QRS complex. An inverted or late P-wave indicates that the impulse was conducted in retrograde (backward) fashion. Clinically, a premature atrial or junctional complex may be palpated as a "skipped" or early beat during pulse taking, or the patient may perceive a palpitation or skipped beat. Otherwise, these arrhythmias are usually of little clinical significance (Brown and Jacobson, 1988).

A more serious supraventricular arrhythmia is supraventricular tachycardia, or SVT. In this arrhythmia, the heart rate is rapid, exceeding 150 BPM. The tachycardia may be sustained, lasting hours or even days, or may be "paroxysmal" (PSVT), appearing

abruptly and spontaneously reconverting to the previous rhythm within seconds or minutes. The P-wave is often not visible, making assessment of atrial or junctional origin difficult, but the duration of the QRS complexes occurs within an appropriate interval. The R-R interval, however, is markedly shortened. Figure 11-13 demonstrates supraventricular tachycardia at a rate of 190 BPM. Other related forms of SVT include paroxysmal atrial tachycardia (PAT) and multifocal atrial tachycardia (MAT). Clinically, patients with SVT may perceive a "racing" heart rate, which may be quite distressing. At very rapid heart rates, for example, greater than 170 BPM, diastolic ventricular filling time is markedly reduced, which may cause hemodynamic compromise. Symptoms associated with inadequate cardiac output, such as dizziness, lightheadedness, and syncope may ensue. Some individuals with SVT remain asymptomatic; the rhythm being detected incidentally, for example, during routine pulse or telemetry monitoring.

Atrial fibrillation is the most common, clinically encountered arrhythmia, seen in more than 5% of patients over age 69. (National Heart, Lung and Blood Institute, Working group on atrial fibrillation, 1993) Atrial fibrillation is characterized by inconsistent, irregular R-R intervals with an absence of true P-waves. P-waves may be replaced by multiple, fibrillatory F-waves of varying configuration. This arrhythmia signifies that there is no established sinus or atrial pacemaker, rather that many impulses are simultaneously generated from multiple locations within the atria. The

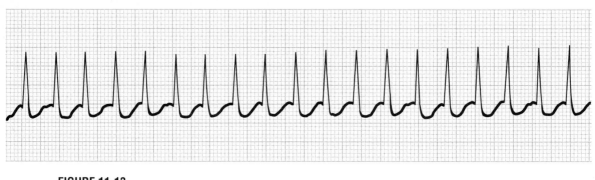

FIGURE 11-13
Supraventricular tachycardia.

atria, therefore, are not pumping effectively which, in turn, may impair ventricular contraction. This is because of the loss of the additional ventricular filling supplied by atrial contraction. Impulses do conduct through the AV junction to the ventricles; however, this occurs inconsistently resulting in the irregular R-R interval. The ventricular response to atrial fibrillation is important. A rapid ventricular response, resulting in tachycardia, may cause hemodynamic compromise with associated symptoms or poor activity tolerance. Of additional clinical significance is the association between atrial fibrillation and embolic cerebrovascular accidents. Figure 11-7 illustrates atrial fibrillation with a "controlled," that is, less than 100 BPM, ventricular response. Pulse monitoring of an individual in atrial fibrillation reveals an irregularly irregular pattern.

Another arrhythmia that is characterized by abnormal atrial activity is atrial flutter, seen in Figure 11-14. In this rhythm, P-waves are replaced by F-waves that have a distinctive morphology often referred to as a "saw tooth" or "picket fence" appearance. Of clinical importance is the ratio of atrial to ventricular conduction and whether or not the patient is hemodynamically stable (Brown and Jacobson, 1988).

Because the intrinsic rate of spontaneous depolarization of the AV node is less than that of the SA node, spontaneous AV node depolarization is normally prevented. However, in the absence of an atrial impulse the AV node depolarizes spontaneously and generates an impulse that then is conducted to the ventricles. Thus in junctional rhythm or nodal rhythm

(Figure 11-15), the QRS complex is not preceded by a P-wave. The AV node may generate an isolated "escape" beat, or it may take over as the heart's pacemaker. Sustained nodal or junctional rhythm is usually between 40 and 60 BPM, corresponding with the inherent rate of spontaneous AV node depolarization.

Ventricular Arrhythmias

Ventricular arrhythmias result from spontaneous depolarization of a region within ventricular myocardium; a region outside the normal pathway for impulse generation. For this reason, the site of impulse generation is called an ectopic focus. Ventricular arrhythmias may be distinguished from supraventricular arrhythmias, in that the QRS duration of a ventricular arrhythmia is longer than normal 0.12 seconds. The appearance of ventricular arrhythmias may be characterized as being "wide and weird." It is important to point out that not all rhythms with a QRS duration greater than 0.11 seconds represent ectopic ventricular beats; some widened QRS rhythms result from disturbances of impulse conduction within the ventricles, rather than from impulse generation within the ventricles.

The reason for the widening of the QRS complex resulting from ventricular impulse conduction disturbance or impulse generation is apparent when one considers the normal conduction of a sinus impulse within the ventricles. An impulse normally is rapidly conducted to ventricular myocardium via the Purkinje's

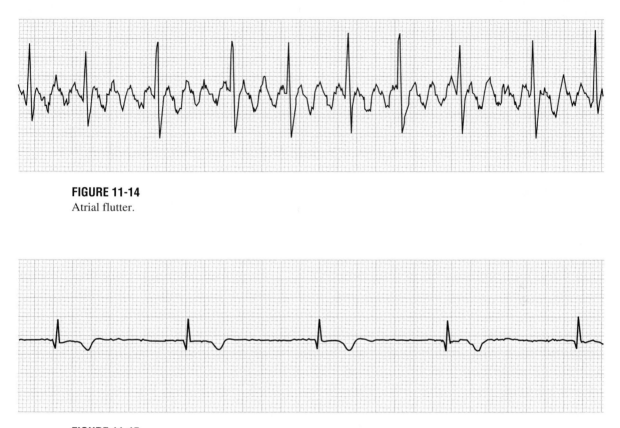

FIGURE 11-14
Atrial flutter.

FIGURE 11-15
Junctional rhythm.

fibers. This assures that the impulse reaches all regions of ventricular myocardium in a timely fashion, with subsequent coordinated depolarization and contraction. Within ventricular myocardium itself, however, propagation of the depolarization wave proceeds more slowly, as a result of the syncytial arrangement of myocardial cells.

An impulse generated within the ventricles, outside the normal conduction pathways, initially depolarizes surrounding local myocardium. The depolarization wave then spreads outward from that focus, but is propagated at a slower velocity. Ventricular contraction, in this case, is not coordinated; some regions contract well before the depolarization wave reaches regions remote from the ectopic focus. It follows that the ventricular ejection of blood is reduced

during an ectopic beat (Figure 11-16). An ECG rhythm (bottom) is recorded simultaneously with the record of arterial blood pressure monitoring (top). The appearance of the "wide and weird" complex results in significant diminution of the corresponding arterial pressure wave.

The most common form of ventricular arrhythmia is a premature ventricular complex, or PVC. In Figure 11-16 the wide and weird QRS complex appears early, interrupting the established rhythm. A pause often follows a PVC, after which the established rhythm resumes. Clinically, a PVC may be perceived by a patient as a "skipped" beat or a palpitation. If pulse monitoring occurs during a PVC, the examiner will likely sense a "skipped" or irregular beat.

PVCs sometimes happen in patterns, occurring at

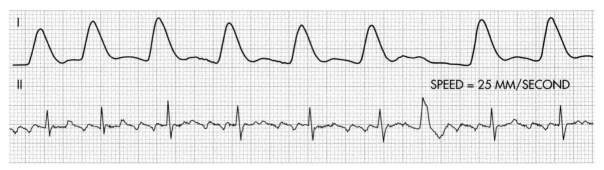

FIGURE 11-16
Diminished arterial pressure wave following a PVC.

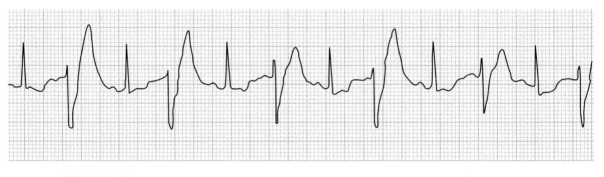

FIGURE 11-17
Ventricular bigeminy.

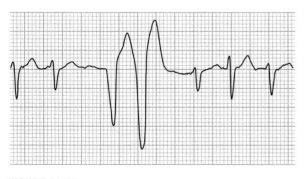

FIGURE 11-18
Ventricular couplet.

regular intervals. A PVC occurs in ventricular bigeminy on every second beat, in ventricular trigeminy on every third beat, and in ventricular quadrigeminy on every fourth beat. Figure 11-17 illustrates ventricular bigeminy. With these rhythms, a regularly irregular pattern may be noted during pulse monitoring. PVCs may also occur twice in succession as a ventricular couplet, seen in Figure 11-18.

PVCs that originate from more than one ectopic focus are termed multifocal PVCs. In this circumstance, the waveforms will have different morphology according to the locations of the ectopic foci. Remember that the positive or negative deflection of the

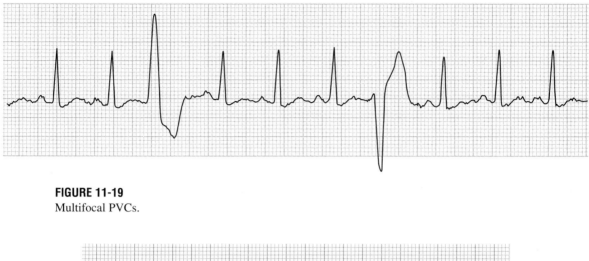

FIGURE 11-19
Multifocal PVCs.

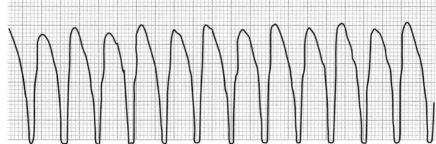

FIGURE 11-20
Ventricular tachycardia.

waveforms depends on the direction of depolarization, as viewed by the lead used for monitoring. In Figure 11-19 the first PVC seen has an initial positive deflection, whereas the second PVC seen has an initial negative deflection. Each of these PVCs comes from a different ectopic focus.

The physical therapists's (PT's) decision-making process in response to observation of ventricular ectopic beats is complex and may not be easily grasped by the entry-level practitioner. Factors such as presence or absence of symptoms, the acuity of the patient, and whether the rhythm is a new finding all influence a clinical response. The presence of a pattern such as bigeminy, couplets, or multifocality is also considered. Further elucidation of clinical responses

to most arrhythmias is beyond the scope of this chapter; however, some arrhythmias demand an immediate response if observed.

Ventricular tachycardia (V-tach, or VT) (Figure 11-20) is defined as three or more consecutive PVCs at a rate greater than 100 BPM (Akhtar, 1990). This is a serious and potentially lethal arrhythmia that may require emergency measures be undertaken. During v-tach all complexes are ventricular in origin. V-tach sometimes occurs in "runs" of three or more ectopic complexes followed by reversion to the baseline rhythm, or it may be sustained. Effective circulation may be preserved, or it may be seriously compromised or absent in sustained v-tach. A patient may be asymptomatic, particularly if only a brief run of

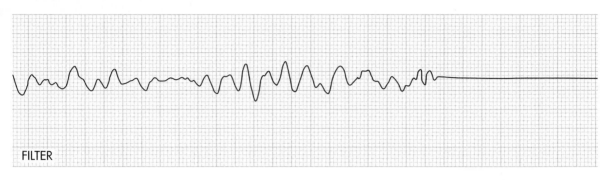

FILTER

FIGURE 11-21
Ventricular fibrillation degenerating into asystole.

v-tach was experienced. If VT is sustained, the patient may be asymptomatic, symptomatic, or unconscious and pulseless. The PT's response depends on the rhythm, regardless of whether it is sustained, and the patient is symptomatic or conscious. Clinical responses range from cessation of activity, ongoing patient observation and immediate notification of a physician to a full code.

Ventricular fibrillation (V-fib, VF) is a lethal arrhythmia accompanied by immediate loss of consciousness and loss of circulation, that is, cardiac arrest. It is characterized by disorganized, simultaneous firing of multiple, ectopic ventricular foci; there is no organized rhythm (Figure 11-21). Effective ventricular contraction ceases and cardiopulmonary resuscitation is indicated until defibrillation is available. Death follows unless defibrillation successfully restores an effective rhythm. Conditions that render the myocardium vulnerable to ventricular fibrillation include v-tach, myocardial ischemia or infarction, dilatation of the heart, hyperkalemia, or electric shock (Guyton, 1991).

If not successfully treated, v-fib may further degenerate into asystole, which indicates complete absence of ventricular electrical activity (Figure 11-21). Asystole may also occur as a primary event. This is known colloquially as "flat line" rhythm. Like ventricular fibrillation, asystole requires that cardiopulmonary resuscitation begin immediately to save the patient's life.

Care must be taken to distinguish an apparent lethal arrhythmia from lead disconnection or movement artifact. Unwary therapists have hastily summoned help on observing v-fib or asystole, only to feel foolish when a lead is reattached to the patient. These arrhythmias are always accompanied by loss of consciousness and pulse; a clinician should assess the patient before taking action. Similarly, during activity or exercise, movement artifact may easily be mistaken for v-tach. By assessing the patient and asking him or her to "hold still," the issue may be quickly resolved.

Conduction Blocks

Conduction blocks are another type of ECG abnormality with which PTs should be familiar. The propagation of a cardiac impulse may be inhibited or terminated along the conduction pathway. Blockage can occur at the sinus node, between the atria and ventricles, or within the ventricular conduction system. Sinus block occurs if the impulse cannot propagate beyond the sinus node. In this case, the AV junction usually takes over as the pacemaker, and a junctional rhythm is seen with the absence of P-waves.

More common are the AV blocks. They are ranked as first-, second-, or third-degree, depending on the extent of delay or obstruction of the cardiac impulse between the atria and ventricles. First-degree AV block is characterized by a prolongation of the P-R interval beyond its normal 0.2 seconds (Figure 11-22). Remember that the P-R interval is measured from the *beginning* of the P-wave to the *beginning* of the QRS complex. Each impulse is delayed between the atria

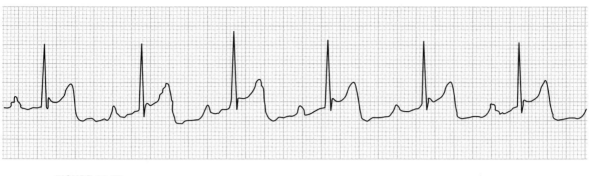

FIGURE 11-22
First degree AV block.

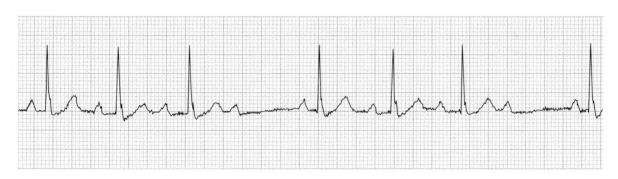

FIGURE 11-23
Second degree AV block, Mobitz type 1.

and ventricles but each eventually reaches the ventricular conduction system resulting in a normal QRS complex. Thus for each P wave, there is a QRS complex; therefore the conduction ratio is 1:1.

Second-degree AV block takes two forms, although in each form, there are some sinus impulses that are not conducted to the ventricles. In second-degree block Mobitz type 1, also known as Wenckebach, the P-R interval lengthens progressively until a P-wave fails to conduct to the ventricles (Figure 11-23). Notice how the first three P-R intervals lengthen until, after the fourth P-wave, a QRS complex fails to appear. The cycle then repeats itself. Second-degree block Mobitz type 2 (Figure 11-24) is characterized by a fixed P-R interval with a "dropped" QRS following every second, third, or fourth

P-wave. The conduction ratio in Figure 11-24 is 3:1, or three P-waves for each QRS complex. Both first- and second-degree AV blocks are considered to be incomplete heart blocks.

Third degree AV block or complete heart block is also known as AV dissociation. In this rhythm (Figure 11-25), P-waves are present, but there is no relationship between P-waves or QRS complexes. P-waves may be superimposed on QRS complexes, but none of the sinus impulses are conducted to the ventricles; the atria and ventricles are contracting independently of each other. In the absence of clinical intervention such as artificial pacing, ventricular depolarization is initiated by a junctional or ventricular pacemaker.

Clinically, AV blocks range in severity from benign,

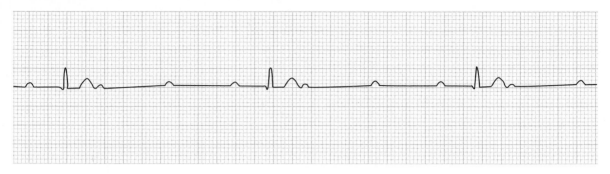

FIGURE 11-24
Second degree AV block, Mobitz type 2.

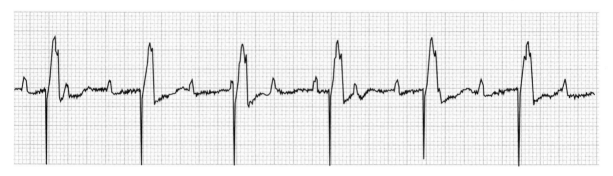

FIGURE 11-25
Third degree AV block with ventricular pacing.

as is usually the case with first degree AV block, to potentially lethal. Whether hemodynamic compromise occurs depends on the extent of impairment of cardiac output caused by too slow of a rate of ventricular contraction (Brown and Jacobson, 1988). Slow rates of ventricular contraction may cause lightheadedness or syncope. In most cases of third degree block, treatment now includes implantation of an artificial pacemaker. In Figure 11-25, the needlelike spikes indicate that an artificial pacemaker is depolarizing the ventricles at a rate of 60 BPM.

MYOCARDIAL ISCHEMIA OR INFARCTION

The ECG provides much more information, beyond that gleaned from arrhythmia analysis. Since PTs

often treat patients with coronary heart disease, information regarding MI or myocardial ischemia is also of interest. Although PTs do not medically diagnose myocardial ischemia or MI, they should have a working knowledge of its electrocardiographic evidence. During myocardial ischemia, blood flow to a portion of myocardium is compromised, resulting in alteration of myocardial metabolism. In MI, a portion of myocardium has died, but an adjacent zone of ischemic myocardial cells endures. These ischemic cells may remain "leaky," and be unable to repolarize. The persistent current flow from the "leaky" region results in a current of injury, which is seen as a shifting of the S-T segment above or below the isoelectric line (Guyton, 1991; Lilly, 1993). S-T segment shift has significant diagnostic value. For exam-

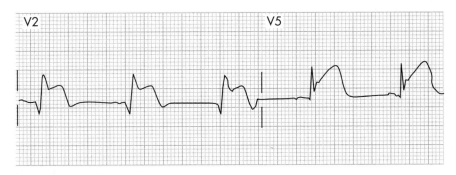

FIGURE 11-26
S-T segment elevation during myocardial infarction.

ple, S-T segment elevation (Figure 11-26) is associated with transmural MI, whereas S-T segment depression is associated with nontransmural or subendocardial MI. Also, the onset of S-T segment depression during activity is often considered diagnostic of myocardial ischemia. Figure 11-27 is an example of exercise-induced S-T segment depression observed in one lead during exercise.

The following is a brief discussion on other abnormalities of the ECG observed in coronary artery disease (CAD). A prominent, pathological Q-wave is indicative of a transmural MI (Lilly, 1993). Indeed, "non-Q" is synonymous with nontransmural concerning MI. The presence of a prominent Q-wave (Figure 11-28) does not, however, distinguish between an old or an acute event.

The T-wave may also undergo changes during myocardial ischemia or MI. During ischemia, for example, the T-wave may invert as a result of prolongation of repolarization (Guyton, 1991). Similarly, during MI, changes in the T-wave may "evolve" with the infarct, at first becoming indistinguishable within an elevated S-T segment, then inverting, then perhaps reverting to original configuration following the passage of time.

CONCLUSION

Understanding the changes in the ECG during ischemia or MI may help PTs integrate all available information to optimize patient evaluation. This knowledge, combined with astute arrhythmia recognition

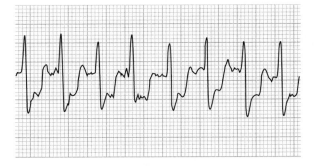
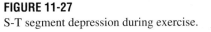

FIGURE 11-27
S-T segment depression during exercise.

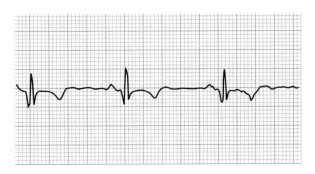

FIGURE 11-28
Significant Q wave.

and symptom assessment, provide entry-level PTs with important tools for management of patients at risk for cardiopulmonary dysfunction.

REVIEW QUESTIONS

1. How may the following dysrhythmias be perceived by a clinician without benefit of ECG monitoring? How may they be perceived by a patient?
   • atrial fibrillation
   • supraventricular tachycardia
   • premature ventricular contractions
   • third degree AV block
   • ventricular fibrillation
2. What determines the clinical significance of an arrhythmia?
3. What property of the SA node allows it to pace the heart? Under what conditions do other portions of the conduction system act as pacemakers?
4. Does an impulse originating within ventricular myocardium generate an effective myocardial contraction? If not, why not?
5. Why is ECG monitoring indicated following myocardial infarction?
6. What event is represented by each of the following:
   • P wave
   • QRS complex
   • T wave
   • U wave
7. What is the possible clinical significance of S-T segment depression, of S-T segment elevation? What symptoms might be anticipated in the presence of those conditions?

References

Akhtar, M. (1990). Clinical spectrum of ventricular tachycardia. *Circulation, 82,* 1561-1573.

American College of Sports Medicine. (1991). *Guidelines for exercise testing and prescription.* (4th ed.). Philadelphia: Lea and Febiger.

Brown, K.R., & Jacobson, S. (1988). *Mastering dysrhythmias: A problem solving guide.* Philadelphia: FA Davis.

Cummins, R.O. (Ed.). (1994). *Textbook of advanced cardiac life support.* Dallas: American Heart Association.

Emergency Cardiac Care Committee and Subcommittees. (1992). Guidelines for cardiopulmonary resuscitation and emergency cardiac care, III: Adult advanced cardiac life support. *Journal of the American Medical Association, 268,* 2199-2241.

Guyton, A.C. (1991). *Textbook of medical physiology.* Philadelphia: WB Saunders.

Lilly, L.S. (1993). *Pathophysiology of heart disease.* Philadelphia: Lea and Febiger.

National Heart Lung and Blood Institute Working group on atrial fibrillation. (1993). Atrial fibrillation: Current understandings and research imperatives. *Journal of American College of Cardiologists, 22,* 1830-1834.

Shih, H.T. (1994). Anatomy of the action potential in the heart. *Texas Heart Institute Journal, 21,* 30-41.

Smith, J.J., & Kampine, J.P. (1990). *Circulatory physiology—the essentials.* Baltimore: Williams and Wilkins.

CHAPTER 12

Multisystem Assessment and Laboratory Investigations

Elizabeth Dean

KEY TERMS

Blood
Endocrine function
Heart
Immune function
Kidneys

Liver
Lungs
Multisystem assessment
Peripheral vascular circulation

INTRODUCTION

The purpose of this chapter is to describe the rationale for multisystem assessment in the patient managed for cardiopulmonary dysfunction and some common laboratory tests related to multisystem assessment. The bases of tests to assess the function of the following organ systems are presented: blood, pulmonary, cardiac, peripheral vascular, renal, endocrine, liver, and immune systems. The information in this chapter is supplemental to the elements of cardiopulmonary and cardiovascular assessment and related laboratory investigations described in Part 2.

The cardiopulmonary system affects and is af-
fected by virtually every organ system in the body. The signs and symptoms of systemic disease can mimic other conditions, including cardiopulmonary dysfunction treated by physical therapists. Therefore the physical therapist must be able to differentiate these presentations to determine what treatment, if any, is indicated, and what treatments may be contraindicated. Knowledge of multisystem function helps confirm a diagnosis, as well as predict a patient's response to treatment and his or her recovery and prognosis. In addition, this information is crucial in refining and modifying treatment prescription. These abilities are particularly important in this era of

professional accountability and with the advent of direct patient access.

RATIONALE FOR MULTISYSTEM ASSESSMENT

The cardiopulmonary system supports cellular respiration and life. Thus every system and every cell in the body is affected by the adequacy of oxygen transport, which is dependent on cardiopulmonary and cardiovascular function. In addition, these systems are affected by virtually every other system in the body. The cardiopulmonary physical therapist (PT) therefore needs thorough knowledge of multisystem function and the interdependence of the organ systems, an ability to assess multisystem function and to integrate this information into a comprehensive and progressive treatment plan.

The lungs and heart are anatomically and physiologically interconnected, and function as a unit to transport oxygen via the peripheral circulation to perfuse and nourish tissues. Tissue homeostasis is dependent on the adequacy of the anatomy and physiology of the blood. The adequacy of peripheral perfusion determines the adequacy of the function of all organ systems in the body. Therefore a knowledge of the failure of the various organ systems can reflect impaired oxygen transport or may identify a threat to oxygen transport.

The elements of laboratory evaluation and testing, as well as normal values, have been compiled from Bauer (1982), Dean (1987), Fishbach (1988), Guyton (1991), Jacobs et al. (1984), Le Fever Kee (1990), Pagana and Pagana (1992), Siest et al. (1985), and Wallach (1986).

ELEMENTS OF MULTISYSTEM ASSESSMENT
Blood

Some common blood tests are summarized in Table 12-1 along with their normal values.

The average blood volume consists of 5 L of blood: 3 L of plasma and 2 L of cells. Plasma is the medium which suspends and transports blood cells. The complete blood count (CBC) is one of the most commonly ordered laboratory procedures. This basic screening test helps to establish the patient's diagnosis, treatment

response, recovery, and prognosis. The CBC includes the red blood cell count (RBC), a variety of red blood cell indices, white blood cell count (WBC), hematocrit (Hct), hemoglobin (Hgb), and platelet count.

Tests of coagulation and hemostasis reflect bleeding pathology, which often involves injury of blood vessels and cells. Damage to the blood vessel wall leads to constriction, a primary mechanism of hemostasis. Circulating platelets adhere to exposed subendothelial tissues, which can predispose thrombus formation.

The fluidity of the blood is regulated by the facilitation and the inhibition of thrombin formation. When these two processes are in balance, the blood has an optimal consistency; it is neither too thick nor too thin. This allows blood to flow optimally through the circulation. Blood vessel injury can disrupt this balance and can promote coagulation.

Disseminated intravascular coagulation (DIC) results from an imbalance between the formation and deposition of fibrin, which leads to the formation of thrombi. The continuous production of thrombin causes depletion of the coagulation factors and bleeding results. Tests used to assess bleeding capacity include thrombin time and fibrin clotting time (partial thromboplastin time [PTT]).

Proteins (amino acids) serve as regulators of metabolism. Much clinical information is obtained by examining and measuring proteins, because proteins regulate many important physiologic functions in the body. Plasma proteins serve as a source of nutrition for the body tissues and function as buffers when combined with hemoglobin.

Albumin, a protein formed in the liver, maintains normal water distribution in the body (colloid osmotic pressure). It transports blood constituents such as ions, pigments, bilirubin, hormones, fatty acids, enzymes, and certain drugs. Approximately 55% of total protein is albumin. The remainder is globulin, which functions in antibody formation, and other plasma proteins (fibrinogen and prothrombin) involved with coagulation.

Lactic acid, a product of carbohydrate metabolism, is produced when cells receive inadequate oxygen in relation to oxygen demand (anaerobic metabolism). When the production of lactic acid exceeds its removal from the blood by the liver, lactic acid accumulates in the blood.

TABLE 12-1

Common Tests of Multisystem Function and Their Normal Values: Blood Tests

TEST		NORMAL VALUES (SI UNITS)
Red blood cell count (RBC)	Men	2.09–2.71 nmol/L
	Women	1.86–2.48 nmol/L
Hemoglobin (Hgb)	Men	8.7–11.2 nmol/L
	Women	7.4–9.9 nmol/L
Hematocrit (Hct)	Men	40% to 54%
	Women	37% to 47%
Platelet count		150,000–350,000/mm^3
Prothrombin time (PT)		10–14 seconds
Partial thromboplastin time (PTT)		60–85 seconds
White blood cell count (WBCC) (Differential WBCC includes counts of neutrophils, eosinophils, basophils, lymphocytes, and monocytes)		5–10 × 103/µl
Erythrocyte sedimentation rate (ESR)	Men	0–15 mm/hr
	Women	0–20 mm/hr
Proteins		
Albumin		38–50 gm/L
Globulin		23–35 gm/L
Fibrinogen		2.0–4.0 gm/L
Lactate	Venous	0.5–2.2 mmol/L
	Arterial	0.5–1.6 mmol/L
Electrolytes (blood)		
Sodium (Na$^+$)		135–148 mmol/L
Potassium (K$^+$)		3.5–5.0 mmol/L
Calcium (Ca^{++})	TOTAL	4.5–5.3 mmol/L
	IONIZED	2.1–2.6 mmol/L
Chloride (Cl$^-$)		98–106 mmol/L
Cholesterol		3.63–6.48 mmol/L
Creatine kinase	Men	0.42–1.51 mmol/s/L
	Women	0.17–1.18 mmol/s/L

NOTE: Normal values may vary depending on the laboratory performing the measurement. Within subject variation occurs from age, and variations in the pre-test standardization procedures.

Cholesterol is used in the production of steroid hormones, bile acids, and cell membranes. Cholesterol is found in muscles, red blood cells, and cell membranes. Low-density and high-density lipoproteins (LDLs and HDLs) transport cholesterol in the blood. High levels of cholesterol are associated with atherosclerosis and increased risk of coronary artery disease (CAD).

Electrolyte assessment is based on the electrolyte constituents of a blood or urine sample. Although present in minute quantities, electrolytes are essential in maintaining normal cellular function and homeostasis. The electrolytes that are routinely studied are sodium, potassium, chloride, calcium, phosphorus, and magnesium.

Pulmonary Function

See Chapters 8 and 14 for a detailed description of the assessment of the pulmonary system and its function.

Cardiac Function

A detailed description of the assessment of the cardiac system and its function appears in Chapters 11 and 14.

Peripheral Vascular Function

Assessment of the peripheral vascular circulation is essential to provide information regarding central and peripheral hemodynamic status, as well as peripheral tissue perfusion. This assessment is essential to establish the integrity of the patient's hemodynamic status at rest and during physical and exercise stress which is associated with most physical therapy treatments. Laboratory tests include segmental blood pressure studies, skin temperature studies, pulse wave analysis, Doppler venous studies, and arteriography. The physical examination corroborates the results of the laboratory investigations and includes the patient's history,

inspection of the integrity of the peripheral circulation particularly to the extremities, palpation to assess peripheral pulses, and auscultation, which can be helpful in detecting bruits or areas of turbulent blood flow associated with arterial stenoses.

Some common tests of peripheral vascular function are summarized in Table 12-2 along with their normal values.

Kidney Function

Urine consists of the end products of cellular metabolism and is produced as large volumes of blood (approximately 25% of the cardiac output [CO]) flow through the kidneys. When the kidneys are compromised, death can ensue within a few days. Although fluid is lost through several routes, the kidneys are primarily responsible for processing and regulating fluid balance in the body.

Urea, the major nonprotein nitrogenous end product of protein catabolism, is measured in the blood as blood urea nitrogen (BUN). The urea is then carried to the kidneys by the blood to be excreted in the urine.

Creatinine is a byproduct in the breakdown of muscle creatine phosphate resulting from energy metabolism. Production of creatinine is constant as long as muscle mass is constant. Kidney dysfunction reduces excretion of creatinine resulting in increased levels of blood creatinine. Analysis of urine for creatinine provides an index of kidney function.

TABLE 12-2
Common Tests of Multisystem Function and Their Normal Values: Tests of Peripheral Vascular Function

TEST	NORMAL VALUES
Skin temperature	Ranges from ambient temperature to 30°C
Ankle systolic pressures	97% of brachial pressure
Peripheral pulses	Apex heart rate
Capillary filling	Instantaneous filling following quick pressure over the nail bed

TABLE 12-3
Common Tests of Multisystem Function and Their Normal Values: Tests of Renal Function

TEST	NORMAL VALUES (SI UNITS)
Blood urea nitrogen (BUN)	3.6–7.1 mmol/L
Creatinine	7.6–30.5 µmol/L

NOTE: Normal values may vary depending on the laboratory performing the measurement. Within subject variation occurs from age, and variations in the pretest standardization procedures.

Increased osmolality stimulates the secretion of anti-diuretic hormone (ADH) that acts on renal tubules. This results in the reabsorption of water, more concentrated urine, and less concentrated serum.

Some common tests of renal function are summarized in Table 12-3 along with their normal values.

Endocrine Function

Endocrine glands are responsible for producing those substances and neuromediators responsible for maintaining homeostasis and enabling the body to adapt when physically and psychologically challenged or perturbed from a resting state. The key endocrine glands are the pancreas, thyroid gland, and the adrenal glands. Endocrine glands regulate metabolism and are responsible for increasing blood flow and pressure, and reducing vascular resistance when metabolic demands increase.

Some common tests of endocrine function are summarized in Table 12-4 along with their normal values.

Pancreatic function and insulin production

Insulin, a hormone produced in the pancreas by the beta cells of the islets of Langerhans, regulates the metabolism of carbohydrates along with liver, adipose tissue, muscle, and other target cells and is responsible for maintaining a constant level of blood glucose. The rate of insulin secretion is determined primarily by the level of blood glucose perfusing the pancreas and is also affected by hormonal status, the autonomic nervous system, nutritional status, smoking, restricted mobility, physical stress such as traumatic insult to the body during illness and injury, and pharmacologic agents.

Amylase is an enzyme produced in the salivary glands, pancreas, and liver, and converts starch to sugar. Inflammation of the pancreas or salivary glands results in more of the enzyme entering the blood. The amylase test is used to diagnose and monitor treatment of acute pancreatitis.

TABLE 12-4

Common Tests of Multisystem Function and Their Normal Values: Tests of Endocrine Function

TEST		NORMAL VALUES (SI UNITS)
Thyroid Function		
Total thyroxine (T4)		65–155 nmol/L
Total triiodothyronine (T3)		1.77–2.93 nmol/L
Adrenal Function		
Epinephrine		0.0–81.9 nmol/24 hr
Norepinephrine		0.0–591 nmol/24 hr
Cortisol	Morning	138–635 nmol/L
	Evening	82–413 nmol/L
Pancreatic Function		
Glucose tolerance test	At 1 hr glucose	1.1–2.75 mmol/L
	At 2 hr glucose	0.2–0.88 mmol/L
Insulin	12 hr fasting	35–145 pmol/L
Amylase	Blood level	25–125 Units/L

NOTE: Normal values may vary depending on the laboratory performing the measurement. Within subject variation occurs from age, and variations in the pretest standardization procedures.

Thyroid

The function of the thyroid gland is to take iodine from the circulating blood, combine it with amino acid tyrosine, and convert it to the thyroid hormones thyroxine (T4), and triiodothyronine (T3). Thyroid hormones have a profound effect on metabolic rate. Increased metabolism causes more rapid use of oxygen than normal and causes greater quantities of metabolic end products to be released from the tissues. These effects cause vasodilatation in most of the body tissues, thus increasing blood flow. Increase in the thyroid hormones increases cardiac output, heart rate, force of cardiac contraction, blood volume, arterial blood pressure, oxygen consumption, and carbon dioxide (CO_2) production, hence an increase in the rate and depth of breathing, increased appetite, food intake and gastrointestinal motility. The thyroid gland also stores T3 and T4 until they are released into the blood stream under the influence of thyroid stimulating hormone (TSH) from the pituitary gland.

Adrenal function

Catecholamines, epinephrine and norepinephrine, are produced by the adrenal medulla of the adrenal glands. Urine samples are used to test for these important vasoactive neurotransmitters in the investigation of various disorders. In addition to their vasoactive properties, the catecholamines are essential in stimulating the sympathetic response in the fight or flight mechanism.

Cortisol is produced by the adrenal cortex of the adrenal glands and is involved with metabolism of carbohydrate, protein, and fat. In addition, it inhibits the action of insulin and thus the uptake of glucose by the cells. The normal secretion of cortisol varies diurnally, that is, high in the morning and low in the evening.

Liver Function

Liver function is especially important in that dysfunction of this organ can be life threatening. The liver has a primary role in carbohydrate and protein metabolism, it produces bile, and is responsible for detoxification of the blood. Its function is assessed

---

TABLE 12-5

Common Tests of Multisystem Function and Their Normal Values: Tests of Liver Function

TEST	NORMAL VALUES (SI UNITS)
Alkaline phosphatase	0.18–0.40 nmol/s/L
Bilirubin (total)	5.1–17.1 µmol/L

NOTE: Normal values may vary depending on the laboratory performing the measurement. Within subject variation occurs from age and variations in the pretest standardization procedures.

TABLE 12-6

Common Tests of Multisystem Function and Their Normal Values: Tests of Immunological Function

Differential White Blood Cell Count

	ABSOLUTE VALUE (No/uL)	RELATIVE VALUE (by Percent)
Neutrophils	3,000-7,000	60-70
Lymphocytes	1,000-4,000	20-40
Monocytes	100-600	2-6
Eosinophils	50-400	1-4
Basophils	25-100	0.5-1

---

with tests of liver enzymes such as amylase and alkaline phosphatase.

Some common tests of hepatic function are summarized in Table 12-5 along with their normal values.

Immunological Function

Immunological function is dependent on the adequacy of the function of several tissues and organs, namely bone marrow, the thymus gland, lymph nodes, and vessels of the lymphatic system, spleen, tonsils, and intestinal lymphoid tissue. Immunological function can break down if insufficient protective immune factors are produced, or the system is overwhelmed by an invading organism for which the body has inappropriate or insufficient resistance.

Some common tests of immunological function are summarized in Table 12-6 along with their normal values. Specific detailed accounts of immmunodiagnostic studies and tests for autoimmune deficiencies are beyond the scope of this chapter but can be reviewed in Fischbach (1988) and Le Fever Kee (1990).

SUMMARY

This chapter described the rationale for multisystem assessment in the patient being managed for cardiopulmonary dysfunction and some common tests of multisystem function. The cardiopulmonary system affects and is affected by virtually every organ system in the body. Thus primary cardiopulmonary dysfunction can lead to multiorgan system complications, and dysfunction of other organ systems can have cardiopulmonary manifestations. In addition, the signs and symptoms of systemic disease can mimic other conditions treated by physical therapists. Therefore the PT must be able to differentiate these presentations to determine whether a pathology will respond to physical therapy management, what treatment is not indicated and what treatments may be contraindicated. Multisystem monitoring provides fundamental information needed to refine and progress the treatment prescription. These abilities are essential in this era of increased professional responsibility and with the advent of direct patient access.

REVIEW QUESTIONS

1. Describe common tests of blood composition.
2. Describe pulmonary function tests.
3. Describe tests of heart function.
4. Describe tests of peripheral vascular function.
5. Desacribe tests of renal function.
6. Describe tests of endocrine function.
7. Describe tests of liver function.
8. Describe tests of immune function.

References

Bauer, J.D. (1982). *Clinical laboratory methods* (9th ed.). St. Louis: Mosby.

Dean, E. (1987). Assessment of the peripheral circulation: An update for practitioners. *The Australian Journal of Physiotherapy, 33,* 164-171.

Fischbach, F. (1988). *A manual of laboratory diagnostic tests* (3rd ed.). Philadelphia: J.B. Lippincott.

Guyton, A.C. (1991). *Textbook of medical physiology* (6th ed.). Philadelphia: W. B. Saunders.

Jacobs, D.S., Kasten, B.L., Demott, W.R., & Wolfson, W.L. (1984). *Laboratory test handbook.* Stow: Lexi-Comp, Inc.

Le Fever Kee, J. (1990). *Handbook of laboratory and diagnostic tests with nursing implications.* Norwalk: Appleton and Lange.

Pagana, K.D., & Pagana, T.J. (1992). *Mosby's diagnostic and laboratory test reference.* St. Louis: Mosby.

Siest, G., Henny, J., Schiele, F., & Yonge, D.S. (1985). *Interpretation of clinical laboratory tests.* Foster City: Biomedical Publications.

Wallach, J. (1986). *Interpretation of diagnostic tests. A synopsis of laboratory medicine.* Boston: Little, Brown.

CHAPTER 13

Special Tests

Gail M. Huber

INTRODUCTION

In assessing the cardiopulmonary patient, the physician uses many tools. The patient interview, physical examination, chest x-ray, and electrocardiogram (ECG) provide information to make a diagnosis. When more information is needed, a variety of invasive and noninvasive tests can be performed. Nuclear medicine offers a variety of tools for evaluation of cardiac and pulmonary function. Echocardiography is a noninvasive method that offers information about the cardiovascular system, including valve function, ventricular performance, and estimation of filling pressures. It is particularly useful with children.

At some point in a patient's workup, the physician may need to use an invasive test. Pulmonary and cardiac angiography is not without risk; however, for evaluating blood flow in the heart and lungs, as well as determining cardiac anatomy, and direct volume and pressure measures, it is without equal. Transesophageal echocardiography is another invasive test. Following the initial assessment of the problem, these same special tests may be used to assist in the determination of appropriate therapy and evaluate prognosis and response to treatment. The noninvasive tests are most important in determining ongoing surgical, interventional, or medical therapy. Physical therapists (PTs) need to understand these invasive and noninvasive tests for several reasons. It is useful to understand how the information is used to make a differential diagnosis and determine treatment. These tests have helped to clarify our understanding of the physiology and pathophysiology of the system. Therapists need to understand the pathophysiological basis for a patient's movement dysfunctions to select the most appropriate treatment strategies. Many special tests can and are being used in research to evaluate treatment interventions. For example, radiolabeled aerosols are used to evaluate mucociliary clearance, providing a method to evaluate the effectiveness of pulmonary hygiene techniques (Miller and O'Doherty, 1992). Clinically, PTs need to use information from the tests to develop a framework for predicting how the patient may respond to a physical therapy intervention. For example, nuclear imaging can provide information about left ventricular ejection fraction. This information helps the PT determine if the patient should be stratified into high-risk or low-risk categories. Monitoring of an exercise session may depend on the risk level, and interpretation of the patient's response to treatment may be effected.

NUCLEAR IMAGING SYSTEMS AND RADIOPHARMACEUTICALS

A general view of how nuclear imaging systems work should help the PT understand some of the differences between the wide variety of tests used today. This area of medicine is experiencing rapid growth and change as technology changes the equipment used to perform the test, the radiopharmaceuticals available, and the computer's increasing ability to analyze data.

Radionuclide imaging allows for the noninvasive acquisition of images from a variety of body tissues. An imaging system requires three basic parts. The first requirement is a radiopharmaceutical that emits gamma radiation and is taken up by the body tissue of interest. Next, a radiation detector or camera is needed. Finally, computers are required to collect and analyze the data.

Radionuclides are elements that are unstable; they gain stability by emitting particles or photons. This is called radioactive decay, and gamma radiation is released. Radionuclides are either cyclotron- or generator-produced. The cyclotron accelerates alpha-particles, deuterons, and protons to energies suitable for the production of the required radionuclide (Kim, 1987). A radionuclide generator is a system of parent and daughter radionuclides in equilibrium. The system is constructed so that the daughter can be re-

moved from time to time for patient use (Kim, 1987). A generator system produces short-lived radionuclides (Iskandrian, 1987).

These elements are often attached to other substrates for transport in the body to the particular tissue of interest. The elements have differing characteristics such as energy output and half-life. Because of their varied distribution in the body tissues, they provide different information.

Detection of the radioactive energy emitted by a specific radiopharmaceutical requires a camera. When certain materials are struck by ionizing radiation, light is emitted. A scintillation detector detects this light. A gamma camera is a scintillation detector able to detect photons exiting the body. It uses a large, collimated crystal monitored by an array of photomultiplier tubes (Kim, 1987). A collimator is a device that allows only those photons traveling in an appropriate direction to reach the crystal. There are several types of collimators: parallel-hole collimators, pinhole collimators, and converging and diverging collimators. The photomultiplier tube records the amount of light from the crystal and converts it into a voltage, that is proportional to the intensity of the light (Kim, 1987).

The camera system is connected to a computer that stores the light images. The computer is able to derive two dimensional images from the data. The computer can also quantify the data and perform a variety of data analyses (Iskandrian, 1987).

Planar Imaging

A single crystal camera (Anger) produces a two dimensional or planar image. Multicrystal cameras (Blau and Blender) also produce planar images but are able to perform fast dynamic imaging used in first pass and gated studies. Planar imaging may be the only option available to obese patients who do not "fit" the single photon emission computed tomography (SPECT) camera.

Tomographic Imaging

If a gamma camera is rotated about the patient and multiple projections obtained, a three-dimensional distribution of tracer is acquired. This is the basis for

SPECT (Kim, 1987). The same gamma-emitting pharmaceuticals are used. Regular gamma cameras or specially designed systems can be used (Iskandrian, 1987). SPECT imaging produces higher spatial resolution (Schwaiger, 1994), and increased sensitivity for coronary artery disease (CAD) over planar images (Beller, 1994). However, attenuation artifacts (absorption of the radioactive energy by other body tissues such that the camera does not detect it) are greater than with planar images, particularly those images involving the inferior wall of the heart in men and the anterior wall in women, and may produce false-positive scans (Schwaiger, 1994). Quality of the images are dependent on the use of stringent quality control measures and experience of the staff. Image quality is also patient-dependent. Patients must be able to lie perfectly still for 15 to 20 minutes, with their hands over their heads, while data are collected.

PTs can identify patients who would have difficulty with arm movements or with remaining still. For these patients, other imaging modalities such as echocardiography may be appropriate.

Positron emission tomography (PET) uses positron-emitting radionuclides. The images obtained by PET can provide information regarding metabolism in lung tissue and cardiac muscle, myocardial perfusion, and myocardial receptor density (Maddahi, 1994). PET is valuable in delineating myocardial areas with reversible and irreversible injury and in assessing the feasibility of surgical revascularization, coronary angioplasty, or thrombolysis with respect to potentially salvageable tissue (Niemeyer, 1992). Many of the radionuclides used in PET scans require a cyclotron for generation and a specialized detection system. PET images offer superior resolution compared with SPECT images (Schwaiger, 1994). PET also allows greater correction for attenuation artifact (Schwaiger, 1994). PET imaging is a newer technology that offers improvement in sensitivity and specificity when compared with SPECT (Mullani, 1992).

PET studies use short scanning times. Protocols can last about 1 hour. The studies can be done at rest or with a pharmacologic stress agent (Schwaiger, 1994). Cost may prohibit the widespread use of this technology.

TESTS OF THE CARDIOVASCULAR SYSTEM
Radionuclide Imaging
Gated/ungated first pass scan

In an ungated first pass study, data are collected on a radiolabeled bolus of blood as it passes through the cardiac chambers. This allows for clear identification of the four cardiac chambers. During gated first pass studies, data are collected at specific periods in the cardiac cycle. Each R-wave of the EKG triggers the acquisition of data, thus the average cycle observed is the compilation of several cycles. Gated equilibrium studies or multiple uptake gated acquisition (MUGA) scans average several hundred cardiac cycles. The quality of the image is best when the patient has a stable sinus rhythm. Patients with irregular heart rates, such as atrial fibrillation have images of poorer quality.

Exercise stress studies

Many of the tests performed using radionuclides are coupled with an exercise test. A treadmill exercise test is performed, and at the peak of exercise, a tracer is injected. Shortly afterward, depending on the tracer, images are acquired. Exercise imaging enhances the identification of ischemic areas. These tests are then often compared with rest studies. Rest/stress or stress/rest protocols can be used.

Pharmacologic stress studies

Many patients are unable to exercise to an intensity sufficient to produce stress on the cardiovascular system. When patients are unable to exercise, pharmacologic agents can be used to dilate the coronary arteries or increase the metabolic demand of the heart. Dipyridimole (Persantine) and adenosine are often used. Pharmacologic stress tests can be coupled with SPECT and PET nuclear imaging techniques or with echocardiography to determine regions of ischemic myocardium suggesting functionally significant blockage in the coronary artery supplying that territory.

Nuclear-derived measurements

Data derived from radionuclide images provide information about perfusion and function. Radionuclides taken up by the myocardium provide a picture of the heart that includes wall thickness and an outline of the chamber. In radionuclide angiography, which includes first pass and gated studies, the blood is highlighted as it passes through the chambers. Qualitative and quantitative measurements can be taken. The most important of these measurements, the ejection fraction (right and left ventricle) is a measure of myocardial function. It is derived from quantitative counts of the ventricular area during diastole and systole (Iskandrian, 1987):

$$\frac{(\text{End-diastolic counts} - \text{End-systolic counts}) \times 100}{\text{End-diastolic counts}}$$

Left ventricular ejection fraction (LVEF) has been shown in several studies (Cass study and the Multicenter Postinfarction Research Group Database) to be highly predictive of 1 year survival (Port, 1994; Maddahi, 1994). Right ventricular ejection fraction (RVEF) has been found to have a wide range of normal values (35% to 75%) (Kinch, 1994) but is not that predictive of function without data about wall motion abnormalities. The strongest radionuclide predictor of outcome is the exercise LVEF. When predicting outcome, multivariate analysis of clinical data, catheterization data and radionuclide measurements have shown that the radionuclide results (exercise LVEF, resting end-diastolic volume, and change in heart rate [HR]) have the same prognostic power as the catheterization data (Port, 1994).

Another important measurement is wall motion. Quantitative and qualitative evaluation of the movement of the myocardium can be made. Wall thickness, and movement are compared with systole and diastole. Assessments are made about akinesia, global or regional hypokinesia, and dyskinesia. Global left ventricular function is a strong predictor of survival. It can help clinicians differentiate a weak heart from one that is stiff, allowing the appropriate treatment. Regional wall function when correlated with knowledge of coronary artery anatomy allows for the identification of potential blockages or areas of infarct. Assessing wall thickness can provide information about hypertrophy or aneurysm but is done more reliably by echocardiography.

Anatomical measurements can be made of chamber size. From these data, chamber volume can be calculated, as well as stroke volume and cardiac output (Table 13-1).

Tests to Evaluate Myocardial Perfusion

Perfusion of the myocardium is a vital factor in the viability and function of the heart. Information about myocardial perfusion is used for diagnostic decisions, treatment decisions and prognosis. Perfusion of the myocardium under rest and exercise conditions is important in the diagnosis of CAD. Efficacy of reperfusion strategies, such as angioplasty and thrombolytic therapy must be evaluated. Identifying tissue that is viable but still at risk is one of the newer applications of myocardial perfusion tests. Information gained from combined perfusion and metabolic studies has helped to increase the understanding of ischemic myocardium. Two types of contractile dysfunction have been delineated. Hibernating myocardium is the result of prolonged ischemia. The contractility of the muscle fiber is effected so that there may appear to be regional wall motion abnormalities. The tissue is alive but not contracting. It is theorized that this is a measure to reduce energy expenditure and ensure myocyte survival. The second condition, myocardial stunning, occurs under conditions of acute ischemia. In this case, there is contractile dysfunction during the acute ischemic episode that persists for some time after perfusion has returned to normal. Both conditions are reversible. Patients demonstrating hibernating myocardium may benefit from revascularization procedures. Patients with stunned myocardium may only require supportive care until contractile function returns. (Schelbert, 1994).

Thallium-201

Thallium-201 is the radioactive isotope most often used in myocardial perfusion studies (Wacker, 1994). It is a cyclotron-produced isotope that emits low-energy radiation (69 to 83 kiloelectron volt [keV]). Administered intravenously, its distribution throughout the body depends on blood flow. Thallium concentrations in the myocardium depend on four processes. First, there is a linear relationship between thallium concentration and coronary blood flow. Second, extraction-transport across the cell membrane depends on active and passive transport mechanisms. Thallium is thought to be transported across the cell membrane through the sodium-potassium ATPase pump (Maddahi, 1994). The third process is washout, also called redistribution. Thal-

TABLE 13–1

Summary of Special Tests of the Cardiopulmonary System

SPECIAL TESTS	CLINICAL FINDINGS
Cardiac Scans *Planar, SPECT, MUGA, First pass*	
Thallium-201 Technitium-99M-sestamibi Technitium teboroxime	Evaluates myocrdial perfusion, used in exercise stress studies and to assess reversibility of defects. Quantitatively can be used to determine: EF, SV, CO, regional function, ventricular volumes, intra-cardiac shunt, valvular regurgitation.
PET Scans	
18-FDG	Assesses myocardial viability by evaluating glucose metabolism. Can identify areas that improve with reperfusion.
11 C acetate	Assesses myocardial viability by evaluating oxidative metabolism. Can identify areas that will improve with reperfusion.
Infarct avid scans	
Technetium-99M-pyrophosphate Indium 111 antimyosin	Identifies areas of infarction by binding with elements released by the death of myocardial tissue.
Pulmonary Scans *Perfusion scan*	
MAB	Identifies regions of decreased pulmonary perfusion, used to identify pulmonary embolism.
Ventilation scan	
99mTc DTPA 133-Xe	Identifies regions of decreased ventilation. Used in conjunction with perfusion scan to identify patients with pulmonary embolism.
Gallium scan	Identification of neoplastic or inflammatory pulmonary lesions
Echocardiography	
M-mode 2-D TEE Doppler	Evaluates myocardial structure. 2-D used in exercise stress studies. Quantitatively measures: chamber size, wall thickness, valve structure and function, pressure and flow through valve, valve area, EF.
Angiography	Quantitative measures of pressure, resistance, flow, O_2 consumption, arteriovenous oxygen difference EF, CO

Abbreviations: EF=ejection fraction, CO=cardiac output, SV=stroke volume

lium enters the cell initially and then is redistributed until an equilibrium is attained based on a net balance between Thallium-201 input through recirculation and intrinsic Thallium washout (Beller, 1994). Finally, concentrations are decay-related, dictated by the half-life of the isotope (Brown, 1994; Iskandrian, 1987).

Thallium-201 images can be qualitatively and quantitatively evaluated. Normally perfused myocardium demonstrates uniform uptake of the tracer. Uniform uptake can occur as long as blockages are less than 50% of the artery. Ischemic but viable myocardium initially appears as areas of decreased uptake, these areas fill in over time, a function of redistribution. Because blood flow is decreased, clearance of Thallium-201 from the defect region is slower (Maddahi, 1994).

In infarcted areas, these defects remain unchanged over time. Qualitative evaluation requires visual inspection of the images. Quantitative evaluation is performed by computer. The computer analyzes the amount of radioactivity taken up in a particular region of interest. It then quantifies this count so that regions can be compared with each other and with normalized data. In this way, unperfused or hypoperfused areas can be identified.

Thallium-201 is used to acquire planar and tomographic images (SPECT) for rest studies, exercise stress studies, and pharmacologic stress studies. The traditional Thallium-201 stress study calls for injection of the tracer at the peak of exercise with collection of the stress data shortly after. The redistribution study is completed 4 hours later. Newer study protocols include reinjection of thallium before the 4-hour redistribution study (Go, 1992) and use in dual-isotope studies (Berman, 1994). Reinjection of thallium and repeat imaging 24 hours after initial study can help identify severely ischemic (greater than 90% blockage) areas, which may take much longer to demonstrate redistribution.

Technetium-99M-sestamibi

New isotopes were approved by the FDA for perfusion imaging in 1990. Technetium (Tc)-99M-sestamibi was developed because of the number of advantages it has over thallium imaging. Sestamibi provides improved SPECT image quality as a result of higher count rates and higher energy, in the 140 keV range. Tc-99M-sestamibi is generator-produced. The isotope has a 6-hour half-life (Berman et al, 1994). Because of the short half-life, higher doses can be injected, and although the percentage of extraction is lower, sestamibi uptake in relation to flow is similar to that of thallium. These factors result in higher count rates, which thus allow the use of gated images and first pass acquisition studies. Higher count rates are preferred when evaluating obese patients. One of the greatest limitations of Tc-99M-sestamibi is that it does not readily redistribute; therefore reversibility of defects cannot be ascertained as well as with thallium. This factor is one reason thallium is much more popular. Two-day protocols or dual isotope protocols can be used to overcome this limitation (Berman, 1994). Lack of redistribution has been exploited in evaluating the impact of thrombolytic therapy

in acute situations. A patient with an acute myocardial infarction (MI) can be injected with tracer, given thrombolytics, stabilized, and scanned 4 hours later. The scan results show myocardial perfusion at the time of injection when the myocardium was ischemic. Later scans demonstrate the new perfusion situation.

Technetium-99M-teboroxime

Another newer isotope is Technetium (Tc)-99M-teboroxime. It is not yet widely accepted because of its rapid washout and visualization problems related to hepatic uptake (Berman et al., 1991; Go, 1992). The half-life for teboroxime is 5 to 6 minutes (Johnson, 1994). It has a myocardial extraction fraction higher than either sestamibi or thallium (Johnson, 1994). Tc-99M-teboroxime uptake parallels myocardial blood flow under both ischemic and nonischemic conditions (Johnson, 1994) and does not appear to rely on active cellular processes.

Because of the short half-life, rapid acquisition imaging systems are required so that the images do not reflect washout. SPECT and first pass studies can be performed but Tc-99M-teboroxime does not permit gated SPECT acquisition (Berman, 1991). Protocols using this isotope are designed to take advantage of the rapid uptake and washout. When used with pharmacologic stress studies, a rest-stress study can be completed within minutes (Johnson, 1994). This may have future application in studying reperfusion following balloon angioplasty or reperfusion therapy with thrombolytic agents (Johnson, 1994). PET tracers are also used to evaluate perfusion and will be discussed below. They include, 13-N ammonia, 82-Rb rubidium, or 15-O water.

Tests to Evaluate Myocardial Viability

Identification of the size of an infarct has traditionally been helpful in determining prognosis. Infarct avid tracers were used. The tracers bind with elements released by necrotic myocardial tissue.

With the development of reperfusion strategies, angioplasty, bypass grafting, and thrombolytic therapy it was noted that areas that appeared to be nonfunctional on perfusion scans regained function once the area regained adequate blood supply. Tests were developed that were able to distinguish these areas of stunned or hibernating myocardium. These tests of myocardial viability often look at metabolism.

According to Maddahi, four different PET approaches have been used for assessment of myocardial viability: (1) perfusion-FDG metabolism imaging, (2) determination of oxidative metabolism with 11-C-acetate, (3) uptake and retention of 82-Rb and (4) the water perfusable tissue index (Maddahi, 1994).

18F-fluoro-deoxyglucose

18F-fluoro-deoxyglucose (FDG) is a glucose analogue that crosses the capillary and sarcolemmal membrane at a rate proportional to that of glucose. It becomes trapped in the myocardium, because it is not a useful substrate in metabolic pathways. FDG distribution is relative to uptake of unlabeled glucose (Maddahi, 1994).

Identification of areas with normal metabolism, altered metabolism or no metabolism is based on the use of glucose as an energy substrate. Normally, perfused myocardial cells use fatty acids for adenosine triphosphate (ATP) production when in a fasting state and use glucose as the primary energy source in the postprandial state. Ischemic myocardium uses glucose in the fasting state and the postprandial state. Infarcted areas show no metabolic activity. Therefore increased uptake of FDG in the postprandial state occurs in both hibernating and normal myocardium, but in the fasting state, it occurs only in the hibernating myocardium. Clinical studies in infarct patients showed that area with persistent thallium-201 perfusion defects have evidence of remaining metabolic activity in 47% of regions when studied with a PET scan, indicating overestimation of irreversible injury. Use of reinjection and late redistribution imaging has significantly lowered this number (Hendel, 1994). The implication derived from this finding is that in areas with perfusion defects, if glucose activity remains, the region is viable (mismatch pattern); conversely, if such activity is absent, the area is likely to be infarcted or necrotic (match pattern) (Niemeyer, 1992). Viewed in functional terms, mismatch simply implies the potential for improvement; match implies no potential for improvement in contractility after successful revascularization (Schelbert, 1994).

11-C-Acetate

Another way to evaluate myocardial viability is to use an isotope that is incorporated into the metabolic pathways related to myocardial oxygen consumption. 11-C-acetate in its activated form, acetyl-CoA, represents the entry point for all metabolic pathways into the tricarboxylic acid cycle, which is tightly coupled to oxidated metabolism. It's advantage over 18-FDG, is that it does not rely on substrate use (i.e., glucose vs. fat metabolism). It accurately reflects oxidative metabolism and can distinguish viable from nonviable myocardium in both acute and chronic ischemic conditions (Bergman, 1994.)

Technetium-99M-pyrophosphate

Technetium-99M-pyrophosphate (TcPyp) identifies areas of myocardial infarction by forming a complex with calcium, which is released when myocardial cells die. TcPyp scans have the best results when obtained 24 to 48 hours postinfarction. This time frame is obviously after reperfusion strategies would have been employed. Sensitivity of this scan is high, but specificity is low, since a number of other processes can result in a positive scan (e.g., myocardial trauma, ventricular aneurysm, and uptake in skeletal structures) (Niemeyer, 1992).

Indium-111-antimyosin

Indium 111 antimyosin is a radiolabled monoclonoal antibody that identifies infarcted myocardial tissue. It binds with myocardial myosin, which is released when the muscle cell dies. It can be used in conjunction with thallium-201 to distinguish infarcted tissue from perfused viable tissue. It is most reliable when performed 48 hours after infarction (Niemeyer, 1992).

Echocardiography

Another noninvasive method of evaluating the heart uses the physical properties of sound. Echocardiography provides information about blood flow, structure, and function of the heart. Motion mode (M-mode) and two-dimensional (2-D) images are highly reliable methods of evaluation. Recent developments of technique and technology include color flow Doppler echo, transesophageal echo, and intravascular echocardiography. These techniques, when used in combination can provide much of the information previously available only by cardiac catheterization (Hartnell, 1994).

Physics of echocardiography

Imaging systems that use ultrasound require a source for generation of the sound wave, a transducer, and a receiver to pick up the reflected sound waves. Sound is absorbed or reflected differentially by specific tissues. Therefore the sound wave reflected from muscle differs from that reflected from vascular space, or valvular structures. Returning signals are converted into electrical signals that generate an image. This is the basis for M-mode and 2-D echo. In M-mode echocardiography, the transducer transmits a single sound wave through the chest wall. A thin slice of the heart, an "ice pick" view, directly under the sound wave, reflects the wave back to the transducer. M-mode, though useful, is rarely used; 2-D is the primary diagnostic mode. In 2-D echocardiography, the transducer is able to pick up a wedge section of the heart. In 2-D the transducer acts as the transmitter and receiver. A "real time" two-dimensional picture of the heart is recorded on videotape. The heart can be viewed in motion, and wall motion can be evaluated.

Doppler echocardiography relies on the Doppler effect to determine velocity. When a sound wave is aimed at moving objects such as red blood cells, the known transmitted frequency and the reflected frequency differ, a phenomenon, known as a frequency shift. The greater the frequency shift the greater the speed of the targeted object (Waggoner and Perez, 1990). The velocity of flow is the terminology used to express Doppler frequency shifts. Both continuous wave and pulsed wave Doppler are used.

Color flow Doppler echocardiography was introduced in the mid-1980s. It is usually superimposed on a two-dimensional image in real time but can be used with M-mode. It is a method that displays anatomic and spatial blood flow velocity estimates with indication of flow direction in real time (Waggoner, 1990). Color is matched based on the direction of flow, and shading is indicative of intensity based on the mean velocity flow estimates (Waggoner and Perez, 1990). It is primarily used to assess the extent of regurgitant jets across "leaky valves," as well as to indicate areas of abnormal shunts such as atrial septal defects. Turbulence created by narrowed valves creates wide color shading.

Measurements derived from echocardiography

Echocardiographic results can be viewed qualitatively and quantitatively. An experienced viewer can analyze the anatomical relationships and structure of the heart, wall motion, valve movement and configuration, and chamber size.

Quantitative measures are calculated from the Doppler frequency shifts. Velocity measures can be used in other equations to estimate pressure and valve area. The modified Bernoulli equation is used to calculate pressure changes around the valve:

$$\Delta P \text{ (mm Hg)} = 4 \times V_{max}^2 \text{ (m/second)},$$
where P is the pressure gradient across the valve and V is the velocity of blood flow through the valve.

These measurements allow calculation of stenotic valve gradients and right-sided filling pressures, valve regurgitation, and ventricular septal defects (Waggoner and Perez, 1990). Valve regurgitation and shunt calculations are more complicated than the Bernoulli equation alone.

Another important quantitative measure is the estimated area of the valve. The continuity equation is used to estimate valve area. It is based on the principle of conservation of mass; that is, in a normal heart, the volume of blood that enters the right atrium should be conserved as it passes through the other chambers. Flow volume at different sites is related to the flow velocity and the cross sectional area of the site. Therefore $A_1 \times V_1 = A_2 \times V_2$, where V_1 is the velocity of flow at one side of the valve and V_2 is the flow velocity at the other side of the valve, and A is the cross-sectional area (Waggoner and Perez, 1990) (Wilson, Vacek, 1990).

Transsophageal echocardiography (TEE)

Because of consistent technical difficulties with transthoracic echocardiography, the technique of transesophageal echo was developed to improve spatial resolution. The technique can obtain M-mode, 2-D, and color flow Doppler images by using a small probe mounted on the tip of a modified gastroscope. The probe is advanced into the esophagus and positioned so that multiple views of the heart are available (Kerber, 1988). Initially, the technique was performed intraoperatively on anesthetized patients and on intubated patients in the intensive care unit. It is now used on awake patients who are mildly sedated (Schneider, 1993). The semiinvasive nature of this test has slowed its adoption. It is most useful in ruling out thrombus or heart valve vegetation as a cause of transient ischemic attack (TIA) or stroke. Especially excellent views of the left atrium and atrial appendage are seen. The atrial appendages cannot be visualized by traditional transthoracic echo. It is also a good assessment of prosthetic valve function.

Cardiac Angiography

The standard with which many of the noninvasive tests are compared is that of cardiac catheterization. It is an invasive test, with a small but serious risk to the patient. Complications include death, stroke, myocardial infarction (MI), bleeding, arterial trauma or thrombus, renal dysfunction, and arrhythmias (Reagan, Boxt, and Katz, 1994). The test is indicated in patients with a high risk of atherosclerotic heart disease whose stress perfusion scans are positive. Patient's with diagnosed CAD with angina, unresponsive to medical therapy, may also need catheterization.

Test Procedure

The cardiac catheterization laboratory requires an x-ray generator tube and image intensifier/cine camera. Data are stored using 35mm file (Reagan, Boxt, and Katz, 1994).

The procedure for cardiac catheterization of the left side of the heart requires the threading of a catheter, guided by fluoroscopy, through the femoral artery or brachial artery to the aorta. Direct measurements of chamber pressures, blood flow, and oxygen saturation can be obtained. When selective coronary arteriography is performed, radiopaque contrast material is injected into the left main or right coronary artery. Cine recordings are made after the injection, and injections are repeated until the entire coronary tree is visualized.

Cardiac ventriculography is when dye is injected into the ventricle and the entire chamber becomes outlined. Several cardiac cycles are recorded on cine. It provides valuable information about global and segmental wall motion, valve motion, and the presence of abnormal anatomy (Grossman, 1986).

TESTS OF THE RESPIRATORY SYSTEM

Unlike the cardiovascular system, special tests of the respiratory system are less commonly used in the initial diagnosis and treatment of disease. This is the result of the generally high quality information obtained from standard x-ray examination when combined with the patient's respiratory symptoms and the results of the physical examination (Lillington, 1987). When further information is needed to refine the diagnosis or treatment decision several tests are available to clinicians. Radionuclide imaging of the chest is useful in the noninvasive evaluation of pulmonary embolism, whereas pulmonary angiography is the invasive but definitive test. A computed tomography (CT) scan of the chest also has a variety of applications (Webb, 1994). Although magnetic resonance imaging (MRI) provides improved tissue contrast in comparison to a CT scan, imaging applications in pulmonary disease continue to suffer from technical limitations (Mayo, 1994).

Bronchoscopy

Bronchoscopy is often used as both a diagnostic and therapeutic treatment modality (Mars and Ciesla, 1993). It allows direct visualization of the trachea and its major subdivisions. Fiberoptic bronchoscopy has virtually replaced bronchography (Lillington, 1987). In fiberoptic bronchoscopy, a flexible tube is inserted into the trachea of mildly sedated patients. This tude is able to enter small brochial subdivisions. Secretions can be removed for evalutaion or as a treatment. It is also possible to obtain biopsy samples using tiny forceps or cell brushings. Bronchoscopy is particularly important in the diagmosis of bronchogenic carcinoma (Price and Wilson, 1986).

RADIONUCLIDE IMAGING
Ventilation-Perfusion Lung Scan

The ventilation-perfusion lung scan is a combination of two separate imaging procedures. It is primarily used in the diagnosis of pulmonary embolism, with limited use for other clinical problems (Lillington, 1987). The perfusion portion requires the injection of radioactive tracer. Technetium-99M-macroaggregated albumin is (almost universally accepted as) the perfusion tracer of choice (Juni and Alavi, 1991). The ventilation scan requires the inhalation of radioactive gas, usually 133-XE gas or Tc-99M-diethylene triamine penta-acetic acid (DTPA) aerosol. Other isotopes can be used for ventilation scanning (e.g. Kr-81M, Xenon-127) but they are more difficult to obtain.

A normal perfusion scan essentially rules out recent pulmonary embolus. If the perfusion scan is abnormal, it is compared with the ventilation scan for match or mismatch of defects. An interpretation scheme is used, such as Biello or Pioped, which classifies the probability of pulmonary embolism into normal, low, intermediate (indeterminate), or high (Juni, 1991; Miller and O'Doherty, 1992). Patients with high probability scans should begin anticoagulation therapy (Juni, 1991). Patients with intermediate (indeterminate) scans may need to have a pulmonary angiogram before beginning treatment (Miller and O'Doherty, 1992).

Miller and O'Doherty (1992) note other applications of ventilation/perfusion scanning to include monitoring of response to radiotherapy and assessment of resectability of bullae. The scan is used to predict whether someone can tolerate a pneumonectomy based on percent flow to the opposite lung and extent of disease present.

Pulmonary Angiography

The diagnosis of pulmonary embolism is the primary indication for pulmonary angiography. It is the gold standard against which ventilation/perfusion scans are compared (Juni, 1992). Contrast dye is injected into the pulmonary circulation through the pulmonary artery. Additional techniques such as balloon occlusion, segmental injections, or increased magnification improve the sensitivity of the test (Lillington, 1987). Interobserver reliability studies performed on the interpretation of pulmonary angiograms are 83% to 86% (Juni, 1992).

Gallium Scintigraphy

Gallium-67-citrate concentrates in neoplastic and inflammatory lesions of the lung (Lillington, 1987). Gallium is more sensitive than normal chest x-ray in identifying infectious and noninfectious inflammatory processes. This is particularly important in identifying opportunistic infections in the immunocompromised patient. In patients with acquired immune deficiency syndrome (AIDS) the sensitivity of gallium scanning for pneumocystis carinii pneumonia approaches 94% to 96% (Kramer and Divgi, 1991). The radioisotope is injected but it takes 48 to 72 hours before imaging can be performed (Miller and O'Doherty, 1992).

Gallium is commonly used in the evaluation of patients with interstitial lung disease; this includes sarcoidosis, amiodarone toxicity, and following cytotoxic therapy with bleiomycin, as well as many other entities (Miller and O'Doherty, 1992). In conjunction with neoplasms, the scan's use is limited to assessing tumor extent (Kramer and Divgi, 1991).

Computed Tomography

A computed tomography (CT) scan of the chest provides a series of cross-sectional x-ray images. Compared with the standard x-ray, it is not commonly used in the initial diagnosis of pulmonary disease. CT scan has been found to be a useful first-line diagnostic tool in the evaluation of mediastinal disease, including mediastinal masses, staging of mediastinal cancers, and identification of cysts (Lillington, 1987).

High-resolution computed tomography (HRCT) has improved the documentation of morphologic changes associated with chronic airflow obstruction. Webb's (1994) review of the application of this new technology identified the utility of this test in a variety of obstructive diseases. HRCT is sensitive in the diagnosis of early emphysema, although rarely used clinically. In cystic disease, such as histiocytosis X and lymphangiomyomatosis, HRCT is able to demonstrate cysts less than 10 mm in diameter, as well as wall thickness.

In the diagnosis of bronchiectasis, HRCT demonstrates a high specificity. It is the procedure of choice after plain chest X-rays. HRCT can discriminate between the three different types of abnormal bronchi seen in bronchiectasis (cylindrical, varicose, and cystic) but again there is little clinical significance (Webb, 1994). It can be used to differentiate lymphangitic spread of cancer versus heart failure when unclear clinically. HRCT also can be used to evaluate clearing of persistent pneumonias. Overall, HRCT has helped clarify disease morphology, but the clinical significance for diagnosis and patient's pulmonary function is less clear.

Magnetic Resonance Imaging

MRI is a technique that does not use radiopharmaceuticals or ionizing radiation. The technique relies on the creation of a powerful magnetic field that causes the hydrogen nuclei in fat and water molecules to resonate, creating magnetic vectors. With specially tuned radio frequency pulses, these vectors are used to create images of the environment of the water and fat molecules. The images are highly dependent on the timing and magnitude of the radio-frequency (Mayo, 1994). Contrast materials (e.g., gadolinium, DTPA) can be used to enhance signal intensity.

MRI is a useful technique in evaluating cardiac structures. It can identify cardiac masses and is the modality of choice for evaluating the pericardium. MRI is secondary to CT in evaluating the mediastinum especially constrictive pericarditis (Mayo, 1994). Evaluation of the lung parenchyma presents unique problems because of respiratory movement and the air tissue interface.

SUMMARY

Many tests are available to identify cardiopulmonary dysfunction. The attending physician determines which tests are appropriate for the patient's particular medical condition. When the tests are completed, results are given, and an evaluation of the results are documented. PTs need to understand the results of the tests and how they will apply to patient function and response to exercise. This understanding applies to the selection of exercise and work loads the PT prescribes for the patient. Until a PT reaches a certain maturity level, as well as a level of understanding and application of the test results to patient treatment, it is highly encouraged that the PT discuss the test and results with the patient's physician. These discussions are excellent opportunities for learning both for the PT and to help the physician understand what physical therapy has to offer the patient with cardiopulmonary dysfunction.

REVIEW QUESTIONS

1. Why is the ejection fraction an important measure of myocardial function?
2. What is the difference between stunned myocardium and hibernating myocardium?
3. Which tests are used to diagnose pulmonary embolism?
4. Which tests can be used to evaluate myocardial viability?
5. Why is echocardiography a good choice for evaluating pediatric cardiac defects?

References

Beller, G. (1994). Myocardial perfusion imaging with thallium-201. *Journal of Nuclear Medicine, 35,* 674-680.

Bergman, S. (1994). Use and limitations of metabolic tracers labeled with positron-emitting radionuclides in the identification of viable myocardium. *Journal of Nuclear Medicine, 35,* (4 suppl), 15s-22s.

Berman, D., Hosen, S., Van Train, K., Germano, G., Maddahi, J., Friedman, J. (1994). Myocardial perfusion imaging with technitium-99M-sestamibi comparative analysis of available imaging protocols. *Journal of Nuclear Medicine, 35,* 681-688.

Berman, D., Kiat, H., Van Train, K., Garcia, E., Friedman, J., & Maddahi, J. (1991). Technetium, 99m sestamibi in the assessment of chronic coronary artery disease. *Seminars in Nuclear Medicine, 21,* 190-212.

Brown, K. (1994). The role of stress redistribution thallium-201 myocardial perfusion imaging in evaluating coronary artery disease and perioperative risk. *Journal of Nuclear Medicine, 35,* 703-706.

Go, R.T., MacIntyre, W.J., Cook, S.A., Neumann, D.R. (1992). Myocardial perfusion imaging in the diagnosis of coronary artery disease. *Current Opinion in Radiology. 4*(4). 23-33.

Grossman, W. (1986) *Cardiac Catheterization and Angiography.* (3rd ed.) Philadelphia: Lea & Febiger.

Hartnell, G. (1994) Developments in Echocardiography. *Radiologic Clinics of North America, 32,* 461-475.

Hendel, R. (1994) Single-photon imaging for the assessment of myocardial viability. *Journal of Nuclear Medicine, 35*(4 suppl), 23s-31s.

Iskandrian, A.S. (1987). *Nuclear cardiac imaging: principles and applications.* Philadelphia: FA Davis.

Johnson, L. (1994) Myocardial perfusion imaging with technetium-99m-teboroxime. *Journal of Nuclear Medicine, 35,* 689-692.

Juni, J., & Alavi, A. (1991). Lung scanning in the diagnosis of pulmonary embolism: the emperor redressed. *Seminars in Nuclear Medicine, 21,* 281-296.

Kerber, R. (Ed.). (1988). *Echocardiography in coronary artery disease.* Mount Kisco, NY: Futura Publishing.

Kim, E. (1987). *Nuclear diagnostic imaging: practical clinical applications.* New York: Macmillan.

Kinch, J., & Ryan, T. (1994). Right ventricular infarction. *New England Journal of Medicine, 330,* 1211-1215.

Kramer, E., & Divgi, C. (1991). Pulmonary applications of nuclear medicine. *Clinics in Chest Medicine 12:1.* 55-75.

Lillington, G. (1987). *A diagnostic approach to chest disease.* Baltimore: Williams and Wilkins.

Maddahi, J., Schelbert, H., Brunken, R., & DiCarli, M. (1994). Role of Thallium-201 and PET imaging in evaluation of myocardial viability and management of patients with coronary artery disease and left ventricular dysfunction. *Journal of Nuclear Medicine, 35,* 707-715.

Mars, M., & Ciesla, N. (1993). Chest physical therapy may have prevented bronchoscopy and exploratory laparatomy-a case report. *Cardiopulmonary Physical Therapy Journal. 4:*1, 4–6.

Mayo, J. (1994). Magnetic resonance imaging of the chest. *Advances in Chest Radiology, 32,* 795-809.

Miller, R.F., & O'Doherty, M.J. (1992). Pulmonary nuclear medicine. *European Journal of Nuclear Medicine, 19,* 355-368.

Mullani, N.A., & Volkow, N.D., (1992). Positron emission tomography instrumentation: a review and update. *American Journal of Physiologic Imaging, 3/4,* 121-135.

Niemeyer, M.G., Van der Wall, E.E., Pauwels, E.K.J., van Dijkman, P.R.M., Blokland, J.A.K., deRoos, A., & Bruschke, A.V.G. (1992). Assessment of acute myocardial infarction by nuclear imaging techniques. *Angiology, 43,* 720-733.

Port, S. (1994). The role of radionuclide ventriculography in the assessment of prognosis in patients with CAD. *Journal of Nuclear Medicine, 35,* 721-725.

Price, S., & Wilson, L. (1986). *Pathophysiology: clinical concepts of disease processes.* New York: McGraw-Hill.

Reagan, K., Boxt, L., & Katz, J. (1994). Introduction to coronary arteriography. *Radiologic Clinics of North America, 32,* 419-433.

Schelbert, H. (1994). Metabolic imaging to assess myocardial viability. *Journal of Nuclear Medicine, 35*(4 suppl), 8s-14s.

Schneider, A., Hsu, T., Schwartz, S., & Pandian, N. (1993). Single, biplane, multiplane, and three dimensional transesophageal echocardiography. *Cardiology Clinics, 11,* 361-387.

Schwaiger, M. (1994). Myocardial perfusion imaging with PET. *Journal of Nuclear Medicine, 35,* 693-698.

Wackers, F.J.T. (1994). Radionuclide evaluation of coronary artery disease in the 1990's. *Cardiology Clinics. 12.* 385-389.

Waggoner, A.D., & Perez, J. (1990). Principles and physics of doppler. *Cardiology Clinics, 12,* 385-389.

Webb, W.R. (1994). High-resolution computed tomography of obstructive lung disease. *Radiologic Clinics of North America, 32,* 745-757.

Wilson, D., & Vacek, J. (1990). Echocardiography. *Postgraduate Medicine. 87.* 191-202.

CHAPTER 14

Clinical Assessment of the Cardiopulmonary System

Susan M. Butler

KEY TERMS

Barrel-chest
Crackles
Cyanosis
Dyspnea
Egophany

Hyperresonant
Resonant
Wheeze
Whispered pectoriloquy

INTRODUCTION

To develop an effective treatment program for the patient with a cardiopulmonary problem, it is essential that a thorough evaluation be performed by the physical therapist (PT). This provides "baseline" data for comparison with subsequent reassessments that occur on a daily basis. Any progress or deterioration in status can then be easily identified with appropriate adjustments made in the treatment plan.

CHART REVIEW/PATIENT INTERVIEW

The first patient contact can be indirect, through the medical chart, or direct, through patient interview. In the inpatient setting, a chart review is the first point of contact, whereas in the outpatient population, the information may be only what is obtainable from the patient. Time management is an ever-present issue in today's era of cost containment and health care reform. Thus a medical chart review should be conducted in an organized fashion. Most PTs develop their own method.

One strategy to chart review is the following sequence:

1. Read the history and physical and admission medical note (i.e., preadmission symptoms).

2. Read the last medical note.

3. *Scan* remainder of chart.

4. Read any reports from medical specialists, consultants, i.e., pulmonologist, neurologist, oncologist.

5. Review any pertinent lab tests. EXAMPLES: chest x-ray, arterial blood gases (ABG's), complete blood count (CBC).

6. Review medications, in particular, pulmonary and cardiac drugs.

7. Review the psychosocial information (i.e., family, architectural barriers).

This last step is crucial in this time of shortened hospital stays. Any detail of the patient's background that would affect discharge planning is crucial to know even on the first day of treatment. Additional information to review that may be helpful and falls into the category of "as time allows" is the documentation of other allied health professionals (i.e., nursing, occupational therapy, speech pathology). Finally, when the initial chart review is finished, a mental picture of the patient should exist, even before the PT steps into the patient's hospital room.

Details regarding the patient interview have been covered in chapter 7. However, there are questions that should be posed to any patient regardless of whether their primary condition is cardiopulmonary. The patient whose referring problem is musculoskeletal or neurologic still must have operational cardiac

and respiratory systems. These questions could include the following: What is the smoking history? Does the patient have a family history of premature coronary artery disease (i.e., a parent or sibling who had a myocardial infarction)? Can the symptoms presented also be signs of a cardiovascular or pulmonary illness? Does the patient have an active versus a sedentary lifestyle? What activities precipitate symptoms? Do these symptoms include breathlessness? The patient should be seen as a human being with multiple organ systems. The patient's problem, whether orthopedic or cardiopulmonary, should not be viewed in isolation. An example is the outpatient with a physical therapy diagnosis of low back pain. When questioned about limiting symptoms, the patient might describe cramping leg pain more suggestive of peripheral vascular disease (PVD).

PHYSICAL EXAMINATION

The traditional components of a chest assessment are **visual inspection, auscultation, percussion,** and **palpation.** The information provided by each of these techniques, when integrated with the patient's history and chart contents, allows the PT to piece together the pieces of the puzzle. For instance, to auscultate breath sounds without observing the symmetry of the chest wall fails to provide the needed clues to the total patient picture; thereby the development of an appropriate plan of care for the patient is made more difficult.

Before each individual component of the assessment is discussed, a review of the pertinent anatomical landmarks and topographical lines is to be discussed. Knowledge of the superficial anatomy and its relationship to the underlying heart and lungs aids the therapist in decision making. The topographical lines allow for more accurate description of the physical findings.

TOPOGRAPHICAL ANATOMIC LANDMARKS

Key anatomical structures include the following:
- **Sternum**
- **Clavicles**

Anatomic Structures

Suprasternal notch—A depression palpable at the tip of the sternum

Sternomanubrial angle—A bony bump where the manubrium meets the body of the sternum; about 5 cm distal to suprasternal notch; also known as *angle of Louis;* palpating lateral to this junction, the *second ribs* is found and thus a reference point for identifying intercostal spaces and successive ribs; also, a superficial marking for where the underlying trachea divides into right and left mainstem bronchi.

Costal angle—The angle formed by the joining of the costal margins with the sternum; normally, no greater than 90 degrees.

Vertebra prominens—The spinous process of the seventh cervical vertebra (C7); allows numbering of thoracic vertebra

- **Suprasternal notch**
- **Sternomanubrial angle (angle of Louis)**
- **Costal angle**
- **Vertebra prominens**

See the box on p. 210 and Figures 14-1 and 14-2 for specific definitions and anterior and lateral views of thorax. Imaginary topographical lines are used to more clearly describe any physical findings (e.g., location of surgical incisions, abnormal breath sounds, etc.) (Figure 14-3).

The anterior view of the thorax has three vertical lines. These are the following:

- *Mid-sternal line* (MSL)—a vertical line bisecting the sternum
- *Mid-clavicular line* (MCL)—lies parallel to the MSL, bisects each clavicle; the lower lung borders cross the sixth rib at the MCL.

Laterally there are three vertical lines, originating in their respective axillary folds:

- *Anterior axillary line* (AAL), *mid-axillary line* (MAL), and *posterior axillary* (PAL)—Like the MCLs, these lines are also bilateral.

  The posterior chest has the following three lines:
- *Vertebral or mid-spinal line*—runs through the spinous processes of the vertebrae.
- *Mid-scapular lines* (MSL)—lie parallel to the mid-spinal lines; bisect inferior angles of scapulae.

VISUAL INSPECTION

Inspection is the foremost element of a chest assessment. Not only should the features of the patient be observed, but also the equipment and any aspect of the patient's surroundings that would contribute to delineating the true picture of that patient. Remember, the PT has speculated a preliminary picture of the patient based on chart review. Now, the ultimate test: how realistic was this initial impression? What are the outward clinical signs that the therapist should

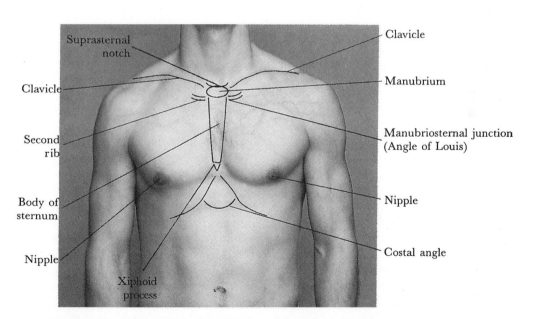

FIGURE 14-1
Topographical landmarks of the chest. (Adapted with permission from Seidel HM et al: *Mosby's guide to physical examination,* ed 3, Boston, 1995, Mosby.)

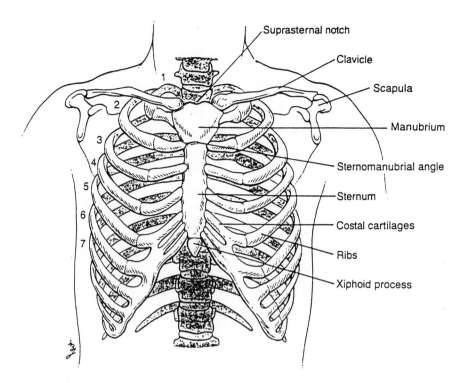

FIGURE 14-2

Anterior view of the thorax. (With permission from Swartz MH: *Textbook of physical diagnoses—history and examination,* ed 2, Philadelphia, 1994, WB Saunders.)

look for? It will be broken down into categories for clarity.

General Appearance

Does the patient appear comfortable? Is there any facial grimacing? Is the patient awake and alert or disoriented? Is there any nasal flaring or pursed-lip breathing? These are signs of respiratory distress. Nasal flaring can be defined as the outward movement of the nares with inspiration (Swartz, 1994). Are the accessory muscles of respiration (i.e, sternocleidomastoid, trapezius) hypertrophied? How is the patient positioned? Is the patient resting comfortably or leaning forward over the bedside table and struggling for breath? What is the patient's build—stocky, thin or cachectic? Is the patient's mobility limited? Can the patient sit unsupported? Should the assessment be performed in stages such as supine or alternate sidelying? Is there any extra equipment in the patient's surroundings? Is the patient wearing supplemental oxygen? Is the oxygen delivered through a nasal cannula or a mask? What is the fraction of inspired oxygen (FiO_2)? Are there any monitoring lines and where are they located. For instance, if an arterial line is present, is it placed in the radial or femoral artery? Are there electrocardiogram (ECG) leads? Is it a "hard line" (directly connected to monitor) vs. telemetry (through radio transmitter)? Are there intravenous (IV) sites? Are these peripheral (antecubital) or central (subclavian or jugular)? Is there a urinary catheter?

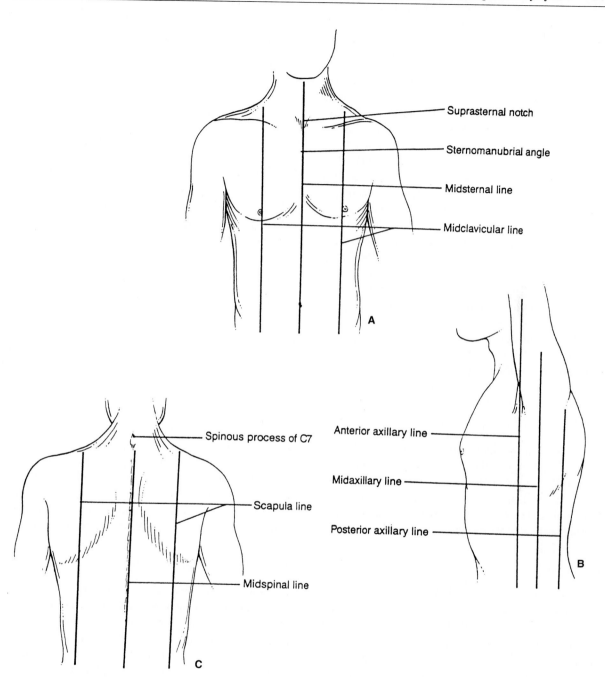

FIGURE 14-3
Imaginary topographical lines. **A,** Anterior view. **B,** Lateral view. **C,** Posterior view. (Adapted with permission from Swartz MH: *Textbook of physical diagnoses—history and examination,* ed 2, Philadelphia, 1994, WB Saunders.)

Skin

Does the skin have a pink, healthy color versus a pallor? Is cyanosis present? Cyanosis is a bluish tinge that can be seen centrally or peripherally. *Central cyanosis* is a result of insufficient gas exchange within the lungs and is not usually seen unless oxygen saturation is less than 80%. A bluish tint may be seen at the mucous membranes (e.g., tongue, lips). *Peripheral cyanosis,* on the other hand, occurs when oxygen extraction at the periphery is excessive. This type is also more associated with low cardiac output states. Areas to observe for peripheral cyanosis might be fingertips, toes, nose, or nail beds. A differentiating feature between central and peripheral cyanosis is that peripheral cyanosis occurs, usually in the cooler body parts such as nail beds and vanishes, usually when the part is warmed. In contrast, central cyanosis does not disappear when the area is warmed.

Are any scars, bruises or ecchymoses observed? Are there reddened areas suggestive of prolonged pressure anywhere? Do the bony landmarks appear more prominent than usual? Are there any signs of trauma to the thorax or any other body parts? Does the skin appear edematous? Does this edema appear to limit joint motion? Are there any surgical incisions, new and old? Do these incisions appear to be healed or seem reddened and swollen? Is there evidence of clubbing of the digits? *Clubbing* can be defined as the loss of angle between the nail bed and the distal interphalangeal joint (Figure 14-4). The cause of clubbing has a variety of theories, including increased perfusion. Its association with arterial oxygen desaturation has been noted, but this is not an exclusive phenomenon. Clubbing has been observed in nonpulmonary diseases such as hepatic fibrosis and Crohn's disease. (George, Light, Matthay, and Matthay, 1990; Seidel, Ball, Dains, and Benedict, 1995; and Swartz, 1994).

Neck

Are the accessory muscles of respirations being recruited for a resting breathing pattern? Do the sternocleidomastoid or trapezius muscles appear prominent? This is an early sign of obstructive lung disease (Swartz, 1994).

Jugular venous distension

The jugular veins empty into the superior vena cava and reflect right-sided heart function. Right atrial pressure (RAP) is evident based on the extent to which the jugular venous pulse (JVP) can be visualized. The more superficial external jugular veins may be seen superior to the clavicles; the internal jugular veins, though larger, lie deep beneath the sternocleidomastoids and are less visible. Jugular venous distention (JVD) can be best seen when the patient lies with the head and neck at an optimal angle of 45 degrees (Figure 14-5). Symmetry of JVD should be noted. The veins are distended bilaterally if there is a cardiac cause such as congestive heart failure (CHF). A unilateral distention is an indication of a localized problem. (Seidel, Ball, Dains, and Benedict, 1995).

CHEST WALL CONFIGURATION

The normal thoracic cage is elliptically shaped when free of disease. The anteroposterior (AP) to lateral diameter is 1:2 or 5:7. The angle of the ribs is less than 90 degrees. The ribs articulate with the vertebra, posteriorly, at a 45-degree angle. The thorax should be observed both anteriorly and posteriorly. With chronic obstructive pulmonary disease (COPD), the ribs become more horizontal and the A-P diameter increases, thus the term *barrel chest* is used. In infants, the chest is round with the anteroposterior and

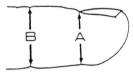

FIGURE 14-4
A, Clubbing of the fingers is best assessed by determining the ratio of the diameter at the base of the nail **B,** to the diameter at the distal interphalangeal joint. This ratio is normally less than 1. (Reprinted with permission from George RB et al: *Chest medicine,* ed 2, Baltimore, 1990, Williams and Wilkins.)

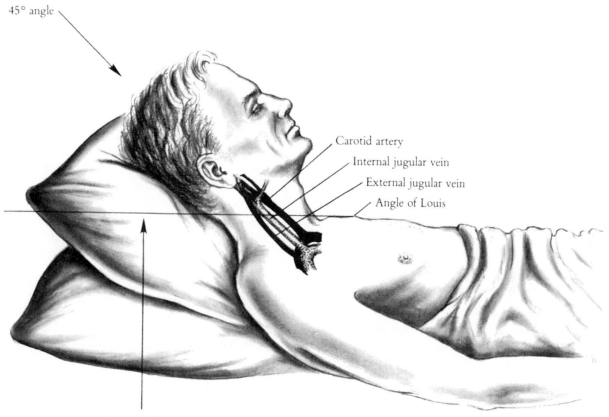

45° angle

Carotid artery

Internal jugular vein

External jugular vein

Angle of Louis

Horizontal line

FIGURE 14-5
Proper positioning to observe jugular venous distention. (Reprinted with permission from Seidel HM et al: *Mosby's guide to physical examination,* ed 3, Boston, 1995, Mosby.)

transverse or lateral diameters of about equal dimensions. As the child grows to adulthood, the chest becomes more elliptical. Again, with the aging process, the chest returns to a more rounded appearance. The increased anteroposterior diameter, in this population, is a result of the multiple factors of decreasing lung compliance, decreased strength of the thoracic and diaphragmatic muscles and skeletal changes of the thoracic spine. The symmetry of the thoracic cage should also be noted. Asymmetry can be the result of structural defects or an underlying intrathoracic

pathology. Again, any asymmetry should be observed from both anterior and posterior views.

Structural defects of the anterior chest may include the following: *pectus excavatum,* or funnel chest—a depressed lower sternum that usually causes restriction only when severe; *pectus carinatum,* or pigeon chest—a prominent upper sternum which does not restrict chest wall movement; and *flail chest*—the chest wall moves inward with inspiration, such as with multiple rib fractures.

Other structural defects are spinal deformities.

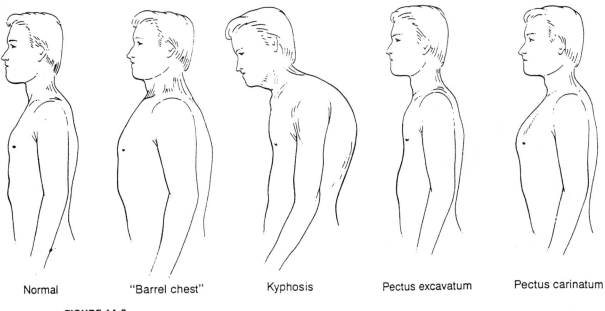

| Normal | "Barrel chest" | Kyphosis | Pectus excavatum | Pectus carinatum |

FIGURE 14-6

Chest wall configurations. (Reprinted with permission from Swartz MH: *Textbook of physical diagnoses—history and examination,* ed 2, Philadelphia, 1994, WB Saunders.)

These are best viewed posteriorly. *Kyphoscoliosis* is one example of how a posterior and lateral spinal deviation can limit chest wall and lung expansion. Another example is a patient with COPD, who usually has a forward head and thoracic kyphosis (Figure 14-6).

BREATHING PATTERN

Respiratory rate normally ranges between 12 and 20 breaths per minute (bpm). *Eupnea* is the term used to describe a normal breathing cycle. *Apnea* is a temporary halt in breathing. *Tachypnea* is a rapid, shallow breathing pattern; this is an indicator of respiratory distress.

Bradypnea exists when respiration is slowed, less than 12 bpm. Causes could be neurologic or metabolic. *Kussmaul's breathing* is an increased rate and depth of respirations and is associated with metabolic acidosis.

Dyspnea describes the sensation of breathlessness or shortness of breath and is seen in cardiopulmonary disorders. The level of dyspnea worsens as the severity of the disease increases. An easy method to document the level of dyspnea is to count the numbers of words that the patient is able to speak per breath. For instance, six-word dyspnea is not as significant as one-word dyspnea. The type of activities that elicit shortness of breath should also be ascertained. For example, is breathlessness precipitated by stair climbing, taking a shower, etc? The "normal" ratio of inspiratory time to expiratory time is 1:2. As the respiratory rate increases this ratio decreases to 1:1. This is seen in respiratory distress, as the patient struggles to breathe in, the expiratory phase is shortened, and a vicious cycle continues. With pursed lip breathing, the idea is to prolong the expiratory phase and slow the breathing pattern.

AUSCULTATION

Auscultation is the art of listening to sounds produced by the body. Lung and heart sounds are the focus of this chapter. Skill in auscultation is dependent on the following four factors:

1. A functional stethoscope
2. Proper technique
3. Knowledge of the different categories of lung sounds: normal, abnormal, and adventitious breath sounds and voice sounds
4. Knowledge of the different categories of heart sounds and murmurs

Stethoscope

A stethoscope need not be fancy to be effective. A PT, skilled in auscultation, can use any basic stethoscope and be able to identify lung sounds. The stethoscope functions more as a filter to the extraneous noises than as an amplifier. A basic stethoscope consists of ear pieces, tubing, and a chestpiece. The bell portion of the chestpiece assesses low-pitched sounds, that is, heart sounds. The diaphragm portion discerns high pitched sounds (Figure 14-7). The tubing should not be so long that sound transmission is not dampened. Length of tubing should be between about 30 cm (12 in) to 55 cm (21 to 22 in). The ear pieces should fit the PT's ears comfortably and allow tuning out of external sounds. Other considerations would be to position the ear pieces anteriorly or forward toward the ear canals. Finally, an aside gained from the author's clinical experience: warming the diaphragm with the hands before placing it on the patient's skin is a first step in developing good patient rapport.

Technique

Environment is another element in the correct performance of auscultation. The room or cubicle should be as quiet as possible. Television and radio should be turned down or off. Any extraneous noises should be minimized or eliminated. This is especially important when auscultation is a new technique for the therapist. The patient should be positioned sitting, if possible, for lung sounds. The anterior, lateral, and posterior aspects of the chest should be auscultated both craniocaudally (apices to bases) and side to side (Figure 14-8). The PT places the diaphragm on the patient's skin so that it lies flat. The patient is instructed to breath in and out through the mouth. A slightly deeper breath than tidal breathing is suggested. A minimum of one breath per bronchopulmonary segment allows for a comparison of the intensity, pitch, and quality of the breath sounds. Movement of the diaphragm from one side to the other side while, at the same time, moving it craniocaudally, enables the PT to compare the right to the left chest. Clothing should be removed and/or draped so that it does not interfere in the assessment of the breath sounds.

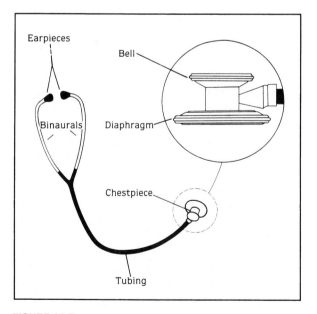

FIGURE 14-7
Stethoscope. (Reprinted with permission from Wilkins RL, Hodgkin JE, Lopez B: *Lung sounds*, St. Louis, 1988, Mosby.)

Chest Sounds

Chest sounds may be divided into these categories:

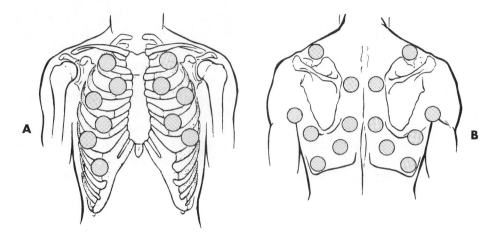

FIGURE 14-8
Stethoscope placement for auscultation of breath sounds. **A,** The chest. **B,** The back. (From Buckingham EB: *A primer of clinical diagnosis,* ed 2, New York, 1979, Harper & Row.)

1. Breath sounds—**normal, abnormal, adventitious**
2. Voice sounds—**egophany, bronchophany, whispered pectoriloquy**
3. Extrapulmonary sounds—**pleural** or friction rubs
4. Heart sounds

Breath Sounds

The terminology of breath sounds given in this chapter is a compilation of multiple resources and clinical experience. Recognition of normal breath sounds is the key to the identification of abnormal and adventitious sounds by offering the listener a point of reference. Normal breath sounds can be broken down into **bronchial, bronchovesicular,** and **vesicular.** The American Thoracic Society (ATS) and the American College of Chest Physicians (ACCP) has attempted to provide standardization of the nomenclature and continues to conduct surveys of health care professionals for use of this terminology in clinical practice.

Bronchial sounds can be described as high-pitched and are heard both in the inspiratory and ex-piratory phase. A distinguishing feature is the pause that exists between the inspiratory and expiratory phases (Figure 14-9). This sound is also described as tracheal as its *normal* location is over the trachea. *Bronchovesicular sounds* are similar in that these are also high-pitched and have an equal inspiratory and expiratory cycles. However, a differentiating feature is the lack of a pause (Figure 14-9). *Bronchovesicular sounds* are heard best wherever the bronchi or central lung tissue is close to the surface. These include superior to the clavicles and suprascapular (apices), and parasternal and interscapular (bronchi). The ATS-AACP, in its 1977 recommendations for pulmonary nomenclature, used the term bronchial to include both bronchial and bronchovesicular sounds. The finite difference is minor (the pause between the inspiratory and expiratory phases). This recommendation is meant to provide uniformity to lung sounds terminology. *Vesicular breath sounds* are heard over the remaining peripheral lung fields. These sounds have primarily an inspiratory component with only the initial one third of the expiratory phase audible. Their intensity is also softer because of the dampening effect of the spongy lung tissue and the cumulative ef-

BRONCHIAL
loud, high pitched; hollow quality; heard over manubrium; louder on expiration; distinct pause between inspiration (I) and expiration (E)

BRONCHOVESICULAR
mixture of bronchial and vesicular; I: E is 1:1; heard over main-stem bronchi -- anteriorly: ICS # 1 and 2, posteriorly: between scapulae

VESICULAR
soft, low pitched; heard over peripheral lung tissue; no pause between I and E; ratio is 3:1

FIGURE 14-9
Normal breath sounds.

fect of the air entry from numerous terminal bronchioles. The idea that vesicular sounds reflect air entry in the alveoli has been disproved. Thus as the therapist auscultates from top to bottom, the breath sounds are quieter at the bases than at the apices. Infants and small children have louder, harsher breath sounds. This is as result of the thinness of the chest wall and the airways being closer to its surface.

Abnormal Breath Sounds

Abnormal breath sounds can be described as when the sound transmission changes as a result of an underlying pathologic process. Sound is filtered by the lung tissues because these organs are air-filled; thus there is dampened sound transmission over the bases versus the apices. On the other hand, sound transmission is enhanced when a liquid or solid is the medium. Certain lung pathologies produce abnormal lung sounds. Abnormal sounds can be divided into three types: *bronchial, decreased,* and *absent.* Bronchial sounds occur in peripheral lung tissue

when it becomes airless—either partially or completely. In a consolidation type of pneumonia, the lung tissue is "airless" because of the complete obstruction of segmental or lobar bronchi by secretions. Sound from the adjacent bronchi is enhanced and becomes more high-pitched and the expiratory component louder and more pronounced. Compression of lung tissue from an extrapulmonary source also produces bronchial sounds. Examples include compression secondary to increased pleural fluid (pleural effusion) or tumor. Tubular breath sounds is a term used synonymously to describe abnormal bronchial breath sounds.

Decreased or absent breath sounds occur when sound transmission is diminished or abolished. Decreased breath sounds are when the normal vesicular sounds are further diminished. Absent sounds are when no sounds are audible. Decreased or absent sounds can be caused by an internal pulmonary pathology or can be secondary to an initially nonpulmonary condition. Hyperinflation caused by emphysema causes decreased sound transmission as a result of the destruction of the acinar units and increased air as a result of loss of normal lung structure. The loss of lung compliance resulting from pulmonary fibrosis also may produce decreased or absent breath sounds. Extrapulmonary causes include tumors, neuromuscular weakness (i.e, muscular dystrophy), and musculoskeletal deformities (i.e., kyphoscoliosis). Pain is a common cause for decreased or absent breath sounds. When the patient attempts to take a deep breath, the volume is limited because of the onset of pain. The etiologic factors of the pain can be varied—from incisional (i.e., midsternotomy) to traumatic (fractured ribs). Given that no underlying pathologies are present, decreased breath sounds may also be a reflection of the depth of respiration and/or the thickness of the chest wall (e.g., in obesity or with the presence of bandages). The skill of auscultation lies in the differentiation between normal and abnormal breath sounds.

Adventitious Breath Sounds

Adventitious breath sounds are the extraneous noises produced over the bronchopulmonary tree and are an indication of an abnormal process or condition. These sounds may be more easily identifiable than abnormal sounds. Adventitious sounds are classified as *crackles* (rales), *rhonchi,* and *wheezes.* Crackles (rales) are described as discontinuous, low-pitched sounds. They occur predominantly during inspiration. The sound of rubbing hair between the fingers or velcro popping simulates crackles. Crackles usually indicate a peripheral airway process. Rhonchi are low-pitched but continuous sounds. These occur both in inspiration *and* expiration. Snoring is a term used to describe its quality. Rhonchi are attributed to an obstructive process in the larger, more central airways. Wheezes are continuous but high-pitched. A hissing or whistling quality is present. Wheezes predominantly occur during expiration and are an indication of bronchospasm (i.e., asthma). However, wheezes can also be caused by the movement of air through secretions, thus inspiratory wheezes can be described.

Extrapulmonary Sounds

An adventitious sound that is nonpulmonary is the *friction rub.* It can be described as a rubbing or leathery sound and occurs during both inspiration and expiration. The sound is produced by the visceral (inner) pleural lining rubbing against the parietal (outer) pleura and is a sign of a primary pleural process such as inflammation or neoplasm. Pain is usually associated with a friction rub.

Voice Sounds

Voice sounds are vibrations produced by the speaking voice as it travels down the tracheobronchial tree and through the lung parenchyma when heard with a stethoscope. These sounds, over the normal lung, are low-pitched and have a muffled or mumbled quality. The transmission of these vocal vibrations can be increased or decreased in the presence of an underlying pulmonary pathologic process. *Bronchophany* describes the phenomenon of increased vocal transmission. Words or letters are louder and clearer. Causes are conditions where there is an increased lung density as in consolidation from pneumonia. The patient is usually asked to repeat "blue moon" or "one, two,

three." *Egophany* is also described when there is increased transmission of the vocal vibrations. In this case, the patient is asked to say "eeee." The underlying process distorts the "e" sound so that an "aaa" sound is heard over the peripheral area by the examiner. Egophany co-exists with bronchophany.

Whispered voice sounds also produce low-pitched vibrations over the chest that are muffled by normal lung parenchyma. *Whispered pectoriloquy* describes when these whispered voice sounds become distinct and clear; "one, two, three" or "ninety-nine" are used to evaluate this sound. Whispered pectoriloquy can be present when bronchophany and egophany are absent. This sign is helpful in identifying smaller or patchy areas of lung consolidation.

Voice sounds are a means of confirmation of the abnormal breath sounds. If a patient with significant atelectasis secondary to compression of lung tissue presents with bronchial breath sounds, then egophany and bronchophany are also audible.

HEART SOUNDS

As with lung sounds, superficial topographical landmarks assist the therapist in auscultation of heart sounds and murmurs. The left ventricular apex is normally located at the MCL in the fifth intercostal space (ICS). The cardiac apex is also known as the *point of maximum impulse (PMI).* There are four reference areas for cardiac auscultation; these do not correspond directly to the underlying cardiac anatomy. On the other hand, these areas do relate to the events arising at the individual cardiac valves. These four areas are defined as the following:

- **aortic:** second ICS, at right sternal border (RSB)
- **pulmonic:** second ICS, at left sternal border (LSB)
- **tricuspid:** fourth and fifth ICS, LSB
- **mitral:** cardiac apex fifth ICS, MCL.

Technique

An environment that is as quiet as possible is recommended. Positions used for cardiac auscultation include the following: supine—used for all areas; left lateral decubitus (sidelying)—listening to cardiac apex or mitral area, bell usually used; and sitting—used for all the areas.

Heart Sounds

The first heart sound (S_1) signifies the closing of the atrioventricular valves. Its duration is 0.10 seconds; it is heard the loudest at the cardiac apex. The two components of S_1 are tricuspid and mitral. Both the diaphragm and the bell of the stethoscope can be used to hear S_1. Its loudness is enhanced by any condition in which the heart is closer to the chest wall (i.e., thin chest wall) or in which there is an increased force to the ventricular contraction (e.g., tachycardia resulting from exercise).

The second heart sound (S_2) represents the closing of the semilunar valves and the end of ventricular systole. Its components are aortic and pulmonic. During expiration, these two components are not distinct, since the time difference in the closure of the valves is less than 30 milliseconds. However, during inspiration, a splitting of S_2 is audible. This physiological split results from the increased venous return to the right heart secondary to the decreased intrathoracic pressure that occurs during inspiration. The pulmonic valve closure is delayed as the right ventricular systolic time is lengthened. A split S_2 is heard normally in children and young adults. The diaphragm of the stethoscope should be used to hear the split. The pulmonic component is the softer sound and is best heard at the LSB, in the second to fourth ICS. The two components may be heard best in the aortic and pulmonic areas, respectively. When the split is heard both phases of respiration, an underlying cardiac abnormality is suspected. Causes may include right bundle branch block and pulmonary hypertension. (Swartz, 1994; Tilkian, Conover, 1993).

Gallops

The third heart sound (S_3) is a faint, low frequency sound and reflects the early (diastolic) ventricular filling that occurs after the atrioventricular valves open. S_3 is normal in children and young adults; however, it is usually abnormal in individuals over age 40. An extra effort must be made to auscultate S_3; the bell of the stethoscope should be used. The ideal position to hear S_3 would be left sidelying; the bell would be placed over the cardiac apex. Causes of a pathological S_3 may include ventricular failure, tachycardia, or mitral regurgitation. "Ken-**TUCK'**-y" is one sound that has been used to approximate the sound sequencing of S_3 in the cardiac cycle (S_1, S_2, S_3).

The fourth heart sound (S_4) signifies the rapid ventricular filling that occurs after atrial contraction. When present, it is heard before S_1. S_4 may be heard in the "normal" trained individual with left ventricular hypertrophy. Location of S_4 is similar to S_3. Its sound can be described as dull because of the sudden motion of stiff ventricles in response to increased atrial contraction. Pathologies eliciting an S_4 may include systemic hypertension, cardiomyopathies, or coarctation of the aorta. "**TENN'**-ess-ee" is a sound that approximates the sound sequencing when S_4 is present (S_4, S_1, S_2).

Murmurs

Cardiac murmurs are the vibrations resulting from turbulent blood flow. These may be described based on position in cardiac cycle (systole, diastole), duration, and loudness. Systolic murmurs occur between S_1 and S_2; diastolic murmurs occur between S_2 and S_1. A continuous murmur starts in S_1 and lasts through S_2 for a portion or all of diastole. The loudness of a murmur is a factor of the velocity of blood flow and the turbulence created through a specific opening such as a valve. Grades **I** to **VI** are described as follows:

- I: faint—requires concentrated effort to hear
- II: faint—audible immediately
- III: louder than II—intermediate intensity
- IV: loud—intermediate intensity; associated with palpable vibration (thrill)
- V: very loud—thrill present
- VI: audible without stethoscope

Murmurs that are Grade III or greater are usually associated with cardiovascular pathology.

MEDIATE PERCUSSION

Mediate or indirect percussion allows the therapist to assess the density of the underlying organs. Striking the chest wall produces vibrations in the underlying structures which, in turn, gives rise to sound waves or percussion tones. The quality of that tone depends on the density of the tissue or organ, that is, it becomes louder over air-filled structures. These tones are described by the following terms:

- **resonant:** loud or high amplitude, low-pitched, longer duration, heard over air-filled organs such as the lungs
- **dull:** low amplitude, medium to high-pitched, short duration, heard over solid organs such as the liver
- **flat:** high-pitched, short duration, heard over muscle mass such as the thigh
- **tympanic:** high-pitched, medium duration, heard over hollow structures such as the stomach
- **hyper-resonant:** very low-pitched, prolonged duration, heard over tissue with decreased density (increased air: tissue ratio); abnormal in adults; heard over lungs with emphysema.

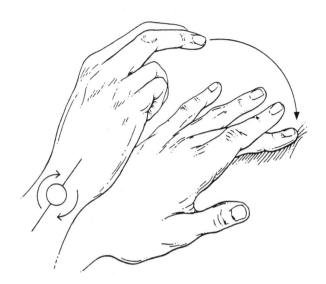

FIGURE 14-10
Mediate percussion technique. (Reprinted with permission from Swartz MH: *Textbook of physical diagnoses—history and examination,* ed 2, Philadelphia, 1994, WB Saunders.)

Technique

The middle finger of the nondominant hand is placed firmly on the chest wall in an intercostal space and parallel to the ribs. The top of the middle finger of the dominant hand strikes the distal phalanx of the stationary hand with a quick, sharp motion. The impetus of the blow comes from the wrist versus the elbow and has been likened to that of a paddle ball player (Swartz, 1994) (Figure 14-10). As with auscultation, the therapist must follow the sequence of apices to bases and side to side so that comparisons can be made. This technique is not usually used in infants, since percussion is too easily transmitted by a small chest.

Diaphragmatic Excursion

Assessment of diaphragmatic movement can be made with mediate percussion. The patient is asked

to breathe deeply and hold that breath. The lowest level of the diaphragm on maximal inspiration coincides with the lowest point where a resonant tone is heard. The patient is then asked to exhale, and mediate percussion is repeated. The lowest area of resonance now moves higher, as the diaphragm ascends with relaxation. The distance between these two points is described as the diaphragmatic excursion; normal is three to five cm (Figure 14-11). Diaphragmatic movement is decreased in patients with COPD.

PALPATION

PTs use palpation in all areas of practice. Touch is an integral part of physical therapy. As part of the chest examination, palpation is used to assess: areas of tenderness and/or abnormalities; chest wall excursion; edema; tactile fremitus; and tracheal deviation.

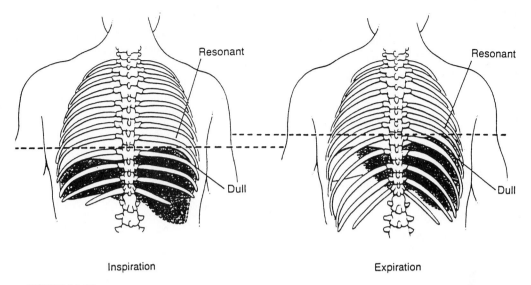

FIGURE 14-11
Diaphragmatic excursion. (Reprinted with permission from Swartz MH: *Textbook of physical diagnoses—history and examination,* ed 2, Philadelphia, 1994, WB Saunders.)

Tenderness

Specific superficial or deep landmarks are identified through palpation. Determination of gross spinal alignment can be performed by tracing the spinous processes in a cephalocaudal direction. Structures can be identified, such as the T-4 vertebra or the sternal angle, which only augment the PTs evaluation. Areas of tenderness can be assessed for degree of discomfort and reproducibility. Differentiation of chest wall discomfort of an organic nature, such as with angina, from that of a musculoskeletal condition may be made through palpation. In a patient complaining of chest pain, angina may be ruled out if the PT can reproduce or increase the discomfort with increased tactile pressure. However, one must also determine that corroborating symptoms (e.g., diaphoresis, tachycardia) are not present. Angina or chest pain secondary to myocardial ischemia usually results from exertion and may be relieved by rest. *Crepitus*

is a crunchy sound often associated with articular structures. However, when bubbles of air occur within subcutaneous tissue, a crackling sensation can be palpated. An air leak from a chest tube site is one cause when crepitus is palpated over the chest wall. Crepitus can also be secondary to a pleural or friction rub.

Edema

Palpation allows the PT to assess peripheral edema. Dependency of body parts can cause swelling from cardiac and noncardiac conditions. Assessment of edema is performed by pressing two fingers into the particular areas for 2 to 3 seconds. If an impression is left once the fingers are removed, then pitting or dependent edema is present. The degree of edema is based on the length of time that the indentation lasts. 1+ is the least; 4+ is the worst.

Chest Wall Excursion

Evaluation of thoracic expansion allows the therapist to observe a "baseline" level by which to measure progress or decline in a patient's condition. Chest wall movement can be restricted unilaterally as a result of lobar pneumonia or a surgical incision. A symmetrical decrease in chest wall motion occurs in the patient with COPD.

The hyperinflation associated with COPD produces an increase in the anteroposterior diameter with a progressive loss of diaphragmatic excursion. Normal chest wall excursion is about 3.25 inches (8.5 cm) in a young adult between 20 to 30 years of age. One method is to use a tape measure at the level of the xiphoid. However, the most common method involves direct hand contact. This technique is performed in all planes and from top to bottom. Symmetry and extent of movement are both noted. Procedures for this method are described in the following:

- *Apical* or *upper lobe motion* (Figure 14-12)
  1. The PT faces the patient. The area to be examined is exposed and draped as needed.
  2. The PT's hands are placed over the anterior chest. The heel of the hand is about the level of the fourth rib and the fingertips reach toward the upper trapezii.
  3. The thumbs lie horizontal at about the level of the sternal angle and meet at the midline, slightly stretching the skin.
  4. The patient is asked to inhale.
  5. The hands should be relaxed to allow for movement beneath.
  6. The symmetry and extent of movement are assessed.

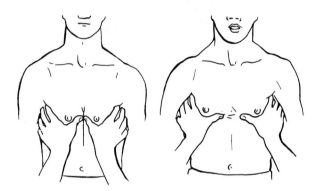

FIGURE 14-13

Evaluation of middle lobe and lingula motion (anterolateral excursion). (From Cherniak RM, et al: *Respiration in health and disease,* ed 2, Philadelphia, 1972, WB Saunders.)

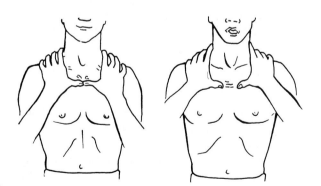

FIGURE 14-12

Evaluation of upper lobe motion. (From Cherniak RM, et al: *Respiration in health and disease,* ed 2, Philadelphia, 1972, WB Saunders.)

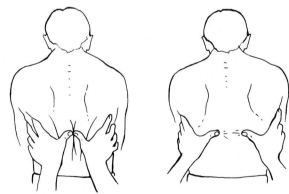

FIGURE 14-14

Evaluation of lower lobe motion (posterior excursion). (From Cherniak RM, et al: *Respiration in health and disease,* ed 2, Philadelphia, 1972, WB Saunders.)

- *Anterolateral* or *middle lobe/lingula motion* (Figure 14-13)
  1. See above.
  2. The PT's hands are placed with the palms distal to the nipple line with the thumbs meeting in the midline. The fingers lie in the posterior auxillary fold.
  3. See steps 4 to 6 above.
- *Posterior excursion/lower lobe motion* (Figure 14-14)
  1. The PT stands behind the patient.
  2. The area to be examined is exposed with draping used as appropriate.
  3. The PTs hands are placed flat on the posterior chest wall at the level of the tenth rib. The thumbs meet at the midline; fingers reaching toward the anterior axillary fold.
  4. See steps 4 to 6 above.

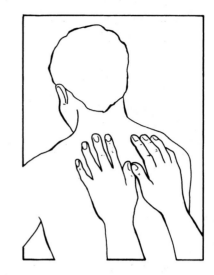

FIGURE 14-15
Evaluation of fremitus, method one.

Tactile Fremitus

Spoken word produces vibration over the chest wall. Voice sounds have been previously discussed under auscultation. With the PTs hands placed on the chest wall, vibrations from spoken words can be felt and are described as *tactile fremitus.* The presence or absence of tactile fremitus provides information on the density of the underlying lungs and thoracic cavity (Swartz, 1994).

Technique (Figures 14-15 and 14-16)

Two methods can be used. The first technique is one in which the therapist uses the palmar surface of one or both hands. The second method involves the use of the ulnar border of one hand. With both techniques, the sequence is, again, cephalocaudal and side to side. In either method, the next step is to ask that the patient speak a predetermined phrase. The two most commonly used are "99" or "one, two, three." A light but firm touch is recommended.

Tracheal Deviation (Figure 14-17)

The trachea's midline position can be examined anteriorly. The PT places an index finger in the medial aspect of the suprasternal notch. This is repeated on the opposite side. An equal distance between the clavicle and the trachea should exist bilaterally. Tracheal deviation may be caused by a pneumothorax, atelectasis or a tumor among other conditions. Whether the deviation will be ipsilateral or contralateral depends on the underlying cause. A right pneumothorax or pleural effusion will deviate the trachea away (toward the left); a left lower lobe atelectasis, however, deviates the trachea toward the affected side, that is, the left.

CASE STUDIES
Case Study One

A 30-year-old man with cystic fibrosis shows symptoms of a one-week history of increased sputum production, loss of appetite, fatigue, and 3-lb. weight loss. The results of the initial chest examination are as follows:

Inspection: Forward head, kyphotic posture, increased anteroposterior diameter, appears thin and fatigued, no dyspnea observed, effective wet cough

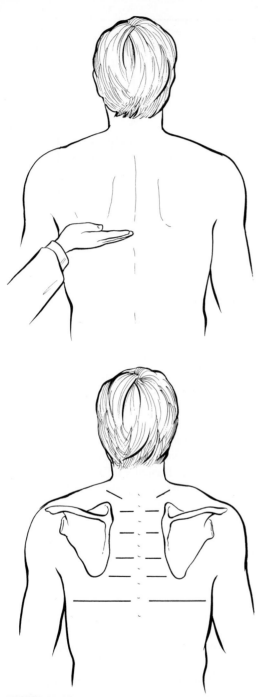

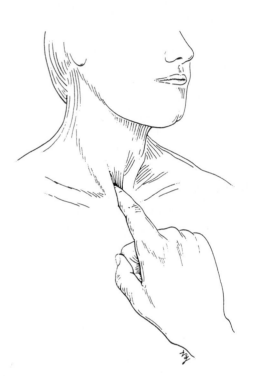

FIGURE 14-17
Technique for determining the position of the trachea.
(With permission from Swartz MH: Textbook of physical
diagnoses-history and examination, ed 2, Philadelphia,
1994, WB Saunders.)

FIGURE 14-16
Technique for evaluating tactile fremitus, method two.
(With permission from Swartz MH: Textbook of physical
diagnoses-history and examination, ed 2, Philadelphia,
1994, WB Saunders.)

Auscultation: Decreased breath sounds with scattered crackles throughout all lung fields, especially over right middle and lower chest

Palpation: Limited chest wall excursion (CWE), especially laterally

Mediate percussion: Dull over right middle and lower chest, especially laterally

Case Study Two

An ll-year-old girl is admitted to Pediatrics with a 4-day history of recurrent fevers, shortness of breath, and lethargy. CXR showed an RML pneumonia.

Inspection: tachypnea; respiratory rate (RR) of 44; Ratio of inspiration to expiration (I:E ratio = 1:1; weak, shallow cough

Auscultation: bronchial over right midanterior chest, egophany also present

Mediate percussion: dull over affected area

Palpation: trachea midline, markedly decreased CWE on right side

Case Study Three

A 72-year-old woman shows symptoms of persistent fevers, left chest wall discomfort, and history of fall 1 week ago. CT scan shows loculated pleural effusion on the left. Left chest tube is inserted for drainage; working diagnosis is empyema. Patient is nonsmoker,

Inspection: RR 30; I:E ratio = 1:2; epidural catheter for pain control

Auscultation: Absent breath sounds halfway up left lower lateral chest wall

Mediate percussion: flat over left lower lateral chest wall

Palpation: trachea deviated to right, decreased

TABLE 14-1				
Differentiation of Common Pulmonary Conditions				
	Inspection	Palpation	Percussion	Auscultation
Emphysema	Increased anteroposterior diameter; use of accessory muscles, thin individual	Decreased tactile fremitus	Increased resonance; decreased excursion of diaphragm	Decreased lung sounds; decreased vocal fremitus
Chronic bronchitis	Possible cyanosis; short, stocky individual	Often normal	Often normal	Early crackles
Pneumonia	Possible cyanosis	Increased tactile fremitus; splinting on affected side	Dull	Late crackles; bronchal breath sounds
Pulmonary embolism	Sudden onset of dyspnea; chest pain	Usually normal	Usually normal	Usually normal
Pneumothorax	Rapid onset	Absent fremitus; trachea may be shifted to other side; may have decreased chest wall excursion on affected side	Hyperresonant	Absent breath sounds
Pleural effusion	May be no outward clinical sign	Decreased fremitus; trachea shifted to other side; decreased chest wall excursion on affected side	Dullness	Absent breath sounds
Atelectasis	Often no outward clinical sign	Decreased fremitus; trachea shifted to same side; decreased chest wall excursion on affected side	Dullness	Absent breath sounds

Adapted with permission from Swartz, MH: *Textbook of physical diagnoses—history and examination,* ed 2, Philadelphia, 1994, WB Saunders.

CWE on left, range of motion of left shoulder joint limited in flexion and abduction at about 90 degrees maximum

See Table 14-1 for a differentiation of diagnoses by the elements of a chest physical examination.

SUMMARY

As demonstrated in the case studies, each element of the chest physical examination contributes to the physical therapist solving the "puzzle" of the individual patient. It is through "putting all the pieces" together that an effective treatment program can be developed.

REVIEW QUESTIONS

1. Describe the sequence for auscultation of lung sounds.
2. State the difference between peripheral and central cyanosis.
3. How are *normal* bronchial breath sounds different from *abnormal* bronchial breath sounds?
4. Name two causes for a pathologic S_3.
5. Name two causes for decreased breath sounds.
6. Formulate a plan for evaluation of a patient with an acute Right Lower Lobe Pneumonia.
7. Which components of the chest physical examination might a physical therapist include in the initial assessment of a geriatric patient with a recent left total hip replacement and a history of COPD?

References

Cherniak, R.M., & Cherniak, L. (1983). *Respiration in health and disease.* (3rd ed.). Philadelphia: WB Saunders.

Fraser, R.G., Pare J.A., Pare, P.D. Frazer, R.S., & Genereux, G.P.: (1988). *Diagnosis of diseases in the chest.* Philadelphia: WB Saunders.

George, R.B., Light, R.W. Matthay, M.A. & Matthay, R.A. (1990). *Chest medicine* (2nd ed.). Baltimore: Williams and Wilkins.

Lehrer, S. (1993). *Understanding lung sounds* (2nd ed.). Philadelphia: WB Saunders.

Mikami, et al: International symposium on lung sounds, *Chest* 92(2):342–345, 1987.

Seidel, H.M., Ball, J.W., Dains, J.E., & Benedict, G.W. (1995). *Mosby's guide to physical examination* (3rd ed.). Boston: Mosby.

Swartz, M.H. (1994). *Textbook of physical diagnoses—history and examination* (2nd ed). Philadelphia: WB Saunders.

Tilkian, A.G., & Conover, M.D. (1993). *Understanding heart sounds and murmurs* (3rd ed.). Philadelphia: WB Saunders.

Wilkins, R.I., Hodgkin, J.E., & Lopez, B. (1988). Lung sounds. St. Louis: Mosby.

Wilkins, et al: Lung sound nomenclature survey, *Chest* 98(4)886–889, 1990.

Willerson, J.T., & Cohn, J.N. (1995). *Cardiovascular medicine.* New York: Churchill Livingstone.

CHAPTER 15

Monitoring Systems in the Intensive Care Unit

Elizabeth Dean

KEY TERMS   Acid base balance   Intraaortic balloon counter pulsation
                 ECG monitoring   Intracardiac pressures
                 Fluid and electrolyte status   Intracranial pressure monitoring
                 Hemodynamic status

INTRODUCTION

The primary goal of the intensive care unit (ICU) team is the achievement of stable cardiopulmonary function and optimal oxygen transport. This chapter presents an introduction to monitoring systems used in the evaluation of cardiopulmonary status in the ICU and describes some related elements of cardiopulmonary regulation that are relevant to assessment and treatment in physical therapy.

ICUs are becoming more specialized. In major hospital centers, units are often exclusively designed and staffed for the management of specific types of conditions e.g., medical, surgical, trauma, burns, and coronary and neonatal care. Although monitoring priorities may differ among intensive care units, the principles are similar and relate either directly or indirectly to the foremost goal of optimizing oxygen transport.

Cardiopulmonary status is often jeopardized with the ICU patient by fluid and electrolyte disturbances and acid-base imbalance. Regulation of these systems and the clinical implications of imbalance are described first with special reference to the ICU patient. The principles of monitoring systems used in assessing cardiopulmonary sufficiency are presented including the electrocardiogram (ECG) monitor, monitors related to left- and right-sided heart function utilizing arterial and venous lines, and the intracranial pressure (ICP) monitor. The intraaortic counter pulsa-

229

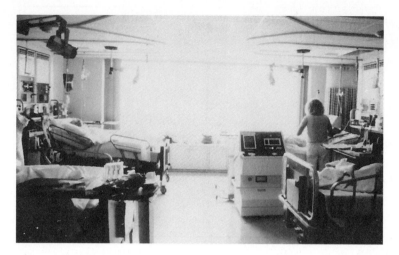

FIGURE 15-1
General view of a typical ICU.

tion technique used to augment myocardial efficiency is also described.

Familiarity with the extensive monitoring facilities in the ICU allays some of the apprehensions the physical therapist (PT) may have working in a critical care. On introduction to the unit, the PT is immediately struck by the high technology atmosphere. Quality care in this setting depends on harnessing the potential of the monitoring equipment to optimize assessment, treatment selection, and effectiveness, as well as reduce untoward risk for the patient.

For further detail on the monitoring topics presented refer to Barrell and Abbass (1978), Burki and Albert (1983), Copel and Stolarik (1991), Cromwell, Weilbell, and Pfeiffer (1980), DeGowin and De-Gowin (1981), and Weidemann, Matthay, and Matthay (1984).

Figure 15-1 illustrates a general view of a typical ICU. A closer view of the patient at bedside indicates to the PT the parameters that are being monitored, and the types of lines, catheters, and leads in place (Figure 15-2). A closer view with the patient's gown removed demonstrates precisely where the various lines, leads, and catheters are positioned, and identifies where caution must be observed. Treatments are modified according to the types and positions of the lines and leads for each individual patient (Figure 15-3).

FLUID AND ELECTROLYTE BALANCE

When the normal regulation of fluid intake, utilization, and excretion are disrupted, fluid, electrolyte, and acid-base imbalances result. Essentially, all medical and surgical conditions threaten these life-dependent mechanisms to some degree. Minor imbalances may be corrected by modification of the patient's nutrition and fluid intake. More major imbalances can be life-threatening and can necessitate prompt medical attention.

Imbalances are reflected as excesses, deficits, or as an abnormal distribution of fluids within the body (Folk-Lighty, 1984; Phipps, Long, and Woods, 1991). Excesses result from increased intake and decreased loss of fluid and electrolytes. Deficits result from abnormal shifts of fluid and electrolytes among the intravascular and extravascular fluid compartments of the body. Excesses occur with kidney dysfunction promoting fluid retention and with respiratory dysfunction promoting carbon dioxide retention. Deficits are commonly associated with reduced intake of fluids and nutrition. Diaphoresis and wounds can also contribute to significant fluid loss. Diarrhea and vomiting drain the gastrointestinal tract of fluid stores. Hemorrhage is always responsible for fluid and electrolyte loss. Deficits may be secondary to fluid entrapment and localized edema within the body, making this source of fluid unavailable for regulation of homeostasis.

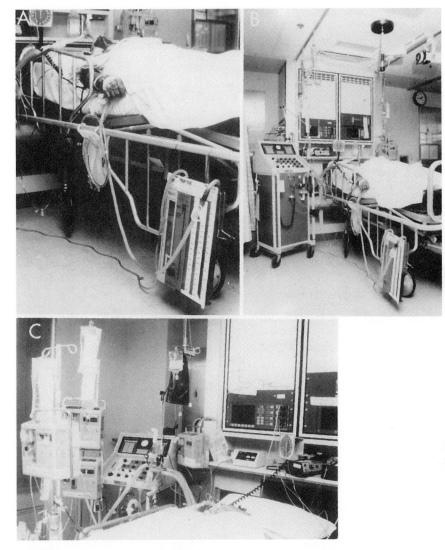

FIGURE 15-2
A and **B,** Closer bedside views of patients in an ICU. Note that with all the equipment, the patient is almost lost. **C,** Note two IV lines with flow monitors. Blood infusion is also being received.

Continued.

Moderate to severe fluid imbalance can be reflected in the systemic blood pressure and jugular venous pressure (CVP). Elevated blood pressure can be indicative of fluid overload, but an intravascular fluid deficit of 15% to 25% must develop before blood pressure drops. The jugular vein becomes distended with fluid overload. Normally, the jugular pulse is not visible 2 cm above the sternal angle when the individual sits at a 45-degree angle. If the jugular pulse is noted, this can be a sign of fluid overload.

Fluid replacement is based on a detailed assessment of the patient's needs. Whole blood is preferred

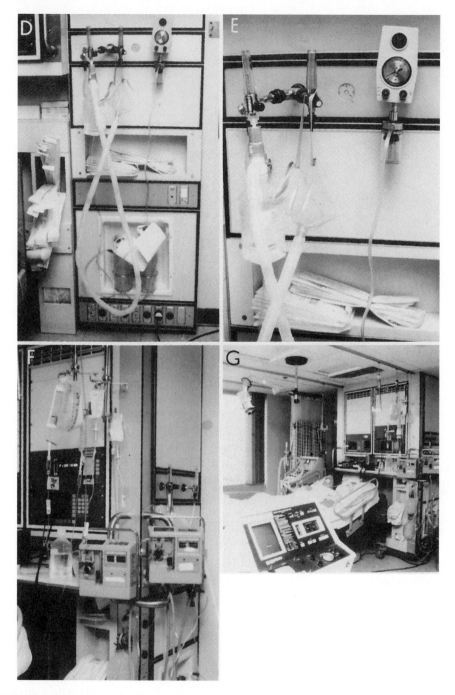

FIGURE 15-2—cont'd

D, Bedside oxygen and suction set-up. **E,** Close-up piped in O_2 and suction units, **F,** Close-up IVs and drip monitoring flow devices (IMED). **G,** Note IABP, ventilator, IVs, organization of unit at the head of the bed. ECG unit overhead, suctioning and airway care equipment at the right of the patient and "Ambu" bag at bedside.

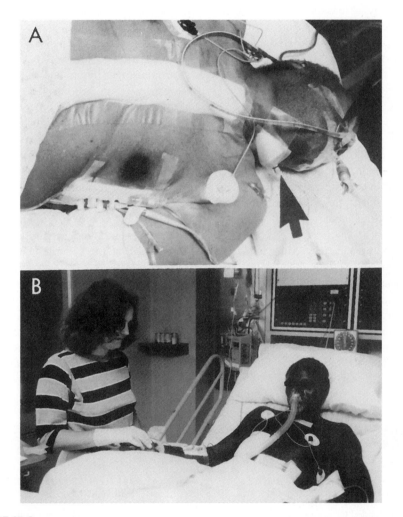

FIGURE 15-3

A, Patient after open heart surgery. Note insert of Swan Ganz, CV tubing connection taped to left chest. On ventilator with oral endotracheal tube, oral airway is in place. Note the nasogastric tube, ECG leads, and dressing covers sternal split incision site. **B,** Patient after open heart surgery. Note ECG leads. Patient is now weaned from ventilator and endotracheal tube; pacemaker wires are held intact at upper abdomen in syringe area. Patient has arterial line in right forearm; Swan Ganz, CVP also removed. Patient is almost ready to leave ICU; he is receiving an aerosol treatment.

to replace blood loss. Plasma, albumin, and plasma volume expanders such as Dextran can be used to substitute for blood loss and to help reestablish blood volume. Albumin and substances such as Dextran increase plasma volume by increasing the osmotic pressure of the blood, hence the reabsorption of fluid from the interstitial space. Low molecular weight Dextran has the added advantage of augmenting capillary blood flow by decreasing blood viscosity, and is therefore particularly useful in treating shock.

Clinical Picture

Excesses and deficits of fluids and electrolytes can be determined on the basis of laboratory determinations of serum levels of the specific electrolytes. Electrolyte levels and hematocrit are decreased with fluid excess (hemodilution) and increased with fluid loss (hemoconcentration).

Excess fluid can be managed by controlled fluid intake, normal diuresis, and diuretic medications. Replacement of fluid and electrolyte losses can be achieved by oral intake, tube feeding, intravenous (IV) infusion, and parenteral hyperalimentation.

Assessment of fluid and electrolyte balance is based on both subjective and objective findings (Table 15-1). At the bedside, the PT must be alert to complaints of headache, thirst, and nausea, as well as changes in dyspnea, skin turgor, and muscle strength. More objective assessment is based on fluid intake, output, and body weight. Fluid balance is so critical to physical well-being and cardiopulmonary sufficiency that fluid input and output records are routinely maintained at bedside. These records also include fluid volume lost in wound drainage, gastrointestinal output, and fluids aspirated from any body cavity (e.g., abdomen and pleural space).

A patient's weight may increase by several pounds before edema is apparent. The dependent areas manifest the first signs of fluid excess. Patients on bed rest show sacral swelling; patients who can sit over the bed or in a chair for prolonged periods tend to show swelling of the feet and hands.

Decreased skin turgor can indicate fluid deficit. Tenting of the skin over the anterior chest in response to pinching may suggest fluid depletion. Wrinkled, toneless skin is more common in younger patients.

Weight loss may be deceptive in the patient on IV fluids, who can be expected to lose a pound a day. This sign should therefore not necessarily be interpreted as underhydration.

The cardiopulmonary assessment can reveal changes in fluid balance. Lung sounds are valuable in identifying fluid overload. Vesicular sounds may be-

TABLE 15-1		
Assessment of Fluid and Electrolyte Imbalance		
AREA	FLUID EXCESS/ELECTROLYTE IMBALANCE	FLUID LOSS/ELECTROLYTE IMBALANCE
Head and neck	Distended neck veins, facial edema	Thirst, dry mucous membranes
Extremities	Dependent edema "pitting," discomfort from weight of bed covers	Muscle weakness, tingling, tetany
Skin	Warm, moist, taut, cool feeling when edematous	Dry, decreased turgor
Respiration	Dyspnea, orthopnea, productive cough, moist breath sounds	Changes in rate and depth of breathing
Circulation	Hypertension, jugular pulse visible at 45-degree sitting angle, atrial dysrhythmias	Pulse rate irregularities, dysrhythmia, postural hypotension, sinus tachycardia
Abdomen	Increased girth, fluid wave	Abdominal cramps

Modified from Phipps WJ, Long BC, Woods NF, editors: Medical-surgical nursing: concepts in clinical practice, ed 4, St. Louis, 1991, Mosby.

come more bronchovesicular in quality. Crackles may increase in coarseness. In the presence of fluid retention involving the pleurae, breath sounds diminish to the bases. Dyspnea and orthopnea may also be symptomatic of fluid excess.

An early sign of congestive heart failure (CHF) with underlying fluid overload is an S_3 gallop (Ken-**TUCK′**-y) caused by rapid ventricular filling.

Vigilance by the PT is essential in all areas of practice and not only the ICU. Fluid imbalance is common in older people and in young children, thus it needs to be watched for on the ward, in the home, and community.

CHEST TUBE DRAINAGE AND FLUID COLLECTION SYSTEMS

Chest tubes are large catheters placed in the pleural cavity to evacuate fluid and air, and to drain into a graduated collection reservoir at bedside (Phipps, Long, Woods, 1991). A typical chest tube drainage

and collection system is shown in Figure 15-4. The removal of thick fluids such as blood and organized exudates with chest tubes is often indicated to prevent entrapment and loculation. Chest tubes are commonly inserted in the sixth intercostal space in the mid or posterior axillary line. Chest tubes inserted into the pleural space are used to evacuate air or exudate. Chest tubes can also be inserted into the mediastinum after open heart surgery, for example, to evacuate blood.

Any collection system is designed to seal the drainage site from the atmosphere and offer minimal resistance to the drainage of fluid and gas. This is accomplished by immersing the end of the collection tube under water (Figure 15-4). This is referred to as an underwater seal system. Additional reservoirs are included to decrease the resistance to fluid leaving the chest. This resistance is greater in a single reservoir system in which the reservoir serves both as the collection receptacle and underwater seal. A third reservoir can be added to the system that is attached

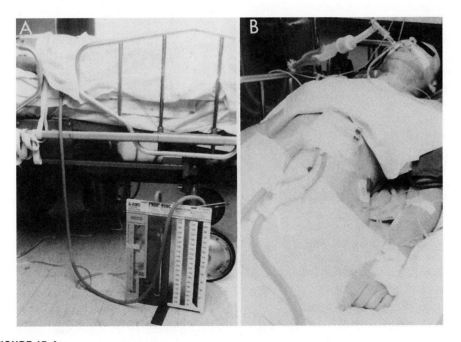

FIGURE 15-4
A, Chest tube drainage. **B,** Anterior view, Mediastinal drains.

to the suction and serves as a pressure regulator. The more elaborate drainage systems are used to precisely measure fluid loss in patients following thoracic and cardiovascular surgery.

The amount of exudate collected in the reservoir is measured every several hours or more often if the patient is losing considerable amounts of fluid or less than the amount predicted. This information is incorporated into the overall fluid balance assessment. In addition, changes in the quantity and quality of exudate should be noted by the PT before, during, and after changes in position and therapeutic interventions.

ACID-BASE BALANCE

Control of acid-base balance in the body is achieved by regulation of hydrogen ion concentration in the body fluids (Guyton, 1991; Shapiro, Peruzzi, and Kozelowski-Templin, 1994). The pH of the body is normally maintained within a range of 7.35 to 7.45, or slightly alkaline. When pH of the blood drops below 7.35, a state of acidosis exists; above 7.45, a state of alkalosis exists. Regulation of pH is vital because even slight deviations from the normal range cause marked changes in the rate of cellular chemical reactions. A pH below 6.8 and above 8 are incompatible with life.

Acid-base balance is controlled by several regulatory buffer systems; primarily carbonic acid-bicarbonate, phosphate, and protein buffer systems. These systems act very quickly to prevent minute-to-minute changes in pH. In compensation, pH is returned to normal primarily by altering the component not primarily affected. If the primary cause is respiratory, the compensating mechanism is metabolic. If the primary cause is metabolic, the compensating mechanism is respiratory. The lungs compensate for metabolic problems over hours, whereas the kidneys compensate for respiratory problems over days (Chapter 9).

Clinical Picture

A guide to the clinical presentation of acid-base imbalances is shown in Table 15-2. Besides the major distinguishing characteristics of acid-base imbalance described in this chapter and elsewhere in this vol-

TABLE 15-2

Signs and Symptoms of Common Acid Base Disturbances

RESPIRATORY ACIDOSIS	METABOLIC ACIDOSIS
Hypercapnia	Bicarbonate deficit
Hypoventilation	Hyperventilation
Headache	Headache
Visual disturbances	Mental dullness
Confusion	Deep respirations
Drowsiness	Stupor
Coma	Coma
Depressed tendon reflexes	Hyperkalemia
Hyperkalemia	Cardia dysrhythmias
Ventricular fibrillation (secondary to hyperkalemia)	(secondary to hyperkalemia)

RESPIRATORY ALKALOSIS	METABOLIC ALKALOSIS
Hypocapnia	Bicarbonate excess
Lightheadedness	Depressed respirations
Numbness/tingling of digits	Mental confusion
Tetany	Dizziness
Convulsions	Numbness/tingling of digits
	Muscle twitching
Hypokalemia	Tetany
Cardiac dysrhythmias (secondary to hypokalemia)	Convulsions
	Hypokalemia
	Cardia dysrhythmias (secondary to hypokalemia)

ume, potassium excess (hyperkalemia) is associated with both respiratory and metabolic acidosis, and neuromuscular hyperexcitability is associated with both respiratory and metabolic alkalosis.

BLOOD GASES

Analysis of the composition of arterial and mixed venous blood provides vital information about respiratory, cardiac, and metabolic function (Ganong, 1993; Snider, 1973; Thomas, Lefrak, Irwin, Fritts, and Caldwell, 1974; Marini, 1987; West, 1995) (see Chapter 9). For this reason, blood gases are usually analyzed daily in the ICU. In cases where the patient's condition is changing for better or worse over a short period of time or a specific treatment response is of interest, blood gases may be analyzed several times daily. With an arterial line in place, frequent blood gas analysis is feasible and not traumatic for the patient. Should the patient be anemic, however, blood loss associated with repeated arterial blood sampling can be detrimental. Thus requests for arterial blood gas analysis need to be particularly stringent in anemic patients.

Arterial saturation (Sao_2) can be readily monitored noninvasively with a noninvasive pulse oximeter. The ear lobe or a finger is initially warmed by rubbing before attachment of the oximeter. Within a couple of minutes, the Sao_2 can be directly read from the monitor. Pulse oximetry is a useful adjunct for routine evaluation of the effectiveness of mechanical ventilation, the effect of anesthesia and treatment response. Continuous estimation of Sao_2 is particularly useful before, during, and after mobilization and exercise, position changes, and other therapeutic interventions. The Sao_2 may appear to be reduced in patients who are anemic, jaundiced, have heavily pigmented skin, or have reduced cardiac output.

Mixed venous oxygen saturation (Svo_2) provides a useful index of oxygen supply and utilization at the tissue level (Copel, and Stolarik, 1991). Svo_2 is highly correlated to tissue oxygen extraction, and thus is a good index of the adequacy of oxygen transport. The Svo_2 is particularly useful as a significant warning sign, a guide to myocardial function, and has been used as a tool to titrate positive end-expiratory pressure support. Normal values of Svo_2 are 75%. Svo_2 values less than 60% or a drop of 10% for several minutes are cause for concern. Excessive Svo2 values in excess of 80% are also cause for concern. High Svo_2 values may occur in patients with left to right shunts, hyperoxia, hypothermia, cyanide toxicity, sepsis, anesthesia, and drug-induced paralysis. Despite its general clinical usefulness, Svo_2 is a nonspecific indicator of the adequacy of oxygen transport, that is, of the balance between oxygen supply and demand. Abnormal Svo_2 values do not indicate precisely where the problem lies; thus other hemodynamic variables need to be considered.

HYPOXEMIA

In health, age and body position are factors that reduce arterial oxygen tension (Oakes, 1988). Arterial oxygen levels diminish with age as a result of reductions in alveolar surface area, pulmonary capillary blood volume and diffusing capacity. Normal PaO_2 levels in older people should exceed 110-0.5 age. In a young adult, Pao_2 ranges from 90 to 100 mm Hg in the upright seated position. In supine, this range is reduced to 85 to 95 mm Hg and in sleeping, to 70 to 85 mm Hg. These values are significant in that in older people, smokers, and people with pathology, these positional effects are accentuated.

Hypoxemia refers to reduced oxygen tension in the blood. Some common signs and symptoms of various degrees of hypoxemia in adults appear in Table 15-3. Although the brain is protected by autoregula-

TABLE 15-3	
Signs and Symptoms of Hypoxemia	
Pao₂	**SIGNS AND SYMPTOMS**
80–100 mm Hg	Normal
60–80 mm Hg	Moderate tachycardia, possible onset of respiratory distress
50–60 mm Hg	Malaise
	Lightheadedness
	Nausea
	Vertigo
	Impaired judgment
	Incoordination
	Restless
	Increased minute ventilation
35–50 mm Hg	Marked confusion
	Cardiac dysrhythmias
	Labored respiration
25–35 mm Hg	Cardiac arrest
	Decreased renal blood flow
	Decreased urine output
	Lactic acidosis
	Poor oxygenation
	Lethargy
	Maximal minute ventilation
	Loss of consciousness
<25 mm Hg	Decreased minute ventilation (secondary to depression of respiratory center)

tory mechanisms, an arterial oxygen tension of 60 mm Hg produces signs of marked depression of the central nervous system (NS) reflecting the extreme sensitivity of cerebral tissue to hypoxia.

Hypoxemia is compensated primarily by increased cardiac output, improved perfusion of vital organs, and polycythemia. Secondary mechanisms of compensation include improved unloading of oxygen as a result of tissue acidosis and anaerobic metabolism, that is, rightward shift to the oxyhemoglobin dissociation curve.

The progressive physiologic deterioration observed at decreasing arterial oxygen levels will occur at higher oxygen levels if any of the major compensating mechanisms for hypoxemia is defective. Even a mild drop in Pao_2 for example, is poorly tolerated by the patient with reduced hemoglobin and impaired cardiac output. Alternatively, the signs and symptoms of hypoxemia may appear at lower arterial oxygen levels, (e.g., in patients with chronic airflow limitation who have adapted to reduced Pao_2 levels).

HYPEROXIA

Mean tissue oxygen tensions rise less than 10 mm Hg when pure oxygen is administered to a healthy subject under normal conditions. Therefore the function of nonpulmonary tissues is little altered. In the lung, high concentrations of oxygen replace nitrogen in poorly ventilated regions. This results in collapse of areas with reduced ventilation perfusion matching. Lung compliance is diminished.

High concentrations of oxygen (inspired oxygen fractions greater than 50%) directly injure bronchial and parenchymal lung tissue. The toxic effect of oxygen is both time and concentration dependent. Very high concentrations of oxygen can be tolerated for up to 48 hours. High concentrations of oxygen in combination with positive pressure breathing can predispose the patient to oxygen toxicity. At concentrations of inspired oxygen less than 50%, clinically detectable oxygen toxicity is unusual regardless of the duration of oxygen therapy.

HYPOCAPNIA

Acute reductions in arterial carbon dioxide levels (hypocapnia) results in alkalosis and diminished cerebral blood flow secondary to cerebral vasoconstriction. The major consequences of abrupt lowering of $Paco_2$ are altered peripheral and central nerve function. Mechanical ventilation may initially cause an abrupt decrease in arterial Pco_2 and lead to a life-threatening situation. In addition to blood gas analy-

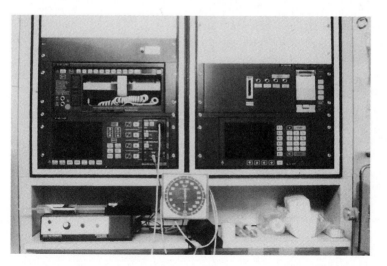

FIGURE 15-5
ECG oscilloscope, printout for ECG. Note defibrillator paddles and BP cuff on shelf.

sis, end tidal CO_2 measurement is useful in that it provides an index of Pa$_{CO_2}$.

HYPERCAPNIA

CO_2, the principal end product of metabolism, is a relative benign gas. CO_2 has a key role in ventilation and in regulating changes in cerebral blood flow, pH, and sympathetic tone. Acute increases in CO_2 (hypercapnia) depress level of consciousness secondary to the effect of acidosis on the nervous system. Similar but slowly developing increases in CO_2, however, are relatively well-tolerated. A high Pa$_{CO_2}$ is suggestive of alveolar hypoventilation, which causes a reduction in alveolar and arterial Po$_2$. Some patients with severe chronic airflow obstruction have been reported to be able to lead relatively normal lives with Pa$_{CO_2}$ in excess of 90 mm Hg if hypoxemia is countered with supplemental oxygen. Acute administration of oxygen to patients with chronic lung disease, however, may be hazardous, because it interferes with the hypoxic drive to breathe observed in these patients.

Acute hypercapnia enhances sympathetic stimulation, causing an increase in cardiac output and in peripheral vascular resistance. These effects may help to offset the effect of excess hydrogen ion on the cardiovascular system, allowing better tolerance of flow pH than with metabolic acidosis of a similar degree. At extreme levels of hypercapnia, muscle twitching and seizures may be observed. Trends in Pa$_{CO_2}$ can be monitored using end tidal CO_2 measurements.

ECG MONITORING

A single channel ECG monitor with an oscilloscope, strip recorder, and digital heart rate display is typically located above the patient at bedside in the ICU (Figure 15-5). The ECG can often be observed both at bedside as well as at a central monitoring console, where the ECGs of all patients being monitored can be observed simultaneously.

The ECG monitor allows for continuous surveillance of the patient regardless of activity. Low and high heart rates are determined below and above which the alarm will be triggered. For routine monitoring in the coronary care unit, a modified chest lead is often used. Three electrodes are positioned on the

chest to provide optimal information regarding changes in rhythm and heart rate, and thereby ensure close patient monitoring. The positive electrode is positioned at the fourth intercostal space at the right sternal border. The negative electrode is positioned at the first intercostal space in the left midclavicular line. The ground electrode used to dissipate electrical interference is often positioned at the first intercostal space in the right midclavicular line, although the ground electrode may be positioned wherever convenient. Other electrode placements may be required, for example, in patients with pacemakers or in patients with chest burns. The electrode wires are usually secured to the patient's gown.

Problems with the monitor usually result from faulty technique, electrical interference, and movement artifact. A thickened baseline can be caused by 60-cycle electrical interference. An erratic signal often results from coughing and movement. The cause of any irregularity must be explained and untoward changes in electrical activity of the myocardium ruled out. It is a dangerous practice for the PT to turn off the ECG alarm system during treatment.

Cardiac dysrhythmias can be broadly categorized into tachdysrhythmias and bradydysrhythmias. Tachydysrhythmias are subdivided into supraventricular and subjunctional tachycardias. Bradydysrhythmias are subdivided into sinus bradycardia, and those related to heart block and conduction abnormalities. The subjunctional tachycardias or ventricular dysrhythmias are life-threatening. Ventricular tachycardia and ventricular fibrillation are medical emergencies requiring immediate recognition and treatment.

The characteristic features of dysrhythmic ECG tracings are illustrated in Chapter 11. PTs specializing in ICU management should be thoroughly familiar with ECG interpretation and the implications of the various dysrhythmias for patient management. For further elaboration of ECG application and interpretation refer to Andreoli, Fowkes, Zipes, and Wallace (1991), Dubin (1989), and Fisher (1981).

Clinical Picture

The clinical picture associated with dysrhythmic activity of the heart depends on the nature of the dysrhythmia, the age and condition of the patient, and

TABLE 15-4

Clinical Picture of Common Dysrhythmias

DYSRHYTHMIA	IN HEALTHY INDIVIDUALS WITH NO UNDERLYING CARDIOVASCULAR DISEASE	IN INDIVIDUALS WITH UNDERLYING CARDIOVASCULAR DISEASE
I. Tachycardias		
A. Supraventricular tachycardia	No symptoms Abrupt onset palpitations, light-headness nausea, fatigue	May precipitate congestive heart failure, acute coronary insufficiency, myocardial infarction, pulmonary edema
1. Sinus tachycardia	Awareness of the heart on exertion or with anxiety	Secondary to some precipitating factor, e.g., fever, electrolyte imbalance, anemia, blood and fluid loss, infection, persistent hypoxemia in COPD, acute MI, congestive heart failure, thyrotoxicosis
2. Paroxysmal atrial tachycardia (PAT)	Prevalent, sudden onset, precipitated by coffee, smoking, and exhaustion	Common supraventricular tachycardia Spontaneous onset of regular palpitations that can last for several hours May be obscured by myocardial insufficiency and CHF in older patients Increased anxiety and report of fatigue
3. Atrial flutter	Rare May be difficult to distinguish from PAT May be precipitated by alcohol, smoking, physical and emotional strain	Rapid regular-irregular rate Suggests block at AV node Atrial flutter waves in jugular venous pulse
4. Atrial fibrillation	Rare, occasionally with alcohol excess in the young	Usually secondary to a variety of cardiac disorders
5. Paroxysmal atrial tachycardia with block	Rare	Common arrhythmia seen with digitalis toxicity
B. Subjunctional	Rare	Usually related to MI, pulmonary embolus, severe CHF Often unconscious, cyanotic, ineffective pulse, blood pressure and respiration
1. Ventricular tachycardia	Rare	Predisposed to ventricular fibrillation
2. Ventricular fibrillation	Rare	Ineffective cardiac output, unconscious, dusky, cardiac arrest threatens
II. Bradycardias		
A. Sinus bradycardia	Physiologic in very fit young adults	In older patients may suggest sinus node and conduction system pathology; can produce syncope or congestive heart failure
B. Heart block	Rare	Hypotension, dizziness, light-headedness, syncope In chronic block with sustained bradycardia, congestive heart failure may be more frequent

TABLE 15-4

Clinical Picture of Common Dysrhythmias

DYSRHYTHMIA	IN HEALTHY INDIVIDUALS WITH NO UNDERLYING CARDIOVASCULAR DISEASE	IN INDIVIDUALS WITH UNDERLYING CARDIOVASCULAR DISEASE
		Most common dysrhythmia iatrogenically produced with digitalis excess
		Associated with numerous cardiac conditions; commonly in age-related degenerative disease in conducting system, inferior and occasionally anterior MIs

specifically the absence or presence of underlying heart disease. Distinguishing clinical features of common atrial and ventricular dysrhythmias are outlined in Table 15-4.

The subjunctional or ventricular dysrhythmias are typically associated with an extremely ill individual. Cyanosis and duskiness of the mucosal linings and periphery may be apparent. The patient is unresponsive, the pulse if ineffective, and spontaneous respirations are likely absent. Defibrillation is initiated to restore an effective, more normal rhythm. The high incidence of myocardial conduction irregularities warrants a defibrillator being present at all times in the ICU for rapid implementation of this common cardioversion procedure by the medical personnel. Ventricular dysrhythmias may be tolerated better if ventricular rate is low, thereby improving cardiac output. Even in this circumstance, however, these dysrhythmias still present an emergency.

The ECG of a patient with a pacemaker will reflect either an imposed fixed or intermittent rhythm and rate depending on whether a fixed rate or demand pacemaker has been inserted.

Intra-Arterial Lines

An arterial line is established by direct arterial puncture, usually of the radial artery. Blood pressure can be measured directly from this line. A digital monitor displays systolic and diastolic blood pressures above the patient at bedside. High and low blood pressure levels are set, above and below which the alarm will sound. Blood gas analysis can be performed routinely with an intraarterial line in place without repeated puncturing of a blood vessel (Figure 15-6).

Pulmonary Artery Balloon Flotation Catheter (Swan Ganz Catheter)

The pulmonary artery balloon floatation catheter or Swan Ganz catheter is designed to provide an accurate and convenient means of hemodynamic assessment in the ICU (Buchbinder, and Ganz, 1976; Forrester, Diamond, McHugh, and Swan, 1971; Swan, 1975). The catheter is usually inserted into the internal jugular vein, the subclavian vein, or a large peripheral arm vein and directed by the flow of blood into the right ventricle and pulmonary artery (see Figure 15-3A (arrow), p. 233). The catheter is securely taped to the patient's arm, which is splinted with an armboard to prevent dislodging. The procedure is generally associated with little risk and discomfort. Some of the complications that have been associated with pulmonary artery catheterization, however, include infection, venous thrombosis, my-

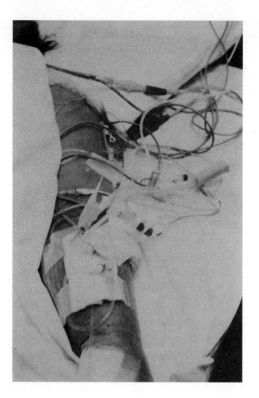

FIGURE 15-6
Intraarterial blood gas line.

ocardial irritation, air embolism, and pulmonary is-chemia or infarct to segmental lung tissue (Puri, Carlson, Bander, and Weil, 1980).

Complex catheters are available for monitoring a variety of parameters. In a two-lumen catheter, the first lumen is used to measure pulmonary artery pressure (PAP) and obtain mixed venous blood samples. The second lumen terminates in a balloon with a volume of less than 1 ml, which is inflated and deflated to obtain pulmonary artery occlusion or wedge pressure (PAOP or PAWP). The average range of the systolic PAP is 20 to 30 mm Hg, and normally reflects right ventricular pressure (RVP). The diastolic PAP ranges from 7 to 12 mm Hg and reflects left ventricular pressure in the absence of pulmonary disease. The average range of PAWP is 8 to 12 mm Hg and gives an estimation of mean left atrial pressure (LAP) and the pressure in the left ventricle (LVP). More elaborate catheters have pacing wires, thermistors for cardiac output determination, and sensors for arterial saturation. Figure 15-7 shows the normal cardiac pressures in each heart chamber. Abnormal cardiopulmonary function may vary these readings.

The PAP increases as a result of elevated pulmonary blood flow, increased pulmonary arteriolar resistance secondary to primary pulmonary hypertension or mitral stenosis, and left ventricular failure. Measurement of PAP and PAWP in particular allows for more prudent management of heart failure and cardiogenic shock.

The PAP, PAWP, and end diastolic LVP are directly related. Impaired left ventricular contractility that compromises normal emptying, (e.g., left ventricular failure, mitral stenosis, or mitral insufficiency), result in an elevated end diastolic LVP, which in turn elevates PAWP and PAP. An end diastolic PAP or PAWP greater than 12 mm Hg is considered abnormal.

The PAP and PAWP are low during hypotension secondary to hypovolemia. Infusion of normal saline, whole blood, or low molecular weight Dextran elevates the blood volume and blood pressure. Restoration of blood volume returns end diastolic PAP and PAWP to normal.

Elevation of the end diastolic PAP secondary to heart failure with pulmonary edema can typically be reduced with appropriate medication. The effectiveness of a drug and its prescription parameters can be assessed by the observed changes in the end diastolic PAP.

Deterioration of cardiovascular status and worsening of the clinical signs and symptoms of heart failure elevate end diastolic PAP and PAWP, decrease cardiac output, decrease arterial and right atrial oxygen tension, and increase the oxygen difference between arterial and venous blood. As the heart pump continues to fail, arterial oxygen tension decreases suggesting abnormal lung function and probably elevated LAP. Pulmonary dysfunction at this stage includes diffusion abnormalities, redistribution of pulmonary blood flow into the less well-ventilated upper lobes, and right to left shunt-

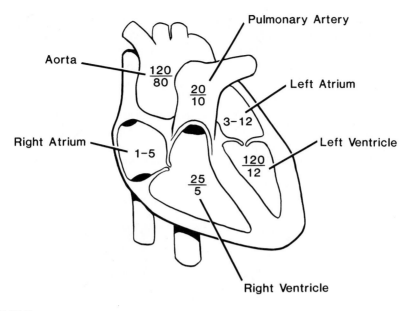

FIGURE 15-7
Normal cardiac pressures in each heart chamber.

ing. All patients with acute infarction or shock have reduced arterial oxygen tension. Pulmonary congestion must be cleared before the patient responds to oxygen administration.

Despite the enormous benefits of direct invasive hemodynamic monitoring to patient assessment and management, the benefits of basic hemodynamic assessment are a fundamental part of the cardiopulmonary assessment regardless of whether the patient has an invasive line in or not (Kirby, Taylor, and Civetta, 1990). Basic hemodynamic monitoring includes heart rate, ECG, blood pressure, and peripheral tissue perfusion.

INTRAVENOUS LINES

IV lines are routinely established in the superficial veins of patients, such as in the hand, usually before admission to the ICU. These lines provide an immediate route for fluids, electrolytes, nutrition, and medications. The specific lines used depend on the patient's individual needs determined by the history, laboratory tests, and physical examination.

MEASUREMENT OF CENTRAL VENOUS PRESSURE

Central venous pressure (CVP) is monitored by means of a venous line or catheter inserted into the subclavian, basilic, jugular or femoral vein (see Figure 15-3A, p. 233). The catheter is advanced to the right atrium by way of the inferior or superior vena cava depending on the site of insertion. Minimal risk of phlebitis or infection is associated with this procedure.

Central venous pressure is the blood pressure measured in the vena cavae or right atrium. Normal CVP is approximately 0 to 5 cm H_2O and 5 to 10 cm H_2O if measured at the sternal notch and midaxillary line, respectively. Essentially the CVP provides information about the adequacy of right-sided heart function, including effective circulating blood volume, effectiveness of the heart as a pump, vascular tone, and venous return. Measurement of CVP is particularly useful in assessing fluid volume and fluid replacement. If the patient has chronic airflow limitation, ventricular ischemia, or infarction, the CVP will reflect changes in pathology rather than fluid volume.

Specifically, CVP provides an index of RAP. The relationship between RAP and end diastolic LVP is unreliable; therefore end diastolic PAP and PAWP are used as the principal indicators of cardiopulmonary sufficiency in patients in failure and shock.

INTRAAORTIC BALLOON COUNTER PULSATION (IABP)

Intraaortic balloon counter pulsation (Figure 15-8) provides mechanical circulatory assistance with the use of an intraaortic balloon. The balloon is inserted into the femoral artery. To maintain proper placement and good circulation, the leg must be extended. The presence of an intraaortic balloon must be taken into consideration whenever the patient is being treated and positioned. Inflation and deflation of the balloon with helium is correlated with the ECG. The intraaortic balloon is deflated during ventricular systole and assists the emptying of the aorta. Stroke volume is potentiated, afterload is reduced (hence, ventricular pressure), and myocardial oxygen delivery enhanced.

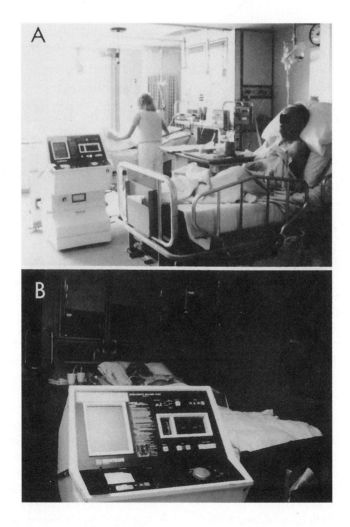

FIGURE 15-8
A, Patient near the window is receiving intraaortic balloon pump (IABP) support. **B,** Close-up of an IABP unit.

The balloon is inflated during diastole, thereby restoring arterial pressure and coronary perfusion. Counterpulsation improves cardiac output, reduces evidence of myocardial ischemia, and reduces ST-segment elevation. Intraaortic balloon counterpulsation is commonly used after open heart surgery, for CHF, medically refractive myocardial ischemia, ventricular septal defects, and left main coronary stenosis in patients who have shock. The intraaortic balloon pump provides protection for the myocardium in many instances until surgery can be performed. Limb ischemia, the most common complication, occurs in 10% to 15% of patients.

Left ventricular assist devices are used postoperatively in patients following open heart surgery who have developed cardiogenic shock and are unresponsive to conventional management. These devices take over the pumping action of the left ventricle and decrease myocardial workload and oxygen consumption. These types of assistive devices may have considerable potential in the management of refractory heart failure.

MEASUREMENT OF INTRACRANIAL PRESSURE

Increased intracranial pressure (ICP) results from many neurological insults including head injury, hypoxic brain damage, or cerebral tumor, and may require surgery. In the adult, the cranial vault is rigid and noncompliant. Increases in the volume of the cranial contents result in an elevated ICP and decreased cerebral perfusion pressure.

Changes in consciousness are the earliest and most sensitive indicators of increased ICP (Borozny, 1987; Luce, 1985). Altered consciousness reflects herniation of the brainstem and compression of the midbrain. Compression of the oculomotor nerve and the pupillo-constrictor fibers results in abnormal pupillary reactions associated with brain damage.

The effect of ICP on blood pressure and pulse is variable. Blood pressure may be elevated secondary to elevated ICP and hypoxia of the vasomotor center. A reflex decrease in pulse occurs as blood pressure rises.

Compression of upper motor neuron pathways interrupts the transmission of impulses to lower motor neurons; progressive muscle weakness results. A contralateral weakened hand grasp, for example, may progress to hemiparesis or hemiplegia. The Babinski sign, hyperreflexia, and rigidity are additional motor signs that provide evidence of decreasing motor function as a result of upper motor neuron involvement.

Herniation can produce incoordinate respirations that are correlated with the level of brainstem compression. Cerebrate rigidity results from tentorial herniation of the upper brainstem. This results in blocking of the motor inhibitory fibers and the familiar extended body posture. Seizures may be present. These neuromuscular changes may further compound existing cardiopulmonary complications in the ICU patient.

Clinically, increased ICP is best detected by altered consciousness, blood pressure, pulse, pupillary responses, movement, temperature, and respiration (Luce, 1985). The ICP monitor provides direct measurement of ICP. A hollow screw is positioned through the skull into the subarachnoid space. The screw is attached to a Luer-Lok, which is connected to a transducer and oscilloscope for continuous monitoring.

The prevention of further increase in ICP and a corresponding reduction in cerebral perfusion pressure is a treatment priority. High ICP and low cerebral perfusion pressure are highly correlated with brain injury. Measures to reduce venous volume are maintained until ICP has stabilized within normal range. Prudent body positioning is used to enhance venous drainage by elevating the bed 15 to 30 degrees and maintaining the head above heart level. Neck flexion is avoided. Fluid intake and output are carefully monitored; the patient may need to be fluid restricted. The Valsalva maneuver is avoided, since intrathoracic pressure and ICP may increase correspondingly.

Normal range of ICP is 0 to 10 mm Hg for adults, and 0 to 5 mm Hg for patients under 6 years of age. The ICP may reach 50 mm Hg in the normal brain; typically, however, this pressure returns to baseline levels instantaneously. In patients with high levels of ICP and low cerebral compliance, extra care must be exercised during routine management and therapy. An ICP elicited by turning or suctioning up to 30 mm Hg may be acceptable provided the pressure drops immediately following removal of the pressure-potentiating stimulus. Patients may be mechanically hyperventilated to keep arterial P_{CO_2} at low levels, since hypercapnia dilates cerebral vessels and hypocapnia constricts them.

To establish whether a patient will tolerate a treatment that requires movement or body positioning, an indication of cerebral compliance is needed. This can be obtained by observing changes in ICP during routine nursing procedures or by titrating small degrees of movement or position change and observe the rate at which the ICP returns to baseline following the challenge. Rapid return to baseline minimizes the risk of reduced cerebral perfusion pressure secondary to the increased ICP. A slow return to baseline or sustained elevation of ICP is consistent with poor cerebral compliance and indicates treatment should be modified or possibly not performed at all depending on the absolute level of the ICP.

ELECTROENCEPHALOGRAM MONITOR

An electroencephalogram, or EEG, provides useful information about gross cerebral functioning and changes in level of consciousness. A single-channel EEG monitor can be readily used in the ICU to reveal evidence of posttraumatic epilepsy when the clinical signs may be inhibited by muscle relaxants. An EEG assessment may also be of some benefit to the PT in assessing the effects of arousal, treatment and sensorimotor stimulation on cerebral function.

SUMMARY

Monitoring cardiopulmonary function and oxygen transport is an essential component of the management of the patient in the ICU. Regulation of homeostasis is disrupted in disease or following medical and surgical interventions. PTs working in the unit require a thorough understanding of homeostatic regulation and monitoring of fluid and electrolyte balance, acid base balance, and blood gases. Physical therapy has an essential role in restoring homeostasis in patients requiring intensive care, using conservative, noninvasive approaches, in addition to averting the musculoskeletal, neuromuscular, and multisystem complications associated with immobility and recumbency. The selection of treatment and the assessment of treatment response must be based upon quantitative evaluation of the parameters affecting oxygen transport and cardiopulmonary function. Meticulous monitoring contributes substantially to more rational management of the ICU patient (i.e., the optimization of physical therapy efficacy, in addition to minimizing deleterious treatment outcomes).

REVIEW QUESTIONS

1. Explain the determinants of fluid and electrolyte balance, and factors that contribute to fluid excesses and deficits.
2. Describe the basis of acid and base balance.
3. Describe the physiological effects of hypoxia and hypercapnia.
4. Explain the physiologic basis of ECG monitoring and common supraventricular and ventricular dysrhythmias.
5. Explain (a) the physiologic basis of the pulmonary artery balloon floatation catheter, and (b) what is represented by altered CVP, RAP (systolic and diastolic), PAP (systolic and diastolic), and the PAOP.
6. Describe the basis of intra aortic balloon counter pulsation.
7. Describe intracranial pressure monitoring, its physiological basis and clinical implications.

References

Andreoli, K. G., Fowkes, V. K., Zipes, D. P., & Wallace, A. G. (Eds.) (1991). *Comprehensive cardiac care* (7th ed.). St. Louis: Mosby.

Barrell, S. E., & Abbas, H. M. (1978). Monitoring during physiotherapy after open heart surgery. *Physiotherapy, 64*(9), 272–273.

Borozny, M. L. (1987). Intracranial hypertension: Implications for the physiotherapist. *Physiotherapy Canada, 39,* 360–366.

Buchbinder, N., & Ganz, W. (1976). Hemodynamic monitoring: Invasive techniques. *Anesthesiology, 45*(2), 146–155.

Burki, N. K., & Albert, R. K. (1983). Noninvasive monitoring of arterial blood gases. A report of the ACCP section on respiratory pathophysiology. *Chest, 83*(4), 666–670.

Copel L. C., & Stolarik, A. (1991). Continuous SvO2 monitoring. A research review. *Dimensions of Critical Care Nursing, 10*, 202–209.

Cromwell, L., Weibell, F. J., & Pfeiffer, E. A. (1980). *Biomedical instrumentation and measurements* (2nd ed.). Englewood Cliffs: Prentice-Hall.

DeGowin, E. L., & DeGowin, R. L. (1981). *Bedside diagnostic examination* (4th ed.). New York: Macmillan.

Dubin, D. (1989). *Rapid interpretation of EKGs,* (4th ed.). Tampa, Fl.: Cover.

Fisher, J. D. (1981). Role of electrophysiologic testing in the diagnosis and treatment of patients with known and suspected bradycardias and tachycardias. *Progress in Cardiovascular Diseases, 24*(1), 25–90.

Folk-Lighty, M. (1984). Solving the puzzles of patients' fluid imbalances. *Nursing, 14*(2), 34–41.

Forrester, J. S., Diamond, G., McHugh, T. J. (1971). Filling pressures in the right and left sides of the heart in acute myocardial infarction: A reappraisal of central-venous-pressure monitoring. *New England Journal of Medicine, 285*(4), 190–193.

Ganong, W. F. (1993). *Review of medical physiology.* (16th ed.). Los Altos: Lange Medical Publications.

Guyton, A. C. (1991). *Textbook of medical physiology* (8th ed.). Philadelphia: WB Saunders.

Kirby, R. R., Taylor, R. W., & Civetta, J. M. (1990). *Pocket Companion Critical Care Immediate Concerns.* Philadelphia: JB Lippincott.

Luce, J. M. (1985). Neurologic monitoring. *Respiratory Care, 30,* 471–479.

Marini, J. J. (1987). *Respiratory medicine and intensive care for the house officer* (2nd ed.). Baltimore: Williams and Wilkins.

Oakes, D. F. (1988). *Clincial practitioners pocket guide to respiratory care.* Old Town: Health Educator Publications.

Phipps, W. J., Long, B. C., & Woods, N. F. (Eds.). (1991). *Medical-surgical nursing: concepts and clinical practice* (4th ed.). St. Louis: Mosby.

Puri, V. K., Carlson, R. W., Bander, J. J., & Weil, M. H. (1980). Complications of vascular catheterization in the critically ill. A prospective study. *Critical Care Medicine. 8*(9), 495–499.

Shapiro, B. A., Peruzzi, W. T., & Kozelowski-Templin, R. (1994). *Clinical application of blood gases* (5th ed.) St. Louis: Mosby.

Snider, G. L. (1973). Interpretation of the arterial oxygen and carbon dioxide partial pressures. A simplified approach for bedside use. *Chest, 63*(5), 801–806.

Swan, H. J. (1975). Second annual SCCM lecture. The role of hemodynamic monitoring in the management of the critically ill. *Critical Care Medicine, 3*(3), 83–89.

Thomas, H. M., 3rd, Lefrak, S. S., Irwin, R. S., Fritts, H. W., Jr., & Caldwell, P. R. (1974). The oxyhemoglobin dissociation curve in health and disease. Role of 2,3-diphosphoglycerate. *American Journal of Medicine, 57*(3), 331–348.

West, J. B. (1995). *Respiratory physiology—the essentials* (5th ed.). Baltimore: Williams and Wilkins.

Wiedemann, H. P., Matthay, M. A., & Matthay, R. A. (1984). Cardiovascular-pulmonary monitoring in the intensive care unit (Part 1). *Chest, 85*(4), 537–549.

PART III

Cardiopulmonary Physical Therapy Interventions

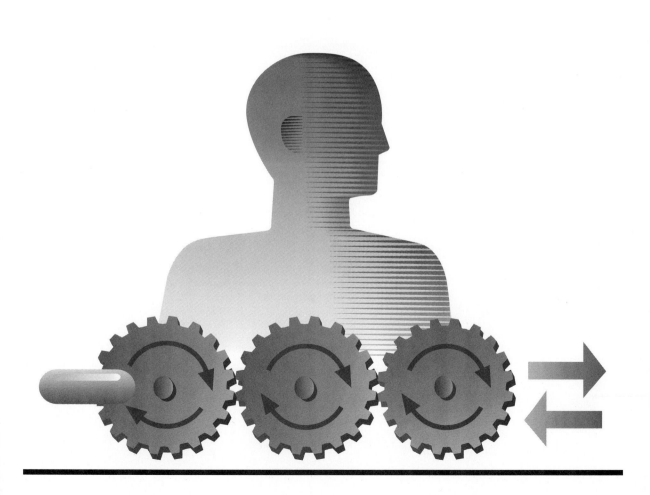

CHAPTER 16

Optimizing Treatment Prescription: Relating Treatment to the Underlying Pathophysiology

Elizabeth Dean

KEY TERMS
Clinical decision making
Extrinsic factors
Intrinsic factors
Oxygen transport deficits
Oxygen transport threats

Pathophysiological factors
Problem definition
Problem list
Restricted mobility and recumbency factors
Treatment prescription

INTRODUCTION

The purpose of this chapter is to provide a basis for clinical decision making and treatment prescription in cardiopulmonary physical therapy (CPPT) for patients ranging from the medically unstable critically ill patient to the medically stable patient with cardiopulmonary dysfunction living in the community. Clinical decision making and treatment prescription is based on the answers to three primary clinical questions related to oxygen transport. With respect to a given patient, the following must be considered:

1. What is the problem?
2. What is the treatment and why?
3. What is the course of treatment?

This chapter focuses on the elements involved in addressing these questions when managing a patient with impaired to threatened oxygen transport. The basic principles for relating CPPT treatment to the patient's underlying pathophysiologic problems (i.e., the pathophysiological mechanisms responsible for impairment of oxygen transport and cardiopulmonary function) are described. A physiologically based treat-

Fundamental Knowledge and Expertise to Critically Problem-Solve Deficits in Oxygen Transport	*Steps in Critical Problem-Solving Deficits in Oxygen Transport*

Fundamental Knowledge and Expertise to Critically Problem-Solve Deficits in Oxygen Transport

Normal cardiopulmonary and cardiovascular anatomy, as well as physiology and how these are affected by normal conditions such as aging and lifestyle habits (e.g., smoking, stress, and the physical environment)

Physiologic adaptation to hypoxia and cardiopulmonary impairment

Cardiopulmonary and cardiovascular pathophysiology and disease processes, and how these affect normal cardiopulmonary and cardiovascular function

Multisystem and integrative pathophysiology that can have a secondary effect on cardiopulmonary function and oxygen transport

Effects of medical, surgical, and nursing procedures on oxygen transport and gas exchange

Investigative laboratory procedures and tests and their effects on cardiopulmonary function

Pharmacological effects on cardiopulmonary function

Steps in Critical Problem-Solving Deficits in Oxygen Transport

1. Determine what factors are specifically contributing to impaired oxygen transport and which steps in the pathway are affected

2. Determine those factors that threaten oxygen transport and the steps in the pathway that are involved

3. Determine the relative magnitude of the effect of each factor either impairing or threatening oxygen transport, and prioritize the importance of each

4. Distinguish those factors that are amenable and those that are not amenable to CPPT in that the latter will modify treatment and affect the monitoring that is needed

5. Given the answers to 1 through 4, select, prioritize, and apply specific treatments prescriptively to address each factor that contributes to cardiopulmonary dysfunction and is amenable to CPPT

---

ment hierarchy is presented, with the premise that physiologic function, including oxygen transport, is optimal when humans are upright and moving. Applying a systematic physiologic approach to the analysis of the patient's problems, with respect to deficits in the oxygen transport pathway, leads directly to the most efficacious treatments. Such an approach provides a basis for modifying or discontinuing treatment based on the use of appropriate treatment outcome measures.

WHAT IS THE PROBLEM?

Oxygen transport is determined by a multitude of factors which affects different steps in the oxygen transport pathway (see Figure 1-1, p. 4) (Chapter 1). For treatment to be directed specifically to the underlying problems, the physical therapist (PT) needs to consider several levels of analysis of the deficits contributing to impaired or threatened oxygen transport. To be proficient in such analysis, the PT must have a thorough knowledge of the multiple factors that contribute to abnormal gas exchange. This knowledge base includes a detailed understanding of the relevant anatomy and physiology, multisystem and integrative pathophysiology, the impact of medical, surgical, and nursing procedures, the effect of various laboratory tests and procedures, and the impact of pharmacological agents on cardiopulmonary function (see box above, at left).

For a given patient, the cardiopulmonary PT prescribes treatment by extracting the relevant information from the history, laboratory tests and investigative procedures, and the assessment (see box above, at right). Problems are prioritized based on the relative magnitude of each one's effect on impairment of oxygen transport. Once the mechanisms for the cardiopulmonary and cardiovascular dysfunction have been identified, specific treatments are selected and prioritized.

The Problem List
Impaired oxygen transport

Two levels of problems need to be identified, namely, functional and physiologic deficits. The functional deficits are those that affect the patient's ability to

Examples of Deficits in and Threats to Steps in the Oxygen Transport Pathway

Central Control of Breathing

Altered central nervous system (CNS) afferent input and control of breathing

Impaired efferent pathways

Pharmacologic depression

Substance abuse depression

Airways

Aspiration related to lack of gastrointestinal (GI) motility

Aspiration secondary to esophageal reflux

Obstruction secondary to airway edema, bronchospasm, or mucus

Inhaled foreign bodies

Lungs

Altered breathing pattern secondary to decreased lung compliance

Ineffective breathing pattern related to decreased diaphragmatic function and increased lung volumes, respiratory muscle weakness, respiratory muscle fatigue, CNS dysfunction, guarding, reflex, fatigue, and respiratory inflammatory process

Ineffective airway clearance related to restricted mobility, immobility, sedation, and pulmonary dysfunction secondary to long smoking history, impaired mucociliary transport, absent cilia, or dyskinesia of cilia, retained secretions, ineffective cough and mucociliary mechanisms, infection, inability to cough efficiently, artificial airway/intubation and endotracheal tube, drug-induced paralysis, and sedation

Large airway obstruction secondary to compliant oropharyngeal structures

Chest wall rigidity and decreased compliance

Loss of normal chest wall excursion movements (pump and bucket handle motions) and capacity to move appropriately in all three planes of motion

Chest wall and spinal deformity

Impaired lung fluid balance and acute lung injury

Blood

Bleeding abnormalities, altered body temperature (hypothermia, hyperthermia), fever, inflammation, hypermetabolism secondary to mediator systems

Altered body temperature related to integumentary disruption

Low hematocrit secondary to GI bleed (more prone to hypoxia)

Anemia

Thrombocytopenia

Disseminated intravascular coagulation

Abnormal clotting factors (i.e., balance between clotting and not clotting, sludging of blood)

Thromboemboli

Bleeding disorders with liver disease; abnormal clotting factors

Continued.

Examples of Deficits in and Threats to Steps in the Oxygen Transport Pathway—cont'd

Gas Exchange

Alveolar collapse, atelectasis, intrapulmonary shunting or pulmonary edema, shallow breathing and tenacious mucus, body position, consolidation and alveolar collapse, ventilation/perfusion mismatch, airway constriction, fluid volume excess, pleural effusions, breathing at low lung volumes, abdominal distension and guarding, ineffective airway clearance, pulmonary microvascular thrombi and altered capillary permeability secondary to circulating mediators, closure of small airways secondary to dynamic airway compression, decreased functional residual capacity, and intrapulmonary shunting, increased lung surface tension

Diffusion defects

Respiratory Muscles

Upper abdominal surgery, weakness, fatigue, neuromuscular disease, ileus related to gastric distension, mechanical dysfunction

Myocardial Perfusion

Coronary artery occlusion

Tachycardia

Potential for cardiac dysrhythmia related to reperfusion

Cardiac dysrhythmia related to myocardial hypoxia

Compression by edema or space-occupying lesions

Heart

Decreased venous return and cardiac output, secondary to volume deficit, ascites, myocardial ischemia, hemorrhage, and coagulopathies

Conduction defects

Mechanical defects

Defects in electromechanical coupling

Abnormal distension characteristics

Abnormal afterload

Blood Pressure

Volume deficit/bleeding

Alteration in peripheral tissue perfusion related to acute myocardial infarction, myocardial depression, maldistribution of blood volume, and altered cellular metabolism

Volume excess

Tissue Perfusion

Impaired cardiac output

Impaired secondary to disseminated microvascular thrombi

Atherosclerosis and thromboembolic events, decreased circulating blood volume, decreased circulating blood volume, decreased vascular integrity, and inflammatory process

Decreased cardiac output related to reduced venous return, impaired right ventricular function, dysrhythmias, increased afterload, and bradycardia

Low oxygen content in the blood

Thromboembolism, vasoconstriction secondary to toxins, sepsis, etc., blood flow alterations and hypermetabolism secondary to mediator systems

Examples of Deficits in and Threats to Steps in the Oxygen Transport Pathway—cont'd

Fluid Volume Excess

Related to excessive intravenous administration

Related to impaired excretion

Apparent hypervolemia secondary to restricted mobility and recumbency (e.g., resulting from hemodynamic instability)

Renal failure

Water intoxication

Therapeutic volume expansion, acute myocardial infarction (MI) and acute renal failure, related to renal retention of sodium and water and increased levels of aldosterone, renin, angiotensin II, and catecholamines

Fluid Volume Deficit

Fluid volume deficit related to volume losses during surgery and inadequate oral intake, blood loss, internal injuries (e.g., hematoma and third spacing phenomenon; hormonal imbalance; increased intestinal motility; vomiting; diarrhea; fluid sequestration in tissues; nasogastric (NG) suction and diarrhea; hypovolemia; sepsis and shock; surface capillary leak and fluid loss as in burns and excoriated wounds; fluid shifts)

Tissue Oxygenation

Multisystem organ failure with altered peripheral tissue perfusion and gas exchange at the cellular level

---

Indirect Factors That Contribute to Oxygen Transport Deficits

Infection

Pulmonary and nonpulmonary infection increase the demands on the oxygen transport system

Cognition

Impaired neurological status and central cardiopulmonary control

Alteration in mental status secondary to inadequate cerebral perfusion with hypotension and cardiogenic shock

Sleep pattern disturbance; altered blood gases and fatigue

Anxiety and agitation related to powerlessness and lack of knowledge, breathlessness, pharmacological paralysis, impaired verbal community secondary to intubation, paralysis etc.

Psychosocial Factors

Anxiety related to the condition, shortness of breath, hospitalization, etc.

Social isolation secondary to impaired communication

Fear and hopelessness

Pain response

Nutrition

Altered nutritional needs secondary to greater need than resting state (i.e., increased caloric need and nutrients associated with illness, inability to ingest food, inability to absorb food)

Restricted ingestion orders of food and water

High caloric needs secondary to infectious process and protein catabolism

perform activities of daily living (ADLs) (e.g., reduced activity or exercise tolerance as a result of reduced peripheral oxygenation, reduced mobility related to deconditioning resulting from resting in bed, extremity or internal injury, anticoagulant therapy, drug-induced paralysis, impaired physical mobility related to muscle weakness and partial paralysis, paralysis, depressed level of consciousness, and anemia).

Physiological deficits are those deficits in oxygen transport, specifically, at the individual steps in the pathway, and oxygen transport overall. Examples of deficits at each step in the pathway appear in the boxes on pp. 253-255.

Threatened oxygen transport

Although the complications of restricted mobility and static body positions are well understood, the precise prescription parameters for mobilization and body positioning to avoid these complications have not been defined in detail. With respect to cardiopulmonary complications, a one- or two- hourly turning regimen is commonly accepted. For the flaccid or comatose patient, range-of-motion (ROM) exercises every several hours facilitates blood flow through dependent areas and enhances alveolar ventilation as well as mobilizes joints and muscles. Antiembolic stockings and pneumatic compression devices are routinely used to minimize circulatory stasis in the legs and the potential for thrombi formation.

The PT has a major role in preventing infection of all types but particularly cardiopulmonary infections. Both cardiopulmonary assessment and treatment involves handling and close physical contact with patients. Thus the risk of nosocomial infection is high in hospitalized patients. Some standard means of preventing infection include meticulous hand washing before and after every patient, and care of invasive lines and catheters. The PT moves and repositions patients often, thus it is essential that lines, leads, and catheters are continuously monitored. The PT must consider when it is appropriate to gown, mask and glove to protect and be protected from the patient adequately.

Factors that contribute to or threaten oxygen transport

Those factors that can impair oxygen transport directly or threaten it fall into four primary categories,

---

Factors That Can Impair Oxygen Transport

1. Cardiopulmonary pathophysiology
     primary (acute, chronic, acute on chronic)
     secondary (chronic, acute on chronic)
   Noncardiopulmonary pathophysiology that impacts upon cardiopulmonary function
2. Immobility—loss of physical exercise stress
   Recumbency—loss of vertical gravitational stress
3. Extrinsic factors (i.e., those related to the patient's care)
4. Intrinsic factors (i.e., those related to the patient)

(see box above), namely, the underlying cardiopulmonary pathophysiology, restricted mobility (loss of physical exercise stress), recumbency (loss of vertical gravitational stress), extrinsic factors (i.e., those related to the patient's care), and intrinsic factors (i.e., those related to the patient). These categories are expanded and explained in detail in Chapter 17.

Restricted mobility and recumbency: special examples of extrinsic factors

Although bed rest can be considered an extrinsic factor (i.e., a therapeutic intervention that contributes to cardiopulmonary dysfunction, the negative sequelae of this intervention are often not fully appreciated clinically based on the widespread use of rest in bed. Therefore to draw to the clinician's attention that the effects of this intervention need to be considered in each patient, the effects of restricted mobility and recumbency are analyzed separately (see Chapters 17 and 18).

Treatment Goals

Once the deficits and threats to oxygen transport have been determined, the goals of treatment fall into three categories: short-term, long-term, and preventive. Short-term treatment goals include the following.

1. To correct or reverse acute cardiopulmonary dysfunction
2. To reduce the rate of deterioration

3. To avoid worsening the patient's condition.

Long-term treatment goals include:

1. To enhance the efficiency of the steps in the oxygen transport pathway overall
2. To enhance the efficiency of those specific steps in the oxygen transport pathway that compensate for impaired steps that may or may not be reversibly affected
3. To maximize oxygen transport capacity to sustain maximal functional activity.

And preventive treatment goals include:

1. To prevent cardiopulmonary dysfunction
2. To prevent multisystem organ complications and nonpulmonary infection that will lead to further restricted movement and recumbency, hence the potential for further deterioration
3. To provide supportive palliative care.

WHAT IS THE TREATMENT AND WHY?
Clinical Decision Making

The basis for clinical decision making in the management of the cardiopulmonary patient is to pair the most efficacious treatments specifically with impaired or threatened steps in the oxygen transport pathway. In addition, the patient spends considerable time between treatments, thus optimal therapeutic effect is dependent on the efficacy of "between treatment" treatments (i.e., teaching the patient to carry out prescriptive treatment whenever possible and eliciting the assistance of the patient's family or nursing staff).

When confined to hospital, many patients spend considerable time recumbent and in restricted body positions, turn and move less frequently, and are upright and moving a smaller proportion of time. Depending on the oxygen transport deficits, the body positions the patient assumes can have a positive, negative or neutral effect on oxygen transport. Thus, the positions the patient assumes and his or her reduced activity levels, must be monitored and any potential ill effects anticipated and countered.

Some examples of some common treatment goals in managing the patient with cardiopulmonary dysfunction are shown in the box above. Specific treatments are identified to address these goals and for each deficit or threat to oxygen transport. Treatment

---

> ### *Common Treatment Goals in the Management of the Patient With Cardiopulmonary Dysfunction*
>
> **OVERALL GOAL:** To optimize or preserve oxygen transport and gas exchange
>
> Treatment directed at specific steps involved
>
> Object to enhance the efficiency of all steps in the pathway
>
> Augment medical management
>
> Coordinate with nursing management (e.g., in critical care)
>
> **Goals Directed at Specific Steps in the Oxygen Transport Pathway**
>
> Maximize air entry and alveolar ventilation (minimize airflow resistance)
>
> Maximize air distribution (optimize lung compliance and chest wall compliance)
>
> Maximize ventilation and perfusion matching
>
> Optimize diffusion
>
> Optimize oxyhemoglobin saturation
>
> Reduce work of breathing (increased resistance, reduced or excessive compliance)
>
> Reduce work of the heart (increased preload, contraction, increased afterload)
>
> Maximize efficiency of heart mechanics
>
> Minimize electrocardiogram (ECG) irregularities (identify factors that contribute to irregularities; anticipate problems)
>
> Optimize blood flow distribution
>
> Optimize oxygen extraction ratio
>
> Reduce excessive or unnecessary energy expenditure
>
> Optimize carbon dioxide (CO_2) removal
>
> Optimize blood volume
>
> Optimize hydration

---

goals and specific treatments are prioritized according to the relative significance of the impact of each on oxygen transport.

A physiologically based treatment hierarchy is shown in the box on p. 258 and 259, and the box on p. 260, top right. The treatment hierarchy is based on

Physiologic Treatment Hierarchy for Treatment of Impaired Oxygen Transport

PREMISE: Position of optimal physiological function is being upright and moving

  I. Mobilization and Exercise

Goal: To elicit an exercise stimulus that addresses one of the three effects on the various steps in the oxygen transport pathway, or some combination

   A. Acute effects

   B. Long-term effect

   C. Preventative effects

 II. Body Positioning

Goal: To elicit a gravitational stimulus that simulates being upright and moving as much as possible i.e., active, active assisted or passive

   A. Hemodynamic effects related to fluid shifts

   B. Cardiopulmonary effects on ventilation and its distribution, perfusion, ventilation, and perfusion matching and gas exchange

 III. Breathing Control Maneuvers

Goal: To augment alveolar ventilation, to facilitate mucociliary transport, and to stimulate coughing

   A. Coordinated breathing with activity and exercise

   B. Spontaneous eucapnic hyperventilation

   C. Maximal tidal breaths and movement in three dimensions

   D. Sustained maximal inspiration

   E. Pursed lip breathing to end tidal expiration

   F. Incentive spirometry

 IV. Coughing Maneuvers

Goal: To facilitate mucociliary clearance with the least effect on dynamic airway compression and adverse cardiovascular effects

   A. Active and spontaneous cough with closed glottis

   B. Active assist (self-supported or by other)

   C. Modified coughing interventions with open glottis (e.g., forced expiratory technique, huff)

  V. Relaxation and Energy Conservation Interventions

Goal: To minimize the work of breathing, of the heart, and oxygen demand overall

   A. Relaxation procedures at rest and during activity

   B. Energy conservation, (i.e., balance of activity to rest, performing activities in an energy) efficient manner, improved movement economy during activity)

   C. Pain control interventions

 VI. ROM Exercises (Cardiopulmonary indications)

Goal: To stimulate alveolar ventilation and alter its distribution

   A. Active

   B. Assisted active

   C. Passive

Continued.

Physiologic Treatment Hierarchy for Treatment of Impaired Oxygen Transport—cont'd

VII. Postural Drainage Positioning

Goal: To facilitate airway clearance using gravitational effects

    A. Bronchopulmonary segmental drainage positions

VIII. Manual Techniques

Goal: To facilitate airway clearance in conjunction with specific body positioning

    A. Autogenic drainage

    B. Manual percussion

    C. Shaking and vibration

    D. Deep breathing and coughing

IX. Suctioning

Goal: To facilitate the removal of airway secretions collected centrally

    A. Open suction system

    B. Closed suction system

    C. Tracheal tickle

    D. Instillation with saline

    E. Use of manual inflation bag (bagging)

the premise that physiologic function, including oxygen transport, is optimal when the human organism is upright and moving. Thus the purpose of the hierarchy is to exploit those treatments that are most physiologic first (i.e., active mobilization and exercise in the upright position). Therefore the hierarchy ranges from the most physiologic interventions, that is, active mobilization and exercise in the upright position, to those interventions that are the least physiologic. The least physiological interventions, (i.e., conventional chest physical therapy techniques such as ROM, postural drainage and percussion) may simulate some of the physiologic effects of being upright and moving; however, their effects are more limited and less scientifically well-substantiated, and affect fewer steps in the oxygen transport pathway. Thus they do not substitute for more physiologic interventions higher up in the treatment hierarchy. All interventions featured in the hierarchy have some role in the management of cardiopulmonary dysfunction, but are recruited in descending order to ensure that the most physiological and efficacious interventions are exploited first.

Treatment Plan

The treatment plan consists of those interventions that will most expediently remediate the problems that have been identified. These interventions are prioritized according to the greatest effect they are predicted to have on remediating the oxygen transport deficit or minimizing any threat to oxygen transport, and on maximizing the benefit-to-risk ratio. Depending on the specific treatment goals and the adequacy of balance between oxygen supply and demand, coordinating physical therapy treatments with other care (e.g., nursing care and certain tests and procedures) is often indicated.

Treatment Prescription

Once the specific pathophysiological problems have been identified, they are differentiated as: (1) those that can be addressed by physical therapy (i.e., noninvasive physical interventions) and (2) those that are not amenable to physical therapy but need to be considered during treatment to determine whether treatment is contraindicated or needs to be modified, and specific outcome and treatment response measures are indicated.

Problems amenable to physical therapy are prioritized, the treatment is indicated for each problem, and its parameters are defined. The treatment goals are identified, that is, to reverse pathophysiological mechanisms contributing to impaired oxygen transport, to compensate for irreversible pathophysiological deficits (improve efficiency of other steps in the oxygen transport pathway), to decelerate deterioration, to avoid making patient worse palliative care/support/comfort, and for prevention. Based on the goal of treatment, the parameters for the treatment prescription are defined. Treatment parameters in the management of a cardiopulmonary patient are shown in the box below.

WHAT IS THE COURSE OF TREATMENT?

Once a treatment has been prescribed, the prescription must be reviewed at each treatment and modified accordingly, that is, change in the prescription parameters, as the patient's condition changes. In addition, the parameters may be modified within a treat-

---

Use of Modalities and Aids

Goal: To incorporate the use of those modalities and aids that enhance the above interventions

Modalities

Treadmill, ergometer, rowing machine

Weights

Pulleys

Nebulizers and aerosols

Flutter valve

BYPAP* and CPAP†

Incentive spirometer

Pharmacologic Agents

Oxygen

Bronchodilators

Antiinflammatories

Mucolytics

Surfactant

Analgesics

---

*Bilevel positive airway pressure
†Continuous positive airway pressure

Parameters of the Treatment Prescription in the Management of the Cardiopulmonary Patient

Define parameters of treatment based on history, laboratory investigations, tests, and assessment

Treatment type

Intensity (if applicable)

Duration

Frequency

Instruct patient in "between treatment" treatment, and if applicable the nurse, a family member, or both

Reassessment every treatment

Modify as necessary within each treatment

Progress between treatments as indicated

Define treatment outcomes

Determine when treatment is to be discontinued

Request for additional supportive information, tests, and investigations as indicated

Predict time course for optimal effects and course of treatment to determine treatment efficacy; modify as necessary

In conjunction with other interventions (e.g., medical, surgical, nursing, respiratory therapy (weaning)) oxygen supplementation, sympathomimetic drugs, ADLs, balance with sleep and rest periods, peak of nutrition and feeds, peak energy times, peak of drug potency and effects (e.g., pain, reduced sedation, reduced neuromuscular blockade)

Assessment and Treatment Outcome Measures Used in the Management of Deficits in Oxygen Transport Pathway

Central Control of Breathing

Central drive to breathe test

Arterial blood gases

Cerebral perfusion

Ambient Air

Partial pressures of O_2, N_2 and CO_2

Air pollution and quality

Humidity

Airways

Clinical assessment including auscultation

Pulmonary function tests

Arterial blood gases

Chest X-ray

Histamine challenge exercise tests

Lungs

Clinical assessment including inspection, percussion, palpation and auscultation

Pulmonary function tests

Ventilation and perfusion scans

Diffusion capacity test

Arterial blood gases

Chest X-ray

Immunulogical status

Respiratory muscle assessment

Assessment of the structure and integrity of chest wall

Lung water studies

Blood

Circulating blood volume and cardiac output

Arterial oxygen content

Venous oxygen content

Plasma volume

Red and white blood cell counts

Protein constituents

Blood—*cont'd*

Platelets

Hemoglobin

Coagulability

Viscosity

Stasis

Hydration

Immunological status

Pulmonary Circulation

Perfusion scan

Pulmonary artery balloon floatation catheter to assess central venous pressure, pulmonary artery pressures, wedge pressure

Heart

Clinical assessment including percussion, palpation, and auscultation

Inspection and clinical observation tests including jugular venous distension test

Heart rate, systolic and diastolic blood pressures, and rate pressure product

ECG

Hemodynamic studies to assess cardiac output, stroke volume, cardiac distensibility, and ejection fraction

Ultrasound procedures to examine mechanical integrity

Scans

Coordination of electromechanical behavior of heart

Coronary artery perfusion studies

Stress test

Hemodynamic monitoring including central venous pressure, pulmonary artery pressures and wedge pressure

Angiography

Chest X-ray

Peripheral Circulation

Clinical assessment

Segmental blood pressures of the extremities

Continued.

Assessment and Treatment Outcome Measures Used in the Management of Deficits in Oxygen Transport Pathway—cont'd

Peripheral Circulation—*cont'd*

Ultrasound studies

Arterial and venous lab studies and investigations

Adequacy and efficiency of lymphatic drainage system of the heart and lungs, and peripheral circulation

Stress test

Tissue

Enzyme studies

Tissue biopsies

Tissue—*cont'd*

Vascularization of tissue

Adequacy and efficiency of arterial and venous tissue

Blood flow

Tissue fluid balance; hydrostatic pressure, oncotic pressure, and lymphatic pressure

Blood work including serum lactates and SvO_2

Tissue oxygenation and pH

Nutritional and hydration status

ment based on the patient's treatment response. The PT also bases the decision when to discontinue a given treatment as well as what overall cardiopulmonary physical therapy to employ, based on treatment response and outcome.

Measures to assess treatment response and outcome are selected that reflect (1) the status of oxygen transport overall, and (2) the integrity of the step or steps in the oxygen transport pathway that were identified as being the primary problems contributing to cardiopulmonary or cardiovascular dysfunction in the original assessment (see box on pp. 261-262.) (see Part II of this text). Cardiopulmonary dysfunction is determined based on the history, assessment and laboratory investigations, such as, pulmonary function testing, breathing pattern, cardiac function testing, fluid balance and renal function, arterial blood gases, arterial saturation, vital signs, and hemodynamic variables, including heart rate and ECG, blood pressure, and rate pressure product. Subjective reports are also clinically relevant, such as subjective ratings of perceived exertion, breathlessness, angina, and fatigue. These same measures are used to detect improved oxygen transport and gas exchange.

Considering that clinical decision making is based largely on the results of tests and measures, it is essential that these measures have certain characteristics. For example, measurements must be objective and their procedures standardized to maximize test validity and reliability. Although PTs specialize in noninvasive assessment procedures as well as treatments, noninvasive measures are prone to imprecision, and hence measurement error and unreliability. It is therefore essential that assessment measurements are performed in a systematic manner according to measurement guidelines to maximize their quality and usefulness in guiding and directing treatment (Chapter 6). Assessment measurements always precede any treatment to ensure that treatment is appropriate, that is, the baseline measurements. Measurements during treatment provides information about the patient's responses, both beneficial and detrimental. This feedback determines the parameters of treatment, and whether the treatment should be modified in some way, or possibly discontinued. The overall treatment response is established by further monitoring and assessment at the termination of treatment, and often at periodic intervals posttreatment so that delayed effects can be monitored. Frequent and periodic measurements over time are referred to as serial measurements and provide useful trend data. The pre- and posttreatment responses and any noteworthy responses during treatment are charted with sufficient information about the procedures that were used, that is, assessment as well as treatment procedures.

PTs often require the results of invasive tests such as blood work or invasive hemodynamic monitoring to establish treatment response and outcome; thus, these need to be requested as required.

SUMMARY

This chapter has provided a framework for clinical problem solving and decision making based on oxygen transport. The process includes diagnosis and treatment prescription in the management of patients with cardiopulmonary dysfunction ranging from the medically unstable critically ill patient to the medically stable patient with cardiopulmonary dysfunction living in the community. The purpose of a systematic approach to clinical decision making is to maximize treatment efficacy and cost effectiveness by focusing on physiological and evidence-based practice. The clinical decision making process involves diagnosis, that is, specific analysis of the patient's problems in relation to the physiology and underling pathophysiology, the contribution of restricted mobility and recumbency, and extrinsic and intrinsic factors. Based on this analysis, treatment interventions and their parameters are prescribed that have the greatest physiological and scientific justification. Treatments and their prescription parameters should have a clear, justifiable rationale. Specific monitoring of the steps in the oxygen transport pathway that are impaired is essential to establish and confirm the diagnoses, determine the most efficacious treatment, evaluate the treatment response, refine and progress the treatment, and determine when to discontinue a given treatment and cardiopulmonary physical therapy overall. The specific components of the treatment prescription include the treatment, its intensity (if applicable), duration, and frequency, as well as its course and progression. A problem-solving approach to patient care has become essential in all health care professions, given the prohibitive cost of such care and the need for all health care to be physiological, evidence-based, cost-effective and ethically justifiable.

REVIEW QUESTIONS

1. Describe the use of the oxygen transport pathway as a conceptual model of cardiopulmonary practice and basis for defining problems related to cardiopulmonary dysfunction.
2. Distinguish between short-term goals, long-term goals and preventive goals of cardiopulmonary physical therapy management.
3. Explain and distinguish the *four* categories of factors (i.e., pathophysiology, restricted mobility and recumbency, extrinsic, and intrinsic) that contribute to cardiopulmonary dysfunction.
4. Describe the factors that need to be considered in treatment prescription.
5. Describe the factors that must be considered in determining the course of treatment.

Bibliography

Barlow, D.H., Hayes, S.C., & Nelson, R.O. (1984). *The scientist practitioner. Research and accountability in clinical and educational settings.* New York: Pergamon Press.

Cutler, P. (1985). *Problem solving in clinical medicine.* (2nd ed.). Baltimore: Williams and Wilkins.

Dantzker, D.R. (1991). *Cardiopulmonary critical care.* (2nd ed.). Philadelphia: WB Saunders.

Dean, E. (1994). Oxygen transport: A physiologically-based conceptual framework for the practice of cardiopulmonary physiotherapy. *Physiotherapy, 80,* 347-355.

Epstein, C.D., & Henning, R.J. (1993). Oxygen transport variables in the identification and treatment of tissue hypoxia. *Heart & Lung, 22,* 328-348.

Goldring, R.M. (1984). Specific defects in cardiopulmonary gas exchange. *American Review of Respiratory Diseases, 129,* S57-S59.

Hillegass, E.A., & Sadowsky, H.S. (1994). Essentials of cardiopulmonary physical therapy. Philadelphia: WB Saunders.

Irwin, S., & Tecklin, J.S. (1995). *Cardiopulmonary physical therapy* (3rd ed.). St. Louis: Mosby.

Patrick, D.F. (1992). Clinical decision making. In Zadai C (Ed.). *Clinics in physical therapy. Pulmonary management in physical therapy.* New York: Churchill Livingstone.

Riegelman, R.K. (1991). *Minimizing medical mistakes.* Boston: Little, Brown.

Schon, D.A. (1983). *The reflective practitioner.* New York: Basic Books.

Wasserman, K., Hansen, J.E., Sue, D.Y., & Whipp, B.J. (1987). *Principles of exercise testing and interpretation.* Philadelphia: Lea & Febiger.

CHAPTER 17

Mobilization and Exercise

Elizabeth Dean

KEY TERMS

Exercise
Metabolic demand
Mobilization
Oxygen transport

Prescription
Recumbency factors
Restricted mobility

INTRODUCTION

The first purpose of this chapter is to define the terms mobilization and exercise and then to review the basis for prescribing mobilization and exercise as *primary* physical therapy treatment interventions to optimize oxygen transport. The three distinct objectives of mobilization and exercise for the purpose of maximizing oxygen transport are described. These include the exploitation of their acute, long-term, and preventive effects. Mobilization or exercise can be prescribed specifically to elicit which of these effects is indicated.

The second purpose of this chapter is to review the negative effects of immobility and reduced exercise stress on multisystem function with special attention to cardiopulmonary and cardiovascular function. Immobility and recumbency are major factors contributing to impaired or threatened oxygen transport in a large proportion of patients. The sequelae of immobility and recumbency adversely affect all steps in the oxygen transport pathway. An understanding of the effects of immobility and reduced exercise stress on normal human physiological function provides the rationale for prescribing exercise for its preventive effects.

DEFINITIONS

Mobilization is defined as the therapeutic and prescriptive application of low-intensity exercise in the management of cardiopulmonary dysfunction usually in acutely ill patients. Primarily, the goal of mobilization is to exploit the *acute* effects of exercise to optimize oxygen transport. Even a relatively low-intensity mobilization stimulus can impose considerable metabolic demand on the patient with cardiopulmonary compromise. In addition, mobilization is performed in the upright position, that is the physiologic position (Chapter 18), whenever possible, to optimize the effects of being upright on central and peripheral hemodynamics and fluid shifts. Thus mobilization is prescribed to elicit both a gravitational stimulus and an exercise stimulus.

Exercise is the term used to describe the therapeutic and prescriptive application of exercise in the management of subacute and chronic cardiopulmonary and cardiovascular dysfunction. Primarily, the goal of exercise is to exploit the cumulative effects of and adaptation to *long-term* exercise and thereby optimize the function of all steps in the oxygen transport pathway.

In addition, mobilization and exercise can be prescribed for their *preventive* effects. In this case, the parameters of the prescription focus on exploiting their multisystemic effects as well as their cardiopulmonary and cardiovascular effects.

BASES FOR THE PRESCRIPTION OF EXERCISE STRESS

The prescription of exercise is fundamental in the management of primary and secondary cardiopulmonary and cardiovascular dysfunction. Exercise science has advanced exponentially over the past 30 years and is a primary basis for cardiopulmonary physical therapy. Guidelines have been developed for prescribing exercise to maximize functional work capacity or aerobic capacity for healthy persons and individuals with chronic heart and lung disease (American College of Sports Medicine, 1994; Belman and Wasserman, 1981; Blair, Painter, Pate, Smith and Taylor, 1988; Froelicher, 1987; Hasson, 1994; Irwin and Tecklin, 1985; Wasserman and Whipp, 1975; Zadai, 1992). Exercise training is based on the findings of a maximum graded exercise test. Submaximal exercise testing is often indicated for patients with severely impaired functional work capacity because of the inherent risks associated with maximal testing (Compton, Eisenman, and Henderson, 1989). Guidelines for submaximal exercise testing, test interpretation and prescription of exercise, however, based on

the submaximal exercise test have been less well-defined (Dean and Ross, 1992a; Dean and Ross, 1993; Shepherd et al, 1968).

The prescription of mobilization and exercise to optimize oxygen transport in the patient with *acute* cardiopulmonary dysfunction has been a relatively neglected area of research compared with exercise prescription in the management of *chronic* cardiopulmonary dysfunction. This is surprising given that "early mobilization" is a key component of cardiopulmonary physical therapy in the management of acutely ill patients. Orlava (1959) was the first to report the beneficial application of mobilization in the management of acute cardiopulmonary compromise, specifically, bronchopulmonary pneumonia. The physiologic literature supports an unequivocal role for therapeutic mobilization to maximize oxygen transport in patients with *acute* cardiopulmonary dysfunction (Dean and Ross, 1992b). Despite this conclusive body of literature, Orlava's work has not been extended significantly in the literature since her work was published more than 35 years ago.

Unlike exercise prescription for the patient with chronic cardiopulmonary and cardiovascular dysfunction, the acute patient cannot be exercise tested in the conventional manner given the risks of an untoward exercise response. Given the profound and direct effects of mobilization and exercise on cardiopulmonary and cardiovascular function, it is essential that the physical therapist be able to identify the specific effects of exercise required and define the optimal therapeutic stimulus, ie, the stimulus that yields the maximal benefit to oxygen transport with the least risk.

Acute and chronic cardiopulmonary and cardiovascular pathology have the additional problem of compromising functional capacity in two important ways. First, in acute illness, the patient tends to be recumbent in bed a greater proportion of time, and second, in both acute and chronic illnesses, the physical activity of the patient is reduced. Recumbency and immobility have physiologically distinct effects on oxygen transport and are the primary determinants of bed rest deconditioning (Chase, Grave, and Rowell, 1966; Convertino, Hung, Goldwater, and DeBusk, 1982; Winslow, 1985). Thus dysfunction of oxygen transport is further exacerbated in patients by the additional factors of recumbency and immobility. The impact of these factors is further exacerbated in smokers, the young, older adults, obese individuals, and patients who are mechanically ventilated.

Even though the prescription of mobilization and exercise for their acute effects is distinct from that for its long-term effects, the efficacy of the acute exercise stimuli needs to be considered in terms of optimizing long-term benefit to oxygen transport as well as the short-term acute effects. Both acute and long-term exercise needs to be prescribed specifically for a given patient given the mechanisms of their underlying pathology (American College of Sports Medicine, 1994). The prescription parameters should include (1) the type or types of mobilization or exercise, (2) specific intensity, (3) duration, and (4) frequency.

These parameters are defined for each type of exercise being prescribed. In addition, (5) the course of the prescription, that is the time over which the prescription is designed to produce its maximum benefit, and (6) the means of progression of the prescription are defined.

Exercise has been reported to have beneficial effects in the management of a multitude of conditions. Its benefits range from enhancing all steps in the oxygen transport pathway to other peripheral and central effects related to virtually every other organ system.

The preventive effects of exercise are central to patient care across all conditions and physical therapy specialties. Exercise is advocated preventively to avoid the deleterious effects of immobility and to provide optimal systemic health protection secondary to cardiopulmonary conditioning.

Mobilization and exercise are the physical therapist's (PT's) "drug" with definable indications, contraindications, and side effects for each patient. The prescriptive parameters are determined by the effects needed to address the patient's underlying problems directly, whenever possible. Mobilization and exercise constitute the most potent and direct interventions affecting oxygen transport that are available to the PT in that, unlike other cardiopulmonary physical therapy interventions, they affect all steps in the oxygen transport pathway. Thus they need to be prescribed specifically as *primary* treatment interventions to remediate cardiopulmonary dysfunction, and their effects exploited first.

OXYGEN TRANSPORT AND METABOLIC DEMAND IN PATIENTS

In health, when individuals have optimal physiological reserve, both the acute and long-term responses to an exercise stimulus can be predicted. Specifically, minute ventilation (VE) and cardiac output (CO), hence oxygen delivery (DO_2), increase commensurate with work rate and oxygen demand.

In patients, whose oxygen transport capacity is reduced or threatened, mobilization and exercise constitute a significant additional metabolic demand that is superimposed on various other factors that contribute to increased metabolic cost (see box on page 268). Hospitalized patients tend to be hypermetabolic. In addition to their basal metabolic demands, their energy demands are increased secondary to such factors as an increased body temperature, healing and repair processes, increased work of breathing and of the heart, and in response to routine interventions and procedures including cardiopulmonary physical therapy. The goal, therefore, in prescribing mobilization and exercise, is to ensure a safety margin wherein the patient's demand for oxygen does not exceed the available supply or delivery. In most situations, this would be indicated clinically by worsening of the patient's oxygen transport objectively and subjectively.

Of the physical therapy related interventions, mobilization, exercise, body positioning, arousal, breathing control maneuvers, coughing, postural drainage, manual techniques, bagging, suctioning and range-of-motion (ROM) exercises can significantly increase oxygen consumption and overall metabolic demand (Dean, Murphy, Parrent, and Rousseau, 1995; Weissmann, Kemper, Damask, Askanazi, Hyman, and Kinney, 1984). Therefore, the capacity of the oxygen transport system to meet the patient's metabolic demands needs to be established in the physical therapy assessment. Can the oxygen transport system support the patient's metabolic demands? If so, what reserve capacity is available to support a mobilization or exercise stimulus? The exercise stimulus is designed to exploit the potential of the reserve capacity. Establishing

---

Factors That Contribute to Increased Metabolic Demand and Oxygen Consumption in Patient Populations

Pathophysiological Factors

Fever (e.g., secondary to an infectious agent or inflammation, surgery, multiple trauma, severe illness)

Thermoregulatory challenges (i.e., too hot or too cold, altered ambient temperature and humidity)

Healing and repairing (i.e., secondary to illness, trauma, surgery)

Combatting infection

Interventions

Response to routine nursing, medical, and physical therapy interventions

Feeding; enterally or parenterally

Physically being handled, e.g., by health care workers

Body positioning

Changing body position, i.e., passive, active assist, or active changes

ROM exercises, i.e., passive, active assist, or active

Mobilization and exercise

Noxious stimulation, e.g., injections, insertion of lines, procedures, neurological checks

Pharmacologic agents

Psychosocial Factors

Social contact, e.g., health care workers, family

Anxiety

Discomfort

Pain

Agitation

Miscellaneous

Noises

Disrupted circadian rhythms when ill, hospitalized or away from daylight

---

the availability of that reserve is essential to optimize the efficacy of the therapeutic exercise stimulus, that is, neither subthreshold or suprathreshold.

Metabolic demand and oxygen uptake are determined by multiple factors. In patients, the effect of arousal, anxiety, pain, and noxious stimulation, in addition to the hypermetabolic demands of recovery, contribute significantly to the energy cost and demand on the oxygen transport system. Thus relaxing and calming patients is a central component of cardiopulmonary physical therapy as these interventions can minimize oxygen demand. Although relaxation, often coupled with analgesia is central to physical therapy management in other settings, relaxation pro-

cedures need to be applied in the management of patients with cardiopulmonary and cardiovascular dysfunction in situations in which agitation, anxiety and pain contribute significantly to increased oxygen demand. This is especially true in intensive care, where oxygen transport is compromised or threatened in most patients (see Chapters 32 and 33).

CELLULAR ENERGETICS IN RESPONSE TO MOBILIZATION AND EXERCISE

The cardiopulmonary unit supports oxygen transport and cellular respiration (Weber, Janicko, Shroff, and Likoff, 1983). Oxygen is continually being used by every cell in the body for oxidative phosphorylation and the synthesis of adenosine triphosphate (ATP). The splitting of a phosphate bond from ATP to form adenosine diphosphate yields a considerable amount of energy for metabolism. The energy for this process comes from the reduction of hydrogen in the formation of water and carbon dioxide, which is the end products of the respiratory or electron transfer chain. These metabolic processes which comprise oxidative phosphorylation, take place in the mitochondria of the cells (Chapter 1).

The balance of oxygen consumption to delivery is precisely regulated to ensure that there is not only an adequate supply of oxygen, but also that under normal resting conditions approximately four times as much oxygen is delivered to the tissues as is used. This safety margin permits the immediate availability of oxygen when the system is perturbed by physical, gravitational, and mental challenges (see Chapter 1).

Anaerobic metabolism occurs during all out short sprint type activities, e.g., hockey, soccer and volley ball. Although PTs tend to focus on aerobic rather than anaerobic training, in conditions where oxygen delivery is significantly compromised, patients may rely on anaerobic metabolism to sustain ATP production and break down to provide energy. Although anaerobic exercise implies that the exercise is performed in the absence of oxygen, anaerobic metabolism provides a short-term means of supporting phosphorylation using substrates other than oxygen to generate and split ATP. If insufficient oxygen is available, the amount of ATP that can be generated anaerobically is limited. Thus this process can only be sustained for a short period. Lactic acid accumulates in the blood during anaerobic metabolism. In healthy, untrained individuals, lactic acid increases exponentially at an exercise intensity of about 55% of maximal aerobic capacity (McArdle, Katch, and Katch, 1994). Anaerobic capacity and specifically the anaerobic threshold can increase with training, however, anaerobic training effects are less significant compared with the training effects achieved with aerobic training.

Anaerobic metabolism is thought to be triggered by tissue hypoxia. The term anaerobic is a misnomer in that oxygen is needed to pay the oxygen debt that it creates. Thus in health, the need for oxygen is de-layed rather than eliminated. In disease states, anaerobic metabolism occurs when a patient's oxygen transport system cannot meet the metabolic demand required, e.g., patients with sepsis and multisystem organ failure. Serum lactate levels are significantly elevated in these patients, resulting in metabolic acidosis, which is extremely unfavorable to the maintenance of homeostasis.

During exercise, the cellular PO_2 is lower than the surrounding interstitial fluid PO_2. Oxygen diffuses rapidly through cell membranes. At the onset of physical exercise, the increased metabolic demand of the muscle and supporting tissues increases the oxygen diffusion gradient. Feedback mechanisms are triggered to increase oxygen delivery, which depends primarily on arterial oxygen content and cardiac output. The first line of defense is the response to an increase in pericellular pH. The concentration of carbon dioxide is increased which, as a result of the decrease in pH, facilitates the dissociation of oxygen from hemoglobin, that is, it shifts the oxyhemoglobin dissociation curve to the right. The cardiac output ($CO = SV \times HR$) increases commensurate with overall metabolic demand. The immediate response to oxygen deficit is an increase in CO to increase oxygen delivery. This averts arterial desaturation which is not normally observed in health even with extreme exertion.

The increase in systemic CO results in increased venous return and pulmonary CO. To oxygenate a greater volume of blood in the lungs, an increased volume of air must be inspired. To effect an increase in VE, tidal volume (VT) and respiratory rate (RR) are increased. At low intensities of exercise, VT increases disproportionately to RR, whereas at moderate to high intensities, VT plateaus and further increases in VE are effected by an increase in RR (Jones and Campbell, 1982). Exercise is associated with a small but significant increase in airway diameter and length of pulmonary structures, hence, a reduction is airway resistance. Zone 2, that is, the zone of greatest ventilation to perfusion (V/Q) matching of the lungs, is increased as a result of pulmonary capillary dilatation and recruitment. Diaphragmatic excursion is enhanced and the distribution of ventilation and perfusion is more uniform throughout the lung, which helps minimize atelectasis and airway closure. Exercise increases the excursion, hence, inflation of the lungs in three planes (i.e., anteroposterior, transverse, and cephalocaudal, particularly in the upright positions).

Rhythmic inflation and deflation of the lungs associated with physical activity has several clinically important physiologic effects. First, this action increases alveolar ventilation by a primary increase in tidal volume. Second, exercise-induced lung motion facilitates lymphatic flow and drainage. Optimal lymphatic drainage is essential to maintain optimal lung fluid balance with the increased volume of blood being processed through the pulmonary circulation and lung parenchyma. This action may explain, in part, the beneficial effect of mobilization on the distribution and function of pulmonary immune factors (Pyne, 1994). The increased movement of the lungs during exercise has a primary effect on mucociliary transport and mucus clearance (Wolff, Dolovich, Obminski, and Newhouse, 1977). Related to its effects on mucociliary transport, physical activity may help minimize bacterial colonization in the airways, hence, reduce the risk of pulmonary infection (Skerrett, Niederman, and Fein, 1989). Finally, lung movement stimulates surfactant production and its distribution over parenchymal tissue. Surfactant is essential for reducing surface tension in the alveoli, maintaining alveolar stability, maintaining lung compliance, thereby, minimizing airway closure and areas of lung collapse.

The heart and peripheral circulation are primed and respond to the increased demands of acute exercise. Hemodynamic adjustments occur immediately with the onset of exercise stress. To maximize the CO available, blood moves from the venous capacitance reservoirs such as the venous compartments of the gut and extremities, particularly the legs. At rest, most of the circulation, 70%, is contained within the highly compliant venous circulation. The Starling Law of the heart regulates the forward movement of blood commensurate with the volume of blood that is received. The heart chambers are normally distensible and adjust to changing volumes of blood returning to the heart and pump more forcefully to eject it through the pulmonary and peripheral circulations.

Muscle enzymes that extract oxygen at the cellular level are also primed and are produced commensurate with chronic metabolic demand.

EFFECTS OF MOBILIZATION AND EXERCISE ON OXYGEN TRANSPORT

In health, optimal function of oxygen transport depends on the integrity of each step in the oxygen transport pathway and the interdependent function of all the steps. As a result of cardiopulmonary and cardiovascular dysfunction, one or more steps in the oxygen transport pathway can be affected. Because of the interdependence of the steps in the pathway and the ability of functional steps to compensate for dysfunctional steps, gross measures of the efficacy of gas exchange and oxygenation can be normal. The number of steps affected by disease and the severity of the disease determines the degree of impairment of oxygen transport overall and the degree to which this is reflected in gross measures of oxygen transport as a whole.

To optimize the capacity of the various steps in the oxygen transport pathway, the oxygen transport system needs to be exposed to two principal stressors: (1) gravitational stress and (2) exercise stress. These stressors are tantamount to life in that they enhance the biochemical, physical and mechanical efficiency of the various steps in the oxygen transport pathway, and the patient's ability to respond rapidly to changes in the physical environment.

The fact that the absence of gravitational stress and exercise stress are the two primary factors contributing to bed rest deconditioning supports the exploitation of both gravitational and exercise stress in remediating cardiopulmonary dysfunction. Therefore mobilization and exercise are the two most physiologic interventions available to the PT for remediating cardiopulmonary dysfunction.

PRESCRIPTION OF MOBILIZATION AND EXERCISE: ACUTE RESPONSES

The clinical decision-making process involved in defining the optimal mobilization and exercise stimulus is multifactorial. Based on the patient's history, history of the present illness, assessment, and results of the lab tests and procedures, the integrity of each step in the oxygen transport pathway is determined, and the integrity of this system overall to preserve arterial oxygenation and pH. The box on p. 271 shows some common conditions associated with acute car-

Acute Pathophysiological Conditions That Benefit From the Acute Effects of Mobilization and Exercise
Atelectasis
Pulmonary consolidation
Pulmonary infiltrates
Bronchopulmonary and lobar pneumonias
Bronchiolitis
Alveolitis
Pleural effusions
Acute lung injury and pulmonary edema
Hemothorax
Pneumothorax
Cardiopulmonary insufficiency
Cardiopulmonary sequelae of surgery
Cardiopulmonary sequelae of immobility

diopulmonary dysfunction for which a rational basis can be made for exploiting the acute effects of mobilization as a primary treatment intervention.

If the patient presents with *acute* cardiopulmonary dysfunction, then primarily the acute effects of mobilization are indicated. These effects are distinct from those that occur on assuming the upright position. The majority of patients benefits most from a mobilization and exercise stimulus when they are in the upright position. The effects of being upright vs. exercise, however, need to be considered separately so that the benefits of their individual and combined contributions can be determined as well as any adverse reactions. The physiological benefits of acute exercise are shown in the box on p. 272. The principal effects that remediate acute cardiopulmonary dysfunction are increased VE secondary to increased VT, RR, or both; improved air flow rates and mucus transport. Cardiac output is increased secondarily to increased stroke volume (SV), heart rate (HR) or both, and increased tissue perfusion. The particular benefits of acute mobilization and exercise that need to be

exploited are directed at each patient's specific pathophysiological deficits. Once the specific effects of acute mobilization or exercise that are needed are identified and matched to the patient's pathophysiology, then the mobilization or exercise stimulus can be prescribed (see box on p. 273).

The increased metabolic demand of acute exercise results in a slight increase in airway diameter, increased VE, alveolar ventilation (VA), VT, RR, air flow rates, CO, SV, HR, blood pressure (BP), rate pressure product (RPP), that is, product of heart rate and systolic blood pressure (RPP is highly correlated with myocardial oxygen consumption, and therefore myocardial work) oxygen consumption (V_{O_2}), and carbon dioxide production (V_{CO_2}). The area of greatest ventilation to perfusion matching in the lungs, zone 2, is increased secondary to increased dilatation and recruitment of pulmonary capillaries (West, 1995).

The hemodynamic benefits of exercise are maximized in the upright position compared with recumbent positions in that exercise alone fails to counter the loss of volume regulating mechanisms associated with recumbency (Sandler, 1986) See Chapter 18 for the effects of position changes.

Mobilization and exercise stimulate the endocrine system. Catecholamines, released to support the cardiovascular system, sustain a given exercise work rate. Increased sympathetic activity secondary to mobilization can help reduce the patient's need for sympathomimetic pharmacologic agents (Bydgeman and Wahren, 1974). Sympathetic nerve stimulation, for example, is increased and sympathetic neurotransmitters are processed more efficiently. This is a significant effect that can be used as a goal for the prescription of mobilization.

Central nervous system (CNS) responses to mobilization include arousal and priming of the various organ systems involved (Browse, 1965).

The prescription of mobilization and exercise to stimulate their acute benefits parallels that of the prescription of exercise for its long-term, central and peripheral aerobic effects. The exercise parameters to achieve long-term adaptations in healthy people have been well-defined by the American College of Sports Medicine (1994) (Table 17-1) and are well-accepted. The individual engages in aerobic exercise at a heart

Acute Physiological Effects of Mobilization and Exercise

Pulmonary System

↑ Regional ventilation

↑ Regional perfusion

↑ Regional diffusion

↑ Zone 2 (i.e., area of ventilation perfusion matching)

↑ Tidal volume

↑ or ↓ Breathing frequency

↑ Minute ventilation

↑ Efficiency of respiratory mechanics

↓ Airflow resistance

↑ Flow rates

↑ Strength and quality of a cough

↑ Mucociliary transport and airway clearance

↑ Distribution and function of pulmonary immune factors

Cardiovascular System

Hemodynamic effects

↑ Venous return

↑ Stroke volume

↑ Heart rate

↑ Myocardial contractility

↑ Stroke volume, heart rate and cardiac output

↑ Coronary perfusion

↑ Circulating blood volume

↑ Chest tube drainage

Peripheral circulatory effects

↓ Peripheral vascular resistance

↑ Peripheral blood flow

↑ Peripheral tissue oxygen extraction

Lymphatic System

↑ Pulmonary lymphatic flow

Lymphatic System—*con't*

↑ Pulmonary lymphatic drainage

Hematologic System

↑ Circulatory transit times

↓ Circulatory stasis

Neurological System

↑ Arousal

↑ Cerebral electrical activity

↑ Stimulus to breathe

↑ Sympathetic stimulation

↑ Postural reflexes

Neuromuscular System

↑ Regional blood flow

↑ Oxygen extraction

Endocrine System

↑ Release, distribution, and degradation of catecholamines

Genitourinary System

↑ Glomerular filtration

↑ Urinary output

Gastrointestinal System

↑ Gut motility

↓ Constipation

Integumentary System

↑ Cutaneous circulation for thermoregulation

Multisystemic Effects

↓ Effects of anesthesia and sedation

↓ Deleterious cardiopulmonary effects of surgery

↓ Risk of loss of gravitational stimulus (when in conjunction with the upright position) and exercise stimulus

---

Clinical Decision Making and Prescription of Acute Mobilization and Exercise

Step 1

Identify ALL factors contributing to deficits in oxygen transport (Chapter 1), that is, those factors contributed to by:

1. The underlying pathophysiology of the disease or condition

2. Immobility and recumbency

3. Extrinsic factors related to the patient's care, and

4. Intrinsic factors related to the individual patient

Step 2

Determine whether mobilization and exercise are indicated, and if so, which form of either will specifically address the oxygen transport deficits identified in Step 1.

Step 3

Match the appropriate mobilization or exercise stimulus to patient's oxygen transport capacity.

EXAMPLES: activities of daily living (ADLs), walking unassisted, standing erect with assist and taking a few steps, transferring from bed to chair*, seated dangling position over bed side, moving in bed†

Step 4

Set the intensity within therapeutic and safe limits of the patient's oxygen transport capacity.

Step 5

Combine the various body positions especially in the erect position with the following maneuvers:

1. Thoracic mobility exercises, that is, flexion, extension, side flexion, and rotation

2. Active, active assist, or passive ROM exercises

3. Breathing control exercises especially coordinated with body movements

4. Coughing, spontaneous and voluntary, supported by self or others

Step 6

Set the duration of the mobilization sessions based on the patient's responses (i.e., changes in measures and indices of oxygen transport) rather than time.

Step 7

Repeat the mobilization session as often as possible based on its beneficial effects and on is being safely tolerated by the patient.

Step 8

Increase the intensity of the mobilization stimulus, duration of the session, or both commensurate with the patient's capacity to maintain optimal oxygen transport when confronted with an increased mobilization stressor, and in the absence of distress; monitored variables to remain within predetermined threshold range.

---

*All sitting positions require upright erect sitting; propped up, semi recumbent, slouched or slumped positions although approximating the upright position are NOT physiologically comparable

†No amount of movement or activity is too small to derive benefits acutely or over long-term

---

TABLE 17-1

Exercise Prescription Parameters to Elicit Long-Term Aerobic Benefits In Healthy Persons

	SPECIFICATIONS
Parameter	
Exercise Type	Rhythmic activity, involving the large muscle groups; the legs, arms or both
Intensity	70% to 85% of the age predicted maximum heart rate or observed maximum heart rate
Duration	20 to 40 minutes
Frequency	Three to five times a week
Course	6 to 8 weeks

Adapted from the American College of Sports Medicine, (1994). Guidelines for exercise testing and prescription. (6th ed.). Philadelphia: Williams and Wilkins.

Mobilization Stimuli
Ambulation—independently, with one or more assisting
Cycle ergometry—lower and upper extremity
ADLs—independently, with one or more assisting
Standing—independently, with one or more assisting
Transferring—independently, with one or more assisting
Dangling—independently, with one or more assisting
Cycle ergometry in bed (lower extremity)
Turning in bed
Bed exercises
Supplemental Aids and Devices for Mobilization
For the patient:
Walking aids, such as crutches, cane, intravenous (IV) pole, wheelchair, orthoses
Weights
Pulleys
Monkey bar
Grab bars
Grab rope
For the PT:
Transfer belts
Mechanical lifts for patients

rate intensity of 70% to 85% of a maximum heart rate, for 20 to 40 times three to five times a week. Aerobic training effects are usually observed within 2 months.

In severely deconditioned individuals and in some patient populations, however, such a prescription would not be realistic, ethical, or indicated. Thus exercise is prescribed that is sufficient to elicit progressive physiological adaptation within defined limits of certain objective and subjective responses, such as perceived exertion, shortness of breath, angina, discomfort/pain, and general fatigue. Considerable research, however, is needed to refine the prescription of mobilization and exercise for their acute effects in patients with acute cardiopulmonary and cardiovascular dysfunction. Furthermore, the specifications for low level exercise needed to affect long-term aerobic adaptation have not been elucidated in detail. However, based on physiological understanding of acute exercise responses and cardiopulmonary pathophysiology, principles for prescribing mobilization for acute cardiopulmonary conditioning can be formulated.

Mobilization Testing

Evaluating a patient's response to a mobilization stimulus can be assessed in two ways. First, the patient can be exposed to a mobilization challenge test. The patient is monitored before, during, and after mobilization activities (see box at left). Relatively low-intensity activities such as bed exercises, moving in bed, changing body position, sitting up, dangling over bed side, transfer to chair, chair exercises, and short walks with assistance, constitute a sufficient stimulus to elicit the acute effects of exercise. The degree of assistance required to perform the activity should be noted, since this significantly influences the patient's individual effort. Second, if the patient's status is unstable and oxygen transport is severely jeopardized, then monitoring a patient during standard care and procedures, such as turning the patient, ADLs, nursing and medical procedures, can provide an indication of the patient's physiological responses to mobilization and the capacity of the oxygen transport system to meet the metabolic demands imposed. No movement is too small. Any movement that is sufficient to perturb the oxygen transport system, no matter how minimal, is sufficient to elicit short- and long-term gains.

Monitoring

Patients for whom mobilization is prescribed require monitoring. Because of the stress to the oxygen transport system that mobilization elicits, the following variables in addition to the oxygen transport variables, are most useful to monitor: heart rate (HR), systolic and diastolic BP, RPP, RR, Sao_2, arterial blood gases, ECG and subjective responses.

Mobilization Prescription

Prescribing a mobilization stimulus for its acute effects parallels the prescription of exercise for its long-term effects with some important differences. In an acute patient, a mobilization or stimulus often results in a greater response gain than such a stimulus in subacute and chronic patients. In addition, to the rapid favorable response an acute patient may have to acute exercise, the patient may exhibit a negative response just as quickly. Thus judicious monitoring of treatment response in these patients is essential.

The scheduling of and preparation for a mobilization session is crucial to the response that can be expected. The following conditions should be adhered to as closely as possible; and their details should be recorded so that any factor that significantly influences the response to treatment can be identified. The patient should be rested, not have eaten heavily

in the previous couple of hours, be as attentive and aroused as possible and be experiencing minimal pain or discomfort. Review of a patient's medication schedule will ensure treatments are well-timed with respect to pain medications, and medications that interfere with a good treatment response, such as narcotics. The patient's clothing should not be restrictive, and any lines, leads, and catheters should not be taut. Any equipment, monitors, and IVs need to be appropriately positioned to avoid disconnections or mishaps. Mobilizing the patient in intensive care requires positioning of the mechanical ventilator and other supports before moving the patient. The PT must prepare personnel before moving a patient particularly if one or more assists are required. Despite the number of persons assisting, the goal is usually to have the patient perform as much of the mobilization activity as possible. Even small degrees of physical movement can provide sufficient stress to the cardiopulmonary system to be beneficial.

The basic components of the mobilization session are comparable to the components of an exercise session described by the American College of Sports Medicine for long-term training effects (Figure 17-1). Wherever possible, the session should include the following components: warm-up, steady-rate, cool-down, and recovery. These components are less distinct when a patient has minimal functional capacity or is being mobilized to remediate acute cardiopulmonary dysfunction. The rhythmic movement of large muscle groups is ideal. Prolonged static maneuvers are usually avoided particularly if the patient is severely ill, because of their disproportionate hemodynamic response. The movements that are usually considered when mobilizing a patient include: turning, sitting up, shifting, transferring, standing and taking some steps. These can be extremely metabolically demanding for patients with significant acute cardiopulmonary dysfunction. Thus pacing the mobilization session allows the patient to rest between stages. The patient is reassured and encouraged to relax and coordinate deep breathing and coughing with the activity. Throughout the session, attention is given to the patient's biomechanical alignment, and postural erectness and stability. Back extension or body positioning minimizes slumping of the chest wall and compromised ventilation. In this way, chest

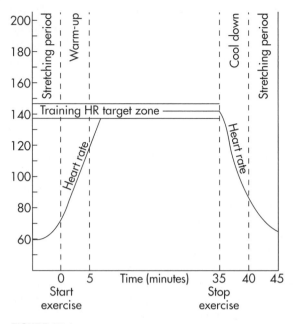

FIGURE 17-1
Components of the exercise training session (i.e., stretching, warmup, training zone, cool down, and stretching.

wall expansion is maximized in three dimensions. The erect position is efficient and requires the least amount of energy to maintain. Less demand is placed on the accessory muscles of respiration in erect sitting, and this effect is enhanced further with leaning forward and support of the arms.

Mobilization Training

With respect to oxygen transport, the purpose of the mobilization session is to elicit the immediate effects of an exercise stimulus, no matter how minimal. The optimal therapeutic dose of the stimulus is based on the patient's presentation and history and the specific parameters are determined by the goals of the treatment and the acute effects of exercise that are indicated. The intensity of mobilization for many patients, for example, is that intensity that elicits optimal tidal volumes and VA, increased breathing frequency and air flow rates, enhanced mucociliary transport, and cough stimulation,

without arterial desaturation, hemodynamic instability, or respiratory distress.

Over time, exposure to an acute exercise stimulus of an appropriate intensity, for an appropriate duration and at an appropriate frequency will stimulate long-term exercise adaptation to that stimulus. Underprescribing the exercise stimulus results in less potent effects and overprescribing results in an excessive, deleterious effect. Although the latter may be tolerated in the short run, the patient's well-being may be jeopardized, such as suboptimal treatment response, overtraining signs and symptoms, and injuries.

The duration of the session and the frequency of sessions should be response-dependent rather than time-dependent. The optimal mobilization threshold, that is, physiological variables increased but not in excess of predetermined acceptable and safe limits, should be maintained for as long as possible within the patient's fatigue and comfort levels, and in the absence of adverse responses. The mobilization session should be repeated as often as the patient can tolerate, that is, exhibits a beneficial response or no deterioration and adequately restores between treatments. Treatment sessions for acute cardiopulmonary dysfunction are usually shorter and more common than for the patient with chronic cardiopulmonary dysfunction. The patient's condition changes rapidly both with respect to improvement as well as deterioration. Progression of mobilization for its immediate acute effects is usually rapid. Progression of exercise for its long-term effects may occur every several weeks whereas progression of mobilization for its acute effects may range from as frequently as every treatment to every few days. Over time, exposure to a progressive mobilization stimulus leads to long-term physiological adaptations throughout the oxygen transport pathway.

Monitoring

The more acute the patient's condition, the more physiologic variables usually need to be recorded. More objective measures are available in special care and intensive care units (ICUs). Subjective responses are also vital components of determining the adequacy of the mobilization stimulus; however, severely ill patients are often unable to respond effectively. Compared with the condition of chronic patients, the condition of acute patients tends to vary more within and between sessions and afterward, which necessitates greater monitoring.

Monitoring needs to be performed continuously for patients for whom acute mobilization has been prescribed. First, a baseline of the patient's resting metabolic state needs to be established. Second, the metabolic responses to stimuli that perturb oxygen transport and the lability of this response needs to be established. Obtaining such a profile provides some indication of the upper limit of the target intensity range for mobilization. The target intensity range can be defined in terms of an upper and lower level of various physiologic variables. The most commonly used are HR, BP, RPP, RR, perceived exertion or breathlessness. Monitoring during nursing procedures and other types of routine care provides an indication of the patient's functional capacity without having to conduct a modified exercise test.

Alternatively, a mobilization or exercise challenge can be given. The patient's response is compared with resting baseline measures. The quality as well as the immediacy of the response is documented. The characteristics of the quality of response is also recorded. Is the response commensurate with the intensity of the exercise stimulus? With cessation of exercise do the responses revert to baseline? If so, how fast? Do the variables return to baseline or remain above baseline?

The variables to be measured depend on the patient (see Chapters 1 and 16). Most commonly, HR, ECG, BP, RPP, RR, and subjective symptoms, are basic measures and indices of exercise response that require no invasive procedures. At the other end of the spectrum is the critically ill patient who has various invasive lines and monitoring equipment, including hemodynamic monitoring and intracranial pressure monitoring. This patient requires more specific and frequent measures of oxygen transport.

Adaptation to an Acute Mobilization Stimulus

When an individual is exposed to repeated exercise stress, that is, of a specific threshold intensity, and for a response-dependent duration and frequency, there is a cumulative adaptive response to that repeated stimulation, or a long-term, training response. In deconditioned individuals with low functional work capacity, or whose oxygen transport system has been compromised by disease, the exercise intensity associated with relatively low-intensity mobilizing activities such as bed exercises, moving in bed, sitting up, dangling over bed side, transferring to chair, chair exercises, and short walks with assistance, constitute a sufficient stimulus for long-term adaptation. However, optimal adaptation only occurs if these activities are prescribed at a requisite intensity, duration, and frequency and the exercise prescription progressed commensurate with the individual's adaptation.

Mobilization activities prescribed to enhance oxygen transport, can be coupled with resistive muscle work to increase muscle strength and endurance (e.g., weights, use of a monkey bar for moving in bed and sitting up, manual resistive exercise, the use of wrist or ankle weights, ergometry, and walking). Coordinating postural, thoracic mobility and upper extremity exercises with inspiratory and expiratory efforts can be effective in stimulating increased VT, and improved ventilation and perfusion matching. Chapters 21 and 22 illustrate how such movement and breathing patterns can be coupled to maximize oxygen transport in neurological patients. Such coordinated exercise, however, can also be used with patients with acute cardiopulmonary conditions. Isometric type exercises, postures that require increased muscle work for stabilization, and activities that elicit the Valsalva maneuver produces disproportionate hemodynamic responses, which could be detrimental. The capacity of the patient to respond appropriately to these loads needs to be established beforehand.

In the management of acute cardiopulmonary dysfunction, the parameters of mobilization stimuli include a relatively low intensity (although often perceived as intense by the patient), short duration, and high frequency of sessions. If the patient is severely compromised (e.g., end-stage heart or lung disease) interrupted or interval training is indicated. This type of training is characterized by either on-off exercise, which allows for rest in between bouts of exercise, or high-low intensity of activity. The volume of work

TABLE 17-2

Relationships Among Mobilization and Exercise Prescription Parameters

Activity and Relative Intensity

	SESSION DURATION	SESSION FREQUENCY
Mobilization activities	5 to 20 min	1 time per 1 to 2 hours to 4 to 6 times per day
Interval continuous aerobic exercise	5 to 20 min	1 time per 1 to 2 hours to 4 to 6 times per day
Continuous aerobic exercise (light)	5 to 20 min	1 time per 1 to 2 hours to 4 to 6 times per day
Continuous aerobic exercise (moderate)	20 to 40 min	2 to 3 times daily to once daily
Continuous aerobic exercise (heavy)	20 to 40 min	Daily to 3 to 5 times per week

that can be achieved in an interrupted protocol by a severely compromised patient, is significantly greater than during continuous activity. With physiological adaptation over time, the exercise period can be increased and the rest period decreased, and possibly eliminated. When high- and low-intensity exercise is alternated the work load can be progressed by either increasing the respective loads in each phase or by increasing the duration of the higher load period. If the patient has low functional work capacity but sufficient physiological reserve, adaptation can be rapid, necessitating small, frequent progressions. As the patient's aerobic capacity increases, the response gains are correspondingly smaller. If the patient has both poor functional capacity and poor physiological reserve capacity, progress would be correspondingly slower and less significant.

When mobilization activities are being prescribed to remediate acute cardiopulmonary dysfunction, particularly in patients in the ICU, extensive and often invasive monitoring is required. This permits detailed assessment, and ongoing metabolic assessment of the patient's treatment responses and recovery. With these supports, mobilization and exercise can be prescribed effectively in these patients. Judicious monitoring minimizes any inherent dangers of either under or over prescribing the intensity of the exercise stimulus (Part II). Special consideration has to be given to the fact that various monitoring leads, lines, and catheters may restrict certain body positions and activities. Such encumbrances, however, do not preclude most activities including ambulation. Moving relatively immobile patients who are tied to their beds with lines and leads is crucial, because it is these patients who benefit significantly from exercise stress and also succumb most severely to its removal.

The goal is to adapt the patient to multiple short mobilization sessions per day, as frequently as once per hour, and progressively increase the intensity of these sessions, reduce the duration and correspondingly reduce the frequency of sessions. Table 17-2 illustrates the inverse relationship between mobilization and exercise intensity, duration, and frequency of the sessions.

Multisystem Effects of Mobilization

Acute exercise affects most organ systems in addition to the cardiopulmonary and cardiovascular systems. The neurological system is primed for activity. To counter postural perturbations, reflexes and postural control adjustments are activated. Blood flow is increased to the working muscles commensurate with the intensity and duration, and therefore overall metabolic demand of the work. The endocrine system also adjusts to largely stimulate the cardiopulmonary and cardiovascular systems through a complex system of neurotransmitters to support the oxygen demands required of the work rate imposed.

PRESCRIPTION OF MOBILIZATION AND EXERCISE: LONG-TERM RESPONSES

In health, the long-term effects of exercise occur in response to a specific and sufficient exercise stimulus to which the individual is exposed for a finite period. With respect to aerobic training or adaptation, the essential

Long-Term Physiologic Effects of Mobilization and Exercise

Cardiopulmonary System

↓ Submaximal minute ventilation

↑ Respiratory muscle strength and endurance

↑ Collateral ventilation

↑ Pulmonary vascularization

Cardiovascular System

↑ Myocardial muscle mass

↑ Myocardial efficiency

Exercise-induced bradycardia

↓ Stroke volume at rest and submaximal work rates

↓ Resting heart rate and blood pressure

↓ Submaximal heart rate, blood pressure, and rate pressure product

↓ Submaximal perceived exertion and breathlessness

↑ Efficiency of thermoregulation

↓ Orthostatic intolerance when performed in the upright position

Hematologic System

↑ Circulating blood volume

↑ Optimize number of red blood cells

↑ Optimize hematocrit

↓ Cholesterol

↓ Blood lipids

Central Nervous System

↑ Sense of well-being

↑ Concentration

Neuromuscular System

Enhanced neuromotor control

↑ Efficiency of postural reflexes associated with type of exercise

↑ Reflex control

↑ Movement efficiency and economy

Musculoskeletal System

↑ Muscle vascularization

↑ Myoglobin

↑ Muscle metabolic enzymes

↑ Glycogen storage capacity

↑ Improved biomechanical efficiency

↑ Movement economy

Muscle hypertrophy

↑ Muscle strength and endurance

↑ Ligament tensile strength

Maintain bone density

Endocrine System

↑ Efficiency of hormone production and degradation to support exercise

Immunological System

↑ Resistance to infection

Integumentary System

↑ Efficiency of skin as a heat exchanger

↑ Sweating efficiency

---

training parameters appear in the box above. As adaptation to the exercise stimulus occurs, each step in the oxygen transport system becomes more efficient facilitating oxygen delivery, uptake and extraction at the cellular level. The long-term effects of aerobic exercise are summarized in the box above. In addition to an increase in maximal oxygen consumption, training results in an exercise-induced bradycardia and increased stroke volume at rest and a reduction in the physiological demands of submaximal work rates. Specifically, ventila-tion and hemodynamic responses to submaximal exercise are decreased. The subjective experience of exercise stress is also reduced. These training effects are commensurate with increases in the efficiency of oxygen transport at each step in the pathway.

As the body adapts to the exercise training stimulus, the intensity needs to be increased to elicit further training benefit. This is the basis for the physiological adaptation to an exercise training stimulus. Depending on the goals of the exercise prescription, a

---

Chronic Pathophysiological Conditions That Benefit From the Long-Term Effects of Mobilization and Exercise

Cardiovascular Conditions

Congenital heart disease

Acquired heart disease

Postsurgical heart conditions

Angina

Hypertension

Hyperlipidemia

Hypercholesterolemia

Congestive heart failure

Heart transplantation

Peripheral vascular disease

Cardiopulmonary Conditions

Chronic obstructive pulmonary disease

Chronic ventilatory failure

Interstitial lung disease

Asthma

Cystic fibrosis

Postthoracotomy conditions

Lung transplantation

Neurological Conditions

Stroke

Parkinson's disease

Quadriplegia

Paraplegia

Cerebral palsy

Down syndrome

Neurological Conditions—*con't*

Multiple sclerosis

Poliomyelitis

Endocrine Conditions

Thyroid dysfunction

Diabetes mellitus

Neoplastic Conditions

Conditions Requiring Organ Transplantation

Pre- and postsurgical stages

Musculoskeletal Conditions

Osteoarthritis

Rheumatoid arthritis

Ankylosing spondylitis

Osteoporosis

Connective Tissue Conditions

Systemic lupus erythematosis

Nutritional Disorders

Obesity

Anorexia

Other Systemic Conditions

Chronic fatigue syndrome

Chronic depression

Alcoholism

Pregnancy

Renal disease

Liver disease

---

decision is made after several weeks whether the exercise intensity needs to be increased to further increase aerobic capacity, or whether a maintenance program is indicated. The training program is progressed by establishing a new exercise intensity usually based on 70% to 85% of the maximal heart rate achieved in a repeat of the initial exercise test.

EXERCISE TESTING AND TRAINING IN PATIENT POPULATIONS

Numerous conditions including nonprimary cardiopulmonary conditions have been shown to benefit from the long-term effects of aerobic exercise (see box above). For each patient, however, with each of these conditions, the exercise prescription

---

Common Indications for Exercise Testing in Patient Populations
Diagnosis
Coronary artery disease and vasospasm
Hyperreactive airway disease
Cardiac vs. pulmonary limitation to exercise
Peripheral vascular disease
Assessment
Maximal functional work capacity
Chest pain
Dyspnea
Endurance
Ability to work
Employment options
Cardiopulmonary and cardiovascular conditioning
Movement economy
Limitations to exercise
Effect of medication
Adequacy of diabetes management
Prescription
Exercise program
Medications

Relative and Absolute Contraindications to Exercise Testing
Absolute Contraindications
Congestive heart failure (CHF)
Acute EKG changes of myocardial ischemia
Unstable angina
Ventricular or dissecting aneurysm
Ventricular tachycardia
Multifocal ectopic beats
Repetitive ventricular ectopic activity
Untreated or refractory tachycardia
Supraventricular arrhythmia
Recent thromboembolic event (pulmonary or other)
Uncontrolled asthma
Uncontrolled heart failure
Pulmonary edema
Uncontrolled hypertension (above 250 mm Hg systolic, 120 mm Hg diastolic)
Acute infections
Relative Contraindications
Recent myocardial infarction (MI) (less than 4 weeks ago)
Aortic valve disease
Severe cardiomegaly
Pulmonary hypertension
Resting tachycardia
Resting electrocardiogram (ECG) abnormalities
Poorly controlled diabetes
Severe electrolyte disturbance
Severe systemic hypertension
Significant conduction disturbance
Complete atrioventricular block
Fixed rate pacemakers
Acute cerebrovascular disease (CVD)
Respiratory failure
Left ventricular failure
Epilepsy

Adapted from Jones, N.L. (1988). Clinical Exercise Testing. (3rd Ed.). Philadelphia: WB Saunders.

differs. Comparable with prescribing mobilization in acute conditions, prescribing exercise for long-term adaptations is based on the patient's presentation, history, premorbid status and conditioning level, lab and investigative reports related to physiologic reserve capacity, the exercise test and the goals of the exercise prescription.

Exercise Testing

Exercise testing no matter how modified can pose a potential risk to the patient, therefore exercise testing must have clear indications, and any contraindications must be ruled out. The indications for exercise testing are numerous (see box above, at left). They range from quantifying maximum functional capacity to as-

TABLE 17-3

Subjective Scales of Exercise Responses Based on the Borg Scale of Rating of Perceived Exertion

	PERCEIVED EXERTION	BREATHLESSNESS	DISCOMFORT/PAIN	FATIGUE
0	Nothing at all	Nothing at all	Nothing at all	Nothing at all
0.5	Very very weak	Very very light	Very very weak	Very very light
1	Very weak	Very light	Very weak	Very light
2	Weak	Light	Weak	Light
3	Moderate	Moderate	Moderate	Moderate
4	Somewhat strong	Somewhat hard	Somewhat strong	Somewhat hard
5	Strong	Hard	Strong	Hard
6				
7	Very strong	Very heavy	Very strong	Very heavy
8				
9				
10	Very very strong	Very very hard	Very very strong	Very very hard
	Maximal	Maximal	Maximal	Maximal

sessing endurance during low level ADLs. Contraindications are classified as either relative or absolute (see box on p. 281, at right). Absolute contraindications prohibit the safe conduction of an exercise test, whereas the presence of relative contraindications requires that the test, protocol, physiological variables monitored, or the end point of the test be modified. Both the indications for the test and any contraindications must be clearly established before performing an exercise test.

The guidelines used to test and train healthy people with no disease states are not directly generalizable to chronic medically-stable patient populations. Because of functional impairments in these patients (e.g., secondary to cardiopulmonary, cardiovascular, neuromuscular, and musculoskeletal dysfunction) exercise testing and training must be modified. Moreover, patients who are physically challenged experience more subjective symptoms in response to exercise compared with healthy people, therefore monitoring the subjective responses to exercise is essential. The Borg scale of rating of perceived exertion can be modified for clinical use to score breathlessness, discomfort, pain, and fatigue (Table 17-3) (Borg, 1970; 1982). If the endpoints of the scale are well-described and understood by the patient, then the ratings can be used to compare the patient's subjective exercise responses over repeated tests.

Depending on the functional impairments and capacity of the patient, the exercise test can be one of various types depending on the objective of testing and potential training. If exercise training is an objective of the exercise test, the activity used in the test should be comparable with that to be used in training. Physiological responses and adaptation to exercise are highly specific to the training stimulus (the specificity of exercise principle). Thus if walking is to be the training activity, the test should be a walking test rather than cycling.

There are numerous variants of standard exercise tests (Table 17-4). These are categorized as continuous and interrupted tests. Continuous tests include maximal and submaximal incremental tests and steady-rate tests, and interrupted tests include maximal interval and submaximal interval tests. Interrupted tests are designed for patients with low functional work capacity who cannot sustain prolonged periods of aerobic exercise. These patients can perform more work over time when the work load is administered in an interrupted or periodic manner. Specifically, the test alternates fixed periods of work and rest, or high and low intensities of exercise. The proportions of work-to-rest or

TABLE 17-4	
Exercise Tests That Can Be Applied to Patient Populations	
TEST TYPE	**INDICATIONS**
Continuous Tests	
Maximal	Generally medically-stable patient
	No significant musculoskeletal abnormalities
	Test maximal functional capacity
	Basis for aerobic exercise program
Incremental	Incremental work rates usually 2 to 5 minutes in duration
Steady-rate	Endurance test at a given work rate; usually a comfortable walking or cycling speed
Submaximal	For patients for whom maximal testing is contraindicated
Incremental	Approximate maximal exercise testing
	Test of near maximal functional capacity or some significant proportion of maximum
Steady-rate	Establish baseline of response to steady-rate exercise usually at 60 to 75% of predicted maximum heart rate
	Establishes an index of endurance, cardiopulmonary conditioning and may give an index of movement economy
Interrupted Tests	
Maximal or Submaximal	Establish level of functional capacity in patients with extremely low functional work capacity
	On-off protocol or high-low intensity protocol, such as 5 min on to 1 min off; alternate high- and low-intensity exercise in cycles, such as 1 minute high to 15 seconds low

high-to-low exercise intensity is set according to the patient's level of impairment. One patient, for example, may be able to tolerate 3 to 5 minutes of relatively high intensity work to 1 to 2 minutes of low-intensity work, whereas another patient may be able to tolerate only 1 minute of low intensity work to 10 to 20 seconds of rest.

For maximal standardization and the capacity to perform more comprehensive monitoring, stationary exercise modalities such as the treadmill, ergometer, or step are recommended. However, there may be indications to perform an exercise test without a modality, such as the 12-minute walk test or some variant like 6 or 3 minutes (McGavin, Gupta, and McHardy, 1976). Standardization of such tests, however, is more difficult. Practice has a significant effect on the results of the 12-minute walk test, thus this test needs to be repeated several times to achieve a valid test. Also, the instructions for this test are less well-standardized clinically compared with those for the

treadmill or ergometer, which jeopardizes stringent test control (Dean and Ross, 1992a).

Like other diagnostic or testing procedures, the validity and reliability of the exercise test depend on the quality of the procedures used. The preexercise test conditions and the preparation and testing procedures need to be standardized (see boxes on pp. 284–285). The test is terminated as soon as the sign or symptom criteria for terminating the test is reached or the criteria for prematurely terminating the test is reached (see box on p. 286). Recording the test conditions and procedures in detail is essential. An example of an exercise test data sheet that can be modified to any testing protocol using an exercise modality is shown in the box on p. 287, at left. Many patients are unable to be exercise tested using a modality. These patients can walk on a marked circuit. An example of an exercise test data sheet is shown in the box on p. 287, at right. Systematic and detailed record-keeping will maximize the test validity and its interpretation as well as ensure

---

Preexercise Test Conditions

Establish the indications for an exercise test.

Determine absolute and relative contraindications to conducting an exercise test.

Ensure patient is free of any acute illnesses including influenza and colds for 48 hours.

Ensure patient understands the purpose of the test and provides signed consent.

Ensure patient has not eaten heavily, has avoided caffeinated beverages and has refrained from smoking for at least 3 hours before testing.

Ensure patient is rested and has not exercised, or is not being excessively exerted for at least 24 hours before testing.

Ensure patient is appropriately dressed, for example, shorts, nonbinding clothes, short-sleeve shirt, socks, running or walking shoes that have proper support, and secured laces or fastenings.

Orthoses should be worn unless the test is evaluating changes in functional capacity with and without an orthosis.

Ensure patient understands the subjective rating scales and is able to read them when held at an appropriate distance.

Select the type of exercise test, the protocol and the exercise test termination criteria beforehand.

Ensure the patient is familiar with and has practiced performing the test or test activity preferably before the test day to reduce arousal, improve movement efficiency, and maximize test validity.

---

that the same procedures are used in follow up tests thereby maximizing the ability to compare test results. It is imperative that retests are conducted comparably in every respect to the original test with respect to patient preparation and the procedures.

Exercise Tests and Protocols

Depending on the functional capacity of the patient, the exercise test can be a continuous maximal, submaximal incremental or steady-rate, or an interrupted maximal or submaximal test. The protocol for the test and the end points to be used in terminating the test are determined beforehand depending on the indications for the test and the objectives. Some commonly used protocols are shown in Figure 17-2 along with a comparison of the energy expenditure of the various work stages in their protocols.

The 12-minute walk test and its variants, 6 minute- and 3 minute-walk tests, were designed to test patients with lung disease (McGavin, Gupta, and McHardy, 1976). These tests have been favored clinically, because they are functional and do not require exercise equipment. However, these tests are often used for patients who have extremely impaired

exercise capacity and are unable to tolerate being tested on an exercise modality. A major disadvantage, therefore is that the patient cannot be as comprehensively monitored. Thus patients need to be selected carefully to undergo a 12-minute walk test or one of its variants.

Knowledge of the patient's functional ability based on verbal report can be useful and can serve as a guideline for determining the exercise test, its parameters, and what the patient's termination criteria should be. Although these verbal reports do not replace an exercise test, they can be used as an adjunct. The oxygen cost diagram is shown in the box on p. 290, at left. This visual analog scale is constructed of a 100 mm line; the high end of the scale represents strenuous activity, that is, walking briskly uphill, and the low end of the scale represents no activity, or sleep. The patient crosses the line at the point where breathlessness does not allow continuation when at the patient's best. Figure 17-3 shows an incremental ladder of workloads associated with step increments in metabolic cost, that is, multiples of resting or near resting metabolic rate (resting metabolic rate = 1 MET, or 3.5 ml O_2/min/kg of body weight). The level of metabolic costs ranges from very light to very

---

Preparation and General Procedures for an Exercise Test

Preparation

Patient changes into exercise clothes and shoes (not new); ensure laces are secure.

If the ergometer is used, the seat-to-pedal distance must be established before the test, and the seat should be adjusted to allow for 15 degrees of knee extension when the foot is lowermost in the pedal in the revolution cycle; the knee must not extend fully.

Patient sits quietly in a supported chair to establish a resting baseline.

Monitors are attached (e.g., heart rate, ECG, blood pressure cuff, pulse oximeter) and the subjective rating scales are explained.

Testing procedures are explained and demonstrated; the patient has an opportunity to answer questions.

General Procedures

Unnecessary conversation and interaction with the patient is kept to a minimum throughout all stages of the test, including postexercise recovery, to optimize the validity of the measurements and the test results overall.

Resting baseline measures are taken over 5 minutes or until they have plateaued.

Patient stands on treadmill or sits erect on cycle ergometer with feet securely strapped into place on the pedals; the metatarsal heads should be positioned comfortably over the pedals.

Patient uses two fingers for balance on one side if possible when walking on the treadmill rather than a hand grip, or if on the ergometer, not the excessively grasp the handle bar.

Additional baseline measures are recorded in this position for 2 to 3 minutes or until the baseline is stable.

The test timer is started.

The warm-up portion of the protocol begins.

The selected protocol is carried out.

Patient is monitored objectively and subjectively at least every couple of minutes throughout all stages of the test, including postexercise recovery.

The test is terminated when the preset exercise test termination criteria or any of the criteria for prematurely terminating an exercise test are reached.

The cooldown begins.

When the cooldown portion of the protocol is complete, the patient moves to the supported chair for the postexercise recovery phase with legs slightly elevated and uncrossed.

Postexercise recovery continues until resting baseline measures have been reached or are within 5% to 10%.

Obtain a report from patient about how patient feels.

Disconnect the monitoring equipment.

Continue to observe patient for any untoward postexercise signs or symptoms.

---

heavy activities. One limitation of such charts on metabolic costs of various activities and exercise is that they can only be used as a rough guide in patients with cardiopulmonary compromise, as they do not take into consideration the increased work of breathing and work of the heart observed in patients with cardiopulmonary dysfunction.

Monitoring

Common variables measured during an exercise test include HR, ECG, systolic and diastolic BP, RPP, RR, Sao_2 and subjective responses such as perceived exertion, breathlessness, discomfort, pain, and fatigue. Measures are taken every few minutes after the patient has been exercising at a given intensity for a few minutes.

Criteria for Prematurely Terminating an Exercise Test

Miscellaneous

Wish of individual for any reason

Failure of monitoring equipment

General Signs and Symptoms

Fatigue

Lightheadedness, confusion, ataxia, pallor, cyanosis, dyspnea, nausea, or peripheral vascular insufficiency

Onset of angina

ECG Signs

Symptomatic supraventricular tachycardia

ST displacement (3 mm) horizontal or downsloping from rest

Ventricular tachycardia

Exercise-induced left bundle branch block

Onset of second- or third-degree atrioventricular block

R=wave on T=wave premature ventricular contractions (one)

Frequent multifocal premature ventricular contractions (frequent runs of three or more)

Atrial fibrillation when absent at rest

Appearance of a Q wave

Cardiovascular Signs

Any fall in blood pressure below the resting level

Exercise hypotension (> 20 mm Hg drop in systolic blood pressure)

Excessive blood pressure increase (systolic $\geq$ 220 or diastolic $\geq$ 110 mm Hg)

Inappropriate bradycardia (drop in heart rate greater than 10 beats/minute with increase or no change in work load)

Adapted from the American College of Sports Medicine, (1994). Guidelines for exercise testing and prescription. (6th ed.). Philadelphia: Williams and Wilkins.

Adapted from Jones, N.L. (1988). Clinical Exercise Testing. (3rd Ed.). Philadelphia: WB Saunders.

Exercise Training Prescription

One of the most common indications for exercise testing is to establish whether a training program is indicated and, if so, what the training parameters should be. The components of exercise training for patients is the same as for healthy people, specifically, selection of the type of exercise, and its intensity, duration, and frequency; and the course of training and its progression. The selection of the type of exercise for training and that used in the exercise test, is based on the objectives of training. The intensity is usually set at some propor-tion of the heart rate response, or some other response, to a maximum or near maximum work rate that was safely tolerated during the exercise test. The training intensity for a patient who is able to tolerate several incremental work stages on a graded exercise test may be optimal between 70% to 85% of the peak heart rate achieved in the test. A patient who is unable to tolerate a couple of increases in work stage, is more likely to benefit from an exercise intensity range of 60% to 75% of the peak heart rate achieved. In some patients, heart rate is an invalid indicator of exercise intensity either

---

**Exercise Test Data Sheet for Treadmill
or Ergometer**

Patient name:

Patient number:

Date:

	Weight (kg)
	Height (cm)
	Body mass index
Reason for test:	FEV_1
	FVC
Type of test:	FEV_1/FVC

- -

Minute	Work rate speed/grade (work/rpm)	HR	BP	RPP	RR	Sao_2	RPE
0							
1							
2							
3							
4							
5							
6							
—							
—							

Review of preexercise checklist

Level of hand support

Use of orthoses: type and side

How often does the patient experience the level of exertion reached in the test (e.g., 1×/week, 1×/month, 3×/day, etc.)

Reason for test termination

NOTE: *Relevant notes and comments include abnormal ECG changes, comments by patient, observations about coordination, and anxiety.

**Exercise Test Data Sheet for a Walk Test
on a Circuit**

Patient name:

Patient number:

Date:

	Weight (kg)
	Height (cm)
	Body mass index
Reason for test:	FEV_1
	FVC
Type of test:	FEV_1/FVC

- -

Minute	Work rate speed/grade (work/rpm)	HR	BP	RPP	RR	Sao_2	RPE
0							
1							
2							
3							
4							
5							
6							
—							
—							

Review of preexercise checklist

Level of hand support

Use of orthoses: type and side

How often does the patient experience the level of exertion reached in the test (e.g., 1×/week, 1×/month, 3×/day, etc.)

Reason for test termination

NOTE: *Relevant notes and comments include abnormal ECG changes, comments by patient, observations about coordination, and anxiety.

Treadmill protocols

Functional class:
- Normal and 1 — Healthy (dependent on age activity); Sedentary healthy
- 2 — Limited
- 3 — Symptomatic
- 4

Bicycle ergometer: 1 Watt = 60 KPDS; For 70 kg body weight (KPDS)

Bruce: 3 = minute stages (mph / %Gr)
Kattus (mph / %Gr)
Balke Ware: %Gr at 3.3 MPH, 1 = minute stages
Ellestad: 3/2/3 = minute stages (mph / %Gr)
USAFSam: 2 = or 3 = minute stages (mph / %Gr)
"Slow" USAFSam (mph / %Gr)
McHenry (mph / %Gr)
Stanford: %Gr at 3 mph; %Gr at 2 mph

METS	O$_2$ cost (ml/kg/min)	Bicycle KPDS (70 kg)	Bruce (mph/%Gr)	Kattus (mph/%Gr)	Balke Ware %Gr	Ellestad (mph/%Gr)	USAFSam (mph/%Gr)	"Slow" USAFSam (mph/%Gr)	McHenry (mph/%Gr)	Stanford %Gr @3 mph	Stanford %Gr @2 mph
16	56.0		5.5/20								
15	52.5		5.0/18								
14	49.0	1500			25						
13	45.5	1350	4.2/16	4/22	24, 23, 22						
12	42.0	1200		4/18	21, 20	6/15					
11	38.5			4/14	19, 18		3.3/25		3.3/21	22.5	
10	35.0	1050	3.4/14	4/10	17, 16	5/15				20.0	
9	31.5	900			15, 14		3.3/20	2/25	3.3/18	17.5	
8	28.0	750			13, 12	5/10			3.3/15	15.0	
7	24.5		2.5/12	3/10	11, 10		3.3/15	2/20	3.3/12	12.5	
6	21.0	600		2/10	9, 8	4/10	3.3/10	2/15	3.3/9	10.0	14
5	17.5	450	1.7/10		7, 6	3/10	3.3/5	2/10	3.3/6	7.5	10.5
4	14.0	300	1.7/5		5, 4	1.7/10	3.3/0	2/5		5.0	7
3	10.5	150			3, 2				2.0/3	2.5	3.5
2	7.0		1.7/0		1		2.0/0	2/0		0.0	
1	3.5										

FIGURE 17-2

Oxygen cost of work stages of some commonly used exercise test protocols. (Reprinted with permission from Froehlicher VF: *Exercise and the heart*, ed 2, Chicago, 1987, Year-Book.)

FIGURE 17-3
Energy cost in METS of activity and exercise.
(From Underhill, SL et al: *Cardiac nursing*, ed 2,
Philadelphia, 1989, JB Lippincott.)

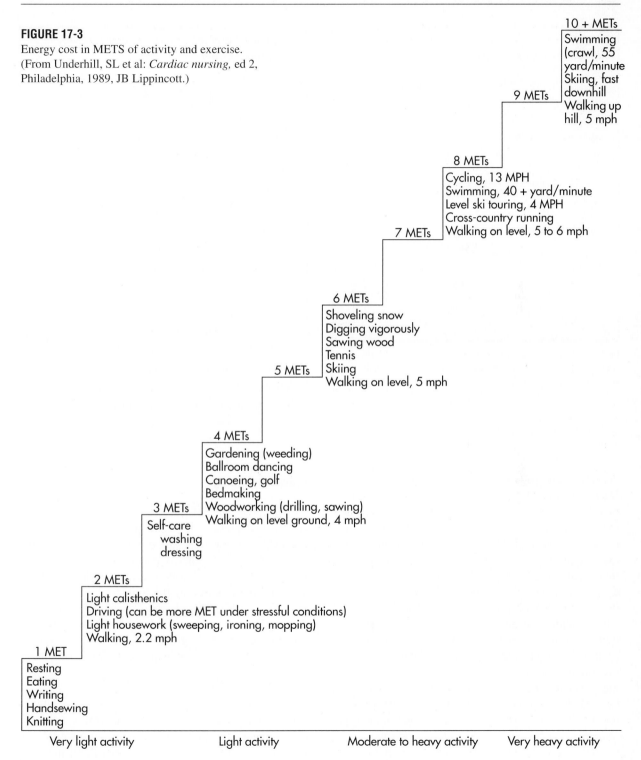

10 + METs
Swimming
(crawl, 55
yard/minute
Skiing, fast
downhill
Walking up
hill, 5 mph

9 METs

8 METs
Cycling, 13 MPH
Swimming, 40 + yard/minute
Level ski touring, 4 MPH
Cross-country running
Walking on level, 5 to 6 mph

7 METs

6 METs
Shoveling snow
Digging vigorously
Sawing wood
Tennis
Skiing
Walking on level, 5 mph

5 METs

4 METs
Gardening (weeding)
Ballroom dancing
Canoeing, golf
Bedmaking
Woodworking (drilling, sawing)
Walking on level ground, 4 mph

3 METs
Self-care
washing
dressing

2 METs
Light calisthenics
Driving (can be more MET under stressful conditions)
Light housework (sweeping, ironing, mopping)
Walking, 2.2 mph

1 MET
Resting
Eating
Writing
Handsewing
Knitting

Very light activity   Light activity   Moderate to heavy activity   Very heavy activity

Oxygen Cost Diagram Used to Assess Breathlessness on Exertion	
Brisk walking uphill	
Medium walking uphill	
	Brisk walking on the level
Slow walking uphill	
	Heavy shopping
	Medium walking
Bedmaking	
	Light shopping
Washing yourself	
	Slow walking on the level
Sitting	
	Standing
	Sleeping
	0

From McGavin CR, Artvinli M, Naoe H, and McHardy GJR: Dyspnea, disability, and distance walked: Comparison of estimates of exercise performance in respiratory disease, *BMJ* 1:822–823, 1978.

Patient's Check List Before Exercise Testing or Training Session
Feeling well over the past 48 hours
No cold or influenza
No temperature
No unaccustomed muscle or joint discomfort or pain
No chest tightness or pain
No unaccustomed breathing difficulty or fatigue
Adequate night's sleep
Have not eaten heavily within past 3 hours
Best time of day
Wearing or using orthoses, walking aids, and devices
Clothing appropriate for exercise conditions, such as indoors or outdoors
Appropriate socks and footwear that is comfortable, well-fitting and secured laces (double-knotted)
Have water within reach
Taken preexercise medications at specified time
Have nitroglycerine within reach (cardiac patients)
Have inhaler within reach (pulmonary patients)
Have sugar supply within reach (diabetics)

because of the pathology or medications (Dean, 1993; Dean and Ross, 1992b). Thus other responses such as blood pressure, arterial saturation, or subjective parameters such as rating of perceived exertion or breathlessness can be used. The duration and frequency of the exercise program are established based on the patient's functional capacity, physiological reserve capacity and exercise responses (see Table 17-2, for general guidelines). Patients with low functional capacities but with adequate physiologic reserve capacity respond to a training stimulus quickly (short training course), thus need to be progressed accordingly. Patients with low functional capacities, however, with limited physiologic reserve capacity, adapt more slowly (long training course). The shorter the training course, the sooner a retest is indicated to progress and reset the training parameters. To ensure that the patient continues to be trained safely and optimally, the training parameters should be progressed based on an exercise retest.

Exercise Training

General procedures

Before an exercise session, the patient needs to review a checklist to ensure that exercise is not contraindicated on that day. This is particularly important for patients whose conditions change rapidly or whose disease course tends to fluctuate, such as multiple sclerosis, cystic fibrosis, and chronic fatigue syndrome. The box above includes guidelines in preparation for exercise testing and training sessions. Such a checklist, however, must be tailored to each patient.

Specific procedures

In the supervised setting, the general procedures used in exercise training are comparable to those used for testing. Specifically, the patient prepares for the training session in a standardized manner, and is monitored according to his or her condition.

The components of the session are the same with respect to a warm-up, cool-down, and recovery. The main part of the exercise program, however, will usually be steady-rate or interrupted exercise. Varying work rates may be indicated for some patients.

In the majority of situations, the goal is to transfer the responsibility of surveillance and monitoring from the PT to the patient. Depending on the patient's pathology and ability to learn how to monitor exercise responses accurately, this process may take varying amounts of time.

Monitoring

For safety reasons and ensuring that the patient is within the target training range of the variables selected to set exercise intensity, the patient must be closely monitored. This is particularly true if the patient has any risk of untoward or adverse reactions to exercise. If patients are considered to be at any risk, then exercise training should only take place in a supervised setting. Stable patients may begin an exercise program in a supervised setting, but with training and education they usually can be transferred to an unsupervised setting. Education includes self monitoring of exercise responses, maintaining exercise intensity within the appropriate limits, and keeping a record of the details of their exercise sessions. When the patient is safely carrying out the exercise program independently in the community some mechanism is needed to follow-up on the patient's progress. If the objective is continued conditioning, then the patient needs to be rescheduled for a retest. If the patient is on a maintenance program, the PT is responsible for reminders about exercise and injury precautions, and notifying the PT or physician if significant adverse effects are observed.

PRESCRIPTION OF MOBILIZATION AND EXERCISE: PREVENTATIVE EFFECTS

Humans are designed to be upright and moving. When they are recumbent and inactive, gravitational stress (the vertical gravitational gradient) and exercise stress are removed. Bed rest is one of the most commonly used yet unquestioned therapeutic practices. Despite its widespread acceptance, the body positions it promotes, namely, being supine and immo-

---

Physiological Consequences of Bed Rest

I. Fluid volume redistribution

　　Decreased plasma and blood volume

　　Decreased total heart and left ventricular volumes

　　Increased hematocrit and hemoglobin

　　Diuresis and natriuresis

II. Muscular inactivity

　　Insulin resistance

　　Loss of muscle mass

　　Loss of muscle endurance

　　Loss of muscle strength

III. Altered distribution of weight and pressure

　　Venous stasis

　　Urine stasis, retention, tendency toward calculus formation

　　Hypercalciuria

　　Bone demineralization

　　Local skin changes

IV. Mixed or unknown etiology

　　Increased heart rate at rest and at all levels of activity

　　Decreased resting and maximum stroke volume

　　Decreased maximum cardiac output

　　Increased venous compliance

　　Increased risk of venous thrombosis and thromboembolism

　　Decreased orthostatic tolerance

　　Cardiovascular deconditioning

　　Decreased $VO_{2\,max}$

　　Anorexia

　　Constipation

　　Increased sensitivity to thermal stimuli; increased sweating and hyperemia

　　Alteration in clearance of some drugs

　　Increased anxiety, hostility, depression

　　Increased auditory threshold

　　Increase in focal point, decreased near point of visual acuity

From Underhill SL, Woods SL, Froehlicher ES, and Halpenny CJ: *Cardiac nursing,* ed 2, Philadelphia, 1989, JB Lippincott.

bile, is nonphysiologic (Chapter 18). The harmful sequelae of this posture have been well-documented (Dean and Ross, 1992b) yet the more severely ill the patient, the more-confined that individual is to the bed, and the greater the risk of multisystem complications (see box on p. 291).

The immediate effects of immobility that are observed are those associated with recumbency; these are followed within 24 to 48 hours by cardiopulmonary and musculoskeletal changes. Within 24 hours, significant fluid shifts occur and blood volume is reduced by 10% to 15%. Within days, these effects can significantly impair oxygen transport. These systemic effects are more profound in premature infants, young and older people, smokers, obese and deconditioned individuals. These effects are further compounded when a patient has either primary or secondary cardiopulmonary and cardiovascular compromise. The less aerobically fit an individual, the less physiological reserve is available in the cardiopulmonary and cardiovascular systems. In the event of a medical or surgical insult, such a patient will have an increased risk of morbidity and mortality than a more fit counterpart. Thus the importance of aerobic fitness cannot be overemphasized.

A primary effect of mobilization and exercise on the cardiopulmonary system is enhanced mucociliary transport and clearance (Wolff, Dolovich, Obminski, and Newhouse, 1977). Frequent body position changes are essential to maintain optimal bronchial hygiene and avoidance of pooling and stagnation of bronchial secretions, hence, airway obstruction and airflow resistance (Chapter 18).

The primary effects of bed rest on the cardiopulmonary system result from recumbency. Pulmonary sequelae of recumbency included reduced lung volumes and capacities, particularly functional residual capacity (FRC), residual volumes (RV) and forced expiratory volumes (FEVs) (Blair and Hickman, 1955; Craig, Wahba, Don, Couture, and Becklake, 1971; Hsu and Hickey, 1976; Powers, 1944; Risser, 1980; Svanberg, 1957). A reduction in FRC in supine position compared with the sitting position has been attributed to both a decrease in thoracic volume and an increase in thoracic blood volume, hence pulmonary venous engorgement (Sjostrand,

1951). Thus alveolar-arterial oxygen difference and arterial oxygen tension are reduced during periods of bed rest (Cardus, 1967; Clauss, Scalabrini, Ray, and Reed, 1968; Ray et al, 1974). Closing volumes are increased precipitating arterial desaturation in recumbent positions.

Cardiovascular sequelae of prolonged recumbency include an increase in resting and submaximal heart rate (Deitrick, Whedon, and Shorr, 1948), a decrease in maximum oxygen uptake (Saltin et al, 1968), and a decrease in total blood volume, plasma volume, and hematocrit (Deitrick et al, 1948; Saltin et al, 1968; Friman, 1979). The combination of an increase in blood viscosity and a decrease in venous blood flow results in an increased risk of thromboemboli (Lentz, 1981; Wenger, 1982).

Musculoskeletal changes that occur with bed rest deconditioning include loss of muscle mass and strength, muscle and ligament shortening, joint contractures, skin lesions, and decubitus ulcers (Rubin, 1988).

CNS changes include slowed electrical activity of the brain, emotional and behavioral changes, slowed reaction times, sleep disturbances, and impaired psychomotor performance (Rubin, 1988; Ryback, Lewis, and Lessard, 1971; Zubeck and MacNeil, 1966).

Metabolic changes that occur during periods of bed rest include reduced insulin sensitivity and glucose intolerance (Mikines, 1991), increased calcium excretion from bone loss and increased nitrogen excretion secondary to protein loss from atrophying muscle (Deitrick et al, 1948; Donaldson, Hulley, and McMillan, 1969; Hulley, Vogel, Donaldson, Bayers, Friedman, and Rosen, 1971).

Bed rest has been associated with a reduction in antibody counts, hence an increased risk of infection (Ahlinder, Birke, Norberg, and Plantin, 1970).

Of clinical significance is the fact that cardiopulmonary and cardiovascular deterioration occur at a faster rate than musculoskeletal deterioration, and that the rate of recovery from the ill effects of bed rest is generally slower than the rate of impairment (Kottke, 1966; Sandler, Popp, and Harrison, 1988).

The negative effects of bed rest are accentuated in older adults (Harper and Lyles, 1988), and are likely to further compound the oxygen transport and other deficits of patients with pathology.

HAZARDS OF BED REST

The literature on the negative sequelae of bed rest has been unequivocal for 50 years (Chobanian, et al., 1974; Dean and Ross, 1992b; Dock, 1944; Harrison, 1944; Ross and Dean, 1989). Thus the use of bed rest as a primary medical intervention requires considerable justification. The recumbent, immobile positions associated with bed rest adversely affect every organ system and particularly compromise oxygen transport by its direct negative effects on the cardiopulmonary and cardiovascular systems. This is particularly significant in that in conventional patient management there is a direct relationship between how sick the patient is and the amount of time confined to bed. In addition, the musculoskeletal and neurological systems are adversely affected.

The cardiovascular sequelae of bed rest primarily include the loss of fluid volume regulating mechanisms, diuresis, and loss of plasma volume. In turn, the hematocrit is increased, and the risk of developing deep vein thromboses and thromboemboli is increased. This is exacerbated by increases in blood viscosity, platelet count, platelet stickiness, plasma fibrinogen (Browse, 1965), and stasis of venous blood flow. The work of the heart is increased in the immobile, recumbent patient as is the work of breathing. The work of the heart is increased as a result of the increased filling pressures and heart rate associated with recumbency, and increased blood viscosity. The work of breathing is increased by the decreased lung volumes secondary to visceral encroachment on the underside of the diaphragm, increased intrathoracic blood volume, and restricted chest wall motion.

With bed rest, the blood vessels of the muscles and splanchnic circulation dilate. With prolonged bed rest, they may lose their ability to constrict. The ability of these vessels to constrict is essential to prevent the pooling of blood and maintain circulating blood volume in the upright position. Thus following bed rest, a patient may feel lightheaded or dizzy, or may faint.

With only a few days of bed rest, skeletal muscle atrophies leading to weakness, discoordination and balance difficulty (Lentz, 1981; Saltin, et al., 1968). With severe weakness, excessive strain may be placed on ligaments and joints. The limited positioning alternatives in bed may contribute to poor pos-

tural alignment, stiffness, and soreness. Bed rest allocates various body parts to being weight bearing. Skin breakdown most commonly occurs over boney prominences such as the sacrum, trochanters, elbows, scapulae, and heels. Muscles imbalance may result from poor postural alignment. Patients are at risk of bone demineralization. Of particular importance in older populations, patients with disabilities, postmenopausal women, and patients on steroids is calcium loss secondary to bed rest or sedentary lifestyle.

Bed rest affects psychological status. Patients may become depressed, sensorily deprived, or develop a psychoneurosis with prolonged bed rest.

The evidence supports the following:

1. Evidence supporting the wide spread use of bed rest as a therapeutic intervention is lacking.
2. Currently the use of bed rest is excessive and nonspecific.
3. Bed rest has multisystem negative effects and therefore must be used judiciously and specifically.
4. Alternative means of managing very ill patients, such as those in the intensive care, must be developed.

ALTERNATIVES TO THE NONSPECIFIC USE OF BED REST

With respect to developing alternative means of managing very ill patients rather than in the recumbent immobile positions, physical therapists need to become vocal in designing furniture and devices that are better suited to the patient's normal physiologic functioning and to the needs of that patient's course of recovery. Such appliances would include a greater number of neurologic and cardiac chairs in ICUs, which enable easy transfer of patients from bed to chair and upright positioning, greater availability of patient-lifting devices, and increased number of orderlies to assist with moving patients.

Rotating beds are electromechanical beds that turn the patient through an arc of about 30 degrees to either side from supine over a 3-minute period (Schimmel, Civetta, and Kirby, 1977). These beds are used for heavy care critically ill patients who are unable to turn themselves or are difficult to turn. Even though studies have shown these beds can enhance oxygenation in severely compromised patients such as patients with adult respiratory distress syndrome (Summer, Curry, Haponik, Nelson, and Elston, 1989; Yarnel, Helbock, and Schwiter, 1986), they need to be used selectively to avoid reliance on passive positioning with the bed vs. more active and active assisted patient positioning.

The use of tilt tables to promote mobilization can be hazardous in that leg movement is minimal. Passive standing on a tilt table constitutes a greater physiological stress than active standing. Upright sitting postures with the legs dependent may elicit greater physiological benefit than passive standing with less risk.

INDICATIONS FOR BED REST

Despite the universal acceptance of bed rest as a medical therapeutic intervention, indications for its therapeutic use have not been documented. Furthermore, considerably more is known about the adverse and potentially life-threatening hazards of bed rest than about its potential benefits. Bed rest should clearly be used as selectively as other medical interventions to ensure that specific benefits are being derived and the multisystemic negative sequelae are being minimized. Many procedures such as surgery are associated with considerable pain, thus being relatively immobile and recumbent in bed is believed to minimize postsurgical discomfort. In some cases, however, relative immobilization rather than confinement to bed may offer the same benefits without the dire risks. Patients who are severely limited are physically supported by a bed and do not have to work against the force of gravity. Minimizing the effects of gravity and the need to weight bear is often indicated in patients following orthopedic surgery. The bed enables a patient with multiple wounds and fractures to be immobilized and supported in a fixed position that is believed to promote healing. Conditions that are associated with edema require minimizing the effect of gravity on the affected limbs. Whether edema can be controlled by localized elevation rather than bed rest must be established. Some conditions particularly in the acute stages to reduce the work of the heart, such as MI, require some activity restriction, thus the use of the bed has been a mainstay of the early man-

agement of such patients. However, 30 years ago restriction to a chair was reported to be significantly more beneficial than restriction to bed in heart disease patients (Levine and Lowe, 1954). Despite this finding, many coronary patients continue to recline in beds rather than chairs. Mobilizing coronary patients and permitting bathroom privileges has also been reported to be less stressful than being confined to bed and having to use a bedpan (Andreoli et al, 1994).

Prescription of an Adequate Stimulus to Elicit the Preventative Effects of Exercise

Although much is known about the protective benefits of cardiopulmonary fitness and conditioning and about the negative effects of bed rest and immobility, little has been documented about defining the appropriate exercise stimulus to optimize the preventive effects of exercise for a given patient. The preventive effects of an exercise stimulus can be defined as that exercise dose that will maintain the patient's conditioning level and prevent deterioration. At present, the prescription of preventative mobilization and exercise is nonspecific. Research is needed to make exercise prescription for the preventative effects of exercise more scientifically based. For example, the following questions need to be answered:

- How do different types of exercise compare with respect to preventative aspects?
- Does exercising in some body positions elicit better preventive effects than other body positions?
- What principles establish which exercise intensity and duration are best?
- What principles establish how often the patient should be mobilized or should perform exercise?

The question arises as to what constitutes an adequate stimulus to maximize the preventive effects of exercise for a given patient. Although the preventive effects of exercise are accepted, this important question has not been adequately researched. Some general practices, however, have become accepted clinically. These include turning patients. The turning frequency that is widely accepted is every 2 hours.

There is no literature, however, to support greater preventive effects turning a patient every 2 hours vs. hourly or every 4 hours. Sitting up and ambulation are two other practices that are also widely used. The timing of these interventions, however, is often based on convenience and what else may be happening with the patient, or on a once or twice daily regimen rather than on a prescriptive basis. Patients who are sitting or walking for preventive reasons often assume suboptimal and even deleterious slumped or malaligned postures. Patients and their caregivers need to be reminded about the importance of proper body position at all times and be provided with appropriately supported chairs, firm bolsters, and adjustable beds that maintain optimal body positions.

Like exercise prescribed for its beneficial acute and long-term effects, exercise to elicit its optimal preventive effects should be prescribed based on the individual (e.g., age; premorbid functional work capacity; the type, distribution, and severity of disease; and within capabilities of patient). Such preventive mobilization or exercise must also be prescribed to avoid any deleterious effects on the patient's overall condition.

Frequent ambulation constitutes preventive exercise. Provided the patient does not require undue monitoring and has been cleared as a risk, preventive exercise can be encouraged by all team members. This role of exercise is quite distinct and separate from the therapeutic interventions of mobilization and exercise for their specific acute and long-term effects that are prescribed for the remediation of acute and chronic cardiopulmonary dysfunction. The application of mobilization and exercise for optimizing oxygen transport is the specific expertise and within the unique domain of the PT.

ASSESSMENT OF MOBILIZATION AND EXERCISE RESPONSES

To prescribe mobilization and exercise for optimal therapeutic effect, resting baseline measures of relevant physiologic oxygen transport responses need to be recorded so that any perturbation of oxygen transport and homeostasis caused by exercise can be identified. Measures that reflect the function of the individual steps in the oxygen transport pathway that are primarily affected, and oxygen transport as a whole, such as oxygen delivery, oxygen consumption, and oxygen extraction at the tissue level, are fundamental. Of considerable clinical relevance is the adequacy of tissue oxygenation; however, to date, there are no clinically expedient means of assessing tissue oxygenation.

SUMMARY

This chapter described three distinct goals associated with the prescription of mobilization and exercise in the management of impaired oxygen transport, namely, to exploit their acute, long-term, and preventive effects.

The PT needs a comprehensive and detailed understanding of how mobilization and exercise have potent and direct effects on oxygen transport acutely, in the long-term, and preventively. The specific mobilization or exercise prescription is based on a comprehensive multisystem assessment and the treatment goals for a given patient. If the acute effects of mobilization or exercise on oxygen transport are indicated, the prescription specifies the parameters of an appropriate mobilization or exercise stimulus, usually, of relatively low intensity, short duration and high frequency. The treatment effects are often immediate. Because treatment responses can be dramatic, the prescription is progressed relatively quickly based on the treatment response measures. Prescribing mobilization to remediate *acute* cardiopulmonary dysfunction requires the same precision and specificity as prescribing exercise for *chronic* cardiopulmonary dysfunction. If the long-term effects of exercise are indicated, the exercise stimulus is defined in an appropriate prescription, i.e., generally higher intensity, longer duration, and less frequent compared with the prescription for the acute effects, and designed to be followed for several weeks or more before significant physiologic adaptation can be observed and progression of the stimulus is indicated. If the preventive effects of mobilization or exercise are required, then the prescription focuses on maximizing these benefits for a given patient by prescribing exercise, that is of sufficient intensity, duration, and frequency, to pre-serve adequate aerobic capacity and endurance for a given patient. The principles for prescribing mobilization and exercise for their optimal preventive effects have not been scientifically elucidated. These three levels of prescription of mobilization and exercise are physiologically distinct and need to be prescribed specifically for each patient.

REVIEW QUESTIONS

1. Distinguish between mobilization and exercise.
2. Distinguish among the prescription of mobilization/exercise for its acute effects, chronic effects, and preventive effects.
3. Describe the differences in the mobilization/exercise prescription parameters (i.e., type of exercise stimulus, intensity, duration, frequency, and course) when prescribing mobilization/exercise for its (1) acute effects, (2) chronic effects, and (3) preventive effects.
4. Explain the effects of mobilization on enhancing the efficiency of oxygen transport.
5. Explain the effects of exercise on enhancing the efficiency of oxygen transport.
6. Describe the negative sequelae of restricted mobility.

References

Ahlinder, S., Birke, G., Norberg, R., Plantin, L.O., and Reizen-stein, P. (1970). Metabolism and distribution of IgG in patients confined to prolonged strict bed rest. *Acta Medica Scandinavica, 187,* 267-270.

American College of Sports Medicine (1994). *Guidelines for Exercise Testing and Prescription* (6th ed.). Philadelphia: Williams & Wilkins.

Andreoli, K.G., Fowkes, V.K., Zipes, D.P., & Wallace, A.G. (eds.). (1991). *Comprehensive Cardiac Care* (7th ed.). St. Louis: Mosby.

Belman, M.J., & Wasserman, K. (1981). Exercise training and testing in patients with chronic obstructive lung disease. *Basics of Respiratory Disease, 10,* 1-6.

Blair, E., & Hickman, J.B. (1995). The effect of change in body position on lung volumes and intrapulmonary gas mixing in normal subjects. *Journal of Clinical Investigation, 34,* 383-389.

Blair, S.N., Painter, P., Pate, R.R., Smith, L. K., & Taylor, C.B. (eds.). (1988). *Resource Manual for Guidelines for Exercise Testing and Training.* Philadelphia: Lea & Febiger.

Borg, G. (1982). Psychophysical basis of perceived exertion. *Medical Science in Sports and Exercise, 14,* 377-381.

Borg, G.A.V. (1970). Psychophysiological bases of perceived exertion. *Scandinavian Journal of Rehabilitation Medicine, 2,* 92-98.

Browse, N.L. (1965). *The Physiology and Pathology of Bed Rest.* Springfield, Ill.: Charles C. Thomas. Publisher.

Bydgeman, S., & Wahren, J. (1974). Influence of body position on the anginal threshold during leg exercise. *European Journal of Clinical Investigation, 4,* 201-206.

Cardus, D. (1967). O2 alveolar-arterial tension differences after 10 days' recumbency in man. *Journal of Applied Physiology, 23,* 934-937.

Chase, G.A., Grave, C., & Rowell, L.B. (1966). Independence of changes in functional and performance capacities attending prolonged bed rest. *Aerospace Medicine, 17,* 1232-1237.

Chobanian, A.V., Lille, R.D., Tercyak, A., Blevins, P. (1974). The metabolic and hemodynamic effects of prolonged bed rest in normal subjects. *Circulation, 49,* 551-559.

Clauss, R.H., Scalabrini, B.Y., Ray, J.F., & Reed, G.E. (1968). Effects of changing body positions upon improved ventilation-perfusion relationships. *Circulation, 37* (Suppl 4), 214-217.

Compton, D.M., Eisenman, P.A., and Henderson, H.L. (1989). Exercise and fitness for persons with disabilities. *Sports Medicine, 7,* 150-162.

Convertino, V.A., Hung, J., Goldwater, D., and DeBusk, R.F. (1982). Cardiovascular responses to exercise in middle-aged men after 10 days of bedrest. *Circulation, 65,* 134-140.

Craig, D.B., Wahba, W.M., Don, H., Couture, J.G., & Becklake, M.R. (1971). "Closing volume" and its relationship to gas exchange in the seated and supine positions. *Journal of Applied Physiology, 31,* 717-721.

Dean, E. (1993). Advances in rehabilitation for older persons with cardiopulmonary dysfunction. In: *Advances in Long-Term Care.* Katz, P.R., Kane, R.L., & Mezey, M.D. (eds.). New York: Springer.

Dean, E., Murphy, S, Parrent, L, and Rousseau, M. (1995). Metabolic consequences of physical therapy in critically-ill patients. Proceedings of the World Confederation of Physical Therapy Congress, Washington, D.C.

Dean, E., & Ross, J. (1992a). Mobilization and exercise conditioning. In: Zadai, C (Ed). *Clinics in Physical Therapy. Pulmonary Management in Physical Therapy.* New York: Churchill Livingstone.

Dean, E., & Ross, J. (1992b). Discordance between cardiopulmonary physiology and physical therapy. Toward a rational basis for practice. *Chest, 101,* 1694-1698.

Dean, E., & Ross, J. (1993). Movement energetics of individuals with a history of poliomyelitis. *Archives of Physical Medicine and Rehabilitation, 74,* 478-483.

Deitrick, J.E., Whedon, G.D., & Shorr, E. (1948). Effects of immobilization upon various metabolic and physiologic functions of normal man. *American Journal of Medicine, 4,* 3-36.

Dock, W. (1944). The evil sequelae of complete bed rest. *Journal of the American Medical Association, 125,* 1083-1085.

Donaldson, C.L., Hulley, S.B., & McMillan A.V. (1969). The effect of prolonged simulated non-gravitational environment on mineral balance in the adult male. *NASA Contact CR-108314,* Moffett Field, CA.

Friman, G. (1979). Effect of clinical bedrest for seven days on physical performance. *Acta Medica Scandinavica, 205,* 389-393.

Froelicher, V.F. (1987). *Exercise and the Heart. Clinical Concepts.* (2nd ed.). Chicago: Year Book Medical Publishers.

Harper, C.M., & Lyles, Y.M. (1988). Physiology and complications of bed rest. *Journal of the American Geriatrics Society, 36,* 1047-1054.

Harrison, T.R. (1944). The abuse of rest as a therapeutic measure for patients with cardiovascular disease. *Journal of the American Medical Association, 125,* 1075-1077.

Hasson, S.M. (ed.) (1994). *Clinical Exercise Physiology.* St. Louis: Mosby.

Hsu, H.O., & Hickey, R.F. (1976). Effect of posture on functional residual capacity postoperatively. *Anesthesiology, 44,* 520-521.

Hulley, S.B., Vogel, J.M. Donaldson, C.L., Bayers, J.M., Friedman, R.J., & Rosen, S.N. (1971). The effect of supplemental oral phosphate on the bone mineral changes during prolonged bedrest. *Journal of Clinical Investigation, 50,* 2506-2518.

Irwin, S., & Tecklin, J.S. (eds.). (1985). *Cardiopulmonary Physical Therapy.* St. Louis: C.V. Mosby.

Jones, N.L., (1982). Clinical Exercise Testing (3rd ed.). Philadelphia: WB Saunders.

Kottke, F.J. (1966). The effects of limitation of activity upon the human body. *Journal of the American Medical Association, 196,* 825-830.

Lentz, M. (1981). Selected aspects of deconditioning secondary to immobilization. *Nursing Clinics of North America, 16,* 729-737.

Levin, S.A., & Lown, B. (1952). 'Armchair' treatment of acute coronary thrombosis. *Journal of the American Medical Association, 148,* 1365-1369.

McArdle, W.D., Katch, F.I., & Katch, V.L. (1994). *Essentials of Exercise Physiology.* Philadelphia: Lea & Febiger.

McGavin, C.R., Artvinli, M., Naoe, H., & McHardy, G.J.R. (1978). Dyspnea, disability, and distance walked: Comparison of estimates of exercise performance in respiratory disease. *British Medical Journal, 2,* 241-243.

McGavin, C.R., Gupta, S.P., & McHardy, G.J.R. (1976). Twelve-minute walking test for assessing disability in chronic bronchitis. *British Medical Journal, 1,* 822-823.

Mikines, K.J. (1991). *Journal of Applied Physiology, 70,* 1245-49.

Orlava, O.E. (1959). Therapeutic physical culture in the complex treatment of pneumonia. *Physical Therapy Review,* 39, 153-160.

Powers, J.H. (1944). The abuse of rest as a therapeutic measure in surgery. *Journal of the American Medical Association, 125,* 1079-1083.

Pyne, D.B. (1994). Regulation of neutrophil function during exercise. *Sports Medicine, 17,* 245-258.

Ray, J.F., Yost, L., Moallem, S., Sanoudos, G.M., Villamena, P., Paredes, R.M., & Clauss, R.H. (1974). Immobility, hypoxemia, and pulmonary arteriovenous shunting. *Archives of Surgery, 109,* 537-541.

Risser, N.L. (1980). Preoperative and postoperative care to prevent pulmonary complications. *Heart and Lung, 9,* 57-67.

Ross, J., & Dean, E. (1989). Integrating physiological principles into the comprehensive management of cardiopulmonary dysfunction. *Physical Therapy, 69,* 255-259.

Rubin, M. (1988). The physiology of bed rest. *American Journal of Nursing, 88,* 50-56.

Ryback, R.S., Lewis, O.F., & Lessard, C.S. (1971). Psychobiologic effects of prolonged bed rest (weightless) in young healthy volunteers. Study II. *Aerospace Medicine, 42,* 529-535.

Saltin, B., Blomqvist, G., Mitchell, J.H., Johnson, B.L., Wildenthal, K., & Chapman, C.B. (1968). Response to exercise after bed rest and after training. *Circulation, 38,* VII:S1-78.

Sandler, H. (1986). Cardiovascular effects of inactivity. In Sandler, H., & Vernikos, J. (eds.). (1956). *Inactivity Physiological Effects.* New York: Academic Press.

Sandler, H., Popp, R.L., & Harrison, D.C. (1988). The hemodynamic effects of repeated bed rest exposure. *Aerospace Medicine, 59,* 1047-1053.

Schimmel, L., Civetta, J.M., & Kirby, R.R. (1977). A new mechanical method to influence pulmonary perfusion in critically ill patients. *Critical Care Medicine, 5,* 277-279.

Shepherd, R.J., et al. Standardization of submaximal exercise test. *Bulletin of the World Health Organization, 38,* 765-775.

Sjostrand, T. (1951). Determination of changes in the intrathoracic blood volume in man. *Acta Physiologica Scandinavica, 22,* 116-128.

Skerrett, S.J., Niederman, M. S., & Fein, A.M. (1989). Respiratory infections and acute lung injury in systemic illness. *Clinics in Chest Medicine, 10,* 469-502.

Summer, W.R., Curry, P., Haponik, E.F., Nelson, S., & Elston, R. (1989). Continuous mechanical turning of intensive care unit patients shortens length of stay in some diagnostic-related groups. *Journal of Critical Care, 4,* 45-53.

Svanberg, L. (1957). Influence of position on the lung volumes, ventilation and circulation in normals. *Scandinavian Journal of Clinical and Laboratory Investigations, 25, 1-195.*

Underhill, S.L., Woods, S.L., Froelicher, E.S.S., & Halpenny, C.J. (1989). *Cardiac Nursing* (2 ed.). Philadelphia: JB Lippincott.

Wasserman, K.L., & Whipp, B.J. (1975). Exercise physiology in health and disease. *American Review of Respiratory Diseases, 112,* 219-249.

Weber, K.T., Janicko, J.S., Shroff, S.G., & Likoff, M.J. (1983). The cardiopulmonary unit: the body's gas transport system. *Clinics in Chest Medicine, 4,* 101-110.

Weissman, C., Kemper, M., Damask, M.C., Askanazi, J., Hyman, A.I., & Kinney, J.M. (1984). Effect of routine intensive care interactions on metabolic rate. *Chest,* 86, 815-818.

Wenger, N.K. (1982). Early ambulation: The physiologic basis revisited. *Advances in Cardiology, 31,* 138-141.

West, J.B. (1995). Respiratory Physiology—The Essentials. Baltimore: Williams & Wilkins.

Winslow, E.H. (1985). Cardiovascular consequences of bed rest. *Heart Lung,* 14, 236-246.

Wolff, R.K., Dolovich, M.B., Obminski, G., & Newhouse, M.T. (1977). Effects of exercise and eucapnic hyperventilation on bronchial clearance in man. *Journal of Applied Physiology, 43,* 46-50.

Yarnel, J.R. Helbock, M., & Schwiter, E.J. (1986). Rotorest kinetic treatment table (Rotobed) in patients with acute respiratory failure. In: Green, B.A., & Summer, W.R. (eds.). *Continuous Oscillating Therapy: Research and Practical Applications.* Miami: University of Miami Press.

Zadai, C.C. (ed). (1992). *Pulmonary Management in Physical Therapy.* New York: Churchill Livingstone.

Zubeck, J.P., & MacNeil, M. (1966). Effects of immobilization: behavioural and EEG changes. *Canadian Journal of Psychology, 20,* 316-336.

CHAPTER 18

Body Positioning

Elizabeth Dean

KEY TERMS   Cardiopulmonary function   Prescriptive body positioning
Gravity   Routine body positioning
Oxygen transport

INTRODUCTION

The purpose of this chapter is threefold. First, therapeutic body positioning, which is prescribed to optimize cardiopulmonary function and oxygen transport is differentiated from routine body positioning. Second, the physiological effects of different body positions and changing body positions on cardiopulmonary function and oxygen transport, are described. And third, the prescription of therapeutic body positioning is described. Body positions that simulate normal physiological effects of gravity and position change on oxygen transport are the priority, that is, being upright and moving. A hierarchy of body positions ranging from the most to the least physiological is presented.

This chapter concentrates on the principles of prescribing therapeutic body positioning and body position changes. The chapter does *not* provide treatment prescriptions, because no specific patient is being considered. Understanding the physiological effects of body position on oxygen transport and how pathophysiology disrupts these normal processes is fundamental to prescribing body positioning. However, an optimal body position can only be prescribed based on consideration of all the factors that impact on oxygen transport, that is, effects of the patient's pathophysiology and its specific presentation in that individual, the effect of immobility, the effect of extrinsic factors related to the patient's care and the effect of intrinsic factors related to the patient (Chapter 18). It is only by an integrated analysis of these factors collectively that (1) the most beneficial body positions can be predicted, (2) the least beneficial body positions can be identified and used minimally, and (3) the appropriate treatment outcome measures can be selected.

GRAVITY AND NORMAL PHYSIOLOGIC FUNCTION: IMPLICATIONS FOR CARDIOPULMONARY PHYSICAL THERAPY

The human is an orthograde animal. From moment to moment, gravity exerts its influence on the human body and importantly on oxygen transport. The combined effects of gravity on the lungs, heart, and peripheral circulation is central to their interdependent function and establishing normal oxygen transport. Knowledge of the effects of gravity on cardiopulmonary function in health and the deleterious effects of pathophysiological states on cardiopulmonary function provide a foundation for the clinical application of body positioning as a *primary* therapeutic intervention to optimize oxygen transport. Because of its potent and direct effect on oxygen transport, therapeutic body positioning is a *primary* noninvasive physical therapy intervention that can augment arterial oxygenation so that invasive, mechanical, and pharmacological forms of respiratory support can be postponed, reduced, or avoided—the singlemost important objective of cardiopulmonary physical therapy.

A patient is continually exposed to gravity, thus every position the patient assumes reflects the effect of gravity on oxygen transport, thus, oxygen transport can be improved, maintained or worsened with changes in body position. Despite being essential to normal cardiopulmonary function, gravity is the principal contributor to significant inhomogeneity of physiological function down the lungs (West, 1995). Figure 18-1 illustrates the effect of this gradient with respect to alveolar ventilation (VA), perfusion (Q), ventilation and perfusion ratio (VA/Q), Pa_{O_2}, P_{CO_2}, P_{N_2}, oxygen content, CO_2 content, pH, and the flow of oxygen and CO_2 in and out of the lungs. Thus the lungs should not be likened to balloons either physiologically or anatomically.

Based on a thorough analysis of all factors contributing to impaired oxygen transport and gas exchange (Chapter 16), those body positions that will have an optimal effect and those that may be deleterious must be discriminated. In this way, a greater proportion of time can be spent in beneficial positions and less time spent in deleterious body positions. When beneficial positions are assumed for too long, however,

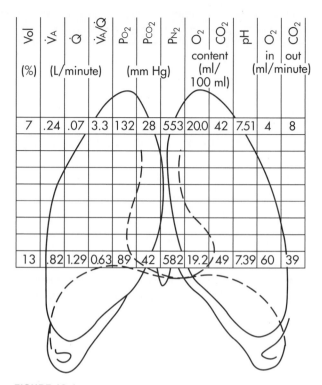

Vol (%)	V̇A (L/minute)	Q̇	V̇A/Q̇	Po₂ (mm Hg)	Pco₂	PN₂	O₂ content (ml/100 ml)	CO₂	pH	O₂ in (ml/minute)	CO₂ out
7	.24	.07	3.3	132	28	553	20.0	42	7.51	4	8
13	.82	1.29	0.63	89	42	582	19.2	49	7.39	60	39

FIGURE 18-1

Regional physiologic differences down the upright lung. VA = alveolar ventilation, Q = perfusion, VA/Q = ventilation perfusion ratio. (Reprinted with permission from West JB: *Respiratory physiology—the essentials,* ed 5, Baltimore, 1995, Williams & Wilkins.)

hydrostatic, gravitational and compression forces acting on the heart, blood volume, lymphatic system, lungs, and chest wall, including the diaphragm, will eventually compromise oxygen transport, and any beneficial effect will be offset. Therefore monitoring is essential to ensure the patient is turned to another position before detrimental effects are observed. Frequent changes in body position and avoidance of prolonged periods in any single position will minimize the risk of diminishing returns, which are inevitable. The time course differs according to pathology, type, severity, and other factors. The duration a patient assumes a body position should be primarily *response-dependent* rather than time-dependent. Knowledge of the deleterious effects of prolonged periods in a single position supports the prescription of both frequent body position changes and extreme consecutive body positions. These perturbations simulate the normal perturbations that the cardiopulmonary and cardiovascular systems are exposed to in health during normal mobility and body position changes. The ability to weigh the relative beneficial and deleterious effects of each possible body position, that is, over 360 degrees in the horizontal plane and 180 degrees in the vertical plane (ranging from 20 degrees head down to 20 degrees lean forward) on a given patient's gas exchange, is critical in prescribing body positioning therapeutically.

PRESCRIPTIVE VS. ROUTINE BODY POSITIONING

The literature supports the benefits of frequent body position changes particularly for the patient who is relatively immobile, severely debilitated, obtunded, breathing at low lung volumes, obese, aged, very young or who has lost the sigh mechanism. The practice of routinely turning patients every 2 hours is widely accepted. This practice is based on the belief that the deleterious consequences associated with assuming a static position for a prolonged period will be prevented. Recent evidence, however, supports that more frequent turning can have greater physiological benefits in critically ill patients (Dean and Suess, 1995) which suggests less severely ill patients may also benefit. The preventive effects of a routine turning regimen are distinct from the acute effects of body positioning on oxygen transport which is the primary focus of this chapter.

PHYSIOLOGICAL EFFECTS OF DIFFERENT BODY POSITIONS

Body positioning has potent and direct effects on most steps of the oxygen transport pathway, thus can be prescribed to elicit these effects specifically. Because humans function optimally when upright and moving, therapeutic interventions that elicit or simulate being upright and moving (i.e., elicit both gravitational and exercise stress) are most justified physiologically. The recumbent supine position, a common position assumed by hospitalized patients, is nonphysiological, therefore deleterious to oxygen transport. The side-lying positions have an effect that is intermediate between upright and supine. The prone position which is under utilized clinically, has such a significant beneficial effect on oxygen transport that a good rationale should be made for *not* incorporating this position into the treatment prescription rather than for using this position.

The indications for therapeutic body positioning and the indications for frequent body position changes to optimize oxygen transport are shown in the boxes on pp. 302–303. For each of the indications listed, an optimally therapeutic body position can be selected for a given patient. A description of the physiological effects of several primary body positions follow, namely, the upright supine, side lying, head down, and prone positions. This information, however, cannot be applied out of context. The specific positions prescribed for a patient are based on a consideration of the multiple factors that impair oxygen transport (Chapter 16) in conjunction with a physiological analysis of the most justifiable positions.

Because of the potent and direct effects of body positioning on various steps in the oxygen transport pathway in health and in disease, it is unknown whether the beneficial effects reported with the use of postural drainage are attributable to enhanced mucociliary transport, or to the direct effect of positioning the good lung down on improving the gas exchange of that lung, by increasing alveolar volume of the affected, nondependent lung, or both. Typically, studies evaluating conventional chest physical therapy, including postural drainage, have failed to control for the direct effect of body positioning on cardiopulmonary function, or for the direct effects of increased arousal and mobilization that occur when changing a patient's body position (Dean, 1994a). This is an extremely serious methodological problem that pervades the literature evaluating conventional chest physical therapy, and one that needs to be considered when interpreting the results of studies on these procedurers. Unless these potent confounding variables are controlled, the degree to which conventional chest physical therapy had a beneficial effect over and above the effects of positioning as well as mobilization and increased arousal cannot be determined (Dean, 1994b).

Indications for Body Positioning To Optimize Oxygen Transport

Cardiopulmonary

↑ Regional alveolar volume

↑ Regional ventilation

↑ Regional perfusion

↑ Regional diffusion

Optimize area of optimal ventilation to perfusion matching

↓ Pulmonary shunting

↑ Lung volumes and capacities particularly, functional residual capacity, vital capacity and tidal volume

↓ Closure of dependent airways

Alter breathing frequency

Alter minute ventilation

Alter position of the hemidiaphragms

↑ Respiratory muscle efficiency

↓ Airway resistance

↑ Lung compliance

↑ Air flow rates

Stimulate cough

↑ Biomechanical efficiency of cough, its strength and productivity

↓ Work of breathing

Improve arterial blood gases, gas exchange and oxygenation

↑ Mucociliary transport and mucus clearance

↓ Gravitational, mechanical and compression forces on the lungs, chest wall, diaphragm and the gut

Facilitate viscerodiaphragmatic breathing

Change the pattern of breathing

Cardiovascular

↓ Preload and afterload

↓ Work of the heart

Improve systolic ejection fraction to pulmonary and systemic circulations

Alter venous return

↓ Gravitational, mechanical and compression forces on the myocardium, great vessels, mediastinal structures, and lymphatic system

Optimize fluid shift from central to dependent areas (extremities) and vice versa to maintain fluid volume regulating mechanisms

Other Systemic Effects

Optimize chest tube drainage

Facilitate urinary drainage

Reduce posturally increased muscle tone

Facilitate patient arousal

Promote relaxation

Promote comfort

Control pain

Promote biomechanically optimal body positions

Intraabdominal pressure

Intracranial pressure

Upright Positions

The physiological position for the human organism is the same as the anatomical position—upright. The upright positions include walking, standing, and sitting. The upright position coupled with movement (e.g., walking and cycling) optimizes oxygen transport to the greatest degree in that ventilation and perfusion are more uniform than without the additional exercise stimulus. The upright standing position maximizes lung volumes and capacities with the exception of closing volume, which is decreased (Svanberg, 1957). Functional residual capacity (FRC), the volume of air remaining in the lungs at the end of a normal expiration, is slightly greater in standing compared with sitting and exceeds that in supine by approximately 50% (Figure 18-2). Maximizing FRC is

Indications for Frequent Changing of Body Position
Cardiopulmonary
Alter chest wall configuration
Shift distribution of alveolar volume
Shift distribution of ventilation
Shift distribution of perfusion
Shift distribution of diffusion
Shift distribution of ventilation to perfusion matching
Shift mechanical physical compression of the heart on adjacent alveoli
Shift position of the heart thereby alter chamber end disastolic filling pressures, preload, afterload, and work of the heart
Shift distribution of mucus transport and accumulation
Stimulate effective and productive cough
Facilitate lymphatic drainage
Perturb pattern of monotonous tidal ventilation
Alter breathing pattern
Shift gravitational, mechanical and compression forces on the lungs, chest wall, diaphragm, and the gut
Simulate normal inflation-deflation sigh cycles
Shift intraabdominal pressure
Cardiovascular
Shift gravitational, mechanical, and compression forces on the myocardium, great vessels, mediastinal structures, and lymphatic system
Stimulate fluid volume shifts particularly to the dependent limbs
Other Systemic Effects
Optimize chest tube drainage
Promote urinary drainage
Shift abnormal postural tone patterns
Alter arousal state
Promote relaxation
Promote comfort
Control of pain
Prevent skin breakdown, risk of infection, and resulting positioning limitations
Limit lying on a preferred side

associated with reduced airway closure and maximal arterial oxygenation (Hsu and Hickey, 1976; Ray et al, 1974). Figure 18-3 illustrates the relationship of FRC and closing capacity as a function of age. Because of age-related changes, closing capacity of the dependent airways increases with age; this effect is further accentuated with recumbency. Airway closure is evident in supine in the healthy 45-year-old person, and in the upright position in the healthy 65-year-old person (Leblanc, Ruff, and Milic-Emili, 1970). These effects are further accentuated in patient populations, thus the upright position is favored and the supine position should be minimized to prevent airway closure and impaired gas exchange.

With respect to pulmonary function testing, the upright sitting position with legs dependent is the standard reference position (American Thoracic Society, 1987). When upright, the diameter of the main airways increases slightly. If the airways are obstructed even small degrees of airway narrowing induced by recumbency can result in significant airway resistance (Figure 18-4). The vertical gravitational gradient is maximal when upright, the anteroposterior dimension of the chest wall is the greatest, and compression of the heart and lungs is minimal (Weber, Janicki, Shroff, and Likoff, 1983). The shortened position of the diaphragmatic fibers is countered by an increase in the neural drive to breathe in the upright position (Druz and Sharp, 1982).

The distribution of ventilation is determined primarily by the effect of gravity, which changes down the lung due to the anatomical position and suspension of the lungs within the chest. At FRC in the upright position, the intrapleural pressures at the apex is -10 cm H_2O and at the base -2.5 cm H_2O (Figure 18-5). The intrapleural pressure is less negative in the base because of the weight of the lung. Because of the greater negative intrapleural pressure in the apices, thus low compliance, these lung units have a larger initial volume, thus smaller volume changes occur during respiration. Because the lung units at the base have a smaller initial volume, thus high compliance, larger volume changes occur during respiration. Therefore depending on their relative position with respect to gravity, different regions of the lung are at different parts of the pressure volume curve.

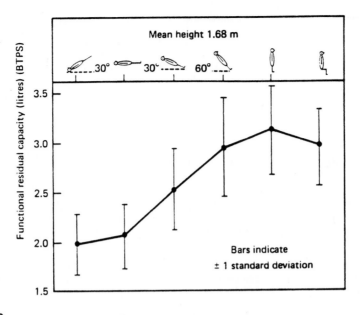

FIGURE 18-2
Changes in functional residual capacity in various body positions. (Data reprinted with permission from Nunn JF: Applied respiratory physiology, London, 1987, Butterworths.)

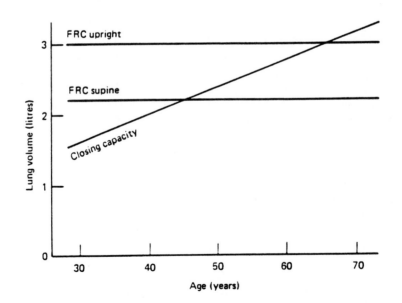

FIGURE 18-3
Functional residual capacity (FRC) and closing capacity as a function of age. (Data reprinted with permission from Nunn JF: Applied respiratory physiology, London, 1987, Butterworths.)

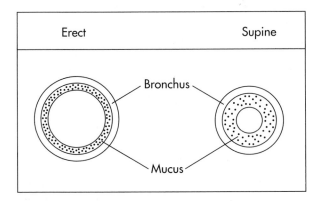

FIGURE 18-4

Effect of body position on bronchiolar diameter. (Reprinted with permission from Browse NL: The physiology and pathology of bed rest, Springfield, Ill. 1965, Charles C. Thomas.)

A common clinical concern is the patient breathing at low lung volumes (e.g., the patient in pain, the surgical patient with thoracic or abdominal incisions, older and younger patients, obese patients, pregnant patients, patients with gastrointestinal dysfunction such as paralytic ileus and ascites, organomegaly, intrathoracic and intraabdominal masses, patients who are malnourished, mechanical ventilated patients and patients with spinal cord injuries. Breathing at low lung volumes reverses the normal intrapleural pressure gradient such that in the upright lung the apices have a negative intrapleural pressure compared with the bases, which have a positive intrapleural pressure, that is, exceeds airway pressure (Figure 18-6). This results in the apices being more compliant, thus better ventilated than the bases. The bases are prone to airway closure in patients breathing at low lung volumes.

Another factor that reverses the normal intrapleural pressure gradient is mechanical ventilation. Despite its necessity in the management of patients in respiratory failure, mechanical ventilation contributes to hypoxemia in several ways. First, it reverses the normal intrapleural pressure gradient so that the uppermost lung fields are preferentially ventilated. Because the dependent lung fields are preferentially perfused, ventilation perfusion mismatch is promoted. Positive pressure ventilation has the additional com-

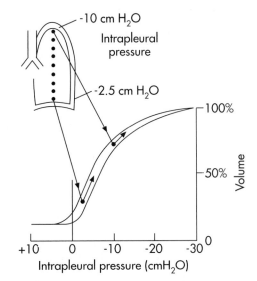

FIGURE 18-5

Schematic of the regional differences in ventilation down the upright lung. (Reprinted with permission from West JB: *Ventilation/ bloodflow and gas exchange,* ed 4, Oxford, 1985, Blackwell Scientific.)

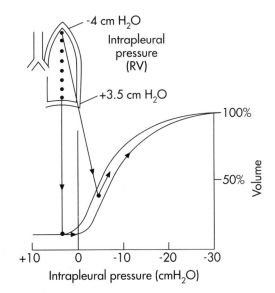

FIGURE 18-6

Schematic of the regional differences in ventilation at low lung volumes. (Reprinted with permission from West JB: *Ventilation/ bloodflow and gas exchange,* ed 4, Oxford, 1985, Blackwell Scientific.)

plication of increasing intrathoracic pressure and reducing venous return and cardiac output. These factors in addition to the negative pressure required to open the inspiratory valve can increase the work of breathing associated with mechanical ventilation (Cane, Shapiro, and Davison, 1990; Rivara, Artucio, Arcos, and Hiriart, 1984).

Although gravity is the primary determinant of *interregional* differences in the distribution of ventilation in the healthy lung, *intraregional* differences, secondary to differences in compliance and resistance of contiguous lung units, also contribute (Ross, Dean, and Abboud, 1992). These effects are exaggerated in patient populations (Bates, 1989).

The distribution of perfusion down the upright lung is also primarily gravity dependent (Figure 18-7). The pressures affecting blood flow through the pulmonary capillaries and resulting in the typical uneven distribution of blood flow are alveolar pressure, and the arterial and venous pressures. Zone 1, at the apex, alveolar pressure predominates arterial and venous pressures, thus has minimal to no blood flow. Zone 2, in the midzone, reflects the blood flow from

the recruitment of pulmonary vessels. Arterial pressure exceeds alveolar pressure and blood flow. Zone 3, in the lower area of the lung, reflects the blood flow from the distension of pulmonary vessels; arterial and venous pressures exceed alveolar pressure. And, zone 4 (not illustrated) in the most dependent portion of the lung has minimal to no pulmonary blood flow because of interstitial pressure acting on the pulmonary blood vessels creating a compression force (West, 1995).

Ventilation (V) and perfusion (Q) matching reflects the interfacing of the distributons of V and Q down the upright lung. Both V and Q increase down the upright lung; however, V increases disproportionately more than Q (Figure 18-8). As a result, the optimal area for V/Q matching is in the mid zone where the ratio is about 1.0 (West, 1985).

The upright position is associated with significant hemodynamic effects. These effects reflect primarily the central blood volume that is shifted from the thoracic compartment to the dependent venous compartments on assuming the upright position from supine (Blomqvist and Stone, 1963; Gauer and Thron, 1965;

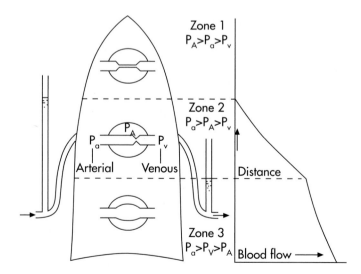

FIGURE 18-7
Schematic of pressures affecting the pulmonary capilaries and blood flow. (Reprinted with permission from West JB: *Ventilation/bloodflow and gas exchange,* ed 4, Oxford, 1985, Blackwell Scientific.)

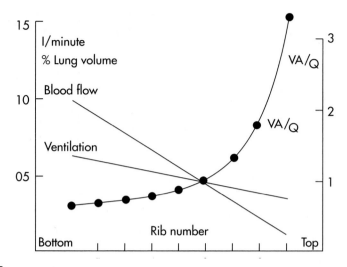

FIGURE 18-8
Distributions of ventilation and blood flow down the upright lung and the distribution of ventilation perfusion matching down the upright lung. (Reprinted with permission from West JB: *Ventilation/bloodflow and gas exchange,* ed 4, Oxford, 1985, Blackwell Scientific.)

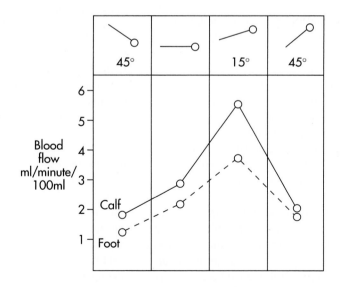

FIGURE 18-9
Effect of body position on peripheral blood flow. (Reprinted with permission from Browse NL: *The physiology and pathology of bed rest,* Springfield, Ill., 1965, Charles C. Thomas.)

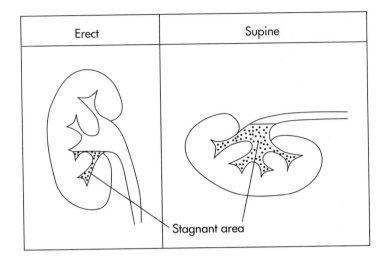

FIGURE 18-10
Effect of body position on drainage from the pelvis of the kidney. (Reprinted with permission from Browse NL: The physiology and pathology of bed rest, Springfield, Ill., 1965, Charles C. Thomas.)

Sandler, 1986). End diastolic and stroke volumes are decreased, which results in a compensatory increase in heart rate (Thandani and Parker, 1978). Cardiac output is correspondingly decreased. The net effect of these physiological changes is a reduction in myocardial work (Langou, Wolfson, Olson, and Cohen, 1977). This finding in corroborated by the observation that anginal threshold is increased in cardiac patients in this position (Prakash, Parmely, Dikshit, Forrester, and Swan, 1973). Peripheral vascular resistance increases and blood flow decreases, with the assumption of the upright position greater than 45 degrees to offset dependent fluid shifts and potential blood pressure drop (Figure 18-9). Another important effect of body position on fluid volume is the promotion of urinary drainage from the renal pelvi to the bladder in the upright positions as a result of the reduced area for urinary stasis in this position compared with supine (Figure 18-10). Optimal renal function is essential in preserving normal hemodynamic status.

Supine Position

The supine position is clearly not a physiological position for humans unless sleeping, and is physiologically the least justifiable position for ill patients regardless of whether they exhibit cardiopulmonary dysfunction (Dock, 1944; Moreno and Lyons, 1961; Powers, 1944; Winslow, 1985). The nonspecific use and overwhelming acceptance of bed rest has developed historically over the past 130 years. In the mid-1800s, that internal organs could be rested as a therapeutic intervention comparable with immobilizing and resting injuries of the limbs was the prevailing medical philosophy. The injudicious application and overuse of bed rest to cure all medical problems was critically challenged by Harrison (1944) and Browse (1965). Although there has been a significant decrease in use of prolonged periods of bed rest based on innumerable studies of the negative sequelae of bed rest over the past several decades (Dean and Ross, 1992b), the merits of bed rest as a therapeutic modality and the parameters for its prescription, that is, indications and specifications to achieve healing and recovery without deterioration, have not been scientifically established. This void in our scientific knowledge seems incongruous given the exponential rate of medical research and advances over the years in understanding obscure diseases and treatments. Because recumbency in bed is nonphysiologic and therefore associated with dire side effects, rest in bed needs to be as scientifically investigated and judiciously prescribed as any medication.

The supine position alters the chest wall configuration, the anteroposterior position of the hemidiaphragms, the intrathoracic pressure, and the intraabdominal pressure secondary to the shifting of the abdominal viscera in this position (Behrakis, Baydur, Jaeger, and Milic-Emili, 1983; Craig, Wahba, Don, Couture, and Becklake, 1971; Don, Craig, Wahba, and Couture, 1971; Druz and Sharp, 1981; Klingstedt et al, 1990; Roussos, Fukuchi, Macklem, and Engel, 1976; Saaki, Hida, and Takishima, 1977). The normal anteroposterior configuration becomes more transverse. The hemidiaphragms are displaced cephalad, which significantly reduces FRC in this position (Hsu and Hickey, 1976). Excess secretions tend to pool on the dependent side of the airway. Thus the upper side may dry out, exposing the patient to infection and obstruction (Fig. 18-11).

An increase in intrathoracic blood volume also contributes to a reduction in FRC, lung compliance, and increased airway resistance in the supine position (Nunn, 1987; Sjostrand, 1951). Collectively, these effects predispose the patient to airway closure and an increase in the work of breathing. Although a healthy person can accommodate to these physiological changes, a healthy person does not assume this position for prolonged periods without shifting. A hospitalized patient, however, is less likely to adapt to these immediate changes and their long-term effects. In addition, they may be less responsive to the need to shift position or unable to respond to afferent stimuli prompting a need to change position. These effects are accentuated in older people whose arterial oxygen tensions progressively diminish with age (Ward, Tolas, Benveniste, Hansen, and Bonica, 1966; Nunn, 1987).

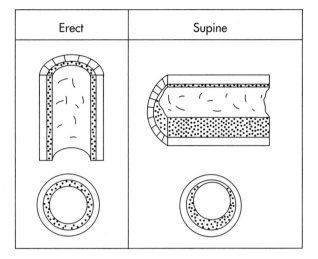

FIGURE 18-11
Effect of body position on the distribution of mucus within the bronchi. (Reprinted with permission from Browse NL: The physiology and pathology of bed rest, Springfield, Ill., 1965, Charles C. Thomas.)

Several significant cardiovascular changes occur on assuming the supine position. A central shift of blood volume from the extremities to the central circulation initiates orthostatism (Sandler, 1986). This fluid shift increases both the preload and afterload of the right side of the heart. This increased volume tends to distort the interventricular septum, and reduces left ventricular volume and preload. Prefaut and Engel (1981) observed that hypoxic vasoconstriction secondary to closure of the dependent airways in the supine position contributed to preferential perfusion of the nondependent lung zones. The relatively increased central blood volume inhibits the release of antidiuretic hormone. Ten to 15 percent of fluid is lost within 24 hours (Sandler, 1986), which can manifest clinically as cardiac underfilling, orthostatic intolerance, and a negative fluid balance (Dean and Ross, 1992a).

Because of a reduction in the vertical gravitational gradient, and therefore the intrapleural pressure gradient of the lung in supine, the distribution of V/Q matching appears more uniform and evenly matched in the supine position (Bates, 1989). These changes,

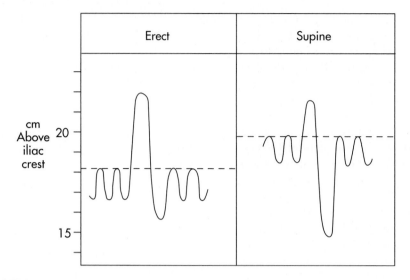

FIGURE 18-12
Effect of body position on the level and movements of the diaphragm during respiration.
(Reprinted with permission from Browse NL: The physiology and pathology of bed rest,
Springfield, Ill., 1965, Charles C. Thomas.)

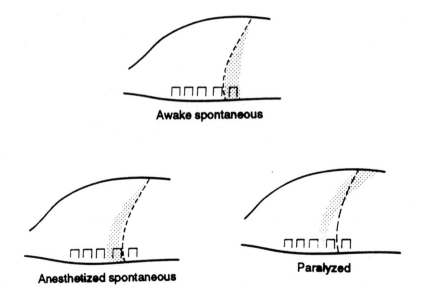

FIGURE 18-13
Position of the diaphragm in an awake spontaneously breathing subject, and in an anesthetized
subject with and without paralysis. The broken line is the end-expiratory position of the diaphragm
in the awake state in the supine position. The shaded area shows the excursion of the diaphragm
during inspiration and expiration.
(From Froese AB, Bryan AC: Effects of anesthesia and paralysis on diaphragmatic mechanics in
man. *Anesthesiology* 41:242-255.)

however, must be considered in conjunction with other changes associated with supine, namely reduced FRC, reduced vital capacity, reduced flow rates, increased area of dependent lung, and increased closure of the dependent airways. These deleterious factors offset any theoretical benefit of the supine position on V/Q matching (Ross and Dean, 1992).

The position of the diaphragm and its function, is dependent on body position. Figure 18-12 illustrates the effect on body position on the level and movement of the diaphragm. In the supine position, the resting level of the diaphragm is influenced differentially by anesthesia and neuromuscular blockade (Froese and Bryan, 1974). Figure 18-13 illustrates these effects. In the spontaneously breathing subject, the excursion of the diaphragm is greater posteriorly because the dependent viscera beneath the posterior portion of the diaphragm. During anesthesia with or without paralysis, the diaphragm ascends 2 cm into the chest. When paralysis is induced, the loss of diaphragmatic tone results in greater excursion of the nondependent rather than the dependent part of the diaphragm.

Side-Lying Positions

Compared with the supine position, side lying is more physiological, thus a more justifiable position in terms of its therapeutic benefit (Hurewitz, Susskind, and Harold, 1985; Ibanez, Raurich, Abizanda, Claramonte, Ibanez, and Bergada, 1981; Ross and Dean, 1992; Roussos, Martin, and Engel, 1977). The side-lying position accentuates anteroposterior expansion at the expense of transverse excursion of the dependent chest wall. In this position, the dependent hemidiaphragm is displaced cephalad because of the compression of the viscera beneath it. This results in a greater excursion during respiration, and greater contribution to ventilation of that lung and to gas exchange as a whole. The FRC in side lying falls between that in upright and supine. Similarly, compared with supine, compliance is increased, resistance is reduced, and the work of breathing reduced, whereas these are reversed when comparing this position with upright. Figure 18-14 illustrates the difference in lung volumes between maximal inspiration and FRC in a spontaneously breathing subject in

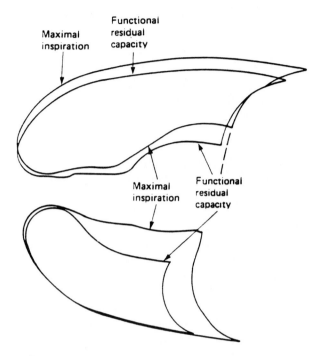

FIGURE 18-14
Outlines of the lungs at two lung volumes in a conscious spontaneously breathing subject in the right side-lying position. (Reprinted with permission from Nunn JF: Applied respiratory physiology, London, 1987, Butterworths.)

right side lying. Although effective ventilation is enhanced to the dependent lung, inspiratory lung volume and FRC are significantly reduced.

There is evidence to suggest that side lying results in increased end diastolic ventricular pressure on the dependent side secondary to compression of the viscera beneath the diaphragm, and reduced lung compliance on that side (Lange, Katz, McBride, Moore, and Hillis, 1988). Although such changes can be readily accommodated in health, for the patient with compromised oxygen transport, they may impair gas exchange further.

Optimal V/Q matching occurs in the upper one third of each lung in the side lying position (Kaneko, Milic-Emili, Dolovich, Dawson, and Bates, 1966). The total area therefore for optimal V/Q matching is likely greater than that in the upright position, which contributes to an improved V/Q matching. These apparent improvements, however, are offset by reduced lung volumes and air flow rates in this position.

In both healthy people and patients, arterial oxygen tension is greater in side lying compared with supine (Clauss, Scalabrini, Ray, and Reed, 1968). This is true both for patients receiving supplemental oxygen as well as those who are not. Thus sidelying can be used to enhance the efficiency of oxygen transport and thereby minimize or avoid the use of supplemental oxygen. Arterial blood gases are improved in patients with unilateral lung disease (Remolina, Khan, Santiago, and Edleman, 1981; Sonnenblick, Meltzer, and Rosin, 1983) when positioned with the good lung down and worsened with the affected lung down. When lung pathology is bilateral, arterial blood gases are improved when patients lie on the right side compared with the left. This can be explained by the greater size of the right lung and the reduced compression of the heart on the lung in this position compared with left side lying (Dean, 1985; Zach, Pontoppidan, and Kazemi, 1974).

Head Down Position

The head down position augments oxygen transport in some patients by improving pulmonary mechanics. Patients with chronic airflow limitation, for example, tend to have hyperinflated chests and flattened diaphragms in which the contraction of the diaphragm is inefficient because of the position of its muscle fibers on the length tension curve. The head down position causes the viscera to be displaced cephalad beneath the diaphragm. The diaphragm is positioned more normally and rests at a higher and more mechanically efficient position in the chest (Barach and Beck, 1954; De Troyer, 1983). In this position, patients may experience relief from dyspnea, reduced accessory muscle use, reduced upper chest breathing patterns and reduced minute ventilation. Patients with pathology to the bases may also benefit from the head down position in that this position favors gas exchange in the more functional upper lung fields and promotes alveolar distension of bases, which are uppermost in the head down position. Other patients, however, such as those with respiratory muscle fatigue may have increased respiratory distress in this position due to the resistive loading of the diaphragm from the weight of the viscera beneath.

Prone Position

There is considerable physiological justification for the use of the prone position to enhance arterial oxygenation and reduce the work of breathing in patients with cardiopulmonary dysfunction. Specifically, the prone position increases arterial oxygen tension, tidal volume and lung compliance (Albert, Leasa, Sanderson, Robertson, and Hlastala, 1987; Schwartz, Fenner, and Wolfsdorf, 1975; Wagaman, Shutack, Moomjiam, Schwartz, Shaffer, and Fox, 1979). These benefits have also been observed in critically ill patients (Langer, Mascheroni, Marcolin, and Gattinoni, 1988). In one study (Douglas, Rehder, Beynen, Sessler, and Marsh, 1977), supplemental oxygen was reduced in four out of five mechanically ventilated patients whose positioning regimen included the prone abdomen-free position. The two common variants of the prone position are prone abdomen-restricted and abdomen-free. Prone abdomen-restricted refers to lying prone with the abdomen in contact with the bed, whereas in the prone abdomen-free position the patient's hips and chest are elevated so that the abdomen is free.

While both prone positions augment gas exchange, the prone abdomen-free position, comparable with the hands and knees position (Mellins, 1974), enhances lung compliance, tidal volume, FRC and diaphragmatic excursion to a greater degree. Although patients in respiratory failure have been shown to benefit significantly from the prone position, certain precautions must be observed. The patient must be positioned so that all pressure points particularly on the head and face, and stress on the mechanical ventilator tubing and circuitry is minimized. The patient should be monitored continuously and not be unattended. A semiprone position can provide many of the physiological benefits of a full prone position, and minimize some of the risks, particularly in mechanically ventilated patients and patients with cervical spine pathology. In addition, the semiprone position simulates the prone abdomen-free position. The semiprone position may be more conservative, safer, and comfortable for the patient who is severely ill, potentially hemodynamically unstable, older, or who has a protruding abdomen.

For patients who are not able to be effectively mobilized some variant of the prone position is even more important. Excessive recumbency, particularly in patients who are being positioned through a restricted arc (e.g., supine and one-quarter turns to either side) needs to be offst by some variant of the prone position and this position needs to be incorporated often. Inevitably, patients exposed to a restricted arc of positioning will develop atelectasis in the dependent lung fields. The only means of preventing and countering compression and hydrostatically induced atelectasis is by placing those dependent areas uppermost.

The time course for the development of such hydrostatic complications is dependent on the patient. Although objective measures of oxygen transport and the adequacy of the steps in the oxygen transport pathway are essential to monitor, functional changes will likely precede the appearance of objective changes.

PHYSIOLOGIC EFFECTS OF FREQUENT CHANGES IN BODY POSITION

The box on p. 303 lists some of the significant physiological effects of frequent changes in body position that are largely mediated through their effects on respiratory mechanics, cardiac mechanics, airway closure, mucociliary transport, lymphatic drainage, and altered neural activation of the diaphragm. These effects resulting from the change in position are distinct from the benefits derived from a particular body position. The benefits of changing position can be enhanced by moving to an extreme position, ie, moving from supine to prone compared with supine to side lying. Extreme body position changes simulate, but do not replace, the physiological "stir-up" and perturbations that occur with normal mobility and being upright. When the "stir-up" regimen was originally proposed, Dripps and Waters (1941) did not appreciate fully its physiological implications. The net effect of changing body position is a "stirring up" of the constituent distributions of ventilation, perfusion, and ventilation and perfusion matching. Areas of dependent atelectasis, physiologic dead space and shunting, and mucus distribution are dramatically shifted. The "stir-up" correspondingly stimulates lymphatic drainage, surfactant production and distribution, and the distribution and function of pulmonary immune factors (Pyne, 1994). Frequent physical perturbations also inhibit bacterial colonization (Skerrett, Niederman, and Fein, 1989). Frequent body position changes redistribute compression forces acting on the diaphragm, myocardium, and mediastinal structures, and the compression of the lungs by the myocardium and mediastinal structures.

Frequent body position changes have significant effects on stimulating the patient and increasing arousal and a more wakeful state (Figure 18-15). The more upright the patient is positioned the greater the neurological arousal and greater the stimulus to breathe; this effect is augmented by encouraging the patient to be self-supporting. Concomitant with an increase in arousal, the patient is stimulated to take deeper breaths, and hence increase alveolar ventilation. When body positioning is coupled with mobilization, vasodilatation, and recruitment of the pulmonary capillaries is stimulated, which in turn improves the even distributions of ventilation and perfusion, and hence augments V/Q matching.

PRESCRIPTION OF THERAPEUTIC BODY POSITIONS AND BODY POSITION CHANGES

Prescription of body positioning is based on an analysis of the factors that contribute to impaired oxygen transport. Specific positions are selected to simulate as closely as possible the physiologic function of the normal healthy upright cardiopulmonary unit, and the perturbations and "stirring up" that occurs in the cardiopulmonary system during normal mobility and being upright. A hierarchy of body positioning alternatives based on the physiologic justification of the various positions, appears in the box on p. 314. These positions range from the most to the least physiologic. The hierarchy is based on the premise that oxygen transport is optimal when upright and moving. Mobilization in the upright position increases tidal

---

Physiological Hierarchy of Body Positions

Most Physiologic Therapeutic Body Positions

Normally moving upright in a 1 G gravitational field and exposed to a range of body positions and body position changes over the course of several hours

Relaxed erect standing (not too prolonged)

Erect sitting (self supported or with assist) with feet moving (e.g., active, active assisted or passive cycling motion)

Erect sitting (self-supported or with assist) with feet dependent

Lean forward sitting with arms supported and feet dependent

≥ 45 degree sitting with legs dependent

Erect long sitting (legs non dependent)

< 45 degrees sitting (legs non dependent)

Prone and semiprone/side lying

Supine

Least Physiological Therapeutic Body Positions
Provisos

The upright erect position implies the back, head and neck are vertical and aligned with flexion only at the hips; the patient is not slumped or recumbent.

The less able the patient is to assist in positioning the greater the need for more extreme positions and greater the turning frequency.

If the patient is totally unable to move, that is, in coma or paralyzed, extreme body positions are also indicated if not contraindicated because of hemodynamic instability or increased intracerebral pressure. The upright position is used as much as possible provided the patient is physically supported for safety and monitored in terms of treatment response. Passive standing on a tilt table is hemodynamically questionable; preferably patients should be placed in a high Fowler's position with legs positioned dependently using the knee breaks in the bed.

Regimens of 360-degree horizontal turning and 180-degree vertical turning (ranging from 20 degrees head down to 20 degrees lean forward) are used unless contraindicated. Positioning through a maximal arc simulates as closely as possible three dimensional movement of the chest wall during normal respiration.

---

volume, respiratory rate, and hence minute volume, flow rates, mucociliary transport, and clearance, and enhances the efficiency and effectiveness of airway clearance and coughing. Thus incorporating active movement into the body position change is optimal.

Despite the well-documented benefits of the judicious application of therapeutic body positioning to enhance oxygen transport, it does not replace the more physiological intervention of mobilization and exercise to maximize oxygen transport. Rather, once the effects of mobilization/exercise have been exploited maximally, then body positioning is the next best physiological approximation to a mobilized up-

right state. Furthermore, even the mobilized patient can benefit from therapeutic body positioning between mobilization sessions.

Body position needs first to be exploited when coupled with movement followed by the erect sitting positions with legs dependent. Figure 18-16 illustrates several variants of the sitting position. Each of these positions has distinct effects on oxygen transport, thus the specific upright position has to be prescribed specifically as the supported and "propped up" positions in bed do substitute for upright erect sitting. These variants only have a role when the patient will deteriorate by attempting to position in the

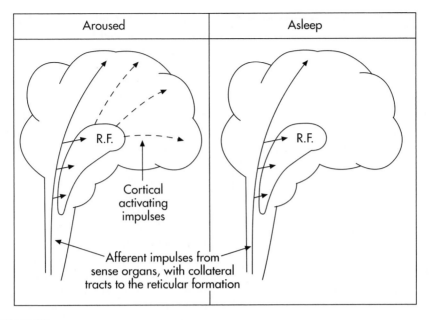

FIGURE 18-15
Effect of arousal on cerebral activity. (Reprinted with permission from Browse NL: The physiology and pathology of bed rest, Springfield, Ill., 1965, Charles C. Thomas.)

upright erect position, or the patient immediately deteriorates once in the position. Sitting with the feet down is preferable to long sit because of the hemodynamic benefits associated with this position. Sitting up in bed fails to position the patient in a perfectly vertical upright position. Fowler's position in bed can be maximized and the use of knee breaks in the bed provides a gravitational stimulus to the circulating blood volume.

A major difficulty with positioning patients in bed is the tendency to lose the position. Patients lose optimal positions in bed very quickly and thus need to be monitored to ensure the specific positions are maintained. Pillows should not be used to maintain a body position, since these are easily compressed and shifted. Blankets and sheets tightly rolled and secured with tape, and specially made bolsters are considerably more effective in maintaining a patient's body position.

Although there is a role for modified positions, such as half side lying these positions are often overused at the expense of full turns to each side, or prone or semiprone positions. Patients can be positioned safely, with appropriate supervision and monitoring, and comfortably in these full positions by observing the normal precautions of passive positioning.

A common practice is to progressively turn patients in one-quarter turns, such as supine to side lying and back to supine and so forth. However, the use of extreme positions and extreme position changes may yield greater benefit with respect to the degree of perturbation and "stir-up" elicited (Piehl and Brown, 1977). Extreme position changes result in significant alterations in the distributions of V, Q, and V and Q matching. Mucociliary transport is stimulated, and secretion accumulation and stagnation is minimized. In addition, the more extreme the body position, the greater degree of arousal stimulated particularly in the upright positions, which is essential in critically ill patients.

Another important consideration is the time course of changes in oxygen transport with positions and position changes. There are three plausible out-

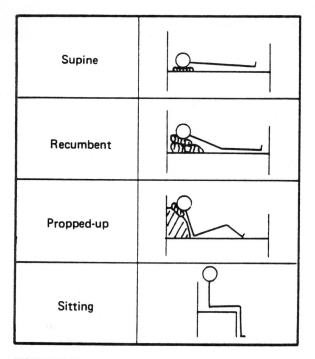

Supine	
Recumbent	
Propped-up	
Sitting	

FIGURE 18-16

Approximations of the upright position from supine. The recumbent and propped-up positons are not comparable physiologically to the upright sitting position. (Reprinted with permission from Browse NL: The physiology and pathology of bed rest, Springfield, Ill., 1965, Charles C. Thomas.)

comes: a favorable response, no response, an unfavorable response. With the passage of time, all three outcomes will deteriorate. The specific time depends on the multitude of factors contributing to impaired oxygen transport.

Because of the significant changes that can be expected with positioning and positioning changes, the physical therapist (PT) has a prime therapeutic opportunity to assess and treat the patient before, during, and after position changes.

Mechanical Body Positioning

Mechanical turning beds such as the Rotobed® have significant benefits on oxygen transport in severely ill patients (Brackett and Condon, 1984; Fink, Helsmoortel, Stein, Lee, and Cohn, 1990; Gentillelo, Thompson, Tonnesen, 1988; Gonzalez-Arias, Goldberg, Baumgartner, Hoopes, and Rubin, 1983; Kelley, Vibulsrest, Bell, and Duncan, 1987; Meinig, Leininger, and Heckman, 1986; Summer, Curry, Haponik, Nelson, & Elston, 1989). These beds are indicated for patients who are moderately hemodynamically unstable and on neuromuscular blockers, and thus tolerate manual turns poorly. Such turning frames are contraindicated, however, for patients who are less ill. Even for those patients who require multiple assistants and extra caution and time to turn and position effectively, these issues should never deny a patient a much needed treatment with proven efficacy.

The benefit of these beds on oxygen transport in critically ill patients has implications for the management of less critically ill patients. The continuous mechanical rotation of the Rotobed® can be simulated by increasing the frequency and arc of positions when manually positioning patients.

PRACTICAL CONSIDERATIONS IN POSITIONING PATIENTS

Prescriptive body positioning takes a significant amount of the PTs time as well as other team members' time. Such prescriptive positioning is based on clear indications and well-defined parameters; it is not to be confused with 'routine' positioning. For any hospitalized patient who is recumbent and inactive compared with being out of hospital, body positioning is a 24 hour concern, ie, a concern both during treatment and between treatments. Such patients are at risk of impaired oxygen transport.

Despite the time and labor involved in turning a patient to prone, particularly if mechanically ventilated, the benefits of this position outweigh the time and effort required to prone a patient even for short periods. Given the considerable benefits that can be derived from the prone position, a good case needs to be made for not turning a patient prone. Frequently, therapeutic body positioning can be effectively coordinated with nursing interventions and other procedures.

Extreme body positions and body position changes are the goal. However, when these are less feasible, modified positions may be used. Even though the greatest benefits will be derived from extreme changes as these simulate the normal range of changes the human body is exposed to in health, small changes can be effective in altering intrapleural gradients slightly so that previously closed alveoli will be opened even though previously opened ones may be prone to closure. Although modified positions and small degrees of position change should not be relied upon their effects should not be minimized in patients for whom extreme positions are contraindicated. Before and after every position change are prime opportunities to assess the patient, and to encourage deep breathing and coughing, or suction the patient as indicated.

Another important consideration is the time course of change in oxygen transport with positions and position changes. There are three possible outcomes: a favorable response, no response, an unfavorable response. With the passage of time, all these outcomes will deteriorate. The specific time depends on the multitude of factors that contribute to the patient's oxygen transport and the patient's responses.

MONITORING THE RESPONSE TO A BODY POSITION OR POSITION CHANGES

The prescriptive parameters of body positioning and body position changes include the positions selected, the duration spent in each position, the sequence of position changes, the cycle of all positions, and position changes overall. Because a patient necessarily assumes a body position at all times, positioning patients between treatments can contribute as much to the overall treatment response as the treatment itself as the patient is likely to spend more time in the between-treatment positions than in the within-treatment positions.

The duration and frequency of the positions and the frequency of body position changes are response-dependent rather than time-dependent. Monitoring is the basis for defining and modifying the body positioning prescription. The physiological variables to be monitored depend on the patient's specific presentation, cardiopulmonary dysfunction, and its severity and distribution. Monitoring of the noncritically ill pa-

tient includes subjective and objective evaluation of indices of the adequacy of oxygen transport (Part II). Among the most important are oxygen delivery, oxygen consumption, oxygen extraction, and gas exchange indicators such as the A-aO_2 difference and PaO_2/PAO_2. Subjectively, the patient's facial expression, respiratory distress, dyspnea, anxiety, discomfort and pain are assessed. Objectively, heart rate, blood pressure, respiratory rate, SaO_2, flow rates, beside spirometry are readily assessed. The appropriate standardization and procedures need to be used to ensure that the measures are both valid and reliable (see Chapter 6). Because physiological variables are changing from moment to moment, serial measures over a period of time should be taken to establish an average value rather than using peak or discrete measures which may misrepresent a treatment effect.

In order to interpret and compare various measures, the FiO_2 and any change in FIO_2 must be recorded. The use of the ratio PaO_2/FIO_2 enables comparison of gas exchange within and between patients when patients FiO_2s differ or are changed (Dean and Ross, 1992c). Similarly, for mechanically ventilated patients, any changes in the ventilatory parameters must also be noted, in addition to other interventions that have a direct effect on oxygen transport. Only in this way will the clinician be able to conclude within reasonable doubt that the position or position change was instrumental in enhancing cardiopulmonary function.

Measures are recorded before (pretreatment baseline), during, and at periodic intervals following the treatment. A valid stable pretreatment baseline is essential to determine the therapeutic effect of a given position on oxygen transport. Variables monitored during the treatment are focused on ensuring that the treatment is having a beneficial effect, in addition to its not having any deleterious effect on the patient subjectively or with respect to any parameter of oxygen transport. As long as beneficial effects are being recorded a position can be safely maintained, however, diminishing returns can be expected as the period becomes prolonged. Patients maintained in static positions for more than one to two hours need to be monitored closely. A position change is physiologically defensible after this duration rather than the risk of diminishing returns and potentially worsening the patient's condition.

Although sicker than a noncritically ill counterpart, the critically ill patient has the advantage of having more monitoring lines in place. These lines give access to several measures and indices of oxygen transport, and certain hemodynamic and pulmonary variables are available continuously.

In summary, the prescription of therapeutic body positions is based on a detailed analysis of each patient's unique presentation and the factors contributing to impairment of oxygen transport or threatening it. Then those positions that are predicted to result in the best therapeutic outcome are selected and applied, and those that are predicted to lead to an adverse result are used minimally and with appropriate monitoring. Monitoring is an essential component to body position prescription in that it confirms the prediction of beneficial and deleterious positions, establishes when a position change is indicated, and helps the PT anticipate the point of diminishing returns of any given body positions. The specific physiological variables monitored are those that reflect the steps in the oxygen transport pathway that are most affected in a given patient.

SUMMARY

The purpose of this chapter was to differentiate routine and therapeutic body positioning designed to optimize oxygen transport. The physiological effects of different body positions and changing body positions on cardiopulmonary and cardiovascular function and oxygen transport, were described. The primary goal is to strive toward the physiological position for optimizing oxygen transport, that is, upright and preferably moving. Issues related to optimizing the prescription of therapeutic body positioning and monitoring treatment outcome were presented.

This chapter focused on the physiological effects of body positioning, an intervention that has well-documented, direct and potent effects on oxygen transport. Establishing a clear rationale for prescribing a specific body position or body position changes is essential. The rationale, however, is based on multiple other factors in addition to the physiological consider-

ations presented. Thus this chapter has presented principles that must be considered in the decision-making process behind the prescription of therapeutic body positioning, rather than a treatment prescription for a given patient.

REVIEW QUESTIONS

1. Describe the effects of gravity on cardiopulmonary function and oxygen transport.
2. Distinguish between prescriptive and routine body positioning.
3. In reference to the seated upright position, describe the effects of different body positions (i.e., supine, side lying, head down, and prone) on cardiopulmonary function and oxygen transport in health.
4. In reference to the seated upright position, describe the effects of different body positions (i.e., supine, side lying, head down, and prone) on cardiopulmonary function and oxygen transport in disease.
5. Explain how a physiologically ideal body position with respect to oxygen transport can be deleterious over time.
6. Distinguish between the prescription of therapeutic body positions and frequency of body position changes.
7. Describe the principles of monitoring oxygen transport variables during body positioning.

References

Albert, R.K., Leasa, D., Sanderson, M., Robertson, H.T., & Hlastala, P. (1987). The prone position improves arterial oxygenation and reduces shunt in oleic-acid induced acute lung injury. *American Review of Respiratory Diseases, 135,* 628-633.

American Thoracic Society. Standardization of spirometry. 1987 Update. *American Review of Respiratory Diseases, 136,* 1285-1298.

Barach, A.L., & Beck, G.J. (1954). Ventilatory effects of head-down position in pulmonary emphysema. *American Journal of Medicine, 16,* 55-60.

Bates, D.V. (1989). *Respiratory Function in Disease* (3rd ed.). Philadelphia: W.Bates, D.V. (1989). *Respiratory Function in Disease* (3rd ed.). Philadelphia: W. B. Saunders.

Behrakis, P.K., Baydur, A., Jaeger, M.J., & Milic-Emili, J. (1983). Lung mechanics in sitting and horizontal body positions. *Chest, 83,* 643-646.

Blomqvist, C.G., & Stone, H.L. (1963). Cardiovascular adjustments to gravitational stress. In: Shepherd, J.T., & Abboud, F.M. (eds.). *Handbook of Physiology.* Section 2: Circulation, vol. 2, Bethesda: American Physiological Society.

Brackett, T.O., & Condon, N. (1984). Comparison of the wedge turning frame and kinetic treatment table in the acute care of spinal cord injury patients. *Surgical Neurology, 22,* 53-56.

Browse, N.L. (1965). *The Physiology and Pathology of Bed Rest.* Springfield: C.C. Thomas.

Cane, R.D., Shapiro, B.A., & Davison, R. (1990). *Case Studies in Critical Care Medicine.* Chicago: Year Book Medical Publishers.

Clauss, R.H., Scalabrini, B.Y., Ray, J.F., & Reed, G.E. (1968). Effects of changing body position upon improved ventilation-perfusion relationships. *Circulation, 37* (Suppl 2), 214-217.

Craig, D.B., Wahba, W.M., Don, H.F., Couture, J.G., & Becklake, M.R. (1971). 'Closing volume' and its relationship to gas exchange in seated and supine positions. *Journal of Applied Physiology, 31,* 717-721.

Dean, E. (1985). Effect of body position on pulmonary function. *Physical Therapy, 65,* 613-618.

Dean, E. (1994a). Invited commentary to 'Are incentive spirometry, intermittent positive pressure breathing, and deep breathing exercises effective in the prevention of postoperative pulmonary complications after upper abdominal surgery? A systematic overview and meta-analysis'. *Physical Therapy, 74,* 10-15.

Dean, E. (199b). Tightening up physical therapy practice: The confounding variable—friend or foe? (Editorial). *Physiotherapy Canada, 46,* 77-78.

Dean, E., & Ross, J. (1992a). Mobilization and exercise conditioning. In: Zadai, C.C. (ed.). *Clinics in Physical Therapy. Pulmonary Management in Physical Therapy.* New York: Churchill Livingstone.

Dean, E., & Ross, J. (1992b). Discordance between cardiopulmonary physiology and physical therapy. Toward a rational basis for practice. *Chest, 101,* 1694-1698.

Dean, E., & Ross, J. (1992c). Oxygen transport: The basis for contemporary cardiopulmonary physical therapy and its optimization with body positioning and mobilization. *Physical Therapy Practice, 1,* 34-44.

Dean, E., & Suess, J. (1995). Relationship of frequency of body position changes and oxygen transport in ARDS patients. Submitted for publication.

De Troyer, A. (1983). Mechanical role of the abdominal muscles in relation to posture. *Respiratory Physiology, 53,* 341-353.

Dock, W. (1944). The evil sequelae of complete bed rest. *Journal of the American Medical Association, 125,* 1083-1085.

Don H.F., Craig, D.B., Wahba, W.M., & Couture, J.G. (1971). The measurement of gas trapped in the lungs at functional residual capacity and the effect of posture. *Anesthesiology, 35,* 582-590.

Douglas, W.W., Rehder, K., Beynen, F.M., Sessler, A.D., & Marsh, H.M. (1977). Improved oxygenation in patients with acute respiratory failure: The prone position. *American Review of Respiratory Diseases, 115,* 559-566.

Dripps, R.D., Waters, R.M. (1941). Nursing care of surgical patients. I. The 'stir-up'. *American Journal of Nursing, 41,* 530-534.

Druz, W.S., & Sharp, J.T. (1981). Activity of respiratory muscles in upright and recumbent humans. *Journal of Applied Physiology, 51,* 1552-1561.

Druz, W.S. & Sharp, J.T. (1982). Electrical and mechanical activity of the diaphragm accompanying body position in severe chronic obstructive pulmonary disease. *American Review of Respiratory Diseases, 125,* 275-280.

Fink, M.P., Helsmoortel, C.M., Stein, K.L., Lee, P.C., & Cohn, S.M. (1990). The efficacy of an oscillating bed in the prevention of lower respiratory tract infection in critically ill victims of blunt trauma. A prospective study. *Chest, 97,* 132-137.

Froese, A.B., & Bryan, A.C. (1974). Effects of anesthesia and paralysis on diaphragmatic mechanics in man. *Anesthesiology, 41,* 242-255.

Gauer, O.H., & Thron, H.L. (1965). Postural changes in the circulation. In: Hamilton, W.F. (ed.). *Handbook of Physiology,* Washington: American Physiological Society.

Gentillelo, L., Thompson, D.A., & Tonnesen, A.S. (1988). Effect of a rotating bed on the incidence of pulmonary complications in critically ill patients. *Critical Care Medicine, 16,* 783-786.

Gonzalez-Arias, S.M., Goldberg, M.L., Baumgartner, R., Hoopes, D., & Rubin, B. (1983). Analysis of the effect of kinetic therapy on intracranial pressure in comatose neurosurgical patients. *Neurosurgery, 13,* 654-656.

Harrison, T.R. (1944). The abuse of rest as a therapeutic measure for patients with cardiovascular disease. *Journal of the American Medical Association, 125,* 1075-1077.

Hsu, H.O., & Hickey, R.F. (1976). Effect of posture on functional residual capacity postoperatively. *Anesthesiology, 44,* 520-521.

Hurewitz, A.N., Susskind, H., & Harold, W.H. (1985). Obesity alters regional variation in lateral decubitus position. *Journal of Applied Physiology, 59,* 774-783.

Ibanez, J., Raurich, J.M., Abizanda, R., Claramonte, R., Ibanez, P., & Bergada, J. (1981). The effect of lateral position on gas exchange in patients with unilateral lung disease during mechanical ventilation. *Intensive Care Medicine, 7,* 231-234.

Kaneko, K., Milic-Emili, J., Dolovich, M.B., Dawson, A., & Bates, D.V. (1966). Regional distribution of ventilation and perfusion as a function of body position. *Journal of Applied Physiology, 21,* 767-777.

Kelley, R.E., Vibulsrest, S., Bell, L., & Duncan, R.C. (1987). Evaluation of kinetic therapy in the prevention of complications of prolonged bed rest secondary to stroke. *Stroke, 18,* 638-642.

Klingstedt, C., et al. (1990). Ventilation-perfusion relationships and atelectasis formation in the supine and lateral positions during conventional mechanical and differential ventilation. *Acta Anaesthesiologica Scandinavica, 34,* 421-429.

Lange, R.A., Katz, J., McBride, W., Moore, D.M., & Hillis, L.D. (1988). Effects of supine and lateral positions on cardiac output and intracardiac pressures. *American Journal of Cardiology, 62,* 330-333.

Langer, M., Mascheroni, D., Marcolin, R., & Gattinoni, L. (1988). The prone position in ARDS patients. *Chest, 94,* 103-107.

Langou, R.A., Wolfson, S., Olson, E.G., & Cohen, L.S. (1977). Effect of orthostatic postural changes on myocardial oxygen demands. *American Journal of Cardiology, 39,* 418-421.

Leblanc, P., Ruff, F., & Milic-Emili, J. (1970). Effects of age and body position on airway closure in man. *Journal of Applied Physiology, 28,* 448-451.

Meinig, R.P., Leininger, P.A., & Heckman, J.D. (1986). Forces in patients treated in conventional and oscillating hospital beds. *Clinical Orthopedics and Related Research, 210,* 166-172.

Mellins, R.B. (1974). Pulmonary physiotherapy in the pediatric age group. *American Review of Respiratory Diseases, 110* (Suppl. 1), 137-142.

Moreno, F., & Lyons, H.A. (1961). Effect of body posture on lung volumes. *Journal of Applied Physiology, 16,* 27-29.

Nunn, J.F. (1987). *Applied Respiratory Physiology.* London: Butterworths.

Piehl, M.A., & Brown, R.S. (1977). Use of extreme position changes in acute respiratory failure. *Critical Care Medicine, 4,* 13-14.

Powers, J.H. (1944). The abuse of rest as the therapeutic measure in surgery. *Journal of the American Medical Association, 125,* 1079-1083.

Prakash, R., Parmely, W.W., Dikshit, K., Forrester, J., Swan, H.J. (1973). Hemodynamic effects of postural changes in patients with acute myocardial infarction. Chest, 64, 7-9.

Prefaut, C.H., & Engel, L.A. (1981). Vertical distribution of perfusion and inspired gas in supine man. *Respiratory Physiology, 43,* 209-219.

Pyne, D.B. (1994). Regulation of neutrophil function during exercise. *Sports Medicine, 17,* 245-258.

Ray, J.F., et al. (1974). Immobility, hypoxemia, and pulmonary arteriovenous shunting. *Archives of Surgery, 109,* 537-541.

Remolina, C., Khan, A.U., Santiago, T.V., & Edelman, N.H. (1981). Positional hypoxemia in unilateral lung disease. *New England Journal of Medicine, 304,* 523-526.

Rivara, D., Artucio, H., Arcos, J., & Hiriart, C. (1984). Positional hypoxemia during artificial ventilation. *Critical Care Medicine, 12,* 436-438.

Ross, J., & Dean, E. (1989). Integrating physiologic principles into the comprehensive management of cardiopulmonary dysfunction. *Physical Therapy, 69,* 255-259.

Ross, J., & Dean, E. (1992). Body positioning. In: Zadai, C.C. (ed.). *Clinics in Physical Therapy, Pulmonary Management in Physical Therapy.* New York: Churchill Livingstone.

Ross, J., Dean, E., & Abboud, R.T. (1992). The effect of postural drainage positioning on ventilation homogeneity in healthy subjects. *Physical Therapy, 72,* 794-799.

Roussos, C.H., Fukuchi, Y., Macklem, P.T., & Engel, L.A. (1976). Influence on diaphragmatic contraction on ventilation distribution in horizontal man. *Journal of Applied Physiology, 40,* 417-424.

Roussos, C.H., Martin, R.R., & Engel, L.A. (1977). Diaphragmatic contraction and the gradient of alveolar expansion in the lateral posture. *Journal of Applied Physiology, 43,* 32-38.

Sandler, H. (1986). Cardiovascular effects of inactivity. In: Sandler, H., & Vernikos, J. (eds.), *Inactivity: Physiological Effects.* Orlando: Academic Press.

Sasaki, H., Hida, W., & Takishima, T. (1977). Influence of body position on dynamic compliance in young subjects. *Journal of Applied Physiology, 42,* 706-710.

Scharf, S.M., & Cassidy, S.S. (Eds.). (1989). *Heart-Lung Interactions in Health and Disease.* New York: Marcel Dekker.

Schwartz, F.C.M., Fenner, A., & Wolfsdorf, J. (1975). The influence of body position on pulmonary function in low birthweight babies. *South African Medical Journal, 49,* 79-84.

Sjostrand, T. (1951). Determination of changes in the intrathoracic blood volume in man. *Acta Physiologica Scandinavica, 22,* 116-128.

Skerrett, S.J., Niederman, M.S., & Fein, A.M. (1989). Respiratory infections and acute lung injury in systemic illness. *Clinics in Chest Medicine, 10,* 469-502.

Sonneblick, M., Meltzer, E., & Rosin, A.J. (1983). Body positional effect on gas exchange in unilaeral pleural effusion. *Chest, 83,* 784-786.

Summer, W.R., Curry, P., Haponik, E.F., Nelson, S., & Elston, R. (1989). Continuous mechanical turning of intensive care patients shortens length of stay in some diagnostic-related groups. Journal of Critical Care, 4, 45-53.

Svanberg, L. (1957). Influence of posture on lung volumes, ventilation and circulation of normals. *Scandinavian Journal of Clinical Laboratory Investigations, 25,* 1-195.

Thandani, U., & Parker, J.O. (1978). Hemodynamics at rest and during supine and sitting bicycle exercise in normal subjects. *American Journal of Cardiology, 41,* 52-58.

Wagaman, M.J., Shutaack, J.G., Moomjiam, A.S., Schwartz, J.G., Shaffer, T.H., & Fox, W.W. (1979). Improved oxygenation and lung compliance with prone positioning of neonates. *Journal of Pediatrics, 94,* 787-791.

Ward, R.J., Tolas, A.G., Benveniste, R.J., Hansen, J.M., & Bonica, J.J. (1966). Effect of posture on normal arterial blood gas tensions in the aged. *Geriatrics, 21,* 139-143.

Weber, K.T., Janicki, J.S., Shroff, S.G., & Likoff, M.J. (1983). The cardiopulmonary unit: The body's gas exchange system. *Clinics in Chest Medicine, 4,* 101-110.

West, J.B. (1985). *Ventilation/Blood Flow and Gas Exchange* (4th ed.). Oxford: Blackwell Scientific Publications.

West, J.B. (1995). *Respiratory Physiology—The Essentials* (5th ed.). Baltimore: Williams & Wilkins.

Winslow, E.H. (1985). Cardiovascular consequences of bed rest. *Heart Lung, 14,* 236-246.

Zach, M.B., Pontoppidan, H., & Kazemi, H. (1974). The effect of lateral positions on gas exchange in pulmonary disease. *American Review of Respiratory Diseases, 110,* 49-53.

CHAPTER 19

Physiological Basis for Airway Clearance Techniques

Anne Mejia Downs

INTRODUCTION

Techniques for assisting the mobilization of secretions from the airways have long been advocated for use in the patient with an impairment in mucociliary clearance or an ineffective cough mechanism. The goals of this therapy are to reduce airway obstruction, improve mucociliary clearance and ventilation, and optimize gas exchange.

Airway clearance techniques have been referred to in the literature in a variety of ways, including chest physiotherapy, chest physical therapy, bronchial drainage, postural drainage therapy, and bronchial hygiene.

Research studying the results of airway clearance are often difficult to evaluate because the components of a given treatment have not been standardized. Availability of equipment or education about a technique as well as cultural differences in its application confound the results. Differences in the outcome measures for a given technique also occur—some studies use wet or dry (dehydrated) sputum volume or radioaerosol clearance, whereas other studies use pulmonary function tests, radiographic evidence or arterial blood gases to asses the effectiveness of an airway clearance technique. Although a treatment has been shown to be effective in one cross section of patients with pulmonary disease, care must be taken not to generalize the effectiveness of the treatment across other groups of patients or differing time frame (acute vs. chronic). The majority of secretion clearance research has been focused on patients with cystic fibrosis, as the need for ongoing secretion removal is apparent in this population.

Recently the "gold standard" of airway clearance, namely a combination of postural drainage, percussion, and vibration with cough, has been challenged (Lapin, 1994). The indications for routine airway clearance with certain diagnoses have been questioned and the conditions leading to effective application have been examined. Postural drainage and percussion has been shown to be ineffective in some cases, and in fact, to be detrimental to the pulmonary status of some patients. Caregivers have also been shown to suffer from the performance of percussion—repetitive motion injuries of the wrists have been documented as a result of regular performance of percussion (Ford, Godreau, Burns, 1991, MMWR Publication 1989).

Alternate techniques have arisen out of the need to find effective methods for those patients not responsive or not tolerant of traditional methods. A desire to increase compliance with airway clearance (Currie, 1986), especially in those patients approaching adolescence and adulthood has led to an investigation of more independent techniques. Many of these techniques have been practiced for years in European countries, but are more recently being introduced to practitioners in the United States.

It is important to remember, however, that secretion clearance is but one step to take toward realizing effective gas exchange in the complex oxygen transport pathway (Dean, 1992). Airway clearance, when indicated, should be integrated into a total approach to optimize oxygen transport.

INDICATIONS FOR AIRWAY CLEARANCE

Oxygen transport is the primary purpose of the cardiopulmonary system (see Chapter 1). Ventilation of the alveoli is an important step in the oxygen transport chain that allows optimal delivery of oxygen to the tissues. Several medical and surgical conditions may interfere with this process. Retained secretions or mucus plugs in the airways may interfere with the exchange of oxygen. The secretions need to be mobilized from the peripheral or smaller airways to the larger, more central airways where they may be removed by coughing or suction.

The following conditions are indications for airway clearance:

1. Cystic fibrosis—In this multisystem genetic disease, copious (often purulent), thick secretions and mucus plugs block the peripheral and central airways. Even infants diagnosed with cystic fibrosis, whether symptomatic or not, show evidence of small airway obstruction in the form of bronchial mucus casts (Wood, 1989). Recurrent bacterial infections combined with this mucus hypersecretion in the lungs leads to destruction of the bronchial walls, or bronchiectasis. Airway clearance continues to be an important therapy in the treatment of cystic fibrosis. This practice is supported by evidence of deteriorating lung function when regular treatments of postural drainage and percussion have been stopped (Desmond, 1983, Reisman, 1988).

2. Bronchiectasis—This condition results in a breakdown of the elastic tissue in the bronchial walls, causing severe dilation. Inflamed mucosa and copious, purulent secretions are present in this condition. Airway clearance has been shown to benefit patients with bronchiectasis in the mobilization of sputum (Mazzocco, 1985, Gallon, 1991).

3. Atelectasis—This condition is caused by the collapse of an alveolar segment, often by retained secretions. It is a documented sequela of patients who have undergone surgery under general anesthesia, especially thoracic or abdominal surgery. Airway clearance techniques are indicated where atelectasis is suspected to be caused by mucus plugging (Marini, 1979, Hammon, 1981).

4. Respiratory muscle weakness—Many patients with neurological or metastatic diseases or general debilitation, tend to hypoventilate or have an increased work of breathing. They are unable to

maintain adequate control of respiratory secretions and often have a weak, ineffective cough (Massery, 1987). This is especially true in patients with diminished diaphragm innervation resulting from spinal cord injuries (Wetzel, 1990).

5. Mechanical ventilation—Patients on ventilatory support for any reason, including obtunded or comatose patients, are at risk for atelectasis and are unable to independently manage their secretions (Dickman, 1987).

6. Neonatal respiratory distress syndrome—These infants are born lacking surfactant in the lungs, which results in atelectasis. Airway clearance techniques may be useful in clearing secretions and preventing atelectasis but must be monitored carefully in this population (Finer, 1978).

7. Asthma—This condition is characterized by the presence of hyperreactive airways and mucus plugging. Airway clearance techniques may be beneficial to assist with the mobilization of mucus plugs but are not helpful in treating uncomplicated acute exacerbations (Eid, 1991).

Chest physical therapy techniques appear not to be beneficial in the treatment of patients with pneumonia or chronic bronchitis without large amounts of secretion production. No differences were found with the inclusion of postural drainage and percussion in these populations (Britton, 1985; Sutton, 1982; Rochester, 1980; Wollmer, 1985).

Viral bronchiolitis is an asthma-like lung disease occurring in infants less than 2 years of age. These patients do not appear to benefit from airway clearance techniques (Webb, 1985).

Also of little benefit, and possibly harmful, is the inclusion of chest physical therapy in the routine care of postoperative patients without extensive secretions (Eid, 1991). Even in patients with a history of lung disease, the use of airway clearance techniques have failed to affect the incidence of atelectasis as a postoperative complication (Torrington, 1984).

Postural Drainage

Postural drainage (PD) is a passive technique, in which the patient is placed in positions that allow the bronchopulmonary tree to be drained with the assistance of gravity (Figure 19-1). Positioning the patient to enable gravity to assist the flow of bronchial secretions from the airways has been a standard treatment for some time in patients with retained secretions (Zadai, 1981).

Knowledge of the anatomy of the tracheobronchial tree is vital to an effective treatment. Each lobe to be drained must be aligned so that gravity can mobilize the secretions from the periphery to the larger, more central airways. The mechanism of postural drainage is considered to be a direct effect of gravity on bronchial secretions, although a study by Lannefors (1992) observing that gravity influences regional lung ventilation and volume suggested these other mechanisms are also involved.

Postural drainage (also known as bronchial drainage) has been shown to be effective in mobilizing secretions in patients with cystic fibrosis (Wong, 1977, Lorin, 1971), bronchiectasis (Mazzacco, 1985), and other pulmonary diseases (Bateman, 1981; Zausmer, 1968). Other treatments such as percussion, vibration, and the active breathing cycle (ACB) technique may be used while the patient is in postural drainage positions.

There are many contraindications to optimal positioning for PD, especially the head down or Trendelenberg positions required for the lower lobes.

Percussion

Percussion, sometimes referred to as chest clapping, is a traditional approach to secretion mobilization. A rhythmical force is applied with cupped hands to the patient's thorax over the involved lung segments with the aim of dislodging or loosening bronchial secretions. This technique is performed with the patient in postural drainage positions and requires a caregiver to administer. In the United States, percussion in conjunction with postural drainage continues to be a mainstay of treatment of the person with pulmonary disease, especially in neonates or patients who are unresponsive.

The proposed mechanism of action of percussion is the transmission of a wave of energy through the chest wall into the lung. The resulting motion loosens secretions from the bronchial wall and

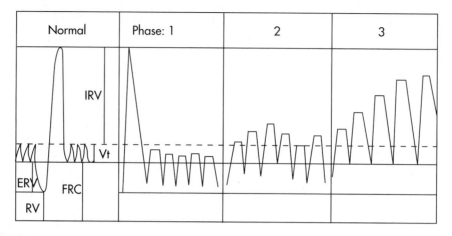

FIGURE 19-1

Phases of autogenic drainage shown on a spirogram of a normal person. Phase 1: unstick phase 2: collect, phase 3: evacuate. (VT = tidal volume, ERV = expiratory reserve volume, RV = reserve volume, FRC = Punctual residual capacity, IRV = inspriatory reserve volume; IRV + VT + ERV = vital capacity)

moves them proximally where ciliary motion and cough (or suction) can remove them. The combination of postural drainage and percussion has been shown to be effective in secretion removal (Denton, 1962; May, 1979, Radford, 1982). A study by Rossman et al. (1982) is in disagreement, finding that mechanical percussion did not enhance postural drainage in secretion removal.

A handheld mechanical percussor may be used by a caregiver to decrease fatigue or by the patient for self-administration of percussion. The effectiveness of mechanical versus manual percussion has been studied. Maxwell and Redmond (1979) found mechanical percussion equivalent to manual percussion in affecting removal of secretions. This is supported by Pryor et al. (1979) in patients using the forced expiration technique, although there was a significant increase in pulmonary function with manual techniques (Pryor, Parker, and Webber, 1981).

There are many contraindications to percussion. If the patient's pulmonary status is of greater concern than the relative contraindications, it may be decided to modify and administer the treatment.

Vibration

Vibration is a sustained cocontraction of the upper extremities of a caregiver to produce a vibratory force that is transmitted to the thorax over the involved lung segment. Vibration is applied throughout exhalation concurrently with mild compression to the chest wall. Vibration is often applied in postural drainage positions following percussion to the area. A mechanical vibrator may be used by the patient or a caregiver in place of manual vibration.

Vibration is proposed to enhance mucociliary transport from the periphery of the lung fields to the larger airways. Since vibration is used in conjunction with PD and percussion, many studies do not separate out the effects of vibration from the other components. In fact in multiple studies, the techniques of PD, percussion, and vibration are described as a single entity and referred to as chest physical therapy (CPT), pulmonary therapy, or postural drainage therapy.

Pavia (1976) demonstrated a higher, though not statistically significant, rate of secretion clearance and sputum production with vibration. However, this study was conducted with subjects in an upright position only, not a replication of the use of vibration clinically.

Mackenzie et al. (1980) used measurement of total lung/thorax compliance to assess the effect of secretion clearance. Significant improvement in total lung/thorax compliance was demonstrated after treatment with postural drainage, percussion, and vibration in mechanically ventilated patients. Feldman et al. (1979) demonstrated improved ventilatory function by showing a significant improvement in expiratory flows at lung volumes in patients receiving postural drainage, percussion, vibration, and coughing.

Shaking

Shaking consists of a bouncing maneuver sometimes referred to as "rib springing" against the thoracic wall in a rhythmic fashion throughout exhalation. A concurrent pressure is given to the chest wall, compressing the thorax. Shaking is similar in application to vibration, with shaking being on one end of the spectrum in application of force, and vibration being on the opposite end, supplying a gentler amount of pressure. Many variations exist throughout the spectrum between these techniques. Shaking may be used in place of percussion or intermittently with percussion and vibration. Shaking may be used in postural drainage positions and requires the assistance of a caregiver.

Shaking is proposed to work in the same manner as vibration, mobilizing secretions to the central, larger airways from the lung periphery. Since the compressive force to the thorax is greater, producing increased chest wall displacement, the stretch to the respiratory muscles may produce an increased inspiratory effort and lung volume (Levenson, 1992).

The same relative contraindications for percussion should be observed for shaking, since it does involve application of force to the thorax.

Manual Hyperinflation

This technique is used on patients with an endotracheal or tracheostomy tube that can be attached to a manual ventilation bag. One caregiver uses the bag to hyperinflate the lungs with a slow, deep inspiration and after a short inspiratory pause, provides a quick release to allow rapid exhalation. A second caregiver

applies shaking or vibration at the very beginning of exhalation to mobilize secretions. The timing of this sequence is important to achieve the desired effect (Webber, 1988). It has been likened to simulation of a cough—deep inspiration, pause, and forceful exhalation. Saline may be instilled into the airway at the beginning of the cycle, with suctioning a component at the end of treatment of each side. Manual hyperventilation is performed in postural drainage positions and requires two competent caregivers to perform.

The inspiration provided by the manual ventilation bag, which is deeper than the patient could generate, promotes aeration of the alveoli. The compression of the thorax augments the high expiratory flow rate from the bag, accelerating the movement of the secretions from the smaller airways to the larger bronchi (Clement, 1968).

Clement (1968) reports this method of airway clearance enables patients to be maintained on ventilators for long periods with normal lung function. It has been demonstrated that hyperinflation and suction in the treatment of atelectasis was enhanced by the addition of positioning and vibrations (Stiller, 1990).

Active Cycle of Breathing

Thompson (1973) in New Zealand described clearing bronchial secretions in patients with asthma by a technique of forced expirations and diaphragmatic breathing. British physiotherapists have modified the technique and further described it in the literature, first as the forced expiration technique (FET) (Pryor, 1979) and later as the ACB technique (Webber and Pryor, 1993).

As described by Webber and Pryor (1993), the ACB consists of repeated cycles of three ventilatory phases: breathing control, thoracic expansion exercises, and the FET. Breathing control is described as gentle tidal volume breathing with relaxation of the upper chest and shoulders. The thoracic expansion phase consists of deep inspiration, and may be accompanied by percussion or vibration performed by a caregiver or the patient. This phase helps to loosen secretions. The forced expiration technique involves one or two huffs (forced expirations). Webber and Pryor (1993) report huffing from a mid-lung volume (a medium sized breath in) and continued down to low-lung volume will move secretions from the peripheral to the upper airways. Upper airway secretions may be cleared by a huff from high lung volume (a deep breath in). The ACB may be performed in the sitting position, but has been shown to be more effective in gravity assisted (postural drainage) positions (Steven, 1992).

The period of breathing control is essential between the other phases to prevent bronchospasm (Lapin, 1990). The period of thoracic expansion, which increases lung volume, promotes collateral ventilation, allowing air to get behind secretions and assist in their mobilization (Prasad 1993). Mead et al. (1967) described the physiological theory of "equal pressure point," which is the basis for the FET. The equal pressure point (EPP) is the point in the airways where the pressure is equal to the pleural pressure. The forced expiratory maneuver produces compression of the airway peripherally to the EPP. A huff from high lung volume causes compression within the trachea and bronchi to move secretions from these larger airways. A huff continued to low lung volume shifts the EPP more peripherally to move more peripheral secretions (Webber, 1988).

The ACB technique may be performed by a patient independent of a caregiver. FET performed by patients independently has been shown to clear more sputum in a shorter amount of time than PD with self-percussion combined with percussion and shaking by a physical therapist (PT) (Pryor, 1979). Improvement in pulmonary function (Webber, 1986) and sputum clearance (Sutton, 1983) have been demonstrated in patients with cystic fibrosis who incorporated the FET into their postural drainage treatments.

Because huffing has been shown to stabilize collapsible bronchial walls, it increases the expiratory flow in patients with obstruction without causing airway collapse (Hietpas, 1979). Another benefit of this technique lies in its ability to maintain oxygen saturation. The decrease in oxygen saturation that has been demonstrated with postural drainage and percussion has been prevented with the use of the ACB technique (Pryor, 1990). Hassani et al. (1994) has recently shown that unproductive cough and FET resulted in the movement of secretions proximally from all regions of

the lung in patients with mild hyposecretion. This suggests that FET might help avoid prolonged retention of secretions even in patients who produce little sputum.

Autogenic Drainage

Autogenic drainage (AD) or "self-drainage" was introduced by Chevaillier in Belgium in 1967 for treatment of asthmatic patients. He observed that during sleep, as well as playing and laughing during the day, mucus was mobilized better than during PD and clapping. AD is an antidyspnea technique based on quiet expirations in a relaxed state without use of postural drainage positions (Chevaillier, 1992).

AD uses diaphragmatic breathing to mobilize secretions by varying expiratory airflow. It consists of three phases: (1) breathing at low-lung volumes to "unstick" the peripheral secretions, (2) breathing at low- to mid-lung volume (tidal volume) to collect the mucus in the middle airways, and (3) breathing at mid- to high-lung volumes to evacuate the mucus from the central airways (Chevaillier, 1984). The patient is seated in a relaxed position and exhales actively with the mouth and glottis open and listens for the movement of mucus while avoiding a wheeze. The phases in the AD technique are depicted in Figure 19-1.

The physiology of AD's three phases has been explained eloquently by Shoni (1989). The first phase starts with an inspiration, followed by a breath hold to ensure equal filling of lung segments by collateral filling, and then a deep exhalation into the expiratory reserve volume range. By lowering mid-tidal volume below functional residual capacity level, secretions from peripheral lung regions are mobilized by compression of peripheral alveolar ducts. Mid-expiratory tidal volume is lowered in the range of normal expiratory reserve volume. The second phase of AD consists of tidal volume breathing so that breathing is changed gradually from expiratory reserve volume into the inspiratory reserve volume range to mobilize secretions from the apical parts of the lungs. The velocity of the airflow must be adjusted at each level of inspiration so that the maximal expiratory airflow is reached without being high enough to cause collapse of the airways. Flow volume curves show that higher flows of longer duration can be achieved with AD (Dab, 1979), demonstrating that mucus can be moved further and at a faster rate. The third phase consists of deeper inspiration into the inspiratory reserve volume, with huffing often used to help in evacuating the mobilized secretions. Control of airflow during this final phase is essential to avoid uncontrolled, unproductive coughing.

The Belgian method has been modified by German practioners to use a combination of diaphragmatic and costosternal breathing in a treatment that is not delineated into phases (David, 1991). The patient varies his or her mid-tidal volume in a passive exhalation followed by an active exhalation through pursed lips or through the nose. The German method includes other maneuvers in conjunction with autogenic drainage, including inhalation therapy, FET, chest wall exercises, and sports.

Autogenic drainage has been compared with positive expiratory pressure and PD with percussion/vibration. More sputum was produced with AD in patients with hyperreactive airways (Davidson, 1988). In a 2-year crossover trial, AD was found to be as effective as conventional CPT among patients with cystic fibrosis for improving pulmonary function (Davidson, 1992). However, patients exhibited a strong preference for AD, increasing the likelihood of compliance. Miller (1993) showed greater clearance of inhaled radioisotope with AD vs. the ACB technique, with no significant differences in sputum weight, spirometry, or transcutaneous oxygen saturation. Giles (1993) also studied oxygen (O_2) saturation in AD and found an increase in O_2 saturation with AD over PD with percussion and greater sputum recovery with AD.

The learning of AD requires tactile and auditory feedback and continued modifications of the patient's technique is necessary, at least initially, to achieve a good result. AD takes considerable time to learn and requires a great deal of cooperation from the patient. Therefore it is not suitable for the very young or distractable patient.

Positive Expiratory Pressure

The development and utilization of positive expiratory pressure (PEP) breathing came about in the 1980s in Denmark and is now widely used in Europe with increasing acceptance in the United States.

The application of PEP consists of a mask or mouthpiece connected to a one-way breathing valve to which expiratory resistors are attached. This results in positive pressure in the airways during exhalation. A manometer in the circuit determines and monitors the correct pressure generated by the patient. A patient uses PEP in a cycle of about 10 breaths at tidal volume with slightly active expiration followed by huffing or coughing to expectorate secretions (Falk and Kelstrup, 1993).

High- or low-pressure PEP may be prescribed. In low-pressure PEP, the resistance is regulated to achieve 10 to 20 cms of water pressure during expiration. The pressure should be sustainable during only slightly active expiration. The prescription for high pressure PEP requires the patient to perform forced vital capacity maneuvers through the range of expiratory resistances with the mask connected to a spirometer. The appropriate resistor is one that produces a flow volume curve demonstrating a maximal forced vital capacity, good plateau, and no curvilinearity (Prasad, 1993). In general, the range of pressure generated with high pressure PEP is 50 to 120 cms of water pressure. Low-pressure PEP is used more often, as it offers equal effectiveness at a lower risk of pneumothorax.

It is theorized that PEP allows more air to enter through collateral channels, allowing reinflation of collapsed alveoli. Pressure is built up distal to an obstruction, promoting the movement of secretions towards the larger airways (Anderson, 1979; Groth, 1985). Airway stability is maintained with PEP promoting improved ventilation and gas exchange, as well as airway clearance (Hardy, 1994). Supplemental oxygen can be supplied during treatment with PEP and nebulized medication has been shown to be effectively delivered with this treatment as well (Anderson, 1982).

PEP has been shown to benefit patients at risk for postoperative atelectasis but has also gained wide practice in the area of airway clearance, especially for patients with cystic fibrosis (Malhmeister, 1991). Numerous studies have demonstrated PEP's effectiveness. Tyrrell (1986) has shown the PEP mask to be as effective as conventional physiotherapy over a 1 month period with no difference in pulmonary function. Falk (1984, 1993) demonstrated increased sputum production and clearance with the use of PEP over FET alone. However, Hofmeyer (1986) found FET produced a greater quantity of sputum without the addition of PEP. Oberwaldner (1986) evaluated lung function during 10 months of regular treatments with high-pressure PEP and found reduced pulmonary hyperinflation and airway instability and higher flow rates with PEP vs. conventional CPT. These improvements in lung function deteriorated only 2 months after a return to conventional CPT. A study by Plfeger et al. (1992) compared PEP to AD and found that PEP produced the highest amount of sputum and an increase in lung function when added to both techniques. Finally, decreased duration of hospitalization has been cited as a benefit of PEP for airway clearance (Simonova, 1992).

Increased independence for the patient and presumably, better compliance have been cited as advantages of this technique. However, frequent assessment of patient technique and appropriate level of resistance is recommended (Lapin, 1990). A PEP mouthpiece (Resistex) has recently been FDA approved, but the PEP mask has not yet been approved by the FDA.

A form of PEP in combination with high frequency oscillation is available in a device developed in Switzerland, which is quickly gaining popularity in the United States. The Flutter™ VRP1 (VarioRaw SA, Aubonne, Switzerland) is a handheld device that interrupts the expiratory flow and decreases the collapsability of the airways. The pipe-like device consists of a steel ball, a plastic cone, a perforated cover, and a mouthpiece. The patient completes about 10 to 15 deep breaths keeping the cheeks flat while the Flutter™ is tilted to achieve the maximum effects of the vibration in the chest. This is followed by huffing to eliminate the airway secretions.

Exhalation through the Flutter™ device causes airway vibrations and oscillating endobronchial pressures (Althaus, 1993) to ease the expectoration of mucus. The PEP maintained by the Flutter™ (5 to 35 cms of water pressure) prevents dynamic airway compression and improves airflow acceleration. Therefore the improvement in expectoration is based on the increase in airway diameter, as well as on the improvement in airflow acceleration (Schibler, 1992).

Recently approved by the FDA for use by patients with cystic fibrosis, the Flutter™ continues to be the focus of study in the United States. Konstan et al. (1994) compared the amount of sputum expectorated with use of the Flutter™ vs. vigorous voluntary cough vs. PD, percussion and vibration. More than three times the amount of sputum was produced by subjects with cystic fibrosis using the Flutter™ than with the other two methods and no adverse effects were reported. Ambrosino (1991) has reported success in the treatment of COPD patients with the device.

Reports in the European literature advocate the use of the Flutter™ for airway clearance (Althaus, 1989). In comparison with AD, the Flutter™ was found to be equal in amount of mucus expectoration (Lindemann, 1992). When compared with the PEP-mask, the Flutter™ showed a small increase in spirometry, whereas the PEP-mask did not, but the two techniques were otherwise comparable (Schw. Med. Wschr. 1989).

The advantages of the Flutter™ device lie in its portability and ease of learning. Young children can be taught to use the device effectively, and because of its small size, it can easily be used for multiple treatments throughout the day.

High Frequency Chest Compression

Efforts aimed at mucus clearance by creating a differential air flow rate, that is, greater expiratory than inspiratory flow rate, led to the development of a high frequency chest compression (HFCC) system. Hansen and Warwick (1990) designed a large-volume variable frequency air-pulse delivery system to be used by patients with obstructive lung disease to promote mucus clearance.

The ThAIRapy™ Vest (American Biosystems, Inc.) system consists of an inflatable fitted vest connected to an air-pulse generator by flexible tubing. This device provides oscillation of the entire thoracic cavity at varying frequencies (5 to 25 Hz) and is used while sitting upright. The lung volume expired tends to increase with lower frequencies (less than 10 to 12 Hz), whereas the flow rates tend to increase with higher frequencies (12 to 20 Hz). Three frequencies are selected for large volume and three for high flows. Each frequency is used for 3 to 5 minutes with continuous aerosolized medication or saline to assist secretion mobilization (Warwick, 1992).

Two probable mechanisms of action have been offered to explain the significant increase in sputum mobilization (Klous, 1994). The first mechanism proposes that oscillatory airflow leads to changes in the consistency of mucus, which result in increased sputum mobilization. Significant decreases in mucus viscoelasticity were observed during administration of oscillatory airflow (Tomkiewicz et al, 1994). The second mechanism proposes that the difference between the expiratory and inspiratory velocities produces shear forces strong enough to move mucus. Chang et al. (1988) demonstrated that nonsymmetrical airflow (peak expiratory flow rates greater than inspiratory flow rates) could be a significant factor leading to enhanced mucus clearance during the administration of HFCC. Each chest compression produces a transient flow pulse similar to that observed during coughing and by using those flows with the greatest rates and volumes, sufficient force is obtained to move mucus in the airway (Warwick, 1991).

High frequency chest wall compression has been shown to increase mucus clearance rates in dogs, with the most pronounced effect in the 11 to 15 Hz frequency range (King, 1983). Radford et al. (1982) used bronchoscopy to demonstrate a marked increase in speed and flow of mucus by oscillations at even higher frequencies not attainable by manual percussion. Results of short-term use of the ThAIRapy™ vest have been mixed, but show HFCC to be at least as effective as conventional CPT. Robinson (1992) showed no significant improvement or deterioration of lung function with its use. In two different studies, Kluft (1992) and Faverio (1994) demonstrated increased wet and dry sputum weights using HFCC vs. manual CPT, and Arens (1993) showed similar dry sputum weight, but an increase in wet sputum weight and a significant improvement in pulmonary function with HFCC vs. conventional CPT. One 2-year study showed improved lung function and greater sputum production in subjects with cystic fibrosis with the use of HFCC vs. manual CPT (Warwick, 1991). No adverse effects were observed with long-term use of the ThAIRapy™ vest.

Hospitalized patients with acute exacerbation of their lung disease have been shown to tolerate HFCC well (Burnett, 1993), and safety and tolerance of this method has been demonstrated in long-term mechanically ventilated patients (Whitman, 1993).

Expense of the apparatus may be a significant deterrent to its use; it is more costly than other mechanical aids for airway clearance. However, in a study of HFCC users insured by Blue Cross and Blue Shield, a 49% reduction in health care costs was shown in the year following initial use of the vest as compared with the year prior to HFCC use (Ohnsorg, 1994). The impact of the use of the HFCC device in a hospital department was analyzed with a substantial savings resulting from therapy self-administration (Klous, 1993).

Exercise

In addition to its many effects on health and well-being, exercise has been shown to assist in secretion clearance. It has been suggested that exercise can replace all or part of a conventional chest physiotherapy routine in some patients or at some stages of lung disease (Zach, 1982; Andreasson, 1987; Cerny, 1989).

Exercise increases mucociliary transport in patients with chronic bronchitis (Oldenberg, 1979). Higher transpulmonary pressure with aerobic exercise may open closed bronchi as well as increase collateral ventilation to allow mucus to be moved (Andreasson, 1987). It has also been shown that exercise induced hyperventilation is more effective than eucapnic hyperventilation in mobilizing bronchial secretions (Wolff, 1977). The contribution of expiratory airflow and exercise-induced coughing are other factors in more effective secretion removal.

Some studies conclude that exercise alone is not sufficient and recommend its use to complement other forms of airway clearance. Airway clearance using PD and FET was shown to be more effective than exercise with a cycle ergometer at inducing sputum expectoration (Salh, et al, 1989). Results from Bilton et al (1992) demonstrated that any modality which included the ACB technique in PD positions alone or in combination with exercise is better than exercise alone at clearing sputum.

Other studies have suggested that some forms of exercise may serve as a replacement for chest physiotherapy, citing a lack of decrease in lung function following the cessation of CPT and continuing with an exercise program (Zach, 1984; Andreasson, 1987). In hospitalized patients with cystic fibrosis, no significant change in pulmonary function was reported when exercise was substituted for two treatments of PD, percussion and vibration, and the weight of sputum produced was equivalent (Cerny, 1989).

When mucous clearance was studied, no significant differences were found between exercise on a cycle ergometer, postural drainage, and PEP mask breathing (Lannefors, 1992). Increases in sputum expectoration on exercise vs. nonexercise days have been reported (Zach, 1981; Baldwin, 1994). For patients with cystic fibrosis who demonstrate compliance with an exercise program alone or in addition to another form of secretion mobilization, there is evidence of positive prognostic value (Nixon, 1992).

It is difficult to compare these studies across the board; however, because the mode and length of exercise differs, as does the measurement of effectiveness of airway clearance. Exercise as an airway clearance technique is not suitable for the very young (less than 4 to 5 years of age), patients with neuromuscular limitations, or patients with severely limited exercise tolerance. Moreover, the potential need for supplemental oxygen during exercise should be monitored. Nonetheless, evidence suggests that an exercise program, in addition to clearing secretions, may decrease morbidity and mortality by improving exercise capacity (Lapin, 1993).

Contraindications/Precautions to Airway Clearance

General precautions and contraindications to postural drainage positioning

It is essential that the therapist and the health care team discuss treatment priorities. A decision to use postural drainage might be made despite a contraindication, if the benefits were thought to outweigh the risks in a particular case.

For example, it is known that use of the Trendelenburg (head down) position increases intracranial pressure in neurosurgical patients (Humberstone,

1990). However, if the patient develops atelectasis, the stress of respiratory embarrassment may also increase intracranial pressure. In this instance, the decision may be made to tip the patient to clear the atelectasis and then subsequently return to a modified conservative regimen (Frownfelter, 1987).

A fall in arterial O_2 saturation has been reported with the use of postural drainage from additional in chest physiotherapy, although the effects of PD were not separated techniques (Selsby, 1990; Huseby,

---

Contraindications for Postural Drainage
All Positions Are Contraindicated for the Following:
Intracranial pressure (ICP) > 20 mm Hg
Head and neck injury until stabilized
Active hemorrhage with hemodynamic instability
Recent spinal surgery (e.g., laminectomy) or acute spinal injury
Active hemoptysis
Empyema
Bronchopleural fistula
Pulmonary edema associated with congestive heart failure (CHF)
Large pleural effusions
Pulmonary embolism
Aged, confused, or anxious patients
Rib fracture, with or without flail chest
Surgical wound or healing tissue
Trendelenburg Position is Contraindicated for the Following:
Patients in whom increased ICP is to be avoided
Uncontrolled hypertension
Distended abdomen
Esophageal surgery
Recent gross hemoptysis related to recent lung carcinoma
Uncontrolled airway at risk for aspiration

AARC Clinical Practice Guideline. (1991). Postural drainage therapy. *Respiratory Care, 36* (12), 1418–1426.

1976). Therefore O_2 saturation levels should be monitored during treatment, most importantly in those patients with known low PaO_2 values.

Caution must also be used in treating the patient with end-stage lung disease in postural drainage positions because of the risk of hemoptysis (Hammon, 1979; Stern, 1978).

Decreased cardiac output (Laws, 1969; Barrell, 1978) has been associated with chest physiotherapy treatment; however, the effects of postural drainage were not separated from those of percussion and vibration.

In the pediatric population, some experts recommend caution with the position used to treat the anterior lower lobes because of the risk of gastroesophageal reflux. The box on p. 330 summarizes the precautions and contraindications for postural drainage.

General contraindications and precautions to external manipulation of the thorax

In patients who are very young, who have limited ability to cooperate, or who are not compliant with other airway clearance techniques, percussion, shaking, and vibration offer a method to dislodge retained secretions. Because of the force transmitted to the thoracic cage with these techniques, there are many precautions and contraindications to consider. The therapist should not make this decision alone, but needs direction from the medical team. Chest physiotherapy is not a completely benign procedure and should not be performed in the absence of good indications (McDonnell, 1986).

Percussion has been shown to contribute to a fall in PaO_2 in acutely ill patients (Connors, 1980), especially in patients with cardiovascular instability (Gormenzano, 1972) and in neonates (Fox, 1978). The factor that seems most associated with or predictive of the effect is the baseline or before-therapy PaO_2 (McDonnell, 1986).

Cardiac arrhythmias have been associated with chest percussion for bronchial drainage (Hammon, 1981). Huseby (1976) hypothesizes that hypoxemia may be the underlying mechanism of CPT-caused cardiac arrhythmias.

Patients with hyperreactive airways (e.g., asthma)

show an intolerance for percussion as part of chest physiotherapy. Campbell et al. (1975) demonstrated a fall in FEV_1 associated with percussion that was not evident when percussion was omitted. Administration of a bronchodilator before treatment with percussion abolished the fall in FEV_1. Wheezing has also been associated with percussion and vibration in patients with cystic fibrosis and COPD (Tecklin, 1975; Feldman, 1979).

The box below summarizes the precautions and contraindications for external manipulation of the thorax associated with percussion, shaking, and high frequency chest compression. Vibration involves less force to the thorax and may be better tolerated than the aforementioned techniques. A nebulized bronchodilator may be administered during a treatment of high frequency chest compression to avoid the consequences of hyperreactive airways.

Other precautions

Manual hyperinflation has been shown to cause significant depression of cardiac output in patients who

---

> ### *Contraindications to External Manipulation of the Thorax*
>
> **In Addition to Contraindications for Postural Drainage:**
>
> Subcutaneous emphysema
>
> Recent epidural spinal infusion or spinal anesthesia
>
> Recent skin grafts, or flaps, on the thorax
>
> Burns, open wounds, and skin infections of the thorax
>
> Recently placed pacemaker
>
> Suspected pulmonary tuberculosis
>
> Lung contusion
>
> Bronchospasm
>
> Osteomyelitis of the ribs
>
> Osteoporosis
>
> Coagulopathy
>
> Complaint of chest-wall pain

AARC Clinical Practice Guideline. (1991). Postural drainage therapy. *Respiratory Care, 36* (12), 1418–1426.

are unable to compensate hemodynamically with lit-tle cardiac reserve (Clement, 1968; Laws, 1969). Sig-nificant and deleterious increases in ICP have also been demonstrated (Garradd, 1986). Webber (1988) offers these additional contraindications to manual hyperinflation: severe hypoxemia with few bronchial secretions as in ARDS, acute pulmonary edema, air leak (e.g., pneumothorax), severe bronchospasm as in acute asthma, and hemoptysis.

The use of PEP for airway clearance carries an in-creased risk of pneumothorax (Oberwaldner, 1986). Bronchodilator premedication should be considered when applying PEP in patients who show clinical and/or physiological signs of airway hyperreactivity (Pfleger, 1992).

The increased airflow produced by the huff cough, as in the ACB technique, may aggravate bron-chospasm (Hietpas, 1979). Additionally, Hietpas cau-tions that spontaneous explosive coughing may be precipitated by the movement of secretions into the larger airways by the huff cough.

Several precautions must be observed when using exercise as a form of airway clearance. Desaturation has been shown to occur with exercise in people with pulmonary disease (Lane, 1987; Henke, 1984), and therefore it becomes prudent to monitor oxygen satu-ration, providing supplemental oxygen for the exer-cise period when indicated. Exercise-induced bron-chospasm must also be considered when pulmonary compromise is seen with exercise, especially with higher intensity exercise (Godfrey, 1975). When indi-cated, it is recommended to provide an inhaled bron-chodilator 20 to 30 minutes before exercise to allevi-ate this symptom (Orenstein, 1985). Andreasson (1987) reports a risk of pneumothorax in conjunction with exercise in those patients with extensive bullae.

Factors Affecting Selection of Airway Clearance Techniques

In the pulmonary population, lack of compliance in performing airway clearance on a regular basis has been well documented (Currie, 1986; Passero, 1981; Muszynski-Kwan, 1988; Litt, 1980). The problem is worse in the adolescent group. Litt (1980) has also shown that the complexity and increased duration of

---

Factors to Be Considered When Selecting an Airway Clearance Technique

Motivation

Patient's goals

Physician/caregiver's goals

Effectiveness (of considered technique)

Patient's age

Patient's ability to concentrate

Ease (of learning and of teaching)

Skill of therapists/teachers

Fatigue or work required

Need for assistants or equipment

Limitations of technique based on disease type and severity

Costs (direct and indirect)

Desirability of combining methods

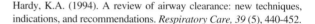

Hardy, K.A. (1994). A review of airway clearance: new techniques, indications, and recommendations. *Respiratory Care, 39* (5), 440-452.

a prescribed treatment has a negative influence on pa-tient adherence. It has been suggested that enhanced compliance might be achieved if the treatment were specifically tailored to the individual patient's needs with regard to clinical status, family functioning, and family concerns. Negotiation between the patient and the caregiver to agree on follow-through with the pre-scribed treatment regimen is also effective (Shultz, 1980). For this reason, it is imperative to consider multiple factors in the recommendation of a specific technique of airway clearance, especially in the pa-tient with a chronic disease (see box above).

The age of the patient will affect the usefulness of a particular technique. Infants and very young chil-dren are limited to conventional physical therapy (postural drainage, percussion, and vibration), since they are not able to cooperate with other methods of airway clearance. After the age of 3 or 4, a youngster may be taught huffing and breathing control, and as-sisted with the ACB technique. A vest for use with HFCC is now available for children as young as 2 or 3 years of age. PEP, Flutter™ and exercise also are suitable for this age group, depending on the child's attention span and cooperation. Children 12 years of age and older are capable of using any of the airway clearance techniques, including AD, which requires more concentration than a younger child is typically able to exhibit.

The lack of an assistant to provide airway clearance is a factor that prompts many patients to seek methods other than postural drainage and percussion. HFCC, PEP, Flutter™, ACB, exercise and AD are techniques that provide independence from a caregiver. These methods have been chosen by adults living on their own, students away at school, and adolescents eager for independence. For optimal results, each technique's effectiveness must be regularly reevaluated by a health care team member skilled in the area of airway clearance after it has been agreed that a patient exhibits independence in a given technique.

The clinical status of the patient during each hospital admission must be evaluated to determine the appropriateness of an ACT. For example, airway hyperreactivity might be worsened by PD and percussion, and care must also be taken when using ACB in this case. HFCC, Flutter™, and exercise should be preceded with an inhaled bronchodilator in this case, and PEP can be performed concurrently with bronchodilator administration. AD lends itself well to use by patients with airway hyperreactivity.

Gastroesophageal reflux prohibits patients from performing airway clearance in conventional PD positions. In this instance, AD, Flutter™, PEP, HFCC, and exercise, or ACB in upright positions, are the preferred treatments. In infants or neurologically impaired patients where PD and percussion is the treatment of choice, modified PD positions are used and sufficient time allowed between a feeding and a treatment with PD.

The severity of a patient's lung disease will affect the choice of ACT. Specifically, a patient with end-stage lung disease or an acute exacerbation might not have the required energy level to carry out an active airway clearance technique such as AD or PEP effectively. A more passive technique would be appropriate, at least temporarily. Also a marked decrease in PFT's limits the airflow control necessary for AD, Flutter™, or PEP.

Accessibility of equipment or trained personnel limits the use of some airway clearance techniques. Many of these techniques are new or not available to many health care centers, especially in the United States, since they were pioneered in Europe. Proper instruction and review of a patient's technique is imperative to achieve optimal results, and in the case of PEP, the reassessment of resistance is recommended. In the case of AD, the method is limited by the number of instructors available to teach the technique to patients and requires a great deal of time on the part of the health care team member to learn. The patient must possess motivation and the time to learn the technique and be willing to "fine tune" the technique with the therapist periodically.

In this area of cost containment, the financial requirements of a technique must also be taken into consideration, especially in the case of a chronic condition. The availability of any given method then, could be determined by the insurance coverage or additional financial resources of the patient. If several methods prove to be equally effective, it would be prudent to select the methods requiring the least expense. Although the most common form of airway clearance in the United States continues to be postural drainage and percussion by a caregiver, this often proves to be quite expensive, especially if a family member is not available for ongoing home treatments. The equipment needed for ACTs varies. The generator required for HFCC is expensive to purchase or rent on a monthly basis. Mechanical percussors or vibrators are moderately priced, and PEP and the Flutter™ valve are the least expensive of those techniques requiring equipment. A patient independently using ACB or AD consumes the least financial resources.

Ultimately, the regular use of a particular ACT by a patient is governed by personal belief in the effectiveness of the method for his or her own disease process, the manner in which the method affects the patient family's life habits, and the patient's willingness to use the technique on a daily basis. Compliance is ultimately the best measure of any airway clearance technique's effectiveness.

Clinical outcome measures to assess the effectiveness of an airway clearance technique can be followed during clinical appointments or periods of hospitalization. Radiographic changes, arterial blood gas values, O_2 saturation, and pulmonary function tests may demonstrate adequate airway clearance or the need to reassess the appropriateness of the technique or the application of it by the patient. Though it is difficult to quantify, many patients subjectively rely on amount of sputum production to guide their choice of secretion clearance method. This measure provides immediate feedback to the patient without visiting the hospital or clinic.

SUMMARY

The goals of airway clearance are to decrease airway obstruction, improve secretion clearance, and improve ventilation and gas exchange. Routine application of airway clearance techniques in many conditions has not been shown to be effective in achieving these goals. ACTs are not without side effects or complications; routine use of these methods is not recommended without clear indications.

Indications for ACTs have been divided into those for acute illness and chronic disease states. In acute illness, traditional chest physical therapy, that is, PD, percussion, and vibration, has been shown to be beneficial in patients with copious secretions and in the treatment of atelectasis (Kiriloff, 1985). For patients with cystic fibrosis, treatment with PEP and exercise in conjunction with PD, percussion, and vibration were also shown to be effective in an acute exacerbation (Boyd, 1994). Acute asthma, bronchitis, and pneumonia without copious secretions, bronchiolitis, and routine postoperative conditions were not shown to benefit from PD, percussion, and vibration (Sutton, 1982; Eid, 1991).

In chronic disease states, patients with cystic fibrosis and bronchiectasis were found to benefit from PD, percussion, and vibration (Kiriloff, 1985). Positive expiratory pressure and exercise were also shown to be effective in the chronic management of patients with cystic fibrosis (Boyd, 1994).

In those patients for whom traditional chest physical therapy is not effective, the caregiver must consider many factors in recommending an alternate form of airway clearance. Age of the patient is a prime factor in the appropriateness of a selected technique. For infants, PD, percussion, and vibration remain the mainstay of secretion clearance. In older children, the active cycle of breathing may be initiated, positive expiratory pressure and Flutter™ may be taught, and high frequency chest compression is available for children after about age 3 or 4. Exercise should be included in treatment as well. Children 12 years of age or older and adults have the complete range of airway clearance techniques at their disposal, including autogenic drainage.

Treatments aimed at secretion clearance require an individualized approach to tailor the treatment to the patient's condition and lifestyle, to continuously reevaluate the patient's status, and to monitor the response to treatment.

Acceptance of the specific treatment technique by the patient and family is paramount; compliance is the key to achieving effective treatment, especially in chronic lung disease.

Further research in the area of airway clearance is certainly needed. Studies with consistent application of techniques, similar outcome measures, and consistent study design will assist practitioners in evaluating and recommending a given technique of airway clearance.

REVIEW QUESTIONS

1. What kinds of pulmonary conditions would *not* be likely to benefit from ACTs?
2. Which ACTs would be the easiest (for the therapist and the patient) to incorporate into a routine of conventional PD and percussion?
3. What possible factors could be considered a contraindication to chest percussion with PD in a trauma or postoperative patient?
4. What factors might make it difficult for a patient to accept a new method of airway clearance?
5. Which ACTs would be most appropriate during an acute exacerbation of a pulmonary disease?

References

AARC Clinical Practice Guideline. (1991). Postural drainage therapy. *Respiratory Care,* 36 (12), 1418-1426.

Althaus, P., et al. (1989). The bronchial hygiene assisted by the Flutter VRP1 (module regulator of a positive pressure oscillation expiration). *European Respiratory Journal, 2 (8),* 693.

Althaus, P. (1993). Oscillating PEP. In Bronchial Hypersecretion: Current Chest Physiotherapy In Cystic Fibrosis (CF), Published by International Committee for CF (IPC/CF).

Ambrosino, N., et al. (1991). Clinical evaluation of a new device for home chest physiotherapy in nonhypersecretive COPD patients. *American Review Respiratory Diseases,* 143 (4), 260.

Andersen, J.B., Qvist, J., Kann, T. (1979). Recruiting collapsed lung through collateral channels with positive end-expiratory pressure. *Scandanavian Journal Respiratory Diseases, 60,* 260-266.

Andersen, J.B., Klausen, N.O. (1982). A new mode of administration of nebulized bronchodilator in severe bronchospasm. *European Respiratory Journal suppl.* 63, 119, 97-100.

Andreasson, B., et al. (1987). Long-term effects of physical exercise on working capacity and pulmonary function in cystic fibrosis. *Acta Pediatrics of Scandanavian, 76,* 70-75.

Arens, R., et al. (1993). Comparative efficacy of high frequency chest compression and conventional chest physiotherapy in hospitalized patients with cystic fibrosis. *Pediatric Pulmonol, suppl. 9,* 239.

Baldwin, D.R. (1994). Effect of addition of exercise to chest physiotherapy on sputum expectoration and lung function in adults with cystic fibrosis. *Respiratory Medicine, 88,* 49-53.

Barrell, S.E., Abbas, H.M. (1978). Monitoring during physiotherapy after open heart surgery. *Physiotherapy, 64,* 272-273.

Bateman, J., et al. (1981). Is cough as effective as chest physiotherapy in the removal of excessive tracheobronchial secretions? *Thorax, 36,* 683-687.

Bilton, D., et al. (1992). The benefits of exercise combined with physiotherapy in the treatment of adults with cystic fibrosis. *Respiratory Medicine, 86,* 507-511.

Boyd, S., et al. (1994). Evaluation of the literature on the effectiveness of physical therapy modalities in the management of children with cystic fibrosis. *Pediatric Physical Therapy,* 70-74.

Britton, S., Bejstedt, M., Vedin, L. (1985). Chest physiotherapy in primary pneumonia. *British Medical Journal, 290 (8),* 1703-1704.

Burnett, M., et al. (1993). Comparative efficacy of manual chest physiotherapy and a high-frequency chest compression vest in treatment of cystic fibrosis. Abstract presented at ATS International Conference, San Francisco.

Campbell, A.H., O'Connell, J.M., Wilson, F. (1975). The effect of chest physiotherapy upon the FEV1 in chronic bronchitis. *Medical Journal Australia,* 1, 33-35.

Cerny, F.J. (1989). Relative effects of bronchial drainage and exercise for in-hospital care of patients with cystic fibrosis. *Physical Therapy,* 69, 633-639.334

Chang, H.K., Weber, M.E., King, M. (1988). Mucus transport by high-frequency nonsymmetrical oscillatory airflow. *Journal of Applied Physiology,* 65 (3), 1203-1209.

Chevaillier, J. (1992). Airway clearance techniques. Course Presented at Sixth Annual North American Cystic Fibrosis Conference, Dallas.

Clement, A.J., Hubsch, S.K. (1968). Chest Physiotherapy by the 'bag squeezing' method: A guide to technique. *Physiotherapy,* 54, 355-359.

Connors, A.F., et al. (1980). Chest physical therapy: The immediate effect on oxygenation in acutely ill patients. Chest, 78, 559-564.

Currie, D.C. (1986). Practice, problems and compliance with postural drainage: A survey of chronic sputum producers. *British Journal of Diseases of the Chest,* 80, 249-253.

Dab, I., Alexander, F. (1979). The mechanism of autogenic drainage studied with flow volume curves. *Mon Paed,* 10, 50-53.

David, A. (1991). Autogenic drainage-the German approach. In Pryor, J. (Ed.), *Respiratory Care.* Edinburgh: Churchill Livingstone.

Davidson, N.G.T., et al. (1988). Physiotherapy in cystic fibrosis: A comparative trial of PEP, AD, and conventional percussion and drainage techniques. Abstracted in *Pediatric Pulmonol,* suppl. 2, 132.

Davidson, A.G.F., et al. (1992). Long-term comparative trial of conventional percussion and drainage physiotherapy versus AD in cystic fibrosis. Abstracted in *Pediatric Pulmonology, suppl.* 8, 235.

Dean, E., Ross, J. (1992). Discordance between cardiopulmonary-Physiologyogy and physical therapy. *Chest,* 101, 1694-98.

Denton, R. (1962). Bronchial secretions in cystic fibrosis. *American Review of RespiratoryDisease,* 86, 41-46.

Desmond, K., et al. (1983). Immediate and long-term effects of chest physical therapy in patients with cystic fibrosis. *Journal of Pediatrics,* 103, 538-542.

Dickman, C., Wilchynski, J.A. (1987). Respiratory failure. In Frownfelter, D. (Ed.): Chest Physical Therapy and Pulmonary Rehabilitation (2nd Ed.) Chicago: Year-Book Medical Publishers, Inc.

Eid, N., et al. (1991). Chest physiotherapy in review. *Respiratory Care, 36 (4),* 270-282.

Falk, M., et al. (1984). Improving the ketchup bottle method with PEP, PEP in cystic fibrosis. *European Journal of Respiratory-Disease,* 65, 423-32.

Falk, M., et al. (1993). Short-term effects of PEP and the FET on mucus clearance and lung function in cystic fibrosis. Abstracted in *Pediatric Pulmonology,* suppl. 9, 241.

Falk, M., Kelstrup, M. (1993). PEP. In Bronchial Hypersecretion: Current Chest Physiotherapy in cystic fibrosis (CF). Published by International Physiotherapy Committee for Cystic Fibrosis (IPC/CF).

Faverio, L., et al. (1994). A comparison of bronchial drainage treatments in patients with cystic fibrosis. Abstract presented at ALA/ATS International Conference, Boston.

Feldman, J., Traver, G.A., Taussig, L.M. (1979). Maximal expiratory flows after postural drainage. American Review of Respiratory Disease, 119, 239-245.

Finer, N., Boyd, J. (1978). Chest physiotherapy in the neonate: A controlled study. *Pediatrics,* 61, 282-285.

Ford, R.M., Godreau, K.M., Burns, D.M. (1991). Carpal tunnel syndrome as a manifestation of cumulative trauma disorder in respiratory care practitioners. Abstracted in *Respiratory Care, 36.*

Frownfelter, D. (1987). Postural drainage. In Frownfelter, D. (Ed.), Chest Physical Therapy and Pulmonary Rehabilitation 2nd Ed. (271-287). Chicago: Year Book Medical Publishers, Inc.

Fox, W.W., Schwartz, J.G., Shaffer, T.H. (1978). Pulmonary physiotherapy in neonates: Physiologyogic changes and respiratory management. *Journal of Pediatrics, 92,* 977-981.

Gallon, A. (1991). Evaluation of chest percussion in the treatment of patients with copious sputum production. *Respiratory Medicine, 85,* 45-51.

Garradd, J., Bullock, M. (1986). The effect of respiratory therapy on intracranial pressure in ventilated neurosurgical patients. Aust Journal Physiol, 32(2), 107-111.

Giles, D.R., Acurso, F.J., Wagener, J.S. (1993). Acute effects of PD and clapping versus AD on oxygen saturation and sputum recovery in cystic fibrosis. Abstracted in *Pediatric Pulmonology,* suppl. 9, 252.

Godfrey, S., Silverman, M., Anderson, S. (1975). The use of the treadmill for assessing exercise induced asthma and the effect of varying the severity and duration of exercise. *Pediatrics,* 56(suppl), 893-898.

Gormenzano, J., Branthwaite, M.A. (1972). Pulmonary physiotherapy with assisted ventilation. *Anaesthesia,* 27, 249-257.

Groth, S., et al. (1985). PEP (PEP-mask) physiotherapy improves ventilation and reduces volume of trapped gas in cystic fibrosis. *Bulletin of European Physiopathology and Respiratory,* 21, 339-343.

Hammon, W.E., Martin, R.J. (1979). Fatal pulmonary hemorrhage associated with chest physical therapy. *Physical Therapy,* 59, 1247-1248.

Hammon, W.E., Martin, R.J. (1981). Chest physical therapy for acute atelectasis. *Physical Therapy,* 61(2), 217-220.

Hansen, L.G., Warwick, W.J. (1990). High-frequency chest compression system to aid in clearance of mucus from the lung. BioMed Instr Technol, 24, 289-294.

Hardy, K.A. (1994). A review of airway clearance: New techniques, indications, and recommendations. *Respiratory Care, 39 (5),* 440-452.

Hasani, A., et al. (1994). Regional mucus transport following unproductive cough and FET in patients with airways obstruction. *Chest,* 105, 1420-1425.

Hietpas, B.G., Roth, R.D., Jensen, W.M. (1979). Huff coughing and airway patency. *European Journal of Respiratory of Disease,* 24, 710-713.

Henke, K.G., Orenstein, D.M. (1984). Oxygen saturation during exercise in cystic fibrosis. *American Review of Respirator Diseases,* 129, 708-711.

Hofmeyer, J.L., Webber, B.A., Hodson, M.E. (1986). Evaluation of PEP as an adjunct to chest physiotherapy in the treatment of cystic fibrosis. *Thorax, 41,* 951-954.

Humberstone, N. (1990). Respiratory assessment and treatment. In Irwin, S., Tecklin, J.S. (Eds.), *Cardiopulmonary Physical Therapy,* 2nd Ed. (pp. 283-321). St. Louis: Mosby.

Huseby, J., et al. (1976). Oxygenation during chest physiotherapy. Abstracted in *Chest, 70,* 430.

King, M., et al. (1983). Enhanced tracheal mucus clearance with high frequency chest wall compression. *American Review of Respiratory Disease,* 128, 511-515.

Kirifoff, L.H., et al. (1985). Does chest physical therapy work? *Chest,* 88, (3) 436-444.

Klous, D., et al. (1993). Chest vest and cystic fibrosis: Better care for patients. *Advanced Respiratory Care Management, 3,* 44-50.

Klous, D.R. (1994). High-frequency chest wall oscillation: Principles and applications. Published by American Biosystems, Inc., St. Paul.

Kluft, J., et al. (1992). Comparison of bronchial drainage treatments by sputum quantification. Abstracted in Pediatric Pulmonol, Suppl. 8, 238.

Konstan, M.W., Stern, R.C., Doershuk, C.F. (1994). Efficacy of the Flutter device for airway mucus clearance in patients with cystic fibrosis. *Journal of Pediatrics,* 124, 689-693.

Lane, R., et al. (1987). Arterial oxygen saturation and breath issues in patients with cardiovascular disease. Clin Sci, 72, 693-698.

Lannefors, L., Wollmer, P. (1992). Mucus clearance with three chest physiotherapy regimes in cystic fibrosis: A comparison between postural drainage, PEP, and physical exercise. *European Respiratory Journal,* 5, 748-753.

Lapin, A. (1990). Physical therapy in cystic fibrosis: A review. *Cardiopulmonary Physical Therapy, 1 (3),* 11-12.

Lapin, C.D. (1993). Is exercise a substitute for airway clearance techniques? Symposium presented at Seventh Annual North American Cystic Fibrosis Conference, Dallas.

Lapin, C.D. (1994). Conventional postural drainage and percussion. Is this still the gold standard?—Against. *Pediatric Pulmonology,* suppl. 10, 87-88.

Laws, A.K., McIntyre, R.W. (1969). Chest physiotherapy: A physiological assessment during intermittent positive pressure ventilation in respiratory failure. *Can Anaes Soc Journal,* 16(6), 487-493.

Levenson, C.R. (1992). Breathing Exercises. In Zadai, C.C. (Ed.) Pulmonary Management in Physical Therapy. New York: Churchill Livingstone.

Lindemann, H. (1992). Evaluation of VRP1 physiotherapy. *Pneumology,* 46, 626-630.

Litt, I.F., Cushey, W.R. (1980). Compliance with medical regimens during adolescence. *Pediatric Clinics of North America,* 27, 3-15.

Lorin, M.I., Denning, C.R. (1971). Evaluation of postural drainage by measurement of sputum volume and consistency. *American Journal of Physical Medicine,* 50 (5), 215-219.

MacKenzie, C.F., et al. (1980). Changes in total lung/thorax compliance following chest physiotherapy. Anes and Anal, 59 (3), 207-210.

Mahlmeister, M.J., et al. (1991). Positive-expiratory-pressure mask therapy: Theoretical and practical considerations and a review of the literature. *Respiratory Care, 36 (11),* 1218-1229.

Marini, J.J., Pierson, D.J., Hudson, L.D. (1979). Acute lobar atelectasis: A prospective comparison of fiberoptic bronchoscopy and respiratory therapy. *American Review of RespiratoryDiseases, 119,* 971-978.

Massery, M. (1987). Respiratory rehabilitation secondary to neurological deficits: Understanding the deficits. In Frownfelter, D. (Ed.), Chest Physical Therapy and Pulmonary Rehabilitation (Second Ed.). Chicago: Year Book Medical Publisher, Inc.

Maxwell, M., Redmond, A. (1979). Comparative trial of manual and mechanical percussion technique with gravity-assisted bronchial drainage in patients with cystic fibrosis. *Archives of Diseases of the Childhood, 54,* 542-544.

May, D.B., Munt, P.W. (1979). Physiologic effects of chest percussion and postural drainage in patients with stable chronic bronchitis. *Chest, 75,* 29-32.

Mazzocco, M.C., et al. (1985). Chest percussion and postural drainage in patients with bronchiectasis. *Chest, 88 (3),* 361-363.

McDonnell, T., McNicholas, W.T., Fitzgerald, M.X. (1986). Hypoxaemia during chest physiotherapy in patients with cystic fibrosis. *Irish Journal of Medical Sciences, 155,* 345-348.

Mead, J., et al. (1967). Significance of the relationship between lung recoil and maximum expiratory flow. Journal Applied Physical, 22, 95.

Miller, S., et al. (1993). Chest physiotherapy in cystic fibrosis (CF): A comparative study of autogenic drainage (AD) and active cycle of breathing technique (ACBT)(formerly FET). Abstracted in Pediatric Pulmonol, suppl. 9, 240.

MMWR Publication From the Centers For Disease Control (CDC). (1989). Occupational disease surveillance: Carpal tunnel syndrome. *JAMA, 282 (7),* 886-889.

Muszynski-Kwan, A.T., Perlman, R., Rivington-Law, B.A. (1988). Compliance with and effectiveness of chest physiotherapy in cystic fibrosis: A review. *Physiology of Canada,* 40 (1), 28-32.

Nixon, P.A. (1992). The prognostic value of exercise testing in patients with cystic fibrosis. *New England Journal of Medicine,* 327, 1785-1788.

Oberwaldner, B., Evans, J.C., Zach, M.S. (1986). Forced expirations against a variable resistance: A new chest physiotherapy method in cystic fibrosis. *Pediatric Pulmonology, 2,* 358-367.

Ohnsorg, F. (1994). A cost analysis of high-frequency chest wall oscillation in cystic fibrosis. Abstract presented at the ALA/ATS International Conference, Boston.

Oldenberg, F.A., et al. (1979). Effects of postural drainage, exercise, and cough on mucus clearance in chronic bronchitis. *American Review of Respiratory of Diseases,* 120, 739-745.

Orenstein, D.M., et al. (1985). Exercise conditioning in children with asthma. *Journal of Pediatrics,* 106, 556-560.

Passero, M.A., Remor, B., Salomon, J. (1981). Patient-reported compliance with cystic fibrosis therapy. *Clinics of Pediatrics,* 20, 265-268.

Pavia, D., Thomson, M.L., Phillipakos, D. (1976). A preliminary study of the effect of a vibrating pad on bronchial clearance. *American Review of RespiratoryDiseases,* 113, 92-96.

Pfleger, A., et al. (1992). Self-administered chest physiotherapy in cystic fibrosis: A comparative study of high-pressure PEP and autogenic drainage. *Lung, 170,* 323-330.

Prasad, S.A. (1993). Current concepts in physiotherapy. *Journal of the Royal Society of Medicine,* 86, suppl. 20, 23-29.

Pryor, J.A., et al. (1979). Evaluation of the forced expiration technique as an adjunct to postural drainage in treatment of cystic fibrosis. *British Medical of Journal,* 18, 417-418.

Pryor, J.A., Parker, R.A., Webber, B.A. (1981). A comparison of mechanical and manual percussion as adjuncts to postural drainage in the treatment of cystic fibrosis in adolescents and adults. *Physiotherapy, 67 (5),* 140-141.

Pryor, J.A., Webber, B.A., Hodson, M.E. (1990). Effect of chest physiotherapy on oxygen saturation in patients with cystic fibrosis, 45, 77.

Radford, R., et al. (1982). A rational basis for percussion-augmented mucociliary clearance. *Respiratory Care, 27,* 556-563.

Reisman, J., et al. (1988). Role of conventional therapy in cystic fibrosis. *Journal of Pediatrics,* 113, 632-636.

Robinson, C., Hernried, L. (1992). Evaluation of a high frequency chest compression device in cystic fibrosis. Abstracted in Pediatric Pulmonol, Suppl. 8, 255.

Rochester, D.F., Goldberg, S.K. (1980). Techniques of respiratory physical therapy. *American Review of Respiratory Diseases, 122,* 133-146.

Rossman, C.M., et al. (1982). Effect of chest physiotherapy on the removal of mucus in patients with cystic fibrosis. *American Review of Respiratory Diseases, 126,* 131-135.

Salh, W., et al. (1989). Effect of exercise and physiotherapy in aiding sputum expectoration in adults with cystic fibrosis. *Thorax,* 44, 1006-1008.

Schibler, A., Casaulta, C., Kraemer, R. (1992). Rational of oscillatory breathing as chest physiotherapy performed by the Flutter in patients with cystic fibrosis (CF). Abstracted in *Pediatric Pulmonology,* suppl. 8, 244.

Selsby, D., Jones, J.G. (1990). Some physiological and clinical aspects of chest physiotherapy. *British Journal of Anaesthesia,* 64, 621-631.

Shoni, M.H. (1989). Autogenic drainage: A modern approach to physiotherapy in cystic fibrosis. *Journal Royal Soc Medicine,* suppl. 16, 82, 32-37.

Shultz, K. (1980). Compliance with therapeutic regimens in pediatricics: a review of implications for social work practice. *Social Work Health Care, 5(3),* 267-278.

Simonova, O., et al. (1992). PEP-mask therapy in complex treatment of cystic fibrosis patients. Abstracted in *Pediatric Pulmonology,* suppl. 8, 245.

Stern, R.C., et al. (1978). Treatment and prognosis of massive hemoptysis in cystic fibrosis. *American Review of RespiratoryDiseases,* 117, 825-829.

Steven, M.H., et al. (1992). Physiotherapy versus cough alone in the treatment of cystic fibrosis. New Zealand *Journal Physiotherapy, 20* (2), 31-37.

Stiller, K., et al. (1990). Acute lobar atelectasis: A comparison of two chest physiotherapy regimens. *Chest, 98,* 1336-1340.

Sutton, P.P., et al. (1982). Chest Physiotherapy: A review. *European Journal of Respiratory Diseases, 63,* 188-201.

Sutton, P.P., et al. (1983). Assessment of the forced expiration technique, postural drainage and directed coughing in chest physiotherapy. *European Journal of Respiratory Diseases, 64,* 62-68.

Tecklin, J.S., Holsclaw, D.S. (1975). Evaluation of bronchial drainage in patients with cystic fibrosis. *Physical Therapy, 55,* 1081-1084.

Thompson, B.J. (1973). The physiotherapist's role in the rehabilitation of the asthmatic. *New Zealand Journal of Physiotherapy, 4,* 11-16.

Tomkiewicz, R., Bivij, A., King, M. (1994). Rheologic studies regarding high frequency chest compression (HFCC) and improvements of mucus clearance in cystic fibrosis. Abstract presented at ATS International Conference, Boston.

Torrington, K., Sorenson, D., Sherwood, L. (1984). Postoperative chest percussion with postural drainage in obese patients following gastric stapling. *Chest, 86,* 891-895.

Tyrrell, J.C., Hill, E.J., Martin, J. (1986). Face mask physiotherapy in cystic fibrosis. *Archives of Diseases of the Childhood. 61,* 598-611.

Warwick, W.J., Hansen, L.G. (1991). The long-term effect of high-frequency chest compression therapy on pulmonary complications of cystic fibrosis. *Pediatric Pulmonology. 11,* 265-271.

Warwick, W.J. (1992). Airway clearance by high frequency chest compression. Symposium presented at Sixth Annual North American Cystic Fibrosis Conference, Washington, D.C.

Webb, M.S.C., et al. (1985). Chest physiotherapy in acute bronchiolitis. *Archives of Diseases of the Childhood. 60,* 1078-1079.

Webber, B.A., et al. (1986). Effect of postural drainage, incorporating the FET, on pulmonary function in cystic fibrosis. *British Journal of Diseases of the Chest, 80,* 353-359.

Webber, B.A. (1988). Is postural drainage necessary? Paper Presented at Tenth International Cystic Fibrosis Conference, Sydney.

Webber, B.A. (1988). Physiotherapy for patients receiving mechanical ventilation. In Webber, B.A. (Ed.) The Brompton Hospital Guide to Chest Physiotherapy (Fifth Ed.). Oxford, Blackwell Scientific Publications.

Webber, B., Pryor, J. (1993). Active cycle of breathing techniques. In Bronchial Hypersecretion: Current Chest Physiotherapy in Cystic Fibrosis (CF). Published by International Physiotherapy Committee for Cystic Fibrosis (IPC/CF).

Webber, B.A., Pryor, J. A. (1993). Physiotherapy skills: techniques and adjuncts. In Physiotherapy for Respiratory and Cardiac Problems. Edinburgh: Churchill Livingstone.

Wetzel. J.L., et al. (1990). Respiratory rehabilitation of the patient with a spinal cord injury. In Irwin, S., Tecklin, J.S. (Eds.), Cardiopulmonary Physical Therapy (Second Edition). St. Louis: C V Mosby Co.

Whitman, J., et al. (1993). Preliminary evaluation of high-frequency chest compression for secretion clearance in mechanically ventilated patients. *Respiratory Care,* 38 (10), 1081-1087.

Wolff, R.K., et al. (1977). Effects of exercise and eucapnic hyperventilation on bronchial clearance in man. *Journal of Applied Physiology: Respiratory Environment Exercise Physiol, 43,* 46-50.

Wollmer, P., et al. (1985). Inefficiency of chest percussion in the physical therapy of chronic bronchitis. *European Journal of Respiratory Disease, 66,* 233-239.

Wong, J.W., et al. (1977). Effects of gravity in tracheal transport rates in normal subjects and in patients with cystic fibrosis. *Pediatricics, 60,* 146-152.

Wood, R.E. (1989). Treatment of cystic fibrosis lung disease in the first two years. Pediatric Pulmonol, 4, 685-690.

Zach, M., Oberwaldner, B., Hausler, F. (1982). Cystic fibrosis: physical exercise versus chest physiotherapy. *Archives of Diseases of the Childhood. 57,* 587-589.

Zadai, C.C. (1981). Physical therapy for the acutely ill medical patient. *Physical Therapy, 61 (12),* 1746-1753.

Zausmer, E. (1968). Bronchial drainage: Evidence supporting the procedures. *Physical Therapy, 48,* 586-591.

CHAPTER 20

Clinical Application of Airway Clearance Techniques

Anne Mejia Downs

KEY TERMS

Active cycle of breathing technique (ACBT)
Airway clearance techniques (ACTs)
Autogenic drainage (AD)
Dynamic air therapy bed
Flutter™
Forced expiratory technique (FET)
High frequency chest compression (HFCC)

Manual hyperventilation
Percussion
Postive expiratory pressure (PEP)
Postural drainage (PD)
Shaking
Trendelenburg
Vibration

INTRODUCTION

Oxygen transport from the lungs to body tissues can be limited in patients that possess an ineffective cough or an impairment of normal mechanisms of mucociliary clearance. The caregiver must augment these mechanisms using the array of techniques available for airway clearance. Each technique has a physiological basis for improving the mobilization of secretions. The caregiver must consider the pathophysiology and the symptoms of the disease, the availability of the technique to the patient, and the patient's acceptance of the technique in prescribing an optimal method of airway clearance.

The previous chapter addressed the physiological basis of each technique, the history of its use, and research to establish its effectiveness. This chapter provides an introduction to the application of these techniques to patients and addresses the benefits and liabilities of each technique.

Airway clearance techniques differ with respect to equipment needs, the skill level required to perform them, and their usefulness with various clinical problems. Matching a patient with an appropriate method or combination of methods may increase effectiveness, reduce complications, and promote adherence to the long-term treatment.

UTILIZATION OF AIRWAY CLEARANCE TECHNIQUES

This section will deal with the application of airway clearance techniques (ACTs) with specific instructions for patient treatment. Contraindications and precautions for each ACT are addressed in Chapter 21. This section will speak to practical concerns regarding patient care.

Preparation for any secretion removal technique should include evaluation of the patient's pulmonary status (see Chapter 15) so that measures may be compared before and after a treatment is completed. A physical examination, including inspection, palpation, measurement of vital signs, and chest auscultation provides assessment of a treatment's effectiveness. Laboratory tests including chest x-ray, arterial blood gas measurements, and pulmonary function studies should be reviewed, since these may be used as measures of treatment effectiveness.

Scheduling an optimal time for patient treatment must take into account several factors. At least 1 half hour to 1 hour should be allowed for the completion of tube feedings or meals. The inhalation of bronchodilator medications should take place before airway clearance maneuvers. Inhaled antibiotics are best scheduled after airway clearance has taken place for optimal deposition of medication. Adequate pain control is necessary to receive a patient's best effort and cooperation with a treatment. It is also important to have all necessary equipment and personnel available at the start of the treatment.

POSTURAL DRAINAGE

Postural drainage (PD) is accomplished by positioning the patient so that the position of the lung segment to be drained allows gravity to have its greatest effect (see Figures 20-1 through 20-5). Modified positions are used when a precaution or relative contraindication to the ideal position exists. For example, if an increase in intracranial pressure is a concern, the head of the bed should remain flat instead of being tipped into Trendelenburg (head down) position.

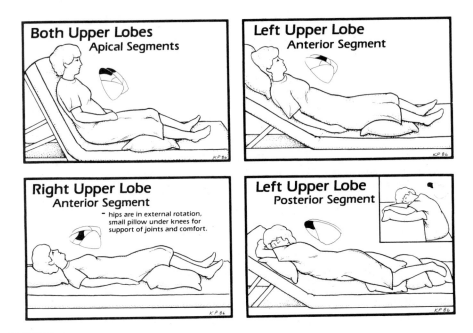

FIGURE 20-1
Upper lobes.

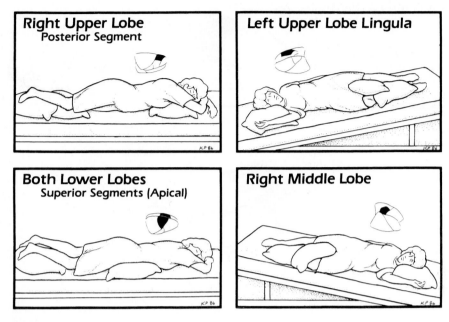

FIGURE 20-2
Upper, middle, and lower lobes.

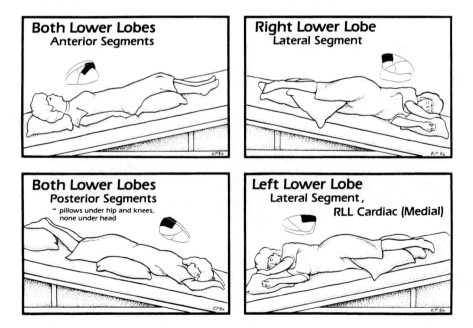

FIGURE 20-3
Lower lobes.

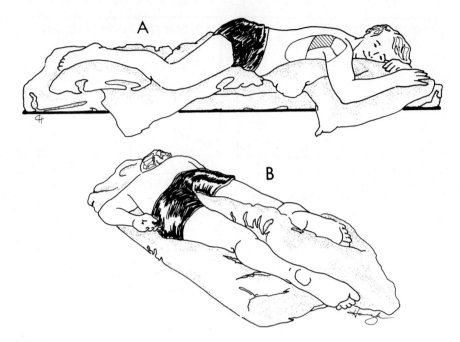

FIGURE 20-4
A, right upper lobe—posterior segment (anterior view—patient positioned three-fourths prone).
B, right upper lobe—posterior segment (posterior view). NOTE: Upper extremities toward prone,
underneath arm pulled free from under patient's body. This position may also be a modified
position for right lower lobe posterior segment.

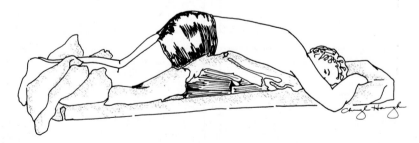

FIGURE 20-5
Both lower lobes—posterior segments (shown using telelphone books or pillows for home use). A
beanbag chair is also helpful for home treatments.

Equipment Required For Postural Drainage

1. For the hospitalized patient, there exists a variety of beds that employ manual or electric devices to position the patient. Air therapy beds, most often used in the intensive care unit (ICU), are valuable aids allowing ease of positioning, especially in large or unresponsive patients.
2. Make use of pillows or bedrolls to support body parts or relieve pressure areas.
3. For home treatment, aids in positioning might include pillows, a slant board (or ironing board if the patient is small), a foam wedge, sofa cushions, or a bean bag chair.

Preparation for Postural Drainage

1. Nebulized bronchodilators before PD may facilitate the mobilization of sputum.
2. An adequate intake of fluids (if allowed) decreases the viscosity of the secretions, allowing easier mobilization.
3. Become familiar with the workings of the model of bed the patient is occupying, especially the movement of the bed into the Trendelenberg position.
4. In the ICU, it is imperative to be familiar with the multiple lines, leads, and tubes attached to the patient. Allow enough slack from each device to position a patient for postural drainage.
5. Make sure there are enough personnel to position the patient with as little stress to both patient and staff as possible (Frownfelter, 1987).
6. Have suctioning equipment ready to remove secretions from an artificial airway or the patient's oral or nasal cavity after the treatment.

Treatment with PD

1. After determining the lobe of the lung to be treated, position the patient in the appropriate position, using pillows or bed rolls as needed to support the patient comfortably in the position indicated. See figures 20-1 through 20-5, p. 340-342.
2. If postural drainage is used exclusively, each position should be maintained for 5 to 10 minutes, if tolerated, or longer when focusing on a specific lobe. Extended times in a position may be used by coordinating the positioning with nursing care for skin pressure relief. If postural drainage is used in conjunction with another technique, the time in each position may be decreased. For example, if percussion and vibration are performed while the patient is in each PD position, 3 to 5 minutes is sufficient.
3. A patient who requires close monitoring should not be left unattended in a Trendelenberg position, but this may be appropriate if patients are alert and able to reposition themselves.
4. It is not necessary to treat each affected lung segment during each treatment; this may prove to be too fatiguing for the patient. The most affected lobes should be addressed with the first treatment of the day, with the other affected areas addressed at a subsequent treatment.
5. The patient should be encouraged to take deep breaths and cough after the treatment and if possible after each position. Having the patient sit upright or lean forward optimizes this effort (Frownfelter, 1987).
6. Secretions may not be mobilized immediately after the treatment but possibly 1 half hour to 1 hour later. The patient should be thus informed and requested to clear secretions then. The nurse or family member should be included in this aspect of treatment, especially with difficult patients who need such encouragement (Frownfelter, 1987).

Advantages and Disadvantages of PD

PD is relatively easy to learn; the patient and/or caregiver must be familiar with the appropriate positioning for the affected lung fields. Treatment in the hospital may be coordinated with other patient activities—positioning for skin pressure relief, bathing, or positioning for a test or procedure. Home treatment may be coordinated with activities such as reading or watching television.

However, for many patients, optimal PD positions will be contraindicated for a variety of reasons (see Chapter 21). Compliance with PD may be reduced because of the length of the treatment, especially in

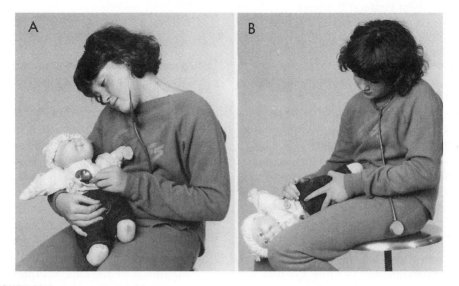

FIGURE 20-6
A and **B,** If children are able to role play the treatment, they will better understand what is expected and be more cooperative with therapy.

the pediatric population, who will require considerable distractions to maintain a desired position.

The cost of the equipment required for PD is minimal; inexpensive items may be used for home treatment. However, the cost of a caregiver's time to provide the treatment, especially in the case of a chronic disease, may be substantial. A family member may be willing to learn the procedure, which would provide a benefit in terms of expense, as well as flexibility in scheduling (Figure 20-6).

PERCUSSION

Percussion is performed with the aim of loosening retained secretions from the airways so they may be removed by suctioning or expectoration. A rhythmical force is provided by clapping the caregiver's cupped hands against the thorax over the affected lung segment, trapping air between the patient's thorax and the caregiver's hands (Figure 20-7). It is performed during both the inspiratory and expiratory phases of

breathing. Percussion is used in postural drainage positions for increased effectiveness (Sutton, 1985; Bateman, 1979) and may also be used during the active cycle of breathing (ACB) technique.

Equipment Required for Percussion

1. The only equipment required for manual percussion is the caregiver's cupped hands to deliver the force to mobilize secretions.
2. For the adult and older pediatric population, electric or pneumatic percussors that mechanically simulate percussion are available. This enables a patient to apply self-percussion more effectively. Several models have variable frequencies of percussion, as well as different levels of intensity.
3. Several devices may be used to provide percussion to infants: padded rubber nipples, pediatric anaesthesia masks, padded medicine cups, or the bell end of a stethoscope.

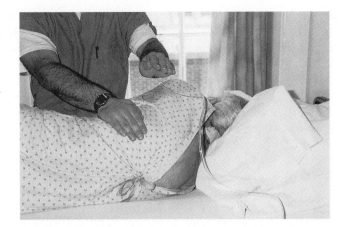

FIGURE 20-7
Chest percussion.

Preparation for Percussion

1. Placing the patient in appropriate PD positions (as the patient's condition allows) enhances the effect of percussion.
2. Place a thin towel or hospital gown over the patient's skin where the percussion is to be applied. The force of percussion over bare skin may be uncomfortable; on the other hand, padding that is too thick absorbs the percussion without benefit to the patient.
3. Adjust the level of the bed so that proper body mechanics may be used during the treatment. Fatigue or injury of the caregiver may be the result of lengthy or numerous treatments if proper body mechanics are ignored.

Treatment With Percussion

1. Position the hand in a cup with the fingers and thumb adducted. It is important to maintain this cupped position with the hands throughout the treatment, while letting the wrists, arms, and shoulders stay relaxed.
2. The sound of percussion should be a hollow sound as opposed to a slapping sound. If ery-

thema occurs with percussion, it is usually a result of slapping or not trapping enough air between the hand and the chest wall (Imle, 1989).
3. An even, steady rhythm will best be tolerated by the patient, and the rate of manual percussion is normally between 100 and 480 times per minute (Imle, 1989).
4. The force applied to the chest wall from each hand should be equal. If the nondominant hand is not able to keep up with the dominant hand, the rate should be slowed to match that of the slower hand. It might also be helpful to start with the nondominant hand and let the dominant hand match the nondominant (Frownfelter, 1987). The force does not have to be excessive to be effective; the amount of force should be adapted to the patient's comfort.
5. If the size of an infant does not allow use of a full hand, percussion may be done manually with four fingers cupped, three fingers with the middle finger "tented," or the thenar and hypothenar surfaces of the hand (Crane, 1990).
6. Hand position should be such that percussion does not occur over bony prominences. The spinous processes of the vertebrae, the spine of

the scapula, and the clavicle should all be avoided. Percussion over the floating ribs should also be avoided, since these ribs have only a single attachment.

7. Percussion should not be performed over breast tissue. This would produce discomfort and diminish the effectiveness of the treatment. In the case of very large breasts, it may be necessary to move the breast out of the way with one hand and percuss with the other hand.

8. A patient may be taught to perform one-handed self-percussion to those areas that can be reached comfortably, either manually or with a mechanical percussor. This does however, virtually preclude the treatment of the posterior lung segments.

Advantages and Disadvantages of Percussion

The addition of percussion to a PD treatment may enhance secretion clearance and shorten the treatment. Patients often find the rhythm soothing and are relaxed and sedated by percussion, especially young children and infants.

Patients with chronic lung disease, who have used PD and percussion for many years and have found it effective, are reluctant to try an alternative method of airway clearance. Compliance with this method is dependent on the availability of a family member or other caregiver to provide the treatment. Mechanical percussors allow the patients more independence or decrease fatigue of a caregiver, and are especially useful in patients requiring ongoing treatment at home.

Percussion is not well-tolerated by many patients postoperatively without adequate pain control. The force of percussion is also a threat to patients with osteoporosis or coagulopathy. Other contraindications are listed in Chapter 21. Percussion has been associated with a fall in oxygen saturation, which can be eliminated with concurrent thoracic expansion exercises and pauses for breathing control (Pryor, 1990).

Delivering percussion for extended periods on an ongoing basis can result in injury to the caregiver, whether a family member or a health care provider. Repetitive motion injuries of the upper extremities may occur in long-term delivery of percussion for airway clearance.

The expense of a mechanical device for percussion is minimal compared with the ongoing cost of a caregiver to provide percussion and PD in the hospital setting or a home care situation. In the case of young children or unresponsive patients, there are few choices for airway clearance. For other populations, however, a more independent method would also prove to be more cost-effective if adequate compliance was achieved.

VIBRATION/SHAKING

The techniques of vibration and shaking are on opposite ends of a spectrum. Vibration involves a gentle, high frequency force, whereas shaking is more vigorous in nature. Vibration and shaking are performed with the aim of moving secretions from the lung periphery to the larger airways where they may be suctioned or expectorated. Vibration is performed by co-contracting all the muscles in the caregiver's upper extremities to cause a vibration while applying pressure to the chest wall with the hands. Shaking is a stronger bouncing maneuver, which also supplies a concurrent, compressive force to the chest wall.

Like percussion, vibration and shaking are used in conjunction with PD positioning. Unlike percussion, they are performed only during the expiratory phase of breathing, starting with peak inspiration and continuing until the end of expiration. The compressive forces follow the movement of the chest wall.

Equipment Required for Vibration/Shaking

1. For manual techniques, the only equipment required is the caregiver's hands.
2. Mechanical vibrators are available to administer the treatment and are useful for self-treatment by a patient or to reduce fatigue in the caregiver.
3. For infants, a padded electric toothbrush is an alternative (Crane, 1990).

Preparation for Vibration/Shaking

1. Place the patient in the appropriate PD position or modified position as the patient's status allows.
2. Place a thin towel or hospital gown over the

patient's skin. The material should not be thick enough to absorb the effect of the vibration or shaking.

3. Proper body position of the caregiver is important to deliver an effective treatment and to decrease caregiver fatigue.

Treatment with Vibration/Shaking

1. *Conventional chest physical therapy* is often referred to as a combination of postural drainage and percussion, vibration, or shaking.

2. For shaking, with the patient in the appropriate PD position, place your hands over the lobe of the lung to be treated and instruct the patient to take in a deep breath. At the peak of inspiration, apply a slow (approximately 2 times per second), rhythmic bouncing pressure to the chest wall until the end of expiration. The hands follow the movement of the chest as the air is exhaled.

3. For vibration, the hands may be placed side by side or on top of one another as shown in Figures 20-8 and 20-9. As with shaking, the patient is instructed to take in a deep breath while in a proper PD position. A gentle but steady cocontraction of the upper extremities is performed to vibrate the chest wall, beginning at the peak of inspiration and following the movement of chest deflation.

4. If the patient is mechanically ventilated, the previously described techniques must be timed with ventilator-controlled exhalation.

5. If the patient has a rapid respiratory rate, either voluntary or ventilator-controlled, it may be necessary to apply vibration or shaking only during every other exhalation.

6. The frequency of manual vibration is between 12 and 20 Hz; shaking is 2 Hz (Gormezano, 1972; Bateman, 1981).

7. A mobile chest wall is necessary to apply a compressive force without causing discomfort. If a patient has limited chest wall movement, vibration will probably be tolerated better than shaking.

8. Mechanical vibrators may be used by patients themselves, realizing that limited attention can be paid to the posterior portions of the lungs.

Advantages/Disadvantages of Vibration/Shaking

The use of vibration or shaking with PD may enhance the mobilization of secretions. Shaking or vibration may be better tolerated than percussion, especially in the postsurgical patient.

Manual vibration and shaking allows the caregiver to assess the pattern and depth of respiration. The stretch on the muscles of respiration during expiration may encourage a deeper inspiration to follow. A

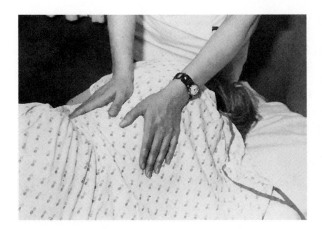

FIGURE 20-8
Vibration—hands positioned on both sides of the chest.

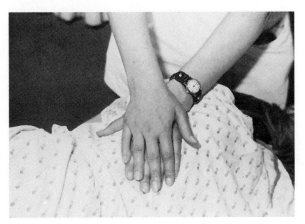

FIGURE 20-9
Vibration—hand placement one on top of the other.

mechanical vibrator, more commonly used with pediatric patients, may be preferred by a caregiver to deliver long-term airway clearance.

The patient cannot apply these techniques herself, except in a limited manner with a mechanical vibrator, so compliance and regular administration of vibration depends on caregiver availability.

The same contraindications for percussion apply, since compression to the thorax is involved with shaking and vibration. The technique of vibration is less constrained by these contraindications than is shaking.

MANUAL HYPERINFLATION

The technique of manual hyperinflation is used in patients with an artificial airway, who are mechanically ventilated or who have a tracheostomy. This method of airway clearance promotes mobilization of secretions and reinflates collapsed areas of lung. Two caregivers are necessary to provide this treatment and the coordination between these two people is key to achieving satisfactory results. This technique is shown in Figure 20-10.

Equipment Required for Manual Hyperinflation

1. A manual ventilation bag, such as the Ambu, attached to an oxygen source is needed for lung inflation. A positive-end expiratory pressure (PEEP) valve may be attached. This is recommended when greater than 10 cm PEEP is being used for mechanical ventilation (Webber, 1993).
2. A second trained caregiver is necessary to provide shaking or vibration in an appropriate sequence with lung inflation.
3. Normal saline should be available for installation into the airways to assist with loosening secretions.

Preparation for Manual Hyperinflation

1. It may be necessary to premedicate the patient with a sedative or analgesic so that airway clearance may be better tolerated.
2. The two caregivers providing the treatment should be positioned on opposite sides of the bed to allow greater freedom of movement and

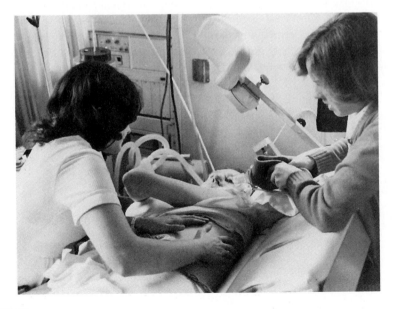

FIGURE 20-10
Simulated cough using self-inflating bag and chest compression with vibration.

improved observation of the patient's response to treatment.

3. Normal saline (2 to 3 mL) may be used before hyperinflation to assist with loosening, thick secretions (Webber, 1993).
4. The positions for treatment will be primarily side-lying with the head of the bed flat or slightly elevated to patient tolerance.

Treatment With Manual Hyperinflation

1. One caregiver squeezes the manual ventilation bag slowly to inflate the lungs. A pause is maintained momentarily at the peak of inflation to allow collateral ventilation to fill underexpanded areas of the lung. Release of the bag should be rapid, resulting in a high expiratory flow rate (Clement, 1968).
2. A second caregiver provides thoracic compression with shaking or vibration to assist with the mobilization of secretions. The compression phase should begin just before the inflation pressure has been released and continue until the end of the expiratory phase.
3. In a patient who is breathing spontaneously, "bag squeezing" with the manual ventilation bag should be timed to augment the patient's inspiratory effort, making vibration more effective (Imle, 1989).
4. After about six cycles of inspiration/expiration, the patient's airway is suctioned using sterile technique. The length of treatment is individualized and depends on the amount of secretions present in the airways and the areas of the lungs affected.
5. Manual hyperinflation may be performed with intubated infants or children using an appropriately sized ventilation bag. Care must be taken to apply slow inflation, so as to avoid a high peak inspiratory pressure, which carries the risk of barotrauma (Webber, 1993).
6. When manual hyperinflation is contraindicated, shaking or vibration may be timed with the expiratory phase of the ventilator without additional inflation during inspiration (Webber, 1988).

Advantages/Disadvantages of Manual Hyperinflation

Manual hyperinflation may be helpful in managing airway secretions in those patients requiring long-term mechanical ventilation. In this patient population, the choice of airway clearance techniques is limited, especially when the patient is unresponsive. Manual hyperinflation simulates a cough by augmenting the inspiratory effort, momentarily maintaining a maximal inspiratory hold, and causing an increased expiratory flow.

However, hyperinflation has the potential to cause significant barotrauma. There are a number of contraindications to this technique including unstable hemodynamics, pulmonary edema, air leak, and severe bronchospasm (Webber, 1988). In addition, it is not appropriate for infants with increased pulmonary resistance requiring high inflation pressures or in preterm infants at risk of pneumothorax (Webber, 1993). Other contraindications are discussed in Chapter 21.

Thus manual hyperinflation requires two well-trained caregivers. This may be its biggest disadvantage.

ACTIVE CYCLE OF BREATHING TECHNIQUE

The active cycle of breathing (ACB) technique involves three phases repeated in cycles: breathing control, thoracic expansion, and the forced expiratory technique (FET). This method encourages active participation of the patient and has been shown to be as effective when performed by the patient alone as with the aid of a caregiver (Pryor, 1979). Postural drainage positions may be used in conjunction with ACB technique. This method of airway clearance may be used with some children as young as 3 or 4 years of age. The sequence of ACB technique is shown in the box on p. 350.

Equipment Required for ACB Technique

1. The only equipment required for this manual technique is the patient's or caregiver's hands to percuss or shake/vibrate the chest wall during the thoracic expansion phase.
2. Mechanical percussors or vibrators may be used during the thoracic expansion phase, either for self-percussion by the patient or for use by the caregiver.

ACB Technique

- Breathing control

    Diaphragmatic breathing at normal tidal volume

- 3-4 Thoracic expansion exercises

    Deep inhalation with relaxed exhalation at vital capacity

    with or without chest percussion

- Breathing control

- Three to four thoracic expansion exercises

- Breathing control

- Forced expiratory technique

    One to two huffs at mid to low lung volume

    Abdominal muscle contraction to produce forced exhalation

- Breathing control

Adapted from Webber, B., Pryor, J. (1993). Physiotherapy skills: techniques and adjuncts. In Webber, B. Pryor, J. (eds.). (1993). *Physiotherapy for respiratory and cardiac problems.* Churchill Livingstone: Edinburgh.

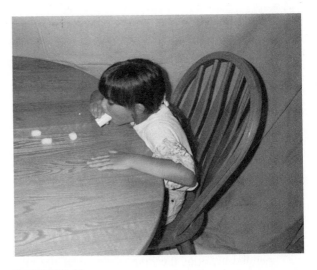

FIGURE 20-11
Peak flow meter mouthpiece.

3. If PD positions are used, equipment for positioning will be required.
4. To teach the huffing maneuver (part of the FET), it may be helpful to use a peak flow meter mouthpiece to keep the mouth and glottis open (Figure 20-11). Young children may be taught games of huffing at cotton balls or tissue to improve the technique (Webber, 1993). To help them focus on the expiratory maneuver, small children may also be taught to flap their arms to their lateral chest as they perform the huff, a technique referred to as the "chicken breath" (Mahlmeister, 1991).

Preparation for ACB Technique

1. Treatment of two or three productive areas during one session may be tolerated by most patients.
2. The patient is positioned or positions herself in a PD position to stimulate drainage of a pro-

ductive area of the lungs. The entire treatment may also be done in the sitting position.

3. A minimum of 10 minutes in any productive position may be necessary to clear a patient with a moderate amount of secretions. Patients after surgery or with minimal secretions may not require as much time, and very ill patients may fatigue before optimal treatment is given (Webber, 1993).

Treatment With the Active Cycle of Breathing Technique

1. *Breathing control*—The patient is instructed to breathe in a relaxed manner using normal tidal volume. The upper chest and shoulders should remain relaxed and the lower chest and abdomen should be active. The phase of breathing control should last as long as the patient requires to relax and to prepare for the next phases, usually 5 to 10 seconds.
2. *Thoracic expansion*—The emphasis during this phase is on inspiration. The patient is instructed to take in a deep breath to inspiratory reserve;

Ineffective Huffing	*Effective Huffing*
• Mouth half or almost closed	• Mouth open, O-shaped to keep glottis open
• Expiration always starting from high lung volume	• Forced expiration
• Abdominal muscles not used	From mid to low lung volume moves peripheral secretions
• Sound more like hissing or blowing	from high to mid lung volume moves proximal secretions
• Mouth shaped as for "E" sound	• Muscles of the chest wall and abdomen contract.
• Incorrect quality of expiration	• Sound is like a sigh, but forced.
• Too vigorous or long, producing paroxysmal coughing	• Rate of expiratory flow varies with the following:
• Too gentle	The individual
• Too short	The disease
• "Catching" or "grunting" at the back of the throat	The degree of airflow obstruction
	• Crackles heard if excess secretions are present

From Partridge, et al, *Physiotherapy,* March 1989, Vol. 75, No.3

expiration is passive and relaxed. The caregiver or the patient may place a hand over the area of the thorax being treated to further encourage increased chest wall movement.

3. Chest percussion, shaking, or vibration may be performed in combination with thoracic expansion as the patient exhales. For surgical patients or those with lung collapse, a breath hold or a sniff at the end of inspiration encourages collateral ventilation to assist with reexpansion of the lung.

4. *FET:* This phase consists of huffing interspersed with breathing control. A huff is a rapid, forced exhalation but not with maximal effort. This maneuver can be compared with fogging a pair of eyeglasses with warm breath so they may be cleaned. Unlike a cough in which the glottis is closed, a huff requires the glottis to remain open. In an effective huff, the muscles of the abdomen should contract to provide greater expiratory force. Other characteristics of effective vs ineffective huffing are shown in the boxes above.

5. Two different levels of huffing are characterized in the FET. To mobilize secretions from peripheral airways, a huff after a medium-sized breath in will be effective. This huff will be longer and quieter. To clear secretions that have reached the larger, proximal airways, a huff after a deep breath in will be effective. This huff will be shorter and louder.

6. The patient must pause for breathing control after one or two huffs. This will prevent any increase in airflow obstruction.

7. The ACB technique may be adapted to the individual patient's needs. If secretions are tenacious, two cycles of the thoracic expansion phase may be necessary to loosen secretions before the FET can follow. In a patient with bronchospasm or unstable airways, the period of breathing control may be as long as 10 to 20 seconds (Webber, 1993). After surgery, the patient may be shown how to support the incision with their hands during the FET to achieve sufficient expiratory force.

8. When a huff from a medium-sized inspiration through complete expiration is nonproductive and dry sounding for two cycles in a row, the treatment may be concluded (Pryor, 1991).

Advantages and Disadvantages of ACB Technique

Incorporation of the ACB technique into a treatment of PD and percussion allows the patient to participate actively in a secretion mobilization treatment and offers the prospect of independently managing airway clearance. The ACB may be introduced at 3 or 4 years of age, with a child becoming independent in the technique at 8 to 10 years of age.

The technique may be adapted for patients with gastroesophageal reflux, bronchospasm, and an acute exacerbation of their pulmonary disease. A decrease in oxygen saturation caused by chest percussion may be avoided by using the ACB technique (Pryor, 1990). When the technique is performed independently, the cost of using ACB technique for the long term is minimal.

However, in young children and in extremely ill adults, a caregiver will be necessary to assist the patient with this technique. An assistant will also be re-quired for the patient in whom percussion or shaking during the thoracic expansion phase increases the effectiveness of the treatment.

Care must be taken to adapt the ACB technique for patients with hyperreactive airways or after surgery. This individual approach will be helpful with all patients using the technique to optimize effectiveness.

AUTOGENIC DRAINAGE

Autogenic drainage (AD) is a breathing technique that uses expiratory airflow to mobilize bronchial secretions. It is a self-drainage method that is performed independently by the patient in the sitting position. AD consists of three phases: (1) the "unsticking" phase, which loosens secretions in the peripheral airways, (2) the "collecting" phase, which moves the secretions to the larger, more central airways, and (3) the "evacuating" phase, which results in the removal of the secretions. This technique of airway clearance requires much patience and concentration to learn and is therefore not suitable for young children. It is ideal, however, for the adolescent or adult who prefers an independent method.

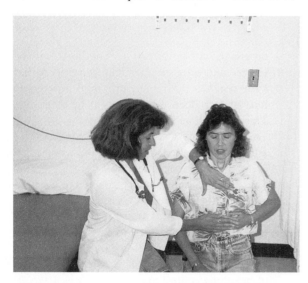

FIGURE 20-12
Autogenic drainage: German method. Autogenic drainage shown on a spirogram of a normal person. The method is not divided into separate phases. (Vt=tidal volume, ERV=expiratory reserve volume, RV=reserve volume, FRC=functional residual capacity, IRV=inspiratory reserve volume, IRV + Vt + ERV = vital capacity). (From David, A. (1991). Autogenic drainage—the German approach. In Pryor, J. (Ed.), *Respiratory Care,* Edinburgh: Churchill Livingstone.)

Equipment Required for AD

1. No equipment is needed for a patient to perform the technique of AD. The patient must possess good proprioceptive, tactile, and auditory perception of the mucus moving; this feedback makes it possible to adjust the technique of AD.
2. To teach this method to a patient, a caregiver requires keen tactile and auditory senses to coach a patient to move between the phases by listening to and feeling the location and the quality of the secretions.

Preparation for AD

1. The patient should be seated upright in a chair with a back for support. The surroundings should be devoid of distractions, allowing the patient to concentrate on the breathing technique.
2. The upper airways (nose and throat) should be cleared of secretions by huffing or blowing the nose.

3. The caregiver should be seated to the side and slightly behind the patient, close enough to hear the patient's breathing. One hand should be placed to feel the work of the abdominal muscles and the other hand placed on the upper chest (see Figure 20-12).

Treatment With Autogenic Drainage

1. In all phases, inhalation should be done slowly, though the nose if possible, using the diaphragm or lower chest. A 2- to 3-second breath hold should follow, allowing collateral ventilation to get air behind the secretions.
2. Exhalation should occur through the mouth with the glottis open, causing the secretions to be heard. The vibrations of the mucus may also be felt with the hand placed on the upper chest. The frequency of these vibrations reveals their location. High frequencies mean that the secretions are located in the small airways; low frequencies mean that the secretions have moved to the large airways (Chevaillier, 1992).
3. *The unsticking phase*—This phase mobilizes mucus from the periphery of the lungs by lowering the mid-tidal volume below the functional residual capacity level (Schoni, 1989). In practice, inspiration is followed by a deep expiration into the expiratory reserve volume. The patient attempts to exhale as far into the expiratory reserve volume as possible, contracting the abdominal muscles to achieve this. This low lung volume breathing continues until the mucus is loosened and starts to move into the larger airways.
4. *The collecting phase:* This phase collects the mucus in the middle airways by increasing the lung volume over the unsticking phase. Tidal volume breathing is then changed gradually from expiratory reserve volume toward the inspiratory reserve volume range (Schoni, 1989) so that the lungs are expanded more with each inspiration. The patient increases both inspiration and expiration to move a greater volume of air. This low to middle lung volume breathing continues until the sound of the mucus decreases, signaling its movement into the central airways to be evacuated.
5. *The evacuating phase*—In this phase, the patient increases inspiration into the inspiratory reserve volume range. This middle-to-high lung volume breathing continues until the secretions are in the trachea and are ready to be expectorated. The collected mucus can be evacuated by a stronger expiration or a high-volume huff. Nonproductive coughing should be avoided, since it may result in collapse of airways.
6. Compression of the airways should be avoided. If wheezing is heard, the expiratory flow rate must be decreased. Beginners may have to use pursed lips to avoid airway compression (Chevaillier, 1992). Instructing the patient to roll the tongue (if possible) may assist in controlling the expiratory flow rate.
7. A German modification of AD resulted from the observation that many patients had difficulty breathing in the expiratory reserve volume range. In the simplified procedure, the patient begins by varying the mid-tidal volume without excessive effort. After a passive but rapid expiration, an actively performed expiration follows, achieving exhalation to a low expiratory reserve volume (David, 1991). See Figure 9-1, p. 155. for the difference between the two methods of AD.
8. The duration of each phase of AD depends on the location of the secretions. The duration of a session depends on the amount and viscosity of the secretions. A patient who is experienced in autogenic drainage will clear secretions in a shorter amount of time than a beginner. An average treatment will be 30 to 45 minutes in length.

Advantages and Disadvantages of AD

After instruction in the technique of AD has been completed, it may be performed independently by patients over 12 years of age and requires no additional equipment. Since it does not require the use of postural drainage positions, it is appropriate for patients with gastroesophageal reflux. It is also recommended for use in patients with airway hyperreactivity (Pfleger, 1992).

Although it is widely used in Europe, the use of AD in the United States is limited by the lack of trained caregivers but is growing in popularity.

To learn this technique, patients must demonstrate good self-discipline and possess the ability to concentrate. This method takes more practice than others. A patient must also be available for periodic reevaluation and refinement of the technique.

AD is not the treatment of choice for a patient who is unmotivated or uncooperative, and the study of flow volume curves suggests that AD would not be appropriate for small children even if they are cooperative (Dab, 1979).

The period of hospitalization for an acute pulmonary exacerbation is a difficult time for a patient to learn AD. In fact, patients who are skilled in the technique choose a more passive (less energy-consuming) form of airway clearance at such a time until they return to their baseline pulmonary status.

POSITIVE EXPIRATORY PRESSURE

Positive expiratory pressure (PEP) creates a back pressure to stent the airways open during exhalation and promotes collateral ventilation, allowing pressure to build up distal to the obstruction. This method of airway clearance prevents collapse of the airways, which eases the mobilization of secretions from the periphery toward the central airways. A mask or mouthpiece apparatus provides a controlled resistance (10 to 20 cm water pressure) to exhalation and requires a slightly active expiration; tidal volume inspiration is unimpeded.

A variation of positive expiratory pressure, known as high-pressure PEP, uses the same mask apparatus but at much higher levels of pressure (50 to 120 cm water pressure). Inspiration is performed to total lung capacity; this is followed by a forced expiratory maneuver against the PEP mask.

A form of intermittent PEP is provided by a device called the Flutter™. This pipe like device provides (1) positive expiratory pressure, (2) oscillation of the airways (at frequencies of 6 to 20 Hz) and (3) accelerated expiratory flow rates to loosen secretions and move them centrally.

PEP is performed in the upright position and can be used during acute episodes, as well as chronic pulmonary conditions. Children over 4 years of age may be instructed in the technique, and PEP may provide an independent method of airway clearance in older children and adults.

Equipment Required For Positive Expiratory Pressure

1. A PEP mask is manufactured by Astra Tech in Denmark, but is not approved by the Federal Department of Agriculture (FDA) and is not available in the United States. However, a self-made PEP mask system may be assembled using a soft ventilation mask, a T-piece, a one-way valve, and resistors of various sizes or an adjustable resistor valve (Figure 20-13). The mask should fit tightly but comfortably over the mouth and nose.

2. Another form of PEP delivery consists of a mouthpiece attached to a one way valve (for use with noseclips) with adjustable expiratory resistance. The Resistex™ valve (from Mercury Medical, Clearwater, Fla.) has recently been FDA-approved.

3. A manometer is placed proximal to the resistor in the initial stages of instruction in the use of PEP. First, the manometer helps to determine and monitor the appropriate level of resistance needed for the patient to achieve 10 to 20 cm of water pressure throughout exhalation. Secondly, the visual display of the manometer serves as feedback to assist the patient in mastering the technique (Mahlmeister, 1991).

4. Aerosol medication by nebulizer or metered dose inhaler may be placed inline to be delivered simultaneously with PEP for airway clearance. Deposition of medication improves with PEP (Andersen, 1982; Frischnecht-Christensen, 1991).

5. Supplemental oxygen may also be placed inline for patients who are hypoxic.

6. With high-pressure PEP mask therapy, spirometry is used to determine the appropriate resis-

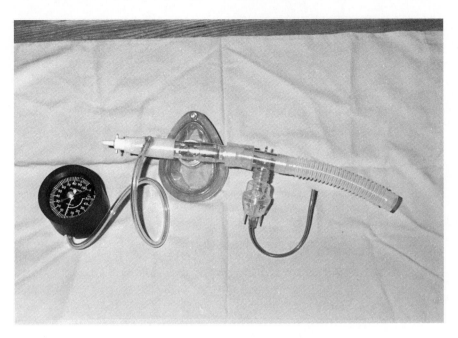

FIGURE 20-13
Self-made PEP mask system.

tance for each patient individually.

7. The Flutter™ VRP1 valve (from VarioRaw, Switzerland), recently FDA-approved, is marked in the United States (by Scandipharm Pharmacy, Birmingham, Ala.). It is a pipe-like device consisting of a mouthpiece, a plastic cone, a steel ball, and a perforated plastic cover.

8. The PEP mask, mouthpiece, and the Flutter™ should be cleaned regularly with hot, soapy water. The one-way valve should be cleaned with hot water only; soap may cause it to stick or become brittle. In the hospital, the equipment will need to be sterilized according to infection control recommendations.

Preparation for PEP

1. For PEP therapy, the patient should be seated upright with elbows resting on a table. Use of a mask may require securing the device with both hands for a tight seal (Figure 20-14).

2. If aerosolized medication is to be used simultaneously, the patient should be instructed in how to stop the flow of the aerosol when the mask or mouthpiece is removed during the PEP treatment session.

3. To determine the correct level of resistance for low-pressure PEP, the patient inhales using tidal volume and exhales actively into the mask/mouthpiece. Different resistors are tested (or the resistor valve is adjusted) while the level of PEP is monitored on the manometer. The resistance is gradually decreased until the PEP level supplying 10 to 20 cm of water pressure has been identified (Falk 1993). Mahlmeister (1991) reports most patients achieve this pressure range with flow resistors of 2.5 to 4.0 mm in diameter. Selection of the proper resistor produces the desired inspiratory to expiratory ratio of 1:3 to 1:4 (Mahlmeister, 1991). The use of too great a resistance will create too low a pressure or an increased respi-

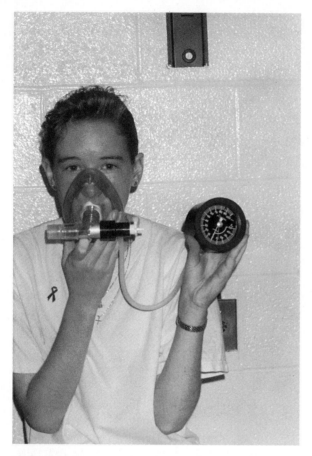

FIGURE 20-14
Preparation for PEP therapy.

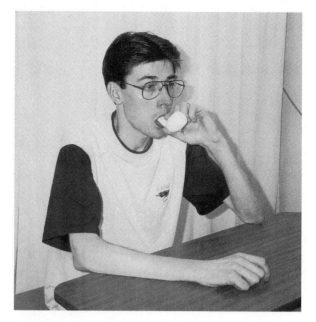

FIGURE 20-15
Use of Flutter (R) valve.

ratory rate, whereas too small of a resistor will create too high a pressure or a slow respiratory rate (McIlwaine, 1993).

4. For high-pressure PEP, appropriate resistance is determined by connecting the outlet of the PEP mask to a spirometer. Forced vital capacity maneuvers are performed through different expiratory resistors. The resistor producing the highest forced vital capacity through the PEP mask is selected for continued use (Oberwaldner, 1986).

5. To use the Flutter™ valve, the patient should be seated upright (Figure 20-15). The full effects of the vibration induced by the Flutter™ may be received by changing the angle of the device. Movement of the Flutter™ upward increases the

pressure and frequency while movement of the device downward results in lower pressure and frequency (Althaus, 1993). The Flutter™ reaches frequencies of between 6 and 20 Hz.

Treatment With PEP

1. The patient should be instructed to breathe into the mask or mouthpiece to tidal volume using the lower chest and abdomen. Exhalation into the mask or mouthpiece should be slightly active but not forced.

2. The patient continues breathing into the mask or mouthpiece for 10 to 15 breaths, using a normal respiratory rate. Initially, the patient and caregiver monitor the effort by means of the manometer, ensuring that a pressure of 10 to 20 cms of water pressure is achieved throughout exhalation. After the technique is mastered with the appropriate resistor, the manometer may be removed from the system. The appropriate resistance should be rechecked periodically during clinical visits or periods of hospitalization.

> ### Technique for Using Flutter™
>
> - Inhale deeply and hold breath for 2 to 3 seconds.
>
> - Place Flutter™ in mouth and, keeping cheeks as stiff as possible, exhale through Flutter™ adjusting the degree of tilt to maximize vibrations.
>
> - Exhalation need not be forced. Patient best determines "speed" of exhalation.
>
> - Perform multiple exhalations through the Flutter™ (usually 5 to 15) with breath hold to maximize mobilization of mucus.
>
> - *After performing multiple "loosening" breaths, increase depth of breath and speed of exhalation through Flutter™ to precipitate coughing and mucus expectoration.*
>
> - Repeat entire sequence until "clear."

For more information about Flutter™, contact Sandipharm; 22 Inverness Center Parkway; Birmingham, AL 35242; (205) 991-8085,

3. After a series of 10 to 15 breaths, the mask is removed from the face and the patient performs a series of huffs (and coughing if necessary) to expectorate any mucus that has been mobilized.

4. The series of PEP breaths followed by huffs should be repeated about four to six times. The total treatment lasts about 15 to 20 minutes and should be repeated twice to three times during the day. The frequency and duration of the treatment must be individualized for each patient. During periods of pulmonary exacerbation, patients are encouraged to increase the frequency of PEP treatments, rather than extending the length of individual sessions (Mahlmeister, 1991).

5. The procedure for use of high-pressure PEP differs from that of low-pressure PEP. The expiratory pressure used in this method usually ranges between 50 and 120 cms of water pressure. The patient breathes in and out through the mask at tidal volume for 6 to 10 breaths, then inspiration is done to total lung capacity and a forced expiratory maneuver is performed

against the PEP mask. This is repeated until all the mucus is mobilized (McIlwaine, 1993).

6. The recommended procedure for use of the Flutter™ is shown in the box at left. The device is held horizontally with the lips tightly around the mouthpiece. After a deep inspiration through the nose, the breath is held for 2 to 3 seconds before exhaling deeply through the Flutter™. The cheeks must be kept flat and to use the abdominal muscles for effective exhalation. The vibration of the chest may be palpated by the patient and caregiver to provide feedback as to the optimal angle of the device. A Flutter™ session consists of 10 to 15 breaths followed by huffing (this may be done into the device), with a session lasting about 15 to 20 minutes. To avoid dizziness due to hyperventilation, a patient should refrain from forced exhalation. It may be necessary to pause every 5 to 10 exhalations before resuming the session (Althaus, 1993).

Advantages and Disadvantages of PEP

PEP therapy does not possess some of the limitations of conventional PD and percussion for secretion clearance and is therefore applicable to a wider patient population. It is relatively easy to learn in one or two sessions, and may be applied equally to the pediatric and adult populations. PEP is appropriate for use in hospitalized patients, as well as long-term use at home.

The expense of the equipment is minimal and once the patient is competent in the technique, it provides independence (except for small children). All of the PEP devices (the Flutter™ in particular) are quite portable, making airway clearance easier to perform during travel or when away from home during the day.

Although rare, pneumothorax has been reported with high-pressure PEP (Oberwaldner, 1986). A decision to use PEP should be carefully evaluated in cases of acute sinusitis, ear infection, epistaxis, recent oral or facial surgery or injury (Mahlmeister, 1991). For PEP therapy to be effective, a patient should be able to cooperate and actively participate with the treatment. Pfleger (1992) recommends that patients with airway hyperreactivity should take a bronchodilator premedication before the use of PEP.

Low-pressure PEP is more commonly used in North America, because it is felt to be as effective, easier, and safer to use and monitor than high-pressure PEP. In those patients in whom PEP is an appropriate airway clearance technique, a high degree of acceptance has been shown (Falk, 1984; Steen, 1991). This may translate into better adherence in the long term.

HIGH FREQUENCY CHEST COMPRESSION

The ThAIRapy® (from American Biosystems, Inc., St. Paul, Minn.) system of high frequency chest compression (HFCC) (also referred to as high frequency chest wall oscillation) consists of a vest linked to an air-pulse generator. Figure 20-16 shows a patient using HFCC. Although the sensation of the device is somewhat akin to mechanical percussion, it differs significantly in its mechanism of action. HFCC works by differential airflow, that is, the expiratory flow rate is higher than the inspiratory flow rate, allowing the mucus to be transported from the periphery to the central airways for expectoration. HFCC has also been shown to decrease the viscosity of mucus, making it easier to mobilize.

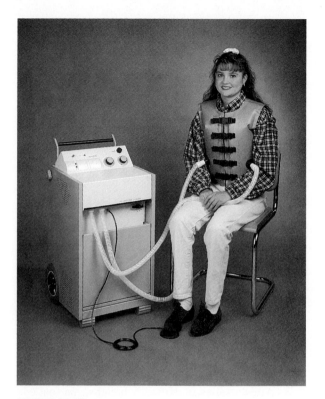

FIGURE 20-16
Patient using high frequency chest compression.

Equipment Required for High Frequency Chest Compression

1. The air-pulse generator, required for a treatment of HFCC, weighs just over 100 lbs, but can be wheeled from one room to another.
2. The inflatable vest is constructed to fit over the entire thorax and should extend to the top of the thigh when the patient is sitting upright. Five different sizes are available (from child to large adult). For use in a hospital setting, adjustable vests are available, which are fitted to subsequent patients with velcro straps.
3. Simultaneous use of an aerosolized medication or saline is recommended throughout the treatment. This humidifies the air to counteract the drying effect of the increased airflow.

Preparation for HFCC

1. The patient should be seated upright in a chair. The vest should fit properly, but breathing should not feel restricted while the vest is deflated. A single layer of clothing should be worn under the vest.
2. The pressure control setting should be adjusted to either the high or the low setting according to patient comfort.
3. The foot/hand control may be placed on the floor to be activated by stepping on it, or placed under the thigh to be activated by leaning onto it, or pressed with the hand.

Treatment With HFCC

1. The treatment should progress through different frequencies, from low (7 to 10 Hz) to medium (10 to 15 Hz) and then to high (15 to 25 Hz), to achieve both higher flow rates and increased lung volume. Warwick (1991) reported that the

frequencies associated with the highest flow rates were usually greater than 13 Hz, whereas those associated with the largest volume were usually less than 10 Hz.

2. The recommended protocol (American Biosystems, Inc., 1994) gives the option of intermittent or continuous use. For the intermittent (only on exhalation) method, the patient should inhale deeply and depress the foot/hand control at peak inspiration. Exhalation should be passive and relaxed while the vest is pulsating. For the continuous method, the foot/hand control should be depressed while breathing normally. At least once per minute, the patient should inhale to total lung capacity.

3. The average length of time spent at each frequency is 3 to 5 minutes, but this will vary according to patient tolerance, amount, and consistency of secretions, and the phase of the patient's illness (acute or chronic).

4. After treatment at each frequency for the prescribed length of time, the foot/hand control should be released and the patient instructed to huff or cough to clear loosened secretions. The control is adjusted to the next prescribed frequency, and the procedure is repeated.

5. HFCC has been used on a smaller scale with patients requiring long-term mechanical ventilation. Whitman et al. (1993) found use of the ThAIRapy™ vest to be safe and effective, and resulted in time savings over conventional PD and percussion.

6. Patients requiring central intravenous (IV) access such as a Porta-cath or Hickman are able to use the ThAIRapy™ Vest with sufficient padding (such as a foam doughnut pillow) to relieve pressure around the access site.

Advantages and Disadvantages of HFCC

This method of airway clearance allows independence and is easy to learn in a short period. The ThAIRapy® Vest is now designed to accommodate children as young as 3 years of age, and a vest may be custom-made for very large or obese adults. HFCC is appropriate with those patients in whom PD positions are contraindicated, and it has been used successfully in reclining patients who are unable to tolerate the upright sitting position.

Use of HFCC may result in time savings at home as well as in a hospital or long-term care facility. Nebulized medications are administered concurrently with the airway clearance treatment, and all lobes of the lungs are treated simultaneously. The amount of time for patient contact required for a hospital caregiver is much less with this method than with conventional PD and percussion.

A disadvantage of this method of airway clearance is the cost of the equipment. A monthly rental fee is reimbursed by most insurance companies. However, a study by Ohnsorg (1994) demonstrated a decline in total health care costs for the year after the ThAIRapy® Vest was put into use by 11 patients. A study of the impact of the device in a hospital setting (Klous, 1993) showed a substantial savings as a result of therapy self-administration. A disadvantage of HFCC is its lack of portability. Although the device can be readily moved from room to room in the house, it does not accommodate use away from home.

In those patients for whom it is appropriate (and reimbursable), HFCC is an effective method of airway clearance. It provides independence for long-term use at home as well as for acute exacerbations in the hospital.

EXERCISE FOR AIRWAY CLEARANCE

A regular program of exercise has been shown to improve many variables in patients with lung disease. Peak oxygen consumption, maximal work capacity, respiratory muscle endurance, and exercise tolerance all improve with an exercise program (Orenstein, 1981, Andreasson, 1987). Secretion clearance is also improved with exercise (Zach, 1981; Oldenburg, 1979). Based on improvement in pulmonary function, exercise has been recommended as a replacement, partial or complete, for conventional chest physical therapy (PD and percussion) (Zach, 1982; Cerny, 1989; Andreasson, 1987).

Exercise for secretion clearance has focused on aerobic or endurance exercise to increase ventilation. The many forms of exercise must be adapted to the individual patient's status and abilities.

Equipment Required For Exercise

1. A walking program requires nothing more than a suitable pair of shoes and a safe location.
2. The following exercise equipment may be suitable for a patient who is beginning an exercise program: treadmill, bicycle ergometer, mini-trampoline, or arm ergometer.
3. For more accomplished exercisers or patients with a higher exercise tolerance, equipment may include a stair climber, cross-country ski machine, or rowing machine.
4. Tools to monitor a patient's response to exercise include a blood pressure monitor, heart rate monitor, pulse oximeter, and a scale to measure patient's level of perceived exertion (Figure 20-17).

6
7   Very, very light
8
9   Very light
1
0   Fairly light
1
1   Somewhat hard
1
2   Hard
1
3   Very hard
1
4   Very, very hard
1

FIGURE 20-17
Perceived exertion scale. (From Borg, G., 1982. Psychophysical basis of perceived exertion, Med Sci Sports Exer, 14(5), 377.)

5. Supplemental oxygen and oxygen delivery supplies will be necessary for those patients who demonstrate oxygen desaturation during exercise.

Preparation for Exercise

1. Patients with hyperreactive airways should be premedicated with a prescribed bronchodilator before exercise.
2. Baseline vital signs should be recorded before beginning the exercise. In a home setting, patients should be knowledgeable in pulse taking and estimating their level of perceived exertion. For those patients who require closer monitoring, a pulse oximeter may be rented from an oxygen supply company.

Treatment With Exercise

1. The principles of an exercise prescription addressing intensity, duration, and frequency, as well as principles of warm up and cool down are addressed in Chapter 24 and should be followed when using exercise as a form of airway clearance. Individualizing an exercise program for each patient is important.
2. Patients in the hospital for an acute exacerbation may not be able to perform endurance exercise for the first couple of days. They should be started slowly and progressed as tolerated. Monitoring of heart rate, blood pressure, oxygen saturation, respiratory rate, and level of perceived exertion at periods before and during exercise, and during recovery, will allow titration of the workload and duration for optimal performance.
3. The patient should be instructed in huffing or coughing (productive, not prolonged) to expectorate secretions as they are loosened.
4. A regular, consistent program of exercise must be scheduled around the patient's daily activities to achieve adherence (e.g., walking the dog, sports at school, stopping by the health club after work).

TABLE 20-1								
Airway Clearance Techniques Applied to Patients								
TYPE	**INDEPENDENCE**	**EQUIPMENT NEEDED**	**AGE**			**REFLUX PRESENT**	**SEVERE EXACERBATION**	**REACTIVE AIRWAYS**
			<4	**>4**	**>12**			
Traditional CPT*	No	PD board percussor	Yes	Yes	Yes	Modified	Modified	May cause bronchospasm
HFCC	Yes	Vest and generator	No	Yes	Yes	Yes	Yes	May include bronchodilator
PEP	Yes	Mask or mouthpiece	No	Yes	Yes	Yes	Yes	May include bronchodilator
ACB Technique	Yes	PD board	No	Yes	Yes	Modified	Modified	Needs care
AD	Yes	None	No	No	Yes	Yes	No	Good results
Exercise	Yes	Variety	No	Yes	Yes	Yes	No	Bronchodilator Premedication

*Includes postural drainage, percussion, shaking, vibration, and coughing.
Modified from Maggie McIlwaine, 1993, unpublished.

Advantages and Disadvantages of Exercise For Airway Clearance

Exercise has the advantage of being the only airway clearance technique that is performed regularly by people without lung disease. This factor that makes it appealing to those patients who do not want to call attention to their differences from their peers. Exercise may improve self-esteem, a sense of well-being, and quality of life. The level of exercise tolerance in patients with cystic fibrosis has been demonstrated to be of prognostic value (Nixon, 1992).

Because the amount or frequency of exercise required to achieve its benefits would not be tolerated by many patients, it is often recommended as an adjunct to other forms of airway clearance. This is particularly true during an acute exacerbation when activity tolerance is limited, or in infants or patients with neurological or muscular limitations.

Care must be taken in prescribing exercise to patients with hyperreactive airways or with a tendency toward oxygen desaturation. Use of bronchodilator medication and supplemental oxygen delivery may be necessary to achieve exercise tolerance, but these patients require close monitoring as well.

Andreasson (1987) observed that regular contact with a caregiver seems to be necessary for successful exercise training as does family support, especially in young children. Compliance will also be affected by a patient's preference for a particular activity, scheduling conflicts, and commitment by friends and family members.

SELECTION OF AIRWAY CLEARANCE TECHNIQUES

The process of prescribing an appropriate technique for secretion mobilization should be ongoing, with periodic reevaluation of the method and its effects on the patient. Because of the low compliance reported with conventional chest physical therapy (Passero, 1981), it is necessary for caregivers to address the many factors that may alter a patient's adherence to a particular method. These factors include the availability of both the caregiver to teach the technique and the patient to learn it; the effectiveness of the technique (subjective and objective); support for the technique from family, friends, and health care personnel; and the cost of the treatment. Table 20-1 summarizes factors that influence the choice of an airway clearance technique.

AVAILABILITY

Many techniques of airway clearance are new to health care providers in the United States although they have been used in Europe for some time. Use of a method may be limited by the lack of caregivers trained to instruct patients in a particular technique. This is especially true for AD, which takes longer for a caregiver to learn to teach than does use of the Flutter™ or ThAIRapy™ Vest. The ACB technique is easily incorporated into conventional chest physical therapy by learning the FET and modifying the use of percussion or shaking. Manual hyperinflation, on the other hand, because of increased precautions for its use, requires more study and observation before implementation. Exercise for airway clearance may be out of the realm of a caregiver who is trained in respiratory care but not exercise therapy.

The patient's availability must also be taken into consideration. An outpatient clinic visit does not lend itself to instruction in AD, but instruction in PEP, ACB technique, HFCC, or Flutter™ can be initiated, with further training during return visits. On the other hand, if a patient is admitted for exacerbation of a pulmonary disease, the patient is a captive audience for instruction of AD or a home exercise program once the acute stage has passed.

Reevaluation of any airway clearance technique is key to its success. The patient and caregiver must be available to demonstrate and review the technique periodically so that modifications can be made. A change in a patient's level of independence or motivation, a decline or marked improvement in pulmonary status, or a decrease in the effectiveness of a technique all necessitate reevaluation of the current method.

EFFECTIVENESS

The prime consideration in selecting a technique is the effectiveness of the technique measured both subjectively and objectively. Objective measures include: pulmonary function studies, chest x-rays, blood gas values, changes in mechanical ventilator settings, changes in auscultation, and quantity of sputum produced. A patient's response to treatment can be evaluated by changes in heart rate, respiratory rate, oxygen saturation, and level of fatigue.

A patient's subjective response to the treatment has implications for adherence to any technique. The ease of sputum mobilization and the quantity of sputum are useful feedback for a patient. How much effort the treatment requires, or more importantly, how much energy remains after completion of the treatment, will affect the patient's willingness to continue.

Complications that occur as a result of a technique or precautions to be observed must guide a patient and caregiver to find an alternate technique in many instances. A patient hospitalized with an acute pulmonary exacerbation may need to be assisted with a more passive method of secretion clearance until the patient's condition allows a return to a more independent technique. A patient with hyperreactive airways may find that bronchospasm renders percussion ineffective. The presence of gastroesophageal reflux may force the decision to use a technique which can be performed in an upright position. Sinus surgery may make use of a PEP mask intolerable. Placement of a chest tube may necessitate a temporary replacement for HFCC.

SUPPORT

When airway clearance must take place on a daily basis, it becomes necessary to accommodate a patient's schedule. A patient may have a preference for the most effective treatment performed in the shortest amount of time. A patient may also be interested in performing another activity during the airway clearance treatment: AD or Flutter™ may be performed while riding in a car (as a passenger); HFCC can be conducted while studying for an examination; and while running on a treadmill or during percussion by an assistant, a patient can be watching the news.

Many patients adopt a multifaceted approach to secretion clearance, becoming adept at several methods and using them as conditions dictate. Patients who use AD or exercise primarily will need to use an alternate form of airway clearance during an acute exacerbation of an illness. Use of HFCC at home may necessitate use of a more portable technique when away from home for long periods. Patients who rely on an assistant to perform percussion may need to learn a more independent method for occasions when the assistant is not available.

In a home where more than one family member requires ongoing airway clearance, as can be the case for parents of children with cystic fibrosis, spending the least amount of time for the greatest benefit becomes of primary importance. For an infant or young child, performance of secretion mobilization must be carried out by an adult. As the child grows older and the choices of a technique increase, close supervision remains necessary. In the adolescent, even when physical assistance is no longer required, emotional support from family and friends is paramount to continued success with a technique. Finally, the support received from health care providers is vital to the patient's motivation to continue with a technique, or to learn a new one.

COST

In this age of health reform, especially in long-term care or chronic disease, cost of a treatment must be considered. The initial cost of equipment, replacement costs, and the expense of assistance required, all figure into the total cost of treatment.

The generator for HFCC is the most costly piece of equipment presented here, but replacement should not be necessary. The vest itself should not require replacement except for growth of a child. PEP masks and mouthpieces, and the Flutter™ are relatively inexpensive, with replacement of equipment expected to occur occasionally during a lifetime of use (more often for a one-way valve in a self-made PEP). AD and ACB require no equipment.

Payment of a trained assistant for home use of postural drainage and percussion when family support is not available is at great expense. Depending on the duration and frequency of treatment, this cost may outweigh that for other airway clearance techniques on a long-term basis.

Often the choice of an airway clearance technique is limited by the reimbursement available for equipment or assistance. Nonetheless, the caregiver must strike a balance between economic and clinical considerations in choosing a mode of therapy.

FUTURE TRENDS IN AIRWAY CLEARANCE

A recent resurgence of interest in airway clearance has led to the introduction of additional techniques.

The effectiveness of these newer techniques compared with more established methods are just beginning to be studied. Health care providers have anecdotally reported their effectiveness, but long term, well-designed studies are needed.

INTRAPULMONARY PERCUSSIVE VENTILATOR (IPV)

The intrapulmonary percussive ventilator (IPV) (from Percussionaire Corp., Sandpoint, Idaho) is an airway clearance device that simultaneously delivers aerosolized solution and intrathoracic percussion (Homnick, 1994). The functional component in the IPV is an apparatus known as the phasitron. The phasitron was originally developed by Bird in 1979 for the volumetric diffusive respiration (VDR) ventilator. It is used with thermally injured patients in place of conventional mechanical ventilation. The VDR ventilator functions by accumulation of subtidal volume breaths, which build to an oscillatory equilibrium that is followed by passive exhalation (Rodenberg, 1992). Figure 20-18 shows a VDR ventilator waveform.

In the IPV, the phasitron provides high-frequency impulses during inspiration, and positive expiratory pressure maintained throughout passive exhalation. The pressure generated is 10 to 30 cms. of water pressure. Treatment with IPV is titrated for patient comfort and visible thoracic movement.

Homnick et al. (1994) performed a 6-month study using the IPV for airway clearance in patients with cystic fibrosis. No significant differences were demonstrated in pulmonary function studies, body weight, use of antibiotics, or hospital days between the IPV and conventional chest physical therapy group. Three fourths of the patients estimated increased sputum production with IPV and satisfaction was high for comfort and independence.

DYNAMIC AIR THERAPY BED

The EFICA CC™ Dynamic Air Therapy® bed (from HILLROM, Batesville, Indiana) is used in hospitalized patients, primarily in an intensive care setting. The modes available from the bed are continuous lateral rotation, percussion, vibration, and the ability to position the patient in postural drainage positions. Use of the bed demands less time of the caregivers

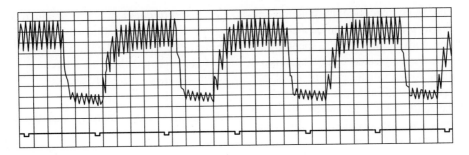

FIGURE 20-18
VDR ventilator waveform. (From Rodeberg, D.A., (1992). Decreased pulmonary barotrauma with the use of volumetric diffusive respiration in pediatric patients with burns: The 1992 Moyer Award, *Journal of Burn Care Rehabilitation 13,* 506–511.)

for hands on airway clearance treatment.

A small pilot study by Samuelson et al. (1994) compared the bed to manual percussion and postural drainage in adult patients with cystic fibrosis. Patients were randomized to receive four treatments a day with either the Dynamic Air Therapy® bed or manual chest physical therapy for 1 week and then switched to the other modality for an additional week. Outcome measures included pulmonary function studies, 6-minute walk distance, dyspnea score, and a Quality of Well Being Scale. Both therapies demonstrated a positive effect from baseline, but a significant improvement was found only in the 6-minute walk distance of those patients treated with the bed therapy first.

Studies on more appropriate patient populations, especially nonambulatory, critically ill patients, for whom the Dynamic Air Therapy® beds are generally prescribed, are necessary to demonstrate the most effective use of this expensive equipment.

SUMMARY

Numerous airway clearance techniques have been shown to reduce obstruction, enhance mucociliary clearance, and improve ventilation, accomplishing the goal of improved oxygen transport. Their effectiveness has been demonstrated in controlled situations and evaluated with sophisticated equipment. Caregivers must incorporate this information into the real life situations presented by patients and choose a technique or combination of techniques that best suits each patient's needs.

An individualized approach to airway clearance requires consideration of the multitude of variables, both physiological, psychological, and practical that affect a patient's response to treatment. Health care providers are challenged to keep abreast of techniques and their modifications to best provide for the patient's needs.

The role of the caregiver involves more than technical expertise. The caregiver is uniquely positioned to simplify medical language for a patient and encourage adherence to airway clearance. Support of a treatment by a health care provider can increase the benefit derived from the treatment.

Further study is needed to compare and standardize techniques, follow long-term outcomes, and establish optimal treatment guidelines. This information will assist both patients and caregivers to maximize treatment with airway clearance techniques.

REVIEW QUESTIONS

1. Which ACTs can be performed without acquiring additional equipment?
2. Are there any ACTs that are *not* suitable for use in an intensive care unit?
3. What are the airway clearance methods most suited for instructing a patient/family in during a single outpatient clinic visit?

4. What outcome measures do you have at your disposal for evaluating the effectiveness of airway clearance?

5. How would you encourage adherence of a prescribed method of airway clearance in:
   - a fiercely independent adolescent with a spinal cord injury?
   - a 3 year old newly diagnosed with cystic fibrosis?
   - an older patient with bronchiectasis?

References

Althaus, P. (1993). Oscillating PEP. In Bronchial Hypersecretion: Current Chest Physiotherapy in Cystic Fibrosis (CF), Published by International Committee for CF (IPC/CF).

Andersen, J.B., Klausen, N.O. (1982). A new mode of administration of nebulized bronchodilator in severe bronchospasm. *European Journal of Respiratory Diseases, suppl. 63,* 119, 97-100.

Andreasson, B., et al. (1987). Long-term effects of physical exercise on working capacity and pulmonary function in cystic fibrosis. *Acta Paediatr Scand,* 76, 70-75.21-38.

Bateman, J., et al. (1979). Regional lung clearance of excessive bronchial secretions during chest physical therapy in patients with stable chronic airways obstruction. *Lancet, 1,* 294-297.

Bateman, J., et al. (1981). Is cough as effective as chest physiotherapy in the removal of excessive tracheobronchial secretions? *Thorax, 36,* 683-687.

Cerny, F.J. (1989). Relative effects of bronchial drainage and exercise for in-hospital care of patients with cystic fibrosis. *Physical Therapy,* 69, 633-639.

Chevaillier, J. (1992). Airway clearance techniques. Course Presented at Sixth Annual North American Cystic Fibrosis Conference, Dallas.

Clement, A.J., Hubsch, S.K. (1968). Chest physiotherapy by the 'bag squeezing' method: A guide to technique. *Physiotherapy,* 54, 355-359.

Crane, L.D. (1990). Physical therapy for the neonate with respiratory disease. In Irwin, S, Tecklin, JS, (Eds.), *Cardiopulmonary Physical Therapy* (pp. 409-410). St. Louis: Mosby.

Dab, I., Alexander, F. (1979). The mechanism of autogenic drainage studied with flow volume curves. *Mon Paed,* 10, 50-53.

David, A. (1991). Autogenic drainage-the German approach. In Pryor, J (Ed.), Respiratory Care. Edinburgh: Churchill Livingstone.

Falk, M., et al. (1984). Improving the ketchup bottle method with PEP, PEP in cystic fibrosis. *European Journal of Respiratory Diseases, 65,* 423-32.

Frownfelter D. (1987). Postural drainage. In Frownfelter, D. (Ed.). *Chest Physical Therapy and Pulmonary Rehabilitation* (2nd Ed.) (265-290). Chicago: Year Book Medical Publishers.

Frischknecht-Christensen E., Norregaard, O., Dahl, R. (1991). Treatment of bronchial asthma with terbutaline inhaled by conespacer combined with positive expiratory pressure mask. *Chest, 100 (2),* 317-321.

Gormenzano, J., Branthwaite, M.A. (1972). Pulmonary physiotherapy with assisted ventilation. *Anaesthesia, 27,* 249-257.

Homnick, D., Spillers, C., White, F. (1994). The intrapulmonary percussive ventilator compared to standard aerosol therapy and chest physiotherapy in the treatment of patients with cystic fibrosis. Abstracted in *Pediatr Pulmonology,* Suppl. 10, 266.

Imle, P.C., (1989). Percussion and vibration. In Mackenzie, (Ed.). *Chest Physical Therapy in the Intensive Care Unit, 2nd Ed.* (pp. 134-152). Baltimore: Williams & Wilkins.

Klous, D., et al. (1993). Chest vest and cystic fibrosis: Better care for patients. *Advanced Respiratory Care Management,* 3, 44-50.

Klous, D.R. (1994) *High-frequency chest wall oscillation: Principles and applications.* Published by American Biosystems, Inc., St. Paul. 626-630.

Mahlmeister, M.J., et al. (1991). Positive-expiratory-pressure mask therapy: Theoretical and practical considerations and a review of the literature. *Respiratory Care, 36 (11),* 1218-1229.

McIlwaine, M. (1993). Airway clearance techniques (ACT) Refresher Class. Presented at Seventh Annual North American Cystic Fibrosis Conference, Dallas.

Nixon, P.A. (1992). The prognostic value of exercise testing in patients with cystic fibrosis. *New England Journal of Medicine,* 327, 1785-1788.

Oberwaldner, B., Evans, J.C., Zach, M.S. (1986). Forced expirations against a variable resistance: A new chest physiotherapy method in cystic fibrosis. *Pediatr Pulmonology,* 2, 358-367.

Ohnsorg, F. (1994). A cost analysis of high-frequency chest wall oscillation in cystic fibrosis. Abstract presented at the ALA/ATS International Conference, Boston.

Oldenberg, F.A., et al. (1979). Effects of postural drainage, exercise, and cough on mucus clearance in chronic bronchitis. *American Review of Respiratory Diseases, 120,* 739-745.

Orenstein, D.M., et al. (1981). Exercise conditioning and cardiopulmonary fitness in cystic fibrosis. *Chest, 80 (4),* 392-398.

Passero, M.A., Remor, B., Salomon, J. (1981). Patient-reported compliance with cystic fibrosis therapy. *Clinical Pediatrics, 20,* 265-268.

Pfleger, A., et al. (1992). Self-administered chest physiotherapy in cystic fibrosis: A comparative study of high-pressure PEP and autogenic drainage. *Lung, 170,* 323-330.

Pryor, J.A., et al. (1979). Evaluation of the forced expiration technique as an adjunct to postural drainage in treatment of cystic fibrosis. *British Medical Journal, 18,* 417-418.

Pryor, J.A., Webber B.A., Hodson, M.E. (1990). Effect of chest physiotherapy on oxygen saturation in patients with cystic fibrosis, 45, 77.

Pryor, J.A. (1991). The forced expiration technique. In Pryor, J.A. (Ed.), *Respiratory Care* (pp. 79-100). Edinburgh: Churchill Livingstone.

Rodeberg, D.A., et al. (1992). Decreased pulmonary barotrauma with the use of volumetric diffusive respiration in pediatric patients with burns: The 1992 Moyer Award. *Journal of Burn Care Rehabilitation,* 13, 506-511.

Samuelson, W., Woodward, F., Lowe, V. (1994). Utility of a dynamic air therapy bed vs. conventional chest physiotherapy in adult CF patients. Abstracted in *Pediatr Pulmonology, Suppl. 10,* 266.

Schoni, M.H. (1989). Autogenic drainage: A modern approach to physiotherapy in cystic fibrosis. *Journal of the Royal Society of Medicine, suppl. 16, 82,* 32-37.

Steen, H.F., et al. (1991). Evaluation of the PEP mask in cystic fibrosis. *Acta Paediatr Scand, 80* (1), 51-56.

Sutton, P.P., et al. (1985). Assessment of percussion, vibratory-shaking and breathing exercise in chest physical therapy. *European Journal of Respiratory Diseases, 66,* 147-152.

Warwick, W.J., Hansen, LG (1991). The long-term effect of high-frequency chest compression therapy on pulmonary complications of cystic fibrosis. *Pediatr Pulmonol, 11,* 265-271.

Webber, B.A. (1988). Physiotherapy for patients receiving mechanical ventilation. In Webber, B.A. (Ed.) *The Brompton Hospital Guide to Chest Physiotherapy (Fifth Ed.).* Oxford: Blackwell Scientific Publications.

Webber, B., Pryor, J. (1993). Active cycle of breathing techniques. In Bronchial Hypersecretion: Current Chest Physiotherapy in Cystic Fibrosis (CF). Published by International Physiotherapy Committee for Cystic Fibrosis (IPC/CF).

Webber, B.A., Pryor, J.A. (1993). Physiotherapy skills: techniques and adjuncts. In *Physiotherapy for Respiratory and Cardiac Problems.* Edinburgh: Churchill Livingstone.

Whitman, J., et al. (1993). Preliminary evaluation of high-frequency chest compression for secretion clearance in mechanically ventilated patients. *Respiratory Care, 38 (10),* 1081-1087.

Zach, M.S., Purrer, B., Oberwaldner B. (1981). Effect of swimming on forced expiration and sputum clearance in cystic fibrosis. *Lancet, 11,* 1201-1203.

Zach, M., Oberwaldner, B., Hausler, F. (1982). Cystic fibrosis: physical exercise versus chest physiotherapy. *Archives of Diseases of the Child, 57,* 587-589.

CHAPTER 21

Facilitating Airway Clearance With Coughing Techniques

Mary Massery
Donna Frownfelter

KEY TERMS

Airway clearance deficits
Assisted cough
Complications with coughing
Cough
Cough pump
Cough stages

Mucous blanket
Reflex cough
Smokers cough
Swallowing disturbance
Throat clearing

INTRODUCTION

Cough truly serves many purposes: a therapeutic technique, a diagnostic signpost, and a social necessity. If it didn't already exist, we would have to invent it.

    Glen A. Lillington, MD

The cough is an interesting phenomenon. A cough can either be a reflex or a voluntary action. Generally, in healthy individuals a cough is rarely heard unless the person has a cold or an irritant is inhaled and a sneeze or a cough ensues to evacuate the foreign body. The mucociliary escalator functions to clear secretions and inhaled particulate matter. Unless the mucus is very thick, such as in individuals with dehydration, inhalation of a foreign body, or a bolus of food goes "down the wrong hole" or into the trachea rather than the esophagus, a cough is not the usual mechanism to clear mucus.

A nervous cough or throat clearing may also signal that the airways are irritated, mucus is not clearing normally, or the person is in an uncomfortable situation. This is something to be aware of especially when treating asthmatics, patients with cystic fibrosis, or patients with psychological problems.

In reality the mucous blanket and the cough mechanism are the two ways the lungs have of providing airway clearance under normal everyday circumstances.

367

It is interesting how many people are unaware of their coughing. For example, when asked if they cough, smokers with typical morning and ongoing smoker's coughs will deny that they do. Spouses will chime in, "He coughs and hacks all the time." An individual might constantly clear his or her throat and swallow mucus but will claim to be unproductive of mucus and free of coughing. It is important for therapists to be aware of both the reflex and voluntary nature of their patients' coughs.

Frequent coughing or throat clearing may also indicate other problems than airway clearance deficits. For example, a patient may have postnasal drip from a sinus infection or allergy. When the mucus drips down into the back of the throat, it can cause a reflex cough to clear it. Other causes include bronchogenic carcinoma, nervousness, and smoking. In a pediatric patient, a foreign body or object inserted or inspired into the nose or airway should be ruled out.

Cigarette smoking paralyzes the cilia so airway clearance is altered. It has been noted that for every cigarette an individual smokes the cilia are paralyzed for approximately 20 minutes. Many individuals are chain smokers and light up one cigarette after the other. Consequently, coughing is the only means of clearing the lungs. This is understandable when a smoker coughs up a large amount of mucus in the early morning on arising. After sleeping for hours the individual's cilia are able to clear secretions; a cough assists in airway clearance. During the day the smoker who chain smokes must cough regularly to clear secretions because the cilia are paralyzed by the smoke.

COUGH PUMP

One must appreciate the complexity and intricacy of the cough pump. Mucus is transported up against gravity by the mucous blanket and propelled cephalad by the action of the cough.

In general the cough is most effective at high expiratory flow rates and at high volumes. The cough is of limited value beyond the sixth or seventh generation of airway branching. Consequently when a patient has a lower lobe pneumonia or atelectasis, coughing alone will not clear the retained secretions.

Airway clearance techniques, such as postural drainage, autogenic drainage, or active cycles of breathing, need to be used to mobilize the secretions to the area where the cough will be effective (see Chapter 20).

COUGH ASSOCIATED WITH EATING OR DRINKING

If a cough is associated with eating or drinking or taking medications, the patient should be evaluated for a swallowing disturbance. This usually consists of a "cookie swallow," a fluoroscopy study where the patient is given barium or a variety of consistency liquids and solids to swallow and observed to see if aspiration into the respiratory tract occurs. Patients may have dysfunction after a cerebrovascular accident (CVA) or prolonged intubation or because high placement of a tracheostomy tube inhibits the proper function of the larynx during swallowing. Speech language pathologists working with patients with dysphagia can help patients learn techniques to prevent aspiration. They also help the patient and spouse (significant other) to understand cognitively proper positioning (usually sitting up in semi-Fowler's) and proper head and neck position (usually chin tuck and slight neck flexion) during swallowing. If a patient has dysphagia and cannot or will not follow a safe swallowing retraining program and continues to choke and aspirate food and liquid, aspiration pneumonia will occur and can lead to the patient's condition deteriorating and even to death. In a situation such as this, alternative feeding would need to be considered.

COMPLICATIONS OF COUGHING

The act of coughing can be hazardous to the patient. A patient should never be asked to cough repeatedly as a routine part of treatment. The irritation and possible narrowing of the airways during the forced exhalation may cause bronchospasm. If a patient is sounding dry and unproductive, do not encourage frequent coughing. This is especially true in patients with asthma.

If a patient demonstrates retained secretions on x-ray, encourage hydration (drinking water), use airway clearance mobilization techniques, and carefully evaluate the cough. Instruct the patient in controlled coughing when mucus is felt in the throat or upper airways. The patient may try to cough in a controlled fashion after a postural drainage session or use the forced expiratory technique. The forced expiratory technique uses midlong volume ventilation followed by one to two huffs, which can include chest compression with the arms. Forced coughing can also increase blood pressure and lower cardiac output. *Tussive syncopy* can occur when a patient goes into a series of coughs in which the intrathoracic pressure becomes so high that venous return to the heart is impaired. The cardiac output falls and the patient becomes very dizzy, progressing to unconsciousness. Care must be exercised, especially with patients with primary lung disease; they must learn to control their coughing to prevent untoward side effects.

Stages of Cough

There are four stages involved in producing an effective cough (Linder, 1993). The first stage requires inspiring enough air to provide the volume necessary for a forceful cough. Generally, adequate inspiratory volumes for a cough are noted to be at least 60% of the predicted vital capacity for that individual. The second stage involves closing of the glottis (vocal folds) to prepare for the abdominal and intercostal muscles to produce positive intrathoracic pressure distal to the glottis. The third stage is the active contraction of these muscles. The fourth and final stage involves opening of the glottis and forcefully expelling the air. The patient should be able to cough three to six times per expiratory effort. A minimal threshold of a FEV_1 (forced expiratory volume in 1 second) of at least 60% of the patient's actual vital capacity is a good indicator of adequate muscle strength necessary for effective expulsion (Figure 21-1). During a cough, alveolar, pleural, and subglottal pressures may rise as much as 200 cm H_2O (Bach, 1993; Jaeger, 1993; Linder, 1993).

COUGH EVALUATION

How do you assess whether a patient's cough is effective? The answer appears to be obvious: ask the patient to cough. However, the obvious answer often

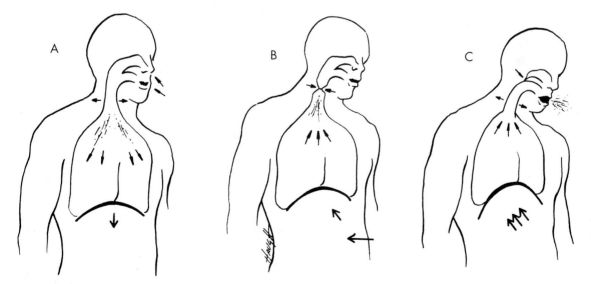

FIGURE 21-1

Cough mechanics. **A,** Stage 1: adequate inspiration. **B,** Stage 2: glottal closure; Stage 3: building up of intrathoracic and intraabdominal pressure. **C,** Stage 4: glottal opening and expulsion.

does not adequately analyze the functional performance of a cough, especially for a neurologically impaired patient. The clinician must first take time to set up the patient for successful evaluation of their cough. Guidelines for setting up the patient follow:

1. Do not ask the patient to cough in whatever posture you happen to find him or her in. Ask, "What position do you like to cough in when you feel the need to cough?" Then ask the patient to assume that posture, or assist him or her in assuming a posture as close to the preferred posture as possible. Listen closely to his or her answers. A patient should spontaneously choose a posture that lends itself to trunk flexion, which is necessary for effective expulsion and airway protection. A red flag or inappropriate choice would be a preference for coughing while supine, which involves the opposite: trunk extension and poor mechanical alignment for airway protection.

2. Now the patient is ready to demonstrate coughing. Do not make the mistake of asking a patient to "show me a cough" or he or she may simply "show you" a cough. It may not be the way the patient coughs to clear secretions. Instead continue to set the patient up for success by asking him or her to "show me how you would cough if you had secretions in your chest and you felt the need to cough them out." With these instructions you are asking the patient to show you something functional not theoretical.

Cough effectiveness can now be accurately assessed. Guidelines for objective evaluation with pulmonary function tests have been indicted. This section focuses on analyzing the movement during all four stages. An effective cough should maximize the function of each individual stage. Thus the clinician should see a deep inspiratory effort paired with trunk extension, a momentary hold, and then a series of expiratory coughs on a single breath while the patient moves into trunk flexion.

Stage 1: Adequate Inspiration

Did the patient spontaneously inspire a deep breath before coughing or did he or she cough regardless of the inspiration or expiration cycle? Did the patient spontaneously use trunk extension, an upward eye gaze, or the arms to augment the inspiratory effort? Did the patient take enough time to fully inspire before coughing? If the patient inspires adequately, he or she should be able to sustain two to six coughs per expiratory effort for a cascade effect. Neurologically impaired patients who have inadequate inspiratory efforts usually present with only one or two coughs per breath and generally produce a quieter cough (Hoffman, 1987).

Stage 2: Glottal Closure

Did the patient hold his or her breath at the peak of inspiration before the expulsion phase or did the patient go directly from inspiration to expiration? Did you hear a cough or a huff? A huff (or a complete absence of a hold between inspiration and expiration), when the patient intended to give you a cough, is an indication of insufficient glottal closure. This can result from a wide variety of situations including glottal edema after prolonged intubation, partial or full paralysis of the vocal folds, hemiparesis of the vocal folds, or timing or sequencing difficulty secondary to brain injuries to name a few. A complete lack of glottal closure will not produce any cough sound because the vocal folds are not approximating.

Stage 3: Building up of Intrathoracic and Intraabdominal Pressure

Did you see active contraction of the intercostal and abdominal muscles? Did the patient spontaneously move into trunk flexion during this phase? Did the cough have a low resonant sound? Inadequate force is usually heard as a higher pitch cough, often called a *throaty cough.* The sound is quieter overall and does not produce as many coughs per expiratory effort. It is sometimes associated with neck extension rather than flexion as the patient attempts to clear the upper airway only. The air appears to leak out rather than being propelled out of the larynx during the cough. Like inadequate lung volumes, inadequate pressure also prevents the patient from coughing more than once or twice on one expiratory effort.

Stage 4: Glottal Opening and Expulsion

Timing of the opening of the glottis and forcefully expelling the air is directly tied into the function of the third stage. During expulsion, does the patient appear to gag before successfully allowing the air to be expelled? Does the patient seem to get stuck holding his or her breath? Deficiencies in this area are often related to brain injuries and coordination difficulties. The opposite can also occur. Some patients will get stuck at the end of expulsion, especially those with severe neurological impairments or bronchospasms and may have difficulty initiating the next inspiratory effort.

PATIENT INSTRUCTION

When working with patients, especially those with primary pulmonary disease or primary disease superimposed on secondary disease (i.e., a patient with a CVA and asthma), there are some helpful techniques to make secretion mobilization more effective.

Patients with asthma tend to go into an expiratory wheeze when they force and prolong exhalation. This can lead to bronchospasm and respiratory distress. The patient can be taught a pump cough, a variation on a huff technique. A huff may be used when patients have had an endotracheal tube in for an extended time. The vocal folds are swollen and irritated. Consequently, they will not close and form a tight seal to build up pressure and cough. The patient is instructed to huff rather than cough to mobilize secretions. It is done with more open vocal folds, a low sound, and less effort, yet it is quite effective in mobilization of secretions.

The pump cough extends the huff and is more effective. The patient is instructed to take three short huffs and follow it with three short, easy coughs at lower lung volume, not deep breaths or deep lung volumes. Three or four sequences are done . . . huff, huff, huff, cough, cough, cough, huff, huff, huff, cough, cough, cough, huff, huff, huff, cough, cough, cough. Usually if secretions are present a spontaneous cough might occur or the secretions will mobilize with the small cough.

Patients with emphysema have overdistended lungs and difficulty with exhalation. Do not instruct the patient to take a deep breath and cough because this can cause more air trapping, which does not facilitate expulsion of secretions. Patients will be more effective trying to take controlled small or medium breaths followed by huffs or a small series of coughs. The active cycles of breathing and forced expiratory pressure technique is also a good choice for these patients.

Several ideas are presented because the therapist needs a bag of tricks. Some techniques work well for some patients and not for others. Try several with each patient and let him or her determine what works best.

Another variation that decreases stress on the patient is to use a series of coughs starting with a small breath and a small cough, then a medium breath and a medium cough, then a larger breath and a large cough. This is a good technique to use with postoperative patients, who get fatigued trying to maximally cough each time.

For patients with transient or permanent neuromuscular weakness or paralysis, further instructions may be necessary (Jaeger, 1993; Braun, 1984). These patients must use every physical trait to maximize the function of each stage of the cough (see Figure 21-1, p. 369, and the box on p. 372). Physically assisting these patients during the expulsion stage of the cough only addresses one aspect (Slack, 1994; Fishburn, 1990). Care must be taken to look at all four stages to maximize the airway clearance potential of any assistive cough technique. First, the patient must be positioned for success. The beginning of any cough requires trunk extension or inspiratory movement to maximize inhalation, whereas the expulsion stage requires trunk flexion or expiratory movement to maximize exhalation (Massery, 1994). Thus for any given posture, the clinician must assess the following: (1) whether the posture allows for both trunk movements, (2) whether flexion and extension are possible, which movement is more important for that particular patient, and whether that posture facilitates this occurrence, (3) how gravity is effecting the patient's muscle strength and function in this posture, and (4) whether the patient can still protect the airway in this posture. When these questions are answered satisfactorily, the clinician is ready to instruct the patient in the act of coughing.

> *Positioning and Patient Instruction to Improve Cough Effectiveness*
>
> - Position the patient for success, especially in regard to trunk alignment.
> - Maximize inspiratory phase through verbal cues, positioning, and active arm movement.
> - Improve hold stage through verbal cues and positioning.
> - Maximize intrathoracic and intraabdominal pressures with muscle contractions, physical assist, or trunk movement.
> - Instruct the patient in appropriate timing and trunk movements for expulsion.
> - Make the procedure physically active on the patient's part.

An example may provide the best illustration of these instructions. A clinician may pick a modified sitting position for a patient with generalized weakness (e.g., incomplete spinal cord injury, developmental delay, or temporary weakness or exhaustion after a medical or surgical procedure). The patient looks slumped, so the clinician places a lumbar support (e.g., a lumbar roll, a towel, or a pillow) behind the lower back to increase trunk extension in that position. The patient is asked if he or she is comfortable and if he or she can swallow safely. Next the clinician tries to maximize the first cough stage by asking the patient to take in a deep breath. Observing that the patient did not appear to take in as deep a breath as the clinician perceived capable, the clinician adds further instructions such as the following: (1) "Look upward while you inhale." (2) "Raise both of your arms up over your head as high as you can while you inhale," (3) "Squeeze your shoulders back while you inhale." (4) "Straighten or extend your back while you inhale." For those with more limited arm function, apply appropriate ventilatory strategies detailed in Chapter 22. Very subtle movements can then be requested, such as the following: (1) "Bring your arms up and out while you inhale." (2) "Rotate your arms outward while you inhale." (3) "Turn your forearm up while you inhale." Although less dramatic than the larger movements de-

scribed previously, these subtle motions may significantly increase the patient's inspiratory effort and provide a more active means for the patient to participate in his or her own coughing program.

Stage two involves closing the glottis. For some patients with weakness or timing problems, a sharp loud command to "hold it" at the peak of inspiration, may be sufficient to facilitate closure. Remember to allow enough time for the patient to take in a deep inspiratory effort before asking them to "hold." Some clinicians rush the first phase, by saying in quick succession: "take a deep breath and hold it," thus unintentionally limiting the time of the inspiratory effort. A more appropriate verbal cue would be: "take a deep breath in . . .in. . .in. . .in. . . , and now hold it," allowing adequate time for the patient to inhale.

Stages three and four (building up pressure and expulsion) are discussed together because their timing is interdependent. The patient now needs to move into trunk flexion, with or without the clinician's assistance, to maximize expulsion. For those patients who can assist, they can be asked to do the opposite of stage one: (1) "Look down while you cough." (2) "Pull both of your arms down to your hips as you cough." (3) "Roll your shoulders forward while you cough." (4) "Bend your trunk forward while you cough." Likewise, patients with more limited arm function can be asked to do the following: (1) "Squeeze your arms to your chest while coughing." (2) "Roll your shoulders and arms inward while coughing." (3) "Turn your hands down while coughing."

In this manner the clinician has used every conceivable resource to maximize a voluntary cough. Even the weakest cough can be made more effective by applying the following simple concepts: (1) position for success, (2) maximize inhalation first, (3) ask for a breath hold, (4) encourage maximal intrathoracic and intraabdominal pressures, (5) instruct the patient in appropriate timing and trunk movements for expulsion, and (6) make the procedure as active as possible for the patient. However, even with excellent instructions, many neurological patients require the clinician's physical assistance to inhale deeper or to exhale more forcefully because of muscle weakness or paralysis (MacLean, 1989).

ACTIVE ASSISTED COUGH TECHNIQUES

If after instruction and modification in the patient's cough as described previously, the patient still can not produce an effective cough, then one of the following assistive cough techniques may be appropriate. However, a patient who needs some assistance to improve a cough is not excused from an active role in coughing. Keep the act of coughing as active as possible for each patient, whether that is accomplished by adding a few verbal cues to improve overall timing or posture while the patient independently performs the cough, or whether it is accomplished by adding eye gazes for a very weak patient who cannot move the upper extremities and breathes with the assistance of a ventilator. Encourage the patient to be responsible for his or her own care by teaching the concepts involved in producing an effective cough (Estenne, 1990). In that manner, you will help the patient develop the problem solving skills necessary for modifications later. Modify and develop additional techniques on the principles presented thus far. See the box below for techniques presented in this chapter.

Manually Assisted Techniques

Costophrenic assist

The first assistive cough technique, the costophrenic assist, can be used in any posture. After assessing the most appropriate position for the patient (most often sitting or sidelying) and giving the patient instructions to maximize all four coughing stages, the thera-

pist places his or her hands on the costophrenic angles of the rib cage (Figure 21-2). At the end of the patient's next exhalation, the therapist applies a quick manual stretch down and in toward the patient's navel to facilitate a stronger diaphragmatic and intercostal muscle contraction during the succeeding inhalation. The therapist can also apply a series of repeated contractions from proprioceptive neuromuscular facilitation (PNF approach (Sullivan, 1982). throughout inspiration to facilitate maximal inhalation. The patient may assist the maneuver by actively using his or her upper extremities, head and neck, eyes, trunk, or all of the above to maximize the inspiratory phase. The patient is then asked to "hold it." Just a moment before asking the patient to actively cough, the therapist applies strong pressure through his or her hands, again down and in toward the navel. In this manner the therapist is assisting both the build up of intrathoracic pressure and the force of expiration. Of course, the patient would also actively participate by using his or her arms, trunk, or other body parts throughout the entire procedure (see Chapter 22).

This technique's obvious use would be for patients with weak or paralyzed intercostal or abdominal muscles. The therapist must remember to evaluate the effect of gravity and posture in each position for the appropriateness of this technique (Massery, 1987). It is

---

Assisted Cough Techniques
Manually assisted techniques
1. Costophrenic assist
2. Heimlich-type or abdominal thrust assist
3. Anterior chest compression assist
4. Counterrotation assist
Self-assisted techniques
1. Prone on elbows head flexion self-assisted cough
2. Long-sitting self-assisted coughs
3. Short-sitting self-assisted coughs
4. Hands-knees rocking self-assisted cough
5. Standing self-assisted coughs

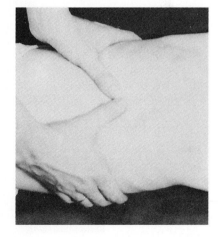

FIGURE 21-2
Assisted cough techniques in supine position; costophrenic assist.

helpful for lower airway clearance but does not directly assist in upper chest clearance unless the patient is able to move his or her upper body independently while the therapist assists the lower chest. This technique is easy to learn and teach and can usually be used from the acute phase through the patient's rehabilitation phase, thus accounting for its popularity.

Heimlich-type assist or abdominal thrust assist

The second technique, the Heimlich-type assist or an abdominal thrust, requires the therapist to place the heel of his or her hand at about the level of the patient's navel, taking care to avoid direct placement on the lower ribs (Figure 21-3). After appropriate positioning, the patient is instructed to "take in a deep breath and hold it." Unfortunately, manual facilitation of inhalation is not feasible with this technique. As the patient is instructed to cough, the therapist quickly pushes up and in, under the diaphgram with the heel of his or her hand, as in a Heimlich choking maneuver. The patient is instructed to assist with appropriate trunk movements to the best of his or her ability. Technically, this procedure is very effective at forcefully expelling the air (Braun, 1984), as in a cough, but it can be extremely uncomfortable for the patient because of (1) its concentrated area of contact, (2) the abrupt nature, which may elicit an undesired high neuromuscular tone response or worse when combined with the sensory input that the therapist's manual contacts supply, (3) the force, which may cause an abdominal herniation. Because of its limited usefulness, the Heimlich type of assist or abdominal thrust should only be used when the patient does not respond to other techniques and the need to produce an effective cough is imminent. Patients with low neuromuscular tone or flaccid abdominal muscles fare best with this procedure.

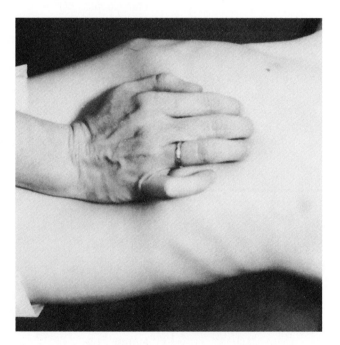

FIGURE 21-3
Hand position for Heimlich-type assist or abdominal thrust.

The therapist can simultaneously use both of the above techniques in sidelying. If the patient is hemiplegic or suffered from an unilateral lung or thorax disease or trauma, emphasizing one side of the thorax over the other may be an appropriate focus during airway clearance treatments. One upper extremity is used to perform the Heimlich-type of assist while the other does an unilateral costophrenic assist. In this manner the therapist can compress simultaneously all three planes of ventilation in the lower chest. The possibilities of combining techniques and positions are almost endless once the therapist understands the principles on which they were developed.

Anterior chest compression assist

The third assistive cough is called the *anterior chest compression assist,* since it compresses both the upper and lower anterior chest during the coughing maneuver. This is the first single technique thus far to address the compression needs of the upper and lower chest in one maneuver. The therapist puts one arm across the patient's pectoralis region to compress the upper chest and the other arm is either placed parallel on the lower chest or abdomen (Figure 21-4) or placed like in the Heimlich type of maneuver (Figure 21-5). The commands are the same as in the other techniques. Because of the direct manual contact on the chest, inspiration can be easily facilitated first, followed by a "hold." Thus the therapist can readily enhance the first two cough stages. The therapist then applies a quick force through both arms to simulate the force necessary during the expulsion phase. The directions of the force are (1) down and back on the upper chest, and (2) up and back on the lower chest or abdominal arm. Performed together the compression force from both arms makes the letter V.

The anterior chest compression technique is more effective than the costophrenic assist for patients with very weak chest wall muscles because of the added compression of the upper anterior chest wall. These authors have found sidelying or 3/4 supine position to be the most effective position for this technique. However, the anterior chest compression technique is not appropriate for patients with a cavus condition of the upper anterior chest because it promotes further collapsing of the anterior chest wall.

Counterrotation assist

The most effective assistive cough for the widest cross-section of neurological patients, in these authors' clinical experience, is the fourth and final method described in sidelying, the counterrotation assist. The positioning and procedures required for the counterrotation technique are described in detail in chapter 22 and apply for both the patient and the therapist (Figure 21-6). The therapist should recall that orthopedic precautions of the spine, rib cage, shoulder, and pelvis still persist for this technique.

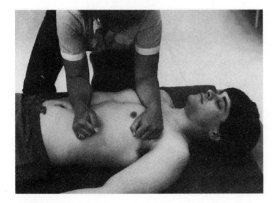

FIGURE 21-4
Assistive cough techniques in supine position; variation of the anterior chest compression assist.

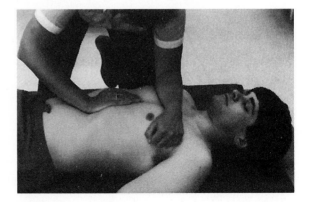

FIGURE 21-5
Assistive cough techniques in supine position; variation of the anterior chest compression assist.

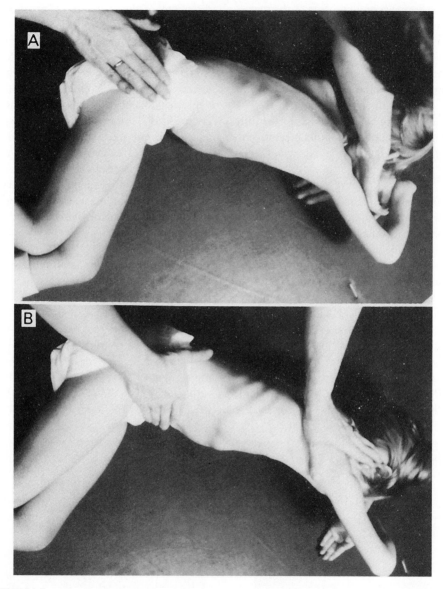

FIGURE 21-6
Counterrotation assist; **A,** Hand placement during expulsion phase; **B,** Hand placement during inspiration phase.

The therapist begins by following the patient's breathing cycle with his or her hands positioned over the patient's shoulder and pelvis (see Figure 21-6). The therapist then gently assists the patient in inhalation and exhalation to promote better overall ventilation. This sequence is generally repeated for three to five cycles or until the patient appears to have achieved good ventilation to all lung segments.

At this point, the patient is ready to begin the coughing phase of the procedure. The patient is asked to take in as deep a breath as possible with the therapist assisting the patient in chest expansion (see Figure 21-6, *B*). The patient is then instructed to "hold it" at the end of maximal inspiration. The patient is then commanded to cough out as hard as possible while the therapist quickly and forcefully compresses the chest with his or her hands in their flexion phase positions (see Figure 21-6, *A*).

The importance of following a true diagonal plane of facilitation during both the flexion and extension phases of this technique cannot be overemphasized. Failure to do so will result in shifting of the air within the chest cavity rather than the desired forcing out. This air shifting can occur to varying degrees, when the upper and lower chest are not used together, as in all the other assistive cough techniques. When done properly, the counterrotation assist is the only one to rapidly close off the chest cavity in all three planes of ventilation in all areas of the chest. Unless the patient voluntarily closes his or her glottis, it is impossible to withhold the air from being forcefully expelled. However, a common mistake made by the therapist is pulling the patient back into trunk extension during the expulsion phase rather than into trunk flexion. A good rule of thumb: if you can see your patient's face when you are applying the compression force, you have pulled them into extension. The head and neck should stay forward and flexed, thus only a facial profile should be seen.

Other effects of counterrotation make this procedure particularly beneficial to patients with low levels of cognitive functioning.

1. The rotation component is a natural inhibitor of high tone. Thus this is the least likely of all techniques discussed so far to elicit an increase in abnormal tone during the coughing phase. In fact the opposite usually prevails. Gentle rota-

tion before passively coughing in a comatose patient can reduce high tone and frequently reduce a high respiratory rate. Both of these reduce the possibility of the patient keeping his or her glottis closed during the expulsion phase.
2. Counterrotation is an excellent mobilizer for a tight chest, which in itself can facilitate spontaneous deeper breaths. Tidal volumes (TVs) can therefore be increased for many patients by mobilizing the chest walls.
3. Finally, rotation can be a vestibular stimulator and may assist in arousing the patient cognitively, allowing him or her to take a more active role in the procedure.

The true beauty of the technique is the fact that no active participation on the part of the patient is required for success. Incoherent or unresponsive patients, such as those patients with low functioning following a head trauma, CVA, or cerebral palsy, will still demonstrate good secretion clearance with this technique. The mechanics of the procedure dictate that the air within the lungs be rapidly and forcefully expelled regardless of the patient's level of active participation. Obviously, patient participation is desirable to clear secretions even more effectively and for teaching the patient to eventually clear his or her own secretions, but it is not critical.

Clinical experience has demonstrated with patients who have extremely tenacious secretions, use of vibration instead of quick chest compression during the cough itself may be more effective. This prolongs the cough phase and gives the secretions time to be moved along the bronchi for successful expulsion. These patients may also require a series of three or four cough cycles before clearing most of their secretions. In general, patients from all the diagnostic groups discussed thus far with or without good cognitive functioning are appropriate for this procedure. The majority of them find it to be the most comfortable and effective assistive means of expectorating secretions.

Self-assisted Techniques

The coughing techniques discussed in this section are intended to be used as self-assisted procedures, thus usually taught later in a patient's rehabilitation process. Five different techniques will be presented in detail. Suggestions for variations are included. All self-assisted cough techniques can start out as physically assisted techniques; however, because they are more active and require greater gross motor movement, they lend themselves to self-assisted techniques.

Prone on elbows head flexion self-assisted cough

Prone is not frequently used as a posture for coughing because the position itself inhibits full use of the diaphragm by preventing lower anterior chest and abdominal excursion following a neurologic insult. This forces the patient to use an alternate breathing pattern that facilitates greater accessory muscle use. Because this change in breathing patterns often occurs spontaneously, prone on elbows can be an effective posture for promoting spontaneous use of the accessory muscles in a more difficult activity (coughing). However, without the full use of the diaphragm, the resultant cough will be weaker than in other postures. Prone on elbows should not be the exclusive posture for assisting a cough. After mastering the timing of the procedure, most patients move back to another posture, usually sitting or sidelying, and to other techniques to

capitalize on the functional increase in chest expansion and compression abilities. For the population of patients who can assume a prone on elbows posture independently (i.e., some patients with tetraplegia), this technique may be used functionally. Here, they can assist their own coughs when the need arises, rather than wait for someone to assist them in a position change.

The head flexion assist requires good use of head and neck musculature, seen in patients sustaining a spinal level injury below C_4 (e.g., spinal cord injuries (SCIs), spina bifida). It can be used either as a self-assisted or therapist-assisted procedure, using the principles of trunk extension to facilitate inspiration and trunk flexion to facilitate expiration. With the patient prone on elbows, the therapist instructs him or her to bring the head and neck up and back as far as possible, breathing in maximally (Figure 21-7). The patient is then instructed to cough out as hard as possible while throwing the head forward and down (Figure 21-8). This head-and-neck pattern can be initially assisted by the therapist to establish the desired movement pattern, and gradually progressed to a resisted pattern to promote increased accessory muscle participation and to strengthen those muscle groups.

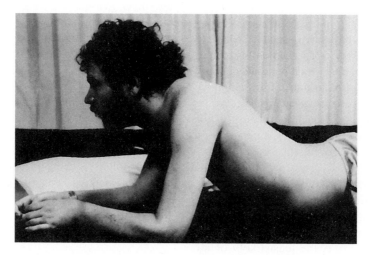

FIGURE 21-7
Head flexion assistive cough in prone on elbows; extension and inspiratory phase.

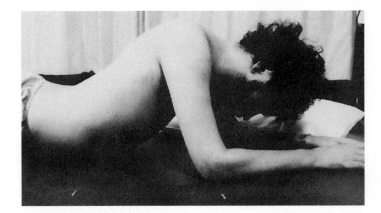

FIGURE 21-8
Head flexion assistive cough in prone on elbows; flexion and coughing phase.

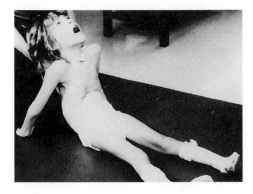

FIGURE 21-9
Tetraplegic–self-assisted cough in long sitting: maximizing the inspiration phase.

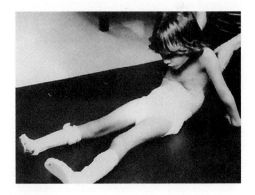

FIGURE 21-10
Tetraplegic–self-assisted cough in long sitting: maximizing the expiration or coughing phase.

Long-sitting self-assisted cough

For the first procedure, tetraplegic–long-sitting self-assist, the patient is positioned on a mat in a long-sitting posture (legs straight out in front of the patient) and with upper extremity support. The therapist instructs the patient to extend his or her body backward while inhaling maximally (Figure 21-9). The therapist then tells the patient to cough as the patient throws his or her upper body forward into a completely flexed posture, using shoulder internal rotation if possible (Figure 21-10). Once again, the extension aspect of the procedure is used to maximize

inhalation, whereas the flexion aspect is used to maximize expiration. The self-directed chest compression occurs mainly on the superior-inferior plane of ventilation only.

The second procedure, the paraplegic–long-sit assist, uses the same principles as the techniques described for the tetraplegic–long-sit assist. These patients have active spinal extension musculature and can achieve greater trunk extension and flexion safely, achieving greater chest expansion before the cough and greater chest compression on a superior-inferior plane during the cough. The patient positions his or her upper extremities in a butterfly position or

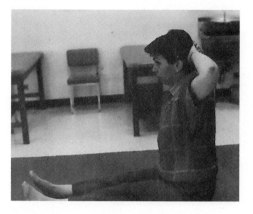

FIGURE 21-11
Paraplegic–self-assisted cough in long-sitting: inspiration.

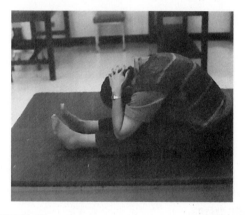

FIGURE 21-12
Paraplegic–self-assisted cough in long-sitting: expiration.

uses elbow retraction, depending on the level of injury (Figure 21-11). During the flexion phase, patients throw themselves onto their legs, thereby compressing both the upper and lower chest (Figure 21-12). This can be taught very successfully to patients with paraplegia, provided they do not have an interfering tone problems. If the patient lacks hip flexion or is worried about bony contact or skin injury, place a pillow (or two as needed) on the legs. This will limit the hip flexion and minimize trauma from the quick thrust onto the legs.

Short-sitting self-assisted cough

The third assistive cough in sitting, the short-sitting self-assist, is typically performed in a wheelchair or over the edge of a bed. The patient is instructed to place one hand over the other at the wrist and place them in his or her lap. As in the previous technique, the patient is then asked to extend his trunk backward while inhaling maximally, followed by a strong voluntary cough. During the cough, the patient pulls his or her hands up and under the diaphragm, resembling the motion of a Heimlich maneuver (Figure 21-13). The hands mimic the abdominal muscles, which would ordinarily contract to push the intestinal contents up and under the diaphragm to aid its recoil ability. This short-sitting technique uses the diaphragm more substantially than the long-sitting procedure and is therefore generally more effective as an assistive cough. It is an effective self-assisted method for patients who have weak diaphragms or abdominal musculature. Most SCI or spina bifida patients, C_5 or below, can successfully learn this technique. Tetraplegics usually require trunk support from their wheelchairs to perform it independently and safely, whereas most paraplegics can perform it from an unsupported short-sitting position. Patients who lack good upper-extremity coordination, such as many Parkinson's and multiple sclerosis (MS) patients, cannot perform the procedure quickly or forcefully enough to make it effective and usually require assistance from another person.

Variations on all sitting techniques can be readily made. Use the concepts explained in the introduction to cough techniques to develop techniques that work for your patients. For example, in a wheelchair, ask your patient to lift his or her arms up while inhaling, hold, and then cough while he or she throws the arms down toward feet or lap using maximum trunk flexion. (Use a seat belt for safety.) Another idea is to have the patient hook one arm on a push handle of the wheelchair, move the other upper extremity up and back (as in a PNF D_2 pattern), watch the patient's moving hand to maximize trunk rotation, inhale during the movement, hold, and again cough as he or she throws trunk and upper extremity down toward opposite knee. When devising the most appropriate self-assisted cough for your patient, remember to look for combination of trunk, upper extremity, head, neck, and eye patterns that will maximize all four phases of the cough.

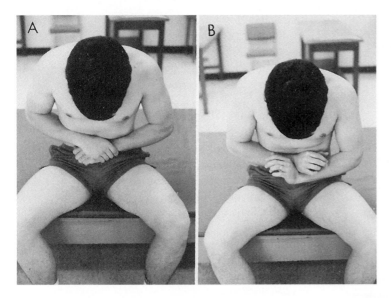

FIGURE 21-13
Assisted cough in short sitting. **A,** Hand position for patient with good hand function; **B,** Hand position for patients with only wrist function.

Hands-knees rocking self-assisted cough

The last assistive cough to be discussed is performed most frequently as a multipurpose activity to increase the patient's balance, strength, coordination, and functional use of breathing patterns (including quiet breathing and coughing) simultaneously. The patient assumes an all-fours position (hands-knees). He or she is then instructed to rock forward, looking up and breathing in as he or she moves to a fully extended posture (Figure 21-14). After this, the patient is told to cough out as he or she quickly rocks backward to the heels with a flexed head and neck (Figure 21-15). Once again, the importance of flexion and extension components of a cough are noted. The rocking can be done with or without a therapist's assistance. For patients with generalized or spotty weakness throughout (e.g., some SCI, head traumas, Parkinson's, MS, cerebral palsy, or spina bifida patients), this method is perfect for incorporating many functional goals into a single activity. It can help prepare them for more challenging respiratory activities that they will undoubtedly meet after their discharge from a rehabilitation center.

For patients with limited lower-extremity range of movement or skin concerns associated with a quick force, a pillow can be placed on the lower legs, thus restricting knee flexion and preventing direct contact of bony prominences.

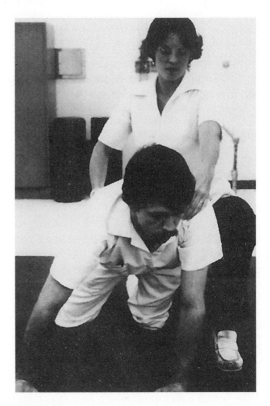

FIGURE 21-14
Assisted cough in hands-knees position; extension or inspiratory phase.

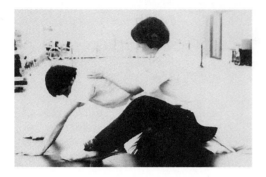

FIGURE 21-15
Assisted cough in hands-knees position; flexion or coughing phase.

Standing self-assisted cough

Standing uses the same concepts and can be readily used for self-assisted coughs, provided the patient has adequate standing balance and/or upper extremity support. Use any technique previously described and modify for this higher developmental posture. Combinations of trunk, head, and extremity movements during the cough maneuver is almost endless, thus specific techniques are not itemized.

SUMMARY

In all postures and in all techniques, both for assisted and self-assisted coughs, the importance of initial positioning and ventilatory strategies is of utmost importance to the success of the airway clearance technique. There is an effective idea waiting to be incorporated for all patients to improve their cough, from the tiniest postural change to full body movements and physical assists. Be creative in applying the concepts to all patient populations.

REVIEW QUESTIONS

1. What is the purpose of a cough?
2. What are the two mechanisms for airway clearance?
3. Why would a therapist assist a patient to cough?
4. What techniques are most effective to assist coughing?
5. What is a smoker's cough, and why does it occur?
6. What are the stages of a cough?
7. What should the therapist interpret when a patient's cough is associated with eating or drinking?
8. What effect does coughing have on the blood pressure and cardiac output?
9. What special techniques can be taught to asthmatic patients to mobilize secreations?
10. What manual techniques are most effective in spinal cord patients?

References

Bach, J.R. (1993). Comparison of peak expiratory flows with manually assisted and unassisted coughing techniques. *Chest 104(5):*1553–62.

Braun, S.R., Giovannoni, R., & O'Connor, M. (1984). Improving cough in patients with spinal cord injury. *American Journal of Physical Medicine 63(1):*1–10.

Estenne, M., Detroyer, A. (1990). Cough in tetraplegic subjects: an active process. *Annals of Internal Medicine 12(1):*22–28.

Fishburn, M.J., Marino, R.J., & Dittuno, J.F. (1990). Atelectasis and pneumonia in acute spinal cord injury *Archives of Physical Medicine and Rehabilitation 71:*197–200.

Hoffman, L.A. (1987). Ineffective airway clerarance related to neuromuscular dysfunction. *Nursing Clinics of North America 22(1):*151–66.

Jaeger, R.J., Turba, R.M., Yarkony, G.M., & Roth, E.J. (1993). Cough in spinal cord injured patients: comparison of three methods to produce cough. *Archives of Physical Medicine and Rehabilitation 74:*1358–61.

Linder, S.H. (1993). Functional electrical stimulation to enhance cough in quadriplegia. *Chest 103(1):*166–9.

MacLean, D., Drummond, C., & Macpherson, C., et al. (1989). Maximum expiratory airflow during chest physiotherapy on ventilated patients before and after the application of an abdominal binder. *Intensive Care Medicine 5:*396–399.

Massery, M.P. (1987). An innovative approach to assistive cough techniques. Topics in *Acute Care Trauma Rehabilitation (3):*73–85.

Massery, M.P. (1994).. What's positioning got to do with it? *Neurology Report 18(3):*11–14.

Slack, R.S., Shucart, W. (1994). Respiratory dysfunction with traumatic injury to the central nervous system. *Clinics in Chest Medicine 15(4):*739–49.

Sullivan, R.E., Markos, P.D., & Minor, A.D. (1982). An integrated approach to therapeutic exercise: Theory and clinical application. Reston, Va.: Reston Publishing.

CHAPTER 22

Facilitating Ventilation Patterns and Breathing Strategies

Mary Massery
Donna Frownfelter

KEY TERMS

Controlled breathing
Diaphragmatic breathing pattern
Jacobsen's progressive relaxation

Ventilatory strategies
Work of breathing

INTRODUCTION

Attaining optimal ventilatory patterns requires the use of a variety of techniques. Some are passive in nature, such as passive positioning of the patient or application of an abdominal binder for better diaphragmatic positioning. Some require very active participation on the part of the therapist and/or patient, such as in assisted-cough techniques or in glossopharyngeal breathing instruction. Other techniques are subtly incorporated into the patient's total physical rehabilitation program, requiring little overt attention to the patient's respiratory performance, such as when using ventilatory strategies. All of these diverse aspects of treatment play an important role in the total development of a successful respiratory rehabilitation program for the neuromuscular and musculoskeletal pa-

tient. No single technique is appropriate in all cases. Sound clinical judgment and experience must be exercised when applying these ideas with each patient. It is the hope of these authors that the techniques identified in this chapter will stimulate the clinician's creative talents, and that they will extrapolate and improve on the techniques according to specific patient population needs. See the box on next page for specific areas covered in the chapter.

POSITIONING CONCERNS

All patients spend some portion of the day in a horizontal position for rest or sleep. Using this opportunity to assist the patient in passive drainage of lung secretions is a natural beginning in the development of a pa-

383

Categories of Therapeutic Interventions Presented in this Chapter to Optimize Ventilation Patterns

1. Positioning concerns
2. Ventilatory and movement strategies
3. Manual facilitation techniques
   - Facilitating controlled breathing patterns (diaphragmatic)
   - Mobilizing the thorax
   - Facilitating upper chest breathing patterns (accessory muscles)
   - Promoting symmetrical breathing patterns (unilateral dysfunction)
   - Reducing high respiratory rates
4. Glossopharyngeal breathing
5. Enhancing phonation skills

---

tient's long-term respiratory program. Specific postural drainage positions are covered extensively in this book (see Chapter 21). Using a combination of these positions in your patient's bed position rotation, in the hospital, or at home can help to achieve multiple goals. First, they can assist the patients in clearing secretions passively that they may have difficulty performing actively. Second, these position changes provide for skin relief and better circulation. Finally, they assist in retarding the development of joint contractures or other musculoskeletal abnormalities. A four-position rotation (i.e., supine, prone, side-to-side) is usually an effective and reasonable means of incorporating these goals into a long-term prophylactic program.

Simple adaptations may make ventilation easier in each of these postures. For example, in supine, placing the arms up over the patient's head facilitates greater anterior upper chest expansion. Likewise, positioning the pelvis in a slight posterior tilt facilitates more diaphragmatic excursion. See Chapter 40 for more detailed explanations. Observation of all precautions and contraindications to passive positioning is still warranted.

Just as passive positioning of the patient in bed helps to maintain bronchial hygiene and improve ventilation potential, passive positioning of the patient's skeletal frame in an upright posture (sitting, standing) helps to maximize the patient's mechanical advantage of breathing. For example, patients with spinal cord injuries (SCIs) resulting in tetraplegia will be unable to support their intestinal contents properly under the diaphragm to allow for maximal expansion of the chest in all three planes of ventilation (see Chapter 37). Use of an abdominal support from the iliac crest to the base of the xiphoid process provides positive pressure support to restore intestinal positioning in an upright position (Figure 22-1). Research has documented well the significant improvements in vital capacity, inspiratory capacity, and tidal volume in sitting with use of a strong abdominal support. These binders have also been used in nursing care to provide for better circulation and in the prevention of hypotension.

The abdominal binder's value in cosmesis may be underrated. Many of these neurological patients were once normal, healthy individuals with high self-esteem who took great pride in their appearances. They now present with a protruding belly (the anterior and inferior shift of the intestines resulting from flaccid abdominal muscles), which may be psychologically disturbing to them. Thus the use of a binder may greatly aid in the restoration of that person's self-esteem, which should be a high-priority goal in any rehabilitation program.

A rigid type of abdominal support can be used when the vertebral column and the abdominal viscera need support. These are called *body jackets* or *total contact thoracic lumbar sacral orthosis* (TLSOs). (Figure 22-2). A TLSO is a rigid trunk support molded individually to the shape of the patient's entire trunk from the axilla down to the pubis. It is made up of two separate front and back pieces, with an anterior cutout in the abdomen to allow for normal diaphragmatic displacement of the viscera. Many of these jackets also use a strong elastic support across the cutout to allow for diaphragmatic motion but to minimize excessive displacement of the abdominal contents. This is very appropriate for the growing

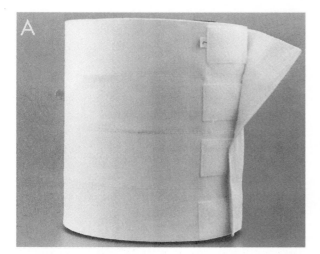

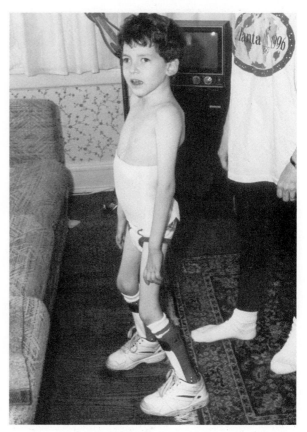

FIGURE 22-1
A, Abdominal binder—Velcro fastener. **B,** placement of abdominal binder.

child who needs more spinal stability or the completely flaccid tetraplegic patient who may also require the same support. Because head and neck positioning are so interdependent on trunk positioning, a body jacket may be the difference to these patients between being dependent or independent in an upright posture. It may result in significantly better head control, eye contact, longer phonation, and possibly better articulation. However, because it limits trunk movement, its usefulness for each patient must be assessed carefully.

Logically, the next consideration under passive respiratory techniques is proper wheelchair positioning. Optimal performance in respiratory functioning, as well as many other areas of rehabilitation, depends on good alignment of the body against the forces of gravity. Symmetry must be strived for through the use of a body jacket, lateral trunk supports in the wheelchair, abdominal binders, or some other means (Figure 22-3). This is especially important for patients with hemiplegia where habitual asymmetrical posturing leads to musculoskeletal problems later. Symmetrical breathing patterns and uniform aeration of all lung segments are augmented by careful upright positioning. Therefore everything from the type of neck support to the height and width of the arm rests to the length and type of the foot supports must be carefully analyzed for each patient.

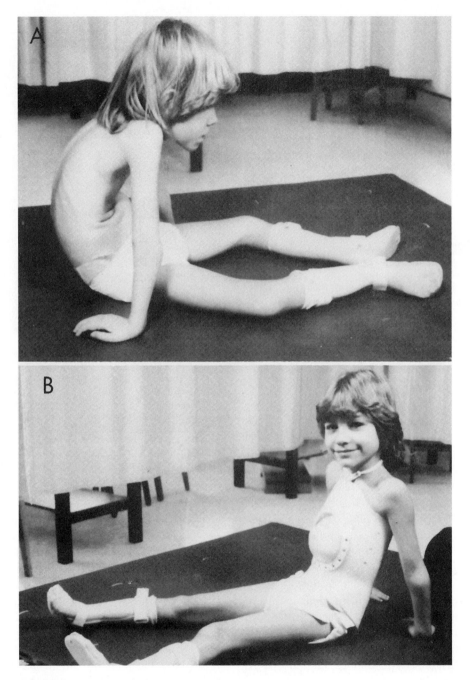

FIGURE 22-2
A, patient with C5 congenital tetraplegia independent long sitting. **B,** long sitting with body jacket support. Note changes in head position and eye contact, hip alignment, and shoulder rotation.

VENTILATORY AND MOVEMENT STRATEGIES FOR IMPROVING FUNCTIONAL OUTCOMES

Once the patient is positioned for success, motor activities should be introduced that improve the patient's ventilatory support, or the therapist should capitalize on the patient's good ventilatory support to improve the motor activity. Using ventilatory strategies to improve motor performance or movement strategies to improve ventilation performance enables patients to achieve their functional goals sooner than other patients; patients also get sick less often. Gener-

ally, these simple concepts take no more than 1 to 2 additional minutes of therapy, with no additional equipment costs other than a few extra pillows or towels. Therefore time or money are not mitigating factors. However, these ideas do require the practitioner to look carefully at the patient before beginning any therapy, asking "Have I positioned my patient for respiratory success?" "Am I simply treating the patient in whatever position I found them in?" and "Have I carefully chosen my verbal cues to include a respiratory response and a functional response?" The practitioner must actively include respiration in every single activity to help the patient understand that breathing transcends all activities. See the box below for a summary of the most important ventilatory-movement strategies.

Incorporating Simple Therapy Tasks
Inspiration

After the patient has been carefully positioned for respiratory success, as described previously, begin the patient's therapy or daily-living activities. From an anatomical perspective, the pattern of inspiration is naturally associated with the following: (1) trunk extension, (2) shoulder flexion, abduction, and external rotation movements, and (3) an upward eye gaze. Expiration is logically associated with the opposite: (1) trunk flexion, (2) shoulder extension, adduction, and internal rotation movements, and (3) a downward

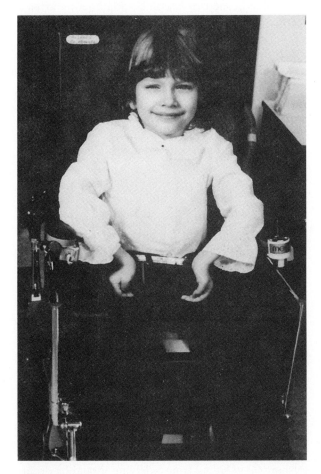

FIGURE 22-3
Wheelchair alignment considerations.

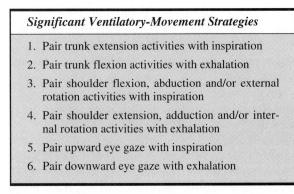

Significant Ventilatory-Movement Strategies

1. Pair trunk extension activities with inspiration
2. Pair trunk flexion activities with exhalation
3. Pair shoulder flexion, abduction and/or external rotation activities with inspiration
4. Pair shoulder extension, adduction and/or internal rotation activities with exhalation
5. Pair upward eye gaze with inspiration
6. Pair downward eye gaze with exhalation

eye gaze. Accordingly then, the simple task of passive range of movement (ROM) can easily include the active goal of increasing ventilation by asking the patient to breathe in and look up every time his or her arm is raised up into shoulder flexion. This encourages the patient to breathe in when his or her chest wall muscles are being maximally stretched and the ribs are naturally opening up, causing both activities to be more successful. It also begins to teach the patient to use ventilatory strategies to optimize potential functional movement, such as in reaching up to a kitchen cabinet.

Expiration

Likewise, active or passive exhalation should be coordinated with the reverse upper extremity ROM pattern (i.e., the arm returning from flexion back to the patient's side). This can be done using all types of exhalation patterns, including the following: (1) passive quiet exhalation, (2) forceful exhalation as in blowing, coughing, or pursed-lips exhalation, or (3) vocalization patterns. Thus the therapist may ask the patient to slowly count out loud to 10 while the arm is being returned to his or her side. Subconsciously, the patient learns to correlate exhalation with shoulder extension while simultaneously learning a much more complex idea—that of controlling his or her rate and volume of expiration by including deliberate speech during exhalation maneuvers.

To improve exhalation potential, increase the patient's relative trunk flexion alignment. While still supine and performing upper-extremity ROM, this can be simply accomplished by asking the patient to lift his or her head and watch the hand as it returns to his or her side, which increases abdominal and intercostal activation, or by increasing knee flexion, which increases posterior pelvic tilting and trunk flexion. Pairing trunk flexion with exhalation completes the ventilatory-trunk movement strategy.

Combining positioning with respiratory verbal cues, as described in ROM activities, changes passive upper-extremity ROM exercises to dynamic upper-extremity ROM exercises. It encourages increased inspiratory and expiratory capacities, develops early functional motor planning strategies, and facilitates trunk mobility. In this manner the patient has the opportunity to learn from the beginning of his or her rehabilitation process that movement and breathing go hand in hand. Clinically, incorporating appropriate breathing patterns with movement early in the rehabilitation process discourages the development of Valsalva patterns or shallow breathing patterns when the motor activities become more difficult and complex.

Dynamic Activities

Inhalation promotes trunk extension and exhalation promotes trunk flexion and vice versa. This basic theme occurs naturally in all motor activities but may have ceased to become spontaneous after a neuromuscular or musculoskeletal insult. Valsalva maneuvers during transitional movements, such as rolling or coming to sitting or standing, are often noted with these patients. By teaching them strategies that incorporate breathing into their motor plans for all motor activities, Valsalva patterns can be eliminated or minimized while simultaneously promoting better cardiac function.

Every activity of daily living cannot be described in this book, however, suggestions for typical gross motor activities using ventilatory strategies as a means to improve these motor tasks are presented. Extrapolation of these concepts to all other motor activities should be carefully analyzed by each therapist for each individual patient.

Rolling

Ask patients to attempt to roll and assess whether they tend to move with trunk extension or flexion to begin the roll. If they roll with a trunk extension pattern ask them to breathe in while they roll and to look up. If they roll with trunk flexion as their primary movement pattern, instruct them to roll while blowing out and tucking their chin. In doing so, patients work with, not against, natural whole patterns of movements to increase the likelihood of success.

Coming up to sitting

Pushing up to sitting from sidelying should be evaluated in much the same manner. If patients are more effective in coming upright when using trunk extension, have them inhale as they push up to sitting.

Asking them to "look up" as they move will reinforce the upper chest movements through the use of the symmetrical tonic neck reflex (STNR). If they have more success pushing up with trunk flexion, have them blow out and tuck the chin while moving.

Dressing

Dressing activities can benefit from the same concepts. While putting on lower-extremity items such as pants, socks, and shoes in a long sitting position, have the patient first take in a deep breath while extending his or her trunk. Then have the patient blow out, huff out, or cough while flexing the trunk to reach his or her toes. This combines the functional daily task of dressing with improving breath control, trunk control, and airway-clearance techniques.

Upper-extremity dressing and upper-extremity exercising can incorporate the same ideas. All movements should be coordinated with harmonious chest wall movements to maximize upper-extremity tasks. Thus every time the arm is moving up above 90 degrees of shoulder flexion, the patient should be asked to breathe in, allowing for the normal shoulder/rib cage rhythm to occur. Full shoulder flexion requires opening of the intercostal spacing and the separation of the individual ribs. Many neurological patients have lost the intrinsic mobility of the chest wall and thus may have lost some functional shoulder ROM as well. Not pairing inspiration with shoulder flexion is likely to limit the patient's shoulder ROM to approximately 140 to 150 degrees. It may also encourage Valsalva maneuvers during the activity and may cause more shoulder pain.

Coming up to standing

Coming up to standing requires both trunk movements, thus the patient should initiate the forward trunk lean with exhalation and initiate the standing phase with inhalation and neck extension. Active neck extension during assumption of standing not only facilitates greater inhalation but, along with the influence of the tonic labyrinthine reflex (TLR), facilitates more significant contractions of the trunk and hip extensors. Clinically, this often results in a more noticeable upright posture and may make the difference between an assisted standing pivot transfer and an independent one. Returning to sitting should be accompanied with slow controlled exhalation, such as in pursed-lips blowing or counting out loud, to maximize the body's controlled descent into gravity's influence.

FACILITATING A CONTROLLED DIAPHRAGMATIC BREATHING PATTERN

Why would a therapist want to change a patient's breathing pattern? The answer is simple—when the pattern being used is ineffective. Patients generally use a pattern of breathing that is the most efficient for them.

A healthy person uses approximately 5% of the total oxygen consumption for the muscular work of breathing and 10% of their vital capacity. Consequently, breathing at rest is generally perceived as effortless under normal conditions.

However, in patients that physical therapists evaluate and treat (often after surgery, respiratory disease, or dysfunction secondary to neurological insult or injury), the vital capacity may be significantly decreased and the oxygen consumption may be greatly increased resulting from the use of accessory muscles or the extra effort needed to breath or cough. In the example of a patient with tetraplegia the vital capacity may be reduced to 1000 to 1500 ml. If the normal tidal volume (normal volume of breathing) is 500 ml that would mean that with each breath the patient would use 33% to 50% of his or her vital capacity (maximal inspiration followed by maximal exhalation). This would greatly increase the oxygen consumption just for normal quiet breathing. The patient would have little pulmonary reserve. During exercise or stress, the patient would have an increased subjective feeling of shortness of breath (dyspnea) and feel an increase in their work of breathing. There are specific terms to describe breathing patterns, the most common are listed in the box on p. 390 at top. Also see the box on p. 390 at bottom for indications for teaching controlled-breathing techniques.

It should be appreciated that breathing comfortably and in control is associated with wellness and a sense of ease. Even in normal individuals who are under stress and have increased work levels we are more cognizant of the increase in work of breathing. For a patient that is struggling with every breath and wonders how he or she will get through the day, ven-

---

Breathing Pattern Terminology

Eupnea—Normal breathing, repeated rhythmic inspiratory-expiratory cycles

Hyperpnea—Increased breathing, usually refers to increased tidal volume with or without increased frequency

Polypnea, tachypnea—Increased frequency of breathing

Hyperventilation—Increased alveolar ventilation in relation to metabolic rate (an increase in alveolar ventilation seen is a decrease in the arterial P_{CO_2})

Hypoventilation—Decreased alveolar ventilation in relation to metabolic rate (a decrease in alveolar ventilation) seen as an increase in P_{CO_2}

Apnea—Cessation of respiration in the resting expiratory position

Dyspnea—The patient's subjective feeling of shortness of breath

Apneusis—Cessation of respiration in the inspiratory position

Apneustic breathing—Apneusis interrupted periodically by exhalation

Cheyne-Stokes respiration—Cycles of gradually increasing tidal volume followed by gradually decreasing tidal volume (usually followed by an apneic period)

Biot's respiration—Sequences of uniformly deep gasps and apnea, followed by deep gasps

Adapted from Comroe, J. H., Jr. (1974). *Physiology of respiration,* (2nd ed). St. Louis: Mosby.

Indications for Teaching Controlled-Breathing Techniques

Patients with any or the following:

- Pulmonary dysfunction either primary or secondary causes
- Pain from surgery, trauma, or disease
- Apprehension or nervousness
- Bronchospasm or impending bronchospasm in asthma
- Airway clearance dysfunction
- Restriction of inspiration resulting from musculoskeletal dysfunction such as scoliosis, kyphoscoliosis, pectus excavatum, obesity, pregnancy, pulmonary pathology such as fibrosis, scarring from radiation therapy, neurological weakness such as spinal cord injury, Parkinson's disease, or myasthenia gravis
- Congestive heart failure, pulmonary edema, or pulmonary emboli
- Rib fractures
- Ventilated patients on assist control or intermittent mandatory ventilation (IMV)
- Metabolic disturbances that have a compensatory respiratory response
- Debilitated or bedridden patients that tend to have constant volume ventilation, retain secretions, and are prone to pneumonia and atelectasis from poor airway clearance

> ### *Goals of Teaching Controlled-Breathing Techniques*
>
> - To decrease the work of breathing
> - To improve alveolar ventilation
> - To improve airway clearance by improving cough
> - To increase strength, coordination, and efficiency of respiratory muscles
> - To teach the patient how to respond to and control breathing
> - To assist in relaxation
> - To mobilize and maintain mobility of the thorax
> - To enable patients to feel self-control and confidence in managing disease or dysfunction

tilatory strategies and breathing-control techniques can be the key to maximizing potential. See the box above for a list of goals in teaching controlled-breathing techniques.

Breathing control has long been used in yoga to focus and promote meditation. This is a key to maximizing rehabilitation. If you can not breathe you cannot function! It is of primary importance to assess the patient's breathing at rest and during exercise. We often hold our breath with exertion, especially with new activities. We must assess the cardiopulmonary and neuromuscular response to each new activity.

CONSIDERATIONS FOR TEACHING BREATHING CONTROL TO PATIENT'S WITH PRIMARY VERSUS SECONDARY PULMONARY DYSFUNCTION

Patients with primary lung disease, such as emphysema, asthma, bronchitis, or cystic fibrosis, present a much different picture than patients with spinal cord injury, Parkinson's disease, myasthenia gravis, or Guillain-Barré syndrome.

In general, patients with primary lung disease use their accessory muscles and greatly increase the work of breathing secondary to the shortness of breath or coughing. They often complain that they have more difficulty "getting air out," which demonstrates the decreased expiratory flow rates noted on pulmonary function tests. The goal with these patients is to teach them to relax the neck and chest accessory muscles and use more diaphragmatic breathing to reduce the work of breathing in combination with relaxed pursed-lip breathing on exhalation. Their treatment programs focus on energy conservation and pacing activity with breath control.

However, with secondary pulmonary dysfunction patients, such as spinal cord injury, there is a more restrictive component to inspiration. In this case, they may have accessory muscles intact, but they are not using them to faciliate deep breathing or coughing. They may have a strong diaphragmatic breath but the upper chest collapses on inspiration (paradoxical breathing, see Chapter 37). In these cases the goal is to teach them to use the accessory muscles to balance the upper and lower chest. This facilitates an increase in vital capacity to prevent atelectasis and pneumonia by increasing the volume of ventilation and improving the cough mechanism.

The choice of appropriate ventilatory strategies depends on the patient's individual problem. The following questions should be considered when evaluating patients:

- Does the patient have more difficulty in inspiration or exhalation?
- Is there a normal sequence to inspiration (i.e., abdominal wall rises, then mid chest, then upper chest, with a full inspiration? Or does the chest sink and the abdomen rise on inspiration?
- Does the patient appear to be working hard to breathe? Is the patient using the accessory muscles to an extreme?
- Does the patient have trouble coughing or speaking a normal volume and for the normal length of sentences?
- Is ventilation the limiting factor in accomplishing an activity (i.e., transfer, gait, or bed mobility)?

Patients with primary pulmonary disease generally benefit from ventilatory strategies that relax the accessory muscles and facilitate relaxed diaphragmatic breathing.

On the other hand, patients with secondary pulmonary dysfunction usually benefit from the balanced use of the diaphragm and accessory muscles to increase vital capacity and breath support for activities.

Diaphragmatic Facilitation Techniques
1. Relaxation technique
2. Repatterning techniques
• Relaxed pursed-lip breathing
• Exhalation, hold, and inhalation
3. Sniffing
4. Diaphragmatic scoop technique
5. Lateral costal facilitation technique
6. Upper chest inhibiting technique
7. Normal timing technique

FACILITATING DIAPHRAGMATIC BREATHING

This section is laid out starting with the easiest intervention to facilitate diaphragmatic breathing and progressing to specific inhibition and facilitation techniques.

See the box above for a summary of methods to facilitate diaphragmatic ventilation patterns.

DIAPHRAGMATIC CONTROLLED BREATHING

Diaphragmatic breathing is the normal mode of respiration. The diaphragm and intercostals are the normal muscles of quiet inspiration. When evaluating a patient's breathing pattern, the use of accessory muscles during quiet breathing should be noted; the patient with primary pulmonary disease should be instructed in relaxation of the accessory muscles to decrease the work of breathing. In a patient with a spinal cord injury or other neuromuscular disorders, these muscles may assist in balancing ventilation and may be useful in increasing vital capacity, and improving the ability to cough, improving breath support for speaking, and increasing potential for functional activities.

In general, controlled diaphragmatic breathing needs to be emphasized in each posture and with all therapeutic activities. Carry-over is not necessarily present. If the patient is only shown the pattern in supine, it may not carry over to sitting or during a sliding-board transfer when the activity becomes difficult. A helpful sequence to use might be teaching the breathing pattern in sidelying, supine, sitting, standing, walking, stairs climbing, and other functional activities, especially with chronic

obstructive pulmonary disease (COPD) patients.

Neurologically impaired patients need modification with their activity levels and capabilities.

POSITIONING CONCERNS
Position of Pelvis

The first step in facilitating any breathing pattern is to position the patient for respiratory success. The details are discussed in this chapter and Chapter 40. Often the patient's posture and pelvic position has a dramatic effect on breathing. In general, a slight, relative posterior tilt of the pelvis facilitates diaphragmatic breathing and a relative anterior tilt facilitates opening of the anterior chest and upper chest breathing. It is helpful to see what difference a slight, relative change in pelvic position will do to the patient's ability to ventilate. This is especially true with secondary pulmonary problems related to neurological and neuromuscular dysfunction.

RELAXATION OF UPPER CHEST AND SHOULDERS

Jacobsen's progressive relaxation exercises are familiar to physical therapists. Jacobsen proposed that a maximal muscle contraction would yield a maximal muscle relaxation. This technique can be applied to the upper chest and shoulders. The therapist places his or her hands on the patient's shoulder girdle. The patient is asked to shrug his or her shoulders up into the therapist's hands and hold it. "Don't let me push your shoulders down," is the therapist's command. Then, "Let your shoulders relax, let them go." The emphasis is on the relaxation phase. Verbal commands can be very important with this procedure. A strong command to, "Raise your shoulders into my hands" is followed by a quiet, more relaxed, "Now relax and let them go," repeating quietly, "That's it, let them go, feel them relax." Sometimes the relaxation activity is all that it takes to resume a more natural pattern of breathing and you can move on to other therapeutic activity. If the patient starts to use accessory muscles again the technique is repeated. The patient learns to feel the difference between tension and relaxation of the shoulders and can self-monitor and perform the relaxation independently.

REPATTERNING TECHNIQUE

If a patient needs more support to gain control of breathing and is experiencing shortness of breath, a simple repatterning technique is very beneficial. An example might be an asthmatic patient with a high respiratory rate who is feeling panicky. When the patient is asked why he or she is breathing so fast the reply will usually be, "I am not getting enough air, I can't catch my breath." The patient is asked to start with exhalation. "Try to blow out easily with your lips pursed. Don't force it just let it come out." By doing this, the respiratory rate will automatically be decreased. When the patient feels some control of this step, then ask him or her to "hold the breath at the top of inspiration just for a second or two." Make sure the patient does not hold his or her breath and bear down as in a Valsalva maneuver. Lastly, ask the patient to take a slow breath in, hold it, and let it go through pursed lips. Patients often learn that when they are short of breath, this technique will help them gain control, making them feel less panicky.

Sniffing

If working toward a generalized controlled-breathing pattern does not improve the patient's ventilatory pattern adequately, a technique that more specifically addresses the need to initiate breathing from the diaphragm can be attempted. Sniffing is a simple and effective means of teaching increased diaphragmatic breathing. Sniffing is primarily diaphragmatic breathing by nature. Use this technique first when attempting more specific diaphragmatic training with all patients who are capable of attempting sniffing because of its simplicity.

As with all procedures, the most important step is the first step: position the patient appropriately to increase the likelihood of increased diaphragmatic breathing resulting from musculoskeletal alignment. This includes the following: (1) choosing a gravity-eliminated position, such as sidelying, or a gravity-assisted position, such as supported semi-Fowler's sitting (supported spine), (2) choosing a relatively posteriorly tilted pelvis with flexed knees, (3) choosing the arms to be down below 90 degrees of flexion (in relative shoulder extension, adduction, and internal rotation), and (4) choosing to use a pillow or pillows under the head. (For details on positioning, see Chapter 40.) For each patient, choices will be different (i.e., the amount of knee flexion or the number of pillows). Find the right combination of positioning characteristics that best facilitates diaphragmatic movement for that particular patient. In this manner the therapist sets up the patient for respiratory success before beginning the manual or verbal techniques.

Now, begin the technique. Ask the patient to place his or her hands on their stomach for increased proprioceptive feedback and the relative extension, adduction, and internal rotation position of the shoulders. In a quiet melodic voice, ask the patient to "sniff in 3 times." Note if the patient demonstrates more abdominal rise and/or lower chest expansion. If so, draw attention to this fact. During exhalation, tell the patient to "let it out slow," which helps to inadvertently slow the respiratory rate (RR) and often encourages some relaxation. Progress the training by asking the patient to "now sniff in twice." Do you still see greater diaphragmatic excursion and less upper chest excursion? If so, continue by asking for "one long slow sniff." If successful, the therapist should follow with: "now do it quieter," then "now do it slower," "even quieter," and so forth. By this time, the patient should be demonstrating an easy onset, slow RR, diaphragmatic pattern with relaxed shoulders.

Clinical experience has shown this technique is highly successful with about 80% of patients who have primary pulmonary pathologies or neurological impairments. The key to success seems to stem from the relaxed tones and words that the therapist uses, which decrease anxiety and imply relaxation and not "effort." Once the pattern has been established, the patient can easily be instructed to go through the training as needed independently. The sequence (in whole or in part) may be appropriate for patients before getting out of bed if they become anxious and demonstrate excessive upper chest breathing during this activity. For other patients, it may be appropriate before or during eating or before climbing stairs. Obviously, the application of this technique will be individualized for each patient, depending on the deficits.

PROCEDURE FOR TEACHING CONTROLLED DIAPHRAGMATIC BREATHING (SCOOP TECHNIQUE)

Minimal patient instruction is necessary to facilitate diaphragmatic breathing using the scoop technique. It allows the patient to feel the breathing pattern, then it is brought to the patient's cognitive awareness. The patient then learns to self-cue to incorporate the breathing pattern.

The following is a suggested sequence:

1. Position the patient for success, generally in a sidelying position with the bed in semi-Fowler's or supine in semi-Fowler's with a bend in the knees to achieve a relative posterior pelvic tilt and relax the abdominal muscles.

2. Place your hand on the patient's abdomen at the level of the umbilicus. Tell the patient you want to feel his or her breathing. Follow the patient's breathing pattern for a few cycles until you are in his or her rhythm. Do not invade the patient's breathing pattern rather, at first, follow their movement.

3. After the normal rate at the end of the patient's exhalation, give a slow stretch and "scoop" your hand up and under the anterior thorax as shown in Figure 22-4. The command, "Breathe into my hand," is given as the slow scoop stretch is done.

4. As the "scoop stretch" is performed instruct the patient to, "breathe into my hand" during the inspiration. Give a scoop at the end of exhalation with each breath. The verbal command can be effectively replaced with audible breathing to facilitate the ventilatory pattern if verbal cues are ineffective or inappropriate.

5. After achieving some success, it is helpful to call the patient's attention to the awareness of the breathing pattern. For example, the therapist can ask, "Can you feel how your abdomen rises as you breathe in?"

6. The patient's hand can be placed on the abdomen with the therapist's hand on top. Reinforce the breathing pattern, then remove your hand and allow the patient to independently feel the ventilatory pattern (Figure 22-5).

A few things should be taken into consideration. Try not to have patients take too many deep breaths; they may begin to feel light-headed because they may hy-

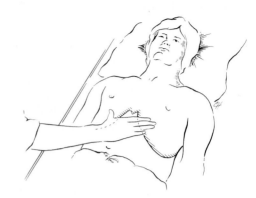

FIGURE 22-4
Therapist's hand placement for diaphragmatic breathing.

perventilate and blow off too much CO_2. The fact that they are breathing more with their diaphragms is the important consideration. Note also the position of the pelvis and trunk.

When the patient has mastered the breathing pattern in sidelying, try supine. Then progress to sitting (Figure 22-6), standing (Figure 22-7), walking (Figure 22-8), and finally stairs (Figure 22-9). Each developmental position increases the difficulty in performing diaphragmatic breathing. In sidelying or supine the patient is fully supported. The sidelying position is especially good for initially teaching diaphragmatic breathing because the diaphragm is in a gravity-eliminated position. In supine the patient must breathe up against gravity. However, as we progress to sitting, the patient must now provide trunk support and maintain stability up against gravity, as well as relax the shoulders. In standing the entire body must be supported, and when walking or stairs are added, the element of breathing coordination really comes into play.

Coordination of breathing for walking involves being careful not to allow patients to breath hold. They need to keep inspiration and exhalation regular at least at a ratio of 1·1, preferably exhaling a little longer.

In general the preferred pattern for patients with primary pulmonary dysfunction is as follows: (1) Pause at the base of the stairs to gain control. (2) Have the patient take a breath in and move as he or she exhales up one stair. (3) The patient then pauses to inspire and exhales as he or she walks up one stair. (4) The patient

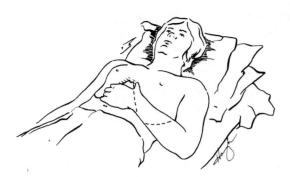

FIGURE 22-5
The patient is encouraged to continue practicing diaphragmatic breathing to become aware of his breathing pattern. this is usually the first position of the diaphragmatic breathing teaching sequence.

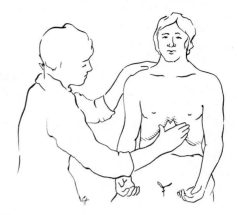

FIGURE 2-6
The patient advances to the sitting position for breathing retraining. Note the relaxed position of the patient's shoulders and hands.

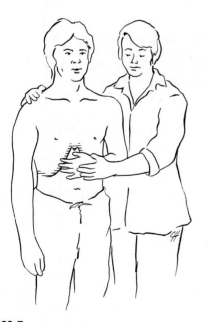

FIGURE 22-7
The third position in the sequence is standing. Full-length mirrors are helpful at this point.

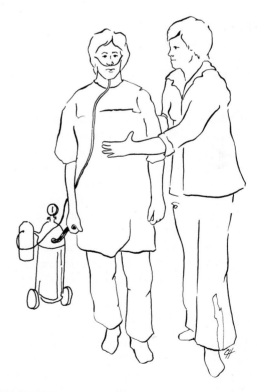

FIGURE 22-8
Walking is the fourth stage of retraining. The patient is encouraged to relax, control his breathing, take long steps and *slow* down.

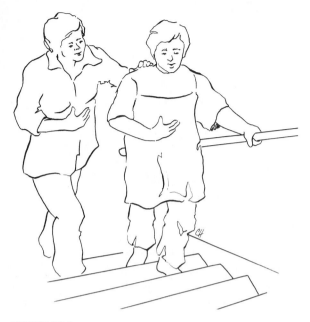

FIGURE 22-9
Stairs are important, especially if the patient has them at home. He is instructed to pause slightly as he breathes in and to exhale as he climbs one to two stairs.

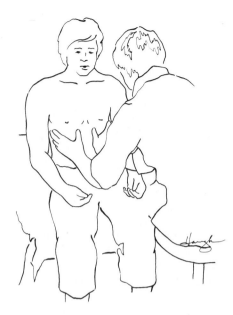

FIGURE 22-10
Bilateral lower lobe expansion (this also facilitates diaphragmatic movement).

should be encouraged to use the handrail and pace his or her movement slowly and with breath control.

In general neuromuscular patients with lower-extremity weakness may benefit from inspiration while ascending stairs and exhalation during descent. Going downstairs is an eccentric muscle pattern and exhalation is a relative eccentric contraction of the diaphragm.

Refer to the section on ventilation and movement strategies on p. 387 of this chapter to determine appropriate incorporation of breathing in functional tasks.

LATERAL COSTAL BREATHING

Lateral costal breathing also facilitates diaphragmatic excusion. This may be done bilaterally as in Figures 22-10, 22-11, 22-12, 22-13, and 22-14 or unilaterally as in Figures 22-15, 22-16, and 22-17. Lower chest lateral costal expansion facilitates diaphragmatic and intercostal breathing where the mid chest will recruit primarily intercostal activity.

Upper Chest Inhibition

If all other manual facilitation techniques cease to produce the desired increase in diaphragmatic breathing, then inhibiting the upper chest during inhalation may be effective.

Again, position the patient appropriately. These authors usually choose sidelying or 3/4 supine. Begin by facilitating the diaphragm, usually with the diaphragm scoop. Slowly bring your other arm across the upper chest at about the level of the sternal angle. Leave it there for a couple of respiratory cycles without applying any pressure to feel the upper chest's movement.

After assessing this movement, gently allow your arm to follow the upper chest back to its resting position when the patient exhales. Now on the patient's next inspiratory effort, do not move your arm's position. Thus your arm position will apply pressure or resistance to the expansion of the upper chest. This gentle pressure will cause postural inhibition to the anterior and superior movement of the upper chest.

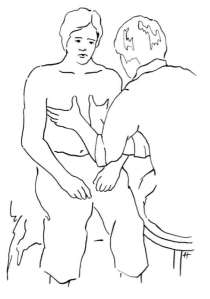

FIGURE 22-11
Bilateral midchest expansion exercise.

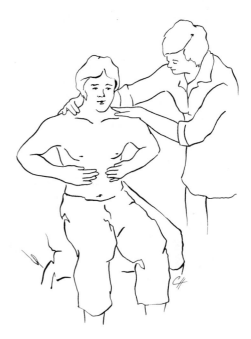

FIGURE 22-12
Self-assisted bilateral chest expansion exercise. Keep the patient's shoulders relaxed.

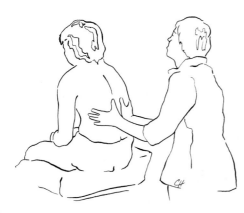

FIGURE 22-13
Bilateral posterior chest expansion exercise.

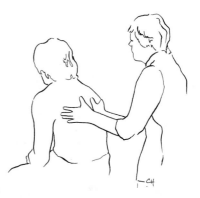

FIGURE 22-14
Bilateral posterior chest expansion exercise.

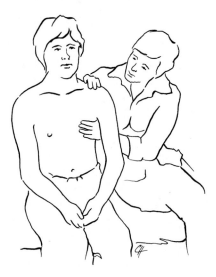

FIGURE 22-15
Unilateral (segmental) breathing, left mid-lung field.

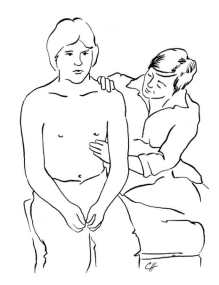

FIGURE 22-16
Unilateral (segmental) breathing emphasizing the left lower lobe. Note that the patient's shoulder must remain down, with hands placed on ulnar border or palm up in his lap.

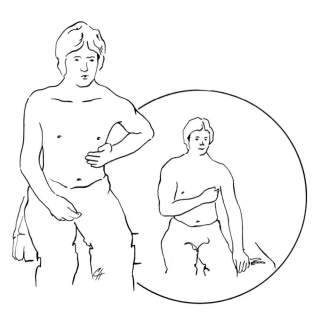

FIGURE 22-17
The patient can perform unilateral (segmental) breathing by placing either hand on the side of the chest to be emphasized. The patient can also perform mid-chest expansion by moving his hand up.

After each expiratory cycle, add more pressure until the patient subconsciously increases the lower chest breathing out of necessity.

When you note more diaphragmatic and/or lower intercostal muscle excursion, verbally note this to the patient. Ask the patient to try to reproduce this pattern. With your other arm continue to facilitate the desired response, such as with the diaphragm scoop. Slowly, during each of the next series of inhalation, release your inhibition as the patient tries to maintain the improved lower chest breathing pattern. If the patient is only partially successful, the inhibition can be partially reapplied to assist the patient. If the patient becomes anxious because the therapist's inhibition is preventing upper chest breathing, then decrease the inhibition to a comfortable level. This technique should never cause an increase in anxiety or it will only encourage more upper chest breathing rather than less.

Normal Timing

During normal quiet inspiration (controlled breathing), the diaphragm contracts, which is seen outwardly as a gentle rise of the abdomen. The second movement is seen as lateral costal expansion of the lower chest and usually to a lesser extent, lower anterior chest expansion. Lastly, the upper chest rises slightly in primarily a superior-anterior plane with less lateral expansion noted. A normal timing technique adapted from the physical therapy approach of proprioceptive neuromuscular facilitation (PNF) can help the patient work on this sequence. After the patient has learned to initiate inspiration with his or her diaphragm and lower chest wall muscles more consistently, this technique can help to put the whole sequence together. The diaphragm continues to be the primary mover, but the other accessory muscles are encouraged to do what they should do, which is to assist the diaphragm for better overall ventilation.

Generally, the patient is positioned symmetrically in either supine or supported sitting with a neutral pelvic position. The therapist waits until the end of an expiratory cycle and then, using the hand placement of the diaphragm scoop, asks the patient to breathe in "here." With the other hand, the therapist moves up

the chest wall to the lower sternum and touches the patient with the instructions again to "now breathe here." Finally, the therapist uses the first hand to move up to the upper sternum (usually around the level of the sternal angle) and asks the patient to "now breathe here." It is important that the therapist smoothly transitions from one hand to the next to assist the patient in developing a smooth motor transition from one area of the chest to the other. The manual cues provide tactile cuing rather than true motor facilitation. Because of this, the normal timing sequence is obviously a more-advanced technique intended for use after achieving initial diaphragmatic training success.

MOBILIZING THE THORAX

For some patients, controlled breathing alone may not alleviate the inefficient ventilatory patterns even with utilization of good positioning and appropriate ventilatory strategies. The thorax itself may be incapable of moving freely enough to allow for adequate chest wall excursion necessary for that breathing pattern. For example, a patient with a spinal cord injury who is demonstrating an excessive diaphragmatic pattern that is unbalanced by the normal neuromuscular support of the intercostal and abdominal muscles can breathe using minimal chest wall expansion. This is often noted as belly breathing. It may be necessary to mobilize individual rib segments to gain the potential for chest wall expansion in all three planes of ventilation before facilitating a specific breathing pattern. If the potential for movement is not there, then the breathing pattern cannot change. Likewise, a patient with primary pulmonary dysfunction undergoing chest surgery, or a patient suffering from an acute chest trauma, may also find the rib cage stiff or sore and thus limited in its potential expansion. All three of these patients may benefit from the inclusion of rib cage mobilization in their therapy programs. The rib cage musculoskeletal limitation may be secondary to muscular atrophy, spasticity, or pain. Thus patients with either primary pulmonary dysfunction or secondary pulmonary dysfunction can benefit from the concept of chest mobilization.

It is beyond the scope of this textbook to detail all

Techniques to Mobilize the Thorax

1. Use of towel or pillow rolls to mechanically open up the anterior or lateral chest wall
2. Use of upper extremity patterns to facilitate opening of individual rib segments
3. Counterrotation of the trunk
4. Use of ventilatory-movement strategies to facilitate opening of the entire thorax
5. Specific rib mobilization to free up an individual segment
6. Myofascial release techniques to free up restrictive connective tissue on and around the thorax
7. Soft tissue release techniques to lengthen individual tight muscles

---

the numerous techniques involved in musculoskeletal mobilization of the thorax, however, some simple techniques and suggestions for further study are presented. See the box above for a summary of mobilization techniques.

Once again the therapist should note that the initial step in achieving success begins with positioning considerations. Starting in supine, anterior chest wall mobility can be improved by placing a vertical towel roll down the length of the thoracic spine and allowing gravity to pull the shoulders back to the bed. In this position, the anterior chest is opened up, placing the intercostal and pectoralis muscles on stretch for easier facilitation of upper chest expansion.

In sidelying, the lateral aspect of the chest can be passively mobilized with gravity's assistance by placing a towel roll(s) or pillow(s) under the lower chest (ribs 8 to 10) on the weight-bearing side. To determine an appropriate amount of sidebending, make sure that the patient's shoulder and pelvis are still in direct contact with the surface even with the towel roll(s) in place. This maximizes the stretch on the chest without placing the patient in a position that is too advanced for his or her present chest wall mobility. Patients vary from tolerating only a single thin towel roll up to tolerating three pillows under the lower ribs.

In both postures, active or passive stretching can be added after positioning for success. In supine, ask the patient to bring the arms directly up over his or

her head (shoulder flexion), as far as possible while watching his or her hands. Using the appropriate ventilatory strategy, the patient is also instructed to inhale during this movement. Because full shoulder flexion and inspiration both require opening of the individual rib segments, pairing them in this gravity-assisted position will promote a greater passive chest wall stretch then either technique alone. If straight flexion is not a viable option, use a butterfly position, raising the arms up in shoulder flexion, abduction, and external rotation with elbows bent (like butterfly wings), again pairing this with voluntary maximal inspiration and upward eye gaze. Pairing inspiration and shoulder flexion maximizes the stretch on the chest and encourages better ventilatory strategies.

In sidelying, ask the patient to bring his or her arm up in straight flexion to maximize anterior chest expansion or to move the arm into abduction to maximize the lateral costal expansion. Pair either movement with inspiration and upward eye gaze. If upper extremity movement is not possible, the therapist can passively use counterrotation of the trunk to mobilize the chest while in the sidelying over the towel or pillow roll. Continue to ask for active eye gazing.

The same concepts can be used in upright postures, such as sitting or standing. Use a vertical towel roll again along the thoracic spine either along the back of a chair (wheelchair) or along the wall. Move the patient's arms passively or actively up into the most flexion or butterfly ROM possible. The patient will get a significantly greater stretch to the anterior chest wall using the towel roll than without it. Precautions apply for patients with musculoskeletal problems along the spine and for patients with impaired skin-tolerance.

If these general mobilizing techniques do not produce adequate chest wall mobility to allow for freer breathing patterns to occur, then more specific techniques need to be considered including the following: (1) specific rib mobilization, (2) myofascial release to tight connective tissues (e.g., scar tissue secondary to surgical or traumatic areas), and/or (3) soft tissue release of tight muscle groups (neurological patients often present with tightness in the pectoralis, intercostal, and quadratus lumborum muscles groups, whereas orthopedic patients tend to have more tightness in the neck and back muscles). Use the positioning and ventilatory strategies previously suggested (e.g., sidelying over a towel roll) during these specific interventions to maximize the potential gains in chest wall mobility. It is beyond the scope of this textbook to detail all the numerous techniques involved in musculoskeletal mobilization and release of the thorax. These three interventions are intended as suggestions for further study in outside texts.

FACILITATING ACCESSORY MUSCLES IN VENTILATION

If the patient is still not demonstrating an optimal breathing pattern after facilitating a preferred breathing pattern through appropriate positioning, appropriate ventilatory strategies, chest wall mobilization, and diaphragmatic retraining, then specific facilatory or inhibitory techniques should be initiated to the accessory muscles of ventilation. Specific techniques are discussed here in detail. See the box above for a summary.

Because the diaphragm normally supplies the bulk of the inspired air during quiet breathing, diaphragmatic breathing is the preferred pattern of breathing. However, after some neurological insults, strictly diaphragmatic breathing may not be possible or even preferred. Unlike pulmonary rehabilitation programs for chronic lung or asthmatic patients, where diaphragmatic breathing is almost always encouraged and use of accessory muscles discouraged, restoration of independent, efficient breathing patterns for the neurologically impaired patient may require the regular use of accessory muscles.

Positioning continues to be the single most important aspect of all ventilatory facilitation techniques. If your patient is positioned for success, the probability of a successful response is much more likely. By assessing the patient's head, upper-extremity, trunk, pelvic, and lower-extremity positioning before every activity or technique, the therapist is empowered to use mechanical positioning and gravity to the patient's advantage rather than to a disadvantage. For example, a slightly posteriorly tilted pelvis tends to facilitate diaphragmatic breathing, whereas a slightly anteriorly tilted pelvis tends to facilitate upper chest breathing. Thus when facilitating more accessory

---

Accessory Muscle Facilitation Techniques

1. Pectoralis facilitation
2. Sternocleidomastoid and scalenes facilitation
3. Trapezius facilitation
4. Diaphragm inhibiting technique
   - Manual inhibition
   - Postural inhibition
5. Lateral costal facilitation
6. Serratus push-up

---

muscle breathing, the patient would be put in an advantageous posture by slightly anteriorly tilting the pelvis. In supine, this could be as simple as decreasing the amount of knee flexion that is present or using a small towel roll under the lumbar spine.

Pectoralis Facilitation

The pectoralis muscle group is a powerful anterior and lateral expander of the upper chest and can substitute quite effectively for paralyzed intercostal muscles in the upper chest when trained to do so. Training usually begins in either modified sidelying or supine. To increase the use of this muscle during inspiration, the therapist should place his or her hand in the same direction as the contracting muscle fibers. Specific proprioceptive input is very important when facilitating a muscle, thus make sure the hand is diagonally placed on the upper thorax (Figure 22-18).

The heel of the therapist's hand should be near the sternum and the fingers aligned up and out toward the shoulder. The patient is then asked to breathe into the therapist's hands while the therapist applies a quick manual stretch (as in repeated contractions PNF) to the muscle fibers (down and in toward the sternum). This elicits the quick stretch reflex of the muscle and simultaneously provides added sensory input, which facilitates a stronger and more specific muscle contraction. To emphasize an increase in lateral expansion, facilitation should gradually be transferred from the sternal area out toward the therapist's finger tips by the patient's shoulder. Unlike in the case of facilitating a more diaphragmatic pattern, verbal cues

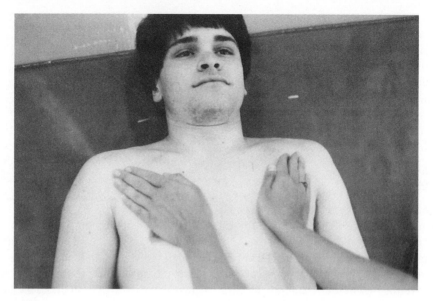

FIGURE 22-18
Hand placement for facilitation of the pectoralis muscles for upper chest breathing.

should be strong and demanding to elicit a stronger maximal voluntary effort.

Sternocleidomastoid and Scalene Facilitation

This same principle can be applied to the sternocleidomastoid and scalene muscles. In supine, therapists need only change the angle of their hand alignment to more specifically facilitate the sternocleidomastoid and scalene muscles. Turning the hands parallel to the trunk so that the fingers are pointing up toward the neck rather than pointing out toward the shoulder, the therapist applies the same quick stretch and uses the same verbal cues. The altered hand position now specifically facilitates the sternocleidomastoid and scalene muscles and secondarily influences the pectoralis muscles. The sternocleidomastoid and scalene muscles primarily expand the chest in a superior and anterior plane, whereas the pectoralis muscles expand the chest in primarily a lateral and anterior plane, thus accounting for the slight difference in the facilitation positioning.

Trapezius Facilitation

The trapezius muscle assists in superior expansion of the chest. Facilitation can be initiated in supine or sidelying positions to decrease the resistance from gravity. It can be progressed to an upright posture in which the patient would have to work against gravity.

Placing the hands over the tops of the patient's shoulders, the therapist quick stretches the trapezius in a downward direction to facilitate a stronger elevation response. Repeated contractions can be added to facilitate the contraction throughout the full ROM. Obviously, the shoulder shrug motion should be paired with inhalation and upward eye gaze to maximize the facilitation response.

Inhibition of the Diaphragm

Two techniques are described to inhibit the excessive use of the diaphragm during inspiration. Ideally, the therapist is venturing to balance the use of accessory muscles, especially the intercostal, sternocleidomastoid, scalenes, and trapezius muscles with the diaphragm's contraction. This is done to prevent paradoxical movements of the chest, or worse, to prevent adverse musculoskeletal changes in the chest wall, such as a pectus excuvatum that can result from muscle imbalance.

Inhibiting the diaphragm may be necessary during breathing retraining for some patients with spinal cord injuries, polio, spina bifida, developmental delays, head traumas, and cerebral palsy. The diaphragm may be too weak to produce an adequate tidal volume or vital capacity without the assistance of accessory muscles. In these cases the diaphragm-inhibiting technique is used to encourage the use of the accessory muscles to assist in independent voluntary ventilation. Patients learn to use their weakened diaphragm muscles in concert with intact accessory muscles. Not only does this allow for an increased tidal volume and vital capacity, but it also provides better aeration of all lung segments and better mobilization of the entire thorax.

In contrast to the first reason that this technique may be used, an unusually strong diaphragm, acting without support from surrounding musculature, specifically the intercostals and abdominal muscles, may also need to be inhibited. For example, a paraplegic or lower level tetraplegic patient with an intact diaphragm but absent abdominal and intercostal muscles may demonstrate a paradoxical breathing pattern (see compensatory breathing patterns, Chapter 37). In this case the accessory muscles must be encouraged to keep the diaphragm in check, attempting to avoid the development of a pectus excuvatum. The goal of this breathing retraining method is to stop the paradoxical movements of the upper chest during inspiration by balancing the use of the upper and lower chest. In some cases, spastic intercostal muscles, like in some spinal cord injury situations, may intercede to prevent this paradoxical movement by maintaining the upper chest's position during inspiration in spite of the negative pressure within the chest and gravity's influence on top of the chest. Balancing the chest's movements should produce an increase in tidal volume and vital capacity potential and mobilize a greater portion of the chest, just as the technique does in the first case presented.

To perform the diaphragm-inhibiting technique, the patient is positioned supine, semi-sitting or side-lying with the top arm positioned overhead or pulled back at the waist to open up the upper chest. If tolerated, remove pillows from under his or her head, anteriorly tilt the pelvis and assess patient's airway safety by checking if he or she can still swallow comfortably. The heel of the therapist's hand is placed lightly on the patient's abdomen at about the level of the umbilicus. No instructions are given to the patient at this point. As the patient begins to exhale a normal breath of air, the therapist gently allows the heel of his or her hand to move up and in toward the central tendon of the patient's diaphragm (see Figure 22-4, p. 394). When expiration for that breath is completed, the therapist strictly maintains the hand position in that shortened expiratory position. During the following inspiratory phase, the diaphragm will experience some gentle resistance to its inferior descent, causing inhibition to its full ROM. On the next expiration, the technique is repeated with the therapist carefully pushing the heel of his or her hand further up and in, maintaining greater inhibition during each inspiratory phase. After two or three ventilatory cycles, a patient usually begins to subconsciously alter his or her breathing pattern to include more upper chest expansion to reconcile the diaphragm's transient inability to produce enough chest expansion to yield an adequate tidal volume. The therapist should carefully observe which accessory muscles the patient spontaneously chooses. Are they used symmetrically? What is the general quality of the movement? Is the onset harsh or smooth? Does the patient appear fatigued or uncoordinated?

It is not until this point that the therapist should verbally acknowledge any alteration of the patient's breathing pattern. Without changing his or her hand position, the therapist tells the patient what it is that he or she likes about the new breathing pattern (e.g., balance between upper and lower chest expansion or less paradoxical motion of the sternum). Then the patient is asked if he or she notices any difference from before, bringing this breathing pattern to a conscious level. Only after some orientation to this pattern, usually no more than 4 to 6 breathing cycles in the full inhibiting pattern, should the therapist begin to grad-

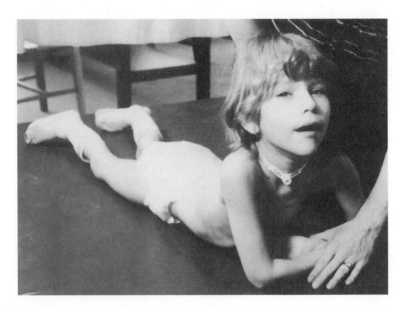

FIGURE 22-19
Diaphragm inhibiting in prone on elbows position.

ually release the pressure being applied.

While slowly releasing pressure with each cycle of inspiration, the therapist asks the patient to attempt cognitively to reproduce the desired pattern. It should take the same number of cycles to release the pressure as it did to apply it. This technique easily allows for gradations of inhibition, from full inhibition, where the patient is forced to use upper accessory muscles or risk becoming short of breath, to barely a proprioceptive reminder to change his or her breathing pattern. It also allows for gradation of inhibition while the patient is learning to assume control over the new breathing pattern. If during the releasing phase of this technique the patient begins to lose control over the new pattern, the therapist can gently reapply some pressure during the next expiratory phase to help the patient regain that control. At that point, the therapist can release or reapply pressure as necessary until the desired pattern is obtained and full release of pressure is completed.

This technique is particularly effective with patients who are having difficulty cognitively altering their own breathing pattern, such as with small children, brain-damaged patients, or slow motor learners, because it requires no cognitive effort until success has

already been achieved. Extra care must be taken not to initiate any applied pressure quickly because of the likelihood of eliciting unwanted abdominal contractions or spasticity or eliciting a stronger diaphragmatic contraction resulting from the quick stretch reflex. The technique should never be painful. The therapist must keep his or her hand on the abdomen, not the rib cage, to properly influence the diaphragm. This technique can be progressed by changing postures, which requires greater trunk control. Can the patient still maintain the overall pattern? Can the patient breathe without paradoxical movements against gravity?

The second technique is for the more advanced patient and simply presents a physical block to diaphragmatic excursion. The patient is positioned in a prone-on-elbows position (Figure 22-19). With most severely neurologically impaired patients, the lower chest will be in direct contact with the surface, so lower anterior and inferior expansion is inhibited and lateral costal expansion is limited. The upper chest is positioned in extension and the upper extremities are fixated, optimizing the length-tension relationship of the anterior and superior accessory muscles for easy facilitation. In addition, anterior excursion of the upper chest is now in a gravity-assisted posture. Through the use of head and neck pat-

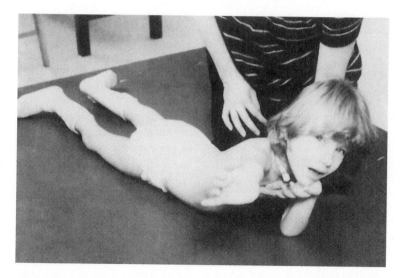

FIGURE 22-20
Static-dynamic upper extremity activities in prone on elbows to encourage upper chest accessory muscle participation.

terns, such as in PNF diagonals, or static-dynamic activities, such as in weight shifting to one supporting limb while reaching out with the other extremity, the therapist can readily facilitate greater upper chest breathing (Figure 22-20). These are the same patterns the therapist can use to achieve other goals, such as increased head and neck control, increased shoulder stability, or increased upper body balance. Therefore, by helping the patients to coordinate movement goals with ventilatory patterns, it becomes more likely that the patients will incorporate these patterns functionally into daily activities. This is the ultimate goal of any ventilatory retraining procedure.

The manual diaphragm-inhibiting technique is usually less threatening to the patient than the prone-on-elbows-inhibition technique. Prone on elbows itself can inhibit the diaphragm so completely for neurological patients lacking spinal extensors that they become extremely short of breath. Consequently, do not position the patients in this more demanding posture until success appears likely.

Serratus Push-up

Facilitating greater posterior chest expansion can be achieved in a prone-on-elbows position. Gravity is now assisting anterior excursion of the chest and resisting posterior excursion. To emphasize the serratus anterior muscle's role in posterior expansion, the patient is instructed to perform an upper body push-up (with or without the therapist's assistance). The serratus anterior muscle causes lateral scapular movement thereby facilitating maximal posterior excursion of the thorax. The patient is instructed to take a deep breath in during the push-up and to exhale the air (passively or forcefully) when returning to the starting position. Forceful exhalation in this activity can be used as a forerunner to effective cough retraining. Gentle or controlled exhalation can be used to encourage greater breath support for vocalization or for eccentric trunk muscle training.

Emphasizing posterior chest expansion during inhalation is the only occasion where inspiration would be paired with trunk flexion. In all other inspiratory situations, inspiration is paired with trunk extension, and exhalation is paired with trunk flexion.

PATIENTS WITH ASYMMETRICAL DYSFUNCTION

Patients with asymmetrical weakness need a different approach from the controlled or upper chest breathing

---

> *Promoting Symmetrical Ventilatory Function for Patients With Asymmetrical Deficits*
>
> 1. Use of positioning to achieve more symmetrical alignment of the chest and trunk in both reclining and upright postures
> 2. Use of postural inhibition to the stronger or uninvolved side to promote greater chest wall expansion on the weaker or involved side
> 3. Timing for emphasis technique to promote active symmetrical breathing anywhere in the thorax

patterns presented previously. These patients need facilitation to the weaker side to promote symmetrical chest wall expansion in both the upper and lower chest. See the box above for a summary of techniques.

Symmetrical Positioning

Symmetrical ventilatory patterns may be effortlessly achieved by altering the patient's position in each posture to maximize the chest wall's potential to move in a symmetrical pattern. This is especially true in an upright position in which asymmetry is generally more pronounced. For example, hemiplegic patients may lean toward their involved side in sitting because of weakness or spasticity. Likewise, after thoracic surgery, a primary pulmonary patient may lean toward the surgical side to avoid pain caused by chest movement around the incision. Both situations cause asymmetrical breathing patterns and decrease ventilation on the involved side. Improving chest wall alignment may alleviate the ventilatory deficit on the involved side.

Postural Inhibition

For some patients, more aggressive positioning must be used to achieve greater chest wall excursion and ventilation on the involved side. This can be accomplished by inhibiting the chest wall movements on the uninvolved or stronger side. Usually, the best posture in which to achieve this inhibition is sidelying. When the patient lies on his or her uninvolved

side with his or her arms positioned down below 90 degrees of shoulder flexion, lateral chest expansion into that side becomes inhibited because of the physical barrier. This forces the patient to find another way to meet his or her ventilatory needs, which indirectly facilitates chest expansion on the opposite side (the uppermost side). The therapist can then supply sensory and motor input through his or her hands to the patient's upper, middle, or lower chest on the involved or weaker side to facilitate increased ventilation on that side. Early in the rehabilitation process or soon after thoracic surgery, the patient may have difficulty performing lateral chest expansion against gravity in sidelying (gravity-resisted movement). If so, position the patient in a 3/4-supine position to lessen the workload imposed by gravity. Gradually, work the patient up to a full sidelying posture to achieve the greatest strengthening benefits.

Timing for Emphasis

Another technique to promote symmetrical chest wall movements is performed in numerous postures, such as supine, sitting, or standing. The therapist places his or her hand symmetrically on the lower lateral chest wall, on the mid chest, or on the upper anterior chest wall. At the end of exhalation, the therapist gives a quick stretch on the muscles being touched to facilitate a deep inspiratory effort in that area of the chest. Immediately after both sides begin to move into an inspiratory pattern, the therapist manually blocks (or inhibits) expansion of the chest on the stronger side while giving continued quick stretches on the weaker side. This facilitates greater expansion on the weak side by use of an overflow response. This technique, adapted from the PNFs timing for emphasis technique, uses the strength of the stronger side to facilitate movement on the weaker side. It can be applied to any area of the chest where symmetrical movements should be the norm.

REDUCING RESPIRATORY RATES

In addition to altering breathing patterns through facilitation and inhibition techniques, reducing respiratory rates (RR) may also be necessary before arriving at an efficient breathing pattern for some patients. See the box below for a summary of techniques. Many neurological patients with high neuromuscular tone increase their RR to compensate for a decrease in their tidal volumes (TV) or because of brain-stem impairments to the respiratory centers. In addition, many patients who are anxious, such as asthmatic, orthopedic, or surgical patients experiencing pain, may also demonstrate an excessively high RR. Attempting to restore ventilatory efficiency may require increasing TV while concurrently decreasing RR.

Previous Facilitation Techniques

The techniques previously described in this chapter promote an increase in TV by improving the overall ventilatory patterns and often cause a secondary reduction in RR. See sections on controlled breathing, mobilizing the thorax, and upper chest breathing facilitation.

Counterrotation

The technique described next is specifically developed to promote a lower RR. The counterrotation technique reduces high neuromuscular tone and increases thoracic mobility, thus often resulting in an increase in TV and simultaneous reduction in RR. These authors have found this technique to be extremely effective for the following: (1) patients with decreased cognitive functioning after a neurological insult or after surgery, (2) very young children because there are no verbal cues, or (3) patients with high neuromuscular tone. As described in Chapter 21, it can also be easily adapted as a very effective as-

---

Techniques to Reduce High Respiratory Rates
1. Previous techniques that increased tidal volume
2. Counterrotation technique
3. Butterfly technique in sitting
• Straight planes
• Counterrotation
4. Relaxed pursed lip breathing with inspiratory and expiratory pauses

---

sisted cough technique. One medical contraindication for this technique is bony instability of the spine because of its rotary nature.

In bed or on a mat, place the patient in sidelying with knees bent and arms resting comfortably out in front of the head or shoulders. In this technique the higher the upper extremities can be placed within a comfort zone, the better the result. Relaxed positioning of the patient is essential to the success of this technique, thus position the patient in an open yet comfortable position. Normalizing neuromuscular tone is the first step in attempting to decrease a high RR. Patient discomfort is likely to elicit increased tone and an increased RR.

The therapist's own position is also important because it directs the force that is applied to the patient's chest. Initially, the therapist needs to stand behind the patient, perpendicular to his or her trunk. If the patient is lying on the left side, the therapist places his or her left hand on the patient's shoulder and his or her right hand on the patient's hip. The therapist then leaves his or her hands in place and simply follows the patient's respiratory cycle. This allows the therapist to assess the patient's subjective rate and rhythm and the patient's overall neuromuscular tone. Only after this assessment should the clinician begin the active phase of the technique. Using a PNF technique called *rhythmic initiation,* the patient is gently log-rolled in a small ROM in sidelying. The rolling is gradually increased achieving more ROM from sidelying toward prone. This progression of movement generally reduces high tone, which usually makes the second phase of the technique more effective.

During this phase, the therapist needs to audibly duplicate the patient's RR. As the patient moves into greater rolling ROM and begins to slow his or her RR, the therapist needs to use the patient's audible cuing as a facilitator for establishing a slower RR. Thus the therapist begins by having the patient establish the audible RR and then the therapist slowly takes over. Audible cues can be very strong facilitators of ventilatory rhythms.

Phase two requires the therapist to slowly change his or her position. Transitioning to a diagonal posture, the therapist now stands or half kneels behind the patient near his or her hips, turning diagonal to the patient until facing the patient's head at roughly at 45-degree angle. The hand placement begins to get more specific. Assume again that the patient is side-lying on the left. At the beginning of the expiratory cycle, the therapist's left hand slowly glides over the patient's shoulder on the right pectoral region, with care being taken not to unintentionally use the thumb or finger tips, and the right hand slowly glides back to the patient's right gluteal fossa (the hollow of the buttocks) (Figure 21-6, *A,* (p. 376). The therapist can then manually compress the rib cage in all three planes of ventilation at the end of exhalation by gently pulling the shoulder back and down, while simultaneously pushing the hip up and forward. This movement promotes more complete exhalation.

When the patient begins the next inspiration, the therapist switches hand placement to capitalize on the improved potential for TV. The therapist's left hand slides back to the patient's right scapula, and the therapist's right hand slides forward just anterior to the patient's right iliac crest (see Figure 21-6, *B,* p. 376). As the patient inhales, the therapist slowly stretches the chest to maximize inspiration volumes (TVs). The therapist's left hand pushes the scapula (or the thorax if the scapula is unstable) up and away from the spine and the right hand pulls the pelvis back and down to maximize all three planes of ventilation, resulting in greater inspiration. The therapist should use the flat or heel of the hand whenever possible to avoid unintentional patient discomfort and to maximize the facilitated area.

Initially, the therapist begins and ends the respiratory cycle according to the patient's RR. However, as the patient's tone is relaxed and increased TVs are promoted through the effects of counterrotation, the therapist gradually slows the rate of rotation down, giving the patient audible breathing cues to also facilitate a slower RR. The patient generally accommodates to a slower RR as the therapist gains more control over the patient's breathing pattern. With many patients, the results can be marked. If the patient can cognitively follow commands, he or she can be alerted to this change and encouraged to assist in voluntarily breathing at the slower rate.

The therapist can progress the technique by decreasing the manual input. The last facilitation to be removed should be the audible cues. As with the diaphragm-inhibiting technique, the therapist can reestablish control quickly if needed by simply reapplying stronger manual input. If the patient has an extremely fast RR (i.e., 50 to 60 breaths/min), the facilitation can be applied every 2 to 3 breaths so as not to fatigue the patient or therapist.

It should be apparent that this technique need not be used exclusively for respiratory goals but rather can be incorporated into the patient's total rehabilitation program. It is a natural precursor to active rolling or it can be used as a vestibular stimulator.

Butterfly Technique

If the patient has greater motor control, an upright version of this technique may be appropriate. In unsupported sitting, stand behind or in front of the patient, depending on his or her balance needs, and ask the patient to bring his or her arms up into a butterfly posture or assist his or her arms up to this posture. Starting from a comfortable ROM position for that patient, begin to audibly breathe with the patient's RR. When the patient inhales, raise the arms up into slightly more shoulder flexion. When the patient exhales, lower the arms slightly. Slowly begin to move in greater and greater increments of range, all the while breathing out loud with your patient. Through your audible breathing cues, begin to "ask" your patient to slow down the RR and take deeper slower breaths. The use of the following concurrent ventilatory strategies promotes deeper inhalations and exhalations: (1) shoulder flexion and trunk extension paired with inspiration and (2) shoulder extension and trunk flexion paired with exhalation. Thus it becomes possible and probable for the patient to increase his or her TV and decrease RR.

As in the previous technique, the therapist begins by breathing out loud at the patient's pace and transitions to breathing audibly at a slower, more desirable pace. The patient picks up on this subtle cuing and subconsciously reduces his or her own RR even if they cannot follow verbal commands.

This technique can be modified to encourage more intercostal and oblique abdominal muscle contractions by using a diagonal rather than a straight plane

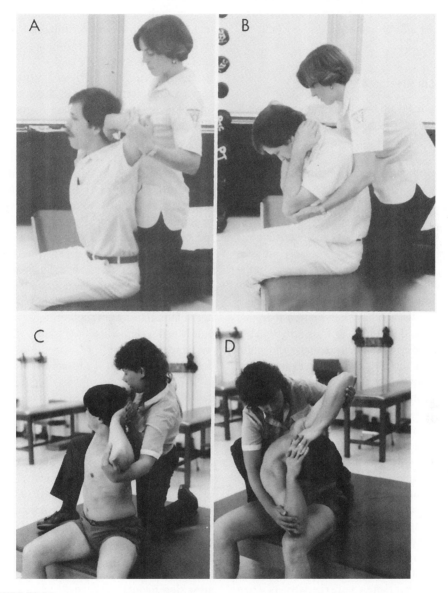

FIGURE 22-21
A, butterfly technique facilitating inspiration; **B,** butterfly technique facilitating exhaltation;
C, butterfly with trunk rotation facilitating inspiration. All three planes of respiration are stretched
on the patients right side. **D,** butterfly with trunk rotation facilitating exhaltation. All planes
compressed on the right side.

of movement. Have the patient look up and over one shoulder as he or she breathes in and brings arms up and behind his or her head. Then have the patient look down and away toward the opposite knee as he or she breathes out and brings arms down to the opposite knee (Figure 22-21).

Relaxed Pursed-Lip Breathing

Use of a relaxed pursed-lip breathing pattern as previously described under "Facilitating a controlled breathing pattern," is also a technique to reduce RR. By prolonging the expiratory phase through pursed lips, the patient secondarily decreases his or her RR.

GLOSSOPHARYNGEAL BREATHING

A small population of neurological patients requires more than just promoting the use of accessory muscles or changing RR to meet basic ventilatory needs. In the last decade, more high-level SCIs (above C4) have survived the initial trauma because of advances in medical technology. However, the rehabilitation therapist is then faced with the difficult task of restoring quality of life. For these patients, as well as many old polio patients, mastery of the glossopharyngeal breathing (GPB) technique allows for greater voluntary ventilation, which many patients state does improve the quality of their lives. This augmented breathing pattern allows patients to regain some control over their lives and to regain control over their ventilation, which was lost as a result of high neurological insults.

GPB is a technique developed in the 1950s by polio patients looking for a way to reduce their dependence on the iron lung for ventilation. It was found that by using the lips, soft palate, mouth, tongue, pharynx, and larynx, a patient could actually inhale enough air to sustain life without mechanical ventilation. Only intact cranial nerves are required. This method is sometimes referred to as *frog breathing* because it uses the principles of inspiration common to the frog. The patient learns to create a pocket of negative pressure within the buccal (mouth) cavity by maximizing that internal space, thereby causing the outside air to rush in. At that point, the patient closes off the entrance (the lips) and proceeds to force the air back and down the throat with a stroking maneuver of the tongue, pharynx, and larynx.

Research has consistently shown that use of this technique with severely impaired neurological patients can increase pulmonary functions significantly, especially for TV and VC. If GPB is the only means of ventilation off of a ventilator or phrenic nerve stimulator, mastery of this technique is critical to a patient's survival in case of mechanical failure. All attempts should be made to successfully teach GPB to this patient population.

A clinical example may help to illustrate its usefulness. A 14-year-old male sustained a C1 complete SCI while racing in front of a train. After he was medically stable, two phrenic nerve stimulators were implanted in his chest. The patient had no nonassisted means of ventilation. Neuromuscularly, the patient had limited use of one trapezius, sternocleidomastoid, and intrinsic neck muscles. The patient and family feared that long-term nursing home placement would be inevitable because of their fear of his phrenic nerve stimulator malfunctioning or a battery wearing out, causing immediate respiratory distress. The family believed it could not bear the psychological burden placed on them if the patient went home to live. GPB instruction was suggested and began slowly because the patient stated that he learned motor skills slowly. After a painstaking 2-month period, the patient learned to breathe without the use of his phrenic nerve stimulator for 3 to 5 minutes before fatiguing and hypoventilating. Within the next 1 to 2 months, this same patient learned to breathe for up to 2 hours off of his stimulator, using GPB only. To the staff's surprise, he even learned to talk and operate his sip-and-puff wheelchair while using GPB. The patient was then successfully discharged to his home. This does not imply that this was the only factor considered in his discharge planning, but it was perhaps the most significant.

Instruction in GPB takes time and concentration. It is best to start off in small time blocks of 10 to 15 minutes because it can be very fatiguing. However, it is important to successful learning of the technique that the patient gets consistent, preferably daily training. Once the patient has mastered the technique, practice sessions can be lengthened considerably, and the patient can be taught self-monitoring techniques. Specific goals of GPB training must be explained to the patient before the beginning of treatment to gain his or her support and cooperation. In addition to providing the ventilator-or stimulator-dependent patient with a TV necessary for gaining independence from mechanical assists, GPB has many other benefits. For the tetraplegic patient who has a partially intact diaphragm (C3 to C4) or the loss of essential accessory muscles (C5 to C8), GPB can accomplish the following: (1) increase VC to produce a more effective cough, (2) assist in a longer and stronger phonation effort, and (3) act as an internal mobilizer of the chest wall.

The muscles used in this technique do not have the same internal proprioceptive, sensory, or visual feedback mechanisms as the trunk and limb muscles. Thus necessary adjustments in the technique are sometimes difficult to see or feel. The patient cannot see his or her tongue pushing the air back or truly feel the pharynx swallowing the air into the lungs, so the therapist's external feedback system is very influential. Use of a mirror can greatly enhance the visual component of feedback. Small changes, like adjustments in posture or a suggestion of another sound to imitate, may be all that is needed for the patient to learn the stroking maneuver correctly. Success in GPB can be assessed objectively with a spirometer and a pulse oximeter. For those patients incapable of breathing independently, any TV reading will indicate successful intake of air. For patients who are not ventilator dependent, a VC reading that is greater than 5% over the baseline indicates successful use of GPB. Lower-level tetraplegics, C5 to C8, have demonstrated increases in VC by as much as 70% to 100%.

Therapists can monitor their own successes with this technique by taking VC readings with and without GPB or by subjective analyses. Maximal inhalation, followed by three or four successful GPB strokes, will cause a feeling that the chest will burst if an attempt is made to inhale more air. Likewise, a sensation of "needing to cough" is another subjective indication of successful GPB. However, a feeling of indigestion is usually indicative of swallowed air in the stomach instead of the lungs.

During the initial treatment session, the therapist demonstrates to the patient what a stroking maneuver looks like several times to give an idea of the motion required. The therapist continues to mimic the pattern as the patient attempts to duplicate it. This gives the patient an active model to mimic and decreases feelings of uneasiness surrounding the necessary but somewhat silly facial grimaces. If the patient is able to breathe independently, his or her ability to breath hold and to close off the nasal passageway should be checked because air leakage is a common cause of failure. The patient is then instructed to take in a maximal inspiration before attempting the stroking maneuvers to eliminate the possibility of using other accessory muscles during the technique.

If possible, position the patient in an upright or at least a symmetrical position. Specifically, the patients are instructed to bring their jaws down and then forward as if reaching their bottom lip up for a carrot dangling just in front and above the upper lip (Figure 22-22, A). Slight cervical hyperextension is necessary to allow for maximal temporal mandibular joint (TMJ) excursion. (A contraindication for this technique is a TMJ disorder.) The lips should be shaped as if they were to make the sound "oop." The patient is then told to close the mouth, reaching the bottom lip up to the top lip (see Figure 22-22, B). The tongue and jaw are drawn back toward the throat, with the mouth and tongue formation of the word *up* or the sound "ell" (see Figure 22-22, B). The lower jaw is moving in roughly a rectangular pattern. Most patients learn the stroking maneuvers by making the sounds at first, as they become more proficient, the sounds and excessive head and neck motions diminish. Often, the students (patients) outperform the teacher (therapist), because through consistent use, they learn all of its finer subtleties.

Although this technique can be broken down into several stages as it has been here for the purpose of description, most of the literature cautions the therapist against it. (Zumwalt, Adkins, Dail, and Affeldt, 1956). Simple, minimal instructions seem to accomplish more, perhaps because the continuity of movement is so essential to the success of the inhalation. Specific instructions can be given later if necessary.

Common problems encountered with GPB instruction are as follows: (1) an open nasal passage or glot-

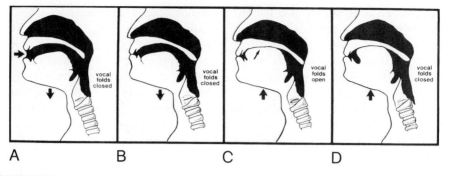

FIGURE 22-22

Glossopharyngeal breathing; **A,** mouth opened to draw in air; **B,** jaw closed to entrap the air; **C,** air pushed back with tongue into trachea; **D,** vocal folds closed to prevent passive air leaks. Entire maneuver is then repeated.

tis that allows the air to escape, (2) a feeling of indigestion indicating that the air is being swallowed into the esophagus rather than the trachea, (3) incorrect shape of the mouth as the air is being drawn in, usually not puckered enough, (4) uncoordinated backward movement of the tongue, (5) inadequate jaw mobility, TMJ dysfunction, or decreased cervical ROM, or (6) incorrect sounds while performing the technique, such as the word *gulp* or an "em" sound. Avoiding any instruction for the tongue seems to produce better results. Concentrate on assisting the patient in learning the external physical movements.

Tolerance to GPB can be increased when mastery of a single stroke becomes consistent. For patients using it as an assist to their own voluntary ventilation, 3 to 4 strokes on top of a maximal inspiration is usually sufficient. Ventilator- or stimulator-dependent patients may need to use as many as 10 to 14 strokes per breath. These figures should be used only as rough guidelines. Each patient will use a slightly different technique with a different number of strokes, with the only important factor being a method that works for them. Fatigue with long trials of GPB can be monitored effectively with an oximeter. The oxygen saturation level should stay above 90% to maintain adequate PaO_2 levels. For example, if the patient begins the GPB session with an oxygen saturation level in the upper 90s, fatigue can be monitored and anticipated by watching if the oxygen levels decrease. If the lev-

els begin to fall to the mid 90s and then the low 90s, you can anticipate when they will reach 90%. At that point, end the GPB training and put the patient back on the previous ventilatory support system. Oximetry not only allows for accurate monitoring but also provides a means for an objective means for monitoring progress over time. In addition, a spirometer objectively measures improvements in VC using GPB. It gives the patients concrete indications of success or failure with the technique.

ENHANCING VOCALIZATION SKILLS

In contrast to procedures that assist the patient in inhalation, procedures intended to improve a patient's phonation skill must focus on elongating the expiration phase. Coughing is a gross-motor skill that relies more on force than fine control of the ventilatory muscles for its effectiveness. Conversely, phonation requires precise, fine-motor control of these muscles and the vocal folds to provide a consistent air flow through the larynx. Both are expiration activities and depend on the preceding inspiration for optimal performance; however, coughing uses concentric contractions of the expiratory muscles to force the air out, and quiet talking uses primarily eccentric contractions of the inspiratory muscles to slowly release the air during expiration. Because of these differences, procedures to improve coughing and phonation will be different in focus. See the box above for a summary of techniques. Coughing is covered in detail in Chapter 21.

Because the patient's TV and total inspiratory capacity are the power source for phonation, they become important concerns in a phonation program. Generally, a normal TV is adequate for conversational speech. However, larger volumes of air, thus greater inspiratory capacities, are required for singing, loud talking, or professional speaking. Therefore the breathing pattern facilitation techniques described previously in this chapter are ideal before instructing the patient in better expiration control. For example, facilitating diaphragmatic and/or accessory muscle breathing techniques, along with the use of quick stretches or repeated contractions, can facilitate the desired deeper inhalation.

Positioning Concerns

Consistent with all previous techniques, the first aspect of improving breath support for vocalization is to optimize the patient's position. The vocal folds have an ideal muscle length-tension relationship when the head is in a neutral chin tuck. In addition, an open anterior chest wall will allow for the greatest potential for chest wall excursion and thus the largest VC. Use the previously described suggestions for positioning to determine if your particular patient needs positioning to encourage a more diaphragmatic, upper chest, or unilateral breathing pattern.

Manual Techniques

Several simple techniques can be used to improve eccentric control of the diaphragm and intercostal muscles in preparation for speech. Vibration or shaking to the lower chest during expiration assists in a slower, more controlled recoil of the diaphragm. Why this occurs is not fully understood. It may be that the sensory and proprioceptive stimulation that the vibration or shaking provides augments the patient's concentration on those muscles resulting in longer phonation. The patient is instructed to phonate an "ah" or "oh" sound for as long as possible. The therapist simultaneously vibrates the patient's chest with an even and gentle force throughout and slightly beyond the full expiration phase, placing his or her hands on the lateral costal borders of the thorax, the mid chest, or on the pectoral area, depending on which area of the chest needs the most help in controlling exhalation. This is very different from the rapid, forceful pressure that is applied to the patient's chest when promoting a deep cough. Be certain that the patients understand this important difference. The therapist must stress to the patients that they should not let air escape before vocalization and that they should try to keep the voice intensity consistent throughout the procedure. This will promote slow eccentric release of the inspiratory muscles during the entire course of the vocalization. Progress can be readily monitored by timing the patient's vocalization, before, during, and after this technique. About 10 to 12 seconds of vocalization, or 8 to 10 syllables per breath, is generally considered adequate for functional use in speech.

For children, this technique can be modified. The child is asked to say "ah" or "oh" for as long as possible while the therapist percusses or taps lightly with his or her hands on the child's upper or lower chest so as to produce a series of staccato sounds. Most children enjoy the new sound that this makes and will try repeatedly to phonate longer and louder to accentuate the different intensities.

Therapeutically, this requires them to take a deeper inhalation before vocalizing, followed by an elongated expiratory phase, both of which are necessary for functional speech. As the child becomes more adept at it, the therapist can apply more pronounced clapping over the chest, accomplishing a wider range of voice intensities and doubling as a means of percussion for postural drainage.

Eccentric Resistance Techniques

More specific facilitation can be used to increase breath support. Ideally, the patient is positioned symmetrically in supine or supported sitting, allowing for maximal chest wall expansion. The patient is instructed to visualize his or her chest being pulled up toward the ceiling and held there. They are then told to vocalize slowly trying not to let the chest "fall." Meanwhile, the therapist is applying consistent pressure to the patient's chest to try to force a quicker exhalation. The patient is told to resist this motion by trying to control and prolong expiration. Like the antagonistic reversal technique described in PNF, the therapist is resisting the patient's attempt to eccentrically contract and control the trunk muscles. This strengthens the eccentric phase of exhalation and promotes greater breath control for vocalization.

The same concept can be applied to functional tasks. Moving into gravity, that is, coming down to sitting from a standing posture, lying down from a sitting posture, and bringing an arm down from reaching into a higher cabinet, all require eccentric control of the muscles involved in that activity to slow the body's descent into gravity's influence. Because quiet speech uses a similar muscular contraction, teaching the patient to count out loud or to otherwise vocalize when performing an overall eccentric activity usually improves both activities. For example, the patient can be instructed to reach up to a high shelf or cabinet while inhaling. Then, using gravity to provide the eccentric resistance, the patient is asked to bring his or her arm back down to his or her lap or side while slowly counting out loud and controlling the rate of

the arm's descent. The activity can be progressed several ways. The activity can include lifting something heavy off the shelf and controlling it along with the arm and trunk while lowering the object or weight to a table or to the patient's lap. Or the postural demands of the activity can be increased. The patient can still lift the heavy object or weight but he or she can now be required to do this in standing, which increases the demands on the musculoskeletal system.

Verbal Techniques

Speech activities that do not require a therapist's physical assistance can be done in a group or individual setting. Singing, for instance, promotes strong and prolonged vocalization with maximal inspiration, which is a significant goal in a phonation program. Similarly, whistling promotes long, even exhalations but is nonverbal. Both are easily incorporated into a group activity on the nursing floor, in therapy or in the community.

Along recreational lines, games that promote controlled blowing further the refinement of motor control over the respiratory muscles. This can be accomplished by blowing bubbles, especially large ones, blowing out candles, especially trick candles, blowing a ping-pong ball through a maze, or by blowing air hockey discs across the table rather than pushing them. Patients with musical inclinations should be encouraged to learn to play wind or brass instruments where refined breath control is mandatory for success. Obviously, the possibilities for recreational use are endless, and simply require imagination on the part of the therapist.

Further refinement of breath control for speech can be promoted by interrupting the outgoing air flow. Functional speech is a series of vocal stops and starts. This procedure is geared toward improving functional communication skills. The therapist tells the patient to take a deep breath and then to count out loud to 100. After a few numbers, the patient is told to "hold it." He or she is then told to start up where he or she left off, with the therapist periodically interrupting. Because this activity requires the patient to stop and start the inhalation and exhalation phases at will in all aspects of the ventilatory cycle, it is more advanced and should be used only after some control of exhalation has been mastered.

SUMMARY

In summary, use of appropriate choices in positioning together with use of an appropriate ventilatory and movement strategy for any given task will make the success of that task all the more likely. If these simple, time-efficient methods of facilitation do not produce adequate ventilatory changes by themselves, it is then appropriate to add on the next layer of facilitation—manual facilitation techniques. Specifically, the techniques that are described in this chapter assist in facilitating the following: (1) greater diaphragmatic breathing patterns (or controlled breathing), (2) increased chest wall mobility, (3) greater accessory muscle breathing patterns (or primarily upper chest breathing), (4) increased symmetrical breathing patterns (unilateral disorders), (5) reduction in high respiratory rates, (6) auxillary techniques GBP, and (7) improved phonation support. Obviously, not all techniques would be appropriate for any single patient. It is up to the therapist to determine which techniques would best address their patients' deficits.

In conclusion, positioning has everything to do with increasing ventilation potential and functional skills. From the beginning of the patient's respiratory program, optimizing ventilation and breath control through passive and active positioning techniques should be used by all medical disciplines, not just physical therapy. As the patients progress, the clinician can and should, assist them in developing better and more efficient movement strategies for higher level activities by coordinating appropriate breathing patterns, such as trunk extension-inhalation or trunk flexion-exhalation strategies, into all activities. After these quick and easy suggestions are used, a therapist who is exposed to numerous manual facilitation ideas and techniques to promote more effective and efficient breathing patterns can now choose an appropriate intervention. In some cases, increasing diaphragmatic breathing may be the desired outcome. For other patients, increased upper chest breathing or increased movements on one side of the chest may be

more desirable. Some may benefit even more from techniques to reduce the high RR or to mobilize the thorax. For a select patient population, instruction in GPB may be necessary to support breathing off of mechanical ventilatory support. Lastly, the therapist can now choose to use techniques to improve the patient in developing adequate breath support for vocalization and communication.

It is these authors' hope that the therapist now understands how widespread the influence of effective ventilation can be on a patient's recovery from disease or trauma. Understanding that facilitating effective ventilation goes far beyond the old diaphragmatic exercises, therapists can be empowered to incorporate other techniques and strategies to get their patients healthier quicker and to assist them in reaching their greatest rehabilitation potential.

REVIEW QUESTIONS

1. Why would a therapist want to try to change a patient's breathing pattern?
2. How can ventilatory strategies be incorporated into a treatment session?
3. When would a therapist not teach diaphragmatic breathing?
4. What is the role of relaxation in breathing control?
5. When would a therapist consider teaching the patient to use his upper chest more in breathing?
6. When would a unilateral breathing pattern be taught?

Bibliography

Andreasson, B. Jonson, B., & Kornfralt, R. et al. (1987). Long-term effects of physical exercise on working capacity and pulmonary function in cystic fibrosis. *Acta Paediatrica Scandanavia 76(1):*70–75.

Atrice, M. , Backus, D.A., Gonter, M. & Morrison, S. (1993). Acute physical therapy management of individuals with spinal cord injury. *Orthopedics & Physical Therapy Clinics of North America 2(1):*53–70.

Bach, J.R. (1991). New approaches in the rehabilitation of the traumatic high level quadriplegic. *American Journal of Physical Medicine and Rehabilitation 1991;70(1):*13–9.

Boughton, A., & Ciesla, N. (1986). Physical therapy management of the head-injured patient in the intensive care unit. *Topics in Acute Care Trauma Rehabilitation 1(1):*1–18.

Boehme, R. (1992). Assessment and treatment of the respiratory system for breathing, sound production and trunk control. *Teamtalk 2(4):*2–8.

Braun, N.T. (1982). Force-length relationship of the normal human diaphragm. *Journal of Applied Physiology 53:*405–412.

Brown, J.C. Swank, S.M. Matta, J. & Farras, D.M. (1984). Late spinal deformity in quadriplegic children and adolescents. *Journal of Pediatric Orthopedics 4(4):*456–61.

Cash, J. (1977). *Neurology for physiotherapists.* (Ed. 2). London: JB Lippincott.

Cheshire, D.J., Flack, W.J. (1979). The use of operant conditioning techniques in the respiratory rehabilitation of the tetraplegic. *Paraplegia 16:*162–74.

Clough, P. (1983). Glossopharyngeal breathing: it's application with a traumatic quadriplegic patient. *Archives of Physical Medicine Rehabilitation 64:*384–85.

Delgado, H.R. et al. Chest wall and abdominal motion during exercise in patients with chronic obstructive pulmonary disease, *American Review of Respiratory Disorders,* 126:200, 1982.

DeTroyer, A. (1983). Mechanical action of the abdominal muscles. *Bull Eur Physiopathol Respir 19:*575.

DeTroyer, A., etr al. (1985). Mechanics of intercostal space and actions of external and internal intercostal muscles. *J. Clinics Invest 5:*85–87.

Druz, W.S., & Sharp, J.T. Electrical and Mechanical Activity of the Diaphragm Accompanying Body Position in Severe Chronic Obstructive Pulmonary Disease. *American Review Respiratory Disorders,* 125:275, 1982.

Estenne, M., & DeTroyer, A. (1990). Cough in tetraplegic subjects: an active process. *Annals of Internal Medicine 112(1):*22–28.

Fishburn, M.J., Marino, R.J., & Ditunno, J.F. (1990). Atelectasis and pneumonia in acute spinal cord injury. *Archives of Physical Medicine Rehabilitation 71:*197–200.

Goldman, J.M., et al. (1986. Effect of abdominal binders on breathing in tetraplegic patients. *Thorax 41(12):*940–5.

Gross, D., et al. (1980). The effect of training on strength and endurance of the diaphragm in quadriplegia. *American Journal of Medicine 68:*27–35.

Hapy, M.J. (1992). Wheelchair seating and positioning: options and solutions. *Physical Therapy Forum* issue:4–8.

Hixon, T.J. (1991). *Respiratory function in speech and song.* San Diego: Singular Publishing Group.

Hornstein, S., & Ledsome, J. (1986). Ventilatory muscle training in acute quadriplegia. *Physiotherapy* Canada *38(3):*145–49.

Huss, D. (1987. Seating for spinal cord clients. In *Proceedings of the Third International Seating Symposium,* Memphis, Tenn.: 209–22.

Imle, P., Boughton, A.C. (1987). The physical therapist's role in the early management of acute spinal cord injury. *Topics in Acute Care Trauma Rehabilitation 1(3):*32–47.

Jasper, M., Kruger, M. Ectors, P., & Sergysels, R. (1986). Unilateral chest wall paradoxical motion mimicking a flail chest in a patient with hemilateral C7 spinal injury. *Intensive Care Medicine 12(6):*396–98.

Johnson, E.W., Reynolds, H.T., & Staugh, D. (1985). Duchenne muscular dystrophy: a case of prolonged survival. *Archives of Physical Medicine and Rehabilitation 66(4):*260–1.

Kendall, F.P. McCreary, E.K. & Provance, P.G. (1993). Muscles testing and function. Baltimore: Williams and Wilkins.

MacLean, D., et al. (1989). Maximum expiratory airflow during chest physiotherapy on ventilated patients before and after the application of an abdominal binder. *Intensive Care Medicine 15(6):*396–39.

Mahler, D. A., Therapeutic Strategies in Mahler, D.A. (Ed.) (1990). Dyspnea New York: Futura Publishing, 231– 263.

Maloney, F.P. (1979). Pulmonary function in quadriplegia: effects of a corset. *Archives of Physical Medicine Rehabilitation 60:*261–65.

Martinez, F.J. (1991). Couser, J.I. (1991). Celli BR: Respiratory response to arm elevation in patients with chronic airflow obstruction. *American Review of Respiratory Diseases* 143:476, 1991.

Massery, M.P. (1994). What's positioning got to do with it? *Neurol Report 18(3):*11–14.

Mazza, F.G., DiMarco, A.F., Altose, M.D., & Strohl, K.P. (1984). The flow-volume loop during glossopharyngeal breathing. *Chest 85(5):*638–40.

Mellin, G., Harjula, R. 1987). Lung function in relation to thoracic spinal mobility and kyphosis, *Scandanavian Journal of Rehabilitation Medicine* 1987;19(2):89–92.

Micheli, J. (1985). The use of the modified Boston orthosis sytem for back pain: Clinical indications. *J Ortho Pros* 39:41–46.

Montero, J.C., Feldman, D.J., & Montero, D. (1967). Effects on glossopharyngeal breathing on respiratory function after cervical cord transection. *Archives of Physical Medicine and Rehabilitation 48:*650–53.

Mueller, R.E., Petty, T.L., & filley, G.F. (1970). Ventilation and arterial blood gas changes induced by pursed lips breathing. *Journal of Applied Physiology 28:*784, 1970.

Roa, J., Epstein, S., Preslin, E., Shannon, T. & Celli, kB. (1991). Work of breathing and ventilatory muscle recruitment during pursed lips breathing in patients with chronic airway obstruction. *American Review of Respiratory Disorders 143:* pA 77.

Rood, M.S. (1962). The use of sensory receptors to activate, facilitate and inhibit motor response. In Sattely, G. *Approaches to the Treatment of Patients with Neuromuscular Dysfunction.* 3rd Internal Congress World Confederation of Occupational Therapists.

Saumarez, R.C. (1986). An analysis of possible movements of human upper rib cage. *Journal of Applied Physiology (2):*678–689.

Scheitzer, J.A., (1994). Specific breathing exercises for the patients with quadriplegia. *Physical Therapy Practice* 1994;3(2):109–122.

Shaffer, T.H., Wolfson, M.R., & Bhutani, V.K. Respiratory msucle function, assessment and training. Phys Ther 1981;61:1711–23.

Sharp, J.T., Drutz, W.S., Moisan, T., Foster, J., Machnach, W. (1980). Postural Relief of Dyspnea in Severe Chronic Obstructive Pulmonary Disease. *American Review of Respiratory Disoders* 122:201.

Sivak, E.D., Gipson, W.T., & Hanson, M.R. Long-term management of respiratory failure in amyotrophic lateral sclerosis. *Annals of Neurology* 1982;12:18–23.

Sullivan, P.E., Markos, P.D., & Minor, A.D. (1982). *An integrated approach to therapeutic exercise: Theory and clinical application.* Reston, Va.:Reston Publishing.

Zumwalt, M., Adkins, H.V., Dail, C.W., & Affeldt, J.E. Glossopharyngeal breathing. *Physical Therapy Review* 1956;36(7):455–459.

CHAPTER 23

Exercise Testing and Training: Primary Cardiopulmonary Dysfunction

Susan K. Ludwick

KEY TERMS

Arteriovenous-oxygen difference (a-v_{O_2} difference)
Cardiac output (Q)
Forced expiratory volume in 1 second (FEV_1)

Forced vital capacity (FVC)
Minute ventilation ($\dot{V}E$)
Oxygen consumption ($\dot{V}_{O_2}$)
Stroke volume (SV)
Tidal volume (TV)

INTRODUCTION

Shortness of breath, especially with activity, is very common in patients who have cardiopulmonary diseases. Shortness of breath can be quick in onset or of a chronic nature. One of the results of shortness of breath, especially when it is of a chronic nature, is the vicious cycle of deconditioning it causes in patients. Eventually, these individuals may become deconditioned to the point that activities of daily living usually taken for granted, such as washing up in the morning, may be overwhelmingly fatiguing. Physical therapists need to understand the underlying mechanisms of shortness of breath, evaluate their patients appropriately given their limitations, and then be able to devise therapy programs that would keep these individuals active within the limits of their disease in order for them to maintain certain levels of independence.

LUNG DISEASE

In individuals without lung disease the cardiovascular system normally limits maximal aerobic exercise. Typically, maximal oxygen consumption ($\dot{V}_{O_2}$) may be limited by the heart's inability to increase its cardiac output (Q) either by an inability to increase heart rate (HR) or stroke volume (SV) or by an inability to provide adequate oxygen delivery to exercising skeletal muscle represented by the arteriovenous-oxygen difference (a–vo_2difference). This relationship of Vo_2 to Q is represented by the Fick equation:

$$Vo_2 = Q \times a - vo_2 \text{ difference}$$

However, patients with lung disease may be limited in their exercise capacity for several reasons. They may be limited by altered lung mechanics, impaired gas exchange, development of pulmonary hypertension, or respiratory muscle fatigue. Each of these factors make traditional cardiovascular evaluation of exercise capacity inadequate, since these patients are limited by their breathing and not by their cardiovascular systems.

Altered Lung Mechanics

One of the characteristics of obstructive lung disease is the destruction of elastic tissue in the lung. The destruction of elastic tissue prevents normal recoil of lung tissue on expiration. Therefore it is difficult for patients to empty their lungs. This coupled with the tendency for bronchial walls to collapse contributes to air trapping. This results in lung hyperinflation. With exercise, our bodies require an increase in oxygen uptake to perform more work. Minute ventilation increases in order for oxygen uptake to improve. We know that minute ventilation is the product of tidal volume and respiratory rate (TV × RR = V_E. If respiratory rate increases as a natural response to an increase in exercise, it may not allow enough time for lungs to adequately empty and fill again if elastic tissue is destroyed. Therefore tidal volume cannot adequately increase with increases in exercise intensity. The result is that minute ventilation will not increase in proportion to exercise. If minute ventilation does not increase as required, then oxygen consumption and, therefore, amount of work will be effected.

Patients with restricture lung disease will have stiffer lungs that are resistant to expansion on inspiration. The patient will have to work harder to maintain pressures for adequate lung expansion and ventilation. Eventually all lung volumes and capacities become decreased.

Impaired Gas Exchange

During exercise, there needs to be a balance of ventilation to perfusion (V/Q) in the lungs for adequate blood oxygenation to occur. In patients with airways disease, underventilation of the lungs could occur because of elastic tissue destruction. Underventilation results in V/Q mismatches (low V/Q ratio). Hypoxemia occurs as a result.

Pulmonary Hypertension

In normal individuals, there is typically an increase in the diameter and in the number of blood vessels with exercise. However, in patients with lung disease, there may be a decrease in the number and/or in the distensibility of blood vessels. This results in the increase of pulmonary vascular resistance. An increase in the pulmonary vascular resistance contributes to a decrease in left ventricular filling. If there is a decrease in left ventricular filling, then there will be a decrease in cardiac output, which would limit the ability to do work.

Respiratory Muscle Fatigue

Respiratory muscles in a normal individual consume little oxygen at rest or with moderately increased ventilation during activity. With exercise, oxygen consumption increases greatly. However, a patient with lung disease would have an increase in ventilatory muscle oxygen consumption up to 40% of the total body oxygen consumption. The respiratory muscles may not be able to keep up with the total demand and would start to fatigue (see Chapter 25). Another contributing factor in respiratory muscle fatigue is the musculoskeletal deformity that many of these individuals develop with the disease processes. Muscle fibers need to be at an optimal length to work efficiently for adequate force generation to perform work. However, with musculoskeletal deformity, these fibers may be placed at lengths that make it difficult for efficient work to be done. Eventually, they fatigue because of inadequate force generation needed to support the work of breathing.

Clinically, patients with obstructive lung disease show breathing patterns that are slower and deeper at rest and with exercise. Specifically, longer expiratory cycles are observed because of the extra effort these patients make to empty their lungs before inspiration. Patients with restrictive lung disease have a pattern of rapid, shallow breathing in an effort to maintain adequate minute ventilation in the face of decreased lung capacities.

HEART DISEASE

Patients with acute or chronic cardiac failure or valvular heart disease have elevated pulmonary venous pressures. This develops into interstitial edema. Therefore the lungs are said to be "wet," their compliance is decreased, and the work of breathing is elevated.

Clinically, these patients have pulmonary rales on auscultation. They adopt rapid, shallow breathing patterns to minimize respiratory muscle work. These patients, as with patients with chronic lung disease, will have ventilatory responses to exercise, depending on the severity of the disease.

Assessment

Before starting the actual exercise assessment, it is important to get an idea of the patient's activity level and what activities cause shortness of breath. How far can the patient walk before becoming short of breath? Can the patient tolerate walking outside? Is he or she only able to walk comfortably to get about inside a house or apartment? Can the patient walk up stairs? Does dressing, taking a bath or shower, or combing hair cause shortness of breath? Can the patient do his or her own grocery shopping? Is the patient able to do any heavy housework, such as vacuuming or bed making? Is the patient able to make his or her own meals?

If aerobic capacity is limited because of either cardiac or ventilatory limitations, how can we functionally assess exercise capacity without the use of expensive testing equipment? Traditional methods of measuring maximal oxygen uptake, including treadmill testing, may have limited usefulness because oxygen uptake for the pulmonary patient, as explained before, is limited by ventilation. Anaerobic threshold, which is defined as the highest oxygen consumption during exercise above which a sustained lactic acidosis occurs, is useful in measuring exercise tolerance in normals. However, it is not particularly useful with patients, since peak exercise levels may be below the anaerobic threshold. Some have looked at the measurements of FEV_1 and FVC to predict exercise capacity. However, the literature has shown that there is no correlation between these measurements of lung mechanics and exercise capacity. It makes more sense to define exercise capacity by evaluating the patient's functional exercise capacity. This can be done by using timed walking distances. The 12-minute walk as defined by Kenneth Cooper has been adapted by McGavin, Gupta, and McHardy (1976) for use with patients that have chronic bronchitis. This test is also useful in determining exercise capacity in other patient populations as well. This evaluation is useful because it correlates with VO_2 as measured on the treadmill. However, results are reported in terms of distance walked and not in how much oxygen was consumed. Therefore it gives a more functional picture of exercise tolerance since it uses a familiar activity. If 12 minutes is too long for some patients, 3- and 6-minute walks are just as useful. These walking tests are simple to implement and use simple measurement devices. Patients can also use them as methods to monitor their own progress.

To assess patients using the 12-minute walk, one must simply instruct the patient to walk as far as possible in 12 minutes. It is not absolutely necessary to walk without stopping. The patient may slow down or even stop to take a short rest if needed. The only required equipment is a stopwatch and a measured corridor.

UPPER-EXTREMITY VERSUS LOWER-EXTREMITY ACTIVITY

Up to this point, we have discussed exercise assessments in reference to lower-extremity activity. However, shortness of breath may be of even earlier onset when performing routine activities of daily living involving upper extremities (i.e., grooming, lifting, and carrying). This in fact may be the most frustrating limitation to patients, since these are the types of activities that we normally take for granted in our everyday lives. When patients begin to have difficulty performing these activities, they feel a loss of control in their lives. It is important to note that the exercise responses to these activities are different and should be assessed separately from walking.

Celli, Rassulo, and Make (1986) have reported the appearance of dyssynchronous thoracoabdominal movement when comparing arm activity with leg activity. Early fatigue was observed to occur despite lower heart rates, minute ventilation, and oxygen uptake when compared with leg work. It was hypothesized that exercise limitation during arm activity was probably because of a smaller contribution of accessory muscles to the work of breathing, since these muscles must contribute to postural support of the upper extremity during activity. Despite these limitations in upper-extremity exercise tolerance, improvements have been demonstrated after an exercise training program.

Upper-extremity assessments may be considered two ways. They can be either supported or unsupported (Criner and Celli, 1988). Supported assessments would be those that may involve the use of an upper-extremity ergometer. Unsupported assessments would include those activities involving reaching. Since activities of daily living involve combing hair, washing, dressing, and reaching at various heights, assessments imitating these things would be most useful. One such test that could be used would involve repetitive reaching at a height level to the head. Reaching up with a light object of approximately 1 pound may imitate reaching up to kitchen cupboards to put away groceries. Counting the number of repetitions and timing the activity would give a functional picture of upper-body activity tolerance.

BREATHING

Patients who have pulmonary diseases have limited ventilatory reserves, which manifests as shortness of breath. The degree of the shortness of breath may depend on the severity of the lung disease. Normally, during quiet breathing, average pleural pressures surrounding the large airways are typically negative, whereas intraluminal pressures are more positive. These positive pressures keep the airways open dur-

ing expiration. There are no compressive forces working to narrow the airways. However, in patients with airflow limitation, the work of breathing is shifted to the muscles of expiration. Therefore expiration becomes a more active process, resulting in the generation of more positive pleural pressures compressing the airways. Closing off of airways creates the feeling of shortness of breath. An important yet simple technique that can be taught to patients is the practice of purse-lipped breathing to control shortness of breath. By having the patient expire through pursed lips, a back pressure is created in the airways that helps to keep them from collapsing despite the positive pleural pressures down on them. This is a useful technique that can be used at rest and during exercise to slow down respiratory rate, increase tidal volume, and increase blood oxygenation.

When evaluating exercise tolerance with patients, it is important to assess the work of breathing. Borg (1982) has developed two scales that can help to quantify dyspnea. In our facility, we have used a simple scale of 1 to 4 to describe shortness of breath (see boxes below and on p. 421). On our scale, a score of 1 would represent baseline (comfortable) breathing. A score of 4 would represent shortness of breath so severe that one is not able to talk. Since exercise limitation is more closely related to ventilatory rather than

The 15 Point RPE Scale	
6	
7	VERY, VERY LIGHT
8	
9	VERY LIGHT
10	
11	FAIRLY LIGHT
12	
13	SOMEWHAT HARD
14	
15	HARD
16	
17	VERY HARD
18	
19	VERY, VERY HARD
20	

Borg, G. (1982). Psychological Bases of Perceived Exertion, *Medicine and Science in Sports and Exercise, 14*, 378.

The 10 Point RPE Scale	
0	NOTHING AT ALL
0.5	VERY, VERY WEAK
1	VERY WEAK
2	WEAK
3	MODERATE
4	SOMEWHAT STRONG
5	STRONG
6	
7	VERY STRONG
8	
9	
10	VERY, VERY STRONG
-	MAXIMAL

Borg, G. (1982). Psychological Bases of Perceived Exertion, *Medicine and Science in Sports and Exercise, 14*, 380.

cardiovascular limitation, monitoring heart rate is not an accurate measure of exercise intensity. Asking patients to quantify their dyspnea is much more reliable.

EXERCISE GUIDELINES

After evaluating your patient's exercise capacity, the exercise program can be developed. Structuring the program with the warm-up, training, and cool-down phases should be done.

Before starting exercise, purse-lipped breathing should be taught since this should be used throughout the exercise session to control shortness of breath. Instruction for teaching this technique could be as follows: patients should be instructed to take a relaxed breath in through their noses. The breaths should be relaxed. They should not be forced. Exhalation should be through pursed lips as if to blow out a candle. Again, expiration should not be forced.

Warm-up

The exercise program should always start with warm-up exercises. Chair exercises are desirable, since sitting up to exercise can help conserve energy that the patient will need for the training portion. Mixing upper and lower body exercises should be done. Examples of these exercises include arm scissoring,

reaching over the head, marching while sitting, knee extension, and stretching hamstrings with the leg being stretched propped on another chair in front. Exercises should be timed with purse-lipped breathing to pace the exercise comfortably and control shortness of breath. An example of this would be:

Start with your arms stretched forward at shoulder height. Breathe in through your nose while bringing your outstretched arms out to either side. Blow out through pursed lips while bringing your arms back to the front and crossing them in a scissoring manner. Repeat 10 times.

Adding scapular retraction exercises to stretch out pectorals (i.e., pinching scapulas together) is helpful since these patients spend many of their days in forward flexion types of postures. These exercises help with posture and help to increase lung expansion with inspiration.

Training Phase

After completing the warm-up exercises, patients may now start their walks. The patients should practice their purse-lipped breathing during their walking. Walking for 12 minutes at a comfortable pace to keep breathing at a level 3 should be the goal. Rest periods are acceptable during the 12-minute time. Another goal could be to minimize rest periods to the points where a patient could walk for 12 minutes nonstop.

The upper-body exercise session could consist of low-resistance, high-repetition exercises combined with purse-lipped breathing to help with shortness of breath. These exercises could consist of PNF patterns or of ring shifting, for example, at a level just above the shoulder. Light weights could be added as a progression in addition to adding repetitions.

Cool Down

The cool-down period would consist of repeating the warm-up exercises at a pace where breathing would be brought down to baseline.

Frequency

Patients should exercise at least three to four times per week.

Intensity

Patients should exercise so that their breathing guides how hard they are working. We advocate that patients work no higher than a level 3. After the cool-down period, breathing should be at baseline.

Termination of Exercise Testing or Training

Several signs or symptoms will alert the therapist that the session should be stopped. This chapter focuses on typical clinical situations not using electrocardiographic (ECG) or sophisticated monitoring systems. Consequently patient response must be watched closely, such as facial appearance of discomfort, increased use of accessory muscles; in addition, blood pressure, heart rate, and pulse oximeter readings are very important. Exercise should be terminated in any of the following situations:

- Patient requests
- Chest pain occurs or increases from patient's normal
- Patient appears pale and skin is diaphoretic
- Blood pressure is extremely elevated or drops with exercise
- Patient complains of leg cramping
- Oxygen saturation drops below 90%
- Patient complains of dizziness
- Patient's coordination is affected by increased muscle weakness and fatigue with prolonged exercise

TRADITIONAL EXERCISE TESTING

For those patients without shortness of breath from lung disease or cardiac failure who could tolerate more vigorous exercise, there are more traditional methods of exercise testing that are useful in assessing exercise capacity. The primary modalities used are bicycle ergometry and treadmill testing. There are advantages and disadvantages to both. ECG monitoring and blood pressure readings may be more easily obtained if a patient is tested on a bicycle. However, the disadvantage to this modality is that this is not as familiar an activity to some patients as walking. Therefore maximal heart rates may not be achieved because of leg fatigue. Treadmill testing is more commonly used because walking and running are more natural activities. A patient is more likely to reach his or her maximum oxygen consumption and heart rate. However, ECG recordings tend to have more artifact and blood pressure recordings are more difficult to obtain at high intensities. If treadmill testing is the modality of choice, there are several different testing protocols that use different combinations of grade elevation and belt speed. The type of treadmill test used depends on the fitness level of the patient and the reason for doing the test. For example, certain testing protocols may be used to test initial aerobic fitness levels in asymptomatic individuals and athletes and then for assessing the effects of their training programs. Another type of treadmill test may be used to help diagnose cardiac disease. The two most commonly used protocols are the Bruce and Bakke exercise tests. They have normative data from which functional aerobic impairment can be calculated.

Energy Conservation and Work Simplification

Working with energy conservation and work simplification techniques is an important component of cardiopulmonary training. An analysis of the patient's work practices and suggestions for modification with the goal of achieving increased functionality in everyday life needs to be stressed. A brief description of some of these techniques is provided to help the physical therapist reinforce these practices to patients.

Since most individuals have been accustomed to a faster paced life, pacing is a basic concept worth discussing with patients. Daily activities were probably done quickly. First and foremost, it is important to slow down when walking or climbing stairs. Patients will not be as tired and out of breath when reaching their destinations. Rest periods should be planned during the day. If wasting time is a concern while taking a break, reading a book or doing some handwork may make this time more worthwhile.

Using a cart to carry items is quite helpful. Using upper-extremity activity while carrying items increases oxygen consumption when walking. If oxygen consumption is increased, ventilatory requirements also will be increased as described previously. Shortness of breath will increase. If a shopping cart is used, leaning on the cart to take a rest will help to keep breathing under control.

Sitting down to work is an energy saver because it saves the legs the work of standing. Standing in the bathroom to shave or wash at the sink can be eliminated by placing a chair in front of the sink or by sitting on the toilet-seat lid. Buying a shower chair helps make washing easier. After coming out of the shower or bath, wrapping up in a terry-cloth robe and sitting on the toilet-seat lid can help the patient catch his or her breath while drying off. An ironing board can be used as an adjustable table. Setting it at low levels can help with meal preparation while sitting.

Organizing work areas can help eliminate unnecessary reaching. Items used most often should be kept at a level between the shoulders and the hips. Heavy appliances can be kept out on counter tops or on the stove so that bending, stooping, and lifting is eliminated. Before cooking, filling the sink with soapy water and putting dirty dishes and utensils in immediately makes clean up easier. A dustpan with a long handle eliminates bending over when sweeping up.

Understanding the development of shortness of breath in individuals with cardiopulmonary disease and then evaluating them appropriately for exercise programs will help these patients improve their functional capacity for activity. Exercise testing and training can range from simple, cost-effective in-home testing to sophisticated use of metabolic carts and equipment for evaluating and training athletes. In addition to improvements in functional capacity, these patients may also show some desensitization to their shortness of breath with an overall improvement in their sense of well-being.

REVIEW QUESTIONS

1. Name and explain four limiting factors of exercise in the patient with COPD.
2. Explain traditional measures of exercise capacity. Which ones are useful for measuring exercise capacity in COPD?
3. Explain the physiological benefits of exercise training with COPD and the perceived mechanisms of improvement.
4. Name the components of a pulmonary rehabilitation program.
5. Name and discuss techniques of energy conservation.

References

American College of Sports Medicine. (1993). *Resource manual for guidelines for exercise testing and prescription* (2nd ed.). Philadelphia: Lea & Febiger.

Belman, M.J. (1989). Exercise in chronic obstructive pulmonary disease, in Franklin, B.A., Gordon, S., & Timmis, G.C. (Eds.). *Exercise in modern medicine*. Baltimore: Williams and Wilkins.

Borg, G. (1982). Psychological Bases of Perceived Exertion, *Medicine and science in sports and exercise, 14,* 378.

Casey, L.C., & Weber, K.T. (1986) Chronic lung disease and chest wall deformities. In Weber, K.T., Janicki, J.S. (Eds.). *Cardiopulmonary exercise testing*. Philadelphia: WB Saunders.

Casciari, R.J., Fairshter, R.D., Morrison, J.T. & Wilson, A.F. (1981). Effects of breathing retraining in patients with chronic obstructive pulmonary disease, *Chest, 79,* 393-398.

Celli, B.R., Rassulo, J., & Make, B.J. (1986). Dyssynchronous breathing during arm but not leg exercise in patients with chronic airflow obstruction, *The New England Journal of Medicine, 314,* 1485-1490.

Criner, G.J., & Celli, B.R. (1988). Effect of unsupported arm exercise of ventilatory muscle recruitment in patients with severe chronic airflow obstruction, *American Review of Respiratory Disease, 138,* 856-861.

McGavin, C.R., Gupta, S.P., & McHardy, G.J.R. (1976). Twelve-minute walking test for assessing disability in chronic bronchitis, *British Medical Journal, 1,* 822-823.

Reis, A.L., Ellis, B., & Hawkins, R.W. (1988). Upper extremity exercise training in chronic obstructive pulmonary disease, *Chest, 93,* 688-692.

Tangri, S., & Woolf, C.R. (1973). The breathing pattern in chronic obstructive lung disease during the performance of some common daily activities, *Chest, 63,* 126-127.

Thoman, R.L., Stroker, G.L., & Ross, J.C. (1966). The efficacy of pursed-lips breathing in patients with chronic obstructive pulmonary disease, *American Review of Respiratory Disease, 93,* 100-106.

Weber, K.T., & Szidon, J.P. (1986) Exertional dyspnea. In Weber, K.T., Janicki, J.S. (Eds.): *Cardiopulmonary exercise testing*. Philadelphia: WB Saunders.

CHAPTER 24

Exercise Testing and Training: Secondary Cardiopulmonary Dysfunction

Phyllis G. Krug

KEY TERMS

Exercise blood gases
Nocturnal ventilation
Oxygen desaturation

Respiratory muscle endurance
Respiratory muscle fatigue
Respiratory muscle strength

INTRODUCTION

When considering the sensation of shortness of breath, one typically pictures someone afflicted with a lung disease, such as asthma, bronchitis, emphysema, or the like. A largely neglected area from the perspective of physical therapy and rehabilitation is that population that develops respiratory limitations secondary to other disease processes.

Secondary respiratory problems are those restrictions arising out of pathology other than primary lung disease. Patients falling into this category present with a vast array of underlying pathologies. Virtually every system in the body can develop a disorder that can have respiratory consequences. It is most efficient to discuss the more common disorders that present themselves clinically. Case studies are presented at the end of the chapter to further elucidate and clarify the process clinically.

Psychological Factors

With respect to shortness of breath, studies related to those with the diagnosis of chronic obstructive lung diseases have shown that people tolerate shortness of breath up to 10 years before seeking medical attention (Black, 1982). The patient usually attributes the symptoms to aging and lack of exercise before considering a medical reason. It has even been documented that patients will curtail activities, social and recreational, before seeking medical advice. By the time medical attention is sought, a damaging cycle has been established (Figure 24-1). The results of inactivity contribute to feelings of inadequacy and poor self image. The inactivity itself fosters and encourages atrophy, not only in the extremities where it is visibly apparent but also in the respiratory muscles. This further adds to the debilitating process, creating secondary weakness and disabilities that are not necessary and are avoidable. These issues are further addressed in the approach to treatment and in the case studies.

EVALUATION

The evaluation begins before the patient arrives. It begins with the information collected from the diagnostic data. Great benefits can be gained from understanding the information, but it is equally essential to recognize its limitations.

Critical Usage of Pulmonary Diagnostic Reports

The diagnostic criteria for secondary cardiopulmonary dysfunction is similar to diagnosis criteria for primary cardiopulmonary dysfunction. In the short

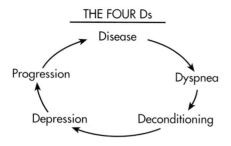

FIGURE 24-1
Flow of progression of respiratory disability. This demonstrates the chronic cyclic pattern that haastens deterioration and death.

review presented here, notes are included to encourage critical analysis of diagnostic material.

Pulmonary function tests

Pulmonary functions tests (PFTs) are used to evaluate flow rates and volume capacities of the lung. Detailed descriptions of these are presented in Chapter 8. Underlying assumptions in these reports are that a patient (1) has cooperated with the testing procedure, (2) has understood the procedure and, (3) has normal respiratory muscle strength to accomplish the test. Let's try and understand the factors that could blur optimal results when taking a pulmonary function test. If a result is produced that shows the patient has poor lung capacity, you could walk away thinking. "Wow, that's a really sick person there, most probably there isn't much I can do to help because he is so restricted in lung capacity." If you look further and investigate the possibilities, you begin to open windows or possibilities for improvement. If there is weakness of the respiratory muscles, then the results obtained reflect the patient's breathing capacity based on weak muscles. This leaves open the option of improving the respiratory muscle strength to see how it may affect the ventilatory capacity. Once you begin to think critically, many windows may become apparent that can provide options for improving the results. For example, if a patient with scoliosis has reduced volume capacity, it is unclear if it is a fixed piece of data or if there is room for improvement from the perspective of posture and strength. The volume and flow measurements of a patient with a lot of secretions would be reduced because of the obstructive nature of the mucus. If that patient was on an aggressive program of postural drainage, would those values improve? Address whether the values obtained in the pulmonary function tests reflect a fixed, irreversible value. The author's clinical experience demonstrates that interventions addressing posture, strength, endurance, and optimal clearance of mucus work to improve values otherwise believed to be unchangeable.

X-ray

The use of x-ray testing is critical in identifying infiltrates, pneumonias, tumors, and obstructions. Yet it too has its limitations and should not be relied on solely to assess a patient's capabilities. Mr. K had a diagnosis of chronic obstructive lung disease with extensive scarring from old tuberculosis. His x-ray was opaque. No viable ventilating lung tissue was seen on the left side. Ausculation with a stethoscope revealed no breath sounds. Yet after months of breathing retraining, thoracolumbar mobilization and soft tissue mobilization, this patient established a most definite improvement in breath sounds on the left side. No improvement was noted in his x-ray. So, our tools are helpful to a point, and we should always give our patient the benefit of the doubt and try.

Auscultation

The stethoscope is effective in identifying many abnormalities within the lung, such as bronchospasm, mucous collection, consolidations, and infiltrates. Yet it is not uncommon to hear perfectly normal breath sounds, and the patient will still report tightness in the chest, wheezing, and even congestion. It is always important to have the patient cough or breathe deeply to increase the flow of air so as to pick up any of these abnormalities. Yet even if this is done and the breath sounds seem normal, always defer to the patient.

Arterial blood gases

Arterial blood gases are designed to measure the level of oxygen, carbon, dioxide, and pH in the arterial blood (see Chapter 9). It reflects how effectively the respiratory system is working in supplying the body with the fuel to carry on the task of living. It is quite common to receive an order for physical therapy including exercise with the information that the blood gases are within normal limits. It is critical to identify if the blood gas values were taken at rest or after exercise. If exercise blood gases are not included in the report, there is no way of knowing how the patient's oxygenation will be affected by activity (desaturation). It is possible to have normal resting blood gases that drop precipitously with activity. This can be a result of limited ventilatory ability or ventilation-perfusion mismatch. It is the responsibility of the therapist of a patient with compromised ventilatory ability to request exercise blood gases or use an oximeter to determine if desaturation is occurring. In discussing exercise blood gases, it should be under-

stood that patients will be more comfortable and probably perform better on equipment that mimic their present life styles. Although the step test that has the patient going up and down a step at a given rate is effective in identifying a change in the blood gases, a patient may feel more comfortable and be able to last longer on either a bicycle or treadmill. Furthermore, during a step test, the patient may fatigue after only a few repetitions. There is more opportunity to evaluate the following: (1) how quickly the gases change, (2) if they improve over time, and (3) the dynamics of breathing mechanics when choosing a modality that the patient may be able to sustain over a longer period of time.

Respiratory muscle strength and endurance

The foundation of the respiratory system's ability to work is the strength and endurance of the respiratory muscles. *Strength and endurance* form the foundation because breathing is an ongoing activity from which the body cannot take a vacation; it requires the endurance to continue without stopping. There are times when the respiratory system requires sudden bursts of increased strength, as is evidenced by the need to cough. Factors predisposing to fatigue are related to muscular ability, ventilatory mechanics, reduction of energy supply by hypoxemia, reduced cardiac output, and malnutrition. The measure of respiratory muscle strength is done via a gauge that measures inspiratory muscle strength and expiratory muscle strength (PI max and PE max). A patient unable to generate 60% to 80% of these values reflects respiratory muscle weakness (Edwards, 1978). A patient who is unable to maintain expected respiratory muscle force with continued or repeated contraction demonstrates the level of respiratory muscle fatigue, which is the precursor of respiratory failure (see box below). A thorough

---

Clinical Signs of Respiratory Muscle Fatigue
Hypoventilation
Rapid shallow breathing
Paradoxical breathing
Increased $Paco_2$

background on a patient includes information on the strength and endurance of the respiratory muscles so that an effective, practical intervention program can be planned. An aggressive exercise program cannot be initiated if a patient is unable to sustain ventilation to properly oxygenate the body. If a patient is in a state of respiratory muscle weakness and is then expected to perform aggressively on a bicycle or treadmill, one can inadvertently push the patient into respiratory fatigue and possibly failure.

History—Critical Listening

In attaining a history from the patient, it is critical to work slowly, so that the patient feels comfortable, and to encourage what could be deemed as simple chatter. After discussing a patient's personal interests, family, and home life you will have the information to recommend an intervention program that will be beneficial for the patient and that the patient will actually do. If it is felt that the patient can improve his or her endurance to be able to walk a mile and the patient is only interested in walking a few blocks, the goals have to be set accordingly. Some therapeutic techniques require a quiet passive posture by the patient. A more tense individual who is pressed for time will not tolerate that kind of intervention. It is therefore crucial to take the time to get the total picture.

From the perspective of the history of respiratory symptomatology, it is common to hear, "I don't know what happened, I was doing just great until I got that cold . . . then it all fell apart." Pursue the investigation, because undoubtedly the history is much longer. The difference is that the patient was able to cope and the presenting situation became excessive. The oxyhemoglobin dissociation curve in Figure 24-2 demonstrates the underlying physiological process (Stoller, 1988). Looking at the S curve, one can see that above 60 mm Hg the curve is fairly flat, and loss or depletion of oxygen above the level can go undetected clinically. However, as the curve demonstrates, there is a critical point around the PaO_2 of 60 where the person will "suddenly" experience severe shortness of breath. In reality the oxygen level was dropping progressively over time but was only critically felt at the drop of the curve. Understanding the progression of the deterioration with shortness of breath can actu-

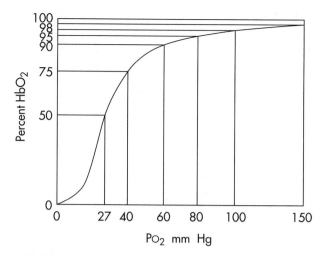

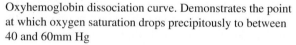

FIGURE 24-2

Oxyhemoglobin dissociation curve. Demonstrates the point at which oxygen saturation drops precipitously to between 40 and 60mm Hg

ally open the perspective of hope for improvement. Because it is not just one system that becomes suddenly ineffective, physical therapists have the latitude to explore the full course of the history and look for the gaps where an intervention can be directed. Has posture changed over time? Has there been progressive weakness? Have activity levels diminished? Were there frequent respiratory infections? Responses to each of these questions can greatly influence factors in a rehabilitation program. If a patient's posture deteriorated over the years, compromising respiratory ability, a program of stretching and strengthening of the postural musculature may provide sufficient space in the thoracic wall for improved lung capacity and oxygenation. It takes a small amount of objective improvement to make a big difference in the quality of life for the individual. Regardless of the underlying cause, attaining a PaO_2 of at least 60 mm Hg is the primary concern.

Because the work of breathing becomes very difficult in primary lung diseases or restrictions secondary to other disease processes, the symptomatic presentations can be quite similar. It very closely simulates the posture of the marathon runner at the end of a run. The runner assumes a bent forward posture, leaning on a wall or gaining support by leaning on the knees (Figure 24-3). This position is optimal for

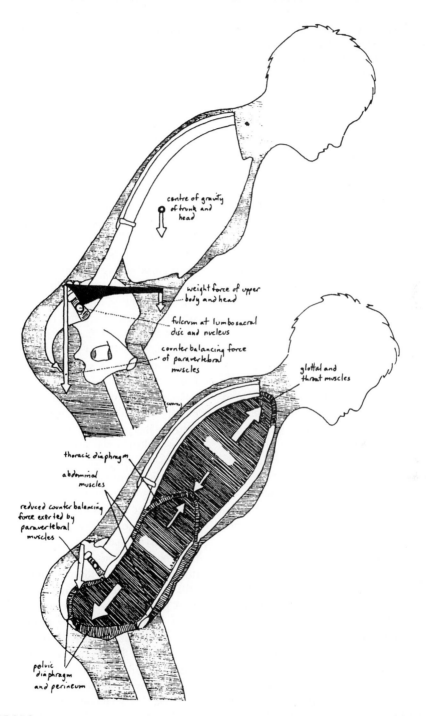

FIGURE 24-3

The flexed forward posture held when experiencing shortness of breath. Similarities between the healthy marathon runner and the person with chronic respiratory difficulty should be considered in reference to muscular, skeletal and pressure changes. (Courtesy of David Gorman, *The Body Moveable*)

enhancing diaphragmatic excursion. After a few moments, the runner will get up and walk away. Unfortunately, the patient experiencing shortness of breath stays in that bent forward position. A patient may stay that way because it is easier to breath or because he or she does not realize the precipitating event has passed. The point of emphasis is that any chronic disease resulting in shortness of breath will have postural effects. Look for limitation in range of motion of the hips and poor mobility of the thorax and the pelvis. This can be evident in a gait pattern that has minimal rotation of the thorax on the pelvis. The stride length will be shortened, with minimal arm swing and an overall stiff, nonfluid gait pattern. The gait pattern of those suffering with chronic shortness of breath and its associated postural changes can be described as walking cinder blocks, implying that the muscles from the neck to the pelvis are fixed and do not allow for normal reciprocal movement.

Exercise Testing

Exercise testing is performed for a variety of reasons. It is a means of (1) gaining baseline information of the patient's activity level, (2) assessing functional ability, (3) prescribing graded-exercise programs, and (4) evaluating cardiovascular ability. The choice of exercise testing should reflect the needs of the patient, the cost-effectiveness of the procedure, and the consideration for the need of extensive diagnostic information and its practical application into the patient's life. The patient's addressed in this chapter are by and large severely limited in their physical abilities because of their underlying disease processes and their secondary respiratory effects. Typically the overall presentation is one of atrophy, deconditioning, and poor mobility that greatly limits the distance walked. The severely limited patient would benefit with a simplified exercise test to identify exercise capacity. When considering the patient with secondary cardiopulmonary restriction, treatment should be aimed at improving the cardiopulmonary status concurrent to the underlying primary process. A few examples can better illustrate this point. The scoliosis patient who has progression of the spinal deformity and secondary pulmonary compromise requires a baseline exercise test to identify exercise capability. It would be premature to begin an exercise training program. The first step would be to address improvement of strength and posture. The goal is directed toward improvement in height, lung capacity, and muscle strength. The baseline data on the exercise test would likely improve. An exercise test subsequent to postural improvement would be a better baseline for an endurance training program.

For the patient with underlying neuromuscular disease, an endurance training program may overfatigue muscle groups and cause damage. Therefore the exercise test, again, is to get a baseline of exercise ability. The therapeutic intervention would be directed toward muscle re-education, postural exercises, and strengthening to help the patient move more efficiently and reduce stress on the affected musculature. The improvement in posture and strength provides a better baseline to sustain an exercise test and subsequent training.

A timed-walk test for a patient with severe limitation would be appropriate. Measure a walkway in 10-foot increments and then time the distance walked for either 6 or 12 minutes. It may be necessary to further modify this test into distance walked for 2 minutes. Instruct the patient to walk as far as possible as fast as possible for the timed segment. Record distance walked. Monitor the blood pressure, heart rate, respiratory rate, ventilatory muscle use, and O_2 saturation.

A patient at a higher level of function may benefit from a more aggressive exercise test that allows for a more accurate level of cardiovascular response to exercise as a baseline for prescription for endurance training. A baseline level is first obtained from the timed-walk test or the patient can walk on the treadmill at 1 to 2 mph, 0% grade for 6 minutes.

A patient whose exercise ability is limited by respiratory factors before the heart rate or blood pressure is even elevated does not require a full-graded exercise test with full ECG, metabolic gas analysis, heart rate, and blood pressure measures. Interest should be more directed toward the following: (1) how far can this person walk, (2) what happens to his breathing pattern and respiratory rate, and (3) does the oxygen saturation drop. Based on this, recommendations can be made for use of supplemental oxygen and possibly more efficient breathing patterns to allow the patient to persevere longer. For example, if a patient has a diffusion problem or a ventilation/perfusion mismatch, it would be helpful to evaluate whether a slower pace would allow the patient to walk longer. Consider enhancing the time allowed for diffusion of the oxygen. It may be found that a slower pace, with attention directed toward deep effective breathing, may yield different values in oxygen saturation and the distance walked. The choice of testing modality should also take place or location into consideration. It seems inappropriate to demand that a severely limited patient being seen in the home undergo extensive graded-exercise testing before recommending an exercise program. The choice of exercise testing should reflect the goals of the patient. If the patient is ready for an aggressive exercise program, then more extensive testing is appropriate. Testing can then progress to stage II. A treadmill *stess test* begins with a speed that is comfortable for the patient—usually between 2 to 3 mph. Work is increased every 3 minutes by either increasing the speed or the incline. It is recommended to increase the speed by 0.5 mph increments, maintain it at a comfortable walking pace, and progress the incline by 2.5% increments after a comfortable pace has been established. *Measurement* of heart rate and blood pressure should be taken at the end of each 3-minute stage and SaO_2 oxygen saturation should be monitored throughout and recorded at the beginning and end of each stage.

The *test is terminated* in the following situations: (1) when the patient reaches 65% to 75% of predicted maximal heart rate, (2) if oxygen saturation drops below 90%, (3) if the blood pressure drops with increasing activity, or (4) the patient experiences symptoms of shortness of breath or muscular discomfort.

If a patient is able to reach 65% of predicted maximum heart rate without cardiopulmonary symptoms, then the patient is capable of exercise conditioning. Oxygen saturation should be above 90%. Below this level requires supplemental oxygen. If the carbon dioxide (CO_2) increases more that 10 torr of resting level, the patient will be limited in exercise potential. Individuals who reach their maximum volume ventilation (MVV) with minimum intensity exercise may have difficulty with an endurance training program.

Exercise Training

Design of an exercise prescription must be individualized and must be prescribed within both useful and achievable levels.

Exercise training should not be limited to a mode of exercise equipment, duration of time, or frequency. A person with a chronic condition has chronic manifestations physically and psychologically. Therapy directed toward the chronic physical changes, that is, postural and overall movement, can result in improved endurance. This perspective should be seriously considered before using precious therapeutic time to put a patient on a treadmill three times per week to measure a heart rate that does not elevate because the patient is too short of breath. The severely limited patient may benefit from general body movement for a duration of 10 to 15 minutes. It could include standing and leaning on a chair and shifting the hips to the rhythm of music. The goal is initially just to move, create a challenge to the cardiorespiratory system, focus on controlled breathing, and show the patient that he or she can sustain movement for prolonged periods. The therapeutic ball has proven to be beneficial. The 65-cm ball is a good size for a patient to sit on (Figure 24-4). It provides support yet allows for movement. Many severely limited patients have been able to sit on a ball shifting their weight from side to side, working on leg strengthening, pelvic and spinal mobility, and challenging the cardiorespiratory system. Once a capable patient becomes interested in a traditional endurance training program, the graded-exercise test can provide the necessary information to prescribe one. The prescription should include intensity, duration, frequency, and modality as follows: (1) *Intensity* is based on 65% to 80% of the predicted heart rate or a level where the patient becomes symptomatic or the oxygen saturation drops to 90%. Consider, for example, an exercise test that is terminated after walking at a speed of 3 mph, at a 5% elevation, 3 minutes into that level. If the limiting factor was shortness of breath with a drop in oxygenation, further testing should be conducted with the use of supplemental oxygen. If the limiting factor was shortness of breath without a drop in oxygen, 2.5 mph at 0% elevation can be used as a 5-minute warm-up, followed by training at 3 mph for up to 15 minutes with 1 minute intervals at 2.5% elevation followed by a cool down of 2.5 mph, 0% elevation, for 5 minutes. (2) *Duration* of exercise is 15 to 30 minutes per session. Initially this can be broken down into interval training where short 1- to 2-minute rest periods can be used progressively, lengthening the intervals until the patient is able to maintain a continuous session. (3) *Frequency* of exercise is three to five times a week on alternate days. (4) *Modality* depends on patient comfort. The target heart rate, or the level before the patient developed symptoms, is used as the training level. Flexibility exercises or slow walking are recommended for warm-up before the endurance exercise program.

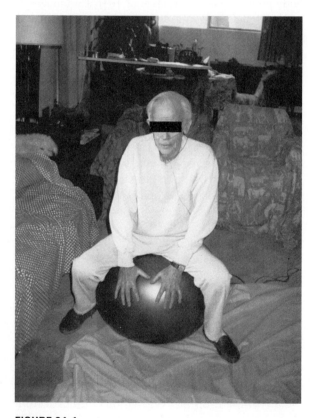

FIGURE 24-4
Therapeutic ball as part of a program of improving mobility and endurance.

Caution is advised in understanding the underlying pathology that resulted in cardiopulmonary limitations. Post polio syndrome is characterized by muscles that were weakened during the initial onset of the disease and more recently report a recurrence of symptoms. Studies have shown that these patients benefit from strengthening and endurance exercise, but extreme caution must be directed toward avoiding overuse (Dean, 1991a; Owen, 1985). The patient will benefit from a carefully considered, judicious exercise program.

SYSTEMATIC APPROACH IN THE REHABILITATION PROCESS
Nocturnal Ventilation—The Role of Rest and the Respiratory Muscles

At this point the therapist is equipped with a vast array of information. The question is how to plan an effective intervention. Clinical experience has shown the importance of first directing attention toward the work of breathing. The literature is filled with discussions about the role of resting the respiratory muscles (Braun, 1983). It is suggested that one of the factors leading to respiratory failure is the respiratory muscles' inability to keep up with the demand of breathing. If we consider the patient with severe scoliosis, the work of breathing is not shared equally by the respiratory muscles because of distortion of the chest wall. In addition, the curvature will add an additional load on the energy expenditure of breathing. Like any muscle in the muscular system, if a load is put on a muscle, it will train and get stronger. Yet, if this goes on for an extended period of time the muscle will be unable to maintain the added work load and the muscle fibers themselves will begin to break down. This process is well understood in the fields of sports medicine and weight training. It is called overuse atrophy. This process also occurs in the respiratory system. In advising a patient in an exercise program, it is critical to be aware of how much we are asking our patients to do. We walk a narrow path between (1) doing nothing and allowing the patient to accept life with the shortness of breath and promote further atrophy and (2) pushing too hard and risking breakdown of the respiratory system. It is the responsibility of the therapist to be aware of the diagnostic and clinical signs of respiratory muscle fatigue.

Diagnostic criteria for respiratory muscle fatigue include the following: (1) increasing pulmonary arterial carbon dioxide ($Paco_2$), (2) reduction of high-frequency signals (greater than 80 Hz) of muscular activity on electromyography studies (EMG) despite continued contraction and dominance of the low-frequency signals (less than 80 Hz), (3) reduction of vital capacity, with decreases in supine VC to 50% of sitting VC, and (4) inspiratory muscle pressure to below 66% of predicted mean.

The clinical signs of respiratory muscle fatigue include the following: (1) paradoxical breathing, (2) increased respiratory rate, and (3) shallow breathing (see box below). First and foremost, we are looking at change from normal. This is where good baseline information is critical. Baseline blood gases, the patient's typical breathing patterns, and the baseline for dyspnea should be considered. This is a critical area

for good clinical judgement. Sometimes the patient has a bad day and just does not do well, other times he or she may be in trouble.

Managing the patient with clinical signs of respiratory fatigue

If the patient has a prescription for oxygen, make sure he or she is using it. Get the patient comfortable and use your hands to guide the body into shifting the work of breathing. This is a very critical factor. In dealing with acute shortness of breath or muscle fatigue the patient undoubtedly will be in a state of panic. Panic complicates the situation by increasing the respiratory rate and consequently reducing tidal volume. The gentle placement of the therapist's hands on the lower rib cage along with a calm, firm, soothing voice can help guide the patient into a more calm, efficient breathing pattern. Studies have shown that tension alone can reduce the expiratory flow rate, so the therapist's role in calming the patient is directly related to improving the breathing pattern (Kotses, 1981).

Resting the respiratory muscles

There is increasing interest in the role of resting the respiratory muscles before it reaches the stage of respiratory fatigue and failure. This is accomplished through nocturnal ventilation using positive- or negative-pressure ventilators (Figures 24-5 and 24-6). The focus is to increase muscle energy supplies and stores. Mechanical ventilation will assume the work of the respiratory muscles and allow them to rest. This may allow the time needed to reverse the factors that led to fatigue. It substantially reduces the oxygen consumption of the respiratory muscles, allowing for more oxygen to reach the other tissues. Studies have shown that after a mean period of approximately 5 months at home on daily 4- to 10-hour ventilatory support, there are significant increases in vital capacity, PI max, and PE max (Marino, 1982). It also showed a reduction in $Paco_2$ along with a reduction in hospitalizations and the number of days hospitalized. The topic of resting the respiratory system adds a different perspective in regard to traditional pulmonary rehabilitation programs promoted. Before

---

Respiratory Muscle Function Assessment
• Pulmonary function test
Effort and strength dependent
• Respiratory muscle strength
PI max—inspiratory pressure
PE max—expiratory pressure
• Respiratory muscle fatigue
60% to 80% PI max
• Respiratory muscle endurance
Maximum volume ventilation
Maximum sustainable ventilation
80% MVV for 5 minutes or 60% MVV for 15 minutes
Fatigue: when Ve (minute ventilation)

NOTE: Inability to reach a predicted value reflects muscle weakness or fatigue.

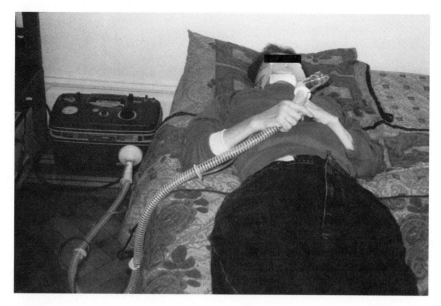

FIGURE 24-5
Positive pressure ventilator used for nocturnal ventilation.

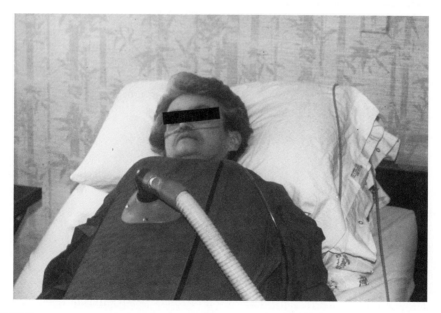

FIGURE 24-6
Negative pressure ventilator used for nocturnal ventilation.

initiating a progressive exercise program or for that matter, any sort of exercise program, it is important to assess the level of respiratory fatigue under which the patient is living. Symptoms, clinical observations, or historical findings that are suggestive of further investigation into the benefit of nocturnal ventilation include sleep disorder, progressive dyspnea, hypercapnia, and dyscoordinate breathing patterns. It has been recommended that a patient be allowed sufficient time to adjust to nocturnal ventilation before advancing into an active exercise program. This decision must be made with medical guidance. It is sometimes recommended that a patient rest on this system for a few months to allow the body to reach a stable level of metabolic rest.

BREATHING TRAINING
Paced Breathing

These techniques are taught regardless of which muscles patient uses to breathe. Because breathing is something we do all day long, it is unfair to expect patients to alter their breathing continuously. Therefore it is helpful to break down breathing into various components. Foremost is coordinating breathing with activity. If a patient is short of breath, he or she needs to know how to get it back. Pursed-lip breathing is an effective means of helping. Pursed-lip breathing works as the center for controlling the respiratory rate and maintains more efficient emptying of the lung. Paced breathing and the rule of thumb are handy tools that help get through daily activities. Breathing has a rhythm of inhale and exhale. Generally, the exhale is longer than the inhale. At rest and with various relaxation techniques, it is possible to greatly extend the length of the exhale. For example, if at rest the person inhales for a count of two, the exhalation might be for a count of four or five. With deeper relaxation the length of the exhalation can be extended to the count of five, six, or even longer. Patients are encouraged to develop and heighten this sense of awareness and begin to coordinate it with activity. The concern is that frequently a person will perform an activity (i.e., bending down to get a shoe, reaching to open a door, washing hair, or lifting a package) and during the activity actually stop breathing or

breath hold. Activities can be divided into two categories. Static activities and rhythmic activities. Static activities are those that are done once. For instance, picking up a shoe. It is done once, until you are ready for the second shoe. The first rule of thumb is to take a breath in before the activity to supply the body with the oxygen it needs, then exhale with the activity. It is simple but it actually helps, and the patient is able to perform an activity with less shortness of breath. The second rule of thumb is to maintain a rhythm with activity. If the activity is washing dishes, vacuuming the carpet, or climbing some stairs, the focus is to maintain a rhythm. That rhythm will change as the activity continues, but the idea is to control it through the purse-lip breathing. For example, climbing stairs may begin with ease and become more difficult with each step. Breathe in on step one and exhale for step two, three, and four. As the activity continues, modify according to the patient's need. It may progress to breathing in on one step and doing the full exhalation on the second step. The patient may still experience shortness of breath but will have better control and get further.

Signs of Improvement

The direction toward improved posture and more efficient quality of movement is a slower process and should be directed in the realm of kinesthetic awareness. If you are working with a patient and find that in a certain posture you observed a better breathing pattern or that with a certain relaxation technique the patient found relief, you want to harness that sensation. Repeat it, use tactile input, have the patient close his or her eyes and imagine it. If the patient has just learned to relax the upper thorax and get a good expansion in the lower thorax, he or she will not be able to walk out of that session and breathe that way continuously. How is this new skill incorporated into a new pattern of breathing? It is effective to stop 20 to 30 times per day, (1) pause, (2) relax the shoulders, (3) focus on the area to expand, (4) do the breathing technique for a few repetitions, and (5) concentrate on it and put it away. The focus of this exercise is not strength training but rather kinesthetic awareness. About 2 weeks of this compulsive stopping, sensing, and being aware is enough time that it becomes the way the patient breathes, becoming incorporated into the patient's pattern of breathing. This obviously will not be successful with someone who mechanically, muscularly, or neurally is incapable of this particular activity. Kinesthetic training can be expanded using the tools of imagery. Too often a patient is taught how to breathe and does so beautifully in the therapy session and then resumes the old pattern after leaving the office. It is a difficult task to incorporate a movement performed in a static stationary position and maintain it during the dynamics of daily life. The power of suggestion and imagery can be used here. This scenario becomes a home exercise program of gaining control of the breathing system. Even if the patient cannot maintain it through the whole process, it is a crucial activity in self-control and minimizes the sense of panic that goes along with activities that result in shortness of breath. It is a very beneficial activity that can then be further advanced while working on a bicycle or treadmill. The underlying emphasis is optimizing the patient's efficiency of movement and breathing and reducing the work of breathing.

OVERVIEW OF THERAPEUTIC OPTIONS

A myriad of therapeutic techniques exist that are viable options in trying to maximize breathing opportunities. It is beyond the scope of this chapter to elaborate on the technique, rationale, and method of all the options appropriate for the population. Once asked by a colleague the appropriate treatments for respiratory patients, I replied, "the same as with any disease process." Evaluate the total situation and plan an intervention that will reduce stress and increase opportunity. If the patient population has developed respiratory problems secondary to an underlying disease, posture, muscle length, muscle strength, and endurance should be considered. The manual therapies are excellent vehicles in gaining access to improvement.

Mobilization: Thorax, Rib Cage, Pelvis, Sacrum, Hip, Shoulders, and Neck

Joint mobilization is a nonthrust manipulation. Pressures may vary from gentle to vigorous but are imparted slowly, as opposed to thrust or high-velocity manipulation. The intent is to regain normal active range of motion, thus improving alignment and stress distribution. The improvement in joint function increases a joint's adaptive potential to mechanical stress and reduces the possibility of re-injury to that joint.

Soft Tissue Therapies

The purpose of soft tissue therapy is to normalize activity of the muscle fibers, restore extensibility, and reduce pain. Soft tissue mobilization includes massage, accupressure, and soft tissue stretching. It uses low-intensity pressure and should not cause pain. If applied properly, its techniques should result in local and general relaxation, and reduction in tone. Myofacial release is a method to normalize myofacial activity, regain tissue extensibility, and reduce pain. It is based on neuroreflexive responses that reduce tissue tension. With the appropriate application of manual contact and the determination of the best point of entry into the musculoskeletal system, a relaxation of tissue tension and decrease in myofascial tightness can be attained.

Neuromuscular Therapy

Proprioceptive neuromuscular facilitation is a method of promoting the response of the neuromuscular mechanisms through stimulation of proprioceptors. The application of a manual stimulus is used to elicit efficient neuromuscular responses. Its primary objective is to develop trunk or proximal stability and control, as well as to coordinate mobility patterns. It can be used to help stabilize vertebral motion and improve spinal movement control.

Muscle energy works under the principle that muscular activity can be used to restore physiological joint motion. It uses active muscle contraction at varying intensities from a precisely controlled position in a specific direction against a distinct counterforce. It is used to mobilize joint restrictions, strengthen weak musculature, stretch tight myofascia, reduce muscle tonus, and improve local circulation.

Positional Release Therapies

Strain/counterstrain is the passive placement of the body in a position of greatest comfort to reduce pain. Relief, if achieved by the reduction and arrest of continuing inappropriate proprioceptive activity, maintains the motion dysfunction. The underlying basis is that every neuromuscular disorder has a palpable point of tenderness and a position that can be obtained for comfort. It is a gentle, nontraumatic type of manipulation that is especially effective when irregular neuromuscular activities have maintained and perpetuated abnormal mechanical stress to tissue. A return to normal length is achieved through positional release of abnormal neuroreflexive activities.

Craniosacral Therapies

Craniosacral therapy is a gentle hands-on method for evaluating and treating problems affecting the craniosacral system. The craniosacral system provides the environment in which your brain and spinal cord develop and function. The palpable parts of the craniosacral system are the bones of the skull, sacrum, and coccyx, which attach to the membranes that enclose the cerebrospinal fluid. Treatment involves the usage of fascial and soft tissue release techniques to detect subtle biological movements. A 10-step protocol is used for evaluating and treating the entire body.

Review

In evaluating the disease process that results in respiratory compromise, it is crucial to recognize the long-term chronic effects on the total body. It is short sighted to limit the focus to the thorax if there is a respiratory problem. Take a step back and look at the total picture and look for those windows of improvement. Some specific techniques have consistently been helpful in helping ease the work of breathing. Both myofacial release techniques and craniosacral therapies focus on the cranium and the sacrum. The mobility of the sacrum and motion of the cranial bones have been shown clinically to be directly related to the ease of breathing. The performance of traction on the sacrum, a gentle hold, provides a release on the thorax. The key is patience. Do not rush

through a treatment. Get comfortable hand contact and feel the tissue soften in your hand, then wait. Watch what happens to the breathing. Hone in on any changes and help the patient become aware of any changes in the pattern of breathing. The diaphragm and thoracic release are also remarkably effective in encouraging greater thoracic expansion. These techniques alone can be effective in relieving wheezing, improving aeration and even mobilizing secretions.

Take the time to explore options. In reference to the cranial bones, restrictions in the movement of the temporal bones has been identified in those suffering with shortness of breath, regardless of diagnosis. The temporal wobble therapy, ear pull, and finger in ear (craniosacral technique) have also been effective in easing the work of breathing. The focus of the therapeutic intervention must be to find some relief from the work of breathing first and then begin a plan of enhancement of relief followed by strengthening of those new found movements. Endurance activities, that is, treadmills, bicycling or walking, are wonderful adjuncts after these important elements have been addressed.

CASE STUDIES
Poliomyelitis with Secondary Severe Kyphoscoliosis

Mr. L is a 65-year-old male with history of poliomyelitis onset at the age of 8 years old. He was left with a total paralysis of his left arm and a severe scoliosis secondary to muscle strength imbalance in the trunk. (Figure 24-7). After recovery from the poliomyelitis, his medical history was unremarkable. He lived independently in a fourth-floor walk-up apartment and worked as a postal clerk until he was admitted in respiratory failure. At that time his oxygen saturation was 80%, his arterial carbon dioxide (Pa_{CO_2}) was 61, and his arterial oxygen level (Pa_{O_2}) was 53. His vital capacity was 1.8 liters—40% of predicted—and his ECG showed right ventricular strain secondary to pulmonary hypertension. Additionally the myocardium was situated in his right cavity secondary to pressure gradients that shifted it from its normal position. His medical management required a tracheostomy and respiratory support with a ventilator and oxygen. He stabilized and was sent for an interim

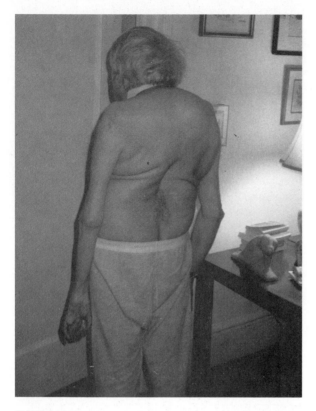

FIGURE 24-7
Patient with history of poliomyelitis and subsequent development of severe scoliosis secondary to muscle imbalances.

of rehabilitation. At that facility he was accidentally extubated and the tracheal area was badly traumatized. The tracheal trauma left the patient comatose for 4 days.

About 2 weeks before the patient's respiratory failure, he was at a dinner with friends, and one of the group videotaped the evening. The tape had invaluable information in it. Firstly, in terms of posture, Mr. L's head was totally sunk into the thoracic cavity leaving him functionally without a neck. Around the dinner table his friends were joking and remarking at how little he was eating. It is even more noteworthy that he even dozed during conversation at the table. The labored breathing, the excessive use of the upper respiratory muscles, the sleepiness, loss of appetite, and lack of energy to eat his meal were all signs of pending respiratory fatigue and failure.

The physical therapy program was problem-oriented and was modified throughout as the patient's needs changed.

Problem 1: Shortness of breath at rest and with activity

Mr. L was instructed in breathing techniques, including paced breathing, pursed-lip breathing, and relaxation exercises to help relax the upper respiratory muscles and encourage deeper, more efficient expansion of the thorax.

Problem 2: Paradoxical breathing pattern

Because of the severity of the curve, the thorax moved in a rotation pattern to the right with the inhale and to the left with the exhale. It was unclear how much of this pattern was due to structural factors or secondary weakness that allowed such severe distortions. A path of exploration was initiated to find potential areas of movement and to further evaluate if there was potential to master those movements. Subtle movements were evoked in the cervical area and initiated a treatment plan of soft tissue mobilization, craniosacral therapy, and strengthening exercises. The window found was that cervical traction allowed Mr. L to increase his head range of motion and he was able to better relax his sternum and allow for breathing from lower down. The terminology of *lower down* is used because it is mechanically impossible for Mr. L to fully use his diaphragm. He was able to recruit other muscle groups, in addition to diaphragmatic, to allow for sufficient thoracic expansion relieving the excessive work of his upper-respiratory muscles.

Aside from the primary paralysis of the left arm, the musculature of the left trunk was also weak and kinesthetically deprived. The term *kinesthetically deprived* refers to the convex part of the curve that was essentially folded inward in total paradoxical motion. Mr. L was totally unaware of that part of his body and had no sense of movement. On soft issue mobilization and tactile input on the left side, the patient began immediately to expand on the left side of the thorax. Because of the severity of the curve, it would be impossible to have normal expansion on the left, but it was unclear if enough force and negative pressure could be generated on the left to enable the patient to (1) shift the myocardium back into the left thoracic cavity, (2) increase his vital capacity enough to reduce his need for oxygen and possibly prevent future respiratory complications. Mr. L began a home program using Theraband, which he looped around his left shoulder and held across his chest with his right hand (Figure 24-8). This position allowed him to grade resistance to scapular adduction, elevation, and depression. He also used weights in trunk exercises. Therapy sessions focused on manual techniques to mobilize the rib cage, stretch the muscles, and release the connective tissue. The technique of the diaphragm and thoracic release were remarkably effective in opening the breathing. This method alone was frequently effective

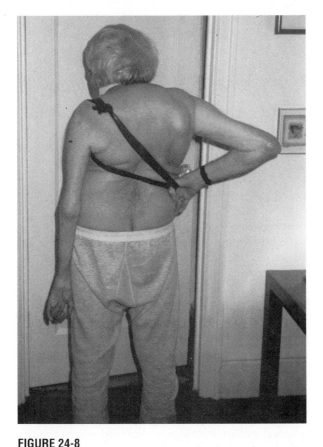

FIGURE 24-8
Creative use of theraband in strengthening of the thoracic musculature.

with the patient reporting "Oh, I am getting more air!" This was easily confirmed; improved aeration was audible with the stethoscope.

Problem 3: Poor endurance

Mr. L had become so deconditioned and anxious at the thought of movement that he was unable to walk even 20 feet. Outdoor ambulation created severe anxiety for which he was receiving psychological therapy. He began a gradual program with walking in place at 2-minute intervals. It is important to note that he was extremely motivated and not only followed his exercise program, but expanded on it (Figure 24-9). He also used the P-Flex respiratory muscle trainer attached to his tracheotomy tube beginning on level 1 for 15-minute intervals, twice a day.

After 1 year on the program, Mr. L grew in height 1 1/4 inches and increased his vital capacity by 700 ml, he no longer required supplementary oxygen, and his myocardium shifted into the left thoracic cavity without any signs of right ventricular strain. His ejection fraction was 45%. He still demonstrated paradoxical motion with respiration, but there was a significant reduction in the amount of sucking in of the lower rib cage on the left with inhalation. Auscultation was remarkable with excellent breath sounds on the left and right and some reduced air movement near the lingula. Mr. L progressed up to walking in place for 25 minutes with 2-pound weights in both hands (he is able to clasp a weight with his paralyzed hand) and attached to both ankles. He gained enough motion in his neck to allow for full range of motion.

Because the pull of gravity will continually work on Mr. L to pull him back into dysfunctional patterns, it is important to keep Mr. L on a program. He is seen once every 2 months to modify and update his exercises and work on his trunk to ensure optimal thoracic capability. Over this extended time other windows have been found working on his sacrum and pelvis. Manual traction, mobilization techniques, and soft tissue releases in these areas all provide for improved thoracic expansion. Hand placement on the sacrum allows for a slow release and relaxation of the upper chest. Manual techniques then followed, encouraging progressively increasing diaphragmatic excursion. Mr. L is able to cue in to changes in his body and work on

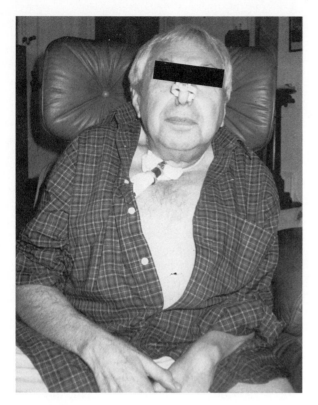

FIGURE 24-9
Respiratory muscle training in patient with tracheotomy.

gaining sensory awareness of the area and aim toward mastery and control of the movement.

Summary of problems

Mr. L benefitted from a program that focused on improving his total potential. He had the benefit of night ventilation so that his body was rested. His total endurance capability was based on finding those windows of improvement. The improvement in alignment and strengthening of the trunk and respiratory muscles provided for maximizing his respiratory capabilities, overall endurance, and quality of life. At this point Mr. L is totally independent. He walks 3 miles per day and goes out with his wife and friends. He has even traveled abroad with a foreign medical supply company providing for his ventilatory needs.

Dystonia With Spasmodic Breathing

Ms. B is a 36-year-old psychologist with the diagnosis of dystonia. She has a 10-year history of torticollis that has been treated with Botox. It is a treatment aimed at paralyzing selective muscle fibers to allow for relief of severe spasms. She presented with recent onset of shortness of breath and inability to get air. On palpation over the lower rib cage and diaphragm, it became evident that there was discoordinate movement of the thoracic musculature. It was unclear whether this was merely discoordinate movement or a function of the dystonia. The technique of diaphragmatic release as demonstrated in craniosacral therapy provided immediate release of the symptom of shortness of breath and reduced the amount of discoordinate movement of the chest wall. Ms. B was taught how to perform the technique on herself and was successful in the exercise. The P-Flex was used to give added resistance to her breathing as a means of extrasensory awareness. It gave her an added awareness of movement of the thoracic wall and a means of controlling it. The final phase of her therapy was mild aerobic activity with the focus of coordinating breathing with movement and increasing overall endurance. She was on a program for 6 months and was followed once per week. Although her symptoms persist sporadically, she is able to catch it in time and gain control of her breathing. According to medical opinion, it is likely that she has the rare progression of respiratory muscle dystonia. It is unclear at this time how this situation will progress, but in the meantime, she has the means of controlling discoordinate movement and breathing with ease.

Postpolio Syndrome

Dr. D is a dentist teaching in a dental school and conducting research in a laboratory. He has a history of poliomyelitis with a possible diagnosis of postpolio syndrome (PPS). Diagnosis is difficult because PPS is characterized by progressive weakness and pain in the musculature that survived the original poliovirus. The underlying mechanism is still unclear; it is suggested that the progression is resultant to long-term overuse and deterioration of surviving muscle fibers. Studies show that the direction of therapy is to unload or rest the overused muscles and shift the work of the musculature. It is difficult in the therapeutic setting to identify the weakness that may be from PPS or weakness from simple aging and inactivity. Great caution is needed in this situation because studies have shown that if the PPS muscles are overworked, it can result in permanent irreversible damage. Dr. D presented with the complaint of cervical pain. On evaluation, it became evident that the pain was related to the cervical lordosis, resulting from the underlying muscle loss aggravated by the stooped posture necessary for his long hours of work in the laboratory. Dr. D primarily relied on his upper respiratory muscles for breathing because of diaphragmatic paralysis and extensive intercostal muscle loss. Dr. D did not have much time available for home exercise or for physical therapy sessions. Exercise prescriptions that would isolate the weak muscles and then focus on repetitive exercises to strengthen them would be problematic because of the threat of tissue damage to muscles affected by PPS. Dr. D was given one exercise to perform twice per day, rolling, to roll from one end of the room to the other and back. He was guided in maintaining control of the trunk musculature throughout the activity. This activity was performed semiregularly for a year with the goal of improving trunk strength and posture. Over the course of the year, endurance exercises were added using a home stationary bicycle. In 1 year, Dr. D grew 1 1/4 inches. He continued to rely on the upper respiratory muscles for breathing, but his overall improved strength and posture left him pain free.

SUMMARY

A multitude of therapeutic options exist for those suffering with respiratory limitations. The presentation of symptomatology of dyspnea is similar in primary lung disease and in secondary cardiopulmonary symptoms. It is crucial to understand the underlying pathology so that the therapeutic intervention and exercise prescription reflect the potential of the patient. Focusing on issues of respiratory muscle fatigue is a primary foundation of rehabilitation potential. Improvement in breathing capacity and overall endurance can be accomplished through techniques to improve posture overall. Endurance training based on graded-exercise tests is an important element in the rehabilitation program but should be placed in perspective to other therapeutic options.

REVIEW QUESTIONS

1. What laboratory data are needed to determine if a patient is a candidate for endurance training?
2. What types of treatment can be beneficial, if a patient is not a candidate for endurance training?
3. What types of interventions can best help a patient enter into a more aggressive exercise program?
4. Is aerobic training limited to treadmill and bicycle? Think about the limitations of these modalities and suggest alternatives.

References

Astrand, P. & Rodahl, K. (1977). *Physical Training. Textbook of work physiology.* New York: McGraw Hill.

Austin, J. (1992). Enhanced respiratory muscular function in normal adults after lessons in proprioceptive musculoskeletal education without exercise. *Chest, 102,* 486–490.

Basmajian, J. (1993). *Rational manual therapies.* Baltimore: Williams & Wilkins.

Black, L. (1982). Early diagnosis of chronic obstructive pulmonary disease. *Mayo Clinic Proceeds 57,* 765–772.

Braun, N. (1983). When should respiratory muscles be exercised? *Chest, 84,*76.

Dean, E. (1991a). Clinical decision making in the management of the late sequelae of poliomyelitis. *Physical Therapy, 71:* 757–761.

Dean, E. (1991b). Effect of modified aerobic training on movement energetics in polio survivor. *Orthopedics, 14,*1243–1246.

Edwards, R. (1978). Physiological analysis of skeletal muscle weakness and fatigue. *Clinical Science and Molecular Medicine, 54,*463.

Feldman, R. (1985). The use of strengthening exercises in postpolio sequelae: methods and results. *Orthopedics, 81,*889–891.

Gorman, D. *The body moveable.* Guelph, Ontario, Canada:Ampersand Printing Co.

Kotses, H. (1981). "Application of biofeedback to the treatment of asthma: a critical review. *Biofeedback and Self Regulation, b,*573–593.

Lisboa, C. (1985). Inspiratory muscle function in patients with severe kyphoscoliosis. *American Review of Respiratory Disease, 132,*48–51.

Marino, W. (1982). Reversal of clinical sequelae of respiratory muscle fatigue by intermittent mechanical ventilation. *American Review of Respiratory Disease, 125,* 85.

Owen, R. (1985). Polio residuals clinic: conditioning exercise program. *Orthopedics, 8,* 882–883.

Shneerson, J. (1978). The Cardio respiratory response to exercise in thoracic scoliosis. *Thorax, 33,* 457–463.

Stoller, J. (1988). *Oxygen therapy techniques—Current respiratory care.* Toronto: BC Della.

Upledger, J. (1992). *Craniosacral therapy.* Washington: Eastland Press.

Weiss, H. (1991). The effect of an exercise program on vital capacity and rib mobility in patients with idiopathic scoliosis. *Spine, 16,* 88–93.

CHAPTER 25

Respiratory Muscle Weakness and Training

Maureen Shekleton
Jean K. Berry
Margaret K. Covey

KEY TERMS Inspiratory muscle training Respiratory muscle fatigue
Muscle endurance Respiratory muscle weakness
Muscle strength Work of breathing

INTRODUCTION

Roussos and Macklem (1982) support the notion of a two-part respiratory system made up of the lungs, which are the gas exchanging organs, and a pump, which ventilates the lungs. The pump is composed of the chest wall, the respiratory muscles, and the nerves and centers in the nervous system that control the respiratory muscles. The respiratory muscles are expected to function continuously throughout life to provide the appropriate level of ventilation for meeting the body's metabolic needs.

Citing the analogy of the heart as the circulatory pump and the consequences of heart failure, Macklem (1982) maintains that the respiratory pump can fail, leading to a condition characterized by hypoventilation and hypercapnia that may ultimately progress to ventilatory failure and death. Causes of respiratory pump failure can be grouped into the following two major categories: (1) those in which the respiratory drive is decreased or the sensitivity and function of the respiratory center is altered (i.e., those that affect the central nervous system control), and (2) those in which the ventilatory response is decreased through impairment of the mechanics of respiration (i.e., those that affect the chest wall or musculature) (Groer and Shekleton, 1989).

The focus of this chapter is on the latter category, and more specifically, on the role of weakness and fatigue of the respiratory muscles as a pathophysiological mechanism seen in many clinical conditions. The view of respiratory muscle fatigue as a cause of ventilatory failure is an idea becoming more widely accepted among pulmonary clinicians (Sharp, 1984). Respiratory muscle fatigue is postulated to be the final common pathway to respiratory failure in all conditions in which the respiratory musculature is affected (Cohen, Zagelbaum, Gross, Roussos, and Macklem, 1982; Grassino, Gross, Macklem, Roussos, and Zagelbaum, (1979); Derenne, Macklem, and Roussos, 1978; Roussos and Macklem, 1982).

Although both the inspiratory and expiratory respiratory muscles are susceptible to fatigue, clinically, concern centers on the inspiratory muscles. The diaphragm is of particular interest. Under normal conditions, the inspiratory muscles including the diaphragm, the external intercostals in the parasternal region, and the scalene muscles are responsible for the active process of breathing, and expiration is a passive process. An analysis of the phenomenon of inspiratory muscle fatigue is presented initially in this chapter. This is followed by a discussion of the identification and management of inspiratory muscle fatigue and its possible prevention through training of the inspiratory muscles.

THE CONCEPT OF INSPIRATORY MUSCLE FATIGUE

It is important to differentiate between muscle weakness and muscle fatigue, although both may lead to hypoventilation (Bryant, Edwards, Faulkner, Hughes, and Roussos, 1979). Muscle weakness refers to a loss in the capacity of a rested muscle to generate force that is chronic situation. Muscle fatigue refers to a loss in the capacity of a muscle under load to develop force or velocity that is reversible by rest (NHLBI Workshop Summary, 1990). Fatigue is an acute loss of contractile force wherein, despite constancy of stimulation, force declines from the initial value. If fatigue is the inability of a muscle to continue to generate a required force, then in the respiratory system, fatigue will be manifested by the inability of the inspiratory muscles to continue to generate the force required to maintain the necessary level of alveolar ventilation to meet the body's metabolic needs. Inspiratory muscle fatigue occurs when inspiratory effort exceeds the capacity of the inspiratory muscles to sustain that effort (Rochester, 1982).

Physiologically, fatigue has been characterized as one of the following three types, depending on its list of origin: central fatigue, transmission fatigue, or contractile fatigue. Central fatigue is due to a decrease in neural drive, which reduces the number of firing frequency of motor units. The resulting force generated by voluntary effort is less than that which can be achieved by electrical stimulation of the motor nerves. If electrical stimulation can restore contractile force or if stimulation and force decline in parallel, central fatigue is present. Transmission fatigue results from an impairment in the transmission of impulses along the nerves or across the neuromuscular junctions. Contractile fatigue results from impairment in the contractile response to neural impulses within an overloaded muscle. Both transmission fatigue and contractile fatigue are classified as peripheral fatigue. Peripheral fatigue is present if force is decreased but electrical stimulation is constant. All three types of fatigue are reversible (Mador, 1991).

Peripheral fatigue can be further categorized according to the selective loss of contractile force that occurs at varying stimulation frequencies. High-frequency fatigue is a selective loss of contractile force at high-stimulation frequencies; low-frequency fatigue is the selective loss of force at low-stimulation frequencies. High-frequency fatigue is thought to be the result of impaired neuromuscular transmission and/or propagation of the muscle action potential. This type of fatigue is seen in myasthenia gravis, during ischemic exercise, with muscle cooling, and with partial curarization. It is reversible in minutes. The mechanism underlying low-frequency fatigue is thought to be impaired excitation-contraction coupling. Recovery from this type of fatigue may take hours to days and possibly longer. Intense dynamic and static muscular activity can lead to low-frequency fatigue (Edwards, 1983; Moxham, 1990).

Mechanisms and Etiology of Fatigue

The major mechanisms thought to be responsible for inspiratory muscle fatigue include an imbalance between energy supply and demand and impaired excitation-activation. Edwards (1983) has proposed a model that accounts for the interaction of both mechanisms in the development of muscle fatigue. He has also proposed the idea that fatigue serves a protective function in that serious irreparable damage may be

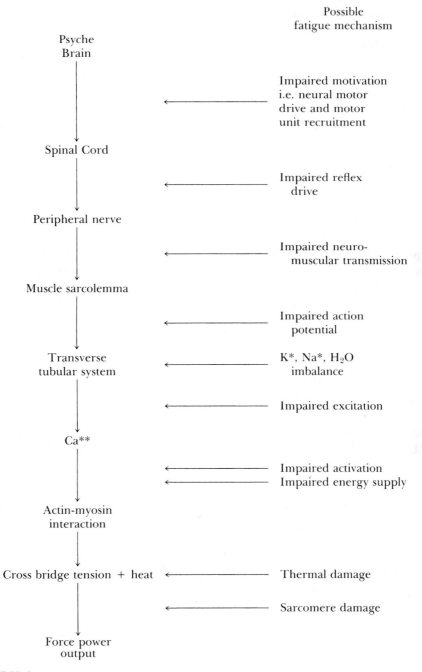

FIGURE 25-1

Chain of command for muscular contraction and the possible mechanisms underlying fatigue. (From Edwards, R.A.T. (1983). Biochemical basis of fatigue in exercise performance: Catasptrophe theory of muscular fatigue. In Knuttgen, H., Vogel, J., Poortmans, J. (Eds.). *Biochemistry of exercise.* Champaign, Ill. Human Kinetics Publishers.).

prevented if the muscle is unable to continue performing beyond a critical point. The central nervous system may exert a protective mechanism to avoid these adverse effects. This idea has persisted and the term *central wisdom* is used to describe the phenomenon (Moxham, 1990) (Figure 25-1, p. 445).

The energy demands of the inspiratory muscles are determined by the work of breathing, the strength and endurance of the respiratory muscles, and the efficiency of the muscles. The work of breathing is the total amount of effort required to expand and contract the lungs. It is determined by the degree of compliance of the lung tissue and the chest wall, the resistance of the airways, the presence of active expiration (normally a passive process), and use of the accessory muscles of respiration. The work of breathing is increased by decreased pulmonary compliance, increased airway resistance, active expiration, and use of the accessory muscles.

Strength and endurance are the fundamental properties of muscle. Strength is defined as the maximal force that a muscle can develop with maximal stimulation. Contractile force is governed by the force-length (length-tension), force-velocity, and force-frequency relationships. Contractile force diminishes in conditions characterized by increased lung volume (hyperinflation), since the muscles are stretched beyond the optimal length to generate maximal force. This stretching of the muscle fibers produces a less desirable length-tension relationship and causes a loss of the zone of apposition, with resulting decrease in strength generation. Strength is also determined by the number and size of individual fibers in a muscle. Strength is adversely affected in conditions in which the size of the fibers is reduced (atrophy) or the number of fibers is reduced (e.g., in malnutrition).

Endurance is defined as the ability to maintain a contraction against a given load and is determined by muscle fiber type, blood supply, and the force and duration of the contraction. Normally, the inspiratory muscles are fatigue resistant. Approximately 75% of the muscle fibers in the adult diaphragm are of the high oxidative, fatigue resistant type (type I and type IIA). In contrast the diaphragm of the neonate contains a relative paucity of type I fibers that have the greatest endurance capacity, and this pattern of fiber distribution is most pronounced in the premature infant. This condition exists in infants for up to a year after birth.

The energy supply to the muscles depends on an intact oxygen transport system, adequate oxygen-carrying capacity of the blood, blood flow, substrate stores and availability, and the efficiency of oxygen uptake and utilization by the muscles. The energy supply to the inspiratory muscles is compromised when cardiac output is reduced, the hemoglobin content of the blood is low, blood flow to the muscles is decreased, or energy substrates are lacking.

Excitation-activation depends on intact, functioning, neuromuscular pathways. Impaired excitation-activation is probably the primary mechanism underlying respiratory muscle weakness and fatigue in the patient with a neuromuscular disorder (Edwards, 1979). Disruption of excitation-activation can occur at any point along this pathway, which Edwards (1983) refers to as a chain of command for muscular contraction. Presented in Figure 25-1 is a list of the possible mechanisms that may lead to fatigue by disrupting the neuromuscular pathway. Impaired excitation of the muscle membrane is probably interrelated with energy metabolism. For example, if the ATP supply to the $Na^+ - K^+$ pump is compromised, an alteration in the Na^+ and K^+ concentrations in the transverse tubular system may result in impaired excitation-contraction coupling.

Although it is difficult to demonstrate the precise mechanisms causing respiratory muscle fatigue in patients, support is found for the concept that central nervous system output is modified to avoid overt fatigue. With extremely high loads imposed on respiratory muscles, patients adopt a rapid shallow pattern of breathing that reduces the work of breathing and can be sustained. Eventually, this pattern of rapid shallow breathing will lead to hypercapnia and acidosis (Moxham, 1990).

In summary, those patients who are at risk for the development of inspiratory muscle fatigue are those in whom energy demands are increased, energy supplies are compromised, or whose neuromuscular chain of command has been disrupted at some point. Patients at highest risk for the development of inspiratory muscle fatigue are those in whom the work of breathing is increased, thus increasing the demands for energy, and those who are experiencing hypoxemia, acidosis, low cardiac output, or any other condition in which the blood supply to the muscle is diminished, thus reducing oxygen supply. Patients whose nutritional status is poor or who are experiencing a catabolic state, such as stress or fever, will have reduced energy stores and may experience muscle fatigue during times of high need.

Assessment of Fatigue

The clinician will most often have to rely on physical signs exhibited by the patient to recognize inspiratory muscle fatigue. Other laboratory methods that would yield more objective evidence of inspiratory muscle fatigue include power spectral analysis of the electromyelogram (EMG), measurement of the maximal relaxation rate, and examination of twitch occlusion pressure.

The following signs are indicative of inspiratory muscle fatigue and are listed in their characteristic order of appearance:

1. Tachypnea
2. Decreased tidal volume
3. Increased P_{CO_2} (which is a late sign)
4. Bradypnea and decreased minute ventilation

Formerly, development of a discoordinated respiratory pattern characterized by inward abdominal movement on inspiration (a sign referred to as *abdominal paradox*) and alternating abdominal and thoracic respiratory patterns (a sign referred to as *respiratory alternans*) were thought to result from respiratory muscle fatigue. Presently, these changes in breathing patterns are thought to result from increases in respiratory load rather than muscle fatigue (Mador, 1991; Tobin, Perez, Guenther, Lodato, and Dantzker, 1987). However, discoordinated respiratory patterns are important clinical signs of respiratory distress and, although they are not specific in their etiology, they are sensitive indicators of important declining respiratory function.

In animals in whom inspiratory muscle fatigue has been experimentally induced the fall in respiratory rate and minute ventilation immediately precedes respiratory arrest and death. This sequence of events has been observed after an initial change in the EMG

power spectrum, which is indicative of muscle fatigue in normal subjects exercised to fatigue, in patients experiencing difficulty being weaned from mechanical ventilation, and in animals in whom fatigue was experimentally induced. When fatigue is present, the ratio of high-to-low frequency power, which can be detected by EMG, shifts as low-frequency power increases and high-frequency power decreases. The difficulty in obtaining an EMG at the bedside and in analyzing the results makes its use in most clinical situations unrealistic at this time.

In summary, rapid shallow breathing is the initial sign of inspiratory muscle fatigue (Yang and Tobin, 1991). The physical signs previously described are reliable and can be used in a clinical situation to determine whether the patient is experiencing inspiratory muscle fatigue.

Treatment of Fatigue

The goals of treating inspiratory fatigue are as follows: (1) restore the balance between energy supply and demand, (2) improve diaphragmatic contractility, and (3) increase the strength and endurance of the inspiratory muscles. The last goal is obviously a more long-term preventive approach, whereas the first two goals apply in the more acute situation when inspiratory muscle fatigue is present.

Energy demands in the patient experiencing fatigue can be decreased by reducing the work of breathing through activities intended to promote compliance, decrease resistance in the lung, chest wall and airways, and promote normal lung volumes and pressures. Energy supplies can be enhanced by ensuring maximal oxygen transport to the tissues and the availability of adequate amounts of oxygen and other energy substrates. Oxygen transport is enhanced by promoting adequate cardiac output, blood flow to the tissues, and oxygen-carrying capacity of the blood. Various forms of respiratory therapy are available to supplement oxygen supplies. Losses of organic and inorganic energy in substrates must be replenished and adequate levels maintained. Nutritional supplementation and administration of electrolytes and inorganic phosphate may be necessary to augment energy supplies. Rest therapy with mechanical ventilation may be required to allow the fatigued muscle to recover and to bring energy supplies and demand into balance.

Much current research is being done in the area of pharmacological interventions to improve diaphragmatic contractility. Aminophylline was initially thought to increase the contractile force of the diaphragm at any given level of activation, but further research indicates that this drug increases muscle energy consumption and potentiates fatigue (Janssens, Reid, Jiang, and Decramer, 1988). Other drugs with inotropic properties are the beta-agonists. Clinical investigation of the potential usefulness and application of these pharmacological agents in inspiratory muscle fatigue is ongoing.

The last goal, that of increasing the strength and endurance of the inspiratory muscles, can be accom-

plished by training the inspiratory muscles in much the same way that athletes train and condition their muscles. Inspiratory muscle training may represent a useful clinical approach to prevent the development of inspiratory muscle fatigue in those patients who are at risk.

INSPIRATORY MUSCLE TRAINING

Inspiratory muscle training (IMT) is currently used in pulmonary rehabilitation to increase the strength and endurance of the inspiratory muscles. Patients with chronic obstructive lung disease experience functional weakness of the respiratory muscles, which can contribute to dyspnea and functional impairment. Theoretically, IMT should reduce dyspnea by improving respiratory muscle function and exercise tol-

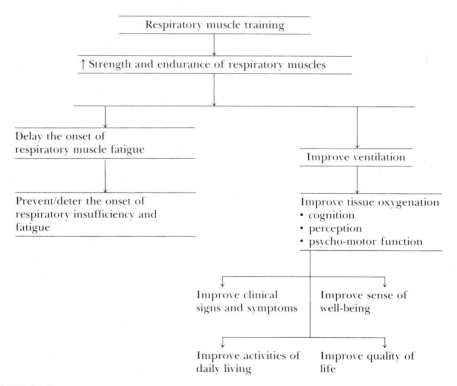

FIGURE 25-2

Conceptual framework for respiratory muscle training. (From Kim M: Respiratory muscle training: Implications for patient care. *Heart and Lung. 13(4)*:333-40).

erance. These effects have yet to be demonstrated in large, controlled studies (Smith, Cook, Guyatt, Madhavan, and Oxman, 1992).

General principles of skeletal muscle training that must be considered when designing and evaluating an IMT program for respiratory patients include overload, specificity, and reversibility. To train a muscle to improve its functional ability, the muscle must be subjected to a stress greater than its usual load (overload), the training must be directed at developing specific functional attributes (e.g., strength or endurance) of the muscle (specificity), and the training must be maintained or function will revert back to pretraining levels (reversibility) (Kim, 1984; Sharp, 1985).

The effects of strength training on the respiratory muscles may include an increase in the size (hypertrophy) and number of the muscle fibers by an increase in protein synthesis by the muscle fibers and a decrease in degradation. Endurance training of the inspiratory muscles is thought to promote an increase in the proportion of fatigue-resistant fibers in the diaphragm, an increase in the metabolic capability of the muscle, and a reduction in the susceptibility of muscle fibers to the deleterious effects of exercise (Leith and Bradley, 1976). Newer evidence suggests an improvement in neuromuscular coordination and efficiency resulting from training (McComas, 1994). Strength training to increase the size and number of myofibrils requires a high load and a slow rate of repetition. Endurance training to increase the metabolic capability of the muscle requires exercise of a sufficient load, speed, and duration, such that cellular concentrations of energy producing substrates drop to minimal levels (Kim, 1984). Endurance training of skeletal muscle has been found to be most effective when brief periods of fatiguing exercise are alternated with periods of rest (Aldrich, 1985) and this concept may be applied to inspiratory muscle training regimes.

Improvement in the strength and endurance of the inspiratory muscles through training has the twofold effect of enhancing the resistance to inspiratory muscle fatigue and improving ventilatory function. The work of breathing is reduced and respiratory reserves are increased. Because the clinical signs and symptoms are diminished, the ultimate outcome for the patient is an improved quality of life. Kim (1984) has

developed a model that outlines the relationship between the effects of a respiratory muscle training and potential patient outcomes (Figure 25-2).

Inspiratory muscle training has been used to successfully increase muscle strength and endurance in healthy volunteers and in patients with chronic air flow limitation (Belman and Mittman, 1980; Larson, Kim, Sharp, and Larson, 1988), cystic fibrosis (Keens, Krastens, et al, 1977). Early Duchenne muscular dystrophy (Wanke et al, 1994), and in those who are quadriplegic (Gross, et al, 1980).

Theoretically IMT in patients experiencing acute respiratory failure should promote improved function of the muscles, and fatigue resistance should facilitate the process of weaning these patients from mechanical ventilation. In conditions requiring full ventilatory support, the respiratory muscles may contract at minimal levels for a period of time, possibly leading to the development of disuse atrophy. As their strength and endurance decrease, the inspiratory muscles will be more prone to fatigue because of the interaction of disuse, the underlying pathophysiological state, and catabolic effects of stress. The ultimate effect of these interacting processes will be difficulty in weaning the patient from the ventilator. An EMG pattern of fatigue has been documented in the ventilatory muscles of neonates who experienced difficulty in weaning (Muller, Gulston, and Gade, 1979). Grassino et al. (1979) found an EMG fatigue pattern in a patient being weaned from mechanical ventilation. Cohen et al. (1982) found an EMG pattern of fatigue in 7 of 12 patients who experienced difficulty during discontinuation of mechanical ventilation. Resolution of the fatigue pattern was observed in those neonates who recovered and in adult patients who were successfully weaned (Andersen, Kann, Rasmussen, Howardy, Mitchell, 1978). There is some evidence that respiratory muscle training may prove to be an important adjunct therapy to facilitate weaning in the patient who requires mechanical ventilation of acute respiratory failure (Aldrich and Karpel, 1985; Aldrich et al, 1989; Shekleton, 1991). However, controlled studies have not been conducted in this patient population.

Two techniques have been used for inspiratory muscle training: isocapnic hyperventilation (also called *isocapnic hyperpnea*) and inspiratory resistive or resistance breathing. Isocapnic hyperventilation is dynamic and is used to increase the endurance of the inspiratory muscles. Expiratory muscles will benefit as well with this technique. Patients are asked to breathe at the highest rate they can manage for 15 to 30 minutes. A rebreathing circuit or the addition of CO_2 to the inspired air must be used with this technique to prevent hypocapnia (Belman, 1981; Belman, and Mittman, 1980). Because of this requirement, the usefulness or this technique will be limited until portable, inexpensive, easy-to-use equipment for home use is developed.

Inspiratory resistive breathing allows both strength and endurance training, since it incorporates both isometric and isotonic exercises. There are two devices available for this purpose, a nonlinear device and a threshold IMT device (Figure 25-3). The nonlinear device has been noted to produce unreliable training loads if the rate of inspiratory flow is not controlled (Guyatt, Keller, Singer, Halcrow, and Newhouse, 1992). With a controlled rate of breathing, patients inspire through a narrow tube that offers a nonlinear airway resistance for one to three daily periods of 15 to 30 minutes. The size of the orifice through which the patient inspires is adjusted to provide a level of resistance that the patient can tolerate without becoming immediately exhausted. In addition, this device is not well suited for stronger patients, since they have difficulty achieving a satisfactory tidal volume with the extremely small orifice at higher loads. With the threshold device, a reliable inspiratory pressure load is provided regardless of airflow rate. The load is adjusted by a nurse therapist, or patient according to a desired percentage of the patient's maximal inspiratory pressure (PI_{max}). Usually, the patient begins training at a low load, equal to about one third of the PI_{max} and progresses slowly in small increments adjusting a screw to alter the tension until the training load reaches 60% of the current PI_{max}. The threshold device delivers a reliable tension because the poppet valve at the end of the device will not open and allow inspiration unless the patient generates the designated negative pressure. Both types of devices are hand held and portable and are easily used and maintained by patients.

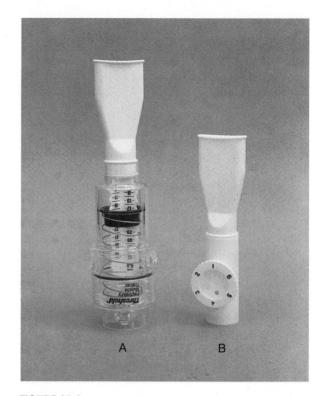

FIGURE 25-3
Handheld resistive breathing training devices. **A,** Threshold; resistance level is altered by tightening screw to increase tension on the spring. **B,** P-Flex; resistance level is altered by changing settings on dial.

Potential outcomes of a training program geared toward increasing inspiratory muscle strength and endurance might include any of the following, depending on the individual patient's conditions and goals of treatment: (1) prevention of acute deterioration of respiratory status and ventilatory failure, (2) improvement of ventilatory function and decrease in the work of breathing, which may lead to an increase in general exercise tolerance and an improved quality of life as tissue oxygenation improves and signs and symptoms are attenuated (Pardy, Pardy, Rivington, Despas, and Macklem, 1981a; 1981b), (3) extension of time before onset of respiratory muscle fatigue, and (4) facilitation of the weaning process in acute respiratory failure patients who are being mechanically ventilated.

SUMMARY

Inspiratory muscle training and conditioning is a newer area of research and treatment for the respiratory patient. As such, further validation of its efficacy and targeting of specific patient populations at greatest risk for loss of inspiratory muscle strength will define its use in pulmonary rehabilitation programs. At this time, inspiratory muscle training looks promising as a means of offering the respiratory patient one possible method of control over disease processes that are most often very debilitating and unrelenting in their course.

REVIEW QUESTIONS

1. What are three types of respiratory muscle fatigue?
2. Name two major mechanisms thought to be responsible for inspiratory muscle fatigue.
3. What factors determine the work of breathing?
4. What is the initial physical sign of inspiratory muscle fatigue?
5. What rehabilitation techniques should be used to increase the strength and endurance of the inspiratory muscles?

References

Aldrich, T. (1985). The application of muscle endurance training techniques to the respiratory muscles in COPD. *Lung, 163,* 15–22.

Aldrich, T. (1984). Inspiratory muscle resistive training in respiratory failure. *Chest, 86*(2), 302.

Aldrich, T.K., Karpel, J.P., Uhrlass, R.M., Sparapani, M.A., Erami, D., Ferranti, R. (1989). Weaning from mechanical ventilation: Adjunctive use of inspiratory muscle resistive training.

Andersen, J., Kann, T., Rasmussen, J.P. , Howardy, P. & Mitchell, J. (1978). Respiratory thoracoabdominal coordination and muscle fatigue in acute respiratory failure. *American Review of Respiratory Diseases, 117* (2), 89.

Belman, M. (1981). Respiratory failure treated by ventilatory muscle training: A report of two cases. *European Journal of Respiratory Diseases, 62,* 391–395.

Bryant, S., Edwards, R., Faulkner, J., Hughes, R.L., & Roussos, C. et al. (1986). Respiratory muscle failure: Fatigue or weakness. *Chest, 89,* (1), 116–124.

Cohen, C., Zagelbaum, G., Gross, D., et al. (1982). Clinical manifestations of inspiratory muscle fatigue. *American Journal of Medicine, 72,* 308–316.

Derenne, J., Macklem, P., Roussos, C. (1978). The respiratory muscles: Mechanics, control, and pathophysiology, Part III. *American Review of Respiratory Diseases, 118,* 581–601.

Edwards, RAT. (1979). The diaphragm as a muscle: Mechanisms underlying fatigue. *American Review of Respiratory Îiseases, 119,* (2 pt 2), 81–84.

Edwards, RAT. (1983). *Biochemistry of Exercise.* Champaign, IL, Human Kinetics Publishers.

Grassino, A., Gross, D., Macklem, P., Roussos, C., & Zagelbaum, C. (1979). Inspiratory muscle fatigue as a factor limiting exercise. *Bulletin European de Physiopathogie Respiratoire, 15,* 105–111.

Groer, M., & Shekleton, M. (1989). *Basic pathophysiology: A holistic approach.* (ed. 3). St. Louis, Mosby.

Gross, D., et al. (1980). The effect of training on strength and endurance of the diaphragm in quadriplegia. *American Journal of Medicine, 68,* 27–35.

Guyatt, G., Keller, J., Singer, J., Halcrow, S., Newhouse, M. (1992). Controlled trial of respiratory muscle training in chronic airflow limitation. *Thorax, 47,* 598–602.

Janssens, Reid Jiang, & Decramer. (1988).

Jardim, J., et al. (1982). Inspiratory muscle conditioning training in chronic obstructive pulmonary disease (COPD) patients. *American Review of Respiratory Diseases, 125,* (pt 2 of 2), 132.

Keens, T., et al. (1977). Ventilatory muscle endurance training in normal subjects and patients with cystic fibrosis. *American Review of Respiratory Diseases, 116,* 853–860.

Kim, M.J. (1984). Respiratory muscle training: Implications for patient care. *Heart and Lung, 13,* (4), 333–340.

Larson, M., Kim, M.J. (1984). Respiratory muscle training with the incentive spirometer resistive breathing device. *Heart and Lung, 13,* (4), 341–345.

Leith, D., Bradley, M. (1976). Ventilatory muscle strength and endurance training. *Journal of Applied Physiology, 41,* 508–516.

Macklem, P. & Roussos, C. (1977). Respiratory muscle fatigue: A cause of respiratory failure? *Clin Sci Mol Med, 53,* 419–422.

Macklem, P.T. (1982). The diaphragm in health and disease. *Journal of Laboratory and Clinical Medicine, 99,* 601–610.

Mador, J.J. (1991). Respiratory muscle fatigue and breathing pattern. *Chest, 100,* 430–435.

Martin, L. (1984). Respiratory muscle function: A clinical study. *Heart and Lung, 13,* 346–348.

McComas, A. (1994). Human neuromuscular adaptations that accompany changes in activity. *Medicine and Science in Sports and Exercise, 26,* 1498–1509.

Muller, N., Gulston, G., Cade, O., et al. (1979). Diaphragmatic muscle fatigue in the newborn. *Journal of Applied Physiology, 46,* 688–695.

Moxham, J. (1990). Respiratory muscle fatigue: mechanisms, evaluation and therapy. *British Journal of Anaesthesia, 65,* 43–53.

National Heart Lung Blood Institute Workshop Summary (1990). Respiratory muscle fatigue: report of the respiratory muscle fatigue workshop group. *American Review of Respiratory Disease, 142,* 474–480.

Pardy, R.L., Rivington, R.N., Despas, P.J., & Macklem, P.T. (1981a). The effects of inspiratory muscle training on exercise performance in chronic airflow limitation. *American Review of Respiratory Diseases, 123,* 26–433.

Pardy, R.L., Rivington, R.N., Despas, P.J., & Macklem, P.T. (1981b). Inspiratory muscle training compared with physiotherapy in patients with chronic airflow limitation. *American Review of Respiratory Diseases, 123,* 421–425.

Rochester, D. (1982). *Fatigue of the diaphragm. Update: Pulmonary diseases and disorders,* New York, McGraw Hill.

Rochester, D., & Braun, N. (1978). The respiratory muscles. *Basics RD, 6,* 20–25.

Roussos, C., & Macklem, P. (1982). The respiratory muscles. *New England Journal of Medicine, 307,* 786–797.

Roussos, C., Fixley, M., Gross, D., et al. (1979). Fatigue of inspiratory muscles and their synergic behavior. *Journal of Applied Physiology, 46,* 897–904.

Sharp, J. (1984). Respiratory muscles. *Current pulmonology,* (Vol. 5), New York, John Wiley & Sons.

Sharp, J. (1985). Therapeutic considerations in respiratory muscle function. *Chest, 88,* 118S–123S.

Shekleton, M.E. (1991). Respiratory muscle conditioning and the work of breathing: A critical balance in the weaning patient. *AACN Clinical Issues in Critical Care Nursing 2 (3):* 405–414.

Smith, K., Cook, D., Guyatt, G., Madhavan, J., & Oxman, A. (1992). Respiratory muscle training in chronic airflow limitation: a meta-analysis. *Amreican Review of Respiratory Disease, 145,* 533–539.

Sonne, L., & Davis, J. (1982). Increased exercise performance in patients with severe COPD following inspiratory resistive training. *Chest, 81,* 436–439.

Tobin, M.K., Perez, W., Guenther, S.M., Lodato, R.F., & Dantzker, D.T. (1987). Does rib cage abdominal paradox signify respiratory muscle fatigue? *Journal of applied Physiology, 63,* 851–860.

Wanke, T., Toifl, K., Mcrkle, M., Formanek, D., Lahrman, H., & Zwick, H. (1994). Inspiratory muscle training in patients with Duchenne muscular dystrophy. *Chest, 105,* 475–482.

Yang, K.L. & Tobin, M., J. (1991). A prospective study of indexes predicting the outcome of trials of weaning from mechanical ventilation. *New England Journal of Medicine, 324,* 1445–1450.

Bibliography

Black, L., & Hyatt, R. (1969). Maximal respiratory pressures: Normal values and relationship to age and sex. *American Review of Respiratory Diseases, 99,* 696–702.

Braun, N. (1984). Respiratory muscle dysfunction. *Heart and Lung, 13,* 327–332.

Braun, N., et al. (1983). When should respiratory muscles be exercised? *Chest, 84,* 76–84.

Derenne, J., Macklem, P., & Roussos, C. (1978). The respiratory muscles: Mechanics, control, and pathophysiology, Part I. American Review of Respiratory Diseases, 118, 119–133.

Nickerson, B., & Keens, T. (k1982). Measuring ventilatory muscle endurance in humans as sustainable inspiratory pressure. *Journal of Applied Physiology, 52,* 768–772.

Roussos, C. (1985). Functions and fatigue of respiratory muscles. *Chest, 88,* 124S–132S.

Roussos, C., & Macklem, P. (1977). Diaphragmatic fatigue in man. *Journal of Applied Physiology 43,* 189–197.

Sharp, J. (1980). Respiratory muscles: A review of old and newer concepts. *Lung, 157,* 185–199.

Tenney, S., Reese, R. (1968). The ability to sustain great breathing efforts. *Respiratory Physiology, 5,* 187–201.

Wyndham, C., et al. (1971). Walk or jog for health. *South African Medical Journal, 45,* 53–57.

CHAPTER 26

Patient Education

Alexandra J. Sciaky

KEY TERMS   Education
Effectiveness
Health behaviors
Learning theory

Methods
Needs assessment
Resources

INTRODUCTION

In cardiopulmonary physical therapy, sound treatment is based on the physiological assessment of the patient. Similarly, effective patient education is based on the learning needs assessment of the patient (Rankin & Stallings, 1990). Cardiopulmonary patient education poses a significant challenge because the physical therapist's duties can range from teaching a hospitalized cardiac patient to do a self pulse check to designing a series of community-based exercise classes for senior citizens with emphysema. Meeting this challenge is important because the benefits of patient education include reduced health-care costs, reduced patient anxiety, increased patient knowledge, satisfaction with care, and increased quality of life. In addition, physical therapists share the responsibility with other health-care providers of ensuring that patients have the opportunity to make informed choices

in their care. Unless effective patient education is implemented this opportunity will be lost.

The overall objective of this chapter* is to provide the clinician with an understanding of the principles and practice of effective patient education. To meet this objective, patient education is defined and pertinent learning theories with examples of how they relate to cardiopulmonary patient education are presented. The learning needs assessment of the patient is explained, followed by a description of patient education methods and materials. Because the effectiveness of patient education efforts are important to evaluate, ways to determine this are addressed. Fi-

---

*The author wishes to thank Jennifer L. Walters, D. Min. and Patricia Wren, MPH for their expertise in education and assistance in preparing this manuscript.

nally, interdisciplinary considerations and educational resources are discussed.

DEFINING PATIENT EDUCATION

Physical therapists believe that patient education is an important part of treatment (Chase, Elkins, Readinger, and Shepard, 1993). The teaching role of the physical therapist has been reported as highly valued by patients as well (Grannis, 1981). According to Bartlett (1985), patient education is "a planned learning experience using a combination of methods such as teaching, counseling, and behavior modification techniques which influence a patient's knowledge and health behavior."

Several factors make patient education unique when compared with other types of teaching. The patient may have limited or no access to the teaching because of financial and/or geographical barriers to health care. The student may lack a sense of well-being because of signs and symptoms of an acute illness, making learning more difficult. The relationship between the teacher and the learner in patient education may be perceived as hierarchical—a medical authority figure instructing a lay person. The student's emotional status may be fearful or anxious, depending on the medical situation. There may be superimposed time constraints, such as length of hospital stay or clinic appointment, which have a direct impact on patient education. All of these factors may pose barriers to learning. As in other types of teaching, however, patient education is information shared in the hope that it will not only be understood but applied in ways that produce the desired changes in health-related behavior.

Objectives

The overall objective of patient education is to affect a durable cognitive improvement that results in a positive change in an individual's or group's health behavior. In many cases the physical therapist must embark on a process to meet this objective in the course of treatment. This process consists of assessing the learning needs of the patient, identifying measurable, realistic objectives, planning and implementing the

---

Patient Education Objectives
1. Enhanced patient-clinician rapport
2. Increased patient knowledge of health disorder/condition
3. Increased adherence to physical therapy treatment plant
4. Decreased health-care costs
5. Increased patient self-efficacy
6. Increased ability to make informed health-care choices

patient education program, and finally evaluating its effectiveness. Specific examples of patient education learning objectives are listed in the box above.

Achieving these objectives will lead to the enjoyment of a host of documented benefits of patient education. These include reduced length of hospital stay (Devine & Cook, 1983), reduced patient anxiety (O'Rourke, Lewin, Whitcross, and Pacey, 1990), improved health-related knowledge (Rowland, Dickinson, Newman, and Ebrahim, 1994), increased quality of life (Manzetti, Hoffman, Sereika, Sciurba, and Griffith, 1994), and improved response to and adherence with medical treatment (Mazzuca, 1982). Patient education has also been shown to empower patients to take more active roles in their health care (Smith, 1987). Patients who are educated partners in their care are able to be smart consumers in the health-care system and adapt more readily to changes in their life styles resulting from illness.

Learning Theory: Concepts Pertinent to Cardiopulmonary Patient Education

The American Physical Therapy Association's Commission on Accreditation of Physical Therapy Education (1990) requires that the graduate physical therapist be able to ". . . apply concepts of teaching and learning theories in designing, implementing and evaluating learning experiences used in the education of patients." Twentieth century behavioral scientists have developed a variety of learning theories and models attempting to explain the complexities of human behavior. Subsequent models have emerged that specifically address health behavior. Although a comprehensive discussion of these models is beyond the scope of this chapter, a list of references for further reading may be found at the end of this chapter. The discussion of the three theoretical concepts which follows is designed to provide the clinician with a rationale for patient education practice in terms of its basis in learning theory. The concepts are social-cognitive theory, the health-belief model, and the behavior-modification approach.

The social-cognitive theory as developed by Bandura (1986) posits that human behavior can be explained and predicted using the following key regulators: incentives, outcome expectations, and efficacy expectations. For example, a myocardial infarction patient perceives value in following the exercise program (incentive). This patient will attempt to exercise if he or she believes his or her current sedentary life style poses a threat to health. The patient also believes exercise will reduce that threat (outcome expectation) and that he or she is personally capable of performing the exercise program (efficacy expectation). Outcome and efficacy expectations directly relate to patients' beliefs about their capabilities and the relationship of their behaviors to successful outcomes. In essence then, behavior is influenced by perceptions that create expectations for similar outcomes over time.

To function competently in a given environment requires a belief in one's ability to attain a certain level of performance. Bandura terms this *self-efficacy* (Bandura, 1977). He argues that perceived self-efficacy influences all aspects of behavior including learning new skills and inhibiting or stopping current behaviors. Self-efficacy has the following four primary determinants: (1) performance accomplishments, the strongest determinant, refers to acting out the desired behavior and mastery over the task, resulting in increased self-efficacy; (2) vicarious experience involves learning through observing the actions of others, especially those with clear, rewarding outcomes; (3) verbal persuasion; and (4) one's physiological state as it relates to perceived ability to perform a given task. For example, a pulmonary rehabilitation program increases a patient's self-efficacy when he or

she successfully completes multiple exercise sessions (performance accomplishments), learns how to deal with dyspnea by consulting fellow program graduates (vicarious experience), receives counseling on energy conservation techniques from the staff (verbal persuasion), and notes that oxygen saturation measured 95% before exercising (physiological state).

The health-belief model, developed in the early 1950s, theorizes that patients are likely to take a health action in the following situations: (1) they believe they are at risk of illness; (2) they believe that the disease poses a serious threat to their lives should they contract it; (3) they desire to avoid illness and believe that certain actions will prevent or reduce the severity of the illness; and (4) they believe that taking the health action is less threatening than the illness itself (Roenstock, 1974). This model was originally developed in an attempt to understand why large numbers of people failed to accept preventative care or screening tests for early disease detection. Subsequent studies have used the model to analyze compliance with regimes for hypertension, asthma, and diabetes (Becker, 1985).

The health-belief model conveys that in the context of health behavior some stimulus or "cue to action" is necessary to initiate the decision-making process. These cues can be internal (i.e., a productive cough) or external (i.e., instructional video tape on pulmonary hygiene techniques). Once the behavior commences, it is understood that many demographic, structural, personal, and social elements are capable of influencing the behavior. In addition, perceived barriers (i.e., unpleasant side effects) may limit or prevent undertaking the recommended behavior.

The behavior-modification approach has its roots in operant-learning theory and consists of techniques that manipulate environmental rewards and punishments in relationship to a specified behavior (Redman, 1993). The theme of this approach is that an individual's behavior can gradually be shaped to meet a set objective. According to Becker (1990), the behavior-modification approach frequently follows a general plan: "identify the problem; describe the problem in behavioral terms; select a target behavior that is measurable; identify the antecedents and consequences of the behavior; set behavioral objectives;

Health Care Contract

Date: _____

Contract Goal: (Specific outcome to be attained)

I, (client's name), agree to (detailed description of required behaviors, time and frequency limitations)

in return for (positive reinforcements contingent upon completion of required behaviors; timing and mode of delivery of reinforcements)

I, (provider's name), agrees to (detailed description of required behaviors, time and frequency limitations)

(Optional) I, (significant other's name), agree to (detailed description of required behaviors, time and frequency limitations)

(Optional) Aversive consequences: (Negative reinforcements for failure to meet minium contract requirements).

We will review the terms of this agreement, and will make my desired modifications, on (date). We hereby agree to abide by the terms of the contract describe above.

Signed: (Client) _____

Signed: (Significant other, if relevant). _____

Signed: (Provider) _____

Contract effective from (Date) _____ to (Date) _____

(From Janz NK, Becker MH, Hartman PE: *Patient Educ Couns* 5(4):165–178, 1984).

devise and implement a behavior change program; and evaluate the program." This plan is very similar to the approach the physical therapist takes on being referred to evaluate and treat a patient. The physical therapist identifies the patient's deficits, describes the problem(s) in functional terms, sets short-term and long-term functional goals, designs a treatment plan to meet those goals, implements the treatment plan and reevaluates the patient. These similarities may facilitate the use of the behavioral-modification approach by physical therapists.

Health-care contracts can be useful in implementing the behavior-modification approach. An example of such a contract may be seen in the box above. The contract should be realistic, measurable, and renewable (Herje, 1980). Specific goals, time frames, behaviors, and contingencies are written in the contract. The clinician and patient discuss, then sign the contract. Positive and negative reinforcements are used to facilitate the desired behaviors in the patient. Ideally, once the contract expires, the patient feels competent and is able to continue the desired behaviors without the external reinforcements.

NEEDS-BASED APPROACH TO PATIENT EDUCATION

The most important aspect of planning for patient education is assessing the learners (Kopper, 1987). The process of patient education requires assessment of the total patient, including an understanding of the psychosocial, socioeconomic, educational, vocational, and cultural qualities of the person (Verstraete and Meier, 1973). Assessing educational needs of the patient allows the physical therapist to determine what the patient needs to know to meet the desired cognitive and behavioral teaching objectives. This assessment also increases patient-teacher rapport and prevents needless repetition of already familiar material.

LEARNING NEEDS ASSESSMENT
Tools

Learning needs can be assessed in a variety of ways. These include patient and family interviews, questionnaires and surveys, written tests, and observation of patient performance (Haggard, 1989). Interviews allow the physical therapist to ask questions directed at determining the patient's view of the illness, including associated beliefs and attitudes. Questionnaires and surveys can be used in conjunction with the interview to document the patient's responses to specific questions about his or her condition. Open-ended questions such as "What are the major problems your illness has caused for you and your family?" elicit more information than a multiple-choice format. Written tests can be helpful in determining what patients already know when the tests are given before any teaching. These tests can also identify problems with reading and comprehension skills. Observing patients as they perform a skill, such as diaphragmatic breathing, reveals whether or not the patient can demonstrate the correct technique. The physical therapist can also pose questions to the patient during the demonstration to determine whether or not the patient knows the rationale for the exercise.

Areas to Assess

The learning needs assessment encompasses the following five major areas: (1) perceptual, (2) cognitive, (3) motor, (4) affective, and (5) environmental (see the box at right). By addressing these five areas, the physical therapist will obtain an accurate picture of the patient's learning abilities, knowledge level, performance skills, attitudes, and cultural influences.

The perceptual area encompasses the learner's ability to receive information via the senses. If the learner's sight, hearing, or sense of touch is impaired, the instructor may need to make modifications so that the information can be received by the learner. The comprehension of symbols, such as numbers, words, or pictures, also needs to be assessed in the perceptual area. The instructor needs to know what meaning the learner attributes to the symbols that will be used in the education program to ensure clarity.

Learning Needs Assessment Areas

Perceptual
    Ability to receive input (vision, hearing, and touch)
    Comprehension of symbols (figures, numbers, words, and pictures)

Cognitive
    Knowledge and analytical skills
    Memory

Motor
    Fine- and gross-motor skills
    Physical adaptations and responses to illness or stimuli

Affective
    Attitudes
    Value-belief system
    Motivation (readiness to learn)

Environmental
    Personal and societal resources
    Amount of instructor contact and setting
    Cultural influences (language, traditions, roles, religion, and life style)

The cognitive area addresses the learner's knowledge and problem-solving skills. The instructor needs to know how much the learner already knows and what needs to be learned. The instructor also needs to know if the learner has any problems with memory. Short- or long-term memory deficits may require that the instructor integrate a prompting system into the education plan.

The patient's fine- and gross-motor skills and functional mobility are covered in the motor area. The instructor needs to be aware of the physiological changes in the patient that affect abilities to perform activities necessary for a given education program. For example, if a support group is being held in a room that is not wheelchair accessible, patients who are wheelchair users will not be able to readily attend.

The affective area comprises the learner's attitudes, beliefs, and readiness to learn. Identifying the learner's value-belief system will assist the instructor in deter-

---

Learning Needs Assessment Survey

Your physical therapist would like to help you learn what you need to know to function as independently as possible and manage your illness/disability. Please answer the following questions to identify your own needs.

Part I.

Name:

Your illness and/or disability is:

1. Do you have any problems seeing or hearing?
2. Do yu have any body areas which are numb (can't feel)?
3. How long have you had this illness/disability?
4. What problems has it caused you?
5. Are you able to care for yourself at home?
6. Are you responsible for the care of any others at home?
7. Do you have someone at home to help you? If so, whom?
8. What questions or concerns do you have?
9. Do you practice a religion? If so, which?
10. The language you understand best is?
11. How much education/schooling have you had?

Part II. There are many different ways to learn. Please read the list of ways to learn below and circle the ones which help you learn best.

Reading materials	Group discussion
Lectures (listening)	By myself
Demonstrations watching)	Games
Videos	Computer programs
Audiotapes (cassettes)	Seminars
Practice/Stimulation (doing)	Role playing
Written tests	Other

Part III. I would like to know more about: (Check all that apply to you.)

____ How to clear mucus from my lungs	____ What causes heart disease
____ How to avoid shortness of breath	____ What I should eat
____ Exercise	____ My medications
____ Monitoring myself	____ Planning my social life
____ What to do if I have chest pain	____ Planning for sexual intimacy
____ What causes lung disease	____ Coping with my feelings

Other things I would like to know:

The three most important things I need to know are:

mining what is important to the learner and facilitate motivation. What the instructor feels is important to learn may not be what the patient feels is important to learn. Identifying what the patient values early will prevent instructor (and patient) frustration later.

Cultural influences and personal and societal resources are included in the environmental area. Being aware of the patient's life style, religion, traditions, roles, and primary language are important for the instructor to assess to individualize the patient's learning experience. Presence or absence of the patient's resources may affect consistency in and access to patient education.

All five of these areas can be addressed with the use of a learning needs assessment survey. See Figure 26-2 for an example. By using a survey in combination with the physical therapy patient evaluation, the therapist can gather all the necessary information to create an optimal patient education experience. The survey in the box on p. 458 consists of three parts, which can be adapted to any patient-care setting. In the pediatric setting, some of the questions could be asked of the parent(s) or rephrased to address elementary-school–aged children. Part I primarily assesses the patient's perception of the illness or disability and its impact on the patient's life. Part II lists a wide variety of teaching methods and asks the patient to indicate which methods are most useful personally. Part III identifies specific topics about which the patient would like to know more. This part is also helpful in alerting the therapist that referrals to other members of the interdisciplinary health-care team may need to be made. For example, if the patient checked off "what I should eat," the therapist should make a referral to the dietician.

Interpretation of Findings

The next important step after gathering information with the learning needs assessment survey is to interpret the findings. The physical therapist must look at the answer to each item on the survey and use that information in the process of designing the content and method for teaching that patient. Interpretation of the survey findings means applying the patient's current health concerns and knowledge deficits to future learning activities. By identifying the patient's needs the physical therapist can then make informed choices in the course of planning and implementing each patient education experience.

Formulation and Prioritization of Goals

As physical therapists set treatment goals for their patients, they should also set educational goals. Treatment goals usually describe functional outcomes (e.g., the patient will perform a stand and pivot transfer from bed to chair, independently) and they are written in behavioral terms. Educational goals should also be written in behavioral terms. For example, "Mr. J will safely perform percussion and postural drainage to Mrs. J's right lower lobe." The stated behavior needs to be measurable in some way. Motor skills can be observed, knowledge skills can be tested, and safety can be documented.

Prioritizing the patient's educational goals in conjunction with treatment goals enhances the therapist's efficiency. Referring again to the learning needs assessment survey (see the box on p. 458) to determine what is important knowledge to the patient will guide the therapist in creating the most appropriate prioritization of goals. Simplicity is usually best. Overwhelming patients with a huge list of items to be accomplished may discourage them before they even start. If the patient's learning needs are very great, start by breaking down the list of goals into smaller groups. Choose the most important goals and try to accomplish them first. If you run into a series of failures, tackle the next group. Build on each success the patient experiences.

EDUCATIONAL METHODS
Method Selection

Using the learning needs assessment survey (see the box on p. 458) will allow the clinician to choose education methods that will facilitate optimal learning in a given patient or group. The patient(s) can self-select the available learning methods that have the greatest learning potential. A combination of methods may be necessary to achieve the educational goals that have been set. If a patient is not sure which methods to indicate, the therapist can base the choice on the other information provided in the survey (e.g., sensory deficits, level of schooling, or type of information desired). Surveys generally require regular updates to ensure that all of the offered methods are listed and the discontinued methods are removed from the list.

Advantages and Disadvantages

Each education method has its own advantages and disadvantages. Table 26-1 shows 13 education methods listed with their key advantages and disadvantages. The table is designed to assist the physical therapist in determining the settings and populations in which the methods will be most useful. This is not a comprehensive list. In fact, some health-education challenges require truly innovative approaches.

In 1988, for example, community health-care providers in Boston were faced with a dilemma. The incidence of acquired immune deficiency syndrome (AIDS) among women of color was increasing and Latino, African-American, and Haitian women were not receiving vital information about how to prevent the transmission of the human immunodeficiency virus (HIV). These communities were largely distrustful of the health-care establishment and were not

TABLE 26-1		
Comparison Chart for Education Methods (Adults and children unless otherwise noted)		
TYPE	**ADVANTAGES**	**DISADVANTAGES**
Reading	Patient can refer back to material. Low effort for instructor.	Requires instructor follow-up for comprehension.
Lecture	Time-efficient for instructor. Cost-efficient.	Low interaction. May pacify rather than engage.
Demonstration	Adds sensory data to learning. Allows for problem solving and modification.	Instructor needs proficiency in skill to be demonstrated.
Video	Access to restricted areas. Portrays events that are infrequent, costly, and difficult to reproduce. Portable.	Noninteractive. May pacify rather than engage. Costly, requiring electronic equipment. Difficult to control quality.
Audiotape	Portable. Useful for sight-impaired learner.	Requires electronic equipment.
Group discussion	Effective use of instructor time. Enlarges pool of real-life experiences. Nonthreatening to some learners. Mutual support possible.	Not as much individual attention given. Group may be hard to control (e.g., too talkative, shy, hostile). Strong facilitator skills needed.
Clubs, camps, and retreats	Draws on community and individual resources. Needs less professional input and time.	Same as above. Some risk of perpetuating myths and false information.
Individual instruction	Instructor can tailor learning to student's needs and desires. More one-on-one time.	Inefficient use of instructor time. Limited pool of experience on which to draw.
Games and directed activities	Helpful for children. Reduces anxiety. Uses repetition. Fun. Unexpected experiences can lead to new understandings or insights.	Scheduling space. Finding participants.
Computer programs	Interactive, self-paced. Large information capacity. Time-efficient for instructor.	Expensive. Special equipment and space needed. May require expert help.
Seminars and workshops	Diversity of instructors and formats. Pool of experts and community resources. Can tailor content broadly or narrowly.	Expense, scheduling, and space.
Role-playing	Trial runs, problem-solving, simulated experiences.	Threatening to some. Can be time-consuming. Instructor needs to be skilled in techniques and dealing with effects on participants.
Oral and written tests	Can provide instructor with evidence of what learner needs to be taught and what has been learned.	Literacy and supplies required, if written. May be time-consuming.

mobilized to stop the spread of HIV. How could they be reached? The Boston Women's AIDS Information Project (BWAIP) trained lay women to educate other women in the places where they congregate, such as beauty salons. Informational brochures, condoms, and posters were distributed in a number of beauty salons in communities where women were at highest risk for contracting HIV. Lay and professional educators would give presentations, show videos, and answer questions of the staff and patrons of these establishments to empower them to disarm myths about AIDS, encourage other women to make appropriate behavior changes, and to make referrals to neighborhood health centers for testing and evaluation.

Teaching young children about their bodies and health may also require unique approaches. In 1993, members of the interdisciplinary team caring for children with cystic fibrosis (CF) at Texas Children's Hospital, Houston, held a CF Education Day for the children and their parents. The children ranged in age from 7 to 11 years old. To teach them about anatomy, a special anatomy apron was fabricated. The apron had life-sized removable "organs" made of stuffed fabric. The children took turns wearing the apron and learned to identify and locate the organs by removing and replacing the apron's heart, lungs, intestines, and pancreas.

By evaluating the advantages and disadvantages of available education methods, the physical therapist can choose the methods that are most effective and use them to their best advantage. Consideration must be given for cost, equipment, scheduling, labor, time, site, flexibility, and reusability. For example, video-taped presentations may be easy for the instructor to schedule, present, and reuse but they can be costly to purchase and require expensive equipment to view.

Content

The specific content of patient education materials and programs should be determined by the needs of the individual or group being taught. However, there are topics common to many cardiopulmonary education efforts. These topics are listed in the box above. The physical therapist can use the topics listed in the table as a checklist to explore the content covered (or to be covered) in a given cardiopulmonary

Cardiopulmonary Patient Education Content
Smoking cessation
Risk-factor modification
Benefits and effects of exercise
Resumption of sexual activity
Normal cardiopulmonary anatomy and physiology
Cardiopulmonary disease process
Airway clearance techniques and suctioning
Energy conservation and pacing techniques
Stress management
Cardiopulmonary resuscitation (CPR)—basic life support
Heart rate, blood pressure, and dyspnea self-monitoring
Nutrition
Medications (schedules, actions, and side effects)
Use of oxygen and other respiratory equipment
Medical procedures (e.g., cardiac catheterization or bronchoscopy)
Community resources
Emergency procedures

education experience. Although the physical therapist may not be responsible for teaching on all these topics, she or he should be familiar with them as they are taught by others on the health-care team. Educational materials on all of these topics have already been developed by a variety of health-care providers, educators, and organizations and may be available for physical therapists' use (see "Interdisciplinary Considerations and Resources").

DETERMINATION OF EFFECTIVENESS

Determining the effectiveness of patient education efforts involves evaluating not only what the patient learned but also how the teacher taught. Sometimes patients learn in spite of educational efforts. As physical therapists, we need to examine how effective we are at teaching and strive to improve our teaching skills just as we strive to improve our treatment skills. Being able to communicate ideas and receive feedback from patients from diverse racial, ethnic, vocational, religious, and generational backgrounds is crucial for physical therapists. We develop rapport with our patients by communicating to them that we have an understanding of their illnesses or disabilities, as they perceive them, and that we plan to integrate their goals or priorities into the treatment plans.

Teacher-Learner Relationship

According to Locke (1986), the primary step to understanding others, is an awareness of one's self. Acknowledging one's own personal values, interests, and biases will significantly increase one's sensitivity toward others. The skilled teacher is aware of her or his own communication style and its limitations and can convey the desire to help despite those limitations.

The teacher-learner relationship that develops between physical therapist and patient largely is due to communication between the two in the context of culture. Communication is a two-way process consisting of verbal and nonverbal messages. The interpretation of these messages depends on the cultural cues operating in the educational setting. Fairchild (1970) defines culture as all social behavior, such as customs, techniques, beliefs, organizations, and regard for material objects, including behaviors transmitted by way of symbols. "The primary mode of transmission of culture is language, which enables people to learn, experience, and share their traditions and customs" (Locke, 1992). In addition, culture can be expressed or experienced via economic and political practices, art, and religion. Health care and medicine have their own cultures. To meet the needs of culturally diverse populations and engage in positive, productive relationships, physical therapists need to operate from a framework of cross-cultural understanding. This understanding and knowledge can then be reflected in patient education efforts.

For example, in a large, urban, acute-care hospital two physical therapy staff members were working together to treat an elderly Jewish woman who was critically ill. The clinicians worked carefully to reposition the woman without disturbing the many tubes and lines that were present. Later the woman expressed that she did not want to have two physical therapy clinicians working with her at the same time. She confided to the nurse that it was because she felt it was too much like the Jewish ritual washing of the body after death, which is traditionally performed by two people. This interpretation of the therapy surprised the physical therapy staff members who treated the woman because they were also Jewish and the thought never occurred to them. The next time the clinicians went to see the woman, they explained why it was necessary for both of them to be present during the treatment. They also encouraged the woman to have other supportive people present and to play her favorite recorded music during the therapy session.

Patient Adherence

The effectiveness of physical therapy treatment, or of any medical treatment, depends on the patient following the health-care provider's recommendations (adherence.) Unfortunately there is often a gap between what the patient is asked to do and what the patient actually does. This gap, or nonadherence, has an incidence rate estimated between 50% to 80% (Meichenbaum and Turk, 1987). Factors affecting patient adherence include knowledge of and course of the illness, complexity of the recommendations, convenience, availability of support system, and the patient's beliefs.

Patient education can improve adherence when the information given includes what behaviors are expected, when they should be performed and what to do should problems arise. Plans for patient education sessions should strive to remove or avoid barriers to patient adherence. These efforts include simplifying and individualizing treatment regimens, fostering collaborative teacher-learner relationships, enlisting family support, making use of interdisciplinary and community resources, and providing continuity of care (Meichenbaum and Turk, 1987). By using an approach that integrates these efforts, the physical therapist can optimize patient adherence to the prescribed physical therapy program.

INTERDISCIPLINARY CONSIDERATIONS AND RESOURCES

The interdisciplinary health-care team has evolved as the complexity and amount of available medical treatments and information has grown. Physical therapists are trained to function as part of an interdisciplinary team and are responsible for learning the areas of responsibility and expertise covered by each member of their team. The team often consists of licensed and nonlicensed health-care providers and may include any or all of the following:

- Physician
- Nurse
- Physical therapist
- Occupational therapist
- Exercise physiologist
- Dietician
- Laboratory technologist
- Pharmacist
- Social worker
- Chaplain or pastoral care associate
- Clinical psychologist
- Speech therapist
- Vocational rehabilitation counselor
- Home-care personnel

All of the above providers may not be present on every team, but their services should be available for patients who need them. By understanding what services and patient education material are provided by each discipline, the physical therapist can reinforce previously presented concepts and avoid giving conflicting information. This also allows the physical therapist to make referrals to the appropriate discipline when other knowledge deficits are identified.

Interdisciplinary team members can also provide the physical therapist with important patient feedback and information. Teaching methods found to be successful with a given patient by the nurse, for example, could be communicated to the physical therapist. The therapist can then use similar methods with that patient for physical therapy education objectives. Communication between team members is enhanced by regular team meetings or rounds and by having a central location to document completed patient education experiences (i.e., the medical record).

Health-related organizations can also be rich resources for patient education information. The American Heart Association and the American Lung Association, for example, have many cardiopulmonary materials available to health-care providers for little or no cost. State public health and local community service agencies may also be sources for printed or audiovisual materials. The Health and Human Services Department of the Federal government has numerous divisions addressing health education. Catalogs listing these publications can be obtained from the Federal Consumer Information Center, Pueblo, Colorado 81009.

Community organizations such as YMCA, YWCA, and the American Red Cross offer a wealth of health-education materials and classes. Many of these agencies also have catalogs of their educational offerings, which can be obtained by telephoning their local offices. Local public, medical, and hospital libraries are also useful for seeking out available health-education materials. Many Chambers of Commerce keep lists of local support groups or clubs, such as Breather's Club or Heartbeats. Regional state colleges or universities have departments dedicated to health education and may have cardiopulmonary materials to share.

SUMMARY

This chapter defined patient education and described selected learning theories as they relate to cardiopulmonary patient education. The evaluation of the patient's learning needs was emphasized and the advantages and disadvantages of a variety of educational methods were discussed. The role of the teacher-learner relationship and patient adherence were explained in reference to the determination of patient education and treatment effectiveness. Finally, interdisciplinary health-care team interactions and resources for patient education materials were considered.

REVIEW QUESTIONS

1. Discuss the benefits of patient education, including impact on health care costs and patient's response to treatment.

2. Define the overall objective of patient education and discuss the potential barriers to learning and ways to minimize them.

3. Explain the rationale for patient education using concepts of adult learning theories or models.

4. Describe the most important aspect of planning for patient education.

5. Discuss the components of a learning needs assessment survey and ways to modify it for specific patient populations.

References

Bandura, A. (1986). *Foundations of thought and action: a social cognitive theory.* Englewood Cliffs, NJ: Prentice-Hall.

Bandura, A. (1977). Self-efficacy: toward a unifying theory of behavioral change. *Psychological Review, 84*(2), 191-215.

Bartlett, E.E. (1985). At last, a definition. *Patient Education Counseling, 7,* 323-324.

Becker, M.H. & Janz, N.K. (1985). The health belief model applied to understanding diabetes regimen compliance. *Diabetes Education, 11,* 41-47.

Becker, M.H. (1990). Theoretical models of adherence and strategies of improving adherence. In S.A. Shumaker, Schron, E.R. & Ockene, J.K., (Eds.), *The handbook of health behavior change* (pp. 26-27). New York: Springer Publishing.

Chase, L., Elkins, J.A., Readinger, J., & Shepard, K.F. (1993). Perceptions of physical therapists toward patient education. *Physical Therapy, 73*(11), 787-95.

Commission of Accreditation of Physical Therapy Education. (1990). *Evaluative criteria for accreditation of educational programs for the preparation of physical therapists.* Alexandria, VA: American Physical Therapy Association.

Devine, E., & Cook, T. (1983). A meta-analysis of effects of psychoeducational interventions on length of post surgical hospital stay. *Nursing Research, 32,* 333-339.

Fairchild, H.P. (Ed.). (1970). *Dictionary of sociology and related sciences.* Totowa, NJ: Rowan & Allanheld.

Grannis, C.J. (1981). The ideal physical therapist as perceived by the elderly patient. *Physical Therapy, 61,* 479-86.

Haggard, A. (1989) *Handbook of patient education.* Rockville, MD: Aspen Publishers.

Herje, P.A. (1980). Hows and whys of patient contracting. *Nursing Education, 5,* 30-34.

Hoffman, S. (1987). Planning for patient teaching based on learning theory, In C.E. Smith (Ed.), *Patient education nurses in partnership with other health professionals* (pp. 159-188). Orlando, FL: Grune & Stratton.

Kopper, J.A. (1987). Assessing knowledge deficit and establishing behavioral objectives. In C.E. Smith (Ed.), Patient education: nurses in partnership with other health professionals (pp. 123-158). Orlando, FL: Grune & Stratton.

Liedekerken, P.C., Jonkers, R., DeHaes, W.F., Kok, G.J., & Saan, J. (Eds.) (1990). *Effectiveness of health education: review and analysis.* Assen, Netherlands: Van Gorcum.

Locke, D.C. (1992). *Increasing multicultural understanding: a comprehensive model.* Newberry Park: Sage Publications.

Locke, D.C. (1986). Cross-cultural counseling issues. In A.J. Palmo & W.J. Weikel et al (Eds.), *Foundations of mental health counseling.* Springfield, IL: Charles C. Thomas.

Manzetti, J.D., Hoffman, L.A., Sereika, S.M., Sciurba, F.C., & Griffith, B.P. (1994). Exercise, education, and quality of life in lung transplant candidates. *Journal of Heart and Lung Transplantation, 13*(2), 297-305.

Mazzuca, S. (1982). Does patient education in chronic disease have therapeutic value. *Journal of Chronic Disease, 35,* 521-529.

Meichenbaum, D., & Turk, D.C. (1987). *Facilitating treatment adherence: a practitioner's guidebook.* New York: Plenum Press.

Miller, P., Johnson, N.L.,Garrett, M.J., Wickoff, R. & McMahon, M. (1982). Health beliefs of and adherence to the medical regimen by patients with ischemic heart disease. *Heart Lung, 11,* 332-339.

O'Rourke, A., Lewin, B., Whitcross, S., & Pacey, W. (1990). The effects of physical exercise training and cardiac education on levels of anxiety and depression in the rehabilitation of CABG patients. *International Disability Studies, 12*(3), 104-6.

Pohl, M.L. (1968). *Teaching function of the nurse practitioner.* Dubuque, IA: Brown.

Rankin, S.H., & Stallings, K.D. (1990). *Patient education: issues, principles and practices.* (2nd ed.). Philadelphia: JB Lippincott.

Redman, B.K. (1993). *The process of patient education.* St. Louis: Mosby.

Roenstock, I.M. (1974). Historical origins of the health belief model. *Health Education Monographs, 2,* 328-335.

Rowland, L. Dickinson, E.T., Newman, P., & Ebrahim, S. (1994). Look After Your Heart Programme: impact on health status, exercise knowledge, attitudes and behavior of retired women in England. *Journal of Epidemiology and Community Health, 48*(2), 123-8.

Smith, C.E. (1987). Nurses' increasing responsibility for patient education. In C.E. Smith (Ed.), *Patient education: nurses in partnership with other health professionals.* Orlando, FL: Grune & Stratton.

Verstaete, M., & Meier, M. (1973). Patient education in a health sciences center. *Minnesota Medicine, 56*(2), 31-35.

Bibliography

Ajzen, I. (1985). From intentions to actions: a theory of planned behavior. In J. Kuhl, & J. Beekman (Eds.), *Action control: from cognition to behavior* (pp. 11-39). New York: Springer-Verlag.

Bandura, A. (1977). *Social learning theory.* Englewood Cliffs, NJ: Prentice-Hall.

Eraker, S.A., Becker, M.H., Strecher, V.J., & Kirscht, J.P. (1985). Smoking behavior, cessation techniques and the health decision model. *American Journal of Medicine, 78,* 817-25.

Fabrega, H. (1973). Toward a model of illness behavior. *Medical Care, 11,* 470-484.

Janz, N.K., & Becker, M.H. (1984). The health belief model: a decade later. *Health Education Quarterly, 11,* 1-47.

Leventhal, H., Meyer, D. & Gutman, M. (1980). The role of theory in the study of compliance to high blood pressure regimens. In R.C. Haynes, M.E. Mattson, & T.O. Engebretson, Jr. (Eds.), *Patient compliance to prescribed antihypertensive medication regimes: a report to the National Heart, Lung, and Blood Institute* (pp. 1-5). (NIH Publication No. 81-2102). Washington, DC: US Department of Health and Human Services.

Marlatt, G.A., & Gordon, J.R. (Eds.). (1985). *Relapse prevention: maintenance strategies in addictive behavior change.* New York: Guilford.

Matarazzo, J.D., Weiss, S.M., Herd, J.A., Miller, N.E., & Weiss, S.M. (Eds.) (1984). *Behavioral health: a handbook of health enhancement and disease prevention.* New York: Wiley.

Melamed, B.G., & Siegel, L.J. (1980). *Behavioral medicine: practical applications in health care.* New York: Springer Publishing.

Stetchen, V.J., Develliis, B.M., Becker, M.H., & Rosenstock, I.M. (1986). The role of self-efficacy in achieving health behavior change. *Health Education Quarterly, 13* 73-92.

PART IV

Guidelines for the Delivery of Cardiopulmonary Physical Therapy: Acute Cardiopulmonary Conditions

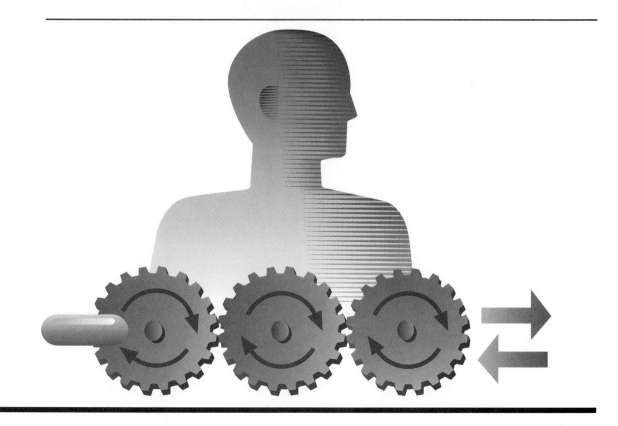

CHAPTER 27

Acute Medical Conditions

Elizabeth Dean
Willy E. Hammon
Lyn Hobson

KEY TERMS

Acute exacerbations of chronic airflow limitation
Alveolar proteinosis
Alveolitis
Asthma
Atelectasis
Bronchiolitis
Bronchitis

Cystic fibrosis
Hypertension
Interstitial pulmonary fibrosis
Pneumonia
Stable angina
Stable myocardial infarction
Tuberculosis

INTRODUCTION

The purpose of this chapter is to review the management of primary cardiopulmonary dysfunction secondary to other medical conditions. Several types of medical conditions are presented to illustrate the principles and basis for cardiopulmonary physical therapy in their management. These principles serve as a guide to problem solving when the practitioner is confronted with pathologies that are not presented. Although conditions are usually classified as either primary lung disease or primary cardiovascular disease, the heart and lungs work synergistically to effect gas exchange and in series with the peripheral vascular circulation to effect cardiac output and tissue perfusion (Dantzker, 1983; Dantzker, 1988; Scharf and Cassidy, 1989; Wasserman and Whipp, 1975). Thus impairment of one organ inevitably has implications for the function of the other organ. In addition, threat to or impairment of oxygen transport has implications for all other organ systems, thus a multisystem approach is essential (see Chapters 1 and 5). The primary pulmonary conditions that are presented include atelectasis, pneumonia, bronchitis, bronchiolitis, alveolitis, alveolar proteinosis, acute exacerbations of chronic airflow limitation, asthma, cystic fibrosis, interstitial pulmonary fibrosis, and tuberculosis. For further epidemiological and pathophysiological detail on these conditions refer to Bates (1989), the Epidemiological Standardization Project of the American Thoracic Society (1989), Luce (1986), Murray and Nadel (1988a), Murray and Nadel (1988b), and West (1987). The primary cardiovascular conditions presented include hypertension, medically stable angina, and uncomplicated myocardial infarction. For further details on these conditions refer to Goldberger (1990), Sokolow, McIlroy, and Cheitlin (1990), and Underhill, Woods, Froelicher, and Halpenny (1989).

Treatment principles are presented that are not intended to be a treatment prescription for a particular patient. The treatment priorities are presented based on the underlying pathology. However, without discussion of a specific patient and knowledge of other significant factors (i.e., the effects of restricted mobility, recumbency, and the effects of extrinsic and intrinsic factors) (Chapter 16), the specific parameters of the treatment prescription cannot be established. Integration of this information is essential for treatment to be specific and maximally efficacious. For specific examples of patient treatment prescriptions refer to the companion text *Clinical case studies in cardiopulmonary physical therapy.*

Atelectasis
Pathophysiology and medical management

Atelectasis refers to partial collapse of lung parenchyma. The pathophysiological mechanisms contributing to atelectasis are multiple (see box on p. 471). These mechanisms include physical compression of the lung tissue (e.g., resulting from increased pleural fluid, pus, pneumothorax, or adjacent areas of lung collapse) or from an obstructed airway (e.g., secretions or tumor) with subsequent reabsorption of oxygen from the trapped air by the pulmonary capillaries resulting in a collapse of the lung tissue distal to the obstruction (i.e., reabsorption atelectasis).

There are two primary forms of atelectasis—microatelectasis and segmental and lobar atelectasis. Microatelectasis is characterized by a diffuse area of lung units that are perfused but not ventilated, hence, right-to-left shunt. Ill and hospitalized patients who are deprived of being regularly upright and moving

have reduced lung volumes and are prone to breathing at low lung volumes and microatelectasis, requiring prophylactic measures to avoid significant effects of atelectasis on oxygen transport and gas exchange. When the conditions for normal lung inflation are removed, alveolar collapse occurs instantaneously.

Microatelectasis is associated with reduced lung compliance because of reduced lung expansion. Mechanically ventilated patients are prone to microatelectasis because the normal mechanics of breathing are violated. In part, this may be explained by restricted mobility, recumbency, and reduced arousal, in addition to reduced functional residual capacity (FRC). Positive end-expiratory pressure (PEEP) is routinely added to minimize these effects. High ventilator system pressure is required to counter reduced lung compliance, which indicates that atelectatic lung tissue it not readily reexpandible.

Microatelectasis is not detected readily with chest x-ray but is on the basis of clinical findings. Nonetheless, microatelectasis can be anticipated in every ill and hospitalized patient whose normal respiratory mechanics are disrupted, and particularly, in recumbent, relatively immobile patients. These effects are further exacerbated in older patients, patients who are overweight, have abdominal masses, spinal deformities, or chest wall asymmetry, smokers, and sedated patients.

Commensurate with its distribution, atelectasis presents with reduced chest wall movement and reduced breath sounds over the involved area. A chest x-ray shows increased density over the involved areas with a shift of the trachea and mediastinum toward the collapsed lung tissue. The patient may be tachypneic and cyanotic because of shunting. Segmental atelectasis results from significant progression of microatelectasis and by obstruction of airways with resorption of gas in the distal lung units of a bronchopulmonary segment or lobe.

The ventilator-dependent patient is predisposed to developing atelectasis because of an unnatural, monotonous breathing pattern, restricted movement, and abnormal and prolonged recumbent body positions. These factors contribute to reduced mucociliary transport, abnormal distribution of pulmonary mucus, and the accumulation of mucus in the dependent lung fields. Furthermore, production of mucus may be in-

Pathophysiological Mechanisms Contributing to Atelectasis

Central Mechanisms

Breathing at low lung volumes (e.g., when in pain or after certain medications)

Inability to generate adequate inspiratory pressure and volume

Central disruption of breathing centers controlling normal periodic and rhythmic breathing pattern

Extramural Mechanisms

Chest wall deformity

Asymmetry of intrathoracic structures

Respiratory muscle weakness (e.g., neuromuscular disease)

Phrenic nerve inhibition (e.g., secondary to upper abdominal or cardiovascular thoracic surgery)

Compression of lung parenchyma secondary to pleural fluid accumulation, blood, plasma, and pus

Compression of lung parenchyma during surgery

Reduced lung expansion secondary to reduced movement

Compression of lung parenchyma secondary to static body positioning

Compression of lung parenchyma secondary to prolonged static body positioning

Mechanical ventilation

Increased alveolar surface tension

Mural Mechanisms

Airway narrowing secondary to increased bronchial smooth muscle tone

Calcification or altered anatomical integrity of airways

Edema of the bronchial wall and epithelium

Intramural Mechanisms

Impaired mucociliary transport

Increased pulmonary secretions

Inspissated pulmonary secretions

Altered distribution of pulmonary secretions

Mucous plug

Space-Occupying Lesions

Exudative and transudative fluid in the lung parenchyma

Foreign-body aspiration

Inflammation

Other Factors

Increased compliance and dynamic airway compression secondary to age-related changes to the lung

Increased time constants because of increased airway resistance, reduced compliance, or both

Splinting or casting of chest wall restricting normal three-dimensional chest wall movement

Pain and altered breathing pattern

Medications including narcotics, sedatives, and relaxants

Oxygen

creased due to tracheostomy or the presence of an endotracheal tube. Mucociliary clearance is further compromised by reduced ciliary activity resulting from high concentrations of oxygen, medication, and loss of an effective cough because of an artificial airway.

The effect of atelectasis on oxygen transport reflects its type and distribution. Hypoxemia, right to left shunt, reduced lung compliance, and increased work of breathing are common clinical manifestations. An increased temperature reflects an inflammatory or infective process and not atelectasis per se.

Principles of physical therapy management

Because it can develop instantaneously when respiratory mechanics are disrupted, microatelectasis should be anticipated and prevented. Those factors that contribute to atelectasis for a given patient are countered accordingly with aggressive prophylactic management (see the box on p. 471).

Once developed, however, atelectasis is treated aggressively. Treatment is primarily directed at reversing the underlying contributing mechanisms whenever possible (Don, Craig, Wahba, and Couture, 1971; Glaister, 1967; Leblanc Ruff, and Milic-Emili, 1970; Lewis, 1980; Ray, Yost, Moallem, Sanoudos, Villamena, and Paredes, 1974; Remolina, Khan, Santiago, and Edelman, 1981). For example, atelectasis resulting from restricted mobility is remediated with mobilization. Atelectasis resulting from prolonged static positioning and monotonous tidal ventilation is managed with mobilization, manipulating body position to increase alveolar volume of the atelectatic area, manipulating body position to optimize alveolar ventilation, or some combination of these interventions. Atelectasis arising from reduced arousal is managed by reducing the causative factors contributing to reduced arousal coupled with frequent sessions of mobilization and the upright position to increase arousal, promote greater tidal volumes and alveolar ventilation, increase zone 2 (area of optimal ventilation and perfusion matching), increase FRC, and minimize closing volume.

Breathing control and coughing maneuvers augment the cardiopulmonary physiological effects of mobilization and body positioning. Coordinating these interventions distributes ventilation more uniformly rather than directing gas to already open alveoli, which will overdistend these units. The distribution of ventilation is primarily altered by body positioning and not by deep breathing (Roussos, Fixley, Geriest, Cosio, Kelly, Martin, and Engely, 1977). Sustained maximal inspiratory efforts may augment alveolar ventilation, however, the parameters for such efforts to be maximally therapeutic have not been studied in detail.

If impaired mucociliary transport or excessive secretions are obstructing airways and contributing to atelectasis, mobilization of pulmonary secretions is the goal that may be affected by mobilization and a "stir-up regimen" (Dripps and Waters, 1941; Ross and Dean, 1989). In addition, postural drainage coordinated with breathing control and coughing maneuvers can facilitate airway clearance. The addition of modified manual techniques may be indicated in some patients.

Pneumonia
Pathophysiology and medical management

Pneumonia is a common cause of morbidity and mortality in the hospitalized patient, particularly in very young and very old patients (Bartelett and Gorbach, 1976). Comparable with other systemic infections, pneumonia results when the normal defense mechanisms of the respiratory system fail to adequately protect the lungs from infection.

Air inspired through the nasal passages is cleansed of particulate matter by filtration (cilia sweep it to the nasopharynx); impaction (irregular contour of the chamber causes particles to rain out); swelling of hygroscopic droplet nuclei, which are either filtered or become impacted; and defense factors located in the mucous blanket, such as immunoglobulins (IgA), lysozymes, polymorphonuclear leukocytes, and specific antibodies. Particles that escape one of these defense mechanisms in the nasopharynx may be prevented from entering the lower airways of the larynx. The mucosa of the larynx is sensitive to chemical irritation or mechanical deformation and responds to this stimuli by producing a cough. The high velocities created by the cough are sufficient to clear several branches of the tracheobronchial tree of particulate matter. The cough reflex is frequently absent or depressed in hosts who are unconscious from drug overdose, epilepsy, alcohol ingestion, or head injury. Patients with artificial airways are more susceptible to infection because all the previously mentioned defense mechanisms are bypassed, causing organisms to be deposited directly in the lower airways. In the lower airways the cough mechanism is rendered ineffective by endotracheal tubes, which prevent approximation of the vocal cords, and by tracheostomy tubes, which cause air to bypass the cords altogether.

The trachea and the tracheobronchial tree to the level of the respiratory bronchioles are protected by the cough reflex, filtration (again by cilia which transport particles to the pharynx), impaction, and chemical factors (IgA). Below the level of the respiratory bronchioles, the cough reflex is ineffective, and filtration and transportation of particles by cilia cannot occur because cilia are absent. The alveolar macrophages play an important role in protecting these airways from particulate matter. Macrophages ingest organisms and transport them to the lymphatic system or higher in the tracheobronchial tree to where cilia can sweep them to the pharynx. This process of phagocytosis can be slowed or stopped by hypoxia, alcohol ingestion, air pollutants, corticosteroids, immunosuppressant agents, starvation, cigarette smoke, and oxygen. Particulate matter may also be removed from the airways below the level of the respiratory bronchioles by postural drainage.

Routes of Infection

A host who has impaired or ineffective defense mechanisms of the respiratory tract becomes susceptible to a variety of organisms. The major routes of infection include airborne organisms, circulation, contiguous infection, and aspiration.

CLASSIFICATION OF PNEUMONIA
Viral Pneumonias

Most respiratory viral infections are contracted by droplets from the respiratory tracts of infected persons. These viruses are responsible for interstitial pneumonias, tracheobronchitis, bronchiolitis, and the common cold. The ciliated cells of the respiratory tract are the most frequent site of infection. They become paralyzed and degenerate with areas of necrosis and desquamation. The mucociliary blanket becomes interrupted because destruction of the cilia leaves a thin layer of nonciliated basal replacement cells. Inflammatory responses cause exudation of fluid and erythrocytes in both the alveolar septae and airways. Congestion and edema become predominant with the formation of intraalveolar hyaline membranes. These changes in the normal mucosal structure and cilia make involved areas of the lung susceptible to superimposed bacterial infections. This is the most common complication seen in viral infections and is usually responsible for the fatalities that occur.

The patient with viral pneumonia presents with fever, dyspnea, loss of appetite, and a persistent nonproductive cough. On auscultation, normal breath sounds are heard throughout both lung fields with scattered inspiratory crackles. X-ray changes range from minor infiltrates to severe bilateral involvement. Consolidation and pleural effusions occur less frequently. Secondary bacterial infections occur frequently, causing patients to develop productive coughs.

Influenza may lead to viral pneumonia in 1% to 5% of cases. Influenza includes acute viral respiratory tract infection, characterized by a sudden onset of headache, myalgia, and fever. The route of infection is by inhalation of airborne particles from an infected person. The incubation period is 24 to 72 hours.

Pulmonary lesions include edema of the respiratory epithelium with necrosis and hemorrhage. At the alveolar level, interstitial edema, proliferation of type I cells, hemorrhage, and an increased number of macrophages are seen. In patients with pneumonia, secondary bacterial infections are frequent and are the cause of most fatalities.

Medical treatment of viral infections is supportive and preventative. Patients should receive vaccines whenever possible to buildup antibodies against specific viruses. Once the patient has contracted the organism, treatment becomes supportive, with rest, salicylates, and high fluid intake being the main treatment priorities. Patients who become more acutely ill with viral pneumonia should be on a vigorous preventative program to lessen the possibility of bacterial infection.

Recovery also depends on good nutrition, hydration, sleep, rest, and reduced stress.

Principles of physical therapy management

Patients may respond to mobilization coordinated with breathing control exercises and positional rotation for enhancing alveolar ventilation, mucociliary transport, and gas exchange overall (Orlava, 1959). Extreme body positions may enhance alveolar volume and ventilation and ventilation and perfusion matching (Dean, 1985; Douglas, Rehder, Beynen, Sessler, and Marsh, 1977; Grimby, 1974; Piehl and Brown, 1976). Vigorous treatment should be initiated at the first sign of a superimposed bacterial infection, which is often accompanied by a productive cough. At this time, the appropriate devices should be prescribed (e.g., ultrasonic or medication nebulizers to loosen secretions). Postural drainage may be indicated in addition to mobilization for airway clearance. Treatments, particularly mobilization, need to be paced to minimize unduly tiring the patient or increasing oxygen demand beyond the patient's capacity to adequately deliver oxygen. Increasing oxygen demands excessively may compromise the patient's gas exchange. Patient education is also fundamental to the treatment that is to be instituted between treatments (i.e., mobilization and positional rotation coordinated with breathing control and coughing maneuvers).

The focus of cardiopulmonary physical therapy in the management of viral pneumonia is to augment alveolar ventilation, increase perfusion, increase diffusion, and improve ventilation and perfusion matching, thereby reducing the threat to oxygen transport and gas exchange. Treatments are prescribed to optimize oxygen transport and gas exchange and to minimize fatigue and lethargy.

Bacterial Pneumonia

Bacterial pneumonia causes the largest number of deaths per year by an infective agent and is the fifth most common cause of all deaths in North America. The patient presents with an abrupt onset of a severe illness characterized by fever, tachypnea, dyspnea, hypoxemia, tachycardia, and a cough producing bloody or purulent sputum. The clinical findings depend on the organism involved and the extent of the pneumonia in the lungs. The infective process may cease with the use of chemotherapeutic agents, aerosols, and physical therapy, or it may spread to contiguous areas, causing pleural effusions and empyemas.

Bacterial pneumonias can occur as either primary or secondary infections. Primary pneumonias arise in otherwise healthy individuals and are usually pneumococcal in origin. Secondary pneumonias occur when the patient's defense system becomes ineffective.

Pneumococcal pneumonia is caused by pneumococcal bacteria, a gram-positive organism. It occurs most frequently in the winter months among adults between 15 and 40 years of age with a predilection for males. Patients present clinically with an abrupt onset of illness characterized by fever, cough, purulent or rust-colored sputum, and pleuritic chest pain over the affected lung field. Physical examination may reveal decreased expansion of the chest over the affected area and muscle splinting. On auscultation, there may be bronchial breath sounds (indicating consolidation), decreased or absent breath sounds, and wheezes or crackles over the affected lung. Chest x-rays may show infiltrates, consolidation, or atelectasis.

There are four stages associated with bacterial infection of lung tissue—engorgement, red hepatization, gray hepatization, and resolution. The engorgement stage occurs within the first few days of infection and is characterized by vascular engorgement, serous exudation, and evidence of bacteria colonization. Red hepatization occurs within 2 to 4 days as a result of diapedesis of the red blood cells. The alveoli are full of polymorphonuclear leukocytes, fibrin, and red blood cells. The organism continues to multiply within the fluid exudate. Areas of consolidation become evident. Gray hepatization occurs within 4 to 8 days and is characterized by evidence of abundant fibrin, decreased polymorphonuclear leukocytes, and dead bacteria. Consolidation continues to be a problem in this stage. Resolution occurs after 8 days as areas of consolidation begin to resolve. Many macrophages are seen and evidence of enzymatic digestion of exudate is present. The affected tissue becomes softer with large amounts of grayish-red fluid present within the alveoli. This process continues for 2 to 3 weeks with the lung gradually assuming a more normal appearance.

Pleural involvement occurs frequently, with the pleural spaces filling with the same type of fluid seen within the alveoli. Resolution is much slower because there are few surfaces available for phagocytosis. Complications that may occur in patients with pneumococcal involvement include empyema, superinfections (occur when large numbers of new organisms invade the lung), abscesses, atelectasis, and delayed resolution (defined as taking more than 4 weeks to resolve).

Treatment of pneumococcal pneumonia involves the use of chemotherapeutic agents, with penicillin being the antibiotic of choice. If the patient is allergic to penicillin, erythromycin or lincomycin is used. Thoracentesis is performed when pleural fluid is present. The patient should also receive ultrasonic nebulization and physical therapy. Supplemental oxygen therapy may be indicated.

Staphlococcal pneumonia is caused by a gram-positive organism. It rarely occurs in the healthy adult but is a frequent cause of pneumonia in children, infants, and patients with chronic lung diseases, especially carcinoma, tuberculosis, and cystic fibrosis. Clinically, the patient presents with the same picture as the patient with pneumococcal pneumonia. There are some differences in the chest x-ray (e.g., patchy areas of infiltrate). Consolidation occurs infrequently in this type of pneumonia. Pleural effusions, empyema, abscesses, bronchopleural fistulas, and pneumatoceles (subpleural cyst-like structures) occur frequently. Treatment includes chemotherapeutic agents, rest, increased fluid intake, ultrasonic nebulization or medication nebulizers, and aggressive physical therapy.

Streptococcal pneumonia is caused by a gram-positive organism, *Streptococcus pyogenes.* It occurs most frequently in very young, very old, and debilitated patients. The clinical picture is very similar to that of staphlococcal pneumonia. Again consolidation is rare and chest x-rays usually show one or more areas of patchy infiltrates. Complications are rare but empyema does occasionally occur. Treatment for this organism

is the same as that for pneumococcal pneumonia.

Hemophilus influenzae pneumonia is caused by a gram-negative organism and occurs primarily in children as bronchiolitis and in adults who have chronic bronchitis. The clinical picture is the same as for the other bacterial pneumonias, with numerous areas of infiltration evident on x-ray. On auscultation, breath sounds are generally good, with crackles heard at the end of inspiration. Treatment of this pneumonia includes chemotherapeutic agents (ampicillin), oxygen, ultrasonic nebulization, and physical therapy.

Other gram-negative organisms causing pneumonia include *Escherichia coli* and *Pseudomonas aeruginosa.* They are seen most frequently in patients with underlying disease, especially pulmonary disease, or in those who are debilitated. They are frequently the cause of superinfections in individuals who have received massive doses of broad-spectrum antibiotics. Clinically these patients present with cough, fever, and dyspnea. On auscultation, crackles, bronchial breathing, and diminished or absent breath sounds can be noted. X-ray changes frequently show bibasilar infiltrates, with the amount of involvement being widely variable. As for other bacterial pneumonias, treatment includes chemotherapeutic agents, ultrasonic nebulization, and physical therapy.

Principles of physical therapy management

The goals of management of bacterial pneumonia include reversing alveolar hypoventilation, increasing perfusion, reducing right-to-left shunt, increasing ventilation and perfusion matching, minimizing the effects of increased mucous production, and optimizing lymphatic drainage. Bacterial pneumonia is frequently associated with increased mucous production. With respect to airway clearance, management focuses on augmenting mucociliary clearance overall, reducing excess mucous accumulation, and reducing mucous stasis. Patients are often mobile and should be encouraged to be so to promote mucociliary transport and enhance lymphatic drainage (Dean and Ross, 1992a; Orlava, 1959; Wolff, Dolovich, Obminski, and Newhouse, 1977). However, the oxygen demands of mobilization and exercise should be well within the patient's capacity to delivery oxygen. These interventions should be prescribed to avoid jeopardizing this balance and unduly fatiguing the patient (Dean and Ross, 1992b). Deep breathing and effective coughing are singularly important maneuvers for clearing airways with special attention to the avoidance of airway closure (Bennett et al., 1990). Prescriptive body positioning can be used to optimize ventilation and perfusion matching (Clauss, Scalabrini, Ray and Reed, 1968; Douglas et al., 1977; Hietpas, Roth and Jensen, 1974; Hasani, Pavia, Agnew, and Clarke, 1991; Ross and Dean, 1992; Ross, Dean, and Abboud, 1992b; Zack, Pontoppidan, and Kazemi, 1974).

Acute Exacerbation of Chronic Bronchitis
Pathophysiology and medical management

Chronic bronchitis is a disease characterized by a cough producing sputum for at least 3 months and for 2 consecutive years. Pathological changes include an increase in the size of the tracheobronchial mucous glands (increased Reid index) and goblet cell hyperplasia. Mucous cell metaplasia of bronchial epithelium results in a decreased number of cilia. Ciliary dysfunction and disruption of the continuity of the mucous blanket are common. In the peripheral airways, bronchiolitis, bronchiolar narrowing, and increased amounts of mucus are observed.

Chronic bronchitis results from long-term irritation of the tracheobronchial tree. The most common cause of irritation is cigarette smoking. Inhaled smoke stimulates the goblet cells and mucous glands to secrete excessive mucus. Smoke also inhibits ciliary action. The hypersecretion of mucus and ciliary damage and dyskinesis lead to impaired mucous transport and a chronic productive cough. The fact that smokers secrete an abnormal amount of mucus increases the risk of respiratory infections and increases the length of the recovery time from these infections. Although smoking is the most common cause of chronic bronchitis, other factors that have been implicated are air pollution, certain occupational environments, and recurrent bronchial infections.

Patients with chronic bronchitis have been referred to as *blue bloaters* because of a tendency to have a dusky appearance and be stocky in build. Although many patients have a high $PaCO_2$, the pH is normalized by renal retention of bicarbonate. Over the long term, the bone marrow produces more red blood cells, leading to polycythemia. The work of the heart is increased due to increased blood viscosity. Long-term hypoxemia leads to increased pulmonary artery pressure and right ventricular hypertrophy.

Patients with chronic bronchitis have tenacious, purulent sputum that is difficult to expectorate. In an exacerbation, usually because of inflammation, infection, or both, they produce even more sputum, which tends to be retained and stagnate. Retained secretions obstruct airways and thus air flow, and reduce alveolar volume. The resulting ventilation and perfusion inequality increases hypoxemia, CO_2 retention, accessory muscle use, metabolic demand, and breathing rate. PaO_2 is further reduced and $PaCO_2$ tends to increase. Hypoxemia and acidemia increase pulmonary vasoconstriction, which increases pulmonary artery pressure and predisposes the patient to right heart failure (cor pulmonale) over time.

A patient having an acute exacerbation of chronic bronchitis tends to have the following characteristics: (1) The patient is often stocky in build and dusky in color. (2) The patient exhibits significant use of accessory muscles of respiration and has audible wheezing or wheezing that is audible on auscultation. (3) Intercostal or sternal retraction of the chest wall may be noted. (4) Edema in the extremities, particularly around the ankles, and neck vein distention reflect decompensated right heart failure. (5) The patient may report that breathing difficulty began with increased amounts of secretions (with a change in their normal color), which is often difficult to expectorate, and increased cough productivity. (6) PaO_2 is reduced, $PaCO_2$ increased, and pH reduced.

Pulmonary function tests indicate reduced vital capacity, FEV_1, maximum voluntary ventilation, and diffusing capacity and increased FRC and residual volume.

Principles of physical therapy management

During an exacerbation requiring hospitalization, these patients are usually treated with intravenous fluids, antibiotics, bronchodilators, and low-flow oxygen. Diuretics and digitalis are often given to treat right heart failure. Airway clearance interventions are selected (i.e., mobilization, body positioning, and postural drainage). These interventions are coordinated with breathing control and coughing maneuvers to facilitate secretion removal and optimize coughing and expectoration, while minimizing dynamic airway compression and alveolar collapse. During recovery, exercise with supplemental oxygen may also benefit the patient. It is important for these patients to avoid bronchial irritants (e.g., cigarette smoking, second-hand smoke, and air pollutants), and to be adequately hydrated to thin secretions to facilitate mucociliary transport and expectoration.

Patients with chronic bronchitis can benefit from a comprehensive rehabilitation program designed specifically for patients with chronic pulmonary disease (Murray, 1993; Oldenburg, Dolovich, Montgomery, and Newhouse, 1979). Specific details of exercise prescription in the management of chronic lung disease and of a comprehensive pulmonary rehabilitation program are described in Chapter 23.

Bronchiolitis
Pathophysiology and medical management

Bronchiolitis results from peripheral airway inflammation. In severe cases the exudate in the peripheral airways becomes organized into a connective tissue plug extending into the peripheral airway. The inflammatory process resembles that in other tissues (i.e., an inflammatory stage followed by a proliferative healing stage). Such inflammation is associated with vascular congestion, increased vascular permeability, formation of exudate, mucous hypersecretion, and shedding of the epithelium. Fluid is exudated out of the circulation onto the alveolar surfaces replacing the surfactant. This in turn increases the surface tension and promotes airway closure. The secretion production associated with airway irritants and inflammation results from the excess mucous production in combination with the inflammatory exudate consisting of fluid protein and cells of the exudate. Airway obstruction results if these substances are not removed. The airway epithelium has the capacity to repair and reline the lumen. A rapid turnover of cells may contribute to cell sloughing and further airway obstruction and a thickened basement membrane. The obstruction associated with bronchiolitis leads to ventilation and perfusion abnormalities and diffusion defect. Clinically, the patient presents with a productive cough. Obliterative bronchiolitis has been reported to be the most significant long-term complication of heart-lung transplantation (Burke, Glanville, Theodore, and Robin, 1987).

Medical management is directed at inflammation control with pharmacological agents, fluid management, and oxygen administration if necessary. Prevention of infection is a priority.

Principles of physical therapy management

The principal pathophysiological defects include ventilation and perfusion inequality and diffusion defect. These defects result from secretions produced by inflammation and increased mucous production and from atelectasis of adjacent alveoli. Physical therapy treatment should promote mucociliary transport and the removal of secretions and mucus to central airways, promote alveolar expansion and ventilation, optimize ventilation and perfusion matching and gas exchange, and reduce the risk of infection.

Bronchiolitis is primarily, although not exclusively, a childhood condition. The effects of inflammation and obstruction in small children are always serious because the anatomical and physiological components of the cardiopulmonary system are smaller, respiratory muscle tone is less well developed, the anatomical configuration of the chest wall is cylindrical, breathing is less efficient until after the age of 2, spontaneous movement and body positioning are more restricted (infants in particular spend more time in nonupright positions), and children are at greater risk of infection (see Chapter 35).

Alveolitis
Pathophysiology and medical management

Bronchioalveolitis is another inflammatory disorder of the peripheral airways that is often associated with an extrinsic allergic reaction. Comparable with bronchiolitis, alveolitis is prevalent in young children. In adults, chronic alveolitis may be a precursor to interstitial pulmonary fibrosis. Acute bouts of alveolitis are reversible, however, chronic inflammation can produce airway narrowing secondary to fibrosis in the alveolar wall and complete obstruction of the airway by organization of the exudate. Chronic inflammation can lead to permanent irreversible parenchymal changes and chronic restrictive lung disease.

Principles of physical therapy management

The principles of physical therapy management are comparable with that for the management of bronchiolitis. Principles of the management of cardiopulmonary dysfunction in children are presented in Chapter 35. Because children and infants in particular are physically immature, the principles of management are different from those for adults.

Alveolar Proteinosis
Pathophysiology and medical management

Alveolar proteinosis is a condition of unknown etiology, characterized by alveoli filled with lipid-rich proteinaceous material and no abnormalities in the alveolar wall, interstitial spaces, conducting airways, or pleural surfaces. Most often it is found in men between 30 and 50 years of age, although it has been reported in both men and women of all ages.

The most common symptoms are progressive dyspnea and weight loss, with cough, hemoptysis, and chest pain reported less frequently. Chest x-rays reveal diffuse bilateral (commonly perihilar) opacities (see Figure 4-10, p. 86). Physical findings include fine inspiratory crackles, dullness to percussion and, in the later stages, cyanosis and clubbing. Pulmonary function studies usually show decreased vital capacity, FRC, and diffusing capacity. Arterial blood gases indicate a low Po_2, especially during exercise, with often normal Pco_2 and pH.

Principles of physical therapy management

One treatment for patients with moderate-to-severe dyspnea on exertion from alveolar proteinosis is bronchopulmonary lavage. The patient is taken to the operating room. After general anesthesia and placement of a Carlen's tube (which isolates each lung), the patient is turned in the lateral decubitus position with the lung to be lavaged downward. The Carlen's tube enables the patient to be ventilated by the uppermost lung while the lower lung is carefully filled with saline to FRC. Then an additional 300 to 500 ml of saline is alternately allowed to run into and out of the lung by gravitational flow. As the saline flows out, manual percussion over the affected lung being lavaged has been reported to increase the amount of proteinaceous material washed from the lung (see Figure 4-11, p. 86). (Hammon, 1987).

Acute Exacerbation of Chronic Airflow Limitation
Pathophysiology and medical management

Emphysema. There are two principal types of emphysema—centrilobular and panlobular. Both types may coexist, however, centrilobular emphysema is 20 times more common than panlobular emphysema. Centrilobular is characterized by destruction of respiratory bronchioles (see Figure 4-1, p. 73), as well as edema, inflammation, and thickened bronchiolar walls. These changes are more common and more marked in the upper portions of the lungs. This form of emphysema is found more often in men than in women, is rare in nonsmokers, and is common among patients with chronic bronchitis. Panlobular emphysema is characterized by destructive enlargement of the alveoli distal to the terminal bronchioles (see Figure 4-1, p. 73). This type of emphysema is also found in patients who have an antitrypsin deficiency. Airway obstruction in these individuals is caused by loss of elastic recoil or radial traction on the bronchioles. When individuals with normal lungs inhale, the airways are stretched open by the enlarging elastic lung, and during exhalation the airways are narrowed due to the decreasing stretch of the lung. However, the lungs of patients with panlobular emphysema have decreased elasticity because of disruption and destruction of surrounding alveolar walls. This in turn leaves the bronchioles unsupported and vulnerable to collapse during exhalation. This form of emphysema can be local or diffuse. Lesions are more common in the bases than the apices and tend to be more prevalent in older people.

Bullae, emphysematous spaces larger than 1 cm in diameter, may be found in patients with emphysema (see Figure 4-2, p. 74). It is thought that they develop from an obstruction of the conducting airways that permits the flow of air into the alveoli during inspiration but does not allow air to flow out again during expiration. This causes the alveoli to become hyperinflated and eventually leads to destruction of the alveolar walls with a resultant enlarged air space in the lung parenchyma. These bullae can be more than 10 cm in diameter and, by compression, can compromise the function of the remaining lung tissue (Figure 4-3, p. 75). If this happens, surgical intervention to remove the bulla is often necessary. Pneumothorax, a serious complication, can result from the rupture of one of these bullae.

Both types of emphysema can lead to chronic chest wall changes. The loss of elastic recoil of the lung parenchyma disturbs the balance between the normal lung recoil pulling the chest wall in and the natural tendency of the chest wall to spring out. This balance is essential in maintaining normal FRC (i.e., the air in the lungs at the end of normal end tidal expiration). Because the residual volume of the lungs is increased, FRC is correspondingly increased. This increase is not functional, however, because it reflects increased dead space. These patients are still prone to dynamic airway compression and airway closure because of the loss of the normal elastic recoil of the lung parenchyma (i.e., increased compliance). This contributes to uneven distribution of ventilation and decreased diffusing capacity. The pressure volume curve is shifted and ventilation is less efficient.

With loss of elastic recoil and the normal tethering of the alveoli maintaining them patent, the chest wall tends to expand outward, thereby contributing to the hyperinflated chest associated with the patient with chronic airflow limitation. The alveolar units are structurally less uniform and the distribution of ventilation becomes even less homogeneous. Inspiratory and expiratory times of the alveolar units also become significantly heterogeneous. The alveoli require long inspiratory filling times (i.e., long time constants). For this reason, the patient with chronic airflow limitation adopts a characteristic breathing pattern in which inspiration and expiration tend to be prolonged. On expiration, the patient may spontaneously adopt a pursed-lip breathing pattern, which is believed to augment alveolar patency and promote collateral ventilation and gas exchange in the lungs by creating positive back pressures (Muller, Petty, and Filley, 1970). In addition, the patient may actively expire to compensate for the loss of the passive elastic recoil that normally empties the lungs at end tidal volume. Overall the work of breathing is increased. As the lungs become more chronically hyperinflated the chest wall becomes increasingly barrel-shaped and rigid. Loss of the normal shape of the chest and bucket and pump handle motions further compromises efficient respiratory mechanics and breathing (Bake, Dempsey, and Grimby, 1976).

The emphysema patient's most common complaint is dyspnea. Physically, these patients appear thin and have an increased anteroposterior chest wall diameter. Depending on disease severity, they breathe using the accessory muscles of inspiration (Chapter 4). These patients may be observed leaning forward, resting their forearms on their knees, or sitting with their arms extended at their sides, pushing down against the bed or chair to elevate their shoulders and improve the effectiveness of the accessory muscles of inspiration.

Emphysema patients have been referred to as *pink puffers* because of the increased respiratory work they must do to maintain relatively normal blood gases. On auscultation, decreased breath sounds can be noted throughout most or all of the lung fields. Radiologically, the emphysema patient has overinflated lungs, flattened hemidiaphragms, and a small, elongated heart (see Figure 4-4, p. 76). Pulmonary function tests show a decreased vital capacity, FEV_1, maximum voluntary ventilation, and a greatly reduced diffusing capacity. The total lung capacity is increased and the residual volume and FRC are even more increased. Arterial blood gases reflect a mildly or moderately lowered PaO_2, a normal or slightly raised $PaCO_2$, and a normal pH. Emphysema patients, unlike patients with chronic bronchitis, tend to develop cardiac insufficiency with progression of the condition, leading to failure at the end stage of the disease (see Figure 4-5, p. 77). At this stage, cardiac hypertrophy may be evident.

Hypoxemia leads to hypoxic pulmonary vasoconstriction, which shunts blood from underventilated to better-ventilated areas of the lung. The afterload against which the right heart has to pump is increased. This elevates the pulmonary artery blood pressure (i.e., pulmonary hypertension). Over the long term, the right heart hypertrophies to work against this increased resistance and eventually may fail (cor pulmonale). Heart enlargement secondary to any cause alters the electrical conduction pattern effecting electromechanical coupling and cardiac output. The altered size and heart position within the chest wall can be detected by ECG changes.

Treatment of emphysema that requires hospitalization often includes intravenous fluids, antibiotics, and low-flow oxygen (Geddes, 1984; Make, 1983). Some patients require bronchodilators, diuretics, and digitalis. Patients with chronic airflow limitation adapt to high $Paco_2$ levels, thus becoming dependent on their hypoxic drives to breathe. Therefore, low flow oxygen is administered to these patients to avoid abolishing their drive to breathe.

The etiology of emphysema is uncertain. The incidence of emphysema increases with age. It is most often found in patients with chronic bronchitis and is significantly more prevalent in smokers than nonsmokers. There appears to be a hereditary factor. Severe panlobular emphysema can develop in patients with an alpha-antitrypsin deficiency relatively early in life even though they never smoked. Repeated lower respiratory tract infections may also play a role in the pathology of emphysema. However, the interrelationship of these and other factors in producing the condition is still not well understood.

Chronic bronchitis and emphysema are marked by a progressive loss of lung function and corresponding cardiac dysfunction. At the end of 5 years, patients with chronic airflow limitation have a death rate four to five times greater than the normal expected value. Death rates reported by various studies depend on the methods of selection of patients, types of diagnostic tests, and other criteria. In general the death rates 5 years after diagnosis are 20% to 55%. The 5-year survival rates based on FEV_1 have been reported as follows: 80% in patients with a FEV_1 greater than 1.2 L, 60% in patients with a FEV_1 close to 1 L, and 40% for patients with a FEV_1 less than 0.75 L. However, if these flow rates are found in patients with complications of resting tachycardia, chronic hypercapnia, and a severely impaired diffusing capacity, the survival rates should be reduced by 25%. Other factors that have been associated with a poor prognosis are cor pulmonale, weight loss, radiological evidence of emphysema, a dyspneic onset, polycythemia, and Hoover's sign (inward movement of the ribs on inspiration).

The most frequent causes of death in patients with airflow limitation are congestive heart failure (secondary to cor pulmonale), respiratory failure, pneumonia, bronchiolitis, and pulmonary embolism.

As emphysema becomes chronic, the hemidiaphragms become more horizontally positioned, placing the muscle fibers at a less efficient position on their length tension curve (Druz and Sharp, 1982). Breathing when the muscle fibers of respiration are mechanically disadvantaged increases the work of breathing and therefore energy demands and oxygen cost. Respiratory muscle weakness and fatigue are serious complications of chronic lung disease that predispose the patient to respiratory muscle failure (Rochester and Arora, 1983) (Chapter 4 and 32).

The net effect of these pathological changes on gas exchange is hypoxemia, hypercapnia, and reduced pH consistent with respiratory acidosis. Long-term respiratory insufficiency leads to chronically impaired oxygen transport and gas exchange. To compensate for hypercapnia, production of bicarbonate is increased to buffer retained CO_2 (i.e., compensated respiratory acidosis). Red blood cell production (i.e., polycythemia) is increased to increase the oxygen-carrying capacity of the blood. The negative effect of polycythemia, however, is increased viscosity of the blood, leading to increased risk of circulatory stasis, thromboses, and increased work of the heart.

Principles of physical therapy management

The patient with emphysema is prone to pulmonary infections and respiratory insufficiency. The clinical picture is hallmarked by alveolar collapse and destruction, ventilation and perfusion mismatching, and diffusion defect. These defects result in impaired or threatened oxygen transport if the physiological compensations are unable to maintain adequate blood gases. Shortness of breath is exacerbated and breathing is labored. Increased work of breathing reflects airway obstruction and inefficiency of respiratory mechanics and the respiratory muscles. Because of long-term airway disease, mucociliary transport is disrupted. Therefore, in the presence of a pulmonary infection and increased production of pulmonary secretions, secretion removal can be a significant problem for the patient.

Specific treatments are prescribed for the patient based on the specific clinical findings (i.e., the type and severity of the cardiopulmonary dysfunction and the presence of infection). Therefore treatments include mobilization coordinated with breathing control and coughing maneuvers, which are effective in enhancing alveolar ventilation, mobilizing secretions, and in ventilation and perfusion matching. Body positioning can be prescribed to alter the distribution of ventilation, to aid mucociliary transport, and to remove pulmonary secretions. Although "pure" emphysema is typically dry, postural drainage positions can facilitate the removal of pulmonary secretions from specific bronchopulmonary segments if indicated. In any given body position, alveolar volume is augmented in the uppermost lung fields and alveolar ventilation is augmented in the lowermost lung fields. The type and extent of pathology will determine the degree of benefit these physiological effects will have on oxygen transport. In addition, body positioning is essential to optimize respiratory mechanics and enhance pulmonary gas exchange, thereby reducing the work of breathing and the work of the heart. The assessment will define the parameters of the treatment prescription that will be effective in relieving the work of breathing and the work of the heart. This information is essential not only for prescribing beneficial positions but also for avoiding deleterious positions. A sitting lean-forward position will assist ventilation secondary to the gravitational effects of the upright position on cardiopulmonary function. If the arms are supported, this position stabilizes the upper chest wall and rib cage, thereby facilitating inspiration. Some patients with horizontal diaphragms and significant respiratory distress benefit from recumbent positions in which the diaphragm is elevated within

the chest wall by the viscera falling against the underside of the diaphragm in this position (i.e., viscerodiaphragmatic breathing) (Barach, 1974). The muscle fibers of the diaphragm are mechanically placed in a more favorable position with respect to their length-tension characteristics. This effect may further be augmented in the head-down position in some patients (Barach and Beck, 1954). Other patients, however, cannot tolerate recumbent positions; in fact, respiratory distress may be increased. If optimal treatment outcome has not been achieved with mobilization and body positioning coordinated with breathing control and coughing maneuvers, conventional physical therapy procedures may offer additional benefit in some patients (e.g., postural drainage and manual techniques).

Because of the tendency toward dynamic airway compression resulting from the highly compliant airways of emphysema patients, open-glottis coughing maneuvers are indicated. Specific outcome measures are recorded before, during, and after treatment to assess short- and long-term treatment effects. In addition, between-treatment treatments are central to maximizing overall treatment efficacy. Thus conveying information effectively and specifically to the patient, nursing staff, and possibly family members is crucial to achieve an optimal treatment outcome.

Comparable with the chronic bronchitis patient, an exercise program for these patients should be prescribed to maximize oxygen transport capacity. Such conditioning may reduce the frequency and severity of subsequent acute exacerbations. In addition, the patient may benefit from other components of a comprehensive pulmonary rehabilitation program.

Acute Exacerbation of Asthma
Pathophysiology and medical management

Asthma is a condition characterized by an increased responsiveness of bronchial smooth muscle to various stimuli and is manifested by widespread narrowing of the airways that changes in severity either spontaneously or as a result of treatment (Hogg, 1984; Rees, 1984). During an asthma attack, the lumen of the airways is narrowed or occluded by a combination of bronchial smooth muscle spasm, inflammation of the mucosa and an overproduction of viscous, tenacious mucus.

Asthma is a widespread disorder affecting 1% of the population. It is common in children under 15 years of age; its prevalence is estimated to be 5% to 15%. It is estimated that 80% of asthmatic children do not have symptoms after the age of 10 years.

Asthma that begins in patients under the age of 35 is usually allergic or extrinsic. These asthma attacks are precipitated when an individual comes into contact with a given substance to which he or she is sensitive, such as pollens or household dust (see the box at right). Often asthmatic patients can be allergic to a number of substances rather than to one or two.

If a patient's first asthma attack occurs after the age of 35, often there is evidence of chronic airway obstruction with intermittent episodes of acute bronchospasm. These individuals, whose attacks are not triggered by specific substances, are referred to as having nonallergic or intrinsic asthma (see box at right). Chronic bronchitis is commonly found in this group, and this is the type of asthma seen in the hospital setting.

The asthmatic patient presents with the following picture during an attack. Lung volumes and expiratory flow rates are reduced, and the distribution of ventilation is less homogeneous (Ross et al., 1992a). The patient has a rapid rate of breathing and uses the accessory respiratory muscles (Figure 4-6, p. 78). The expiratory phase of breathing is prolonged with audible wheezing. The patient may cough frequently, although unproductively, and may complain of tightness in the chest. Radiologically, the lungs may appear hyperinflated or show small atelectatic areas (reabsorption atelectasis). Early in the attack, arterial blood gases reflect slight hypoxemia and a low $PaCO_2$ (from hyperventilation). If the attack progresses, the PO_2 continues to fall as the PCO_2 increases above normal. As obstruction becomes severe, deterioration of the patient is evidenced by a high CO_2, a low PO_2, and a pH of less than 7.3.

Hospitalized asthmatic patients are treated with intravenous fluids, bronchodilators, supplemental oxygen, and corticosteroids. Breathing control in the acute attack relaxes the patient, helps manage the at-

---

Factors That Precipitate Asthmatic Symptoms

Allergic or Extrinsic Asthma

Pollen (especially ragweed)

Animals

Feathers

Molds

Household dust

Food

Nonallergic or Intrinsic Asthma

Inhaled irritants

Cigarette smoke

Dust

Pollution

Chemicals

Weather

High humidity

Cold air

Respiratory infections

Common cold

Bacterial bronchitis

Drugs

Aspirin

Emotions

Stress

Excitement

Exercise

---

tack more effectively, and also provides a means of helping to reduce subsequent attacks. Airway clearance procedures may have a role should the cough become productive. Patients should avoid bronchial irritants and substances that worsen or induce significant bronchospasm or an attack.

An asthmatic attack that persists for several hours and is unresponsive to medical management is referred to as *status asthmaticus*. This condition constitutes a medical emergency, necessitating admission to the intensive care unit (see Chapter 32).

Principles of physical therapy management

The hallmark of an acute exacerbation of asthma is an increased responsiveness of airway smooth muscle to various stimuli (bronchospasm) (i.e., reversible airway obstruction). Although bronchospasm can be a feature of chronic bronchitis and emphysema, the primary cause of airway obstruction in these conditions results from anatomical and physiological changes that are not usually reversible.

Physical therapy is directed at improving gas exchange without aggravating bronchospasm and other symptoms and reversing these when possible. Thus promoting more effective and efficient breathing with relaxed controlled breathing maneuvers and controlled unforced coughing maneuvers in optimal body positions is a priority. Overall oxygen demand, including that associated with an increased work of breathing, needs to be reduced during an exacerbation of asthma. This may require reduced activity, body positioning that improves breathing efficiency, judicious rest and sleep periods, altered diet or restricted diet, adequate hydration, maintaining a thermoneutral environment, rest, reduced arousal, reduced social interaction and excitement, and reduced environmental stimulation. Although general relaxation does not directly relax bronchial smooth muscle, relaxation will assist breathing control, reduce arousal and metabolic demands, and promote more efficient breathing.

Airway narrowing and obstruction is a hallmark of this condition secondary to increased bronchial smooth muscle tone and airway edema. Even small amounts of pulmonary secretions can obstruct the lumen of narrowed airways, which leads to reabsorption atelectasis distal to the site of obstruction, impaired gas exchange, and reduced PaO_2. Thus mucociliary transport is a priority. Mucous clearance can be further impeded by the addition of serous fluid to pulmonary mucus, resulting from airway irritation and inflammation. Cilia are less effective at clearing mucoserous fluid compared with mucus alone. In addition, sheets of ciliated epithelium are shed into the bronchial lumen, further contributing to the stasis of secretions. Thus optimizing the mobilization of secretions and their removal is a priority even in the presence of scant secretions. Interventions that optimize mucociliary transport are selected to minimize exacerbating bronchospasm and further increases in airway resistance.

The primary goals in the management of asthma include reducing airway narrowing, improving alveolar ventilation, reducing the work and energy cost of breathing, reducing hypoxemia or minimizing its threat, and optimizing lung compliance.

Treatment outcome is assessed with indices of oxygen transport overall and of the function of the individual steps in the pathway (Epstein and Henning, 1993). Bedside spirometry, including peak expiratory flow rate, is a sensitive indicator of ensuing compromise in oxygen transport. Some patients use a peak expiratory flow rate meter at home to detect such changes and as an early indicator of the need for medical attention.

Acute Exacerbation of Cystic Fibrosis
Pathophysiology and medical management

Cystic fibrosis (CF) is a complex multisystem disorder transmitted by an autosomal-recessive gene that affects the exocrine glands (Landau, 1973). CF involves all of the major organ systems in the body and is characterized by increased sweat electrolyte content, chronic airflow limitation, ventilation inhomogeneity, and pancreatic insufficiency. Definitive diagnosis of CF includes positive family history, clinical symptoms of poor digestion, growth or recurrent pulmonary infection, and, most importantly, a positive sweat chloride test. Survival has increased dramatically since 1940 when survival was reported to be approximately 2 years of age. In 1980, patients survival was estimated to be 20 years of age and increasing (Hunt and Geddes, 1985). Thus although CF is congenital and manifests in childhood, this condition has now become an adult disorder. Adult patients with CF often have an upper lobe infiltrate, with evidence of atelectasis and bronchiectasis, and chronic staphlococcal infections. The beat frequency of the cilia is often slowed to approximately

3 mm/min, compared with 20 mm/min in age-matched healthy control subjects (Wood, Wanner, Hirsch, and Farrell, 1975). Patients can be categorized into three general groups—those with no significant pulmonary signs, those with pulmonary signs and occasional cough and sputum, and those with pulmonary signs and constant cough and sputum. Those patients in the last group tend to have significantly impaired pulmonary function test results, reduced diffusing capacity, and increased hemoptysis, particularly in the presence of an abnormal chest x-ray and hyperinflation. Airway hyperreactivity appears to be variable.

The A-a gradient for nitrogen reflects lung regions with low ventilation and perfusion ratios. Peripheral airways are often abnormal either anatomically or functionally because of mucous plugging. The lungs of patients with CF may be excessively stiff at maximal lung capacity, with a loss of elastic recoil at low lung volumes (Mansell, Dubrawsky, Levison, Bryan, and Crozier, 1974). Regional ventilation is nonuniform contributing to ventilation and perfusion mismatch and hypoxemia (Cotton, Graham, Mink, and Habbick, 1985; Ross et al., 1992a).

The chronic pulmonary limitation in CF is related to increased secretion of abnormally viscous mucus, impaired mucociliary transport resulting in airway obstruction, bronchiectasis, hyperinflation, infection, and impaired regional ventilatory function, leading to impaired ventilation and perfusion matching and gas exchange. Radiologically, changes are most pronounced in the upper lobes, especially the right upper lobe.

Principles of physical therapy management

Prophylactic cardiopulmonary physical therapy, including facilitation of mucociliary transport and maximizing alveolar ventilation, in conjunction with the judicious use of antibiotics provides effective measures for controlling or slowing the effects of bronchial and bronchiolar obstruction. Involvement of the patient and caregivers in chronic care in the long term is particularly important. Understanding of the pathology and course of CF is essential to modify treatment prescription during exacerbations and remissions of the disease.

The clinical deficits related to oxygen transport include impaired mucociliary transport, increased mucous production, increased difficulty clearing mucus, impaired ventilation and perfusion matching, right-to-left shunt, a diffusion defect, respiratory muscle weakness or fatigue, and reduced cardiopulmonary conditioning (Chatham, Berrow, Beeson, Griffiths, Brough, and Musa, 1994). The increased production of mucus and the difficulty removing mucus increases the risk of bacterial colonization and chronic respiratory infections. These manifestations of CF are worsened with recumbency. Significant postural hypoxemia has been reported in CF patients when moving from sitting to a supine position (Stokes, Wohl, Khaw, and Strieder, 1985). Thus the object of treatment is to optimize oxygen transport and pulmonary gas exchange. Given the pathophysiological deficits in an acute exacerbation of CF, the specific goals are to enhance mucociliary transport, promote airway clearance, optimize alveolar ventilation and therefore gas exchange, maximize the efficiency of oxygen transport overall, and prevent and minimize infection.

Although the degree to which patients with chronic lung conditions, and in particular CF, can respond to aerobic training may be limited, it is essential that their capacity to transport oxygen overall is optimized to compensate for deficits in specific steps of the oxygen transport pathway (Cystic Fibrosis and Physical Activity, *International Journal of Sports Medicine,* 1988; Dean and Ross, 1989). Deconditioning severely impairs oxygen transport. Improved aerobic capacity and cardiopulmonary conditioning is central in the management of CF. Prescriptive aerobic exercise enhances the efficiency of oxygen transport overall by reducing airway resistance by mobilizing secretions, improving the homogeneity of ventilation in the lungs and therefore ventilation and perfusion matching, optimizing oxygen extraction at the tissue level, and increasing respiratory muscle endurance (Keens, Krastins, Wannamaker, Levison, Crozier, and Bryan, 1977; Zach et al., 1992). If optimal conditioning is maintained, oxygen transport is not as compromised during acute exacerbations given the improved efficiency of oxygen transport overall. These effects will be lost, however, as the patient deconditions with restricted mobility and recumbency during the acute episode. Thus it is important that mobility is minimally restricted during an exacerbation (based on the clinical assessment and morbidity) and that exercise conditioning is a mainstay of management between exacerbations. An important additional effect of long-term exercise, which has particular importance for CF patients, is improved immunity (Pyne, 1994; Shepard, Verde, Thomas, and Shek, 1991). This may minimize the risk of infection and perhaps minimize the severity of an infection once acquired.

In severe exacerbations the patient is extremely stressed physiologically, has a significantly increased oxygen consumption, in part because of the increased work of breathing and for the heart, and is prone to arterial desaturation. Thus minimizing undue oxygen demand and fatigue guides the selection of treatment interventions and their parameters in conjunction with stringent monitoring. These patients become hypoxemic and distressed readily. Treatment interventions are selected based on the assessment and the patient's ability to tolerate the treatment and derive optimal benefit. Gradual, paced low-intensity mobilization and frequent body positioning enhance mucociliary transport and airway clearance and maximize the efficiency of the steps in the oxygen transport pathway. Postural drainage can offer additional benefit in these patients if further clearance is required. The addition of manual techniques may be indicated, however, stringent monitoring must be carried out given their potential deleterious effects on gas exchange (Kirilloff, Owens, Rogers, and Mazzocco, 1985; Murray, 1979; Sutton, Pavia, Bateman, and Clarke, 1982).

Forced coughing and expiratory techniques can contribute to airway closure, whereas huffing and other forms of modified coughing with an open glottis minimize airway closure and can be more effective in removing secretions that have accumulated centrally without compromising ventilation and gas exchange (Hietpas et al., 1974; Nunn, Coleman, Sachithanandan, Bergman, and Laws, 1965). Forceful coughing, in which the glottis closes, contributes to airway closure and thus should be avoided, particularly in patients with elevated pulmonary artery pres-

sure, because of the concomitant increase in intrathoracic pressure and strain on the heart and lungs. Patients with CF have severe paroxysms of coughing. This significantly increases intrathoracic pressure, which in turn impedes venous return and cardiac output. Although coughing is an essential mechanism for mucociliary clearance in these patients, the untoward cardiac effects need to be minimized.

Over the past decade, other interventions aimed at secretion clearance in the treatment of CF have included autogenic drainage, the use of the positive expiratory pressure (PEP) mask, and the flutter valve (Pryor, 1993; Webber and Pryor, 1994). Autogenic drainage is based on the theory that the equal pressure point is shifted along the airways by altering the lung volume at which the patient breathes. The patient initially breathes slowly and deliberately at low lung volumes, then at mid and high lung volumes. Breathing at low lung volumes is believed to loosen secretions from the walls of the airways. This is followed by breathing at mid lung volumes, which is believed to help localize and collect the secretions. Finally, breathing at high lung volumes is believed to centralize and facilitate the removal of the secretions with coughing. Thus autogenic drainage may enhance the effectiveness of the patient's cough by manipulating lung volumes and flow rates and controlling coughing to avoid unproductive coughing and wasteful expenditure of energy. The patient is coached by the physical therapist to breathe slowly and deliberately at the volumes set by the therapist who gauges the patient's ventilatory effort and work with the hands around the patient's chest. The patient is not encouraged to breathe below end-expiratory volume and is encouraged to suppress coughing until the expelling phase (i.e., the phase during which the patient is breathing at high lung volumes).

Autogenic drainage may be a useful adjunct for facilitating airway clearance in patients with CF. It is a procedure that patients may use independently and can be applied relatively unobtrusively. It helps optimize the patient's coughing efforts and minimizes the potential for significant airway closure in these patients.

The PEP mask and flutter valve are believed to reduce airway closure and thereby optimize alveolar ventilation and enhance mucociliary clearance in patients with CF.

Acute Exacerbation of Interstitial Pulmonary Fibrosis
Pathophysiology and medical management

Interstitial lung disease has been associated with various occupations and the inhalation of inorganic and organic dusts. Conditions associated with the inhalation of inorganic dusts include silicosis, asbestosis, talc coal dusts, and beryllium. These conditions are most often seen in miners, welders, and construction workers. Workers exposed to organic material, such as fungal spores and plant fibers, may develop a serious pulmonary reaction known as extrinsic allergic alveolitis. Generally, interstitial lung disease is characterized by inflammation of the lung parenchyma, which may resolve completely or progress to fibrosis. Interstitial pulmonary fibrosis results from the deposition of connective tissue after repeated bouts of infection.

The pathophysiological deficits are commensurate with morphological changes of interstitial infiltration and fibrosis, intraalveolar exudate and alveolar replacement (Chung and Dean, 1989) (see Figure 4-12, p. 88). Lung compliance and lung volumes are reduced, expiratory flow at mid lung volume is increased (stiff, inelastic lungs), diffusing capacity is reduced, and hypoxemia can be present in the absence of hypercapnia (Chung and Dean; 1989; Jernudd-Wilhelmsson, Hornblad, and Hedenstierna, 1986). The chest x-ray of a patient with interstitial pulmonary fibrosis secondary to sarcoidosis is shown in Figure 4-12, p. 88. Other changes include increased resting heart rate, pulmonary hypertension, impaired gas exchange, and shortness of breath during exercise and, in some cases, at rest. Symptoms can be reversed by removing the worker from the exposure by a change of employment, by modifying the materials handling process, or by using protective clothing and masks. Repeated exposure to these organic dusts may result in irreversible interstitial fibrosis.

Reaction to fumes and gases can also lead to chronic restrictive patterns of lung disease. Individuals exposed to plastics being heated at high temperatures are also exposed to gases that are toxic to the respiratory system. Chronic pathological changes and impaired gas exchange can result.

Medical management is directed at reducing inflammation, reducing pulmonary hypertension, and increasing arterial oxygenation. Pharmacological management may include corticosteroids for inflammation, immunosuppressive agents, and oxygen therapy. Removing the patient from the work environment contributing to interstitial pulmonary fibrosis is essential in managing the disease and its long-term consequences.

Principles of physical therapy management

The primary clinical manifestations of an acute exacerbation of interstitial pulmonary fibrosis reflect an acute on chronic problem usually resulting from an inflammatory episode, pulmonary infection, or both. The mechanisms responsible include reduced alveolar ventilation, an inflammatory process and its manifestations, potential airway obstruction, and increased work of breathing and of the heart in severe cases. These patients are prone to desaturation during exercise and thus need to be monitored closely.

In mild cases, mobilization increases the homogeneity of ventilation, and ventilation and perfusion matching (Jernudd-Wilhelmsson et al., 1986). Between treatments and in the management of the severely affected patient, body positioning is used to reduce the work of breathing and arousal, maximize alveolar ventilation, maximize ventilation and perfusion matching, and optimize coughing.

Patients with moderate-to-severe interstitial lung disease may desaturate during sleep (Perez-Padilla, West, and Lertzman, 1985) and readily desaturate on physical exertion (Arita, Nishida, and Hiramoto, 1981), thus warranting close monitoring during and between treatments. Increased pulmonary vascular resistance secondary to hypoxic vasoconstriction contributes to increased work of the right heart and potential cardiac insufficiency.

General debility and deconditioning warrant a modified exercise program that can optimize the function of all of the steps in the oxygen transport pathway (Arita et al., 1981; Chung and Dean, 1989).

Tuberculosis

Pathophysiology and medical management

Although the incidence of tuberculosis, a life-long disease, has declined significantly over the past several decades, this disease has been experiencing a resurgence in the industrialized world in recent decades. This may reflect declining sanitation and health standards in some segments of the population and immigration patterns.

Most infections result from inhalation of airborne tubercle bacilli, which triggers an inflammatory response (Luce, 1986). This response includes flooding of the affected area with fluid leukocytes, and later macrophages. The area becomes consolidated and pathologically the condition is considered a tuberculous pneumonia. The infiltrating macrophages become localized and fused, resulting in the characteristic tubercle. Within 2 to 4 weeks, the central part of the lesion necroses. Tuberculosis is associated primarily with pulmonary infection that is comparable with other infectious pneumonias. Tuberculosis, however, is distinct in that it may affect other parts of the body. Symptoms include fatigue, fever, reduced appetite, weight loss, night sweats, hemoptysis, and a cough with small amounts of nonpurulent sputum with pulmonary involvement. The course of the disease is variable. Some lesions heal promptly, whereas other patients experience progression and ensuing death. Other systems that can be involved include brain and meninges, kidney, reproductive system, and bone. In some individuals the disease appears to remit, whereas in others tuberculosis progresses to affect other organ systems or previously dormant foci can be reactivated.

The effects of tuberculosis on pulmonary function are variable, depending on the extent and type of lesions. Lesions may involve the lung parenchyma, the bronchi, the pleurae, and chest wall. Parenchymal involvement can reduce lung volumes, leading to hypoventilation of perfused lung units. Significant disease leads to impaired arterial blood gases, whereas areas of unaffected lung may adequately compensate in milder cases. If fibrosis has occurred, lung compliance will be correspondingly reduced. Airflow resistance may be increased from narrowing or distortion of the bronchioles because of fibrosis. Pleural involvement may result in effusions, empyema, pleural fibrosis, and spontaneous pneumothorax. Unlike parenchymal damage, small amounts of pleural restriction can produce significant changes in pulmonary function. Clinically, patients with significant pleural involvement have significant restrictive disease and correspondingly low lung volumes. The work and energy cost of breathing are markedly increased. Shortness of breath is a common complaint. Comparable with an interstitial pulmonary fibrosis patient, the patient adopts a rapid shallow breathing pattern to reduce the high cost of elastic work of breathing. Thus the dead space tends to be hyperventilated and alveolar hypoventilation results.

In addition to alveolar hypoventilation, lung tissue and pulmonary vascular damage impairs ventilation and perfusion matching and diffusing capacity. In severe cases, hypoxemia and hypercapnia are present. Chronic adaptation includes polycythemia and hypervolemia. Right heart failure may ensue.

The lungs become shrunken and geometrically distorted because of fibrotic changes in the lungs. These changes can lead to kinking and obstruction of the pulmonary blood vessels and maldistribution of pulmonary blood flow, which further compromises ventilation and perfusion matching.

Tuberculosis may be associated with an obstructive component. An increase in airflow resistance comparable with emphysema can be present. This obstruction results from chronic infection, mucosal edema, retained secretions, and bronchospasm.

Antibiotics can be effective in managing the disease such that hospitalization is avoided. If detected early, the prognosis is favorable, provided the patient adheres to the medication schedule and the bacilli do not become resistant to the medications. Surgery may be indicated to resect lung segments that are chronically involved. The extent and severity of the disease determines the course of recovery.

The maintenance of good general health is particularly important in the management, control, and prevention of tuberculosis (e.g., sanitation, balanced diet, sleep, regular exercise, and stress control).

Principles of physical therapy management

Although the acute presentation of tuberculosis is comparable with acute pneumonia (refer to pneumonia section), there are some important differences with respect to physical therapy management. First, tuberculosis is particularly infectious, thus special precautions should be taken by the physical therapist to prevent its spread during its infectious stage. Second, patients are prone to excessive fatigue; treatments should be selected to promote improved oxygen transport without exceeding the patient's capacity to deliver oxygen and without contributing to excessive fatigue. Stimulation of the oxygen transport system with exercise is necessary to avoid the deleterious effects of deconditioning and further compromise of oxygen transport. The patient therefore warrants being monitored closely.

Hypertension

Pathophysiology and medical management

Essential hypertension is the most common type of hypertension (90% of all reported cases) (i.e., of unknown etiology). Generally, hypertension is classified as mild, moderate, or severe. Hypertension is managed pharmacologically with vasodilators (i.e., afterload reducers), diuretics (i.e., volume reducers), and beta-blocking agents (i.e., inotrophic agents). Hypertension is a significant health-care concern in that this condition is frequently associated with heart disease and stroke. Thus its consequences can be dire.

Principles of physical therapy management

Physical therapists treat patients with hypertension as a primary or secondary condition. A prescription of regular aerobic exercise may control hypertension (Froelicher, 1987; Goldberger, 1990). The prescription is based on a consideration of the patient's coexistent problems and general health status. If obesity is a concurrent problem, an exercise program is prescribed to address both concerns.

More frequently, physical therapists treat patients whose hypertension is a secondary condition. Thus, whether the patient is being treated for osteoarthritis, stroke, or cardiopulmonary dysfunction, treatment is modified accordingly. An exercise prescription includes generalized aerobic exercise at an intensity that is optimally therapeutic and not associated with any excessive or untoward hemodynamic responses (Blair, Painter, Pate, Smith, and Taylor, 1988).

Labile hypertensive patients are the most difficult patients to prescribe an exercise program for because of the irregularity of their blood pressure responses. The intensity is modified at each session to accommodate these variations. Because beta-blockers and other medications blunt heart rate responses to exercise, the exercise prescription parameters are defined on the basis of some other objective hemodynamic response or on subjective responses (e.g., the Borg scale of perceived exertion).

The benefits of a modified aerobic exercise prescription include elimination of medication, reduction of medication, and improved pharmacological control on the same dose of medication. In addition, the patient derives all the other multisystem health benefits of exercise. A program of aerobic exercise should be carried out in conjunction with other life-style changes associated with blood pressure control (e.g., nutrition, weight control, stress reduction, and smoking cessation program). Medications should be monitored by the physician during the training program. In addition to exercise having a direct effect on controlling hypertension, the effect of exercise on overall metabolism may alter the absorption and degradation of the medications, which in turn can reduce the prescriptive requirements of that medication. Those types of exercise that are associated with a disproportionate hemodynamic challenge (e.g., static movements and stabilizing postures) are not usually indicated. Rather, aerobic exercise that is rhythmic, involves the large muscles of the legs and possibly the arms, and is performed frequently is indicated (Blair et al., 1988).

Angina

Pathophysiology and medical management

Angina refers to pain resulting from ischemia of the myocardium and often precedes myocardial infarction.

Coronary artery disease is the primary cause of myocardial infarction and is among the leading causes of death in the Western world. Life-style factors including high-fat diet, stress, and low activity levels contribute to atherosclerosis and fat deposition within the coronary blood vessels. When these deposits narrow or totally occlude the vessel lumen, blood flow is restricted or totally obstructed. As the heart continues to demand oxygen and nutrients to work, blood supply needs to be increased. If one or more of the myocardial blood vessels is stenosed, insufficient blood reaches the working myocardial fibers, and ischemia and pain result. Although the classic description of anginal pain is retrosternal vice-like, gripping pain radiating to the left side and down the arm and up into the neck, anginal pain may occur bilaterally anywhere above the umbilicus. Furthermore, patients vary considerably with respect to the degree to which the severity of the pain correlates with the degree of myocardial ischemia and infarction. Thus even apparently minimal chest pain may be associated with significant ischemia and should not be minimized with respect to its clinical significance.

Principles of physical therapy management

The management of patients with heart disease who are hemodynamically unstable and require intensive monitoring to assess and to monitor physical therapy treatment is described in Chapter 32. This chapter addresses the management of the cardiac medical patient who is stable and uncomplicated. Physical therapists must be knowledgeable and proficient in the management of the cardiac patient because these patients are referred with cardiac disease as a primary or secondary problem. Because physical therapy invariably involves physically stressing a patient either with therapeutic exercise or with the application of a therapeutic modality, the physical therapist must address the following questions when managing a patient with heart disease:

1. Does the patient's cardiac status preclude treatment? Why?
2. Is additional information on the patient needed before physical therapy assessment and treatment? What information?
3. How should treatment be modified? Why?
4. Is the patient using antianginal medication appropriately? Is the prescription current? Are there other medications that may influence the patient's cardiopulmonary status and response to treatment? What are they? Does the patient have the antianginal medication present at all times?
5. What physiological parameters should be monitored before, during, and after treatment?
6. What is the patient's knowledge about his or her condition? Can the patient clearly identify what triggers the angina and what makes it worse and better? What life-style changes have been made? What should be reinforced and what education is needed?

A key consideration in the management of any patient with cardiovascular dysfunction is minimizing myocardial strain (Sokolow et al., 1990). Thus mobilization and exercise prescription needs to incorporate an appropriate warm-up, steady-rate, cool-down, and recovery phases, and the type of exercise should be rhythmic and involve the legs (i.e., areas of large muscle mass) and possibly the arms as well. Initially, low-intensity activity that restricts the heart rate to no more than 20 beats above resting heart rate may be indicated to minimize the work of the heart without immobilizing the patient completely. Ejection fraction is not necessarily a good indicator of exercise tolerance because these variables are not well correlated (Dean, 1993). Upper-extremity work alone is more hemodynamically demanding than lower extremity work and thus is prescribed cautiously if at all, at least in the early stage. Exercise or physical activity, involving sustained static postures and isometric muscle contraction, are contraindicated. Breathing should be coordinated with activity such that breath holding and straining are avoided.

A patient with a history of angina, regardless of whether that individual is taking antianginal medications, must be hemodynamically monitored (i.e., heart rate, blood pressure, rate pressure product, and subjective responses).

Patients prone to angina may exhibit symptoms in certain body positions (Lange, Katz, McBride, Moore, and Hillis, 1988; Langou, Wolfson, Olson, and Cohen, 1977; Prakash, Parmley, Dikshit, Forrester, and Swan, 1973). Usually, this reflects an increased workload and increased work of the heart. Recumbent positions increase the mechanical work of the heart by increasing central blood volume (Kaneko, Milic-Emili, Dolovich, Dawson, and Bates, 1966). These patients are not encouraged to lie flat, instead the head of bed is elevated 10 to 15 degrees. Sidelying positions, particularly left sidelying, increase the work of the heart by compressing the heart and impeding ventricular filling and ejection. Patients with impaired oxygen transport and without prior cardiac disease may exhibit myocardial stress and ischemia in these body positions. Thus patients with impaired or threatened oxygenation must be monitored closely, particularly during turning and activities in which oxygen demand is increased and oxygen delivery needs to increase correspondingly.

Uncompliicated Myocardial Infarction
Pathophysiology and medical management

Myocardial infarction commonly referred to as a *heart attack* refers to insufficient myocardial perfusion resulting in a macroscopic area of damage and necrosis of the heart. Infarction results most frequently from narrowing and occlusion of the coronary blood vessels secondary to atherosclerosis. Other causes include occlusion secondary to a thrombus or embolus, reduced blood pressure, or coronary vasospasm. Angina, or ischemic chest pain, often precedes or accompanies a myocardial infarction. Infarctions vary in severity from being silent (i.e., having no characteristic signs and symptoms) and thus going undetected to being fatal. Most infarctions when detected require some hospitalization and monitoring to ensure that the infarction is not evolving further and that the patient is medically stable and in no danger. Chapter 32 describes the management of patients with myocardial infarctions who are admitted to a coronary care unit. This section focuses on the patient with mild heart disease, the medical cardiac patient who is discharged from hospital, the patient who has a history of ischemic heart disease, and the patient who is hospitalized for a condition other than heart disease but develops and is being managed for myocardial ischemia. Judicious movement and body positioning are essential elements in the man-

agement of the myocardial infarction patient (Harrison, 1944). Because these interventions can place significant demands on cardiopulmonary function and oxygen transport, they must be prescribed specifically by physical therapists with considerable knowledge and expertise in the area.

Principles of physical therapy management

Physical therapy stresses patients hemodynamically (Dean, Murphy, Parrent, and Rousseau, 1995). Thus the adequacy of their cardiopulmonary system to effect oxygen transport during and between treatments is essential to establish. The optimal treatment prescription is based on the patient's overall signs and symptoms of coronary insufficiency and hemodynamic instability. The physical therapist must be knowledgeable in detecting inadequate myocardial tissue perfusion and in reducing and preventing myocardial tissue damage. In addition, acute or chronic impaired heart pump function leads to reduced cardiac output and systemic tissue perfusion. Clinical manifestations include reduced mentation, reduced renal function, fatigue, malaise, and moist, cool, and cyanotic skin.

Regardless of whether the patient is being treated in hospital, either on the ward or in the department, or in the private physical therapy clinic, the patient must be hemodynamically monitored. Minimally, heart rate and blood pressure must be taken before, during, and after treatment, along with a subjective rating of anginal chest pain. ECG monitoring is usually continuous in the early stages of the infarction. The object of treatment is to have the patient remain below his or her anginal threshold so that anginal pain is avoided. Breathlessness or rating of perceived exertion may also be used. The rate pressure product (RPP) (i.e., the product of heart rate and systolic blood pressure) is highly correlated with myocardial oxygen uptake and work. Previous stress tests will establish the RPP at which angina occurs and the intensity of the exercise dose should be set at 65% to 80% of this threshold. Patients on beta-blockers have a blunted hemodynamic response to exercise, particularly heart rate responses. Use of ratings of perceived exertion to define the upper and lower limits of an acceptable mobilization stimulus may be indicated in these patients.

In some cases, patients have labile angina (i.e., the onset of angina does not occur reliably at a given RPP). This patient and the patient who reports angina at rest are at higher risk and appropriate precautions must be taken. First, the patient must be assessed to establish that treatment is not precluded (see pertinent questions to be answered before treating a patient with angina). Second, monitoring is essential and may include ECG monitoring. Third, treatments are prescribed below symptom threshold, which is usually consistent with a low exercise intensity in these patients. Comparable with any patient experiencing low functional work capacity, exercise prescribed on an interval schedule enables the patient to achieve a greater volume of work.

Similar to the patient with angina, body positions are selected for the patient with a myocardial infarction that will minimize the work of breathing and of the heart (Sonnenblick, Ross, and Bruanwald, 1968). Significant central fluid shifts are minimized by encouraging the upright position as much as possible to reduce the work of the heart (Levine and Lown, 1952) and by maintaining the head of bed up to 10 to 15 degrees when the patient is recumbent. Patients with elevated intracardiac pressures are less susceptible to orthostatism (Chapter 18).

Comparable with the management of the patient who has a history of angina, body positions, static postures, activities, and respiratory maneuvers associated with increased hemodynamic strain (e.g., breath holding) are avoided.

Relaxation is central in the management of the cardiac patient who is prone to being anxious and apprehensive. Relaxation interventions include autogenic relaxation, progressive relaxation, Benson's relaxation response procedures, biofeedback, and meditation (Underhill et al., 1989). Also, the patient needs to identify and minimize stress triggers and effective individual-specific nonpharmacological relaxants. Relaxation training with or without pharmacological support can be integrated into treatment (Underhill et al., 1989; Webber and Pryor, 1994). Patients with heart disease are often apprehensive and anxious about the intensity of physical activity they can undertake. Thus performing physical activity and exercise while monitored and under the supervision of a physical therapist is often reassuring and gives the patient confidence for performing activity when unsupervised.

The quality and quantity of the patient's sleep and a profile of sleep-wake periods should be reviewed to ensure he or she is deriving maximal benefit. REM sleep with bursts of sympathetic activity during the early hours of the morning may constitute a period of increased risk for the cardiac patient.

Appropriate safety precautions must be taken in all settings where physical therapists practice, given that most physical therapy interventions physically stress patients and that coronary symptoms can occur regardless of whether the patient has a known underlying heart disease. In addition, because the population is aging, physical therapists are treating a growing number of older persons who are known to have a higher prevalence of cardiovascular disease.

Good life-style habits are central to maximizing recovery and improving the long-term prognosis (e.g., good nutrition and hydration, good sleep habits, stress management, and regular physical exercise that is prescribed by the physical therapist) (Underhill et al., 1989).

SUMMARY

The primary acute cardiopulmonary medical conditions that are treated by physical therapists include primary lung dysfunction (i.e., atelectasis, pneumonia, bronchitis, bronchiolitis, alveolitis, alveolar proteinosis, and acute exacerbations of chronic airflow limitation, asthma, cystic fibrosis, interstitial pulmonary fibrosis, and tuberculosis) and primary cardiac disease including hypertension, uncomplicated angina, and myocardial infarction. This chapter focuses on the pathophysiology underlying these disorders and the mechanisms by which they threaten or impair heart-lung interaction and oxygen transport. Thus the basis for the principles of cardiopulmonary physical therapy are described rather than specific treatment prescriptions. Treatment prescription is based on the effects of restricted mobility, recumbency, and extrinsic and intrinsic factors in addition to the underlying pathology. Management is directed at the underlying pathophysiological mechanisms resulting from these four factors wherever possible and secondarily to symptom reduction. To prioritize treatments, the most physiological interventions are exploited foremost because these address multiple steps in the oxygen transport pathway. Less physiological interventions (i.e., conventional cardiopulmonary physical therapy) are instituted after the most physiological interventions have been exploited or in conjunction with these. The challenge of clinical problem solving is determining the optimal treatment prescription that will effect the best results with respect to oxygen transport with the least risk in the shortest period of time.

REVIEW QUESTIONS

1. Describe the primary cardiopulmonary pathophysiology of *acute* atelectasis, pneumonia, bronchitis, bronchiolitis, alveolitis, alveolar proteinosis, acute exacerbations of chronic airflow limitation, asthma, cystic fibrosis, interstitial pulmonary fibrosis, tuberculosis, hypertension, stable angina, and stable myocardial infarction.

2. Relate cardiopulmonary physical therapy treatment interventions to the underlying pathophysiology of *each* of the above acute conditions and provide the *rationale* for your choice.

References

Arita, K.I., Nishida, O., & Hiramoto, T. (1981). Physical exercise in "pulmonary fibrosis". *Hiroshima Journal of Medical Science, 30,* 149-159.

Bake, B., Dempsey, J., & Grimby, G. (1976). Effects of shape changes of the chest wall on distribution of inspired gas. *American Review of Respiratory Disease, 114,* 1113-1120.

Barach, A.L. (1974). Chronic obstructive lung disease: postural relief of dyspnea. *Archives of Physical Medicine and Rehabilitation, 55,* 494-504.

Barach, A.L., & Beck, G.J. (1954). Ventilatory effects of head-down position in pulmonary emphysema. *American Journal of Medicine, 16,* 55-60.

Bartelett, J.G., & Gorbach, S.L. (1976). The triple threat of pneumonia. *Chest, 68,* 4-10.

Bates, D.V. (1989). *Respiratory function in diseases* (3rd ed.). Philadelphia: WB Saunders.

Bennett, W.D., Foster, W.M., & Chapman, W.F. (1990). Cough-enhanced mucus clearance in the normal lung. *Journal of Applied Physiology, 69,* 1670-1675.

Blair, S.N., Painter, P., Pate, R.R., Smith, L.K., & Taylor, C.B. (1988). *Resource manual for guidelines for exercise testing and prescription.* Philadelphia: Lea & Febiger.

Burke, C.M., Glanville, A.R., Theodore, J., & Robin, E.D. (1987). Lung immunogenicity, rejection, and obliterative bronchiolitis. *Chest, 92,* 547-549.

Chatham, K., Berrow, S., Beeson, C., Griffiths, L., Brough, D., & Musa, I. (1994). Inspiratory pressures in adult cystic fibrosis. *Physiotherapy, 80,* 748-752.

Chung, F., & Dean, E. (1989). Pathophysiology and cardiorespiratory consequences of interstitial lung disease—review and clinical implications. *Physical Therapy, 69,* 956-966.

Clauss, R.H., Scalabrini, B.Y., Ray, R.F., & Reed, G.E. (1968). Effects of changing body position upon improved ventilation-perfusion relationships. *Circulation, 37* (Suppl 4), 214-217.

Cotton, D.J., Graham, B.L., Mink, J.T., & Habbick, B.F. (1985). Reduction of the single breath diffusing capacity in cystic fibrosis. *European Journal of Respiratory Diseases, 66,* 173-180.

Cystic fibrosis and physical activity. (1988). *International Journal of Sports Medicine, 9* (Suppl. 1), 1-64.

Dantzker, D.R. (1983). The influence of cardiovascular function on gas exchange. *Clinics in Chest Medicine, 4,* 149-159.

Dantzker, D.R. (1988). Oxygen transport and utilization. *Respiratory Care, 33,* 874-880.

Dean, E. (1985). Effect of body position on pulmonary function. *Physical Therapy, 65,* 613-618.

Dean, E., & Ross, J. (1989). Integrating current literature in the management of cystic fibrosis: a rejoinder. *Physiotherapy Canada, 41,* 46-47.

Dean, E., & Ross, J. (1992a). Oxygen transport. The basis for contemporary cardiopulmonary physical therapy and its optimization with body positioning and mobilization. *Physical Therapy Practice, 1,* 34-44.

Dean, E., & Ross, J. (1992b). Mobilization and exercise conditioning. In C. Zadai (Ed.), *Pulmonary management in physical therapy.* New York: Churchill Livingstone.

Don, H.F., Craig, D.B., Wahba, W.M., & Couture, J.G. (1971). The measurement of gas trapped in the lungs at functional residual capacity and the effects of posture. *Anesthesiology, 35,* 582-590.

Douglas, W.W., Rehder, K., Beynen, F.M., Sessler, A., D., & Marsh, H. M. (1977). Improved oxygenation in patients with acute respiratory failure: the prone position. *American Review of Respiratory Disease, 115,* 559-566.

Dripps, R.D., & Waters, R.M. (1941). Nursing care of the surgical patient. 1. The "stir-up." *American Journal of Nursing, 41,* 23-34.

Druz, W.S., & Sharp, J.T. (1982). Electrical and mechanical activity of the diaphragm accompanying body position in severe chronic obstructive pulmonary disease. *American Review of Respiratory Disease, 125,* 275-280.

Epidemiology Standardization Project. American Thoracic Society. (1989). *American Review of Respiratory Disease, 118,* 1-120.

Epstein, C.D., & Henning, R.J. (1993). Oxygen transport variables in the identification and treatment of tissue hypoxia. *Heart and Lung, 22* 328-348.

Froelicher, V.F. (1987). *Exercise and the heart. Clinical concepts* (2nd ed.). St. Louis: Mosby.

Geddes, D.M. (1984). Chronic airflow obstruction. *Postgraduate Medicine, 60,* 194-200.

Glaister, D.H. (1967). The effect of posture on the distribution of ventilation and blood flow in the normal lung. *Clinical Science, 33,* 391-398.

Goldberger, E. (1990). *Essentials of clinical cardiology.* Philadelphia: J.B. Lippincott.

Grimby, G. (1974). Aspects of lung expansion in relation to pulmonary physiotherapy. *American Review of Respiratory Disease, 110,* 145-153.

Hammon, W.E. (1987). Pathophysiology of chronic pulmonary disease. In D.L. Frownfelter (Ed.), *Chest physical therapy and pulmonary rehabilitation* (2nd ed.). St. Louis: Mosby.

Hasani, A., Pavia, D., Agnew, J.E., & Clarke, S.W. (1991). The effect of unproductive coughing/FET on regional mucus movement in the human lungs. *Respiratory Medicine, 85,* 23-26.

Hietpas, B.G., Roth, R.D., & Jensen, W.M. (1974). Huff coughing and airway patency. *Respiratory Care, 24,* 710.

Hogg, J.C. (1984). The pathology of asthma. *Clinics in Chest Medicine, 5,* 567-571.

Hunt, B., & Geddes, D.M. (1985). Newly diagnosed cystic fibrosis in middle and later life. *Thorax, 40,* 23-26.

Jernudd-Wilhelmsson, Y., Hornblad, Y., & Hedenstierna, G. (1986). Ventilation perfusion relationships in interstitial lung disease. *European Journal of Respiratory Disease, 68,* 39-49.

Kaneko, K., Milic-Emili, J., Dolovich, M.B., Dawson, A., & Bates, D.V. (1966). Regional distribution of ventilation and perfusion as a function of body position. *Journal of Applied Physiology, 21,* 767-777.

Keens, T.G., Krastins, I.R.B., Wannamaker, E.M., Levison, H., Crozier, D.N., & Bryan, A.C. (1977). Ventilatory muscle endurance training in normal subjects and patients with cystic fibrosis. *American Review of Respiratory Disease, 116,* 853-860.

Kirilloff, L.H., Owens, G.R., Rogers, R.M., & Mazzocco, M.C. (1985). Does chest physical therapy work? *Chest, 88,* 436-444.

Landau, L.I., & Phelan, P.D. (1973). The spectrum of cystic fibrosis. *American Review of Respiratory Disease, 108,* 593-602.

Lange, R.A., Katz, J., McBride, W., Moore, D.M., & Hillis, L.D. (1988). Effects of supine and lateral positions on cardiac output and intracardiac pressures. *American Journal of Cardiology, 62,* 330-333.

Langou, R.A., Wolfson, S., Olson, E.G., & Cohen, L.S. (1977). Effects of orthostatic postural changes on myocardial oxygen demands. *American Journal of Cardiology, 39,* 418-421.

Leblanc, P., Ruff, F., & Milic-Emili, J. (1970). Effects of age and body position on "airway closure" in man. *Journal of Applied Physiology, 28,* 448-451.

Lewis, F.R. (1980). Management of atelectasis and pneumonia. *Surgical Clinics of North America, 60,* 1391-1401.

Luce, J.M. (1986). Lung disease of adults. *American Lung Association.*

Make, B. (1983). Medical management of emphysema. *Clinics in Chest Medicine, 4,* 465-482.

Mansell, A., Dubrawsky, C., Levison, H., Bryan, A.C., & Crozier, D.N. (1974). Lung elastic recoil in cystic fibrosis. *American Review of Respiratory Disease, 109,* 190-197.

Muller, R.E., Petty, T.L., & Filley, G.F. (1970). Ventilation and arterial blood gas changes induced by pursed-lip breathing. *Journal of Applied Physiology, 28,* 784-789.

Murray, E. (1993). Anyone for pulmonary rehabilitation? *Physiotherapy, 79,* 705-710.

Murray, J.E., & Nadel, J.A. (1988a). *Textbook of respiratory medicine,* (Part 1). Philadelphia: WB Saunders.

Murray, J.E., & Nadel, J.A. (1988b). *Textbook of respiratory medicine,* (Part 2). Philadelphia: WB Saunders.

Murray, J.E. (1979). The ketchup-bottle method. *New England Journal of Medicine, 300,* 1155-1157.

Nunn, J.F., Coleman, A.J., Sachithanandan, T., Bergman, N.A., & Laws, J.W. (1965). Hypoxaemia and atelectasis produced by forced expiration. *British Journal of Anaesthesia, 37,* 3-12.

Oldenburg, F.A., Dolovich, M.B., Montgomery, J.M., & Newhouse, M.T. (1979). Effects of postural drainage, exercise, and cough on mucus clearance in chronic bronchitis. *American Review of Respiratory Disease, 120,* 739-745.

Orlava, O.E. (1959). Therapeutic physical culture in the complex treatment of pneumonia. *Physical Therapy Review, 39,* 153-160.

Perez-Padilla, R., West, P., & Lertzman, M. (1985). Breathing during sleep in patients with interstitial lung disease. *American Review of Respiratory Disease, 132,* 224-229.

Piehl, M.A., & Brown, R.S. (1976). Use of extreme position changes in acute respiratory failure. *Critical Care Medicine, 4,* 13-14.

Prakash, R., Parmley, W.W., Dikshit, K., Forrester, J., & Swan, H.J. (1973). Hemodynamic effects of postural changes in patients with acute myocardial infarction. *Chest, 64,* 7-9.

Pryor, J.A. (1993). *Respiratory care.* Edinburgh: Churchill Livingstone.

Pyne, D.B. (1994). Regulation of neutrophil function during exercise. *Sports Medicine, 17,* 245-258.

Ray, R.F., Yost, L., Moallem, S. (1974). Immobility, hypoxemia, and pulmonary arteriovenous shunting. *Archives of Surgery, 109,* 537-541.

Rees, J. (1984). ABC of asthma. Definition and diagnosis. *British Medical Journal, 5,* 1370-1372.

Remolina, C., Khan, A.U., Santiago, T.V., & Edelman, N.H. (1981). Positional hypoxemia in unilateral lung disease. *New England Journal of Medicine, 304,* 523-525.

Rochester, D.F., & Arora, N.S. (1983). Respiratory muscle failure. *Medical Clinics of North America, 67,* 573-597.

Ross, J., Bates, D.V., Dean, E., & Abboud, R.T. (1992a). Discordance of airflow limitation and ventilation inhomogeneity in asthma and cystic fibrosis. *Clinical and Investigative Medicine, 15,* 97-102.

Ross, J., & Dean, E. (1989). Integrating physiological principles into the comprehensive management of cardiopulmonary dysfunction. *Physical Therapy, 69,* 255-259.

Ross, J., & Dean, E. (1992). Body positioning. In C. C. Zadai, (Ed.). *Pulmonary management in physical therapy.* New York: Churchill Livingstone.

Ross, J., Dean, E., & Abboud, R.T. (1992b). The effect of postural drainage positioning on ventilation homogeneity in healthy subjects. *Physical Therapy, 72,* 794-799.

Roussos, C.S., Fixley, M., Geriest, J., Cosio, M., Kelly, S., Martin, R.R., & Engel, L.A. (1977). Voluntary factors influencing the distribution of inspired gas. *American Review of Respiratory Disease, 116,* 457-467.

Scharf, S.M., & Cassidy, S.S. (Eds.). (1989). *Heart-lung interactions in health and disease.* New York: Marcel-Dekker.

Shephard, R.J., Verde, T.J., Thomas, S.G., & Shek, P. (1991). Physical activity and the immune system. *Canadian Journal of Sports Science, 16,* 163-185.

Sokolow, M., McIlroy, M.B., & Cheitlin, M.D. (1990). *Clinical cardiology* (5th ed.). Norwalk: Appleton & Lange.

Sonnenblick, E.H., Ross, J. Jr., & Braunwald, E. (1968). Oxygen consumption of the heart. Newer concepts of its multifactorial determination. *American Journal of Cardiology, 22,* 328-336.

Stokes, D.C., Wohl, M.E.B., Khaw, K.T., & Strieder, D.J. (1985). Postural hypoxemia in cystic fibrosis. *Chest, 87,* 785-789.

Sutton, P.P., Pavia, D., Bateman, J.R.M., & Clarke, S.W. (1982). Chest physiotherapy—a review. *European Journal of Respiratory Disease, 63,* 188-201.

Underhill, S.L., Woods, S.L., Froelicher, E.S.S., & Halpenny, C.J. (1989). *Cardiac nursing* (2nd ed.). Philadelphia: JB Lippincott.

Wasserman, K.L., & Whipp, B.J. (1975). Exercise physiology in health and disease. *American Review of Respiratory Disease, 112,* 219-249.

Webber, B.A., & Pryor, J.A. (1994). *Physiotherapy for respiratory and cardiac problems.* Edinburgh: Churchill Livingstone.

West, J.B. (1987). *Pulmonary pathophysiology.* Baltimore: Williams & Wilkins.

Wolff, R.K., Dolovich, M.B., Obminski, G., & Newhouse, M.T. (1977). Effects of exercise and eucapnic hyperventilation on bronchial clearance in man. *Journal of Applied Physiology, 43,* 46-50.

Wood, R.E., Wanner, A., Hirsch, J., & Farrell, P.M. (1975). Tracheal mucociliary transport in patients with cystic fibrosis and its stimulation by terbutlaine. *American Review of Respiratory Disease, 111,* 733-738.

Zach, M., Oberwaldner, B., & Hausler, F. (1982). Cystic fibrosis: physical exercise versus chest physiotherapy. *Archives of Diseases in Children, 57,* 587-589.

Zack, M.B., Pontoppidan, H., & Kazemi, H. (1974). The effect of lateral positions on gas exchange in pulmonary disease. *American Review of Respiratory Disease, 110,* 149-153.

CHAPTER 28

Acute Surgical Conditions

Elizabeth Dean
Maureen Fogel Perlstein
Mary Mathews

K E Y   T E R M S

Anesthesia	Sedation
Cardiovascular surgery	Surgery
Risk factors	Thoracic surgery

INTRODUCTION

The purpose of this chapter is to review the management of cardiopulmonary dysfunction secondary to acute surgical conditions. The cardiopulmonary effects of surgery are described. The two types of surgery that have the greatest impact on cardiopulmonary function, namely, thoracic and cardiovascular surgery, are then presented. These surgeries are particularly invasive and lengthy, require heavy and prolonged anesthesia and sedation, and are associated with increased risk, thus warranting intensive perioperative physical therapy.

The four categories of factors contributing to or threatening oxygen transport are described in Chapter 16. Specifically, these factors include the underlying pathology, restricted mobility, and recumbency, extrinsic factors related to the patient's care and intrinsic factors related to the patient. This chapter examines in detail the extrinsic factors related to surgery and anesthesia and the impact of underlying disease, restricted mobility, recumbency, and intrinsic factors on the effects of surgery and anesthesia.

Treatment principles are presented. These are not intended to be a treatment prescription for a particular

495

patient. The effects of surgery and anesthesia need to be considered in addition to the underlying pathology, the effects of restricted mobility, body position, and intrinsic and extrinsic factors (see Chapter 28). All of these factors must be considered and integrated in the treatment prescription and in defining the precise parameters of the prescription. Such integration is essential for treatment to be specific and maximally efficacious. For specific examples of patient treatment prescriptions refer to the companion text *Clinical case studies in cardiopulmonary physical therapy.*

PERIOPERATIVE COURSE
Surgery and its Cardiopulmonary Consequences

Many factors contribute to perioperative cardiopulmonary dysfunction (see the box at right). Anesthesia and tissue dissection contribute to major changes in lung volume, mechanics, and gas exchange. The extent and duration of these changes increase with the magnitude of the operative procedure and degree of anesthesia required. Anesthesia results in depression of breathing. Thoracic respiratory excursion is significantly reduced. The tone and pattern of contraction of the respiratory muscles, particularly the diaphragm and the intercostal muscles, change, which contributes to many of the secondary cardiopulmonary effects observed after surgery (Muller, Volgyesi, Becker, Bryan, and Bryan, 1979). The loss of end-expiratory diaphragmatic tone causes the diaphragm to ascend into the chest by 2 cm during anesthesia with or without paralysis (Froese and Bryan, 1974). Reductions in functional residual capacity (FRC) are correlated with this change and with altered chest wall configuration and increased thoracic blood volume (Hedenstierna et al., 1985; Hedenstierna, Tokics, Strandberg, Lundquist, and Brismar, 1986). One of the most pervasive and predictable clinical effects observed in the postoperative period is alveolar collapse. Total lung capacity, FRC, and residual volume are significantly decreased. The FRC is reduced by approximately 1 L in supine compared with the erect sitting position (Behrakis, Baydur, Jaeger, and Milic-Emili, 1983; Nunn, 1989) and is further reduced with the induction of anesthesia. Anesthesia, however, fails to reduce FRC in the sitting position (Nunn, 1989).

Surgical Factors That Contribute to Perioperative Cardiopulmonary Dysfunction

Type of surgery

Surgical procedures

Anesthetics (general, with or without intubation, or regional) and sedation

Muscle-relaxant agents and neuromuscular blockade

Supplemental oxygen and humidification

Static body position assumed

Duration of surgery and static body positioning

Incisions

Use of the cardiopulmonary bypass machine (CBM)

Use of the extracorporeal membrane exchanger (ECMO)

Dressings and binders

Splints and fixation devices

Lines and leads

Monitoring devices

Chest tubes placement and number

Catheters

Perioperative pain

Perioperative pain control management

Perioperative fluid balance management

Perioperative blood and plasma transfusions

The consequences of reduced FRC with anesthesia and surgery have significant implications for postoperative complications and the course of recovery. Airway closure occurs with anesthesia and this likely contributes to intrapulmonary shunting. Compression atelectasis of the dependent lung fields occurs during surgery. In addition, compression atelectasis occurs when lung tissue and surrounding structures are being physically manipulated. Although reduced airway caliber in areas of low lung volume can be offset by the airway-dilating effect of many inhaled anesthetics, airway resistance is increased by obstruction of the breathing circuits, valves, and tracheal tubes. The airways may also be obstructed with foreign matter, such as blood and secretions, or from bronchospasm because of irritation of the airways. Because of the decrease in FRC, compliance is decreased and the work of breathing is increased. Hypoxemia secondary to transpulmonary shunting is usually maximal within 72 hours after surgery and often is not completely resolved for several days. Persistent reduction in FRC after surgery delays the restoration of the normal alveolar-arterial oxygen gradient (Alexander, Spence, Parikh, and Stuart, 1973).

A complication of thoracic and upper abdominal surgery, (e.g., cholecystectomy) is irritation or compression trauma of the phrenic nerve. This complication may be more common than expected. Inhibition of the phrenic nerve impairs the contraction of the affected hemidiaphragm, causing it to ascend into the thorax and contribute to atelectasis on that side. This inhibition may last for several days (Dureuil, Viires, and Cantineau, 1986; Ford and Guenter, 1984).

The FIO_2 depends on the mode of 100% oxygen administration. Low-flow nasal oxygen reduces hypoxemia in the absence of hypercapnia and marked transpulmonary shunting in the postoperative patient. Low oxygen flows and low FIO_2s tend to be delivered via nasal cannulae, whereas higher flows can deliver higher FIO_2s via oxygen masks and masks with reservoir bags. FIO_2 and the body position of the patient at the time the blood sample was taken must always be considered when interpreting arterial blood gases. The FIO_2 is selected to provide adequate oxygenation with the lowest oxygen concentration possible.

After surgery the normal pattern of breathing is disrupted. Shallow, monotonous tidal ventilation without normal occasional, spontaneous deep breaths causes alveolar collapse within an hour (Nunn, 1989). Unless resolved, atelectasis becomes increasingly resistant to reinflation within a few hours. This complication is exacerbated in patients receiving narcotics.

Tachypnea and tachycardia are commonly observed with gross atelectasis secondary to hypoventilation. Breath sounds are decreased at the bases, and the coarse wheezes associated with mucus obstructing airflow are heard on auscultation. Large areas of atelectasis are present. Left lower lobe atelectasis is common after cardiac surgery.

If narcotics impair the patient's ability to participate in treatment, analgesia with a less systemic ef-

fect is indicated. Patient controlled analgesia (PCA) is an effective means of having the patient regulate the amount of analgesia he or she is receiving. Intravenous administration prolongs the peak-effect time of analgesics and therefore helps the patient tolerate longer, more intense treatments. Transcutaneous electrical nerve stimulation (TENS) can be a useful adjunct in the management of postoperative pain in some patients. Pain control with TENS may enable the patient to participate more fully in mobilization, deep breathing, coughing, and bed mobility. Research is needed, however, to evaluate this technique in the management of acute pain and define the prescription parameters needed to produce an optimal therapeutic effect. A nonpharmacological, noninvasive means of managing acute pain would be of considerable benefit to patients and would enable them to participate more fully in physical therapy treatments in the absence of untoward side effects often associated with drug administration.

Although sedatives or tranquilizers are prescribed to make the patient more comfortable and to reduce suffering, sedatives, in particular, reduce the patient's arousal and often the ability to cooperate actively with treatment. Thus these medications must be prescribed judiciously to ensure the patient is able to cooperate with physical therapy and other components of care. Oversedation must be avoided if the patient is to derive maximal benefit from cardiopulmonary physical therapy treatments.

Special attention in the postoperative period is given to the prevention or management of cardiopulmonary complications associated with reduced arousal, surgical pain, and restriction of lung capacity and secondary to dressings, binders, and diminished ability to cooperate, move spontaneously, and hyperventilate the lungs periodically. Patients are prone to aspiration in the immediate postoperative period, particularly while the sedation and anesthetic agents are wearing off. This risk is further increased if an airway is required or if an airway and mechanical ventilation is instituted. Postextubation atelectasis must be anticipated and avoided. To minimize this risk, patients are requested not to eat or drink fluids the day before surgery.

Endotracheal intubation and mechanical ventilation are indicated if blood gases fail to improve with conservative management. See Chapter 32 for treatment priorities for a patient during ventilation and the course of weaning from the mechanical ventilator.

The importance of a thorough preoperative assessment and teaching by the physical therapist cannot be overstated. The components of preoperative teaching are summarized in the box below. In cases of elective surgery, preoperative teaching includes a general description of the surgery to be performed, the effect of anesthesia and surgery on cardiopulmonary function, and the systemic effects of restricted mobility and recumbency. The lines, leads, and catheters usually associated with the surgery are explained. The patient is instructed in breathing control maneuvers, supported coughing, chest wall mobility exercises, mobility exercises for the limbs (e.g., hip and knee and foot and ankle exercises), turning in bed, sitting up, transferring, chair sitting, and walking erect postoperatively. In addition, the patient is taught methods of maximizing comfort with body positioning and supporting the surgical incision. If the bed has controls the patient can manipulate, she or he is taught how to make bed adjustments as required. The postoperative course is explained in general terms so the patient can anticipate this period. If the patient is well informed preopera-

tively, he or she will be better oriented and capable of cooperating when waking from anesthetic.

The patient's position is changed frequently in the initial postoperative period. The patient is usually encouraged to change his or her body position frequently, transfer, sit in a chair, and ambulate as soon as possible after surgery. The importance of frequent postural changes and early ambulation in the initial postoperative period are stressed (Dull and Dull, 1983). Early ambulation is a priority in the management of all surgical patients unless contraindicated.

After surgery, the patient is detained in the recovery room until the vital signs have stabilized, there is no apparent internal or external bleeding, and the patient is responding to his or her name. Patients recovering from minor surgery are usually transferred to a ward once discharged from the recovery room. A patient is transferred to the ICU after surgery if complications arise during surgery, if the patient cannot be readily stabilized and requires close monitoring, or if the patient has had more serious surgery such as cranial, cardiovascular thoracic, or emergency surgery, such as that resulting from multiple trauma (Chapter 34).

Patients considered for elective surgery are screened regarding their risks for postoperative complications. The physical therapist is often con-

---

Objectives of the Preoperative Physical Therapy Assessment and Teaching

Develop rapport with patient

Assess the patient and estimate degree of surgical risk (e.g., age, smoking, previous cardiopulmonary dysfunction, neuromuscular dysfunction, musculoskeletal deformity, obesity, substance abuse, pregnancy, nutritional status, and hydration status)

Describe the general preoperative, intraoperative, and postoperative course

Review specific surgical procedures relevant to physical therapy (e.g., anesthesia, type of surgery, body position during surgery, airway, mechanical ventilation, duration, incisions, infusions, drainage systems, chest tubes, and recovery room)

Provide the rationale for, describe, demonstrate, and have the patient practice and provide feedback on the following breathing control maneuvers: maximal inspiratory hold, supported coughing maneuvers, relaxation, bed mobility and positioning, transfers, and mobilization

For patients at risk of postoperative cardiopulmonary dysfunction and complications, review the use of the incentive spirometer and conventional airway clearance interventions (e.g., postural drainage and manual techniques if indicated)

Ask for any questions

sulted by the surgeon to help make a poor-risk patient into a relatively better-risk patient. Patients with upper-respiratory tract infections before surgery may have their surgeries postponed, depending on the type and extent of surgery to be performed, level of anesthesia indicated, and other medical conditions, including cardiopulmonary disease, age, and smoking history. Patients with lower-respiratory tract infections preoperatively constitute a greater operative risk, hence these patients often have their surgeries postponed until the infection has resolved. Patients with chronic cardiopulmonary diseases require a prolonged period of preoperative physical therapy in preparation for surgery. Elective surgery is not usually considered during an exacerbation of chronic lung disease. Even minor surgery may be potentially hazardous for the patient with previous lung disease. The adverse effects of total anesthesia on these patients is magnified because of their reduced pulmonary reserve capacity. Smoking should be discontinued for as long as possible before surgery. The patient is placed on an exercise conditioning program, a regimen of bronchial hygiene, oxygen if necessary, and prophylactic antibiotics. Even patients with extremely low functional work capacity can enhance the efficiency of the steps in the oxygen transport pathway (Chapter 17) with a modified aerobic exercise conditioning program. This preoperative preparation may take one to several weeks, depending on the patient and the indications for surgery.

Rest during the postoperative period is prescribed judiciously as treatment because rest is the time for healing, repair, and restoration. Sleep deprivation impairs recovery and healing. Sleep at night is biologically more restorative than daytime sleep. Thus daytime and nighttime cues are given to restore the patient's circadian rhythms. Although injudicious and excessive recumbency, bedrest, and prolonged periods in any given body position are deleterious, special attention is given to maximizing the amount of quality rest and sleep periods and minimizing disruption of nighttime sleep. Rest needs to be prescribed both within and between treatments. Appropriate rest periods are interspersed within each treatment session, according to the patient's needs to avoid reaching suboptimal, suprathreshold physiological states. Suprathreshold states are associated with an inappropriate balance between oxygen delivery and demand such that the patient becomes compromised (e.g., hemodynamically unstable), cardiopulmonary distress is precipitated, or both).

Preparation for Surgery

To minimize risk and reduce perioperative morbidity and mortality, patients need to be in the best medical and physical condition before anesthesia and surgery. In the case of elective surgery, some patients are prescribed modified aerobic training, smoking cessation, and weight control programs before surgery.

Preoperative teaching is a central component of physical therapy management of the surgical patient. Such teaching establishes rapport with the physical therapist who informs the patient about what to expect before and after surgery. In addition to reviewing the surgical procedures, the physical therapist reviews, and has the patient perform, deep breathing and supported coughing maneuvers, relaxation, bed mobility, positioning, transfers, and mobilization. Preoperative teaching reduces the patient's anxiety and encourages the patient to be as active as possible in her or his recovery. Preoperative teaching reduces postoperative complications and the length of the hospital stay.

There are no strict guidelines about which patients should receive perioperative physical therapy. Although nonthoracic surgeries are generally associated with fewer cardiopulmonary complications (e.g., surgery of the extremities or lower abdomen), patients with preexisting cardiopulmonary, hematological or neuromuscular pathology, or musculoskeletal pathology of the chest wall are at greater risk even in these relative low-risk types of surgeries. In addition, patients are at additional risk if they are older or younger, smoke, or are overweight or pregnant. Thus each surgical patient needs to be assessed individually to establish the degree of relative risk during surgery and the need for perioperative physical therapy. In this way, perioperative complications can be anticipated and avoided or reduced, which is preferable to managing complications once they have developed.

Factors Determining the Effect of Surgery

A patient's response to surgery and the cardiopulmonary complications that may develop depend on many factors (see the box on p. 496). The type of surgery determines the degree of invasiveness, the type or types of anesthetics and sedatives, whether the patient needs to be intubated, the static body position assumed during surgery, the approximate duration of the surgery and period of anesthesia, the incisions that are required, the dressings, the lines, leads, catheters, and monitoring devices needed, the chest tubes, the type and degree of pain, and the need for pain control after surgery.

Pathophysiology

The type and severity of underlying cardiopulmonary dysfunction increases a patient's risk of compromised oxygen transport and gas exchange perioperatively.

Restricted Mobility and Recumbency

Surgery imposes two nonphysiological states on the patient that impact significantly on oxygen transport. These conditions include the following:
1. Restricted mobility
2. Recumbency, specifically a prolonged period of static positioning with the patient breathing at monotonous tidal volumes

Extrinsic Factors

Surgery including the factors in the box on p. 496 are the primary extrinsic factors contributing to cardiopulmonary dysfunction in the perioperative period.

Intrinsic Factors

Intrinsic factors that contribute to cardiopulmonary dysfunction in the surgical patient include a patient's premorbid status (e.g., preexisting cardiopulmonary, renal, endocrine, and hematologic pathology). In addition, life-style factors are significant (i.e., preoperative conditioning level, nutrition, hydration, stress levels, weight, and smoking history).

MAJOR TYPES OF SURGERY
Thoracic Surgery

Thoracic surgery refers to surgery necessitating opening of the chest wall. By convention, this general term usually excludes specialized cardiovascular surgery (i.e., surgery of the heart and great vessels). Thoracic surgery is commonly performed for lung resections secondary to cancer (e.g., pneumonectomy, lobectomy, segmentectomy, and wedge resection). In addition, thoracic surgery is performed to remove an irreversibly damaged area of lung tissue secondary to bronchiectasis, benign tumors, fungal infections, and tuberculosis.

The most common incisions are posterolateral thoracotomy and median sternotomy. The posterolateral thoracotomy procedure requires the patient to assume the sidelying position with the involved side uppermost for the duration of the surgery. The uppermost arm is fully flexed anteriorly. The incision is made through an intercostal space, corresponding to the location of the lesion to be excised. The muscles incised include latissimus dorsi, serratus anterior, external and internal intercostals laterally, and trapezius and rhomboid posteriorly.

At the conclusion of the surgery, chest tubes are placed to evacuate air and fluid from the pleural space by means of an underwater chest tube drainage system. The chest tube and drainage system resolve the pneumothorax created by reestablishing negative pressure in the pleural space and help to reinflate the remaining atelectatic lung tissue. After thoracic surgery, two chest tubes are usually inserted, one at the apex of the lung to evacuate air and one at the base of the lung to drain serosanguinous fluid. The therapist should become familiar with the various drainage systems, how drainage can be facilitated with mobilization and body positioning coordinated with breathing control and supported coughing maneuvers, and certain precautions that need to be observed to avoid impairing drainage or disconnecting the tubing.

Provided the chest tubes are not kinked, there is no contraindication to lying on the side of the chest tubes. Lying on this side, which is usually the side of the surgery and incision, is typically avoided by the patient. Consistent with the adage, "down with the good lung," a patient prefers to lie on the non-surgical side. However, prolonged periods in any position, and particularly, lying on the unaffected side, places these lung fields at risk. To minimize the risk of positional complications and hypoxemia, the patient is encouraged to turn to both sides (Leaver, Conway, and Holgate, 1994; Seaton, Lapp, and Morgan, 1979; Sutton, Pavia, Bateman, and Clarke, 1982). The specific positions and the duration of time spent within each, however, is based on a comprehensive assessment of the patient's condition and the indications and contraindications for each body position.

Patients may appear to splint themselves, thereby restricting chest wall motion, to avoid including pain when moving and deep breathing. They also may resist maximal inspiratory efforts when coughing. Although pain likely contributes to breathing at low lung volumes and ineffective coughing, phrenic nerve inhibition in patients with thoracic and upper abdominal surgeries is likely a more important factor restricting lung expansion than is fully appreciated in many patients (Ford and Guenter, 1984).

Postoperative complaints of pain are both musculoskeletal and pleural in origin. The large number of muscles incised, particularly in the posterolateral thoracotomy incision, combined with the operative position, contributes to the patient's complaints of chest wall pain, shoulder soreness, and restricted movement. Deep breathing and coughing maneuvers may be associated with considerable discomfort after surgery. Pain is accentuated by apprehension and anxiety. Therefore treatments are coordinated with relaxation, noninvasive pain control modalities, and pain medication schedules to elicit the full cooperation of the patient.

Cardiovascular Surgery

Cardiovascular surgery is specialized thoracic surgery involving the heart and great vessels. Because the flow of blood through the cardiopulmonary system is interrupted, the patient is placed on a cardiopulmonary bypass machine or on a machine called an *extracorporeal membrane oxygenator*. Cardiovascular surgery is most commonly performed for coronary artery bypass grafting, valve replacements, and aneurysm repairs. Bypass patients, in whom the saphenous vein is excised for graft material, have the added complication of surgery and wound healing in one leg. Mobility exercises on that leg are often restricted until there is no risk of bleeding or interference with healing. Comparable with the thoracic surgical patient, a cardiovascular patient leaves the operating room with various monitoring lines and leads, intravenous fluid infusions, possible blood or plasma infusions, a Swan-Ganz catheter (Chapter 15), a central venous pressure line, an arterial line, a Foley catheter, and oxygen cannulae.

The preoperative preparation and teaching and the postoperative physical therapy management is intensive. Because of the invasiveness of cardiovascular surgery, patients are usually treated postoperatively in a specialized intensive care unit (Chapter 31). The preoperative and postoperative physical therapy management of patients in the intensive care unit is a specialized area and is described in Chapter 34. Providing the patient with information about what to expect during the perioperative course relieves fear and anxiety. In addition, relaxation procedures can be useful. Patients need to be reassured that their incisions and suture lines will not be disrupted with movement and physical therapy and that supported coughing and supporting themselves when moving will maximize comfort. Until the patient has stabilized, the patient's mobility is restricted to low-intensity mobilization to promote its benefits on gas exchange and reduce metabolic demands and body positioning to optimize alveolar ventilation coordinated with deep breathing and supported coughing maneuvers. Conventional airway clearance interventions (e.g., postural drainage and manual techniques) may be prescribed in the presence of excessive secretions, difficulty in mobilizing secretions, and in the event of productive hydrostatic pneumonia.

Patients undergoing cardiovascular surgery are transferred from the cardiovascular intensive care unit to the ward as quickly as possible. From the ward, these patients should be referred to a physical therapist and a cardiac rehabilitation program in the community for continuity of care and to maximize the functional gains resulting from the surgery. Exercise is prescribed progressively to maximize oxygen transport at each step of the rehabilitation period (i.e., acute, before and immediately after discharge, and long term). The conditioning effects of exercise enable the patient to resume various activities of daily living commensurate with an increasing capacity of the patient's oxygen transport system to meet the demands of these activities. Activities involving straining and isometric contractions are avoided. Weight lifting may be introduced in a long-term rehabilitation program, but the weights are not sufficient to cause strain. Patients with median sternotomy incisions are usually prohibited from using their arms to support themselves when sitting or driving and during activities that may strain the incision site for several weeks or more.

PREOPERATIVE PHYSICAL THERAPY: PRINCIPLES OF MANAGEMENT

Preoperative management includes assessment and preoperative education; the primary components are shown in the box on p. 498. During this time the physical therapist has an opportunity to develop rapport with the patient. The assessment establishes the risk of cardiopulmonary complications and prolonged hospital stay and the type and extent of perioperative physical therapy required. The assessment establishes what the postoperative priorities will be; however, these are modified based on the postoperative assessment. The surgical procedures are described and the effects of surgery and anesthesia and sedation on gas exchange are reviewed so that the patient understands the importance of being actively involved in physical therapy, both during and between treatments after surgery.

POSTOPERATIVE PHYSICAL THERAPY: PRINCIPLES OF MANAGEMENT

The goals of postoperative physical therapy management related to oxygen transport appear in the box at right. It is essential that these goals are addressed between and during treatments. Thus the patient is instructed in mobilization and body positioning coordinated with deep breathing and supported coughing

---

Goals of Postoperative Physical Therapy Related to Oxygen Transport

Maximize arousal

Maximize alveolar volume

Optimize alveolar ventilation

Optimize perfusion

Maximize lung volumes and capacities, especially functional residual capacity

Minimize closing volume

Minimize intrapulmonary shunting

Optimize lung compliance

Optimize mucociliary transport

Optimize mucous clearance

Optimize ventilation and perfusion matching and gas exchange

Maximize expiratory flow rates

Maximize chest tube drainage

Optimize fluid balance systemically (renal function)

Optimize lung water balance and distribution

Promote optimal lymphatic draining

Minimize third spacing and collection of fluid

Minimize the risk of aspiration

Minimize undue work of breathing

Minimize undue work of the heart

Maximize chest wall mobility and movement in three planes

Optimize body and posture alignment when sitting, standing, walking, and recumbent

Optimize circulatory status and tissue perfusion

Optimize peripheral blood flow and velocity

Optimize muscle pump action

Minimize effects of central fluid shifts with recumbency

Maintain fluid-volume regulating mechanisms

Minimize pain nonpharmacologically and coordinate with the patient's pain medications if indicated

Maximize cardiopulmonary endurance

Optimize relaxation

Provide instruction to patient on "between-treatment" treatment maneuvers between treatment sessions, and these interventions should be performed hourly during waking hours (Bennett, Foster, and Chapman, 1990; Blomqvist and Stone, 1983; Bourn and Jenkins, 1992; Hasani, Pavia, Agnew, and Clarke, 1991; Hietpas, Roth, and Jensen, 1974; Orlava, 1959). Pain medications are coordinated as needed with treatments to maximize treatment efficacy.

In addition to goals related to oxygen transport, other important postoperative goals include the following:
1. Maximize joint range of motion
2. Maximize muscle length and ligament integrity with range of motion exercises
3. Maximize patient's ability to perform activities of daily living
4. Maintain or increase general muscle strength and endurance
5. Maintain normal cognitive function to avoid disorientation and hospital-related psychoses.

These goals are achieved with the prescription of general mobility exercise, including hip and knee flexion and extension exercises and foot and ankle exercises. These exercises are performed hourly regardless of whether the patient is sitting in the chair or resting in bed.

Finally, there are important preventative goals (e.g., minimizing the effects of restricted mobility and recumbency on all organ systems) (Chapters 17 and 18). Of particular concern in the surgical patient is the risk of thromboemboli and pulmonary emboli and the risk of pressure points and skin breakdown. Thus mobilization and regular activation of the muscle pumps to minimize circulatory stasis and frequent body-position changes are essential to reduce risks, which can have serious consequences for the patient's recovery. Compression stockings are often put on the patient after surgery. These are not removed other than for cleaning and redistributing pressure until the patient is consistently up and about. These stockings facilitate venous return and increase blood flow and velocity, thereby minimizing the risk of thrombus formation. Should thrombus formation be suspected, an intermittent compression device may need to be attached to the legs to simulate muscle pump action.

Not all patients who have surgery are intubated. Those that are, with the exception of patients undergoing thoracic or cardiovascular surgery, are usually extubated before leaving the operating room or recovery area. Provided no complications develop, most other patients do not require an airway. Patients undergoing major thoracic surgery or cardiovascular surgery remain intubated and mechanically ventilated from several to 24 hours after surgery to minimize the work of breathing and hence the work of the heart to meet the metabolical demands of respiration. These patients are informed that artificial airway and mechanical ventilation enables them to breathe more efficiently initially. A patient is also informed that he or she will not be able to speak while the airway is in place and may have a sore throat after its removal.

Patients are usually aroused and repositioned before leaving the operating room, although this is seldom remembered by patients. Not recalling the immediate postoperative course is common. Patients are likely to be receiving some form of pharmacological analgesia (e.g., morphine). If blood was required intraoperatively, whole blood, packed cells, or plasma may still be infused in the immediate postoperative period or longer. Saline or other solutions are also infused for regulation of fluid balance until the patient is able to drink and eat normally. Once vital signs have stabilized, wounds are stable and not draining, and the patient reasonably alert, the patient is transferred to the ward. The patient is retained in the recovery area should further monitoring be required. If complications develop and oxygen transport and gas exchange threatened, the patient may be transferred to the intensive care unit.

The physical therapist may be consulted to assess and treat the patient as soon as he or she leaves the operating room or while in the recovery room. Most frequently the physical therapist sees the patient once he or she has been transferred to the ward and has been settled. The first 24 hours are critical.

The risk of cardiopulmonary complications is greatest during the perioperative period and diminishes as the patient becomes increasingly upright and mobile. Atelectasis and aspiration after extubation are significant risks for the patient who has been intubated. The goal immediately after extubation is to promote optimal alveolar ventilation, maximize lung volumes and capacities (especially FRC), minimize closing volumes, and maximize expiratory flow rates and hence cough effectiveness. Areas most susceptible to atelectasis are those that may have been physically compressed during surgery (e.g., the left lower lobe of the cardiovascular surgical patient and areas adjacent to a lobectomy or segmentectomy).

Surgery constitutes a significant insult to the body. After the trauma of surgery, anesthesia, sedation, fluid loss, incisions, and the significant energy requirements for healing and repair, patients can be expected to be lethargic and difficult to arouse. The relaxed state induced by anesthesia, sedation, and narcotics increases the risk of aspiration. This risk is exacerbated further in some patients by nausea and vomiting associated with anesthesia and narcotics. Moving and positioning the patient upright whenever possible and interacting with the patient stimulates the reticular activating system making the patient more responsive and aroused. The increased metabolic demands that this requires, along with increased catecholamine release, helps overcome the residual effects of anesthesia, sedation, and muscle relaxants and their threat to oxygen transport, provided the demands are not beyond the capacity of the oxygen transport system to deliver oxygen.

Alternatively, some patients are restless and agitated after the effects of anesthesia have worn off. Hypoxemia can lead to restlessness and agitation. Thus it is important that these patients are not inappropriately sedated. This compounds their need for treatment while making them less able to cooperate with treatment simultaneously (Dripps and Waters, 1941; Ross and Dean, 1989).

At the outset of any treatment, the patient must be aroused as much as possible to cooperate fully and derive the maximal benefit from treatment. The physical therapist interacts continuously with the patient to arouse the patient fully, maintain arousal, stimulate normal cognitive function and orientation, and elicit feedback from the patient to assess the response to treatment. Narcotics depress respiratory status and arousal, and these effects are accentuated in patients whose metabolic states have been disrupted with illness and in older persons. Thus the physical therapist must be vigilant in detecting untoward residual effects of narcotics in the surgical patient.

There are several factors that are particulary important in surgical patients that can affect their sensitivity to narcotic analgesics, such as morphine (Gilman, Goodman, and Gilman, 1990: Malamed, 1989). First, there is considerable intersubject response variability to these agents. Second, older patients can be expected to be more sensitive to narcotics. Three, diverse multisystem pathology has a significant effect on the degradation, absorption, biotransformation, and excretion of morphine. Four, exaggerated effects of morphine have been reported when administered in conjunction with other agents, such as other narcotic analgesics, phenothiazines, tranquilizers, or sedative-hypnotics; in addition, such exaggerated effects have been reported in patients with respiratory depression, hypotension, and sedation and in patients who are unconscious. These situations in which exaggerated drug effects have been reported are commonly encountered in the intensive care setting and can result in unpredictable responses. Finally, the physical dependence and abuse potential of these agents cannot be ignored.

The physical therapist must be familiar with the patient's medications and the medication's indications, side effects, and contraindications. The physical therapist can determine to what extent oxygen transport may be compromised by medication effects, whether some recommendation needs to be made to minimize untoward drug effects on arousal or some other factor that negatively affects oxygen transport and gas exchange. For example, although narcotics are excellent analgesics, they have widespread systemic effects including cardiopulmonary depressant effects, gastrointestinal depressant effects, and muscle relaxant effects—all of which compromise oxygen transport. Thus consideration needs to be given regarding whether other forms of analgesia can be used. Have nonpharmacological means of analgesia been exploited? If pharmacological analgesia is indicated, can analgesics other than narcotics be used? Or at least, can the dose of narcotic be reduced so that satisfactory pain control can be achieved in combination with nonpharmacological interventions?

Mobilization in the upright position coordinated with breathing control and supported coughing maneuvers is encouraged immediately after the patient is first aroused after surgery, unless contraindicated, to help reverse and mitigate reduced arousal, atelectasis, FRC, and impaired mucociliary transport associated with surgery. Mobilization augments cardiopulmonary function (see Chapter 17) particularly when the patient is upright (Levine and Lown, 1952; Lewis, 1980). These beneficial effects are enhanced by improved three-dimensional chest wall motion, improved gut motility, and reduced intraabdominal pressure. Extremity movement during ambulation increases alveolar ventilation, enhances ventilation and perfusion matching by increasing zone 2 of the lungs, and optimizes diffusing capacity. The upright position is essential such that the spine is erect, upper body musculature relaxed, and the chest wall symmetrical. Slouching and leaning particularly to the affected side reduces alveolar ventilation and contributes to uneven distribution of ventilation and areas of atelectasis (Bake, Dempsey, and Grimby, 1976; Don, Craig, Wahba, and Couture, 1971; Glaister, 1967). In addition, if this abnormal posture is maintained, mucociliary transport of the area is impaired and mucus collects and stagnates, increasing the risk of bacterial colonization and infection. Symmetrical posture is monitored at all times (i.e., during ambulation, sitting at bedside, bed mobility exercises, sitting up in bed, and lying in bed). Slouching and favoring the affected side will lead to cardiopulmonary complications and possibly musculoskeletal complications in the short and long term.

Mobilization and active exercise in upright postures whenever possible are prescribed based on the need to enhance multiple steps in the oxygen transport pathway (Dean and Ross, 1992; Ray et al., 1974). The priority is to perform as much activity as possible out of bed and upright (i.e., ambulation, transferring, sitting upright in a chair, and chair exercises with or without hand weights or exercise bands). When in bed, similar devices can be used, including a monkey bar to facilitate moving in bed for patients other than cardiovascular thoracic patients (e.g., the orthopedic patient with extremity fractures and traction). In addition, the use of the monkey bar to perform repetitive bouts of exercise to maintain upper-extremity strength and some general endurance capacity, to relieve pressure and stiffness, and to fa-

cilitate frequent turning. Cycle pedals can be adapted to chairs and recumbent exercise in bed if necessary. Patients whose positioning is restricted with fixation and traction devices require hand, wrist, or ankle weights, and possibly pulleys and other devices, to maintain muscle strength and power. Movements performed with moderately heavy weights for multiple sets (e.g., three sets of 10 repetitions) develop muscle strength. Movements performed with lighter weight for multiple sets (e.g., 5 to 10 sets of 10 repetitions) tend to develop endurance and aerobic capacity. Because of the restrictions imposed by these devices, maintaining joint range is essential (i.e., of the neck, spinal column, and chest wall, as well as the extremities). The rotation component of joint movement is readily compromised, thus this needs to be an integral component of joint range of motion exercises. Proprioceptive neuromuscular facilitation (PNF) movements of the extremities can be beneficial. PNF movements of the chest wall can be coordinated with breathing control and supported coughing maneuvers. Upper body and trunk mobility and strengthening are important goals particularly in the patient with chest wall incisions. The prescription is progressed gradually in the patient with a chest wall incision, particularly in the patient with a median sternotomy who is usually restricted to unresisted, upper-extremity mobility exercises in the first several weeks.

Prescription of body positioning is essential in the management of the surgical patient for two reasons. First, without direction, the patient will tend to assume a deleterious body position (i.e., maintaining a restricted number of body positions that favor the affected side for prolonged periods of time with minimal movement and "stirring up"). Thus once the effects of mobilization have been exploited in a given treatment session, body positions are prescribed for "between-treatment" times that continue to enhance oxygen transport for a given patient and discourage excessive time in deleterious body positions. When not ambulating, patients are encouraged to assume a wide range of body positions (e.g., semi-prone) between treatments, as frequently as possible, (i.e., at least every 1 to 2 hours) (Dean, 1985; Douglas, Rehder, Beynen, Sessler, and Marsh, 1977; Piehl and Brown, 1976; Remolina, Khan, Santiago, and Edel-

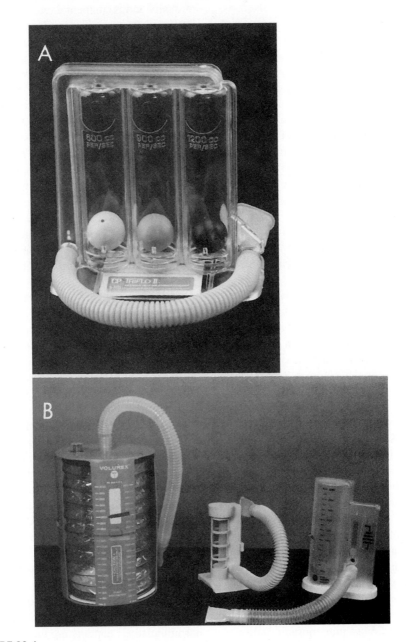

FIGURE 28-1
Incentive spirometers.

man, 1981; Ross and Dean, 1992; Zack, Pontoppidan, and Kazemi, 1974).

Alveoli are likely to remain patent for 1 hour after reinflation. Thus to sustain alveolar inflation and normal FRC, mobilization and body positioning coordinated with breathing control and supported coughing must be carried out frequently (i.e., every 1 to 2 hours) to maintain optimal alveolar volume and distribution of ventilation. Maximal inspiratory maneuvers are coordinated with mobilization and body positioning at least every hour as tolerated. Maximal inspiratory maneuvers alone, however, are unlikely to be effective because the inspiratory pressure may be insufficient to inflate atelectatic alveoli. Rather patent alveoli will tend to be overexpanded. Mobilization and body positioning will directly alter the intrapleural pressure gradient and thereby optimize alveolar expansion (Roussos et al. 1977).

Normal passive expiratory efforts to end tidal volume are encouraged and maximal or forced expiratory efforts are usually avoided to prevent airway closure and potential increase of atelectasis (Hasani et al., 1991; Hietpas et al., 1974; Nunn, Coleman, Sachithanandan, Bergman, and Laws, 1965). Huffing (glottis open) rather than coughing (glottis closed) also minimizes airway closure. There is less risk of bronchospasm than with coughing in which the glottis is closed, transpulmonary pressure is increased, and a compressive phase is involved. If indicated, coughing maneuvers are most effective in the sitting or slightly lean-forward position in which lung volumes and forced expiratory flow are maximized and the respiratory muscles are mechanically advantaged with respect to the length-tension characteristics of the muscle fibers. Airway closure is position-dependent (Chapter 18); therefore the degree of expiration encouraged by the physical therapist should be based on the patient's body position. Airway closure is potentiated in patients who are older, smoke, or are obese and in patients who are in horizontal as opposed to upright body positions.

Mobilization and body positioning coordinated with breathing control and supported coughing maneuvers offer the greatest benefit to oxygen transport in the postoperative patient. Specific benefits are described in Chapters 17 and 18. They include maxi-

mizing FRC, reducing closing volume, maximizing expiratory flow rates, promoting mucociliary transport, promoting airway clearance, optimizing lymphatic drainage, minimizing the effects of increased thoracic blood volume, maintaining fluid-volume regulating mechanisms, and minimizing the work of breathing and of the heart. Sustained maximal inspiration is one intervention that promotes alveolar expansion. Each deep breath is performed to maximal inspiration to total lung capacity with a 3- to 5-second breath hold. This maneuver may reduce pulmonary complications by promoting alveolar inflation and gas exchange. The patient is encouraged to repeat this maneuver several times hourly, and frequently during mobilization, and before, during, and after body-position changes.

Incentive spirometry can be useful in patients who are resistant or unable to cooperate fully with maximal inspiratory efforts (Figure 28-1). Postoperative hypoxemia may be reduced with this technique, which uses the principle of sustained inspiration using a feedback device (either flow or volume feedback) to achieve maximal inflating pressure in the alveoli and maximal inhaled volume. The incentive spirometer can be used independently by the patient. This technique ensures that each inspiration is physiologically optimal and is reproduced precisely from one inspiration to the next. Patients who are surgical risks can benefit from being taught the use of the incentive spirometer during preoperative teaching by the physical therapist to promote better inflation of the lungs with incentive spirometry postoperatively. The patient continues with a regimen of breathing control and coughing maneuvers until full mobility and activities of daily living are resumed.

The application of intermittent positive pressure breathing (IPPB) appears to be less effective for the postoperative patient than previously believed. The details of this modality are described in Chapter 41.

SUMMARY

This chapter reviews the management of cardiopulmonary dysfunction secondary to acute surgical conditions. Surgery and its physiological effects are described. Special reference is made to two specialized types of surgery that have the greatest impact on cardiopulmonary function, namely, thoracic and cardiovascular surgery.

The four categories of factors contributing to or threatening oxygen transport are described in Chapter 16. These factors include pathology, restricted mobility and recumbency, extrinsic factors related to the patient's care, and intrinsic factors related to the patient. This chapter examines in detail those extrinsic factors related to surgery and anesthesia, and the impact of underlying disease, restricted mobility, recumbency and intrinsic factors on the effects of surgery and anesthesia.

In this chapter, treatment principles are presented rather than treatment prescriptions for particular patients. For specific examples of patient treatment prescriptions refer to the companion workbook *Clinical case studies in cardiopulmonary physical therapy.*

REVIEW QUESTIONS

1. Describe the physiological effects of surgery including the specific surgical procedure, the type, depth and duration of anesthesia, sedation, types of respiratory support, static body positioned assumed during surgery, length of surgery, number and type of invasive perioperative procedures, and incisions.
2. Describe surgical risk factors.
3. Relate cardiopulmonary physical therapy treatment interventions to the underlying pathophysiology associated with surgery and those factors listed in Question 1 and provide the *rationale* for your choice.

References

Alexander, J.L., Spence, A.A., Parikh, R.K., & Stuart, B. (1973). The role of airway closure in postoperative hypoxaemia. *British Journal of Anaesthesiology, 59,* 1070-1079.

Bake, B., Dempsey, J., & Grimby, G. (1976). Effects of shape changes of the chest wall on distribution of inspired gas. *American Review of Respiratory Disease, 114,* 1113-1120.

Behrakis, P.K., Baydur, A., Jaeger, M.J., & Milic-Emili, J. (1983). Lung mechanics in sitting and horizontal body positions. *Chest, 83,* 643-646.

Bennett, W.D., Foster, W.M., & Chapman, W.F. (1990). Cough-enhanced mucus clearance in the normal lung. *Journal of Applied Physiology, 69,* 1670-1675.

Blomqvist, C.G., & Stone, H.L. (1983). *Cardiovascular adjustments to gravitational stress. Handbook of physiology* (Vol. 2). Washington, DC: American Physiological Society.

Bourn, J., & Jenkins, S. (1992). Post-operative respiratory physiotherapy. Indications for treatment. *Physiotherapy, 78,* 80-85.

Dean, E. (1985). Effect of body position on pulmonary function. *Physical Therapy, 65,* 613-618.

Dean, E., & Ross, J. (1989). Integrating current literature in the management of cystic fibrosis: a rejoinder. *Physiotherapy Canada, 41,* 46-47.

Dean, E., & Ross, J. (1992). Mobilization and exercise conditioning. In C.C. Zadai (Ed.), *Pulmonary management in physical therapy.* New York: Churchill Livingstone.

Don, H.F., Craig, D.B., Wahba, W.M., & Couture, J.G. (1971). The measurement of gas trapped in the lungs at functional residual capacity and the effects of posture. *Anesthesiology, 35,* 582-590.

Douglas, W.W., Rehder, K., Beynen, F.M., Sessler, A., D., & Marsh, H.M. (1977). Improved oxygenation in patients with acute respiratory failure: the prone position. *American Review of Respiratory Disease, 115,*559-566.

Dripps, R.D., & Waters, R.M. (1941). Nursing care of the surgical patient. 1. The "stir-up." *American Journal of Nursing, 41,* 53-34.

Dull, J. L., & Dull, W.L. (1983). Are maximal inspiratory breathing exercises or incentive spirometry better than early mobilization after cardiopulmonary bypass surgery? *Physical Therapy, 63,* 655-659.

Dureuil, B., (Viires, N., & Cantineau, J.P. (1986). Diaphragmatic contractility after upper abdominal surgery. *Journal of Applied Physiology, 61,* 1775-1780.

Ford, G.T., & Guenter, C.A. (1984). Toward prevention of postoperative complications. *American Review of Respiratory Diseases, 130,* 4-5.

Froese, A.B., & Bryan, A.C. (1974). Effects of anesthesia and paralysis on diaphragmatic mechanics in man. *Anesthesiology, 41,* 242-255.

Glaister, D.H. (1967). The effect of posture on the distribution of ventilation and blood flow in the normal lung. *Clinical Science, 33,* 391-398.

Gilman, A.G., Goodman, L.S., & Gilman, A. (1990). *Goodman and Gilman's the pharmacological basis of therapeutics* (8th ed.). New York: Macmillan Publishing.

Hasani, A., Pavia, D., Agnew, J.E., & Clarke, S.W. (1991). The effect of unproductive coughing/FET on regional mucus movement in the human lungs. *Respiratory Medicine, 85,* 23-26.

Hedenstierna, G., Standberg, A., Brismar, B., Lundquist, H., Svenson, L., & Tokics, L. (1985). Functional residual capacity, thoracoabdominal dimensions and central blood volume during general anesthesia with muscle paralysis and mechanical ventilation. *Anesthesiology, 62,* 247-254.

Hedenstierna, G., Tokics, L., Strandberg, A., Lundquist, H., & Brismar, B. (1986). Correlation of gas exchange impairment to development of atelectasis during anaesthesia and muscle paralysis. *Acta Anaesthesiologica Scandinavica, 30,* 183-191.

Hietpas, B.G., Roth, R.D., & Jensen, W.M. (1974). Huff coughing and airway patency. *Respiratory Care, 24,* 710.

Leaver, H., Conway, J.H., & Holgate, S.T. (1994). The incidence of post-operative hypoxaemia following lobectomy and pneumonectomy: a pilot study. *Physiotherapy, 80,* 521-527.

Levine, R.D. (1984). *Anesthesiology. A manual for medical students.* Philadelphia: J.B. Lippincott Co.

Levine, S.A., & Lown, B. (1952). 'Armchair' treatment of acute coronary thrombosis. *Journal of the American Medical Association, 148,* 1365-1369.

Lewis, F.R. (1980). Management of atelectasis and pneumonia. *Surgical Clinics of North America, 60,* 1391-1401.

Malamed, S.F. (1989). *Sedation. A guide to patient management* (2nd ed.). St. Louis: Mosby.

Muller, N., Volgyesi, G., Becker, L., Bryan, M.H., & Bryan, A. C. (1979). Diaphragmatic muscle tone. *Journal of Applied Physiology, 47,* 279-284.

Nunn, J.F. (1989).The influence of anesthesia on the respiratory system. In K. Reinhart & K. Eyrich, (Eds.), *Clinical aspect of 02 transport and tissue oxygenation.* New York: Springer-Verlag.

Nunn, J.F., Coleman, A.J., Sachithanandan, T., Bergman, N.A., & Laws, J.W. (1965). Hypoxaemia and atelectasis produced by forced expiration. *British Journal of Anaesthesia, 37,* 3-12.

Orlava, O.E. (1959). Therapeutic physical culture in the complex treatment of pneumonia. *Physical Therapy Review, 39,* 153-160.

Piehl, M.A., & Brown, R.S. (1976). Use of extreme position changes in acute respiratory failure. *Critical Care Medicine, 4,* 13-14.

Ray, R. F., Yost, L., Moallem, S., Sanoudos, G.M., Villamena, P., & Paredes, R.M. (1974). Immobility, hypoxemia, and pulmonary arteriovenous shunting. *Archives of Surgery, 109,* 537-541.

Remolina, C., Khan, A.U., Santiago, T.V., & Edelman, N.H. (1981). Positional hypoxemia in unilateral lung disease. *New England Journal of Medicine, 304,* 523-525.

Ross, J., & Dean, E. (1989). Integrating physiological principles into the comprehensive management of cardiopulmonary dysfunction. *Physical Therapy, 69,* 255-259.

Ross, J., & Dean, E. (1992). Body positioning. In C.C. Zadai (Ed.), *Pulmonary management in physical therapy.* New York: Churchill Livingstone.

Roussos, C.S., Fixley, M., Geriest, J., Cosio, M., Kelly, S., Martin, R.R., & Engel, L.A. (1977). Voluntary factors influencing the distribution of inspired gas. *American Review of Respiratory Disease, 116,* 457-467.

Seaton, D., Lapp, N.I., & Morgan, W.K.C. (1979). Effect of body position on gas exchange after thoracotomy. *Thorax, 34,* 518-522.

Sutton, P.P., Pavia, D., Bateman, J.R.M., & Clarke, S.W. (1982). Chest physiotherapy—a review. *European Journal of Respiratory Disease, 63,* 188-201.

Zack, M.B., Pontoppidan, H., & Kazemi, H. (1974). The effect of lateral positions on gas exchange in pulmonary disease. *American Review of Respiratory Disease, 110,* 149-153.

PART V

Guidelines for the Delivery of Cardiopulmonary Physical Therapy: Chronic Cardiopulmonary Conditions

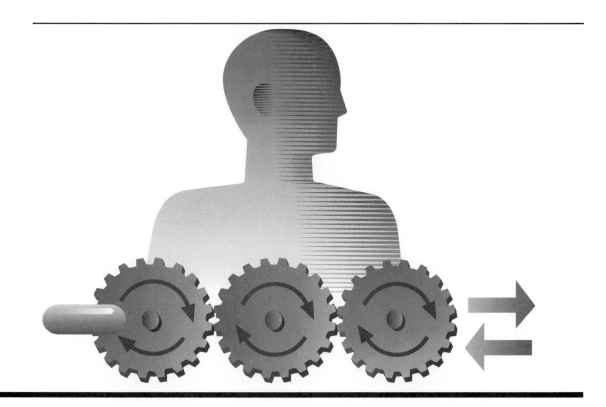

CHAPTER 29

Chronic Primary Cardiopulmonary Dysfunction

Elizabeth Dean
Donna Frownfelter

KEY TERMS

Angina
Asthma
Bronchiectasis
Chronic airflow limitation
Cystic fibrosis
Diabetes

Hypertension
Interstitial pulmonary fibrosis
Lung cancer
Myocardial infarction
Peripheral vascular disease
Valvula heart disease

INTRODUCTION

The purpose of this chapter is to review the pathophysiology, medical management, and physical therapy management of chronic, primary, cardiopulmonary pathology. Because the heart and lungs are interdependent and function as a single unit, primary lung or heart disease must be considered with respect to the other organ and in the context of oxygen transport overall (Dantzker, 1983; Ross and Dean, 1989; Scharf and Cassidy, 1989; Wasserman and Whipp, 1975).

The long-term cardiopulmonary management of chronic lung diseases is presented first. Although

there is no clear line between obstructive and restrictive patterns of lung disease, pathology can be generally defined based on the primary underlying pathophysiological problems. Thus the primary conditions that are presented include obstructive lung disease (i.e., chronic airflow limitation, asthma, bronchiectasis, and cystic fibrosis) and restrictive lung disease (i.e., interstitial pulmonary fibrosis). Lung cancer, which has the characteristics of both obstructive and restrictive patterns of pathology, is also presented.

The long-term cardiopulmonary management of heart disease is then presented with special attention to angina, myocardial infarction, and valvular heart disease. Chronic vascular diseases, including peripheral vascular disease, hypertension, and diabetes, are also presented.

The principles of management of the various chronic primary cardiopulmonary conditions are presented rather than treatment prescriptions, which cannot be discussed without consideration of a specific patient. (For specific examples of patient treatment prescriptions refer to the companion test *Clinical case studies in cardiopulmonary physical therapy.*) In this context the goals of long-term management of each condition are presented, followed by the essential monitoring required, and the primary interventions for maximizing cardiopulmonary function and oxygen transport. The selection of interventions for any given patient is based on the physiological hierarchy. The most physiological interventions are exploited first followed by less physiological interventions and those whose efficacy is less well documented (Chapter 16).

PRIMARY PULMONARY DISEASE

OBSTRUCTIVE PATTERNS

Chronic Airflow Limitation

Chronic airflow limitation is a descriptive term that refers to those disorders that previously have been termed *chronic obstructive pulmonary disease* (e.g., chronic bronchitis, emphysema, bronchiectasis, and cystic fibrosis). Although there may be a reversible component, airflow obstruction associated with these disorders is largely irreversible. The pathophysiology of these conditions is reviewed in detail in Chapter 29.

Bates (1989) described the syndrome of chronic airflow limitation as being caused by four external factors, mediated by four primary tissue responses, and modified by four physiological responses. The principal external causative factors include inhaled irritants, allergens, infectious, and climate. The four principal tissue responses include large airway changes, small airway changes, airway hyperreactivity, bronchiolar damage, and alveolar destruction. The principal physiological responses include a reversible increased airway reactivity component, pulmonary vascular response to alveolar hypoventilation, control of

breathing response to vertilation-perfusion imbalance and hypoxemia, and tissue defenses against elastase.

Decline in pulmonary function and rate of development of the syndrome depend on the combination of causative factors and individual responses to them.

Chronic Bronchitis
Pathophysiology and medical management

Chronic bronchitis is usually associated with a history of smoking and is defined as mucous hypersecretion and cough producing sputum for three months or more over a two-year period (Murray and Nadel, 1988a). Over the first few years of smoking, reversible airways changes occur. Over 10 to 15 years of smoking, mucous hypersecretion and chronic bronchitis become apparent. After 25 to 35 years of smoking, irreversible airway damage and chronic disability occur. Smoking is the major cause of lung cancer. The pathophysiology of chronic bronchitis is reviewed in detail in Chapter 29.

The patient is prone to infection and repeated periods of morbidity. Deterioration of aerobic capacity and functional capacity is related to the severity of the condition. Nutrition and hydration may be impaired particularly in severe cases because of neglect and the excessive energy cost of activities of daily living. Sleep may be irregular, thus the patient's symptoms are worsened (e.g., reduced endurance, fatigue, and lethargy) because of lack of normal physiological restoration from sleep.

The natural history of chronic bronchitis related to smoking includes mucous hypersecretion, reduction in forced expiratory volume (FEV), and increased heterogeneity of the distributions of ventilation, perfusion, ventilation-perfusion matching, and diffusion (West, 1987). General debility and deconditioning ensue.

Smoking contributes to increased mucous production in the small airways, increased mucus in the large airways, respiratory bronchiolitis, reduced elastic recoil, increased airway reactivity, and vascular changes (Bates, 1989). These changes, lead to nonuniformity of time constants in the lung, with consequent inhomogeneous distribution of inspired gas and premature small airway closure, and to nonuniformity of ventilation, perfusion, and diffusion distributions. Although variable among smokers, pulmonary function changes generally correspond to the amount smoked and duration of the smoking history. Over time, the pulmonary function profile becomes increasingly consistent with chronic airflow limitation (i.e., reduced FEV_1 and reduced FEV_1/FVC), however, these are late indicators of pulmonary changes. Signs of uneven distribution of ventilation and increased closing volumes, indicative of small airway involvement, are early pulmonary function changes in smokers. Exercise diffusing capacity is reduced which explains in part the reduced maximal VO_2 of smokers. Dynamic compliance with breathing frequency is also reduced. Residual volume is increased as a percent of total lung capacity. Tracheal mucous velocity is reduced and secretion clearance is impaired. Any patient with a smoking history, regardless of a diagnosis, has some degree of chronic airflow limitation, which must be considered when these patients are receiving medical or surgical care.

The cardiac manifestations of chronic bronchitis stem from airway obstruction, secretion accumulation and reduced capacity to effectively expectorate, polycythemia, low arterial oxygen tensions, and cardiopulmonary deconditioning. Increased airway resistance secondary to obstruction increases oxygen demand and hence the work of breathing. This increased demand is superimposed on an oxygen transport system that is already compromised. The cardiovascular system attempts to compensate for chronically reduced arterial oxygen tension by increasing cardiac output (i.e., stroke volume and heart rate). As blood gases deteriorate, the production of red blood cells increases (i.e., polycythemia) to enhance the oxygen-carrying capacity of the blood. However, polycythemia increases the viscosity of the blood, and in turn, the work of the heart to pump blood to the pulmonary and systemic circulations. Furthermore, viscous blood is prone to circulatory stasis and clotting.

Low arterial oxygen tensions lead to hypoxic pulmonary vasoconstriction and increased pulmonary vascular resistance (i.e., pulmonary hypertension). This also increases the work of the right heart in ejecting blood to the lungs. Chronic overwork of the right ventricle leads to hypertrophy, insufficiency, and eventual failure of the right heart (cor pulmonale). Chronically reduced arterial oxygen levels can in-

crease the demand on the left heart to maintain cardiac output. Similar to right-sided failure, the left heart may become hypertrophied, and over time, may fail.

The significantly increased intrathoracic pressures generated during chronic coughing reduce venous return, cardiac output, and coronary perfusion and increase blood pressure. These effects exert additional myocardial strain, lead to arterial desaturation, and increase the potential for cardiac dysrhythmias.

The complications of chronic bronchitis are exacerbated by cardiopulmonary deconditioning. Despite the pathology, the efficiency of oxygen transport along the steps in the pathway is suboptimal. This reduced efficiency increases the oxygen demands of the patient overall who is unable to adequately supply oxygen.

Pharmacological support in the long-term management of chronic bronchitis includes bronchodilators (e.g., oral, metered-dose inhalant, inhaled powdered, or aerosol), corticosteroids (e.g., oral or inhaled), expectorants, antibiotics, inotropic agents (e.g., digitalis), beta-blockers, antidysrhythmic agents, and diuretics. Patients with chronic lung disease must be monitored closely during exercise given the potential cardiac effects of disease and medications (e.g., beta-blocker agents attenuate the normal hemodynamic responses to exercise and bronchodilators, such as ventolin, elicit tachycardia).

Principles of physical therapy management

The goals of long-term management for the patient with chronic bronchitis include the following:

- Maximize the patient's quality of life, general health, and well-being and hence physiological reserve capacity
- Educate about chronic bronchitis, self-management, effects of smoking, nutrition, weight control, smoking reduction or cessation, other lifestyle factors, medications, infection control, and role of a rehabilitation program
- Facilitate mucociliary transport
- Optimize secretion clearance
- Optimize alveolar ventilation
- Optimize lung volumes and capacities and flow rates
- Optimize ventilation and perfusion matching and gas exchange
- Reduce the work of breathing

- Reduce the work of the heart
- Maximize aerobic capacity and efficiency of oxygen transport
- Optimize physical endurance and exercise capacity
- Optimize general muscle strength and thereby peripheral oxygen extraction

Patient monitoring includes dyspnea, respiratory distress, breathing pattern (depth and frequency), arterial saturation, cyanosis (delayed sign of desaturation), heart rate, blood pressure, and rate pressure product. Patients with cardiac dysfunction or low arteral oxygen tensions require ECG monitoring, particularly during exercise. If supplemental oxygen is used, the FIo_2 administered is recorded. Subjectively, breathlessness is assessed using a modified version of the Borg scale of perceived exertion.

Medication that is needed to maximize treatment response is administered before treatment (e.g., bronchodilators). Knowledge of the type of medication, its administration route, and time to and duration of peak efficacy is essential if treatment is to be maximally efficacious.

The primary interventions for maximizing cardiopulmonary function and oxygen transport in patients with chronic bronchitis include some combination of education, aerobic exercise, strengthening exercises, chest wall mobility exercises, range of motion, body positioning, breathing control and coughing maneuvers, airway clearance techniques, relaxation, activity pacing, and energy conservation. An ergonomic assessment of the patient's work and home environments may be indicated to minimize oxygen demand and energy expenditure in these settings.

The use of supplemental oxygen depends on the severity of the disease. Some patients have no need for supplemental oxygen, some need it only during exercise, and some patients require continuous oxygen with proportionately more delivered during activity and exercise compared with rest. Supplemental oxygen is not usually required until lung damage becomes extreme (i.e., the morphological changes are consistent with the irreversible changes associated with emphysema).

Education is a principal focus of the long-term management of the patient with chronic bronchitis. Education includes the reinforcement of preventative health practices (e.g., smoking reduction and cessation, cold and flu prevention, flu shots, aerobic exercise, strengthening exercises, nutrition, weight control, hydration, pacing of activities, energy conservation, relaxation, and stress management). Chronic bronchitis and emphysema are often associated with sleep disturbances. Obstructive sleep apnea is increasingly prevalent with disease severity. Thus activity and sleep patterns need to be assessed to ensure sleep is maximally restorative and is not contributing to the patient's symptoms. Integral to an exercise prescription is the time of day. Exercise is prescribed when the patient is least fatigued, most energetic, and when performing such a program is most convenient.

Aerobic exercise is an essential component of the long-term management of the patient with chronic bronchitis to optimize the efficiency of oxygen transport overall and mobilize and remove secretions (Oldenburg, Dolovich, Montgomery, and Newhouse, 1979).

Emphysema

Pathophysiology and medical management

Emphysema is associated with a prolonged history of smoking and chronic bronchitis and indicates significant irreversible lung damage. A less common type of emphysema not associated with smoking is alpha-antitrypsin deficiency. Antitrypsin is essential in balancing elastin production and degradation and in preserving optimal lung parenchymal compliance. A deficiency of antitrypsin reduces lung elasticity and contributes to the characteristic increase in lung compliance that is the hallmark of emphysema. The pathophysiology of emphysema is presented in detail in Chapter 4. The principal pathophysiological deficits include irreversible alveolar damage resulting from loss of elastic recoil and the normal tethering of the alveoli, which renders the lung parenchyma excessively compliant and floppy. Excessive distension and dilatation of the terminal bronchioles and destruction of alveoli reduces the surface area for gas exchange. Hence diffusing capacity is correspondingly reduced. The dead space in the lungs and total lung capacity increase significantly. Breathing at normal tidal volume, the patient's airways close beyond that which normally occurs with aging, which contributes to ventilation and perfusion mismatch and hypoxemia. Time constants are altered such that alveolar units are not being evenly ventilated. In its nonacute, chronic stages the primary problems include inadequate and inefficient gas exchange resulting from the structural damage to the lungs and altered respiratory mechanics of the lungs, chest wall, and their interaction. The lungs are hyperinflated, the chest wall becomes rigidly fixed in a hyperinflated position, the normal bucket handle and pump handle motions of the chest wall are impaired, the hemidiaphragms are flattened, the mediastinal structures are shifted, and the heart is displaced and rotated, making its function inefficient (Bake, Dempsey, and Grimby, 1974; Geddes, 1984; Murray and Nadel, 1988a). The normal mucociliary transport system is ineffective because years of smoking destroy the cilia, reduce their number, and alter their configuration and orientation; thus their function is correspondingly obliterated or impaired. In addition, these patients are unable to generate high transpulmonary pressures and forced expiratory flow rates because of altered respiratory mechanics. Consequently, coughing maneuvers are weak and ineffective. The administration of supplemental oxygen is limited because these patients rely on their hypoxic drive to breathe. This life-preserving drive can be attenuated with even moderate levels of oxygen. Thus oxygen administration is limited to low flows. The respiratory muscles are often weak, if not fatigued (Rochester, and Arora, 1983). Overall, patients with emphysema, particularly severe emphysema, tend to be inactive and deconditioned, which further compromises the efficiency of the oxygen transport system and the capacity of other steps in the pathway to compensate.

There are several physiological compensations that occur in response to chronic hypoxemia. Stroke volume and cardiac output are increased. The red blood cell count increases (polycythemia), however, the blood becomes more viscous and requires more work to eject and distribute throughout the body. Thus the stroke work of the heart is further increased. This load on the heart is additional to the increased afterload on the right ventricle because of an increase in pulmonary vascular resistance secondary to hy-

poxic vasoconstriction in the lungs. Over time, the heart becomes enlarged and pumps even less efficiently. In the long-term management of the patient with emphysema, alveolar ventilation, gas exchange, reduced oxygen transport efficiency, and the work of breathing and of the heart are the primary pathophysiological problems. Unlike chronic bronchitis, secretion accumulation may be less problematic in emphysema patients during nonacute periods. Nonetheless, optimizing mucociliary transport is an ongoing concern in that the consequences of mucous retention and infection can be devastating.

Principles of physical therapy management

The goals for long-term management of the patient with emphysema include the following:

- Maximize the patient's quality of life, general health, and well-being and hence physiological reserve capacity
- Educate about emphysema, self-management, smoking reduction and cessation, medications, nutrition, weight control, infection control, and the role of a rehabilitation program
- Optimize alveolar ventilation
- Optimize lung volumes and capacities and flow rates
- Optimize ventilation and perfusion matching
- Reduce the work of breathing
- Reduce the work of the heart
- Maximize aerobic capacity and efficiency of oxygen transport
- Optimize physical endurance and exercise capacity
- Optimize general muscle strength and thereby peripheral oxygen extraction
- Optimize respiratory muscle strength and endurance and overall respiratory muscle efficiency

Education focuses on teaching the patient about emphysema, self-management of the disease, the effect of smoking and smoking cessation, nutrition, weight control, hydration, relaxation, sleep and rest, stress management, activity pacing, energy conservation, and prevention (e.g., cold and flu prevention, flu shots, aerobic exercise, diet, sleep, and stress management).

Comparable with the patient with chronic bronchitis, sleep disturbances are common in the emphysema patient. Activity and sleep patterns are assessed to ensure sleep is maximally restorative. If obstructive sleep apnea is disturbing the patient's sleep, medical intervention is required.

Patient monitoring includes dyspnea, respiratory distress, breathing pattern (depth and frequency), arterial saturation, lightheadedness, discoordination, heart rate, blood pressure, and rate pressure product. Patients with cardiac dysfunction or low arterial oxygen tensions require ECG monitoring particularly during exercise. Subjectively, breathlessness is assessed using a modified version of the Borg scale of perceived exertion.

Medication that is needed to maximize treatment response is administered before treatment (e.g., bronchodilator). Knowledge of the type of medication, its administration route, and time to and duration of peak efficacy is essential if treatment is to be maximally efficacious. When patients are on multiple medications, the interactions and implications on treatment response must be identified.

The primary interventions for maximizing cardiopulmonary function and oxygen transport in patients with emphysema include some combination of education, aerobic exercise, strengthening exercise, ventilatory muscle training (strength and endurance) or ventilatory muscle rest, low flow oxygen, mechanical ventilatory support for home use, chest wall mobility exercises, range of motion exercises, body positioning, breathing control and coughing maneuvers, airway-clearance techniques, relaxation, activity pacing, and energy conservation. An ergonomic assessment of work and home environments may be indicated to minimize oxygen demands in these settings.

The benefits of aerobic and strengthening exercise in the long-term management of airflow limitation to optimize oxygen transport in patients with compromised oxygen delivery is well established (Dean, 1993; Niederman et al., 1991; Ries, Ellis, and Hawkins, 1988; ZuWallack, Patel, Reardon, Clark, and Normandin, 1991). Patients with severe limitations are often unable to exercise at a sufficient intensity to effect aerobic adaptations to the exercise stimulus. Benefits of exercise in these patients may be explained by desensitization of dyspnea, improved movement efficiency and hence movement economy, improved

anaerobic capacity, improved ventilatory muscle strength and endurance, and increased motivation (Belman and Kengregan, 1981; Belman and Wasserman, 1981; Dean, 1993). Exercise intensity is prescribed based on rating of breathlessness (modified Borg scale) (Chapter 17), in conjunction with objective and other subjective responses from the exercise test.

Patients with chronic airflow limitation alter their breathing patterns so that they are breathing on the most metabolically efficient portion of the pressure relaxation curve (Chapter 4 and 29). These patients tend to breathe with prolonged expiratory phases to maximize gas transfer and mixing in the lungs to minimize the effects of altered ventilatory time constants. To facilitate such a breathing pattern, the patient tends to breathe through pursed lips, which may create back pressure to maintain the patency of the airways (Muller, Petty, and Filley, 1970). The metabolical efficiency of the patient's breathing pattern may be improved further by altering breathing mechanics rather than imposing a different breathing pattern that may be suboptimal. Altering breathing mechanics involves manipulating the patient's body position to promote alveolar ventilation, perfusion, and ventilation and perfusion matching.

The increased intrathoracic pressures generated during chronic coughing limit venous return, cardiac output, and coronary perfusion. Blood pressure is also increased. These effects exert additional myocardial strain, lead to arterial desaturation, and increase the potential for cardiac dysrhythmias. Breathing control and coughing maneuvers coupled with body positioning and exercise are instructed such that the work of breathing is minimized (i.e., alveolar ventilation and gas transfer is as efficient as possible), and coughing is also as efficient as possible (i.e., maximally productive with the least energy expenditure).

Physical therapy is one component of a comprehensive rehabilitation program in the long-term management of emphysema. Such a program also needs to include information on health promotion and maintenance, ongoing review and log of medications, respiratory support (e.g., oxygen aerosol therapy, and mechanical ventilatory support), occupational therapy, sexual rehabilitation, psychosocial rehabilitation, and vocational rehabilitation (Dean, 1993; Murray, 1993).

Asthma

Pathophysiology and medical management

Asthma is a common respiratory condition that is characterized by hypersensitivity of the airways to various triggers resulting in reversible airway obstruction (i.e., bronchospasm and bronchial edema (Hogg, 1984; Murray and Nadel, 1988b; Rees, 1984) (Chapter 4). In mild cases, no treatment other than prophylaxis may be needed. In severe cases, asthma can be life threatening. Once affected by the trigger, the airways narrow, increasing the resistance to airflow and reducing oxygen delivery. Breathing through narrowed airways contributes to wheezing, reduced alveolar ventilation, rapid shallow breathing, shortness of breath, increased work of breathing, desaturation, and cyanosis. Increased inhomogeneity of the distribution of ventilation is present in some nonacute asthmatic patients (Ross, Bates, Dean, and Abboud, 1992). Although some triggers may produce mucous hypersecretion, even normal amounts of pulmonary secretions can obstruct narrowed airways leading to atelectasis. Asthma that has well-defined triggers is easier to manage than cases where the triggers are less specific.

Principles of physical therapy management

The goals of long-term management of the patient with asthma include the following:

- Maximize the patient's quality of life, general health, and well-being, and hence physiological reserve capacity
- Educate about asthma, self-management, nutrition, weight control, smoking reduction and cessation, medications and their uses, prevention of asthmatic attacks, and infection control
- Reduce the work of breathing
- Maximize aerobic capacity and efficiency of oxygen transport
- Optimize physical endurance and exercise capacity
- Optimize general muscle strength thereby peripheral oxygen extraction

Patient monitoring includes dyspnea, respiratory distress, breathing pattern (depth and frequency), arterial saturation, cyanosis (delayed sign of desaturation),

heart rate, blood pressure, and rate pressure product. Patients with cardiac dysfunction or low arterial oxygen tensions require ECG monitoring particularly during exercise. Subjectively, breathlessness is assessed using a modified version of the Borg scale of perceived exertion.

Medication that is needed to maximize treatment response is administered before treatment (e.g., bronchodilators and antiinflammatories). Knowledge of the type of medication, its administration route, and time to and duration of peak efficacy is essential if treatment is to be maximally efficacious. When patients are on multiple medications, their interactions and the implications for management must be known.

The primary interventions for maximizing cardiopulmonary function and oxygen transport in patients with asthma include education, aerobic exercise, strengthening exercise, chest wall mobility exercises, range of motion, relaxation, activity pacing, and stress management.

Education is central to self-management of asthma. The patient is taught the basic pathophysiology of the disease and its triggers. Other central topics including preventative health practices are also taught (e.g., cold and flu prevention, flu shots, medication types, administration, and effects, aerobic exercise, nutrition, weight control, hydration, smoking reduction and cessation, relaxation and stress management, and the benefits of an integrative life-long self-management rehabilitation program).

Special mention needs to be made regarding the use of medications and inhalers. These are frequently used unknowledgeably (i.e., the patient is unfamiliar with the basic pharmacokinetics of the medications being used and thus are not delivering optimal effects). In addition, inhalers are often used improperly; therefore the patient does not derive the full benefit of the medication. The instructions provided by the supplier of the inhalers should be strictly followed. There are numerous types of inhalers, all with different applications. By not adhering to the instructions, the patient's time and effort is wasted using the inhaler ineffectively, the patient does not derive the full benefit of the medication, an excessive amount of inhaler may be used to compensate for ineffective application, there may be increased exposure of the patient to the side effects of the medication, and there is considerable economic waste.

A knowledge of the triggers of increased airway sensitivity enables the patient to exert control over bronchospastic attacks. The patient is taught to record the frequency of bronchospastic attacks and identify what triggers and what relieves them. In this way, the patient learns to avoid or minimize their frequency, severity, and duration and minimizes the amount of medication required. These are significant benefits.

The exercise prescription parameters are set below the bronchospasm threshold, which is established based on an exercise test (Chapter 17 and 23). Specialized challenge tests are performed in a pulmonary function laboratory with appropriate medical support. Exercise training enables the patient to determine the balance between optimal aerobic capacity and medication and the optimal physical environment for exercise. Temperature and humidity can have significant effects on work output in asthmatic patients.

Bronchiectasis

Pathophysiology and medical management

Bronchiectasis is characterized by dilatation and anatomical distortion of the airways and obliteration of the peripheral bronchial tree (West, 1987). Bronchiectasis is often the sequelae of prolonged chronic lung infection. The associated inflammation leads to occlusion of the airways, which results in atelactasis of the parenchyma and consequent dilatation of central airways by increased traction on the peribronchial sheath (Bates, 1989). In addition, chronic inflammation weakens the walls of the airways, leading to further dilatation. Fibrotic, connective tissue changes in the wall contribute further to dilatation and airway distortion. These anatomical changes adversely affect normal respiratory mechanics and hence pressure volume characteristics of the lung. The chest wall becomes hyperinflated and assumes the barrel shape associated with chronic airflow limitation. The overall severity of bronchiectasis depends on the number of lung segments involved. There is often some reversible airflow limitation associated with bronchiectasis.

The patient with bronchiectasis has copious tenacious secretions, impaired respiratory mechanics, inefficient breathing pattern, reduced ability to clear secretions, reduced aerobic capacity, and is generally debilitated.

The increased intrathoracic pressures generated during bouts of chronic coughing limit venous return, caridac output, and coronary perfusion. Blood pressure is also increased. These effects exert additional myocardial strain, lead to arterial desaturation, and increase the potential for cardiac dysrhythmias and dysfunction.

Principles of physical therapy management

The goals of long-term management of the patient with bronchiectasis include the following:

- Maximize the patient's quality of life, general health, and well-being and hence physiological reserve capacity and function
- Educate about bronchiectasis, self-management, nutrition, weight control, smoking reduction and cessation, medications and their use, and infection control
- Facilitate mucociliary transport
- Optimize secretion clearance
- Optimize alveolar ventilation
- Optimize lung volumes and capacities and flow rates
- Optimize ventilation and perfusion matching
- Reduce the work of breathing
- Maximize aerobic capacity and efficiency of oxygen transport
- Optimize physical endurance and exercise capacity
- Optimize general muscle strength and thereby peripheral oxygen extraction

Patient monitoring includes dyspnea, respiratory distress, breathing pattern (depth and frequency), arterial saturation, cyanosis (a delayed sign of desaturation), heart rate, blood pressure, and rate pressure product. Patients with cardiac dysfunction or low arterial oxygen tensions require ECG monitoring particularly during exercise. Subjectively, breathlessness is assessed using a modified version of the Borg scale of perceived exertion.

Medication that is needed to maximize treatment

response is administered before treatment. Knowledge of the type of medication, its administration route, and time to and duration of peak efficacy is essential if treatment is to be maximally efficacious.

The primary interventions for maximizing cardiopulmonary function and oxygen transport in patients with bronchiectasis include some combination of education, aerobic exercise, strengthening exercise, chest wall mobility exercises, range of motion exercises, body positioning, breathing control and coughing maneuvers, airway clearance interventions, optimizing rest and sleep, relaxation, pacing, and energy conservation. An ergonomic assessment of the patient's work and home environments may be indicated to maximize function in these settings.

Education is a central component of the patient's long-term self-management rehabilitation program. Preventative health practices are taught (e.g., cold and flu prevention, flu shots, smoking cessation, sleep, aerobic exercise, nutrition, weight control, and hydration, relaxation, stress management, and the long-term benefits of an integrative, rehabilitation program).

Cystic Fibrosis
Pathophysiology and medical management

Cystic fibrosis is a complex exocrine disease that has significant systemic effects (Landau and Phelan, 1973; Murray and Nadel, 1988b). The diesase is congenital and is hallmarked by nutritional deficits contributing to impaired growth and development. Pulmonary function shows progressive decline with commensurate reductions in homogeneity of ventilation and inspiratory pressures (Chatham et al., 1994; Cotton, Graham, Mink, and Habbick, 1985; Ross et al., 1989). Cardiopulmonary involvement can be classified into three groups, namely, no physical signs in the chest, occasional cough and sputum, and constant cough, sputum, and other signs. Patients in each classification can benefit from physical therapy with respect to enhancing oxygen transport. Moderate and severe disease is characterized by significant airflow obstruction secondary to copious, tenacious secretions. In addition, pulmonary hypertension and right heart insufficiency may be manifested and eventual failure may ensue.

Between exacerbations, the medical priorities are to reduce the risk of infection and morbidity and promote optimal health, growth, and development.

Principles of physical therapy management

The goals of long-term management of the patient with cystic fibrosis include the following:
- Maximize the patient's quality of life, general health and well-being, growth and development, and physiological reserve capacity
- Educate the patient and family about cystic fibrosis, self-management, nutrition, prevention of acute exacerbations of the disease, infection control, and medication's uses, modes of administration, pharmacokinetics and times to peak efficacies.
- Facilitate mucociliary transport
- Optimize secretion clearance
- Optimize alveolar ventilation
- Optimize lung volumes and capacities and flow rates
- Optimize ventilation and perfusion matching
- Reduce the work of breathing
- Reduce the work of and strain on the heart
- Maximize aerobic capacity and efficiency of oxygen transport
- Optimize physical endurance and exercise capacity
- Optimize general muscle strength and thereby peripheral oxygen extraction

Patient monitoring includes dyspnea, respiratory distress, breathing pattern (depth and frequency), arterial saturation, cyanosis (a delayed sign of desaturation), heart rate, blood pressure, and rate pressure product. Patients with cardiac dysfunction or low arterial oxygen tensions require ECG monitoring, particularly during exercise. Subjectively, breathlessness is assessed using a modified version of the Borg scale of perceived exertion.

Medication that is needed to maximize treatment response is administered before treatment. Knowledge of the type of medication, its administration route, and time to and duration of peak efficacy is essential if treatment is to be maximally efficacious.

The primary interventions for maximizing cardiopulmonary function and oxygen transport in patients with cystic fibrosis include some combination of education, aerobic exercise, strengthening exercise, ventilatory muscle training (strength and endurance), ventilatory muscle rest, supplemental oxygen, mechanical ventilation for home use, chest wall mobility exercises, range of motion exercises, body positioning, breathing control and coughing maneuvers, airway clearance interventions, relaxation, pacing, and energy conservation.

Education focuses on teaching preventative health practices and infection control (e.g., cold and flu, flu shots, aerobic exercise, nutrition, hydration, relaxation, stress management, activity pacing, and energy conservation).

Physical activity and aerobic exercise need to be integrated early into the life style of the child with cystic fibrosis (Cystic Fibrosis and Physical Activity, International Journal of Sports Medicine, 1988; Keens, Krastins, Wannamaker, Levison, Crozier, and Bryan, 1977; Zach, Oberwaldner, and Hausler, 1992). As much as possible, the child is integrated into activities of his or her peer group. A prescribed aerobic exercise program is designed to optimize the efficiency of oxygen transport at all steps in the pathway and thereby enhance functional capacity overall. Physical activity and aerobic exercise enhances mucociliary transport and mucociliary clearance, maximizes alveolar ventilation and ventilation and perfusion matching, increases ventilatory muscle strength and endurance and airway diameter, and stimulates a productive effective cough. Furthermore, physical activity and exercise have been associated with improved immunity and reduced risks of infection (Pyne, 1994; Shephard, Verde, Thomas, and Shek, 1991). These are significant outcomes for patients with cystic fibrosis who have thick copious secretions.

In addition, breathing control and coughing maneuvers are included as a component of a long-term self-management rehabilitation program. Postural drainage and manual techniques have been the mainstay of airway clearance in the past. Exercise, however, has a primary role in secretion mobilization and as an airway clearance intervention (Dean and Ross, 1989). Breathing control and coughing stategies are coupled with exercise to facilitate secretion clearance. The principles of autogenic

drainage can be integrated into breathing control. This procedure focuses on eliciting coughing when it will be most productive, thereby minimizing less productive, exhaustive coughing. Patients with cystic fibrosis often cough so violently and uncontrollably that it leads to significant arterial desaturation, vomiting, and exhaustion and impedes venous return and cardiac output.

Ventilatory devices such as the positive expiratory pressure (PEP) mask and the flutter valve have shown benefit in some patients with CF with respect to reducing airway closure, clearing secretions, and enhancing gas exchange (Pryor, 1993; Webber and Pryor, 1994). Such aids may be useful adjuncts in some patients, however, they do not replace the multiple benefits of physical activity and exercise on optimizing oxygen transport including mobilizing and removing secretions.

RESTRICTIVE PATTERNS
Interstitial Lung Disease
Pathophysiology and medical management

The pathophysiology of restrictive lung disorders and interstitial lung disease (ILD) in particular is described in Chapter 4. This clasification of lung disease is associated with various occupations and the inhalation of inorganic and organic dust (Chung and Dean, 1989). As the disease progresses, total lung capacity (TLC) and vital capacity (VC) are reduced. Residual volume often remains the same. Maximal flow rates tend to be increased as compliance is reduced. The drive to breathe, breathing frequency, and the ratio of tidal volume to total lung capacity are increased. Glandular hyperplasia may be present, leading to mucous hypersecretion in some patients. Diffusing capacity may be reduced but may only be apparent during exercise (i.e., arterial desaturation and dyspnea). Exercise-induced desaturation and reduction in PaO_2 may also reflect shunt and ventilation and perfusion mismatch (Jernudd-Wilhelmsson, Hornblad, and Hedenstierna, 1986).

Hemodynamic changes may be present (e.g., increased pulmonary artery pressure). Chronically increased pulmonary artery pressures and hence increased pulmonary vascular resistance, lead to increased right ventricular stroke work, hypertrophy, and right ventricular insufficiency. Mixed venous oxygen Po_2 may fall significantly during exercise contributing to arterial hypoxemia.

Principles of physical therapy management

The goals of long-term management of the patient with interstitial lung disease include the following:

- Maximize the patient's quality of life, general health and well-being and hence physiological reserve capacity
- Educate about ILD, self-management, nutrition, weight control, smoking reduction and cessation, medications and their uses, prevention, health promotion, and infection control
- Optimize alveolar ventilation
- Optimize lung volumes and capacities
- Optimize ventilation and perfusion matching
- Optimize mucociliary transport
- Reduce the work of breathing
- Reduce the work of the heart
- Maximize aerobic capacity and efficiency of oxygen transport
- Optimize physical endurance and exercise capacity
- Optimize general muscle strength and thereby peripheral oxygen extraction

Patient monitoring includes dyspnea, respiratory distress, breathing pattern (depth and frequency), arterial saturation, heart rate, blood pressure, and rate pressure product. Patients with cardiac dysfunction or low arterial oxygen tensions require ECG monitoring, particularly during exercise. Subjectively, breathlessness is assessed using a modified version of the Borg scale of perceived exertion.

Medication that is needed to maximize treatment response is administered before treatment. Knowledge of the type of medication, its administration route, and time to and duration of peak efficacy is essential if treatment is to be maximally efficacious.

The primary interventions for maximizing cardiopulmonary function and oxygen transport in patients with interstitial lung disease include some combination of education, aerobic exercise, strengthening exercises, chest wall mobility exercises, range of motion exercises, body positioning, breathing control and coughing maneuvers, relaxation, pacing, and energy conservation. An ergonomic assessment of work and home environments may be indicated to maximize function in these settings.

Education is a central component of a comprehensive rehabilitation program for the management of interstitial lung disease. Education includes information on preventative health practices (e.g., removal from the causative environment, cold and influenza prevention shots, triggers of disease exacerbations and their prevention, smoking, smoking reduction and cessation, nutrition, weight control, hydration, relaxation, activity pacing, and energy conservation).

During aerobic exercise, patients with interstitial lung disease are prone to arterial desaturation (Arita, Nishida, and Hiramoto, 1981). Patients who desaturate during sleep (Perez-Padilla, West, and Lertzman, 1985) require supplemental oxygen during exercise. The intensity of the exercise prescribed is defined by arterial saturation, breathlessness, and work of the heart, in conjunction with other objective responses.

Lung Cancer
Pathophysiology and medical management

Lung cancer is a leading cause of death for men and incidence is increasing for women. Once diagnosed, 80% of patients survive a year. Lung cancer is highly correlated with a history of smoking, and exposure to coal tars, asbestos, and radioactive dusts. The majority of primary malignant tumors are bronchogenic carcinomas. They are centrally located and thus contribute to bronchial obstruction, atelectasis, and pneumonia. Pathophysiologically, lung cancer has features of both obstructive and restrictive lung disease. The patient presents with airway obstruction, dyspnea, cough, and hemoptysis (Murray and Nadel, 1988b). Treatment is limited to surgery, if metastasis has been ruled out, or conservative management with radiation and chemotherapy.

Bronchogenic carcinomas metastasize readily through the circulation and lymphatic channels to other organs including brain, bone, liver, kidneys, and adrenal glands.

If detected early, thoracic surgery may be performed to excise the cancerous tumor (Chapter 28). If inoperable, or in the case of metastases, a patient may be managed at home or in a hospice. Patients are debilitated, often undernourished, fatigued, short of breath, lethargic, depressed, and in pain (Saunders and McCorkle, 1985). Although these patients are often extremely ill, there is a growing trend to manage these patients in the community whenever possible. As the disease progresses, maintaining function and reducing the rate of deterioration become primary goals.

Principles of physical therapy management

The goals of long-term management of the medical patient with lung cancer include the following:

- Maximize the patient's quality of life, general health, and well-being and hence physiological reserve capacity
- Educate the patient and family about the benefits of a palliative program
- Promote self-determination
- Provide supportive care
- Optimize pain control
- Facilitate mucociliary transport
- Optimize scretion clearance
- Optimize alveolar ventilation
- Optimize lung volumes and capacities and flow rates
- Optimize ventilation and perfusion matching
- Reduce the work of breathing
- Maximize aerobic capacity and efficiency of oxygen transport
- Optimize physical endurance and exercise capacity
- Otimize general muscle strength and thereby peripheral oxygen extraction
- Optimize the benefits of sleep and rest
- Minimize the effects of restricted mobility and recumbency

Patient monitoring includes dyspnea, respiratory distress, breathing pattern (depth and frequency), arterial saturation, cyanosis (a delayed sign of desaturation), heart rate, blood pressure, and rate pressure product. Patients who can be mobilized but have cardiac dysfunction or low arterial oxygen tensions require ECG monitoring. Subjectively, breathlessness is assessed using a modified version of the Borg scale of perceived exertion.

Medication that is needed to maximize treatment response is administered before treatment (e.g., analgesics or bronchodilators). Knowledge of the type of medication, its administration route, and time to and duration of peak efficacy is essential if treatment is to be maximally efficacious.

The primary interventions for maximizing cardiopulmonary function and oxygen transport in patients with lung cancer include some combination of education, mobilization, strengthening exercises, chest wall mobility exercises, body positioning, supplemental oxygen, mechanical respiratory support, breathing control and coughing maneuvers, airway clearance interventions, sleep and rest, relaxation, activity pacing, and energy conservation. Treatments are timed whenever possible to coincide with the patients' peak times during the day.

Patients with cancer may benefit from the immunological effects, as well as oxygen transport effects of mobilization and physical activity (Calabrese, 1990). The prescriptive parameters are adjusted each session given the rapid changes in these patients' conditions.

Patients with lung cancer often cough up and expectorate blood in their sputum. The airways need to be as clear as possible to avoid obstruction, atelectasis, risk of infection, and pneumonia. Although airway clearance is an important goal, treatments should avoid contributing significantly to bleeding and blood loss if possible. This blood loss may contribute to anemia and fatigue.

Manual airway clearance interventions may be indicated in some patients. Postural drainage may be coupled with percussion and manual vibration. The impact of manual interventions, however, may contribute to bleeding; thus the patient requires stringent monitoring. Metastases to the thoracic cavity and the ribs in particular may preclude percussion in favor of manual vibration being performed over nonaffected areas. Treatment duration may be limited by the patient's tolerance. Tolerance may be improved by modifying body position or by shortening treatments but increasing their frequency.

PRIMARY CARDIOVASCULAR DISEASE
Angina
Pathophysiology and medical management

Angina pectoris refers to pain resulting from reduced blood flow to the myocardium. Even though usually elicited during exercise, angina may be triggered by stress or, in severe cases, may occur at rest. Atherosclerosis of one or more of the coronary arteries is the principal cause. Coronary vasospasm is a less common cause of angina. The pathophysiology of angina is described in detail in Chapter 4. A history of angina necessitates further examination to establish the severity of the coronary artery occlusion. If severe, the patient is scheduled for coronary bypass surgery (Chapter 28) to restore normal coronary blood flow. The acute and long-term management of the surgical cardiac patient is presented in Chapter 28. In less severe cases, angina is managed conservatively with medications (e.g., sublingual nitroglycerin, nitro patch, education, and physical therapy). After the patient has stabilized, a graded-exercise tolerance test may be conducted under supervision in a cardiac stress testing facility where 12-lead ECG monitoring can be performed. The exercise intensity at which the patient exhibits angina (i.e., the anginal threshold) can be quantified and serve as the basis for the prescription of physical activity and exercise.

The body position in which exercise is performed is important in patients with heart disease. Positions of recumbency increase the volume of fluid shifted from the periphery to the central circulation. This increases venous return and the work of the heart. Thus upright body positions are selected for these patients to minimize cardiac work during exercise and when resting after exercise (Langou, Wolfson, Olson, and Cohen, 1977; Levine and Lown, 1952).

Principles of physical therapy management

Patients may be referred to physical therapy with a history of angina as a primary or as a secondary problem. Regardless, angina is managed with the same care and vigilance given it can be a life-threatening condition. *A patient for whom antianginal medication is prescribed must have the medication present. The medication must not have expired and must be within visible access during treatment.* The physical therapist should examine the medication before treatment to ensure that the expiratory date has not passed and to take responsibility for positioning the medication near the patient for access to it should the patient develop angina during treatment.

The goals of long-term management of the patient with angina include the following:
- Maximize the patient's quality of life, general health, and well-being and hence physiological reserve capacity
- Educate about heart disease, self-management, nutrition, weight control, smoking reduction and cessation, disease prevention, risk factors, medications and their use, physical activity, and exercise
- Maximize aerobic capacity and efficiency of oxygen transport of all steps in the pathway
- Optimize physical endurance and exercise capacity
- Optimize general muscle strength and thereby peripheral oxygen extraction

Patient monitoring includes hemodynamic monitoring (i.e., heart rate, blood pressure, rate pressure product, and dyspnea). Subjective responses to treatment, particularly exercise, should also be recorded (e.g., Borg's rating of perceived exertion). Signs of chest pain, dyspnea, anxiety, lightheadedness, dizziness, disorientation, discoordination, cyanosis, coughing, and chest sound changes (i.e., a gallop) need to be monitored. *Angina is not an acceptable symptom under any circumstance.* Should it occur, however, treatment is immediately discontinued, and emergency measures instituted. Treatments will be safer and more precisely prescribed with continous ECG monitoring. Without ECG monitoring, treatments need to be conservative. If there is any doubt at any time about the hemodynamic stability of a patient and her or his ability to tolerate treatment safely, the patient should be referred to a general practitioner or cardiologist for clearance before being treated.

Medication that is needed to maximize treatment response is administered before treatment. Knowledge of the type of medication, its administration route, time to as well as duration of peak efficacy is essential if treatment is to be maximally efficacious.

For the long-term management of angina, interventions include some combination of education, aerobic exercise, strengthening exercise, chest wall mobility exercises, relaxation, activity pacing, and energy conservation. Education includes information about heart disease and risk factors (i.e., smoking, diet, stress, weight, alcohol, coffee, and being physically active in hot environments) and appropriate preventative strategies (i.e., smoking reduction and cessation, low-fat diet, reduced alcohol comsumption, exercise, relaxation, activity pacing, and stress management).

Patients with angina are at risk of having an infarction; therefore, vigilance and stringent monitoring are needed to detect angina or frank myocardial infarction. These patients are potentially hemodynamically unstable; thus their hemodynamic responses before, during, and after treatment, particularly aerobic and strengthening exercises, should be monitored and recorded. Minimally, heart rate, blood pressure, and rate pressure product should be taken along with the patient's subjective responses to treatment. During physical activity and exercise, heavy lifting, static exercise, straining, and the Valsalva maneuver are avoided, in addition to heavy repetitive upper-extremity work. These activities are associated with a disproportionate hemodynamic response. Physical activity and aerobic exercise are prescribed at a target heart rate or perceived exertion ranges that are below the anginal threshold based on a graded-exercise tolerance text (GXTT) (Chapter 17). Peak exercise tests in cardiac patients that may elicit angina or ST-segment changes are performed in a cardiac stress testing laboratory under the supervision of a cardiologist.

The body position in which aerobic exercise is performed is important in patients with heart disease. Positions of recumbency increase the volume of fluid shifted from the periphery to the central circulation. This increases venous return and the work of the heart. Thus upright body positions are selected for these patients to minimize cardiac work during exercise and during rest after exercise (Langou et al., 1977; Levine and Lown, 1952).

Myocardial Infarction
Pathophysiology and medical management

Angina frequently precedes frank myocardial ischemia and infarction. Myocardial ischemia is reversible, whereas infarction denotes myocardial injury and cell death (i.e., necrosis). Injured myocardial cells either recover or die during the healing period. Thus minimizing further damage and maximizing the healing during this 6-week period is critical. Myocardial infarctions can range from being silent and unnoticed by the patient to being life threatening. They can occur anywhere in the myocardium but occur primarily in the ventricles. The greater the severity, the greater the risk of ventricular insufficiency, acute pulmonary edema, and left ventricular failure. Because myocardial ischemia and infarction impair the pumping action of the heart and thus cardiac output, patients tend to be hypoxemic and in need of oxygen. Even after the oxygen has been discontinued and the myocardium has healed, the patient may continue to be vulnerable hemodynamically. First, the myocardium will have some scarring that will affect both the electrical excitability and the mechanical function of the heart. In addition, the patient may continue to have low normal arterial blood gases. Hypoxemia is lethal in that it triggers dysrhythmias and predisposes tissues to hypoxia. Thus hypoxemia must be avoided. Post myocardial infarction patients are usually discharged home on several medications (e.g., nitroglycerin, calcium antagonists, beta-blockers, and diuretics). Depending on the severity of involvement, patients usually continue to require one or more of these medications over the long term. The need for oxygen is usually short term and restricted to the patient's hospital stay.

Principles of physical therapy management

After discharge from hospital, many post myocardial infarction patients see a physical therapist either privately or through a cardiac rehabilitation program. The majority of patients will remain on a supervised rehabilitation program including an exercise program for 6 to 12 months.

Regardless of the setting, physical therapy includes education, psychosocial support, and a supervised setting for exercising safely and developing confidence during physical exertion. In addition, an exercise program is specifically prescribed for the patient to enhance oxygen transport (i.e., delivery, uptake, and utilization at the tissue level) thereby minimizing the metabolic demand on the heart.

A GXTT is conducted before leaving the hospital or when the patient is enrolled in an exercise program. The time between the exercise test and the exercise prescription and implementation of the exercise program should be minimal. Peak (formerly referred to as maximal) exercise tests are conducted in the presence of a cardiologist and provide the optimal basis for an exercise prescription. Submaximal exercise tests can be conducted by the physical therapist. These can provide the basis for an exercise program, however, the prescription is conservative compared with that based on a peak exercise test. The principles and practice of exercise testing are described in Chapter 17, 23 and 24. Such testing is an art and an exacting science and should be carried out in a rigidly standardized manner to ensure the test results are maximally valid, reliable, and useful.

Comparable with the angina patient and not overt infarction, the following caution must be adhered to with the patient who has a history of myocardial infarction. *A patient for whom antianginal medication is prescribed must have the medication present. The medication must not have expired and must be within visible access during treatment.* The physical therapist should examine the medication before treatment to ensure that the expiratory date has not passed and to take responsibility for positioning the medication near the patient for access to it should the patient develop angina during treatment.

The goals of long-term management of the patient with myocardial infarction include the following:

- Maximize the patient's quality of life, general health, and well-being and hence physiological reserve capacity
- Educate about myocardial infarction, self-management, nutrition, weight control, smoking reduction and cessation, risk factors, disease prevention, medications, life style, activities of daily living, and avoiding static exercise, straining, and the Valsalva maneuver
- Maximize aerobic capacity and efficiency of oxygen transport
- Reduce the work of the heart
- Optimize physical endurance and exercise capacity
- Optimize general muscle strength and thereby peripheral oxygen extraction

Patient monitoring includes hemodynamic monitoring (i.e., heart rate, blood pressure, and rate pressure product). Subjective responses to treatment, particularly exercise, should also be recorded (e.g., Borg's rating of perceived exertion). *Angina is not an acceptable symptom under any circumstance.* Should it occur, however, treatment is immediately discontinued and emergency measures instituted. Treatments will be safer and more precisely prescribed with continuous ECG monitoring. Without ECG monitoring, treatments need to be conservative. If there is any doubt at any time about the hemodynamic stability of a patient and her or his ability to tolerate treatment safely, the patient should be referred to a general practitioner for clearance before being treated.

Medication that is needed to maximize treatment response is administered before treatment (e.g., antiarrhythic agents). Knowledge of the type of medication, its administration route, and time to and duration of peak efficacy is essential if treatment is to be maximally efficacious.

The primary interventions for maximizing cardiopulmonary function and oxygen transport in patients with myocardial infarction include some combination of education, aerobic exercise, strengthening exercises, chest wall mobility exercises, body positioning, breathing control and coughing maneuvers, relaxation, activity pacing, and energy conservation. An ergonomic assessment of both work and home environments may be indicated to minimize myocardial strain.

Education focuses on the teaching the basic pathophysiology of heart disease, its risk factors, and prevention. Health promotion practices are advocated (e.g., smoking reduction and cessation, good nutrition, weight control, hydration, quality rest, and sleep periods). In addition, types of physical activity that impose undue myocardial strain, increase intrathoracic pressure, and restrict venous return and cardiac output, such as heaving lifting, straining, or the Valsalva maneuver, are avoided. The patient is taught to monitor and practice vigilance in monitoring his or her own condition (e.g., new signs of infarction). These patients are potentially hemodynamically unstable and thus their hemodynamic responses before, during, and after treatments, particularly exercise, should be monitored and recorded (i.e., heart rate, blood pressure, and rate pressure product should be taken, along with their subjective responses to treatment).

Peak exercise tests in cardiac patients that may elicit angina or ST-segment changes are performed in a cardiac stress testing laboratory under the supervision of a cardiologist. The parameters of the exercise prescription are set based on a peak exercise test. Intensity is set within a heart rate, oxygen consumption, and exertion range (e.g., 70% to 85%, of the anginal threshold) (Chapter 17).

Aerobic exercise of large muscle groups rather than small muscle groups (e.g., arm ergometry) is selected to minimize the increased hemodynamic demand and strain and the increased work of the heart associated with this type of work. Hot and humid conditions also place additional stress on the heart, thus exercising under these conditions should be avoided.

The body position in which aerobic exercise is performed is important in patients with heart disease. Positions of recumbency increase the volume of fluid shifted from the periphery to the central circulation. This increases venous return and the work of the heart. Thus upright body positions are selected for these patients to minimize cardiac work during exercise and during rest after exercise (Langou et al., l977; Levine and Lown, l952; Prakash, Parmley, Dikshit, Forrester, and Swan, 1973).

Valvular Disease
Pathophysiology and medical management

Valve dysfunction is either congential or acquired and may require treatment as a primary condition or is present as a secondary condition. Any of the heart and pulmonary valves may be affected. Rheumatic fever was a common cause of rheumatic heart disease and in particular mitral valve insufficiency (Goldberger, 1990). Interconnecting lymphatic vessels between the tonsils and the heart are thought to be responsible. Calcification of valves that impairs opening and closing is another example of an acquired valve dysfunction.

Clinically, patients may present with exertional dyspnea, excessive fatigue, palpitations, fluid retention, and orthopnea (Sokolow, McIlroy, and Cheitlin, 1990). These sypmtoms are often relieved when exertion is discontinued.

Prophylactic antibiotics against endocarditis are administered to most patients with significant valvular involvement and in mild disease before procedures such as dental work.

Principles of physical therapy management

The goals of long-term management of the patient with valvular heart disease include the following:
- Maximize the patient's quality of life, general health, and well-being and hence physiological reserve capacity
- Educate about cardiac valvular disease, self-management, nutrition, weight control, smoking reduction and cessation, cardiac risk factors, disease prevention, medications, life style, activities of daily living, and avoiding static exercise, straining, and the Valsalva maneuver
- Maximize aerobic capacity and efficiency of oxygen transport
- Optimize physical endurance and exercise capacity
- Reduce the work of the heart
- Optimize general muscle strength and thereby peripheral oxygen extraction

Physical therapists are involved with the management of patients with valve defects medically, either as a primary or secondary problem, and surgically. After surgery, these patients progress well; the principles of their management are presented in Chapter 28. With respect to the medical management of valve defects, the goal is to optimize oxygen transport in the patient for whom surgery is not indicated either because the defect is not sufficiently severe or because the patient cannot or refuses to undergo surgery. Although the mechanical defect cannot be improved, oxygen transport may be improved with judicious exercise prescription in some patients. The parameters of the exercise prescription are usually moderate in that inappropriate exercise doses can further disrupt the inappropriate balance between oxygen demand and supply and thus further exacerbate symptoms. In addition, there is the potential for further valvular dysfunction if the myocardium is mechanically strained.

The goal of the aerobic exercise prescription is to identify the exercise dose that will optimize the efficiency of other steps in the oxygen transport pathway such that the available oxygen delivered to the peripheral tissues is maximally used without constituting a significant mechanical strain on the heart. Maximizing work output over time is the goal. Thus the severely compromised patient will perform a significantly greater volume of functional work over time with short, frequent sessions of exercise rather than longer, less-frequent sessions.

If the valve defect is a secondary problem, the physical therapist must assess the severity of the defect and its functional consequences. The following questions must be addressed:

1. Does the defect preclude treatment?
2. Does the defect require that treatment be modified, if so, how?
3. What special precautions should be taken?
4. What signs and symptoms would indicate the patient is distressed?
5. What parameters should be monitored?
6. Is the patient taking medications as prescribed? How might these medications alter the patient's response to treatment?
7. Is there any evidence of heart failure? If so, what will the effects of exercise be?
8. If there is no evidence of heart failure at rest, what is the chance that insufficiency will develop with exercise?

Comparable with the management of the patient with a history of angina with or without a history of myocardial infarction, body positions, activities, and respiratory maneuvers that are associated with increased hemodynamic strain are avoided.

Medication that is needed to maximize treatment response is administered before treatment. Knowledge of the type of medication, its administration route, and time to and duration of peak efficacy is essential if treatment is to be maximally efficacious.

These patients are potentially hemodynamically unstable; thus their hemodynamic responses before, during, and after treatments, particularly exercise, should be monitored and recorded. Monitoring includes hemodynamic monitoring (i.e., heart rate, blood pressure, and rate pressure product). Subjective responses to treatment (e.g., rating of perceived exertion) should also be recorded. Signs of dyspnea, chest pain, lightheadedness, dizziness, disorientation, discoordination, cyanosis, coughing, chest sound changes (i.e., a gallop) need to be monitored. Treatments will be safer and more precisely prescribed with continuous ECG monitoring. Without ECG monitoring, treatments need to be conservative. If there is any doubt about the hemodynamic stability of a patient and her or his ability to tolerate treatment safely, the patient should be referred to their general practitioner for clearance before being treated.

The primary interventions for maximizing cardiopulmonary function and oxygen transport in patients with cardiac defects include some combination of education, aerobic exercise, strengthening exercises, chest wall mobility exercises, body positioning, breathing control, coughing maneuvers, relaxation, activity pacing, and energy conservation. An ergonomic assessment of both work and home environments may be indicated to minimize myocardial strain.

Exercise prescription for patients with valvular heart disease is modified to ensure that the energy demand is commensurate with oxygen supply. Otherwise, excessive oxygen demand will worsen the patient's response to physical activity, lead to further distress, and possibly reduced functional capacity. Aerobic exercise of large muscle groups rather than small muscle groups (e.g., arm ergometry) is selected to minimize the increased hemodynamic demand and strain and the increased work of the heart associated with this type of work. As for other types of cardiac conditions, exercising in hot and humid conditions shoud be avoided.

The body position in which aerobic exercise is performed is important in patients with heart disease. Positions of recumbency increase the volume of fluid shifted from the periphery to the central circulation. This increases venous return and the work of the heart. Thus upright body positions are selected for these patients to minimize cardiac work during exercise and during rest after exercise (Langou et al., 1977; Levine and Lown, 1952).

Peripheral Vascular Disease
Patholphysiology and medical management

Peripheral vascular disease results primarily from atherosclerosis and occlusion of the peripheral arteries (e.g., thoracic aorta, femoral artery, and popliteal artery) (Juergens, Spittell, and Fairbairn, 1980). Diabetes mellitus, which can result in microangiopathy and autonomic polyneuropathy, is another contributing factor to peripheral vascular disease in the lower extremities.

Arterial occlusion results in reduced blood flow to the extremities and hence reduced segmental blood pressure distal to the occlusion. In mild cases of arterial stenosis the patient may be asymptomatic because considerable stenosis has to occur before significant reduction in peripheral blood flow. Furthermore, if atheroslerosis develops gradually, collateral circulation may develop sufficiently to offset progressive vessel narrowing. Clinically, the patient presents with complaints of limb pain on exercise, coldness in the affected leg, and possibly numbness (Dean, 1987). The characteristic limb pain results from ischemia and is referred to as intermittent claudication. Mild to moderately severe cases are managed conservatively. Pain at rest is suggestive of severe stenosis and significant reduction of blood flow to the limb. Significantly reduced blood flow leads to ischemia color changes, skin breakdown, ulceration, and eventually gangrene. Bypass surgery is carried to revascularize a threatened limb or in severe cases where gangrene has developed, amputation of the limb is indicated.

Intermittent claudication secondary to mild-to-moderate arterial stenosis can benefit from aerobic exercise, which may stimulate the development of collateral blood vessels around the stenosed vessel. This condition can severely restrict mobility, which reduces function in addition to aerobic capacity and efficient oxygen transport overall.

Patients with peripheral vascular disease from diffuse systemic atherosclerosis can be expected to have stenosis of the coronary arteries even though they may be asymptomatic. These patients are monitored as stringently as cardiac patients.

Principles of physical therapy management

The goals of long-term management of the patient with peripheral vascular disease secondary to atherosclerosis include the following:

- Maximize the patient's quality of life, general health, and well-being and hence physiological reserve capacity

- Educate about atherosclerosis, self-management, nutrition, weight control, smoking reduction and cessation, risk factors, disease prevention, medications, life style, activities of daily living, and avoiding static exercise, straining, and the Valsalva maneuver
- Maximize arobic capacity and efficiency of oxygen transport
- Optimize the work of the heart
- Optimize physical endurance and exercise capacity
- Optimize general muscle strength and thereby peripheral oxygen extraction

The goals of long-term management of the patient with peripheral vascular disease secondary to diabetes mellitus must incorporate both the principles for the managment of the patient with peripheral vascular disease secondary to atherosclerosis and secondary to diabetes mellitus.

Patient monitoring includes hemodynamic monitoring (i.e., heart rate, blood pressure, and rate pressure product). Subjective responses to treatment, particularly exercise, should also be recorded (e.g., pain scale and Borg's rating of perceived exertion). These patients have an increased risk of angina. *Angina is not an acceptable symptom under any circumstance.* Thus patients should be cleared by their physicians or cardiologists before undertaking a therapeutic exercise program. Diabetic patients are potentially hemodynamically unstable; thus their hemodynamic responses before, during, and after treatment, particularly exercise, should be monitored and recorded (i.e., heart rate, blood pressure, and rate pressure product should be taken) along with their subjective responses to exercise (e.g., pain and perceived exertion). If there is any doubt at any time about the hemodynamic stability of a patient and her or his ability to tolerate treatment safely, the patient should be referred to a general practitioner for clearance before being treated or continuation of treatment.

Medication that is needed to maximize treatment response is administered before treatment. Knowledge of the type of medication, its administration route, and time to and duration of peak efficacy is essential if treatment is to be maximally efficacious.

The primary interventions for maximizing cardiopulmonary function and oxygen transport in patients with peripheral vascular disease secondary to atherosclerosis include some combination of education, aerobic exercise, strengthening exercises, relaxation, activity pacing, and energy conservation. An ergonomic assessment of both work and home environments may be indicated to minimize myocardial strain.

Education focuses on teaching the basic pathophysiology of atherosclerosis, its risk factors, and prevention. Health promotion practices are advocated (e.g., smoking reduction and cessation, nutrition, weight control, hydration, quality rest, and sleep periods). In addition, types of physical activity that impose undue myocardial strain, increase intrathoracic pressure, and restict venous return and cardiac output, such as heaving lifting, straining, or the Valsalva maneuver, are avoided. The patient is taught to monitor and practice vigilance in monitoring signs and symptoms of vascular insufficiency in the affected limb and intermittent claudication. Any sign of skin redness in the feet should be monitored closely. In the diabetic patient, any threat of skin breakdown requires medical attention and discontinuation of exercise until medical clearance has been obtained. Patients with peripheral artery disease are taught to take care of their feet particularly before and after exercise. The feet and footwear should be kept clean. The inner surfaces of shoes and socks should be smooth.

During peak exercise tests, patients with peripheral vascular disease secondary to atherosclerosis have an increased risk of angina or ST-segment changes. Such tests therefore should be performed in a peripheral vascular laboratory or cardiac stress testing laboratory under the supervision of a peripheral vascular specialist or cardiologist. The parameters of the exercise prescription are based on a peak exercise test. Walking is the activity/exercise of choice because this activity is most severely limited by intermittent claudication, which has significant implications for function. Intensity of the training stimulus is based on pain rating in conjunction with hemodynamic and other subjective responses. The patient walks at a comfortable, even cadence within her or his pain tolerance (objectively defined on the pain scale) so that limping and gait deviation is avoided.

The body position in which aerobic exercise is performed is important in patients with peripheral vascular disease. Positions of recumbency eliminate the vertical gravitational gradient. This gradient increases blood pressure significantly to the lower extremeites. Therefore the claudication threshold is lowered in recumbent positions. Recumbent positions also increase venous return and the work of the heart. Thus upright body positions are selected for these patients to maximize blood pressure in the lower extremities and to minimize cardiac work during exercise and during rest after exercise (Langou et al., 1977).

Hypertension
Pathophysiology and medical management

Hypertension or high blood pressure is a serious condition. Most patients experience no symptoms; thus adherence to medication regimens is often poor. Approximately 90% of hypertension is termed *essential hypertension* (i.e., no known etiology). Hypertension predisposes a patient to stroke, myocardial infarction, hemorrhage, and infarction of other vital organs (Sokolow, McIlroy, and Cheitlin, 1990). Blood pressure tends to increase with age. With the aging of the population, the incidence of hypertension is increasing. Increased blood pressure results from increased peripheral vascular resistance; therefore medications are prescribed that reduce myocardial afterload and peripheral vascular resistance (Goldberger, 1990).

Patients with existing cardiovascular disease (i.e., hypertension) are at risk for other manifestations. In addition, this population tends to be older and older populations are known to have a higher prevalence of cardiac dysrhythmias. Thus knowledge of cardiac status, including ECG history, should be obtained.

Principles of physical therapy management

Physical therapy contributes to increased metabolical demands and therefore imposes a hemodynamic load resulting in increased heart rate and blood pressure. The assessment should document the history of hypertension, its medical management, and the patient's response. Regardless of the condition being treated, the hypertensive patient's blood pressure must be monitored and treatment modified accordingly. However, blood pressure medications are known to attenuate hemodynamic responses to exercise (Chapter 43) ; thus the limitations of blood pressure measurement must be considered.

A program of aerobic exercise can effectively reduce high blood pressure in some patients (Blair, Painter, Pate, Smith, and Taylor, 1988; Sannerstedt, 1987). The parameters of the exercise prescription needed to control hypertension include an aerobic type of exercise that is rhythmic and involves large muscle groups, an intensity of 60% to 75% of the patient's age predicted maximal heart rate, 60 to 90 minutes in duration, performed 5 to 7 times weekly, for 3 months to achieve an optimal effect. The exercise intensity should be equivalent to a perceived exertion rating of 3 to 5 on the Borg scale (the patient is able to speak while exercising without gasping) provided that blood pressure has not increased excessively. Only modest exercise intensities are prescribed if the patient has extremely high resting blood pressure to ensure that the blood pressure does not rise excessively and is not maintained at a high pressure for a prolonged period. If the patient's hypertension responds to the exercise regimen, exercise needs to be included into the patient's life style in order for the effects to be maintained. In addition to exercise, many patients lose weight, adopt healthier life-style habits, and learn stress management and coping skills concurrently.

The goals of long-term management of the patient with hypertension include the following:

- Maximize the patient's quality of life, general health, and well-being and hence physiological reserve capacity
- Educate about hypertension, self-management, nutrition, weight control, smoking reduction and cessation, risk factors, life-style factors, disease prevention, medications and their applications and side effects
- Maximize aerobic capacity and efficiency of oxygen transport
- Optimize physical endurance and exercise capacity
- Optimize general muscle strength and thereby peripheral oxygen extraction

Patient monitoring includes hemodynamic monitoring (i.e., heart rate, blood pressure, and rate pressure product). Subjective responses to treatment, particularly exercise, should also be recorded. Signs of dyspnea, headache, lighheadedness, dizziness, disorientation, discoordination, cyanosis, coughing, and chest sound changes (i.e., a gallop) need to be monitored. Blood pressure responses that fail to increase with increasing work load and power output may be indicative of congestive heart failure.

Treatments will be safer and more precisely prescribed with contiuous ECG monitoring. Without ECG monitoring, treatments need to be conservative. If there is any doubt about the hemodynamic stability of a patient and her or his ability to tolerate treatment safely, the patient should be referred to a general practitioner or cardiologist for clearance before being treated.

Medication that is needed to maximize treatment response is administered before treatment (i.e., hypertension medications). Knowledge of the type of medication, its administration route, and time to and duration of peak efficacy is essential if treatment is to be maximally efficacious.

The primary interventions in the long-term management of hypertension include education, aerobic exercise, general body strengthening, range of motion, body mechanics, relaxation, stress management, pacing, and energy conservation. The patient is instructed in self-monitoring blood pressure, recording her or his blood pressure and those factors that associated with both high and low pressures, and blood pressure changes after having had medication. Such monitoring enables the patient to self-manage his or her hypertension and thereby reduces the need for medication, if not, eliminate it entirely. Patients, however, should only alter their medications with their physicians' approval. Physical therapists work closely with both hypertensive patients and physicians.

Systemic blood pressure responses to dynamic exercise are greater for upper-extremity than for lower-extremity work (Dean and Ross, 1992). Thus exercise prescription includes aerobic exercise of the large muscle groups to avoid small muscle group work and increasing peripheral vascular resistance and hence hemodynamic work, and the increased exertion, strain, and work of the heart experienced with upper-extremity work. Exercise is also performed in erect and upright rather than recumbent positions to minimize the increased work of the heart secondary to central fluid shifts when the patient is lying in recumbent positions.

Diabetes Mellitus
Pathophysiology and medical management

Diabetes mellitus is a condition associated with impaired insulin metabolism that can result in serious long-term multisystem consequences (Guyton, 1991). The disease is classified as insulin-dependent (IDDM) and non–insulin-dependent diabetes mellitus (NIDDM). Insulin is the carrier responsible for transporting glucose into the cells to undergo oxidation. Juvenile-onset diabetes is frequently the insulin-dependent type, whereas adult onset diabetes often is non–insulin-dependent. The underlying pathophysiology of juvenile and adult-onset diabetes, however, is distinct. Juvenile-onset diabetes results from an inadequate number of islets of Langerhan in the pancreas, which are responsible for insulin production. Adult-onset diabetes, on the other hand, results from reduced insulin sensitivity. In Western industrialized countries, adult-onset diabetes is associated with obesity, inactivity, diet, and stress. In addition, medications can contribute to blood sugar disturbances. The sequelae of diabetes mellitus that frequently result from poor regulation and management of the disease include angiopathy, peripheral neuropathy, autonomical neuropathy, gastrointestinal paresis, visual disturbance, and renal dysfunction (Bannister, 1988; Ewing and Clarke, 1986).

Patients with diabetes mellitus have an accelerated rate of atherosclerotic changes in the vasculature compared with age- and gender-matched nondiabetics. These patients are also prone to peripheral vascular disease secondary to microangiopathy, macroangiopathy, and autonomical neuropathy. Diabetic patients constitute a significant proportion of patients with peripheral vascular disease who require surgical amputation of affected limbs.

Abnormalities of blood sugar metabolism may be observed also in nondiabetic patients. Diabetogenic factors, such as restricted mobility and stress, lead to glucose intolerance and insulin oversecretion (Lipman, 1972). In the nondiabetic patient, these effects can be tolerated over the short term. However, these factors may result in a critical situation for the diabetic patient.

Principles of physical therapy management

Diabetic patients may be referred to a physical therapist for several reasons. First, a newly diagnosed diabetic patient may be referred so that the physical therapist can expose the patient to a quantified exercise stimulus under supervised conditions and thereby help refine the prescription of insulin. Second a patient may be referred for an exercise prescription to help minimize the insulin dose or avoid insulin administration entirely, depending the disease type and severity and the patient's response. Third but most frequently, patients are seen by a physical therapist for the treatment of some other condition and also report diabetes in their histories. A history of diabetes must be considered in the treatment of a patient who is referred for any reason to either improve or at least not contribute to abnormal blood glucose levels and late complications.

Diabetic patients are treated cautiously. Exercise increases metabolical demand commensurate with intensity and hence cellular demand for glucose (Amercan College of Sports Medicine, 1995; Blair et al., 1988). Usually, insulin administration is increased in preparation for exercise. Many active diabetic patients are closely attuned to their dietary and insulin needs, which permits them to be as physically active as nondiabetic individuals. However, the diabetic patients seen by physical therapists are often labile and less well managed. Thus a readily available sugar source must be nearby for insulin regulation when a diabetic patient exercises or when exercising a diabetic patient on a ergometer after anterior cruciate ligament repair in a private clinic.

In addition, diabetic patients may have hemodynamic disturbances because of a autonomic neuropathy and may exhibit impaired fluid-volume regulation during exercise (Bannister, 1988). Patients may experience postural hypotension and become dizzy and lightheaded. In addition, diabetic patients may require a longer cool-down period to adjust hemodynamically after exercise.

Hypoglycemia or low blood sugar is one of the most common complications of diabetes mellitus. This condition results from excess administration of insulin or oral hypoglycemic agent, insufficient food in relation to insulin dose, or an abnormal increase in physical activity or exercise. Hyperglycemia is common in obese patients with adult-onset diabetes. High insulin levels are associated with a higher risk of coronary artery disease. Myocardial infarction and stroke are common causes of death. Another complication is cardiac hypertrophy secondary to hypertension and cardiomyopathy, which predisposes the patient to congestive heart failure. The incidence of peripheral vascular disease is also increased in diabetic patients.

The goals of the long-term management of diabetes mellitus include the following:

- Maximize the patient's quality of life, general health and well-being, and hence physiological reserve capacity
- Educate about diabetes mellitus, self-management, nutrition, weight control, blood sugar regulation and its managment (i.e., the balance between nutrition, diet, exercise, stress and insulin requirements), medications, smoking reduction or cessation, relaxation, stress management, foot care, hygiene, and infection control
- Maximize aerobic capacity and efficiency of oxygen transport
- Optimize physical endurance and exercise capacity
- Optimize general muscle strength and thereby peripheral oxygen extraction

Patient monitoring includes signs and symptoms of hypoglycemia (e.g., lightheadedness, weakness, fatigue, disorientation, and glucose tolerance test) or hyperglycemia (e.g., glucose tolerance test). Hemodynamic responses (i.e., heart rate, blood pressure, and rate pressure product) provide an index of the intensity of an exercise stimulus, however, these responses may be attentuated in the diabetic patient because of the autonomic neuropathy; both parasympathetic and sympathetic neuropathies.

Subjective responses to exercise, including the rating of perceived exertion, may be more valid indicators of exercise intensity than hemodynamic responses in the diabetic patient. The patient is taught to be vigilant in monitoring signs and symptoms of vascular insufficiency in the affected limb. Any sign of skin redness in the feet should be monitored closely. In diabetic patients, any threat of skin breakdown requires medical attention and discontinuation of exercise until medical clearance has been obtained. Healing is considerably delayed in the diabetic foot. Without appropriate attention, infection and potential necrosis can ensue. Patients with peripheral neuropathy are taught to monitor their footwear and socks diligently, to ensure the inner surfaces are clean and smooth before each exercise session, and to check for areas of redness or abrasion of their feet after exercise.

Medication that is needed to maximize treatment response is administered before treatment (e.g., insulin or oral hypoglycemic agents). Knowledge of the type of medication, its administration route, and time to and duration of peak efficacy is essential if treatment is to be maximally efficacious.

The primary interventions in the long-term management of diabetes mellitus include education, maintainance of a log of diet and insulin regimens, activity and exercise, aerobic exercise, strengthening exercises, relaxation, stress management, activity pacing, and energy conservation.

Generally, there are no contraindications to patients with diabetes mellitus being physically active and participating in an exercise program. Daily exercise is advocated for insulin-dependent and non–insulin-dependent diabetic patients to optimize glucose control. The exercise prescription parameters are set at 40% to 85% of peak functional work capacity (American College of Sports Medicine, 1991). If the patient is exercising daily, the exercise parameters are set at the lower end of this range. If the exercise sessions are less frequent (e.g., in the case of a non–insulin-dependent diabetic patient whose blood glucose is well maintained and whose weight is acceptable) the exercise intensity is set at the higher end of this range.

The risk of hypoglycemia can be reduced by observing the following precautions: frequently monitor blood glucose, decrease the insulin dose (in consulting with the physician) or increase carbohydrate intake before exercise, avoid injecting insulin into areas that are active during exercise, avoid exercise during peak insulin activity, consume carbohydrates before, during, and after prolonged aerobic activity, and be knowledgeable about the signs and symptoms of hypoglycemia (American College of Sports Medicine, 1991).

SUMMARY

This chapter reviews the pathophysiology, medical management, and physical therapy management of chronic, primary, cardiopulmonary pathology. Given that the heart and lungs are interdependent and function as a single unit, primary lung or heart disease are considered with respect to the other organ and in the context of oxygen transport overall.

The long-term cardiopulmonary management of chronic lung diseases is presented first. Although there is no clear line between obstructive and restrictive patterns of lung disease, pathology can be generally defined based on the primary underlying pathophysiological problems. Thus the primary conditions presented included obstructive lung disease (i.e., chronic airflow limitation, asthma, bronchiectasis, and cystic fibrosis) and restrictive lung disease (i.e., interstitial pulmonary fibrosis). Lung cancer, which has the characteristics of both obstructive and restrictive patterns of pathology, is also presented.

The long-term cardiopulmonary management of heart disease was then presented with special attention to angina, myocardial infarction, and valvular heart disease. Chronic vascular diseases including peripheral vascular disease, hypertension, and diabetes were also presented.

The principles of management of the various chronic primary cardiopulmonary conditions are presented rather than treatment prescriptions, which cannot be discussed without consideration of a specific patient.

REVIEW QUESTIONS

1. Describe the *chronic* primary cardiopulmonary pathophysiology associated with airflow limitation, asthma, bronchiectasis, cystic fibrosis, interstitial pulmonary fibrosis, lung cancer, angina, myocardial infarction, valvular heart disease, peripheral vascular disease, hypertension, and diabetes.

2. Relate cardiopulmonary physical therapy treatment interventions to the underlying pathophysiology of *each* of the above chronic conditions and provide the *rationale* for your choice.

References

American College of Sports Medicine. (1991). *ACSM's guidelines for exercise testing and prescription* (4th ed.). Philadelphia: Williams & Wilkins.

Arita, K.I., Nishida, O., & Hiramoto, T. (1981). Physical exercise in "pulmonary fibrosis." *Hiroshima Journal of Medical Science, 30,* 149-159.

Bake, B., Dempsey, J., & Grimby, G. (1976). Effects of shape changes of the chest wall on distribution of inspired gas. *American Review of Respiratory Disease, 114,* 1113-1120.

Bannister, R. (1988). *Autonomic failure* (2nd ed.). Oxford: Oxford Medical Publications.

Bates, D.V. (1989). *Respiratory function in diseases.* (3rd ed.). Philadelphia: WB Saunders.

Belman, M.J., & Kendregan, B.A. (1981). Exercise training fails to increase skeletal muscle enzymes in patients with chronic obstructive pulmonary disease. *American Review of Respiratory Diseases, 123,* 256-261.

Belman, M.J., & Wasserman, K. (1981). Exercise training and testing in patients with chronic obstructive pulmonary disease. *Basics of Respiratory Diseases, 10,* 1-6.

Blair, S.N., Painter, P., Pate, R.R., Smith, L.K., & Taylor, C.B. (1988). *Resource manual for guidelines for exercise testing and prescription.* Philadelphia: Lea & Febiger.

Calabrese, L.H. (199). Exercise, immunity, cancer, and infection. In C. Bouchard, R.J. Shepard, T. Stephens, J.R. Sutton, & B.D. McPherson, (Eds.). *Exercise, fitness, and health. A consensus of current knowledge.* Champaign, IL: Human Kinetics Books.

Chatham, K., Berrow, S., Beeson, C., Griffiths, L., Brough, D., & Musa, I. (1994). Inspiratory pressures in adult cystic fibrosis. *Physiotherapy, 80,* 748-752.

Chung, F., & Dean, E. (1989). Pathophysiology and cardiorespiratory consequences of interstitial lung disease—review and clinical implications. *Physical Therapy, 69,* 956-966.

Cotton, D.J., Graham, B.L., Mink, J.T., & Habbick, B.F. (1985). Reduction of the single breath diffusing capacity in cystic fibrosis. *European Journal of Respiratory Diseases, 66,* 173-180.

Cystic fibrosis and physical activity. (1988). International *Journal of Sports Medicine, 9* (Suppl. 1), 1-64.

Dantzker, D.R. (1983). The influence of cardiovascular function on gas exchange. *Clinics in Chest Medicine, 4,* 149-159.

Dean, E. (1987). Assessment of the peripheral circulation: an update for practitioners. *The Australian Journal of Physiotherapy, 33,* 164-172.

Dean, E., & Ross, J. (1989). Integrating current literature in the management of cystic fibrosis: a rejoinder. *Physiotherapy Canada, 41,* 46-47.

Dean, E., & Ross, J. (1992). Mobilization and exercise conditioning. In C. Zadai, (Ed.). *Pulmonary management in physical therapy*. New York: Churchill Livingstone.

Ewing, D.J., & Clarke, B.F. (1986). Autonomic neuropathy: its diagnosis and prognosis. In P.J. Watkins (Ed.). *Clinics in endocrinology and metabolism*. London: WB Saunders.

Froelicher, V.F. (1987). *Exercise and the heart. Clinical concepts*. (2nd ed.). St. Louis: Mosby.

Geddes, D.M. (1984). Chronic airflow obstruction. *Postgraduate Medicine, 60,* 194-200.

Goldberger, E. (1990). *Essentials of clinical cardiology*. Philadelphia: JB Lippincott.

Guyton, A.C. (1991). *Textbook of medical physiology*. (8th ed.). Philadelphia: WB Saunders.

Hogg, J.C. (1984). The pathology of asthma. *Clinics in Chest Medicine, 5,* 567-571.

Jernudd-Wilhelmsson, Y., Hornblad, Y., & Hedenstierna, G. (1986). Ventilation perfusion relationships in interstitial lung disease. *European Journal of Respiratory Disease, 68,* 39-49.

Juergens, J.L., Spittell, J.A., Fairbairn, J.F. (1980). *Peripheral vascular diseases* (5th ed.). Philadelphia: WB Saunders.

Keens, T.G., Krastins, I.R.B., Wannamaker, E.M., Levison, H., Crozier, D.N., & Bryan, A.C. (1977). Ventilatory muscle endurance training in normal subjects and patients with cystic fibrosis. *American Review of Respiratory Disease, 116,* 853-860.

Landau, L.I., & Phelan, P.D. (1973). The spectrum of cystic fibrosis. *American Review of Respiratory Disease, 108,* 593-602.

Langou, R.A., Wolfson, S., Olson, E.G., & Cohen, L.S. (1977). Effects of orthostatic postural changes on myocardial oxygen demands. *American Journal of Cardiology, 39,* 418-421.

Leon, A.S. (1987). Diabetes. In J.S. Skinner (Ed.). *Exercise testing and exercise prescription for special cases. Theoretical basis and clinical application*. Philadelphia: Lea & Febiger.

Lipman, R.L. (1972). Glucose tolerance during decreased physical activity in man. *Diabetes, 21,* 101-105.

Muller, R.E., Petty, T.L., & Filley, G.F. (1970). Ventilation and arterial blood gas changes induced by pursed-lip breathing. *Journal of Applied Physiology, 28,* 784-789.

Murray, E. (1993). Anyone for pulmonary rehabilitation? *Physiotherapy, 79,* 705-710.

Murray, J.E., & Nadel, J.A. (1988a). *Textbook of respiratory medicine*. Part 1. Philadelphia: WB Saunders.

Murray, J.E., & Nadel, J.A. (1988b). *Textbook of respiratory medicine*. Part 2. Philadelphia: WB Saunders.

Niederman, M.S., Clemente, P.H., Fein, A.M., Feinsilver, S.H., Robinson, D.A., Howite, M.S., & Bernstein, M.G. (1991). Benefits of a multidisciplinary pulmonary rehabilitation program: improvements are independent of lung function. *Chest, 99,* 798-804.

Oldenburg, F.A., Dolovich, M.B., Montgomery, J.M., & Newhouse, M.T. (1979). Effects of postural drainage, exercise, and cough on mucus clearance in chronic bronchitis. *American Review of Respiratory Disease, 120,* 739-745.

Perez-Padilla, R., West, P., & Lertzman, M. (1985). Breathing during sleep in patients with interstitial lung disease. *American Review of Respiratory Disease, 132,* 224-229.

Prakash, R., Parmley, W.W., Dikshit, K., Forrester, J., & Swan, H.J. (1973). Hemodynamic effects of postural changes in patients with acute myocardial infarction. *Chest, 64,* 7-9.

Pryor, J.A. (1993). *Respiratory care*. Edinburgh: Churchill Livingstone.

Pyne, D.B. (1994). Regulation of neutrophil function during exercise. *Sports Medicine, 17,* 245-258.

Rees, J. (1984). ABC of asthma. Definition and diagnosis. *British Medical Journal, 5,* 1370-1372.

Ries, A.L., Ellis, B., & Hawkins, R.W. (1988). Upper extremity exercise training in chronic obstructive pulmonary disease. *Chest, 93,* 688-692.

Rochester, D.F., & Arora, N.S. (1983). Respiratory muscle failure. *Medical Clinics of North America, 67,* 573-597.

Ross, J., Bates, D.V., Dean, E., & Abboud, J.T.(1992a). Discordance of airflow limitation and ventilation inhomogeneity in asthma and cystic fibrosis. *Clinical and Investigative Medicine, 15,* 97-102.

Ross, J., & Dean, E. (1989). Integrating physiological principles into the comprehensive management of cardiopulmonary dysfunction. *Physical Therapy, 69,* 255-259.

Sannerstedt, R. (1987). Hypertension. In J.S. Skinner (Ed.). *Exercise testing and exercise prescription for special cases. Theoretical basis and clinical application*. Philadelphia: Lea & Febiger.

Saunders, J.M., & McCorkle, R. (1985). Model of care for persons with progressive cancer. *Journal of Otolaryngology, 14,* 365-378.

Scharf, S.M., & Cassidy, S.S. (Eds.). (1989). *Heart-lung interactions in health and disease*. New York: Marcel Dekker.

Shephard, R.J., Verde, T.J., Thomas, S.G., & Shek, P. (1991). Physical activity and the immune system. *Canadian Journal of Sports Science, 16,* 163-185.

Sokolow, M., McIlroy, M.B., & Cheitlin, M.D. (1990). *Clinical cardiology*. (5th ed.). Norwalk: Appleton & Lange.

Underhill, S.L., Woods, S.L., Froelicher, E.S.S., & Halpenny, C.J. (1989). *Cardiac nursing*. (2nd ed.). Philadelphia: JB Lippincott.

Wasserman, K.L., & Whipp, B.J. (1975). Exercise physiology in health and disease. *American Review of Respiratory Disease, 112,* 219-249.

Webber, B.A., & Pryor, J.A. (1994). *Physiotherapy for respiratory and cardiac problems*. Edinburgh: Churchill Livingstone.

West, J.B. (1987). *Pulmonary pathophysiology*. Baltimore: Williams & Wilkins.

Zach, M., Oberwaldner, B., & Hausler, F. (1982). Cystic fibrosis: Physical exercise versus chest physiotherapy. *Archives of Diseases in Children, 57,* 587-589.

ZuWallack, R.L., Patel, K., Reardon, J.Z., Clark, B.A., & Normandin, E.A. (1991). Predictors of improvement in the 12-minute walking distance following a six-week outpatient pulmonary rehabilitation program. *Chest, 99,* 805-808.

CHAPTER 30

Chronic Secondary Cardiopulmonary Dysfunction

Elizabeth Dean
Donna Frownfelter

KEY TERMS

Ankylosing spondylitis
Cerebral palsy
Chronic renal insufficiency
Hemiplegia
Kyphoscoliosis
Late sequelae of poliomyelitis
Multiple sclerosis

Muscular dystrophy
Osteoporosis
Parkinson's disease
Rheumatoid arthritis
Scleroderma
Spinal cord injury
Systemic lupus erythematosus

INTRODUCTION

The purpose of this chapter is to review the pathophysiology, medical management, and physical therapy management of chronic, secondary cardiopulmonary pathology. Specifically, this chapter addresses chronic cardiopulmonary dysfunction secondary to neuromuscular, musculoskeletal, collagen vascular/connective tissue, and renal dysfunction. The neuromuscular conditions that are presented include muscular dystrophy, hemiplegia, Parkinson's disease, multiple sclerosis, cerebral palsy, spinal cord

injury, and the late sequelae of poliomyelitis. The musculoskeletal conditions that are presented include kyphoscoliosis and osteoporosis. The collagen vascular/connective tissue conditions that are presented include systemic lupus erythematosus, scleroderma, ankylosing spondylitis, and rheumatoid arthritis. Finally, management of the patient with chronic renal insufficiency is presented. The principles of management are presented rather than treatment prescriptions, which cannot be given without consideration of a specific patient. (For specific examples of patient treatment prescriptions refer to the companion text *Clinical case studies in cardiopulmonary physical therapy.*) In this context the goals of long-term management of each condition are presented, followed by the essential monitoring required and the primary interventions for maximizing cardiopulmonary function and oxygen transport. The selection of interventions for any given patient is based on the physiological hierarchy. The most physiological interventions are exploited followed by less physiological interventions and those whose efficacy is less well documented (Chapter 16).

NEUROMUSCULAR CONDITIONS
Muscular Dystrophy
Pathophysiology and medical management

Degenerative neurological and muscular diseases, including Duchenne's muscular dystrophy, lead to respiratory muscle weakness and alveolar hypoventilation (Black and Hyatt, 1971; Braun, Arora, and Rochester, 1983; Inkley, Alderberg, and Vignos, 1974). Vital capacity, forced expiratory volume, airflow rates, and maximum inspiratory and expiratory pressures are reduced. These patients are at risk for the development of atelectasis, impaired mucociliary transport, and pneumonia. In addition, long-term generalized muscular weakness, particularly of the thoracic cavity and abdomen, as well as restricted mobility and confinement to a wheelchair, predispose the patient to thoracic deformities (e.g., scoliosis and dropping of the ribs, and further muscle disuse). Patients with Duchenne's muscular dystrophy are susceptible to dysphagia and upper airway obstruction secondary to gag reflex depression and hypotonia of the pharyngeal structures (Murray and Nadel, 1988a). These factors further compromise or threaten cardiopulmonary function and oxygen transport.

Cardiac dysfunction has also been reported in progressive muscular dystrophy (Moorman et al., 1985; Perloff, de Leon, and O'Doherty, 1966). Although the majority of patients have no clinical evidence of cardiac dysfunction, a high proportion have abnormal ECGs at rest or during exercise and abnormal echocardiography and radionuclide ventriculography showing reduced left ventricular ejection fraction and abnormal ventricular wall motion. Fatty and fibrous tissue infiltrate the myocardium and conduction system and electrical conduction is slowed. Thus subclinical cardiac involvement is prevalent in patients with muscular dystrophy and may explain sudden death in this patient population.

Chronic respiratory muscle weakness is characteristic of muscular dystrophy and other neuromuscular disorders. Because the cardiopulmonary system is seldom stressed due to musculoskeletal dysfunction in these patients, respiratory muscle weakness is seldom detected. Such weakness is significant, however, in that it contributes to several other serious problems, including thoracic mechanical abnormalities, diffuse microatelectasis, reduced lung compliance, a weak cough with impaired mucociliary transport and secretion accumulation, ventilation and perfusion imbalance, and nocturnal hypoxemia (Smith, Calverley, Edwards, Evans, and Campbell, 1987; Smith, Edwards, and Calverley, 1989). Progressive respiratory muscle weakness increases the risk of respiratory muscle fatigue and failure (Macklem and Roussos, 1977).

The severity of disease is not consistently correlated with compromised pulmonary function; thus cardiopulmonary function must be assessed individually in each patient (Hapke, Meek, and Jacobs, 1972). Patients with mild-to-moderate involvement of peripheral muscles may exhibit disproportionate respiratory compromise (Kilburn, Eagan, Sieker, and Heyman, 1959). This may be explained by differential changes in the degree of involvement of the diaphragm and the abdominal and intercostal muscles (Nakano, Bass, Tyler, and Carmel, 1976). Over time, musculoskeletal changes of the chest wall lead to spinal deformity and stiffness with loss of its elastic recoil. Chronic alveolar hypoventilation leads to respiratory insufficiency and the need for ventilatory assistance. With progressive respiratory insufficiency, nocturnal hypoventilation with hypercapnia and hypoxemia develop (Bach, O'Brien, Krotenberg, and Alba, 1987). Nocturnal respiratory support should be considered early to postpone the need for intubation and mechanical ventilation, which is associated with a poor prognostic outcome in patients who have chronically reduced vital capacities and weak cough.

Clinically, patients with muscular dystrophy present with low functional capacity commensurate with the extent of muscle weakness and impaired cardiopulmonary function, including alveolar hypoventilation, orthopnea (shortness of breath, on reclining), impaired mucociliary transport, difficulty clearing secretions, and increased work of breathing. Abdominal muscle strength provides an index of pulmonary function in that it is correlated with vital capacity and expiratory flow rates (Hapke et al., 1972). The significant progressive functional loss associated with Duchenne's muscular dystrophy increases the patient's susceptibility to the sequelae of restricted mobility, including cardiopulmonary deconditioning and reduced efficiency of oxygen transport, circulatory stasis, muscular weakness, and bone loss.

Improved medical management of the complications of myopathies has significantly increased the life expectancy of patients, such as those with Duchenne's muscular dystrophy, over the past 20 years. With advancing age, further complications will arise from age-related changes in cardiopulmonary function (Dean, 1994; Leblanc, Ruff and Milic-Emili, 1970). Thus in the years ahead an increasing number of patients with myopathies will be requiring cardiopulmonary management and prophylaxis.

Principles of physical therapy management

The goals of long-term management for the patient with muscular dystrophy include the following:

- Maximize the patient's quality of life, general health, and well-being and hence physiological reserve capacity
- Educate about cardiopulmonary manifestations of muscle dystrophy, self-management, medications, nutrition, weight control, smoking reduction and cessation, airway protection, infection control, the role of a rehabilitation program, and the eventual need for mechanical ventilatory support
- Optimize alveolar ventilation
- Optimize lung volumes and capacities and flow rates
- Optimize ventilation and perfusion matching and gas exchange
- Protect the airways from aspiration

- Reduce the work of breathing
- Reduce the work of the heart
- Facilitate mucociliary transport
- Optimize secretion clearance
- Maximize aerobic capacity and efficiency of oxygen transport
- Optimize physical endurance and exercise capacity
- Optimize general muscle strength and thereby peripheral oxygen extraction

Patient monitoring includes dyspnea, respiratory distress, breathing pattern (depth and frequency), arterial saturation, cyanosis (delayed sign of desaturation), heart rate, blood pressure, and rate pressure product. Patients with cardiac dysfunction need to be cleared by a cardiologist before starting a rehabilitation program, particularly when it involves a mobilization or exercise program, to refine the prescriptive parameters of the program. If supplemental oxygen is used, the FIO_2 administered is recorded. Subjectively, breathlessness is assessed using a modified version of the Borg scale of perceived exertion. Assessment of nighttime and daytime cardiopulmonary function is needed because respiratory insufficiency often begins with nocturnal hypoxemia in patients with Duchenne's muscular dystrophy.

Medication that is needed to maximize treatment response is administered before treatment. Knowledge of the type of medication, its administration route, and time to and duration of peak efficacy is essential if treatment is to be maximally efficacious.

The primary interventions for maximizing cardiopulmonary function and oxygen transport in patients with muscular dystrophy include some combination of education, mobilization, primarily in the form of functional activities, strengthening exercises, primarily in the form of functional activities (to maintain strength or reduce rate of decline), ventilatory muscle training, postural correction exercises, chest wall mobility exercises, range of motion exercises, deformity prevention, body positioning, breathing control and coughing maneuvers, airway clearance interventions, activity pacing, and energy conservation. An ergonomic assessment of the patient's work and home environments may be indicated to minimize oxygen demand and energy expenditure in these settings. Such an assessment includes review of aids and devices (e.g., wheelchair type, weight, and size and noninvasive mechanical ventilation). Aids and devices are selected to minimize energy demand such that energy is conserved for other activities and undue fatigue is reduced.

The use of supplemental oxygen depends on the severity of the disease. Some patients have no need for supplemental oxygen, some need it only during exercise, and some patients require continuous oxygen with proportionately more delivered during activity and exercise compared with rest.

Education is a principal focus of the long-term management of the patient with muscular dystrophy. Education includes the reinforcement of preventative health practices (e.g., infection control, cold and flu prevention, flu shots, aerobic exercise, strengthening exercises, nutrition, weight control, hydration, pacing of activities, and energy conservation). Weight control is an important goal in patients with chronic neuromuscular diseases because they have the least capacity to compensate for the cardiopulmonary sequelae of obesity (Alexander, 1985). Obstructive sleep apnea is related to hypotonia of the upper airway musculature and obesity. Thus activity and sleep patterns need to be assessed to ensure sleep is maximally restorative and not contributing to the patient's symptoms.

Mobilization is an essential component of the long-term management of the patient with muscular dystrophy to optimize the efficiency of oxygen transport overall and minimize the sequelae of restricted mobility, including circulatory stasis. Maximizing ventilation with mobilization is limited if the patient has severe generalized muscular weakness and increased fatigue. Functional activities provide the basis for the mobilization prescription. Although heavy resistive strengthening exercise has been advocated for these patients (Vignos and Watkins, 1966), a conservative approach, including an exercise program based on functional goals and energy conservation, is more justifiable physiologically. Chest wall mobility exercises include all planes of movement combined with a rotational component. Body positioning to optimize lung volumes and airflow rates is a priority. Breathing control and coughing maneuvers are coupled with body movement and positioning. If mucociliary transport is impaired, leading to secretion accumulation, postural drainage may need to be instituted, coupled with deep breathing and coughing maneuvers.

Although the primary factor contributing to respiratory compromise is respiratory muscle weakness, the capacity of the respiratory muscles to respond to resistive loading is limited. However, ventilatory muscle training may have some role in selected patients, particularly children (Adams and Chandler, 1974; Pardy and Leith, 1984). Improved respiratory muscle endurance and strength may have a generalized effect on functional capacity (Reid and Warren, 1984). Patients with signs of ventilatory muscle fatigue, as opposed to weakness, benefit from ventilatory support at night. Rest of the respiratory muscles at night optimizes their function during the daytime.

Methods of facilitating effective coughing in patients with neuromuscular diseases are extremely important because they constitute life-preserving measures. Supported and unsupported coughing methods are described in detail in Chapters 20 and 21. Patients on noninvasive ventilatory support who are unable to generate adequate peak cough expiratory flow rates can benefit from manual assisted coughing and mechanical insufflation-exsufflation, thereby minimizing the need for endotracheal suctioning (Bach, 1993; Barrach, Beck, Bickerman, and Seanor, 1952). Tracheostomy is delayed as long as possible. Significantly reduced maximal insufflation capacity, however, is an indication for tracheostomy.

Whenever possible, deep breathing and coughing are coupled with chest wall movement to facilitate maximal inflation of the lungs before coughing by increasing pulmonary compliance (Ferris and Pollard, 1960) and maximal exhalation of the lungs during coughing. Body positions are varied and changed frequently to simulate shifts in alveolar volume and ventilation and perfusion that occur with normal movement and body position changes. Glossopharyngeal breathing is a nonmechanical method of assisting ventilation. The patient is taught to use the tongue and pharyngeal muscles to swallow boluses of air past the vocal cords and into the trachea (Bach, Alba, Bodofsky, Curran, and Schultheiss, 1987). The efficiency of training is monitored with spirometry to ensure the patient is able to achieve acceptable vital capacities. Some patients are able to support their ventilation, ventilator-free, for several hours in a day.

One intervention that is prolonging the life of patients with muscular dystrophy, as well as of patients with other progressive neuromuscular diseases, is the use of mechanical ventilatory support (Bach, 1992; Curran, 1981). Home mechanical ventilation provides a noninvasive method of providing positive airway pressure through an oral or nasal mask. This provides considerable advantage over invasive, full body or tracheostomy ventilatory support. Used in conjunction with an insufflation-exsufflation device, pulmonary complications can be minimized and life expectancy increased. Other forms of noninvasive mechanical ventilation include intermittent abdominal pressure ventilation, rocking bed, negative pressure tank ventilator, and chest shell ventilator. The type of ventilation is determined individually based on the indications for ventilation and the patient's status. The use of ventilatory aids as a component of a comprehensive rehabilitation program maintains pulmonary compliance and cough efficacy. Introduction of these devices early will facilitate increased use as the respiratory muscles progressively weaken.

Patients with generalized neuromuscular weakness require prophylactic management given their high risk of developing life-threatening respiratory infections and complications. Prophylaxis should include flu shots, avoiding polluted, smoky environments, smoking reduction and cessation, controlling the types of food eaten and chewing well to avoid choking, and regular deep breathing, frequent movement, and change in body positions (even just shifting and taking some deeper breaths while seated in a wheelchair) to promote mucociliary transport. An optimal time to take deep breaths and to cough is during transfers, which usually are physically exerting and stimulate hyperpnea.

Hemiplegia
Pathophysiology and medical management

Hemiplegia or stroke affects cardiopulmonary function either directly or indirectly (Fugl-Meyer and Grimby, 1984; Griggs and Donohoe, 1982). A cerebral infarct involving the vital centers of the brain can affect cardiopulmonary function. Such infarctions, however, are likely to be lethal. More commonly, after a stroke, chest wall movement and electrical activity on the ipsilateral side are reduced (DeTroyer, DeBeyl, and Thirion, 1981; Fluck, 1966). Facial and pharyngeal weakness contributes to an inability to control oral secretions, swallow effectively, and protect the upper airway. Altered respiratory mechanics and efficiency reflect impaired chest wall movement, asymmetry, and the degree of muscle paresis and spasm.

Patients with hemiplegia have associated problems that contribute to cardiopulmonary dysfunction. These patients tend to be older, hypertensive, and have a high incidence of cardiac dysfunction. Muscle disuse and restricted mobility secondary to hemiplegia lead to reduced cardiopulmonary conditioning and inefficient oxygen transport. Spasticity increases metabolical and oxygen demand. Hemiparesis results in gait deviations, which reduce movement efficiency and movement economy. Reduced movement economy results in an increased energy cost associated with ambulation, which may reduce exercise tolerance because of fatigue (Dean and Ross, 1993). In addition, ambulating with a walking aid is associated with a significantly increased energy cost compared with normal walking. This increased energy cost reduces the patient's exercise tolerance further and increases fatigue.

Principles of physical therapy management

The goals of long-term management for the patient with hemiplegia include the following:
- Maximize the patient's quality of life, general health, and well-being and hence physiological reserve capacity
- Educate about cardiopulmonary manifestations of hemiplegia, self-management, medications, smoking reduction and cessation, nutrition, weight control, and the role of a rehabilitation program
- Optimize alveolar ventilation
- Optimize lung volumes and capacities and flow rates
- Optimize ventilation and perfusion matching and gas exchange
- Reduce the work of breathing

- Reduce the work of the heart
- Protect the airways from aspiration
- Facilitate mucociliary transport
- Optimize secretion clearance
- Maximize aerobic capacity and efficiency of oxygen transport
- Optimize physical endurance and exercise capacity
- Optimize general muscle strength and thereby peripheral oxygen extraction

Patient monitoring includes dyspnea, respiratory distress, breathing pattern (depth, symmetry, and frequency), arterial saturation, cyanosis (delayed sign of desaturation), heart rate, blood pressure, and rate pressure product. Patients with cardiac dysfunction require clearance from a cardiologist before participating in a rehabilitation program and may require ECG monitoring, particularly during exercise. Subjectively, perceived exertion is rated using the Borg scale.

Medication that is needed to maximize treatment response is administered before treatment (e.g., antihypertensive and cardiac medications). Knowledge of the type of medication, its administration route, and time to and duration of peak efficacy is essential if treatment is to be maximally efficacious.

The primary interventions for maximizing cardiopulmonary function and oxygen transport in patients with hemiplegia include some combination of education, aerobic exercise, strengthening exercises, spasticity control, postural correction exercises, gait reeducation, chest wall mobility exercises, range of motion exercises, body positioning, breathing control and coughing maneuvers, airway clearance interventions, activity pacing, and energy conservation. An ergonomic assessment of the patient's work and home environments may be indicated to minimize oxygen demand and energy expenditure in these settings.

Education is a principal focus of the long-term management of the patient with hemiplegia. Education includes the reinforcement of preventative health practices (e.g., infection control, smoking reduction and cessation, cold and flu prevention, flu shots, aerobic exercise, strengthening exercises, gait reeducation, nutrition, weight control, hydration, pacing of activities, and energy conservation). Hemiplegia is often associated with sleep disturbances (e.g., obstructive sleep apnea). Thus activity and sleep patterns need to be assessed to ensure sleep is maximally restorative and not contributing to the patient's symptoms.

Aerobic exercise is an essential component of the long-term management of the patient with hemiplegia to optimize the efficiency of oxygen transport overall. Maximizing ventilation with mobilization is limited if the patient has severe generalized muscular weakness and increased fatigue. Although aggressive mobilization can be supported in these patients (Malouin, Potvin, Prevost, Richards, and Wood-Dauphinee, 1992), appropriate selection of patients for such a regimen, judicious exercise prescription, and monitoring must be instituted to ensure the treatment is optimally therapeutic and poses no risk to a patient in this high-risk group. Chest wall exercises include movement in all planes combined with rotation. Body positioning to optimize lung volumes and airflow rates is a priority. Breathing control and coughing maneuvers are essential and should be coupled with body movement and positioning. Exercise is conducted in the upright positions to minimize the work of the heart and of breathing during physical exertion. Recumbent positions reduce lung volumes and expiratory flow rates, impair respiratory mechanics, increase closing volumes, increase thoracic blood volume, and increase compressive forces on both the lungs and the heart (Dean and Ross, 1992; Ross and Dean, 1992). Thus significant periods and intensities of aerobic exercise should be performed standing or sitting. Lower-extremity work is preferable to upper-extremity work in that the latter is associated with increased hemodynamic stress. Rhythmic exercise of large muscle groups is preferable to static exercise and exercise of small muscle groups, such as the arms, in that it produces smaller hemodynamic effects.

Ambulation or wheelchair locomotion should be as efficient as possible so that the metabolical demand of these functional activities is reduced. Performing these activities inefficiently on a frequent basis contributes to an excessive oxygen demand. The patient expends considerable energy in performing these activities uneconomically, which impairs the patient's tolerance and contributes to excessive fatigue. Conserving energy by performing these activities more economically from an energetic perspective will provide more energy to perform more of these or other activities.

Patients with generalized neuromuscular weakness require prophylactic management given their high risk of developing life-threatening respiratory infections and complications. Prophylaxis should include flu shots, avoiding polluted, smoky environments, smoking reduction and cessation, controlling the types of food eaten and chewing well to avoid choking, and regular deep breathing, frequent movement, and change in body positions (even just shifting and taking some deeper breaths while seated in a wheelchair) to promote mucociliary transport. An optimal time to take deep breaths and to cough is during transfers, which usually are physically exerting and stimulate hyperpnea.

Parkinson's Disease
Pathophysiology and medical management

Parkinson's disease is associated with reduced dopamine in the basal ganglia, resulting in the loss of normal reciprocal inhibitory and facilitatory neuronal input in the execution of smooth coordinated movement (Wilson et al., 1991). The clinical manifestations of the disease include stooped posture, stiffness and slowed motion, fixed masklike expression, and tremor of the limbs. Patients with Parkinson's disease are hypertonic, rigid, and inflexible. Movement initiation is impaired and, once initiated, movement is not fluid. The patient walks with a quick, shuffling gait. These factors contribute to an increased energy cost of movement. Physical activity is restricted and function is compromised, contributing to impaired aerobic capacity, reduced movement efficiency, and hence reduced movement economy.

Although chest wall rigidity and respiratory muscle weakness are associated with a restrictive pattern of lung disease in the Parkinsonian patient (Mehta, Wright, and Kirby, 1978), obstructive type of respiratory dysfunction has been reported (e.g., reduced mid-tidal flow rates, increase airway resistance, impaired distribution of ventilation, and an increase in functional residual capacity) (Neu, Connolly, Schwertley, Ladwig, and Brody, 1966). This obstructive defect may reflect parasympathetic hyperactivity,

which has been associated with the disease. The degree to which these cardiopulmonary manifestations of the disease are offset with anticholinergic drugs, used to treat rest tremor and reverse dystonia, has not been reported.

The upper extremities are rigid and held slightly abducted from the chest wall during locomotion. The rigidity and dyskinesia associated with Parkinson's disease leads to restricted movement and body positioning. The patient becomes deconditioned from disuse. The rigid immobile chest, coupled with reduced body position changes, contributes to cardiopulmonary dysfunction.

Principles of physical therapy management

The goals of long-term management for the patient with Parkinson's disease include the following:
- Maximize the patient's quality of life, general health, and well-being and hence physiological reserve capacity
- Educate about cardiopulmonary manifestations of Parkinson's disease, self-management, smoking reduction and cessation, nutrition, weight control, airway protection, medications, infection control, and the role of a rehabilitation program
- Optimize alveolar ventilation
- Optimize lung volumes and capacities
- Optimize ventilation and perfusion matching and gas exchange
- Reduce the work of breathing
- Reduce the work of the heart
- Protect the airways from aspiration
- Facilitate mucociliary transport
- Maximize aerobic capacity and efficiency of oxygen transport
- Optimize physical endurance and exercise capacity
- Optimize general muscle strength and thereby peripheral oxygen extraction

Patient monitoring includes dyspnea, respiratory distress, breathing pattern (depth and frequency), arterial saturation, heart rate, blood pressure, and rate pressure product. Patients with cardiac dysfunction require ECG monitoring, particularly during exercise. Subjectively, breathlessness is assessed using a modified version of the Borg scale of perceived exertion.

Medication that is needed to maximize treatment response is administered before treatment (e.g., L-dopa). Knowledge of the type of medication, its administration route, and time to and duration of peak efficacy is essential if treatment is to be maximally efficacious. In addition, patients with Parkinson's may be on a beta-blocker to suppress action tremor. Because such medication reduces the heart rate and blood pressure, these patients are prone to orthostatic intolerance. In addition, heart rate and blood pressure responses to treatment and exercises will be less valid.

The primary interventions for maximizing cardiopulmonary function and oxygen transport in patients with Parkinson's disease include some combination of education, aerobic exercise, strengthening exercises, postural correction exercises, gait reeducation, chest wall mobility exercises, range of motion exercises, body positioning, breathing control and coughing maneuvers, activity pacing, and energy conservation. An ergonomic assessment of the patient's work and home environments may be indicated to minimize oxygen demand and energy expenditure in these settings.

Education is a principal focus of the long-term management of the patient with Parkinson's disease. Education includes the reinforcement of preventative health practices (e.g., infection control, airway protection, smoking reduction or cessation, cold and flu prevention, flu shots, aerobic exercise, strengthening exercise, nutrition, weight control, hydration, pacing of activities, and energy conservation).

Aerobic exercise is an essential component of the long-term management of the patient with Parkinson's disease to optimize the efficiency of oxygen transport overall, including maximizing alveolar ventilation and mobilizing secretions, as well as its musculoskeletal benefits. Maximizing ventilation with mobilization is limited by the degree of hypertonicity and rigidity. Chest wall exercises include all planes of movement with a rotational component. Breathing control and coughing maneuvers are essential and should be coupled with body movement and positioning.

Multiple Sclerosis
Pathophysiology and medical management

Multiple sclerosis is a demyelinating disease of the central nervous system. The focal or patchy destruction of myelin sheaths is accompanied by an inflammatory response (McFarlin and McFarland, 1982). The course of the disease consists of a variable number of exacerbations and remissions over the years from early adulthood. Exacerbations are also variable with respect to severity. The neurological deficits include visual disturbance, paresis of one or more limbs, spasticity, discoordination, ataxia, dysarthria, weak, ineffective cough, reduced perception of vibration and position sense, bowel and bladder dysfunction, and sexual dysfunction (Wilson, Braunwald, Isselbacher, Martin, Fauci, and Root, 1991). Breathing disturbances, including diaphragmatic paresis, may occur (Cooper, Trend, and Wiles, 1985). Autonomic disturbance in the form of impaired cardiovascular reflex function at rest and attenuated heart rate and blood pressure responses during exercise are relatively common in patients with multiple sclerosis (Neubauer and Gundersen, 1978; Pentland and Ewing, 1987; Senaratne, Carroll, Warren, and Kappagoda, 1984).

Principles of physical therapy management

The goals of long-term management for the patient with multiple sclerosis include the following:

- Maximize the patient's quality of life, general health, and well-being and hence physiological reserve capacity
- Educate about cardiopulmonary manifestations of multiple sclerosis, self-management, medications, smoking reduction and cessation, nutrition, weight control, infection control, and the role of a rehabilitation program
- Optimize alveolar ventilation
- Optimize lung volumes and capacities and flow rates
- Optimize ventilation and perfusion matching and gas exchange
- Reduce the work of breathing
- Reduce the work of the heart
- Protect the airways from aspiration

- Facilitate mucociliary transport
- Optimize secretion clearance
- Maximize aerobic capacity and efficiency of oxygen transport
- Optimize physical endurance and exercise capacity
- Optimize general muscle strength and thereby peripheral oxygen extraction

Patient monitoring includes dyspnea, respiratory distress, breathing pattern (depth and frequency), arterial saturation, cyanosis (delayed sign of desaturation), heart rate, blood pressure, and rate pressure product. Patients with cardiac dysfunction require ECG monitoring, particularly during exercise. Subjectively, fatigue can be assessed using a modified version of the Borg scale. Perceived exertion is assessed using the Borg scale.

Medication that is needed to maximize treatment response is administered before treatment (e.g., antispasticity medications). Knowledge of the type of medication, its administration route, and time to and duration of peak efficacy is essential if treatment is to be maximally efficacious. In addition, knowledge of the cardiopulmonary side effects of other medications is needed.

The primary interventions for maximizing cardiopulmonary function and oxygen transport in patients with multiple sclerosis include some combination of education, aerobic exercise, strengthening exercises (to maintain or reduce rate of decline), reduce abnormal muscle tone, postural correction exercises, gait reeducation, chest wall mobility exercises, range of motion exercises, body positioning, breathing control and coughing maneuvers, airway clearance interventions, fatigue management, activity pacing and energy conservation. An ergonomic assessment of the patient's work and home environments may be indicated to minimize oxygen demand and energy expenditure in these settings.

Education is a principal focus of the long-term management of the patient with multiple sclerosis. Education includes the reinforcement of preventative health practices (e.g., infection control, cold and flu prevention, flu shots, smoking reduction and cessation, nutrition, weight control, hydration, fatigue management, modified aerobic exercise, modified strengthening exercises, pacing of activities, and energy conservation). Multiple sclerosis is associated with significant fatigue. Thus activity and sleep patterns need to be assessed to ensure sleep is maximally restorative and not contributing to the patient's symptoms. By maintaining a log of activity and rest, the patient can observe relationships between these factors and identify when is the optimal time to rest.

Aerobic exercise is an essential component of the long-term management of the patient with multiple sclerosis to optimize the efficiency of oxygen transport overall. In mild-to-moderate cases the goals of aerobic exercise are to optimize cardiopulmonary conditioning and enhance movement economy. Optimizing cadence of walking or cycling is important to minimize discoordination, energy expenditure, and fatigue and maximize safety. In more severe cases the goal is to maximize ventilation and gas exchange in the patient who has severe generalized muscular weakness, spasm, and excessive fatigue. Subjective parameters (i.e., fatigue and exertion) provide the basis for the intensity of the exercise program in conjunction with objective measures. Parameters, such as intensity and duration, may vary from session to session depending on the patient's general status, which tends to be variable. Aquatic exercise may be an alternative for patients whose discoordination precludes ambulation and cycling or who are troubled by heat. The use of a fan may also enhance the patient's work output.

Chest wall exercises include all planes of movement with a rotational component. Body positioning to optimize lung volumes and airflow rates is a priority. Breathing control and coughing maneuvers are coupled with body movement and positioning. If mucociliary clearance is impaired leading to secretion retention, postural drainage may need to be instituted coupled with deep breathing and coughing maneuvers.

Methods of facilitating effective coughing in patients with neuromuscular diseases are extremely important because they constitute life-preserving measures. Supported and unsupported coughing methods are described in detail in Chapters 20 and 21. Whenever possible, deep breathing and coughing are coordinated with chest wall movement to facilitate maximal inflation of the lungs before coughing and maximal exhalation of the lungs during coughing. Body positions are varied and changed frequently to simulate as much as possible shifts in alveolar volume and ventilation and perfusion that occur with normal movement and body position changes (Ray et al., 1974). In addition, body positioning is used to maximize the patient's coughing efforts.

Patients with generalized neuromuscular weakness require prophylactic management given their high risk of developing life-threatening respiratory infections and complications. Prophylaxis should include flu shots, avoiding polluted, smoky environments, smoking reduction and cessation, controlling the types of food eaten and chewing well to avoid choking, and regular deep breathing, frequent movement, and change in body positions (even just shifting and taking some deeper breaths while seated in a wheelchair) to promote mucociliary transport. An optimal time to take deep breaths and to cough is during transfers, which usually are physically exerting and stimulate hyperpnea.

Cerebral Palsy
Pathophysiology and medical management

Cerebral palsy results from insult to the central nervous system usually before birth (e.g., substance abuse and underoxygenation perinatally) (Wilson et al., 1991). The clinical presentation includes spasticity and residual deformity from severe muscle imbalance, hyperreflexia, and mental retardation. Although there are varying degrees of cerebral palsy severity, patients most frequently seen by physical therapy have significant functional deficits and require long-term care. The loss of motor control and hypertonicity of peripheral muscles often restrict the mobility of patients such that they are wheelchair dependent. Loss of motor function limits physical activity and the exercise stimulus needed to maintain an aerobic stimulus and optimal aerobic capacity. Often coupled with motor deficits are cognitive deficits and mental retardation. These afflictions limit the degree to which the patient can follow instructions, perform treatments, and partic-

ipate actively in a long-term rehabilitation program. Patients with cerebral palsy who are able to ambulate do so at exceptional energy expenditure both with and without walking aids (Campbell and Ball, 1978; Mossberg, Linton, and Friske, 1990). Central neurological deficits, generalized hypertonicity, and musculoskeletal deformity contribute to increased metabolical demand for oxygen and oxygen transport.

Principles of physical therapy management

The goals of long-term management for the patient with cerebral palsy include the following:
- Maximize the patient's quality of life, general health, and well-being and hence physiological reserve capacity
- Educate patient and/or family about cardiopulmonary manifestations of cerebral palsy, self-management, medications, nutrition, weight control, airway protection, infection control, and the role of a rehabilitation program
- Optimize alveolar ventilation
- Optimize lung volumes and capacities and flow rates
- Optimize ventilation and perfusion matching and gas exchange
- Reduce the work of breathing
- Reduce the work of the heart
- Protect the airways from aspiration
- Facilitate mucociliary transport
- Optimize secretion clearance
- Maximize aerobic capacity and efficiency of oxygen transport
- Optimize physical endurance and exercise capacity
- Optimize general muscle strength and thereby peripheral oxygen extraction

Maximizing aerobic capacity and efficiency of oxygen transport and optimizing general muscle strength pertain to the patient with cerebral palsy that is mild in severity. Unfortunately, many patients seen by physical therapists have poorly controlled spasticity and extreme cognitive deficits, which preclude full participation in aerobic and strengthening exercise programs. These patients are at risk for the sequelae of restricted mobility and recumbency.

Patient monitoring includes dyspnea, respiratory distress, breathing pattern (depth and frequency), arterial saturation, cyanosis (delayed sign of desaturation), heart rate, blood pressure, and rate pressure product. Unless mildly affected and not mentally incapacitated, patients with cerebral palsy are less able to provide subjective ratings of treatment response; thus the physical therapist relies particularly on clinical judgment in conjunction with the patient's objective responses to treatment.

Medication that is needed to maximize treatment response is administered before treatment (e.g., antispasticity medications). Knowledge of the type of medication, its administration route, and time to and duration of peak efficacy is essential if treatment is to be maximally efficacious.

The primary interventions for maximizing cardiopulmonary function and oxygen transport in patients with cerebral palsy include some combination of education, mobilization and coordinated activity (aerobic stimulation), strengthening exercises (strength is often difficult to assess and treat because of overwhelming spasticity), chest wall mobility exercises, range of motion exercises, body positioning, breathing control and coughing maneuvers, and airway clearance interventions.

Education is a principal focus of the long-term management of the patient with cerebral palsy. Whenever possible, education is directed at the patient, but it more likely is directed at the parents and care providers. Education includes the reinforcement of preventative health practices (e.g., infection control, cold and flu prevention, flu shots, mobilization, coordinated activity, strengthening exercise, nutrition, weight control, and hydration). Patients with cerebral palsy can be expected to have abnormal sleep patterns. First, central cerebral involvement may affect the periodicity of breathing. During sleep, the effects of such dysfunction are accentuated. Loss of normal periodic breathing and interspersed sighs impairs mucociliary transport. Secretions may accumulate and contribute to airway obstruction and areas of atelectasis. Second, patients with cerebral palsy are unable to reposition themselves during the night in response to both cardiopulmonary and musculoskeletal stimuli. Third,

patients often have poor swallowing and saliva control and thus are prone to aspiration and microatelectasis, particularly when recumbent at night. Inability to reposition themselves at night further increases the risk of aspiration and its sequelae.

Mobilization is an essential component of the long-term management of the patient with cerebral palsy to stimulate aerobic metabolism and optimize the efficiency of oxygen transport overall, including maximizing alveolar ventilation and mobilizing and removing secretions (Wolff, Dolovich, and Obminski, 1977). Maximizing ventilation with mobilization is limited if the patient has generalized spasticity. Furthermore, mobilization stimuli are selected specifically to minimize eliciting further muscle spasm. Prescriptive hydrotherapy and equinotherapy (horseback riding) can provide effective stimulation to the cardiopulmonary system in the multiply handicapped individual and minimize the effects of spasticity. With training, coordination of ambulatory patients can be improved and aerobic energy expenditure reduced (Dresen, de Groot, and Bouman, 1985). In addition, energy is conserved for performing more activity. Chest wall exercises includes all planes of movement with rotation. Body positioning to optimize lung volumes and airflow rates is a priority. Breathing control and coughing maneuvers are essential and should be coupled with body movement and positioning. If mucociliary transport is impaired leading to secretion retention, postural drainage and manual techniques may need to be instituted with appropriate monitoring to ensure they do not have a detrimental effect (Kirilloff, Owens, Rogers, and Mazzacco, 1985).

In this patient population, clearing oral secretions and coughing maneuvers, require special attention. Methods of facilitating effective coughing in patients with neuromuscular diseases are extremely important because they constitute life-preserving measures. Supported and unsupported coughing methods are described in detail in Chapters 20 and 21. Whenever possible, deep breathing and coughing is coupled with chest wall movement to facilitate maximal inflation of the lungs before coughing and maximal exhalation of the lungs during coughing. Body positions are varied and changed frequently to simulate as much as possible shifts in alveolar volume and ventilation and perfusion that occur with normal movement and body position changes. Microaspirations are likely a common occurrence in this patient population, particularly at night. Nighttime positioning must be prescribed for a given patient to minimize aspiration.

Patients with generalized neuromuscular weakness require prophylactic management given their high risk of developing life-threatening respiratory infections and complications. Prophylaxis should include flu shots, avoiding polluted, smoky environments, controlling the types of food eaten and chewing well to avoid choking, stimulation of deep breathing, airway clearance, and frequent movement and change in body positions (even just shifting and eliciting deeper breaths while seated in a wheelchair) to promote mucociliary transport.

Spinal Cord Injury
Pathophysiology and medical management

The cardiopulmonary manifestations and complications of spinal cord injury are directly related to the level of the lesion (Murray and Nadel, 1988b). Cardiopulmonary impairment results from the loss of supraspinal control of the respiratory muscles and the heart below the spinal cord lesion. Loss of diaphragmatic innervation results in ventilator-dependency. Loss of abdominal and intercostal innervation reduces the ability to cough, mucociliary transport, and the ability to clear the airways. Denervation of the heart and orthostatism are less problematic in that the heart's autonomous function and increased responsiveness of the heart and blood vessels to circulating catecholamines adequately compensate. The cough mechanism of quadriplegic patients is ineffective in clearing the airways (Estenne and Gorino, 1992).

Quadriplegic patients are particularly prone to the effects of restricted mobility given the extent of their functional motor loss and sensory deficits, particularly on cardiopulmonary function (Bach, 1991). Mobilization and physical activity are essential for the spinal cord injured patient to maintain optimal cardiopulmonary function and oxygen transport efficiency and the optimal strength and endurance of the respiratory muscles.

Principles of physical therapy management

The goals of long-term management for the patient with spinal cord injury include the following:

- Maximize the patient's quality of life, general health, and well-being and hence physiological reserve capacity
- Educate about cardiopulmonary manifestations of spinal cord injury, self-management, medications, smoking reduction and cessation, nutrition, weight control, infection control, and the role of a rehabilitation program
- Optimize alveolar ventilation
- Optimize lung volumes and capacities and flow rates
- Optimize ventilation and perfusion matching and gas exchange
- Reduce the work of breathing
- Reduce the work of the heart
- Protect the airways from aspiration
- Facilitate mucociliary transport
- Optimize secretion clearance
- Maximize aerobic capacity and efficiency of oxygen transport
- Optimize physical endurance and exercise capacity
- Optimize general muscle strength and thereby peripheral oxygen extraction

Patient monitoring includes dyspnea, respiratory distress, breathing pattern (depth and frequency), arterial saturation, cyanosis (delayed sign of desaturation), heart rate, blood pressure, and rate pressure product. Patients with high spinal cord injuries are somewhat more hemodynamically unstable and have more ECG irregularities than age-matched control individuals; thus their cardiopulmonary status should be monitored during treatment. Subjectively, perceived exertion is monitored using the Borg scale.

Medication that is needed to maximize treatment response is administered before treatment (e.g., antispasticity agents). Knowledge of the type of medication, its administration route, and time to and duration of peak efficacy is essential if treatment is to be maximally efficacious.

The primary interventions for maximizing cardiopulmonary function and oxygen transport in patients with spinal cord injury include some combination of education, aerobic exercise, strengthening exercises (to maintain or reduce rate of decline), postural correction exercises, chest wall mobility exercises, range of motion exercises, body positioning, breathing control and coughing maneuvers, airway clearance interventions, activity pacing, and energy conservation. An ergonomic assessment of the patient's work and home environments may be indicated to minimize oxygen demand and energy expenditure in these settings.

Education is a principal focus of the long-term management of the patient with spinal cord injury. Education includes the reinforcement of preventative health practices (e.g., infection control, cold and flu prevention, flu shots, aerobic exercise, strengthening exercise, nutrition, weight control, hydration, pacing of activities, and energy conservation).

Aerobic exercise is an essential component of the long-term management of the patient with spinal cord injury to optimize the efficiency of oxygen transport overall, including maximizing alveolar ventilation and mobilizing and removing secretions. With higher lesions, exercise is usually confined to upper-extremity work in the form of wheelchair ambulation. Preservation of upper-extremity muscle function and minimization of overuse are primary goals from the outset. Patients can maintain adequate cardiopulmonary conditioning with wheelchair exercise, however, exercise prescription should be conservative to maximize the benefit-to-risk ratio of cardiopulmonary conditioning relying of upper-extremity work. Patients who are able to walk with leg braces and crutches expend considerable energy doing so. A decision needs to be made regarding the benefits of walking at high energy demand vs conserving energy for other activities. Chest wall exercises can be used and should include all planes of movement with a rotational component. Body positioning to optimize lung volumes and airflow rates is a priority. Breathing control and coughing maneuvers are essential and should be coupled with body movement and positioning. Coordination of respiration with aerobic activity and wheeling is taught to maximize work output.

Ventilatory muscle training has a role in the long-term rehabilitation of some patients with high spinal cord lesions. Ventilatory muscle training can increase the strength and endurance of the respiratory muscles (Gross, 1980) and may improve the functional capacity of some patients. A stronger endurance-trained diaphragm will not fatigue as readily as an untrained diaphragm. Standardizing the resistance of the training stimulus alone, however, is not sufficient to produce a training effect. It is essential that flow rate is controlled using a gauge.

Methods of facilitating effective coughing in patients with neuromuscular diseases are extremely important because they constitute life-preserving measures. Supported and unsupported coughing methods are described in detail in Chapters 20 and 21. Whenever possible, deep breathing and coughing is coupled with chest wall movement to facilitate maximal inflation of the lungs before coughing and maximal exhalation of the lungs during coughing. Body positions are varied and changed frequently to simulate as much as possible shifts in alveolar volume and ventilation and perfusion that occur with normal movement and body position changes (Braun, Giovannoni, and O'Connor, 1984).

A comprehensive program includes stretching of the chest wall and passive range of motion exercises of the shoulder girdle. Maximal insufflations are encouraged in optimal body positions. Glossopharyngeal breathing can enable high quadriplegic patients to be freed from mechanical ventilation for hours at a time. Assisted or unassisted coughing is coordinated with deep breathing and rhythmic rocking motion. Manual assisted coughing and mechanical coughing aids, including functional electrical stimulation and insufflation-exsufflation devices, can be useful (Bach, 1991; Linder, 1993). The pneumobelt is a device that can facilitate ventilation without a tracheostomy (Miller, Thomas, and Wilmot, 1988). This device counters loss of abdominal tone and helps preserve normal thoracoabdominal interaction during respiration, which is lost because of reduced rib cage compliance and increased abdominal compliance.

Patients with spinal cord injuries, particularly those with high lesions, require prophylactic management, given their risk of developing life-threatening respiratory infections and complications. Prophylaxis should include flu shots, avoiding polluted, smoky environments, smoking reduction and cessation, controlling the types of food eaten and chewing well to avoid choking, regular deep breathing, airway clearance, and frequent movement and change in body positions (even just shifting and taking some deeper breaths while seated in a wheelchair is beneficial). An optimal time to take deep breaths and to cough is during transfers, which usually are physically exerting and stimulate hyperpnea.

Late Sequelae of Poliomyelitis
Pathophysiology and medical management

The late sequelae of poliomyelitis are reaching epidemic proportions as poliomyelitis survivors from the late epidemic in the 1940s and 1950s reach 35 to 40 years after onset. Three types of poliomyelitis were prevalent during the epidemic in the middle of this century, namely, spinal (the majority of cases), bulbar, and encephalitic. Many survivors are now presenting with disproportionate fatigue, increased weakness, deformity, pain, reduced endurance, and breathing and swallowing problems (Dean, 1991; Howard, Wiles, and Spencer, 1988), and respiratory insufficiency (Lane, Hazleman, and Nichols, 1974). Although cardiopulmonary complications were not associated with the spinal form of poliomyelitis at onset, late-onset breathing and swallowing complications can appear as a late effect of the disease (Dean, Ross, Road, Courtenay, and Madill, 1991). In addition, these patients may be deconditioned and have poor movement economy (i.e., expend excessive energy because of postural deformities) (Dean and Ross, 1993). Thus delayed-onset cardiopulmonary complications, coupled with the effects of overuse and general deconditioning, increases the risk of cardiopulmonary compromise, reduces the ability to recover from these, and increases surgical and anesthetic risk.

Principles of physical therapy management

The goals of long-term management for the patient with the late sequelae of poliomyelitis include the following:

- Maximize the patient's quality of life, general health, and well-being and hence physiological reserve capacity

- Educate about cardiopulmonary manifestations of the late sequelae of poliomyelitis, self-management, medications, smoking reduction or cessation, nutrition, weight control, infection control, orthoses, mobility and ADL aids and devices, and the role of a rehabilitation program
- Optimize alveolar ventilation
- Optimize lung volumes and capacities and flow rates
- Optimize ventilation and perfusion matching and gas exchange
- Reduce the work of breathing
- Reduce the work of the heart
- Protect the airways from aspiration
- Maximize aerobic capacity and efficiency of oxygen transport
- Optimize physical endurance and exercise capacity
- Optimize general muscle strength and thereby peripheral oxygen extraction

Patient monitoring includes dyspnea, respiratory distress, breathing pattern (depth and frequency), arterial saturation, cyanosis (delayed sign of desaturation), heart rate, blood pressure, and rate pressure product. Subjectively, pain, a feature of the late sequelae of poliomyelitis, can be assessed using an analog scale, perceived exertion is assessed using the Borg scale, and fatigue and breathlessness can also be assessed using a modified versions of this scale.

Medication that is needed to maximize treatment response is administered before treatment (e.g., analgesia). Knowledge of the type of medication, its administration route, and time to and duration of peak efficacy is essential if treatment is to be maximally efficacious.

The primary interventions for maximizing cardiopulmonary function and oxygen transport in patients with the late sequelae of poliomyelitis include some combination of education, aerobic exercise, strengthening exercises, postural correction exercises, chest wall mobility exercises, range of motion exercises, body positioning, breathing control and coughing maneuvers, activity pacing, and energy conservation. An ergonomic assessment of the patient's work and home environments may be indicated to minimize oxygen demand and energy expenditure in these settings. Aids and devices are reviewed to optimize energy expenditure (e.g., electric wheelchair or scooter vs manual wheelchair) and to reduce cardiopulmonary distress (e.g., home mechanical ventilation).

Education is a principal focus of the long-term management of the patient with the late sequelae of poliomyelitis. Education includes the reinforcement of preventative health practices (e.g., infection control, cold and flu prevention, flu shots, aerobic exercise, strengthening exercises, nutrition, weight control, hydration, pacing of activities, and energy conservation). Activity and sleep patterns need to be assessed to ensure sleep is maximally restorative and not contributing to the patient's symptoms. Functional work capacity and activity tolerance may be increased by balancing activity to rest, and maintaining fatigue below the patient's critical fatigue threshold, i.e., threshold requiring prolonged recovery time.

Aerobic exercise is an essential component of the long-term management of the patient with the late sequelae of poliomyelitis to optimize the efficiency of oxygen transport overall. The two principal goals of exercise are to optimize cardiopulmonary conditioning and movement economy. Maximizing ventilation with exercise is limited if the patient has severe generalized muscular weakness and increased fatigue. Disproportionate fatigue and other symptoms experienced by patients with the late sequelae of poliomyelitis have been attributed to overwork of affected and unaffected muscles, terminal axon degeneration, and impaired impulse transmission (Dean, 1991). Exercise is therefore prescribed judiciously to provide an optimal aerobic training effect without contributing to further otheruse abuse (i.e., prescriptive parameters based on subjective responses using semi-quantitative scales in conjunction with objective responses). Walking is the most functional type of aerobic exercise, however, aquatic exercise provides a useful medium for patients with lower-extremity paresis who require crutches to walk or are confined to a wheelchair. Reducing physical activity and exercise is indicated in some patients to optimize aerobic and muscle power. The effect of resting affected and unaffected muscles enhances functional capacity.

Methods of facilitating effective coughing in patients with neuromuscular diseases are extremely important because they constitute a life-preserving measure. Supported and unsupported coughing methods are described in detail in Chapters 20 and 21. Whenever possible, deep breathing and coughing is coupled with chest wall movement to facilitate maximal inflation of the lungs before coughing and maximal exhalation of the lungs during coughing. Body positions are varied and changed frequently to simulate as much as possible shifts in alveolar volume and ventilation and perfusion that occur with normal movement and body position changes.

Progressive loss of pulmonary function in patients with ventilatory compromise at onset can lead to respiratory insufficiency. Comparable with other neuromuscular conditions, invasive mechanical ventilation is avoided. Promising alternatives are nasal and oral methods of noninvasive assisted mechanical ventilation (Bach, Alba, and Shin, 1989). In addition, airway clearance can be further assisted with manual assisted coughing, glossopharyngeal breathing, mechanical exsufflation, and mechanical insufflation-exsufflation (Bach et al., 1993).

Poliomyelitis survivors with ventilatory compromise are comparable with other patients with generalized muscle weakness. Of particular concern in this population, however, is the need to establish the role of mobilization and exercise as a first line of defense in the management and prevention of cardiopulmonary dysfunction. However, for those patients whose late effects are due to overuse, additional exercise may be detrimental. Modified mobilization and exercise, however, may be prescribed in an interval schedule (McArdle, Katch, and Katch, 1991) (Chapter 17). The patient exercises for a period of time and then rests or reduces to a lower intensity of exercise to allow the muscles to rest. In addition to the multitude of benefits of mobilization and exercise on oxygen transport overall, these interventions also optimize respiratory muscle strength and endurance. If the patient does not recover within a few hours, the mobilization or exercise stimuli was excessive and should be modified. Chest wall mobility exercises to facilitate breathing and coughing may have a role.

Patients with generalized neuromuscular weakness require prophylactic management, given their high risk of developing life-threatening respiratory infections and complications. Prophylaxis should include flu shots, avoiding polluted, smoky environments, controlling the types of food eaten and chewing well to avoid choking, regular deep breathing, airway clearance, and frequent movement and change in body positions (even just shifting and taking some deeper breaths while seated in a wheelchair is beneficial). An optimal time to take deep breaths and to cough is during transfers, which usually are physically exerting and stimulate hyperpnea.

MUSCULOSKELETAL CONDITIONS
Thoracic Deformities
Pathophysiology and medical management

Respiratory insufficiency can result from abnormalities of the chest wall secondary to congenital deformity, acquired disease, and trauma (Bates, 1989; Murray and Nadel, 1988b). Congenital deformity of the chest wall reduces the mobility of the bony thorax, thereby increasing the work of breathing. Shallow, rapid breathing often results. Minute ventilation is increased at the expense of alveolar ventilation. Severe deformity leads to compression of the mediastinal structures. The heart can be displaced and rotated, impeding its mechanical function. Examples of chronic deformities that impinge on pulmonary function are kyphoscoliosis secondary to poliomyelitis, tuberculous osteomyelitis, and other causes and ankylosing spondylitis. Other examples of deformity include traumatic injury of the vertebral column, ribs, and sternum. Routine cardiopulmonary assessment should include a musculoskeletal examination of the spinal column and thoracic cavity.

Normal pulmonary function and gas exchange depend on symmetry of cardiopulmonary anatomy and physiological function. Asymmetry of the chest wall interferes with normal lung mechanics, regional gradients of ventilation and perfusion in the lungs, and the distribution of inspired gas (Bake, Demsey, and Grimby, 1976; Sinha and Bergofsky, 1972). Significant decrease in lung compliance and increase in work performed against the elastic resistance of the lung are characteristic of kyphoscoliosis. Altered pressure gradients and uneven lung movement during the respiratory cycle may contribute to altered lung water balance and impaired lymphatic drainage. The effects of physiological dead space and shunt may be magnified, producing hypoxemia and hypercapnia. With severe chest deformity, a cycle of respiratory acidosis, pulmonary hypertension, and right heart failure can result in a life-threatening situation.

Principles of physical therapy management

The goals of long-term management for the patient with thoracic deformity include the following:

- Maximize the patient's quality of life, general health, and well-being and hence physiological reserve capacity
- Educate about cardiopulmonary manifestations of thoracic deformity, self-management, medications, nutrition, weight control, infection control, smoking reduction and cessation, and the role of a rehabilitation program
- Optimize alveolar ventilation
- Optimize lung volumes and capacities and flow rates
- Optimize ventilation and perfusion matching and gas exchange
- Reduce the work of breathing
- Reduce the work of the heart
- Protect the airways from aspiration
- Facilitate mucociliary transport
- Optimize secretion clearance
- Maximize aerobic capacity and efficiency of oxygen transport
- Optimize physical endurance and exercise capacity
- Optimize general muscle strength and thereby peripheral oxygen extraction

Patient monitoring includes dyspnea, respiratory distress, breathing pattern (depth and frequency), arterial saturation, cyanosis (delayed sign of desaturation), heart rate, blood pressure, and rate pressure product. Patients with cardiac dysfunction require ECG monitoring particularly during exercise. Subjectively, perceived exertion is assessed using the Borg scale, and breathlessness is assessed using a modified version of this scale.

The primary interventions for maximizing cardiopulmonary function and oxygen transport in patients with thoracic deformity include some combination of education, aerobic exercise, strengthening exercises, postural correction exercises, gait reeducation, chest wall mobility exercises, range of motion exercises, body positioning, breathing control and coughing maneuvers, airway clearance interventions, activity pacing, and energy conservation. An ergonomic assessment of the patient's work and home environments may be indicated to minimize oxygen demand and energy expenditure in these settings.

Education is a principal focus of the long-term management of the patient with thoracic deformity. Education includes the reinforcement of preventative health practices (e.g., infection control, cold and flu prevention, flu shots, smoking reduction or cessation, aerobic exercise, strengthening exercises, nutrition, weight control, and hydration).

Aerobic exercise is an essential component of the long-term management of the patient with thoracic deformity to optimize the efficiency of oxygen transport overall. Maximizing ventilation with exercise in patients with severe deformity may be limited. Optimizing alignment to minimize the cardiopulmonary limitations of the deformity during physical activity, exercise, and rest is a priority. Chest wall exercises include all planes of movement with a rotational component. Body positioning to optimize lung volumes and airflow rates is a priority. Breathing control and coughing maneuvers are essential and should be coupled with body movement and positioning. If mucociliary transport is impaired leading to secretion retention, postural drainage may need to be instituted, coupled with deep breathing and coughing maneuvers.

Ventilatory muscle training may have a role in the management of patients with reduced inspiratory pressures and associated decreases in total lung capacity and hypoxemia.

Methods of facilitating effective coughing in patients with musculoskeletal deformity are extremely important because they constitute life-preserving measures. Supported and unsupported coughing methods are described in detail in Chapters 20 and 21. Whenever possible, deep breathing and coughing is coupled with chest wall movement to facilitate maximal inflation of the lungs before and maximal exhalation during coughing. Body positions are varied and changed frequently to simulate as much as possible shifts in alveolar volume and ventilation and perfusion that occur with normal movement and body position changes.

Patients with chest wall deformities secondary to neuromuscular conditions require prophylactic management given their high risk of developing life-threatening respiratory infections and complications. Prophylaxis should include flu shots, avoiding polluted, smoky environments, smoking reduction and cessation, controlling the types of food eaten and chewing well to avoid choking, regular deep breathing, airway clearance, and frequent movement and change in body positions (even just shifting and taking some deeper breaths while seated in a wheelchair is beneficial). An optimal time to take deep breaths and to cough is during transfers, which usually are physically exerting and stimulate hyperpnea.

Osteoporosis

Pathophysiology and medical management

Osteoporosis is a condition associated with reduced bone mass per unit volume (Smith, Smith, and Gilligan, 1991). Age-related bone loss begins earlier and accelerates faster in women, particularly after menopause, than men. Life-style factors, such as diet, exercise, and smoking, have a significant role in reducing bone mass. Caffeine has also been implicated as a contributing factor to bone loss secondary to increasing urinary calcium loss.

Osteoporosis is classified as idiopathic osteoporosis unassociated with other conditions, osteoporosis associated with other conditions (e.g., malabsorption, calcium deficiency, immobilization, or metabolic bone disease), osteoporosis as a feature of an inherited condition (e.g., osteogenica imperfecta or Marfan's syndrome), and osteoporosis associated with other conditions but the pathogenesis is not understood (e.g., rheumatoid arthritis, alcoholism, diabetes mellitus, or chronic airflow limitation) (Wilson et al., 1991).

The most common clinical features are vertebral pain and spinal deformity resulting from vertebral compression and collapse. Vertebral bodies tend to collapse anteriorly, contributing to cervical lordosis, thoracic kyphosis, postural slumping, and loss of height. Acute episodes may be relieved by restricted mobility. Straining and sudden changes in position can exacerbate an acute episode. Cardiopulmonary complications of osteoporosis are secondary to spinal deformity, chest wall rigidity, and cardiopulmonary deconditioning resulting from restricted mobility.

Osteoporosis is a condition associated with aging and older age groups. The pain of acute episodes leads to periods of restricted mobility and significant cardiopulmonary dysfunction in older persons (Dean, 1993). Exercise that is weight bearing and loads the muscles around bone maintains bone density and decelerates bone loss thus has a central role in preserving bone health. Generally, the growth and remodelling of bone depends highly on the exercise prescription parameters (e.g., type of exercise, intensity, duration, and frequency). Bone mineral content is more closely related to cardiopulmonary conditioning than physical activity level. Furthermore, any detrimental effect of exercise on osteoporosis appears to relate more to malalignment and injury rather than activity itself.

Principles of physical therapy management

The etiology of osteoporosis is diverse; thus management needs to consider the underlying pathophysiology and that several factors may be contributing to the presentation of osteoporosis in the same patient.

The goals of long-term management for the patient with osteoporosis include the following:

- Maximize the patient's quality of life, general health, and well-being and hence physiological reserve capacity
- Educate about cardiopulmonary manifestations of osteoporosis, self-management, medications, nutrition, weight control, smoking reduction and cessation, infection control, and the role of a rehabilitation program
- Optimize alveolar ventilation
- Optimize lung volumes and capacities and flow rates
- Optimize ventilation and perfusion matching and gas exchange
- Facilitate mucociliary transport
- Maximize aerobic capacity and efficiency of oxygen transport
- Optimize physical endurance and exercise capacity
- Optimize general muscle strength and thereby peripheral oxygen extraction

Patient monitoring includes heart rate, blood pressure, and rate pressure product. Patients with cardiac dysfunction require ECG monitoring particularly during exercise. Subjectively, pain and discomfort are assessed with an analog scale or modified Borg scale, and perceived exertion is assessed using the Borg scale.

Medication that is needed to maximize treatment response is administered before treatment (e.g., analgesics). Knowledge of the type of medication, its administration route, and time to and duration of peak efficacy is essential if treatment is to be maximally efficacious.

The primary interventions for maximizing cardiopulmonary function and oxygen transport in patients with osteoporosis include some combination of education, aerobic weight-bearing exercise, strengthening exercises, chest wall mobility exercises, range of motion exercises, activity pacing, and energy conservation. An ergonomic assessment of the patient's work and home environments may be indicated to minimize oxygen demand and energy expenditure in these settings.

Education is a principal focus of the long-term management of the patient with osteoporosis. Education includes the reinforcement of preventative health practices (e.g., infection control, cold and flu prevention, flu shots, smoking reduction and cessation, weight-bearing aerobic exercise, strengthening exercises, range of motion exercises, nutrition, weight control, hydration, pacing of activities, and energy conservation).

Aerobic exercise is an essential component of the long-term management of the patient with osteoporosis to optimize the efficiency of oxygen transport overall. Upright, weight-bearing aerobic exercise is essential to maintain bone density or reduce the rate of bone loss. Maximizing ventilation with exercise is limited if the patient has severe generalized muscular weakness and increased fatigue. Chest wall exercises can be used and should include all planes of movement with a rotational component. Breathing control and coughing maneuvers are essential and should be coupled with body movement and positioning. Straining, Valsalva maneuvers, and jarring activity and exercise are contraindicated.

Methods of facilitating effective coughing in patients with osteoporosis are extremely important because they constitute life-preserving measures. Some patients fracture ribs and vertebrae during coughing. Patients at risk should rely on huffing maneuvers that do not require closing the glottis and do not generate high intrathoracic pressures (Hietpas, Roth, and Jensen, 1979).

COLLAGEN VASCULAR/CONNECTIVE TISSUE DISEASES

Systemic Lupus Erythematosus

Pathophysiology and medical management

Systemic lupus erythematosus (SLE) is a disease characterized by the presence of multiple antibodies that contribute to immunologically mediated tissue inflammation and damage (Segal, Calabrese, Ahmad, Tubbs, and White, 1985). The disease affects the major organ systems, including the central nervous, musculoskeletal, pulmonary, vascular, and renal systems. Symptoms include arthralgic and myalgic stiffness, pain, and fatigue.

The cardiopulmonary manifestations of SLE include atelectasis, resulting from inflammation of the alveolar walls, and perivascular and peribronchial connective tissue, effusions secondary to lung infarction, reduced surface tension, and splinting secondary to pleuritic pain. Other manifestations include pleuritis with or without effusion, pneumonitis, interstitial fibrosis, pulmonary hypertension, diaphragmatic dysfunction, pulmonary hemorrhage, systemic hypertension, myocarditis, constrictive pericarditis, dysrhythmias, tamponade, pericardial pain, arteritis, and defects of the mitral and aortic valves (Dickey and Myers, 1988). Other manifestations that affect cardiopulmonary function include anemia, leukopenia, thrombocytopenia, thrombosis, splenomegaly, ascitis, gastrointestinal bleeding, nephritis, and renal insufficiency (Wilson et al., 1991).

Principles of physical therapy management

The goals of long-term management for the patient with systemic lupus erythematosus (SLE) include the following:

- Maximize the patient's quality of life, general health, and well-being and hence physiological reserve capacity
- Educate about cardiopulmonary manifestations

of SLE, self-management, nutrition, weight control, smoking reduction and cessation, medications, infection control, and the role of a rehabilitation program
- Optimize alveolar ventilation
- Optimize lung volumes and capacities and flow rates
- Optimize ventilation and perfusion matching and gas exchange
- Reduce the work of breathing
- Reduce the work of the heart
- Protect the airways from aspiration
- Facilitate mucociliary transport
- Optimize secretion clearance
- Maximize aerobic capacity and efficiency of oxygen transport
- Optimize physical endurance and exercise capacity
- Optimize general muscle strength and thereby peripheral oxygen extraction

Patient monitoring includes dyspnea, respiratory distress, breathing pattern (depth and frequency), arterial saturation, cyanosis (delayed sign of desaturation), heart rate, blood pressure, and rate pressure product. Patients with cardiac dysfunction should be cleared by a cardiologist before being prescribed an exercise program. Subjectively, discomfort, pain, fatigue, and breathlessness are assessed using analog scales or modified versions of the Borg scale, and perceived exertion is assessed using the Borg scale.

Medication that is needed to maximize treatment response is administered before treatment (e.g., analgesic and antiinflammatory agents). Knowledge of the type of medication, its administration route, and time to and duration of peak efficacy is essential if treatment is to be maximally efficacious.

The primary interventions for maximizing cardiopulmonary function and oxygen transport in patients with SLE include some combination of education, aerobic exercise, strengthening exercises, postural correction exercises, chest wall mobility exercises, range of motion exercises, body positioning, breathing control and coughing maneuvers, airway clearance interventions, activity pacing, and energy conservation. An ergonomic assessment of the patient's work and home environments may be indicated to minimize oxygen demand and energy expenditure in these settings.

Education is a principal focus of the long-term management of the patient with SLE. Education includes the reinforcement of preventative health practices (e.g., infection control, cold and flu prevention, flu shots, smoking reduction or cessation, aerobic exercise, strengthening exercises, nutrition, weight control, hydration, pacing of activities, and energy conservation). An ergonomic assessment of the patient's work and home environments may be indicated to minimize oxygen demand and energy expenditure in these settings.

Aerobic exercise is an essential component of the long-term management of the patient with SLE to optimize the efficiency of oxygen transport overall, including maximizing alveolar ventilation and mobilizing and removing secretions. Parameters of the exercise prescription are based on subjective responses, (e.g., discomfort, pain, breathlessness, and perceived exertion in conjunction with objective responses). Optimal types of aerobic exercise include walking and cycling. Aquatic exercise may be preferable for patients with musculoskeletal involvement that precludes walking and cycling. Chest wall exercises can be used and should include all planes of movement with a rotational component. Body positioning to optimize lung volumes and airflow rates is a priority. Breathing control and coughing maneuvers are essential and should be coupled with body movement and positioning. If mucociliary transport is impaired, leading to secretion retention, postural drainage may need to be instituted, coupled with deep breathing and coughing maneuvers.

Scleroderma

Pathophysiology and medical management

Scleroderma is characterized by the overproduction of collagen and progressive fibrosis of cutaneous and subcutaneous tissues (Gray, 1989). The cardiopulmonary manifestations of this condition result in interstitial pulmonary fibrosis with significantly reduced vital capacity, diffusing capacity, and arterial oxygen tension (Bates, 1989; Wilson et al., 1991). Reduced static compliance is the primary mechanical

deficit. Pulmonary hypertension may be a complicating factor. Broncoalveolar lavage is consistent with an acute inflammatory process. Cardiomyopathy is associated with ischemia, areas of infarction, and myocardial fibrosis (Gray, 1989). Fibrosis of the conduction system predisposes the patient to conduction defects and dysrhythmias. Other cardiopulmonary manifestations include pericarditis with or without effusion and pulmonary and systemic hypertension from renal involvement. Half of patients with scleroderma have renal involvement including intimal hyperphasia, fibrinous necrosis of the afferent arterioles, and thickening of the glomerular basement membrane. Fibrotic changes and stenoses occur in the small arteries and arterioles systemically. Similar changes in the lymphatic vessels may obliterate lymph flow.

Esophageal involvement contributes to regurgitation of gastric contents, which is exacerbated when the patient is recumbent or bends over. Bloating and abdominal discomfort may reflect paralytic ileus and intestinal obstruction. Ascites and fluid accumulation in the gut increases abdominal pressure and encroaches on diaphragmatic motion.

Principles of physical therapy management

The goals of long-term management for the patient with scleroderma include the following:

- Maximize the patient's quality of life, general health, and well-being and hence physiological reserve capacity
- Educate about cardiopulmonary manifestations of scleroderma, self-management, nutrition, weight control, smoking reduction or cessation, medications, infection control, and the role of a rehabilitation program
- Optimize alveolar ventilation
- Optimize lung volumes and capacities and flow rates
- Optimize ventilation and perfusion matching and gas exchange
- Reduce the work of breathing
- Reduce the work of the heart
- Protect the airways from aspiration
- Facilitate mucociliary transport
- Optimize secretion clearance

- Maximize aerobic capacity and efficiency of oxygen transport
- Optimize physical endurance and exercise capacity
- Optimize general muscle strength and thereby peripheral oxygen extraction

Patient monitoring includes dyspnea, respiratory distress, breathing pattern (depth and frequency), arterial saturation, cyanosis (delayed sign of desaturation), heart rate, blood pressure, and rate pressure product. Patients with cardiac dysfunction require ECG monitoring, particularly during exercise. If supplemental oxygen is used, the FIo_2 administered is recorded. Subjectively, breathlessness is assessed using a modified version of the Borg scale of perceived exertion and perceived exertion is assessed using the Borg scale.

Medication that is needed to maximize treatment response is administered before treatment (e.g., immunosuppressive agents and antiplatelet therapy). Knowledge of the type of medication, its administration route, and time to and duration of peak efficacy is essential if treatment is to be maximally efficacious.

The primary interventions for maximizing cardiopulmonary function and oxygen transport in patients with scleroderma include some combination of education, aerobic exercise, strengthening exercises, postural correction exercises, chest wall mobility exercises, range of motion exercises, body positioning, breathing control and coughing maneuvers, airway clearance interventions, activity pacing and energy conservation. An ergonomic assessment of the patient's work and home environments may be indicated to minimize oxygen demand and energy expenditure in these settings.

Patients with esophageal involvement are not treated or exercised immediately after a meal. These patients have frequent small meals, antacids between meals, and do not lie down for a few hours after eating. When recumbent, these patients have the head of bed elevated to minimize the risk of aspiration of gastric contents.

Education is a principal focus of the long-term management of the patient with scleroderma. Education includes the reinforcement of preventive health practices (e.g., infection control, cold and influenza prevention, influenza shots, smoking reduction and cessation, aerobic exercise, strengthening exercise, range-of-motion exercises, nutrition, weight control, hydration, pacing of activities, and energy conservation). An ergonomic assessment of the patient's work and home environments may be indicated to minimize oxygen demand and energy expenditure in these settings.

Aerobic exercise is an essential component of the long-term management of the patient with scleroderma to optimize the efficiency of oxygen transport overall. Chest wall exercises can be used and should include all planes of movement with a rotational component. Body positioning to optimize lung volumes and airflow rates is a priority. Breathing control and coughing maneuvers are essential and should be coupled with body movement and positioning. If mucociliary transport is impaired leading to secretion retention, postural drainage may need to be instituted coupled with deep breathing and coughing maneuvers.

Ankylosing Spondylitis
Pathophysiology and medical management

Ankylosing spondylitis results in reduced total lung capacity, vital capacity, and inspiratory muscle function (Lisboa, Moreno, Fava, Ferreti, and Cruz, 1985; Rosenow, Strimlan, Muhm, and Ferguson, 1977). Ventilatory capacity is preserved given that the respiratory muscles are not involved. The disease results in spinal and chest wall rigidity; thus there is greater reliance on diaphragmatic contribution to ventilation (84%) compared with healthy persons (68%) (Hoeppner, Cockcroft, Dosman, and Cotton, 1984). The patient with ankylosing spondylitis has an increased dependence on diaphragmatic function and therefore is at risk if administered respiratory depressant medications or if he or she undergoes thoracic or upper abdominal surgery (Grimby, Fugl-Meyer, and Blomstrand, 1974).

During exercise, patients with ankylosing spondylitis show minimal chest wall expansion compared with healthy persons (Elliott et al., 1985). Although peak workload is reduced, diaphragmatic fatigue rather than ventilatory capacity, ventilation-perfusion mismatch, or abnormal blood gases is more likely to be the limiting factor.

Principles of physical therapy management

The goals of long-term management for the patient with ankylosing spondylitis include the following:

- Maximize the patient's quality of life, general health, and well-being and hence physiological reserve capacity
- Educate about cardiopulmonary manifestations of ankylosing spondylitis, self-management, nutrition, weight control, infection control, smoking reduction and cessation, and the role of a rehabilitation program
- Optimize alveolar ventilation
- Optimize lung volumes and capacities and flow rates
- Optimize ventilation and perfusion matching and gas exchange
- Facilitate mucociliary transport
- Maximize aerobic capacity and efficiency of oxygen transport
- Optimize physical endurance and exercise capacity
- Optimize general muscle strength and thereby peripheral oxygen extraction

Patient monitoring includes dyspnea, respiratory distress, breathing pattern (depth and frequency), arterial saturation, cyanosis (delayed sign of desaturation), heart rate, blood pressure, and rate pressure product.

The primary interventions for maximizing cardiopulmonary function and oxygen transport in patients with ankylosing spondylitis include some combination of education, exercise, strengthening exercises, ventilatory muscle training, postural correction exercises, gait reeducation, chest wall mobility exercises, range of motion exercises, body positioning, breathing control and coughing maneuvers, pacing, and energy conservation. An ergonomic assessment of the patient's work and home environments may be indicated to minimize oxygen demand and energy expenditure in these settings.

Education is a principal focus of the long-term management of the patient with ankylosing spondylitis. Education includes the reinforcement of preventative health practices (e.g., smoking reduction or cessation, infection control, cold and flu prevention, flu shots, smoking reduction and cessation, aerobic exercise, strengthening exercises, nutrition, weight control, and hydration).

Aerobic exercise is an essential component of the long-term management of the patient with ankylosing spondylitis to optimize the efficiency of oxygen transport overall. Maximizing ventilation with mobilization is limited if the patient has extreme spinal rigidity. Chest wall exercises can be used and should include all planes of movement with a rotational component. Body positioning to optimize lung volumes and airflow rates is a priority. Breathing control and coughing maneuvers are essential and should be coupled with body movement and positioning. Ventilatory muscle training in conjunction with exercise may have some additional benefit in maximizing aerobic capacity.

Rheumatoid Arthritis
Pathophysiology and medical management

Rheumatoid arthritis (RA) is a multisystemic disease that is associated with well-documented cardiopulmonary and cardiovascular effects, including pleuritis with or without effusions, interstitial fibrosis, pulmonary vasculitis, an increased incidence of bronchitis and pneumonia myocarditis, epicarditis, endocarditis, dysrhythmias, neuritis and vasculitis (Ekblom and Nordemar, 1987; Scott, Wise, Hochberg, and Wigley, 1987).

Functional capacity is limited by pain and stiffness in the affected muscles and joints, weakness, the number of joints affected, fatigue, and whether the patient is having an acute episode. Self-limited physical activity and exercise contributes to cardiopulmonary deconditioning. Movement such as walking is often inefficient because of limping. Peak exercise tests are limited by musculoskeletal complaints; thus submaximal tests are more functional in this population. Tests of cardiovascular status must be non–weight-bearing to enable the patient to reach an acceptable stress level without confounding joint pain.

Graded low-intensity aerobic exercise for patients with RA from 15 to 35 minutes three times a week can be sufficient to enhance aerobic capacity (Harkcom, Lampman, Banwell, and Castor, 1985). In addition to improving aerobic capacity, such an exercise prescription results in increased exercise time, reduced affected joint count, improved activities of daily living, reduced joint pain, and general fatigue. Should a joint flare-up occur while the patient is on an exercise program, a few days or weeks of restricted mobility and abstinence from exercise frequently ameliorate the symptoms. Gentle mobilization (preferably weight-bearing), coupled with range of motion exercises during this period, will minimize the negative effects of reduced activity.

Prolonged use of steroids contributes to bone fragility. Thus physical activity and exercise prescriptions are modified accordingly.

Principles of physical therapy management

The goals of long-term management for the patient with RA include the following:

- Maximize the patient's quality of life, general health, and well-being and hence physiological reserve capacity
- Educate about cardiopulmonary manifestations of rheumatoid arthritis, self-management, nutrition, weight control, smoking reduction or cessation, medications, infection control, and the role of a rehabilitation program
- Optimize alveolar ventilation
- Optimize lung volumes and capacities and flow rates
- Optimize ventilation and perfusion matching and gas exchange
- Reduce the work of breathing
- Reduce the work of the heart
- Protect the airways from aspiration
- Facilitate mucociliary transport
- Optimize secretion clearance
- Maximize aerobic capacity and efficiency of oxygen transport
- Optimize physical endurance and exercise capacity
- Optimize general muscle strength and thereby peripheral oxygen extraction

Patient monitoring includes dyspnea, respiratory distress, breathing pattern (depth and frequency), arterial saturation, cyanosis (delayed sign of desaturation), heart rate, blood pressure, and rate pressure product. Subjectively, perceived exertion is assessed using the Borg scale.

Medication that is needed to maximize treatment response is administered before treatment (e.g., steroids, nonsteroidal antiinflammatory drugs, and analgesics). Knowledge of the type of medication, its administration route, and time to and duration of peak efficacy is essential if treatment is to be maximally efficacious. Gentle rhythmic, nonjarring exercise is prescribed, particularly for patients at risk of loss of bone mass secondary to long-term steroid use.

The primary interventions for maximizing cardiopulmonary function and oxygen transport in patients with RA include some combination of education, aerobic exercise, strengthening exercises, postural correction exercises, chest wall mobility exercises, range of motion exercises, body positioning, breathing control and coughing maneuvers, airway clearance interventions, activity pacing, and energy conservation. An ergonomic assessment of the patient's work and home environments may be indicated to minimize oxygen demand and energy expenditure in these settings. A review of mobility aids and devices is carried out to maximize the patient's function and exercise tolerance.

Education is a principal focus of the long-term management of the patient with RA. Education includes the reinforcement of preventative health practices (e.g., infection control, cold and flu prevention, flu shots, smoking reduction or cessation, aerobic exercise, strengthening exercises, range of motion exercises, nutrition, weight control, hydration, pacing of activities, and energy conservation).

Aerobic exercise is an essential component of the long-term management of the patient with RA to optimize the efficiency of oxygen transport overall both with respect to cardiopulmonary conditioning and improving movement economy. Mild-to-moderate exercise during subacute periods can be beneficial. Cycling efficiency of RA patients is comparable with healthy persons. The efficiency of walking, however, is less in RA patients because of limping and associated deformity and pain. Non–weight-bearing exercise is beneficial in patients with severe deformity and pain (e.g., aquatic exercise or water walking). Given the fluctuations in the patient's condition from day to day, exercise prescription is modified frequently to consider the patient's changing condition. Chest wall exercises include all planes of movement with a rotational component. Body positioning to optimize lung volumes and airflow rates is a priority. Breathing control and coughing maneuvers are essential and should be coupled with body movement and positioning.

Chronic Renal Insufficiency
Pathophysiology and medical management

Patients with chronic renal disease have significant systemic complications. Cardiopulmonary manifestations include left ventricular hypertrophy and congestive heart failure secondary to chronic volume and pressure overload (American College of Sports Medicine, 1991). Patients have a high incidence of atherosclerosis, coronary artery disease, glucose intolerance, and diabetes. Also, generalized muscle weakness and fatigue compromises functional work capacity.

Chronically increased fluid volume, although regulated with dialysis, contributes to increased stroke work of the heart and cardiomegaly and hypertension. With respect to pulmonary function, increased fluid volume increases peribronchial fluid and airway closure. After dialysis, the reduction in body weight is related to a reduction in closing volume, increased vital capacity, and forced expiratory flow rates.

The pulmonary-renal syndromes reflect the close relationship between the lungs and kidneys. These syndromes are characterized by altered immunological status, alveolar hemorrhage, interstitial and alveolar inflammation, and pulmonary vascular involvement (Matthay, Bromberg, and Putman, 1980).

The kidneys have a primary role in the production and regulation of certain humoral regulators of metabolism, hemodynamics, fluid balance, and oxygen transport (Rankin and Matthay, 1982). Thus pathology of the kidneys significantly affects those life-sustaining processes.

Principles of physical therapy management

The goals of long-term management for the patient with chronic renal insufficiency include the following:

- Maximize the patient's quality of life, general health, and well-being and hence physiological reserve capacity
- Educate about cardiopulmonary manifestations of renal insufficiency, self-management, medications, nutrition, weight control, infection control, and the role of a rehabilitation program
- Optimize alveolar ventilation
- Optimize lung volumes, capacities, and flow rates
- Optimize ventilation and perfusion matching and gas exchange
- Reduce the work of breathing
- Reduce the work of the heart
- Protect the airways from aspiration
- Facilitate mucociliary transport
- Optimize secretion clearance
- Maximize aerobic capacity and efficiency of oxygen transport
- Optimize physical endurance and exercise capacity
- Optimize general muscle strength and thereby peripheral oxygen extraction

Patient monitoring includes dyspnea, respiratory distress, breathing pattern (depth and frequency), arterial saturation, cyanosis (delayed sign of desaturation), heart rate, blood pressure, and rate pressure product. Subjectively, perceived exertion is assessed using the Borg scale.

Medication that is needed to maximize treatment response is administered before treatment. Knowledge of the type of medication, its administration route, and time to and duration of peak efficacy is essential if treatment is to be maximally efficacious.

The primary interventions for maximizing cardiopulmonary function and oxygen transport in patients with chronic renal insufficiency include some combination of education, aerobic exercise, strengthening exercise, chest wall mobility exercises, range of motion exercise, body positioning, breathing control and coughing maneuvers, airway clearance interventions, activity pacing, and energy conservation. An ergonomic assessment of the patient's work and home environments may be indicated to minimize oxygen demand and energy expenditure in these settings.

Education is a principal focus of the long-term management of the patient with chronic renal insufficiency. Education includes the reinforcement of preventative health practices (e.g., infection control, cold and flu prevention, flu shots, aerobic exercise, strengthening exercises, range of motion exercises, nutrition, weight control, hydration, pacing of activities, and energy conservation.

Aerobic exercise is an essential component of the long-term management of the patient with chronic renal insufficiency to optimize the efficiency of oxygen transport overall. Maximizing ventilation with exercise is limited if the patient has severe generalized muscular weakness and increased fatigue. Maximal oxygen uptake increases in hemodialysis patients along with improvement in other indices of cardiopulmonary conditioning (Painter et al., 1986). Patients may decrease or eliminate the need for antihypertension medications. Exercise carried out during hemodialysis treatment sessions is feasible and safe for appropriate patients. Because hemodialysis treatments require sessions of several hours multiple times weekly, aerobic training (e.g., cycle ergometry) can be effectively incorporated into treatment time (Shallom, Blumenthal, Williams, Murray, and Dennis, 1984; Zabetakis et al., 1982). The exercise prescription of patients with blood glucose abnormalities and coronary artery disease is modified accordingly.

Chest wall exercises can be used and should include all planes of movement with a rotational component. Body positioning to optimize lung volumes and airflow rates is a priority. Breathing control and coughing maneuvers are essential and should be coupled with body movement and positioning.

SUMMARY

This chapter reviews the pathophysiology, medical management, and physical therapy management of chronic, secondary cardiopulmonary pathology. Specifically, this chapter presents chronic cardiopulmonary dysfunction secondary to neuromuscular, musculoskeletal, collagen vascular/connective tissue, and renal dysfunction. The neuromuscular conditions presented include muscular dystrophy, hemiplegia, Parkinson's disease, multiple sclerosis, cerebral palsy, spinal cord injury, and the late sequelae of poliomyelitis. The musculoskeletal conditions presented included kyphoscoliosis and osteoporosis. The collagen vascular/connective tissue conditions presented include systemic lupus erythematosus, scleroderma, ankylosing spondylitis, and rheumatoid arthritis. Finally, management of the patient with chronic renal insufficiency is presented. The principles of management are presented rather than treatment prescriptions, which cannot be given without consideration of a specific patient. In this context the goals of long-term management of each condition were presented, followed by the essential monitoring required, and the primary interventions for maximizing cardiopulmonary function and oxygen transport. The selection of interventions for any given patient is based on the physiological hierarchy. The most physiological interventions are exploited followed by less physiological interventions and those whose efficacy is less well documented.

REVIEW QUESTIONS

1. Describe the *chronic* cardiopulmonary pathophysiology secondary to muscular dystrophy, hemiplegia, parkinson's disease, multiple sclerosis, cerebral palsy, spinal cord injury, late sequelae of poliomyelitis, kyphoscoliosis, osteoporosis, systemic lupus erythematosus, scleroderma, ankylosing spondylitis, rheumatoid arthritis, and chronic renal insufficiency.

2. Relate cardiopulmonary physical therapy treatment interventions to the underlying pathophysiology of *each* of the above chronic conditions and provide the *rationale* for your choice.

References

Adams, M.A., & Chandler, L.S. (1974). Effects of physical therapy program on vital capacity of patients with muscular dystrophy. *Physical Therapy, 54*, 494-496.

Alexander, J.K. (1985). The cardiomyopathy of obesity. *Progress in Cardiovascular Diseases, 28*, 325-334.

American College of Sports Medicine (1991). *Guidelines for exercise testing and prescription* (4th ed.). Philadelphia: Lea & Febiger.

Bach, J.R. (1991). New approaches in the rehabilitation of the traumatic high level quadriplegic. *American Journal of Physical Medicine and Rehabilitation, 70,* 13-19.

Bach, J.R. (1992). Pulmonary rehabilitation considerations for Duchenne muscular dystrophy: The prolongation of life by respiratory muscle aids. *Critical Reviews in Physical and Rehabilitation Medicine, 3,* 239-269.

Bach, J.R. (1993). Mechanical insufflation-exsufflation. Comparison of peak expiratory flows with manually assisted and unassisted coughing techniques. *Chest, 104,* 1553-1562.

Bach, J.R., Alba, A.S., Bodofsky, E., Curran, F.J., & Schultheiss, M. (1987). Glossopharyngeal breathing and noninvasive aids in the management of post-polio respiratory insufficiency. *Birth Defects, 23,* 99-113.

Bach, J.R., Alba, A.S., & Shin, D. (1989). Management alternatives for post-polio respiratory insufficiency. Assisted ventilation by nasal or oral-nasal interface. *American Journal of Physical Medicine and Rehabilitation, 68,* 264-271.

Bach, J.R., O'Brien, J., Krotenberg, R., & Alba, A.S. (1987). Management of end stage respiratory failure in Duchenne muscular dystrophy. *Muscle and Nerve, 10,* 177-182.

Bach, J.R., Smith, W.H., Michaels, J., Saporito, L., Alba, A.S., Dayal, R., & Pan, J. (1993). Airway secretion clearance by mechanical exsufflation for post-poliomyelitis ventilator-assisted individuals. *Archives of Physical Medicine and Rehabilitation, 74,* 170-174.

Bake, B., Dempsey, J., & Grimby, G. (1976). Effects of shape changes of the chest wall on distribution of inspired gas. *American Review of Respiratory Disease, 114,* 1113-1120.

Barrach, A.L., Beck, G.J., Bickerman, H.A., & Seanor, J.H. (1952). Physical methods of stimulating cough mechanisms. Use in poliomyelitis, bronchial asthma, pulmonary emphysema, and bronchiectasis. *Journal of the American Medical Association, 50,* 1380-1385.

Bates, D.V. (1989). *Respiratory function in disease* (3rd ed.). Philadelphia: WB Saunders.

Black, L.F., & Hyatt, R.E. (1971). Maximal static respiratory pressures in generalized neuromuscular disease. *American Review of Respiratory Diseases, 103,* 641-650.

Braun, N.M.T., Arora, N.S., & Rochester, D.F. (1983). Respiratory muscle and pulmonary function in polymyositis and other proximal myopathies. *Thorax, 38,* 616-623.

Braun, S.R., Giovannoni, R., & O'Connor, M. (1984). Improving the cough in patients with spinal cord injury. *American Journal of Physical Medicine, 63,* 1-10.

Campbell, J., & Ball, J. (1978). Energetics of walking in cerebral palsy. *Orthopedic Clinics of North America, 9,* 374-377.

Cooper, C.B., Trend, P.S., & Wiles, C.M. (1985). Severe diaphragm weakness in multiple sclerosis. *Thorax, 40,* 631-632.

Curran, F.J. (1981). Night ventilation to body respirators for patients in chronic respiratory failure due to late stage muscular dystrophy. *Archives of Physical Medicine and Rehabilitation, 62,* 270-274.

Dean, E. (1991). Clinical decision making in the management of the late sequelae of poliomyelitis. *Physical Therapy, 71,* 752-761.

Dean, E. (1993). Advances in rehabilitation for older persons with cardiopulmonary dysfunction. In P.R. Katz, R.L. Kane, & M.D. Mezey (Eds.). *Advances in long-term care.* Vol. 2. New York: Springer Publishing.

Dean, E. (1994). Cardiopulmonary development. In B.R. Bonder, & M.B. Wagner (Eds.). *Functional performance in older adults.* Philadelphia: F.A. Davis.

Dean, E. & Ross, J. (1992). Mobilization and exercise conditioning. In C. Zadai (Ed.). *Pulmonary management in physical therapy.* New York: Churchill Livingstone.

Dean, E., & Ross, J. (1993). Movement energetics of individuals with a history of poliomyelitis. *Archives of Physical Medicine and Rehabilitation, 74,* 478-483.

Dean, E., Ross, J., Road, J.D., Courtenay, L., & Madill, K. (1991). Pulmonary function in individuals with a history of poliomyelitis. *Chest, 100,* 118-123.

DeTroyer, A, De Beyl, T., & Thirion, M. (1981). Function of the respiratory muscles in acute hemiplegia. *American Review of Respiratory Diseases, 123,* 631-632.

Dickey, B.F., & Myers, A.R. (1988). Pulmonary manifestations of collagen-vascular diseases. In A.P. Fishman (Ed.). *Pulmonary diseases and disorders.* New York: McGraw Hill.

Dresen, M.H.W., de Groot, J.R., & Bouman, L.N. (1985). Aerobic energy expenditure of handicapped children after training. *Archives of Physical Medicine and Rehabilitation, 66,* 302-306.

Ekblom, B., & Nordemar, R. (1987). Rheumatoid arthritis. In J. Skinner (Ed.). *Exercise testing and training for special cases.* Philadelphia: Lea & Febiger.

Elliott, C.G., Hill, T.R., Adams, T.E., Crapo, R.O., Nietzeba, R.M., & Gardner, R.M. (1985). Exercise performance of subjects with ankylosing spondylitis and limited chest expansion. *Bulletin of European Physiopathology and Respiration, 21,* 363-368.

Estenne, M., & Gorino, M. (1992). Action of the diaphragm during cough in tetrapelgic subjects. *Journal of Applied Physiology, 72,* 1074-1080.

Ferris, B.G., & Pollard, D.S. (1960). Effect of deep and quiet breathing on pulmonary compliance in man. *Journal of Clinical Investigations, 39,* 143-149.

Fluck, D.C. (1966). Chest movements in hemiplegia. *Clinical Science, 31,* 382-388.

Fugl-Meyer, A.R., & Grimby, G. (1984). Respiration in tetraplegia and in hemiplegia: A review. *International Rehabilitation Medicine, 6,* 186-190.

Gray, I.R. (1989). Cardiovascular manifestations of collagen vascular diseases. In D.G. Julian, A.J. Camm, K.M. Fox, R.J.C. Hall, P.A. Poole-Wilson (Eds.). *Diseases of the heart.* Philadelphia: Bailliere Tindall.

Griggs, R.C., & Donohoe, K.M. (1982). Recognition and management of respiratory insufficiency in neuromuscular disease. *Journal of Chronic Diseases, 35,* 497-500.

Grimby, G., Fugl-Meyer, A.R., & Blomstrand, A. (1974). Partitioning of the contribution of rib cage and abdomen to ventilation in ankylosing spondylitis. *Thorax, 29,* 179-184.

Gross, D. (1980). The effect of training on strength and endurance on the diaphragm in quadriplegia. *American Journal of Medicine, 68,* 27-35.

Hapke, E.J., Meek, J.C., & Jacobs, J. (1972). Pulmonary function in progressive muscular dystrophy. *Chest, 61,* 41-47.

Harkcom, T.M., Lampman, R.M., Banwell, B.F., & Castor, C.W. (1985). Therapeutic value of graded aerobic exercise training in rheumatoid arthritis. *Arthritis and Rheumatism, 28,* 32-39.

Hietpas, B.G., Roth, R.D., & Jensen, W.M. (1979). Huff coughing and airway patency. *Respiratory Care, 24,* 710.

Hoeppner, V.H., Cockcroft, D.W., Dosman, J.A., & Cotton, D.J. (1984). Nighttime ventilation improves respiratory failure in secondary kyphoscoliosis. *American Review of Respiratory Diseases, 129,* 240-243.

Howard, R.S., Wiles, C.M., & Spencer, G.T. (1988). The late sequelae of poliomyelitis. *Quarterly Journal of Medicine, 66,* 219-232.

Inkley, S.R., Alderberg, F.C., & Vignos, P.C. (1974). Pulmonary function in Duchenne muscular dystrophy related to stage of disease. *American Journal of Medicine, 56,* 297-306.

Kilburn, K.H., Eagan, J.T., Sieker, H.O., & Heyman, A. (1959). Cardiopulmonary insufficiency in myotonic and progressive muscular dystrophy. *New England Journal of Medicine, 261,* 1089-1096.

Kirilloff, L.H., Owens, G.R., Rogers, R.M., & Mazacco, M.C. (1985). Does chest physical work? *Chest, 88,* 436-444.

Lane, D.J., Hazleman, B., & Nichols, P.J.R. (1974). Late onset respiratory failure in patients with previous poliomyelitis. *Quarterly Journal of Medicine, 43,* 551-568.

Leblanc, P., Ruff, F., & Milic-Emili, J. (1970). Effects of age and body position on "airway closure" in man. *Journal of Applied Physiology, 28,* 448-451.

Linder, S.H. (1993). Functional electrical stimulation to enhance cough in quadriplegia. *Chest, 103,* 166-169.

Lisboa, C., Moreno, R., Fava, M., Ferreti, R., & Cruz, E. (1985). Inspiratory muscle function in patients with severe kyphoscoliosis. *American Review of Respiratory Diseases, 132,* 48-52.

Macklem, P.T., & Roussos, C.S. (1977). Respiratory muscle fatigue: A cause of respiratory failure? *Clinical Science & Molecular Medicine, 53,* 419-422.

Malouin, F., Potvin, M., Prevost, J., Richards, C.L., & Wood-Dauphinee, S. (1992). Use of an intensive task-oriented gait training program in a series of patients with acute cerebrovascular accidents. *Physical Therapy, 72,* 781-793.

Matthay, R.A., Bromberg, S.I., & Putman, A.M. (1980). Pulmonary-renal syndromes—a review. *Yale Journal of Biology and Medicine, 53,* 497-523.

McArdle, W.D., Katch, F.I., & Katch, V.L. (1991). *Exercise physiology, energy, nutrition, and performance* (3rd ed.). Philadelphia: Lea & Febiger.

McFarlin, D.E., & McFarland, H.F. (1982). Multiple sclerosis. *New England Journal of Medicine, 307,* 1183-1188.

Mehta, A.D., Wright, W.B., & Kirby, B.J. (1978). Ventilatory function in Parkinson's disease. *British Medical Journal, XX,* 1456-1457.

Miller, H.J., Thomas, E., & Wilmot, C.B. (1988). Pneumobelt use among high quadriplegia population. *Archive of Physical Medicine and Rehabilitation, 69,* 369-372.

Moorman, J.R., Coleman, E., Packer, D.L., Kisslo, J.A., Bell, J., Hetlemna, B.D., Stajich, J., & Roses, A.D. (1985). Cardiac involvement in myotonic muscular dystrophy. *Medicine, 64,* 371-387.

Mossberg, K.A., Linton, K.A., Friske, K. (1990). Ankle-foot orthoses: effect of energy expenditure of gait in spastic diplegic children. *Archives of Physical Medicine and Rehabilitation, 71,* 490-494.

Murray, J.F., Nadel, J.A. (1988a). *Textbook of respiratory medicine.* Philadelphia: WB Saunders.

Murray, J.F., Nadel, J.A. (1988b). *Textbook of respiratory medicine.* Philadelphia: WB Saunders.

Nakano, K.K., Bass, H., Tyler, H.R., & Carmel, R.J. (1976). Amyotrophic lateral sclerosis: A study of pulmonary function. *Diseases of the Nervous System, 37,* 32-35.

Neu, H.C., Connolly, J.J., Schwertley, F.W., Ladwig, H.A., & Brody, A.W. (1966). Obstructive respiratory dysfunction in Parkinsonian patients. *American Review of Respiratory Diseases, 95,* 33–47.

Neubauer, B., & Gundersen, H.J.G. (1978). Analysis of heart rate variations in patients with multiple sclerosis. *Journal of Neurology, Neurosurgery, and Psychiatry, 41,* 417-419.

Nunn, J.F., Coleman, A.J., Sachithanandan, T., Bergman, N.A., & Laws, J.W. (1965). Hypoxaemia and atelectasis produced by forced expiration. *British Journal of Anesthesia, 37,* 3-12.

Painter, P.L., Nelson-Worel, J.N., Hill, M.M., Thornbery, D.R., Shelp, W.R., Harrington, A.R., & Weinstein, A.B. (1986). Effects of exercise training during hemodialysis. *Nephron, 43,* 87-92.

Pardy, R.L., & Leith, D.E. (1984). Ventilatory muscle training. *Respiratory Care, 29,* 278-284.

Pentland, B., & Ewing, D.J. (1987). Cardiovascular reflexes in multiple sclerosis. *European Neurology, 26,* 46-50.

Perloff, J.K., de Leon, A.C., & O'Doherty, D. (1966). The cardiomyopathy of progressive muscular dystrophy. *Circulation, 33,* 625-648.

Rankin, J.A., & Matthay, R.A. (1982). Pulmonary renal syndromes. II. Etiology and pathogenesis. *Yale Journal of Biology and Medicine, 55,* 11-26.

Ray, J.F., 3rd, Yost, L., Moallem, S., Sanoudos, G.M., Villamena, Paredes, R.M., & Clauss, R.H. (1974). Immobility, hypoxemia, and pulmonary arteriovenous shunting. *Archives of Surgery, 109,* 537-541.

Rosenow, E.C., Strimlan, C.V., Muhm, J.R., & Ferguson, R.H. (1977). Pleuropulmonary manifestations of ankylosing spondylitis. *Mayo Clinic Proceedings, 52,* 641-649.

Ross, J., & Dean, E. (1992). Body positioning. In C. Zadai (Ed.). *Clinics in physical therapy. Pulmonary management in physical therapy.* New York: Churchill Livingstone.

Scott, T.E., Wise, R.A., Hochberg, M.C., & Wigley, F.M. (1987). HLA-DR4 and pulmonary dysfunction in rheumatoid arthritis. *American Journal of Medicine, 82,* 765-771.

Segal, A.M., Calabrese, L.H., Ahmad, M., Tubbs, R.R., & White, C.S. (1985). The pulmonary manifestations of systemic lupus erythematosus. *Seminars in Arthritis and Rheumatism, 14,* 202-224.

Senaratne, M.P.J., Carroll, D., Warren, K.G,. & Kappagoda, T. (1984). Evidence for cardiovascular autonomic nerve dysfunction in multiple sclerosis. *Journal of Neurology, Neurosurgery, and Psychiatry, 47,* 947-952.

Shallom, R., Blumenthal, J.A., Williams, R.S., McMurray, R.G., & Dennis, V.W. (1984). Feasibility and benefits of exercise training in patients on maintenance dialysis. *Kidney International, 25,* 958-963.

Sinha, R., & Bergofsky, E.H. (1972). Prolonged alteration of lung mechanics in kyphoscoliosis by positive pressure hyperinflation. *American Review of Respiratory Disease, 106,* 47-57.

Smith, P.E.M., Calverley, P.M.A., Edwards, R.H.T., Evans, G.A., & Campbell, E.J.M. (1987). Practical problems in the respiratory care of patients with muscular dystrophy. *New England Journal of Medicine, 316,* 1197-1205.

Smith, P.E.M., Edwards, R.H., & Calverley, P.M.A. (1989). Oxygen treatment of sleep hypoxaemia in Duchenne muscular dystrophy. *Thorax, 44,* 997-1001.

Smith, E.L., Smith, K.A., & Gilligan, C. (1991). Exercise, fitness, osteoarthritis, and osteoporosis. In C. Bouchard, R.J. Shephard, J.R. Sutton, & B.D. McPherson (Eds.). *Exercise, fitness, and health. A consensus of current knowledge.* Champaign: Human Kinetics Books.

Vignos, P.J., & Watkins, M.P. (1966). The effects of exercise in muscular dystrophy. *Journal of the American Medical Association, 197,* 843-848.

Wilson, J.D., Braunwald, E., Isselbacher, K.J., Martin, J.B., Fauci, A.S., & Root, R.K. (Eds). *Harrison's principles of internal medicine* (12th ed.). St. Louis: McGraw Hill.

Wolff, R.K., Dolovich, M.B., Obminski, G., & Newhouse, M.T. (1977). Effects of exercise and eucapnic hyperventilation on bronchial clearance in man. *Journal of Applied Physiology, 43,* 46-50.

Zabetakis, P.M., Gleim, G.W., Pasternack, F.L., Saranitt, A., Nicholas, J.A., & Michelis, M.F. (1982). Long-duration submaximal exercise conditioning in hemodialysis patients. *Clinical Nephrology, 18,* 17-22.

PART VI

Guidelines for the Delivery of Cardiopulmonary Physical Therapy: Intensive Care

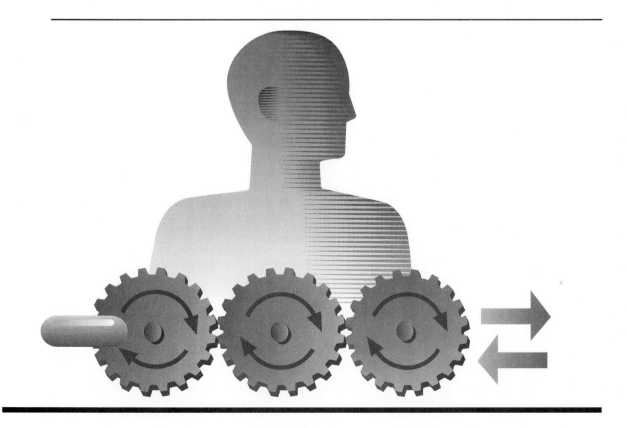

CHAPTER 31

Comprehensive Patient Management in the Intensive Care Unit

Elizabeth Dean

KEY TERMS   Evidence-based practice
Function optimization
Physiological evidence
Prevention

Quality care
Scientific evidence
Treatment goals
Treatment selection and prioritization

INTRODUCTION

Because cardiopulmonary physical therapy in the intensive care unit (ICU) is a specialty in itself, this chapter presents some general aspects of clinical and nonclinical management in this setting. An overview of the general goals of treatment and the rationale for prioritizing treatments according to a physiological hierarchy is described. Both clinical and nonclinical aspects of patient management are presented. Finally, issues related to the management of the dying patient are addressed.

The thrust toward evidence-based practice in health care and the development of conceptual bases for practice have had major implications for cardiopulmonary physical therapy practice in the ICU

(Barlow, Hayes, and Nelson, 1984; Dean, 1985; Dean, 1994a; Hislop, 1975; Ross and Dean, 1989; Schon, 1983; Worthingham, 1960; Zadai, 1986). A superior knowledge of cardiopulmonary physiology, pathophysiology, pharmacology, and multisystem disease and its medical management is essential. Clinical decision making in the ICU and rational management of patients is based on a tripod approach: (1) a knowledge of the underlying pathophysiology and basis for general care, (2) the physiological and scientific evidence for treatment interventions, and (3) clinical experience (Figure 31-1). Quality care is a function of these three areas of knowledge and expertise. Evidence-based practice and excellent problem solving ability will maximize

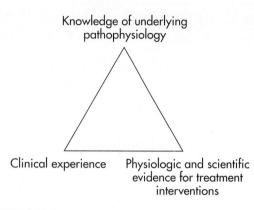

FIGURE 31-1
Tripod approach to patient management.

the benefit-to-risk ratio of cardiopulmonary physical therapy interventions (Riegelman, 1991).

SPECIALIZED EXPERTISE OF THE ICU PHYSICAL THERAPIST

Effective clinical decision making and practice in the ICU demands specialized expertise and skill including advanced, current knowledge in cardiopulmonary and multisystem physiology and pathophysiology, and in medical, surgical, nursing, and pharmacological management (see the box on p. 569). Physical therapists in the ICU need to be first-rate diagnosticians. Given the multitude of factors that contribute to impaired oxygen transport (Dean, 1983; Dean, 1994b; Dean, 1994c), the physical therapist must be able to analyze these to define the patient's specific oxygen transport deficits and problems. Therefore the ICU physical therapist must be capable of integrating large amounts of objective information quickly, interpreting this information, and integrating it to provide the basis for a treatment prescription (i.e., the specific selection, prioritization, and implementation of treatment interventions) (Cutler, 1985). The integration and interpretation of the vast amount of multiorgan system data is perhaps the single most important skill in ICU practice and treatment prescription. With this database, the physical therapist must identify the indications for treatment, contraindications, and optimal timing of interventions. The condition of the ICU patient can change rapidly. The physical

therapist must work within narrow windows of opportunity to effect an optimal treatment response. Treatments are variable with respect to their intensity, duration, and frequency. Usually treatments are short and frequent; thus the maximally beneficial outcome with the least risk to the patient is the objective of every treatment.

GOALS AND GENERAL BASIS OF MANAGEMENT

The ultimate goals of cardiopulmonary physical therapy treatment in the ICU include the following:

1. To have the patient alert and oriented to person, time, and place
2. To have the patient return to premorbid functional level to the greatest extent possible
3. To reduce morbidity, mortality, and length of hospital stay.

As a precursor to achieving these three overriding goals, the immediate goals initially relate to the attainment of optimal oxygen transport and hence cardiopulmonary function and secondly relate to the attainment of optimal musculoskeletal and neurological function. In the ICU the physical therapist must recognize the implications of cardiopulmonary insufficiency on neuromuscular status and that apparent impairment of neuromuscular status in not necessarily indicative of neurological dysfunction. Rather, reduced cardiac output and blood pressure, hypoxemia, hypercapnia, and increased intracranial pressure (ICP) may be indirectly responsible for these changes.

Restricted Mobility and Recumbency

Hospitalization particularly in the ICU is associated with a considerable reduction in mobility (i.e., loss of exercise stimulus), and recumbency (i.e., loss of gravitational stimulus) (see Chapters 17 and 18). These two factors are essential for normal oxygen transport; thus their removal has dire consequences for the patient with or without cardiopulmonary dysfunction.

In terms of a physiological hierarchy of treatment interventions (see Chapter 16), exploiting the physiological effects of acute mobilization, upright positioning, and their combination, are the most physiologically justifiable primary interventions to maximize oxygen transport and prevent its impairment.

Specialized Expertise and Skill of the ICU Physical Therapist
Detailed, comprehensive knowledge of cardiopulmonary physiology and pathophysiology, and pharmacology.
Thorough working knowledge of the monitoring systems routinely used in the ICU and an understanding of the interpretation of the output of these monitoring systems (e.g., ECG, arterial blood gases, fluid and electrolyte balance, hemodynamic monitoring, chest-tube drainage systems, intracranial pressure monitoring). This information is an integral component of the physical therapy assessment of the underlying problems, and for selecting, prioritizing, and progressing or modifying treatment.
Extensive expertise in cardiopulmonary assessment and treatment prescription; preferably a minimum of 2 to 3 years experience in general medicine and surgery.
Detailed understanding of multisystem physiology and pathophysiology and the cardiopulmonary manifestations of systemic disease.
An ability to practice effectively under pressure and in often apparently congested, suboptimal working conditions.
Knowledgeable regarding all emergency procedures including those for respiratory and cardiac arrest, equipment, or power failure.
Knowledgeable regarding the paging system used in the unit for contacting the physical therapist when she or he is out of the unit and out of the hospital. On-call service, 24 hours a day, 7 days a week is a common practice and should be considered in units without this service.
Sensitivity toward each patient's psychosocial situation, culture, and values, and active involvement of the patient and family in clinical decision making whenever feasible.
Superior communication skills (e.g., ability to work cooperatively with other members of the ICU team (see Figure 31-2) and give verbal presentations and discuss patients at rounds).

Recumbency is nonphysiological; it is a position that all too often is to what most patients are injudiciously confined. Changing the position of the body from erect to supine positions results in significant physiological changes, which may jeopardize the patient's already compromised or threatened oxygen transport system (see the box on p. 570, at top left) (see Chapter 18).

The culmination of these deleterious effects offsets the increased homogeneity of ventilation and perfusion and their matching in the supine position. These effects compound the superimposed factors of immobility, recumbency-induced central fluid shifts, prolonged lying without the normal stimulation or will to turn the body, and underlying pathophysiology or trauma that may contribute to impaired cardiopulmonary function and oxygen transport. Theoretically, the more compromised the patient, the greater the priority is to maximize time spent in the upright position in conjunction with exploiting the benefits of acute mobilization.

Specificity of Cardiopulmonary Physical Therapy

Physical therapy interventions must be specifically geared toward the management of each organ system, taking into consideration the pathophysiological basic for the patient's signs and symptoms and rational for each intervention and the physiological and scientific evidence supporting the efficacy of the intervention (Dean and Ross, 1992). Physical therapy provides both therapeutic and prophylactic interventions for the ICU patient. The use of conservative, noninvasive measures is the initial treatment of choice to avert or delay the need for additional invasive monitoring and treatment, supplemental oxygen, pharmacological agents, and the need for intubation and mechanical ventilation. The physical therapist aims toward avoiding, postponing, or reducing the need for respiratory support for as long as possible. In addition, the physical therapist helps to prevent the multitude of side effects of immobility and prolonged confinement to bed. A summary of general information required

Normal Physiological Changes When Changing from the Upright to the Supine Position

Cephalad displacement of the visceral contents and diaphragm

    Compression on the posterior dependent lung fields

Cephalad fluid shift to the central circulation

    Stroke volume and cardiac output

    Total lung capacity

    Vital capacity

    Functional residual capacity

    Residual volume

    Forced expiratory volumes

    Airway resistance

    Closing volumes of small airways

Restriction of chest wall and diaphragmatic excursions

    Arterial oxygen levels

    Cough effectiveness

    Preload and afterload and myocardial work

    Myocardial efficiency

    Sympathetic stimulation and decreased peripheral vascular resistance

General Information Required Before Treating the ICU Patient

Medical and surgical histories

Gender and age

Premorbid status (e.g., life style, ethnicity, culture, work situation, stress, cardiopulmonary conditioning, and oxygen transport reserve capacity)

Smoking history

Hydration and nutritional status: deficiencies, obesity, or asthenia

Recency of onset and course of present condition

Existing or potential medical instability

Indications or necessity for intubation and mechanical ventilation

Invasive monitoring, lines, leads, and catheters

Existence of or potential for complications and multiorgan system failure

Coma

Elevated intracranial pressure (ICP) and the need for ICP monitoring

Risk or presence and site(s) of infection

Quality of sleep and rest periods

Nutritional support during ICU stay

Pain control regimen

General Physical Therapy Goals Toward Function Optimization in the ICU Patient

Maintain or restore adequate alveolar ventilation and perfusion and their matching in nonaffected and affected lung fields and thereby optimize oxygen transport overall

Prolong spontaneous breathing (to the extent that is therapeutically indicated) and thereby avoid, postpone, or minimize need for mechanical ventilation

Minimize the work of breathing

Minimize the work of the heart

Design a positioning schedule to maintain comfort and postural alignment (distinct from therapeutic body positioning to optimize oxygen transport)

Maintain or restore general mobility, strength, endurance, and coordination, within the limitations of the patient's condition and consistent with the patient's anticipated rehabilitation prognosis (distinct from therapeutic mobilization to optimize oxygen transport)

Maximally involve the patient in a daily routine including self-care, changing body position, standing, transferring, sitting in a chair, and ambulating in patients for whom these activities are indicated

Optimize treatment outcome by interfacing physical therapy with the goals and patient-related activities of other team members, coordinating treatments with medication schedules, and treating the patient specifically, based on results of objective monitoring available in the ICU and subjective findings

before treating the ICU patient is presented in the box on p. 570, at top right.

Function Optimization

Function optimization refers to promoting optimal physiological functioning at an organ system level, as well as promoting optimal functioning of the patient as a whole. In critical care, primary goals related to function optimization are initially focused on cardiorespiratory function. With improvement in oxygen transport, increased attention is given to optimal functioning of the patient with respect to self-care, self-positioning, sitting up, and walking. General physical therapy goals related to function optimization are shown in the box on p. 570, at bottom.

Prophylaxis

General aspects of patient care related to physical therapy practice include the role of prophylaxis or prevention. The complications of immobility are de-

scribed in Chapter 17 and relate primarily to the status of the cardiopulmonary, neuromuscular, and musculoskeletal systems. In the ICU the negative physiological effects of immobility are amplified in severely ill and older patients. A primary objective of the physical therapist, therefore, is to avoid or reduce these untoward effects on the patient's recovery and length of stay in the ICU. Specifically, these goals include reducing the deleterious effects of immobility and pathology on cardiopulmonary and neuromuscular function and reducing the risk of deformity and decubiti. The negative sequelae of relative confinement are largely preventable. Particular care must be taken to avoid pressure sores because these significantly increase the risk of infection and deterioration. Physical therapists and nurses need to examine routinely for sites of redness, pressure, and potential skin lesions in every patient, regardless of expected length of stay in the ICU (Stillwell, 1992). The texture of bed coverings, their smoothness, bunching of the bed gown, or irritation from lines and catheters to the patient need to be routinely monitored.

Specific Patient Information Required Before Treating the ICU Patient

Detailed knowledge of the patient's history, including the differential diagnosis on admission to the ICU, and relevant past medical, surgical, and social histories

Detailed understanding and knowledge of the medications administered to the patient, their indications, and side effects, especially those affecting response to physical therapy

Knowledgeable about the stability of vital signs since admission, including heart rate and rhythm, respiration rate and rhythm, blood pressure, skin color, core temperature, and hemodynamic stability

Detailed knowledge of relevant findings of laboratory tests, procedures, and biopsies, including arterial blood gases, blood analysis, fluid and electrolyte balance, ECG, x-ray, thoracentesis, central venous pressure (CVP), left artrial pressure (LAP), pulmonary artery wedge pressure (PAWP), microbiology and biochemistry reports, and urinalysis

If the patient is ventilated, detailed understanding of the rationale for the ventilatory mode and parameters used

With respect to establishing a patient database, do the following: (1) Conduct a thorough, detailed clinical assessment specific to the patient's condition(s), including inspection, palpation, percussion, and auscultation of the chest, as well as a neuromusculoskeletal assessment to rule out any secondary effects of cardiopulmonary dysfunction and to establish rehabilitation prognosis. (2) Establish a physical diagnosis and problem list and prioritize the treatment goals and overall treatment plan. (3) Determine the optimal assessment and treatment outcome measures and be knowledgeable about their interpretation. (4) Conduct serial trend measurements to predict the patient's oxygen transport reserve capacity before treatment and stressing the oxygen transport system

As treatment progresses, record objective and relevant subjective treatment outcome measures and revise treatment goals as indicated by the patient's progress

Preparation for Treating the ICU Patient

Patients in the ICU are generally characterized by some degree of life-threatening medical instability. Before treating a given patient in the ICU, the physical therapist should be thoroughly familiar with the specific information shown in the box on p. 571.

GENERAL CLINICAL ASPECTS OF THE MANAGEMENT OF THE ICU PATIENT
Assessment

The fundamental assessment procedures for the cardiorespiratory system are described in detail in Part Two. Laboratory reports, procedures, sputum culture, and x-rays supplement the findings of inspection, palpation, percussion, and auscultation of the chest. Of particular importance are the blood work, arterial blood gases, ECG, fluid and electrolyte balance, hemodynamic monitoring, and intracranial pressure monitoring. These are the most commonly monitored parameters in the ICU in addition to vital signs—respiration rate, heart rate, temperature, and blood pressure.

Monitoring

Optimal physical therapy treatment depends on optimal use of the monitoring systems available in the ICU. Monitoring systems can be used to establish the indications and contraindications for treatment, parameters of the treatment prescription and progression, in addition to assessing the patient. These are summarized in the box above. Physical therapists need to exploit the considerable amount of objective data available to them in patient management. A thorough knowledge and routine use of monitoring systems for each patient in the ICU cannot be overemphasized in terms of contributing to improved quality of care with less potential risk to the patient.

The monitoring systems described in Chapter 15 provide essential information with respect to the management of the ICU patient. Information regarding acid-base imbalance and fluid and electrolyte balance helps to establish specific treatment goals. The Swan-Ganz catheter in situ gives the pressures for

---

> ### Physical Therapy Uses of Monitoring Systems in the ICU
>
> Establish the indications for and contraindications of cardiopulmonary physical therapy
>
> Define treatment intensity, duration, and frequency for optimal treatment outcome
>
> Determine the appropriateness of response to a specific intervention
>
> Assess the need for supplemental oxygen before, during, and after treatment
>
> Determine appropriate patient positioning between, during, and after treatments
>
> Establish whether the patient is responding negatively to treatment and whether treatment should be discontinued or modified

---

pulmonary artery pressure and wedge pressure, which provide an index of myocardial sufficiency and specifically left heart function. Central venous pressure gives an indication of fluid loading and the ability of the right side of the heart to cope with changes in circulating body fluids. Pressures related to heart function give the physical therapist an indication of pulmonary status and help to determine whether heart dysfunction is affecting lung function, lung dysfunction is affecting heart function, or both. Existing cardiopulmonary stress alerts the physical therapist to appropriately modify workloads or the physical demands of treatment to keep the patient medically stable, avoid undue fatigue, and deterioration.

Changes in ECG may reflect heart disease, lung disease, altered acid base, and electrolyte and fluid balance. The physical therapist is responsible for identifying the patient's heart rhythm and ECG changes that might be expected with improvement or deterioration in oxygen transport, and secondary to medical management, drug intervention and changes in the course of the disease and response to treatment generally.

Pharmacological Agents

The physical therapist needs a thorough knowledge of the common pharmacological agents used in intensive care (Chapter 43). With this knowledge, the physical therapist can augment the effects of these agents and optimize physical therapy treatment response when treatments are coordinated with medication schedules. Most medications have optimal dosages for any given patient, optimal sensitivity, and peak-response time. Most medications have side effects. Side effects may cause deterioration in the patient's condition, create apparent signs and symptoms suggestive of other disorders, or alter response to treatment. The physical therapist therefore needs to identify the medications each patient is taking and their side effects.

Certain medications, such as bronchodilators, sedatives, mucolytic agents, antianginal medications, and analgesics, help the patient to be able to cooperate during treatments. Special consideration must always be given to the different peak-response times of medications used in the ICU. The patient is willing to cooperate more actively in the treatment if pain is reduced, breathing is easier, and mucus is easier to clear. A better treatment effect is therefore more likely. These advantages result in more effective use of the physical therapist's time, and often a shorter, more cost-effective, efficacious treatment.

Certain other medications may prevent close monitoring of patients during exercise and activity. Patients on beta-blocking agents, for example, will not show the normal changes in heart rate and blood pressure in response to exercise. In addition, beta-blockers contribute to fatigue. Caution must therefore be observed when prescribing exercise for these patients. Another classification of drugs called *vasopressor agents* help regulate blood pressure and heart rate. Patients on these agents may also exhibit abnormal exercise responses. Hence monitoring vital signs to assess treatment response may be of limited value for patients on drugs acting on the cardiovascular system.

Narcotics is a commonly used classification of drug used in the ICU and are often administered jointly with sedatives and tranquilizers. Despite their beneficial effects on pain relief, narcotics of any classification of pharmacological agents and particularly in combination with other sedative type drugs antagonize and often prohibit physical therapy treatments because of the patient's reduced arousal, monotonous ventilation, and inability to cooperate with treatment.

In addition, narcotics tend to have significant multisystem effects rather than localized effects. Because physical therapy is the most physiological and noninvasive intervention available to the ICU patient, it behooves the physical therapist to ensure that all other pharmacological agents that are effective and more selective than narcotics in achieving the desired effect have been considered.

TREATMENT PRESCRIPTION IN THE ICU

Physical therapy treatments in the ICU are judiciously selected in a goal-specific manner. As a general guideline, treatments descend in a physiological hierarchy. Mobilization, exercise, and body positioning should be exploited first with respect to their direct and potent effects on oxygen transport overall. At the other end of the hierarchy (i.e., least physiological interventions that have a more limited effect on the steps in the oxygen transport pathway) are conventional interventions, such as manual techniques.

Mobilization and exercise can be prescribed to effect three physiologically distinct outcomes based on their acute effects, their long-term effects, and their preventative effects (see Chapter 17). The treatment prescription needs to focus on which specific effects of mobilization and exercise are required to reverse or mitigate deficits in the oxygen transport pathway or prevent impaired oxygen transport. The treatment prescription is different in each case.

Unlike other patient care areas, the frequency of treatments may range from one to several treatments daily. The frequency depends on the patient's specific treatment goals, the aggressiveness of treatment indicated, interfering related problems and their management, patient cooperation, and tolerance for the physical therapy treatments prescribed. The patient's oxygen reserve capacity needs to be assessed to ensure that the patient can meet the demands of exercise stress. The physical therapist needs to assess the patient's tolerance with respect to duration, intensity, and frequency of treatments, as well as prescribed exercise. Objective and subjective measures of the patient's tolerance to the initial assessment and the observations of other members of the team help to establish this baseline.

Treatment goals and interventions are described in Part III. Interventions frequently used in the ICU include those related to mobilization and exercise, body positioning, breathing control and coughing, mucociliary transport and mucous clearance interventions, such as deep breathing and coughing maneuvers, chest wall mobilization, postural drainage, percussion, vibration, shaking, rib springing, relaxation, body alignment, and general strengthening exercises. These interventions are the mainstay of cardiopulmonary physical therapy. Intensive care physical therapy demands particular skill in selecting, prioritizing, and applying the particular interventions that can effect the optimal treatment outcome in the shortest time in a given critically ill patient. For example, a common scenario in the ICU is the physical therapist's attempting to reduce or reverse the adverse changes observed in blood gases; that is, falling Pa_{O_2} levels and increasing Pa_{CO_2} levels in the patient for whom intubation is being seriously considered if improvement is not observed soon. The focus of treatment for such a patient is delineated into two parts. The physical therapist first focuses on optimizing oxygen transport and cardiopulmonary function of the involved lung fields and second on maintaining optimal cardiopulmonary function of the uninvolved lung fields.

Contraindications and the awareness of potential adverse effects of cardiopulmonary physical therapy are particular concerns in the ICU. The physical therapist needs to be well-versed about these. Treatments need to be modified to achieve an optimal treatment effect without posing a hazard to the patient. Herein lies one of the many challenges of intensive care physical therapy.

Discharge from the ICU

To be recommended for discharge from the ICU, the patient should not require cardiopulmonary physical therapy more than every 4 to 6 hours. The patient should be breathing spontaneously and independently and elicit a cough with or without assistance, preferably one that is effective in clearing secretions. If alert, the patient should be moving purposefully in bed before transfer.

The physical therapist is responsible for documenting the physical therapy treatment priorities and frequent progress notes during the ICU stay in order that the team responsible for the patient after discharge is able to continue management with reduced risk of disruption of care or regression of the patient's condition. The patient should be consulted, if possible, and informed at all times of his or her progress and plans made by the team and family. The patient should be given as many choices as possible about his or her care and be actively involved in long-term planning.

NONCLINICAL ASPECTS OF THE MANAGEMENT OF THE ICU PATIENT
Team Work

Comprehensive patient care in the ICU includes some nonclinical activities. Team work is the essence of optimal patient care, particularly in the ICU. The physical therapist interacts frequently with other team members regarding observations and changes in the patient's condition, treatment goals, and treatment response (Figure 31-2). In addition to providing therapy for patients, the physical therapist is often consulted regarding ambulation, body positioning, lifting, transferring, chair sitting, and self-care.

Infection Control

Personal hygiene and good hygienic practice on the part of the physical therapist cannot be overemphasized. Patients in the ICU are usually prone to infection. Meticulous hand washing with an antiseptic detergent between patients is essential. Soaping for 30 seconds or more with a thorough scrubbing motion and followed by thorough rinsing should be carried out. After contact with infected wounds, saliva, wounds, blood, pus, vomitus, urine, or stool, the physical therapist must be particularly conscientious about washing immediately. Given the concerns regarding HIV infection and AIDS, physical protection, including gowning, gloving, capping, and masking, should be routine.

Recognition of the Patient as a Person

Although constraints do exist in the high technology atmosphere of the ICU, the patient's dignity is observed as much as possible regardless of the reason

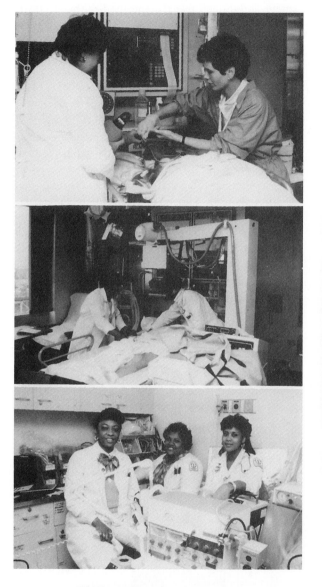

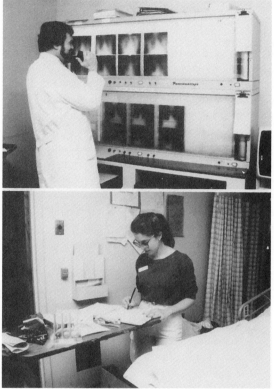

FIGURE 31-2

Team work in the intensive care unit is essential to facilitate communication and patient treatment. **A,** Physical therapist and nurse "bagging" and suctioning the patient. **B,** Two persons positioning for dependent, heavy patients prior to portable chest x-ray. **C,** Respiratory care practitioners. **D,** Radiologist. **E,** Nursing staff.

for admission, the level of consciousness, or belligerent and objectionable behavior directed toward the ICU staff. Gestures, such as using the patient's preferred name, explaining aspects of the patient's care, continually orienting the patient to person, place, time, and day, and having an interpreter available if necessary are widely practiced. A supportive caring atmosphere is created in which the patient is free to make choices and ask questions as much as possible.

ICU as a Healing Environment

The physical environment of the ICU has a profound effect on the patient's recovery independent of the level of care received. Windows with pleasant views, for example, help to orient the patient, and provide a sense of day and night and the passage of time (Figure 31-3). Other benefits include reduced number and types of complications and reduced length of stay in the ICU and in hospital overall. Physical therapists who are involved in the designing of ICUs should consider psychosocial, environmental, technological, and clinical factors.

THE DYING PATIENT

Anticipation of dying and death are traumatic for the patient, family and friends, and the health-care team. The phases of dying (Andreoli, Fowkes, Zipes, and Wallace, 1991; Warner, 1978) that can be anticipated when caring for the dying patient are presented in the box on p. 577.

Principles of physical therapy management

The dying patient and his or her family and friends have special needs that must be included in and in fact constitute an integral part of the patient's overall care. In general the physical comfort and personal hygiene of the patient, as well as the quality of the immediate psychosocial environment, are paramount concerns. Compassion, understanding, and respect for the patient and the family must be forthcoming from the ICU team. The ability to be attentive, comforting, and compassionate are invaluable personal qualities that need to be developed to a high degree in the critical care area. The team needs to attend to how the patient, if sufficiently alert, is dealing with the possibility of dying and take their

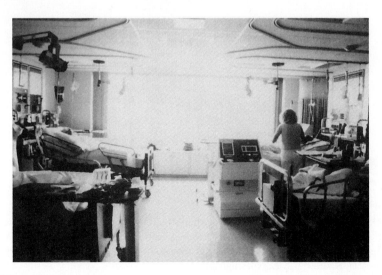

FIGURE 31-3

An overview of an ICU room. Note large window area and openness of room. Windows help patients orient to day and night.

Characteristics of the Dying Patient
Loss of strength, motion, and reflexes in the legs and then in the arms
Failure of the peripheral circulation and profuse sweating, causing body cooling
The dying patient tends to turn toward the light
Decreased sensitivity to touch and deep pressure and pain tends to remain
Often conscious until death
May experience pain, acute loneliness, and fear
May increase spiritual needs, particularly at night
an interval of quiescence just before death

From Andreoli KG, Fowkes VK, Zipes DP, Wallace AG: *Comprehensive cardiac care,* ed 7, St. Louis, 1991, Mosby.

cues from the patient with respect to the role they need to play. If requested by the patient or family, pastoral care services are summoned, preferably before death is imminent.

If life support systems are being continued, the physical therapist may provide treatment to keep the patient as comfortable as possible. Conservative prophylactic cardiopulmonary physical therapy may be provided to reduce the work of breathing. Treatments are kept to a minimum in terms of number and duration if death is inevitable. Range of motion exercises may help to reduce the discomfort of immobility and facilitate nursing management and the basic care of the patient. Analgesics may be continued along with other medications to reduce pain and suffering and maximize comfort. If so, these are prudently timed with treatments if appropriate. In the presence of life supports the patient's needs may have to be anticipated somewhat more than without life supports because they severely limit communication. The dignity and modesty of the patient continue to be observed even after death has occurred.

The patient who has had life supports removed receives the same level of palliative care as the patient with supports. Weakness and wasting may contribute to the fatigue induced by treatment and by coughing. Facilitated and supported coughing may help reduce the effort required to cough productively.

The use of human touch may be the single most important means of communicating with and providing support to the dying patient who may be unable or disinterested in communicating. Supportive touching and handholding may be even more important to the patient on life support systems where these may be experienced as a physical barrier between the patient and those around him or her.

SUMMARY

Cardiopulmonary physical therapy in the ICU is a specialty in itself. The overriding goals pertain to returning the patient to a premorbid level of function and in the process minimize morbidity, mortality, and length of hospital stay. The general goals of critical care are function optimization and prophylaxis. Specific primary goals are defined by the underlying cardiopulmonary pathophysiology and multisystem dysfunction and its sequelae. Specific secondary goals are defined by the presence of or the potential for musculoskeletal and neuromuscular dysfunction. This chapter elaborates on some general aspects of treating ICU patients. The knowledge base and experience of physical therapists working in the area are presented. A broad overview of the objectives of treatment and the rationale for prioritizing treatments according to a physiological hierarchy is described. General clinical and nonclinical aspects of patient management are discussed. Finally, issues related to the management of the dying patient are addressed.

REVIEW QUESTIONS

1. Describe the elements of evidence-based practice in cardiopulmonary physical therapy.
2. Describe the general goals and principles of cardiopulmonary physical therapy in the intensive care unit.
3. Describe the role of monitoring in cardiopulmonary physical therapy care of the critically-ill patient.

References

Andreoli, K.G., Fowkes, V.K., Zipes, D.P., & Wallace, A.G. (1991). *Comprehensive cardiac care.* (7th ed.). St Louis: Mosby.

Barlow, D.H., Hayes, S.C., & Nelson, R.O. (1984). *The scientist practitioner, research and accountability in clinical and education settings.* New York: Permagon Press.

Cutler, P. (1985). *Problem solving in clinical medicine, from data to diagnosis.* (2nd ed.). Baltimore: Williams & Wilkins.

Dean, E. (1983). Research. The right way. *Clinical Management, 3,* 29-33.

Dean, E. (1985). Psychobiological adaptation model for physical therapy practice. *Physical Therapy, 65,* 1061-1068.

Dean, E. (1994a). Oxygen transport: A physiologically-based conceptual framework for the practice of cardiopulmonary physiotherapy. *Physiotherapy, 80,* 347-355.

Dean, E. (1994b). Physiotherapy skills: Positioning and mobilization of the patient. In B.A. Webber & J.A. Pryor, (Eds.). *Physiotherapy for Respiratory and Cardiac Problems.* Edinburgh: Churchill Livingstone.

Dean, E. (1994c). Invited commentary to "Are incentive spirometry, intermittent positive pressure breathing, and deep breathing exercises effective in the prevention of postoperative pulmonary complications after upper abdominal surgery? A systematic overview and meta-analysis." *Physical Therapy, 74,* 10-15.

Dean, E., & Ross, J. (1992). Discordance between cardiopulmonary physiology and physical therapy. *Chest, 101,* 1694-1698.

Hislop, J.H. (1975). Tenth Mary McMillain lecture. The not-so-impossible dream. *Physical Therapy, 55,* 1069-1080.

Riegelman, R.K. (1991). *Minimizing medical mistakes. The art of medical decision making.* Boston: Little, Brown and Company.

Ross, J., & Dean, E. (1989). Integrating physiological principles into the comprehensive management of cardiopulmonary dysfunction. *Physical Therapy, 69,* 255-259.

Schon, D.A. (1983). *The reflective practitioner. How professionals think in action.* New York: Basic Books.

Stillwell, S. (1992). *Mosby's critical care nursing reference.* St Louis: Mosby.

Worthingham, C. (1960). The development of physical therapy as a profession through research and publication. *Physical Therapy, 40,* 573-577.

Zadai, C.C. (1986). Pathokinesiology: The clinical implications from a cardiopulmonary perspective. *Physical Therapy, 66,* 368-371.

Intensive Care Unit Management of Primary Cardiopulmonary Dysfunction

Elizabeth Dean

KEY TERMS

Cardiopulmonary failure
Coronary artery disease
Obstructive lung disease

Primary cardiopulmonary dysfunction
Restrictive lung disease
Status asthmaticus

INTRODUCTION

This chapter presents the principles of cardiopulmonary physical therapy in the management of critically ill patients with primary cardiopulmonary dysfunction that can lead to cardiopulmonary failure. The categories of conditions presented are obstructive lung disease, status asthmaticus, restrictive lung disease, and coronary artery disease (medical and surgical conditions). Each category of condition is presented in two parts. First, the related pathophysiology and pertinent aspects of the medical management of each condition are presented. Second, the principles of physical therapy management are discussed. These are not mutually exclusive for each category because considerable overlap may exist when conditions coexist.

It should be emphasized that these principles are not treatment prescriptions. Rather, each patient must be assessed and treated individually taking into consideration all factors that contribute to impaired oxygen transport (i.e., immobility, recumbency, extrinsic factors related to the patient's care, intrinsic factors related to the patient, and the underlying pathophysiology) (Chapter 1). For examples of treatment prescriptions for specific patients refer to the companion volume to this book entitled *Clinical case studies in cardiopulmonary physical therapy.*

CARDIOPULMONARY FAILURE
Pathophysiology

The heart and lungs work interdependently; thus failure of one organ has significant implications for the

TABLE 32-1

Classification of Respiratory Failure by Cause and Mechanisms

Origin	Drugs	Metabolic	Neoplasms	Infections	Trauma	Other
BRAIN	Narcotics Barbiturates Sedatives Poisons Anesthetics	Hyponatremia Hypocalcemia Hypercapnia Alkalosis Hyperglycemia Myxedema	Primary Metastatic	Meningitis Encephalitis Abscess Bulbar polio	Direct injury Increased pressure	Central alveolar hypoventilation Obstructive sleep apnea
NERVES AND MUSCLES	Curariform drugs Arsenic Aminoglycosides	Hypophosphatemia Hypomagnesemia	Primary Metastatic	Polio Tetanus	Direct injury	Motor neuron disease Myasthenia gravis Multiple sclerosis Muscular dystrophy Guillain-Barré syndrome
UPPER AIRWAY			Tonsillar adenoid hyperplasia Goiter Polyps Malignant tumors	Epiglottitis Laryngotracheitis	Vocal cord paralysis Tracheoma- lacia Cricoarytenoid arthritis Laryngeal edema	
CHEST BELLOWS					Flail chest Burn with keloids	Scleroderma Pleural inter- position (fibrosis, fluid, tumor, air) Spondylitis Scoliosis Kyphosis
CONTRIBUTING FACTORS						Massive obesity Ascites Ileus Pain Recumbency
LOWER AIRWAY AND PARENCHYMA			Malignant Benign	Viral (bronchiolitis, broncho- pneumonia) Bacterial (bronchitis, pneumonia, abscess, bronchiectasis) Fungal Mycoplasma	Contused lung	Bronchospasm Heart failure congestive restric- tive obstructive COPD Respiratory distress syndrome Interstitial lung disease Atelectasis Cystic fibrosis Pulmonary emboli

From Civettia JM, Taylor RW, Kirby RR: *Critical care,* Philadelphia, 1988, JB Lippincott.

function of the other organ (Vincent and Suter, 1987; Weber, Janicki, Shroff, and Likoff, 1983). Insufficiency or failure of the cardiopulmonary system refers to the inability of this system to maintain adequate oxygen and carbon dioxide homeostasis.

Pulmonary failure reflects a gas exchange defect or defect of the ventilatory pump. Table 32-1 shows the classification of pulmonary failure by specific causes and the mechanisms involved. Some common predisposing conditions include primary cardiopulmonary conditions, (e.g., chronic lung disease, overwhelming pneumonia, and myocardial infarction) and secondary cardiopulmonary conditions (e.g., motor neuron diseases, spinal cord injury, stroke, and muscular dystrophy) (Chapter 30). The oxygen and carbon dioxide tensions that have been used to define failure are variable because they depend on factors such as premorbid status, general health, age, prior blood gas profile, and the time frame for the development of failure. Arterial blood gases and pH are essential in the assessment of cardiopulmonary failure, which is usually diagnosed when the PaO_2 falls below 50 to 60 mm Hg and the $PaCO_2$ rises above 50 mm Hg (Shoemaker, Thompson, and Holbrook, 1984).

Primary cardiac failure reflects failure of the myocardium to pump blood to the pulmonary and systemic circulations and maintain adequate tissue perfusion (Austin and Greenfield, 1980). Significant dysfunction of the left ventricle can lead to pulmonary vascular congestion and cardiogenic pulmonary edema (i.e., congestive heart failure) (Matthay, 1985). Diseases of the heart that can lead to failure include significant myocardial damage as a result of infarction or myopathy, valvular heart disease, and congenital defects.

Both primary pulmonary and cardiac failure can be classified into acute and chronic stages. The compensation mechanisms that occur in the two stages are distinct. With adequate physiological compensation, patients can tolerate some degree of chronic failure. Patients with a mild degree of failure can live reasonably independent lives. Moderate failure is significantly more limiting, thus these patients may require home ventilatory support (e.g., supplemental oxygen and nighttime ventilation), and severe failure requires hospitalization and mechanical ventilatory support.

PATIENT WITH OBSTRUCTIVE LUNG DISEASE
Pathophysiology and medical management

Obstructive lung disease can result in ventilatory failure and admission of the patient to the intensive care unit (ICU), or this disease can complicate management if the patient is admitted for other reasons (Boggs and Wooldridge-King, 1993; Underhill, Woods, Froelicher, and Halpenny, 1989). If conservative management fails or is unlikely to improve critically impaired oxygen transport and gas exchange and to adequately remove copious and tenacious secretions, intubation and mechanical ventilation are indicated (Chapter 41). Complicating factors include impaired oxygen delivery, polycythemia, impaired respiratory mechanics secondary to lung damage and increased time constants impairing optimal inhalation and exhalation, flattened hemidiaphragms, rigid

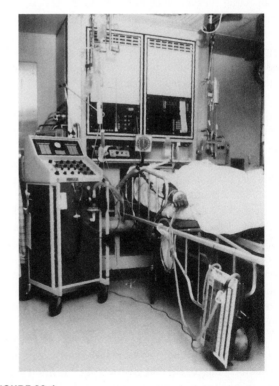

FIGURE 32-1
Patient receiving mechanical ventilation.

barrel-shaped chest wall, increased accessory muscle use and work of breathing, reduced diffusing capacity, impaired mucociliary transport, secretion accumulation, ineffective cough mechanism, increased oxygen consumption, increased work of the heart, and general debility and weakness.

The goal of intubation and mechanical ventilation is to provide an airway and adequate alveolar ventilation, which is based on arterial blood gas analysis. A tidal volume and a respiratory rate that provide satisfactory blood gas and pH values are established and maintained unless the clinical condition changes. The precise regulation of mechanical ventilation helps to restore adequate blood gases and cardiopulmonary function, reduce the work of breathing, rest fatigued ventilatory muscles, and provide an optimal fraction of inspired oxygen (FIo_2) and humidification (Figure 32-1) (Wilson, 1992).

Minute ventilation can be seriously impaired with a leak in the mechanical ventilator circuitry. The tube connecting sites are often the sites of air leakage. Complete disconnection at the endotracheal or tracheostomy connection may occur in those patients with high pulmonary resistance. Close monitoring of the exhaled tidal volume and end tidal carbon dioxide will ensure the patient is receiving sufficient ventilation.

Positive end expiratory pressure (PEEP) is useful in promoting greater opportunity for gas exchange at end-expiration in mechanically ventilated patients. However, venous return, myocardial perfusion, and cardiac output may be impaired during positive pressure ventilation with PEEP administration (Jardin, et al., 1981; Kumar, Pontoppian, Falke, Wilson, and Laver, 1973). Excessive stimulation to cough in these ventilated patients should be avoided because this accentuates the cardiovascular side effects of PEEP. Continuous positive airway pressure (CPAP) can maintain airway patency during spontaneous ventilation. This mode of ventilation, however, seems to be preferred in children, whereas PEEP is used more commonly in adults.

Interference with the gag reflex in the patient with an endotracheal tube increases the risk of aspiration of the oropharyngeal and gastric contents and can result in pneumonitis and pneumonia. Risk of aspiration from the oropharyngeal cavity can be reduced by suctioning through the airway with the cuff of the airway inflated, in addition to suctioning the oropharynx after suctioning via the airway.

Suctioning can be performed frequently in a patient with an artificial airway and is less traumatic. Patients should be suctioned only as indicated because this procedure can produce significant desaturation (up to 60%), particularly in the ventilated patient (Walsh, Vanderwarf, Hoscheit, and Fahey, 1989). Administration of 100% oxygen for 3 minutes before and after suctioning (i.e., hyperoxygenation) minimizes this desaturation effect. This can be accomplished by manually bagging the patient before treatment (i.e., manual hyperventilation) or by presetting the mechanical ventilator (Fell and Cheney, 1971). Risk of aspiration of gastric contents is reduced by the use of a nasogastric tube.

A common cause of acute respiratory failure is advanced chronic airflow limitation (Civetti, Taylor, and Kirby, 1988). The pathophysiological deficits include significant loss of alveolar tissue, increased compliance of alveolar tissue, hyperinflated chest wall, impaired respiratory mechanics, flattened hemidiaphragms, impaired breathing efficiency, and reduced diffusing capacity. Proportional changes in lung volumes and capacities in patients with chronic airway limitation compared with healthy persons are presented in Figure 8-5, p. 150. The primary abnormality is a significantly increased residual volume and inspiratory reserve volume and hence total lung capacity. Failure of oxygen transport ensues secondary to ventilation and perfusion mismatch, ventilatory muscle fatigue, reactive pulmonary hypertension, and right ventricular failure. Correcting the complications of respiratory failure, however, is often more problematic than treating the specific cause. Hypoxemia and hypercapnia are often present. Hypoxemia is usually improved with supplemental oxygen in the absence of significant diffusion defect or shunt.

Cardiovascular complications are among the most prevalent observed in ventilatory failure. Marked hypercapnia (increased arterial P_{CO_2}) with acidemia (reduced pH) can produce extreme vasodilatation and hypotension resulting from the local action on blood vessels (Boggs and Wooldridge-King, 1993). Mild hypercapnia can produce reflex vasoconstriction and hypertension. Occasionally systemic hypertension is observed during weaning from the ventilator with the presence of a moderate degree of hypercapnia.

Right heart failure, cor pulmonale, is a well-known complication of chronic lung disease and congestive heart failure. Both hypoxia and reduced pH cause pulmonary vasoconstriction and an increase in pulmonary artery pressure. Consequently, reversing bronchospasm, hypoxemia, hypercapnia, and acidemia can often reduce pulmonary vasoconstriction, lower pulmonary artery pressure, and thereby improve hemodynamics.

The end stage of respiratory failure results in a progressive increase in airway resistance, work of breathing, oxygen consumption, and carbon dioxide production. In areas of bronchial obstruction, marked alveolar hypoventilation results and ventilation and perfusion are severely mismatched. Hypoxemia and respiratory acidosis produce reactive pulmonary hypertension and further ventilatory failure. Profound carbon dioxide retention, refractory hypoxemia, and respiratory acidemia may terminate in a fatal dysrhythmia (Gibson, Pride, Davis, and Loh, 1977; Macklem and Roussos, 1977; Rochester and Arora, 1983; Vincent and Suter, 1987; Weinstein and Skillman, 1980; Weissman, Kemper, Elwyn, Askanazi, Hyman, and Kinney, 1989).

Acidemia from respiratory causes with a pH of less than 7.25 is often harmful with respect to dysrhythmia production. Conversely, hypoventilation is equally harmful, and pH elevations greater than 7.5 may cause neurological and cardiovascular complications. In acute respiratory failure with profound acidemia, intravenous use of bicarbonate is used to buffer the hydrogen ion concentration until the underlying disorder is corrected. Bicarbonate infusion is guided by frequent pH measurements.

Transport of oxygen and carbon dioxide to and from the tissues depends on adequate pulmonary and systemic circulation. Frequently, blood volume has to be restored by fluids or blood replacement or both. Inotropic agents are used to maintain adequate circulation by augmenting myocardial contractility.

Nutrition

Critically ill patients are hypermetabolical. Metabolical demand and oxygen consumption are increased secondary to healing and repair, increased temperature, altered thermoregulation and after surgery. Patients with chronic cardiopulmonary limitation are often undernourished because of the effort required to purchase food, prepare, and consume it. Furthermore, these patients have an increased oxygen consumption and energy expenditure secondary to the increased work of breathing (Petty, 1985; Rochester and Esau, 1984). Without adequate nutrition, patients incur the effects of deconditioning faster, are debilitated, are less capable of responding optimally to therapy, and are more susceptible to infection. Intravenous hyperalimentation, or external hyperalimentation, is typically instituted early to maintain optimal nutritional status and to avoid excessive physical wasting and deterioration. If a tracheostomy has been performed, the patient is able to eat normally.

Principles of physical therapy management

The principles of management of acute respiratory failure are based on interventions that will enhance oxygen transport (i.e., oxygen delivery, oxygen consumption, and oxygen extraction), and facilitate carbon dioxide removal (Gallagher and Civetta, 1980). Thus the steps of the oxygen transport pathway that have been identified as impaired or threatened by the patient's condition (i.e., immobility, recumbency, and extrinsic and intrinsic factors in addition to the underlying pathophysiology) (Chapter 1) are the focus of treatment. Based on a detailed analysis of these factors, treatments are selected, prioritized, and applied to optimize the steps in the pathway that are affected. These may include treatments to maximize the patency of the airways, increase alveolar ventilation, facilitate mucuciliary transport, facilitate airway clearance, optimize the mechanical position of the diaphragm, optimize ventilation and perfusion matching, optimize pH, eliminate carbon dioxide, optimize peripheral circulation and tissue perfusion, and reduce the work of breathing and of the heart. To optimize oxygen transport, the primary goals of physical therapy management include the following:

1. To improve or maintain arterial oxygen tension (Pa_{O_2}) or prevent its deterioration
2. To improve or maintain arterial oxygen saturation (Sa_{O_2}) or prevent its deterioration
3. To improve or maintain arterial carbon dioxide levels (Pa_{CO_2}) and pH or prevent its deterioration

The means by which these goals are fulfilled depends on each patient's clinical presentation and the specific factors that contribute to cardiopulmonary dysfunction.

Mobilization

Mobilization and ambulation are requisite for normal physiological functioning of the human body (i.e., to stimulate exercise stress and gravitational stress and thereby optimize oxygen transport) (Dean and Ross, 1992b). Although patients in the ICU are encouraged to move, exercise, sit up, stand, sit in chairs, take a few steps, and in some circumstances, ambulate across the unit even if they are ventilated (Mackenzie, Imle, and Ciesla, 1989), therapeutic mobilization is prescribed to exploit its (1) acute effects, (2) the long-term cumulative effects, and (3) the preventive effects (Chapter 17). These effects are physiologically distinct and need to be prescribed specifically to address each patient's problems. With the monitoring capability in the ICU, critically ill patients can move and be moved within safe therapeutic limits.

Given that cardiopulmonary physical therapy is among those activities that are the most metabolically demanding for ICU patients (Dean, Murphy, Parrent and Rousseau, 1995; Weissman and Kemper, 1993; Weissman, Kemper, Damask, Askanazi, Hyman, and Kinney, 1984), the patient's capacity to meet a given increase in oxygen demand must be determined before treatment. Even though cardiopulmonary physical therapy stresses the oxygen transport system as a means of improving the function and efficiency of this system, unnecessary or excessive energy expenditure is undesirable and thus should be minimized. Interventions that can minimize oxygen demand include relaxation, judicious body positioning to facilitate oxygen transport, coordination of treatments with other interventions, scheduling treatments at appropriate times, timing treatments with medications so the maximal effect is achieved, pain control, and coordinating treatments with peak energy periods and around rest periods.

Mobilization and exercise are at the top of the hierarchy of physiological treatments; thus the potent and direct effects of these interventions are exploited first (see Chapter 16). Being moved to (passive) or moving into (active) the upright position promotes improved cardiopulmonary function and gas exchange. Chairs should be available at the side of every ICU bed to provide greater opportunity for the patient to be upright. The benefits of the upright sitting position are different to sitting propped up in bed. Stretcher chairs are particularly useful in reducing the physical labor of lifting patients during transfers. These devices are designed to be positioned under the patient while recumbent in bed and then mechanically configured into a chair. One potential danger, however, is overreliance on these devices. Even minimal ability of the patient to assist with his or her bed mobility and transferring must be exploited, even if the maneuver takes several minutes and multiple assistants. These minimal efforts must be exploited. Without doing so, the patient's oxygen transport system deconditions further, which also reduces the patient's tolerance to be mobilized. What justifies this time and personnel cost is the greater therapeutic outcome that can be expected compared with passive interventions. The fundamental goal is enhanced recovery, reduced suffering, reduced morbidity and mortality, and reduced ICU and hospital stay.

Significant benefit can be gained from standing the ventilated patient, provided there are no absolute contraindications to being upright in terms of cardiopulmonary function, neuromuscular and musculoskeletal status, and skin integrity. Ambulating the ventilated patient is the priority whenever possible (Burns and Jones, 1975; Holton, 1972). The potential risks, however, must be recognized. Mobilization and exercise must be prescribed specifically to ensure that the exercise stimulus is therapeutic (i.e., provides an adequate stressor to the oxygen transport pathway, yet is not hazardous).

Standing and walking even a few steps can be extremely strenuous for the ICU patient with respect to oxygen demand, considering that this patient is hypermetabolical. Such activities need to be introduced gradually and with continuous monitoring to ensure the patient does not exceed the prescribed therapeutic intensity needed to maximize oxygen transport. Standing and walking are coordinated with other aspects of the patient's care and should be carried out in several stages. Monitoring of the ECG and arterial saturation of the critically ill patient performing activities such as standing or walking cannot be overemphasized. By disconnecting these monitors, the physical therapist is working blindly and potentially dangerously because the leads do not reach or because of movement artifact. In anticipation of an increased workload, ventilatory parameters for the ventilated patients may require adjusting. A greater concentration of oxygen should be delivered for at least 3 to 5 minutes before the activity and continued afterward for 10 minutes or so until the patient has recovered from the increased exertion and the heart rate and blood pressure have returned to within 5% to 10% of baseline values.

Active movement has greater therapeutic effect on oxygen transport than assisted or passive movements; thus the benefits of active movements are exploited first. Movement recruiting large muscle groups minimizes the disproportionate hemodynamic stress associated with movement of small muscle groups or movements requiring excessive dynamic stabilization (Hanson and Nagel, 1987). If active movements cannot be performed or excessively stress the oxygen transport system, then active assisted movements are indicated. Passive movements have a role primarily when the patient is paralyzed or so hemodynamically unstable that the patient deteriorates with active movement. With respect to cardiopulmonary benefits, passive movement stimulates changes in ventilatory and circulatory patterns (West, 1995). These can be particularly beneficial in patients who have significant mobility restriction, however, they should not substitute for active and active-assisted movements, which are associated with even greater benefit because they are higher order activities on the physiologically based treatment hierarchy (see Chapter 16).

Body positioning

Body positioning is a potent therapeutic intervention that promotes optimal oxygen transport and gas exchange in two ways; one, from the physiological benefits accrued from the specific positions themselves, and two, from the physiological benefits accrued from physically changing from one position to another (see Chapter 18). Body position can be used preferentially to augment alveolar volume, alveolar ventilation, ventilation and perfusion matching, respiratory mechanics, cough effectiveness, central and peripheral hemodynamics and fluid shifts, mucociliary transport, and secretion clearance (see Chapter 18). Both ventilation and perfusion are enhanced in the inferior lung fields. Thus in postural drainage positions the superior lung being treated is neither preferentially ventilated nor perfused. The less affected lung fields therefore may be contributing more substantially to improving arterial gases. Hence the physical therapist must consider the goals of treatment with respect to pulmonary function in both the involved and less-involved lung fields. During postural drainage, the length of time in a given position needs to be monitored to avoid drainage of secretions into the less involved, functional, inferior lung fields and to avoid the possibility of compression atelectasis in the inferior lung (Dean, 1985; Leblanc, Ruff, and Milic-Emili, 1970).

Although positions can be predicted that will optimize ventilation and perfusion matching, each patient will respond differently, depending on such factors as pathology, age, weight, depth of breathing, and mechanical ventilation (Clauss, Scalabrini, Ray, and Reed, 1968; Ray et al., 1974). Therefore the patient's response to specific positioning must be observed, documented, and objectively monitored with respect to the effect on oxygen transport variables.

Another important goal of body positioning is to potentiate position-dependent fluid shifts to optimize cardiovascular function. For this reason the patient should be positioned upright as often as possible. In addition, there are other beneficial effects of the upright position on pulmonary function (e.g., maximize lung volumes and capacities, minimize alveolar collapse, decrease airway resistance, increase lung compliance and, thereby, reduce ventilator system pressure). To maximize the effect of gravity on promoting fluid shifts, the legs should be positioned dependently at frequent intervals. In a patient who is not self-supporting with or without assistance, fluid shifts can be stimulated with a high Fowler's position coupled with the use of the bed knee-break. Between sessions of therapeutic body positioning, a schedule of four-point turning (supine, left side, prone, right side) is ideal and should be attempted even in the ventilated patient if not strictly contraindicated (Dean, 1994).

Extreme body positions have been reported to have beneficial effects on oxygen transport in patients with acute respiratory failure. The head-down position has been shown to reduce respiratory distress in some patients with obstructive lung disease (Barach and Beck, 1954). The abdominal viscera are displaced cephalad, thereby elevating the typically flattened hemidiaphragms and placing them in a mechanically advantageous position. This effect may be mimicked in other body positions by manual abdominal compression and abdominal binders. In some patients, however, the additional load imposed by the increased intraabdominal pressure on the underside of the diaphragm may inadvertently increase the work of breathing and increase respiratory distress. The prone position has been reported to be beneficial in patients with acute respiratory failure (Douglas, Rehder, Beynen, Sessler, and Marsh, 1977; Piehl and Brown, 1976). A variant of the prone position, semi-prone, may be more beneficial in some patients by reducing intraabdominal pressure. In addition, the semi-prone position may be safer and more comfortable for the mechanically ventilated patient. The prescription of any body positioning must be based on its anticipated benefits on oxygen transport. The more extreme positions should be introduced in progressive stages and the patient's response monitored to ensure the response is favorable.

Supplemental oxygen

Supplemental oxygen is usually administered continuously, whether the patient is ventilated or not, to maintain Pao_2 level within an optimal range (Dantzker, 1991). Oxygen concentrations can be increased before postural drainage and treatment to help compensate for any physical stress imposed by treatment. Oxygen, however, should always be increased to 100% and inspired for at least 3 minutes before and after suctioning. Should arterial desaturation be apparent during treatment, oxygen may need to be increased. If the patient is spontaneously breathing without oxygen, supplemental oxygen may also be indicated during treatment to avoid desaturation in some patients. Oxygen administration must be knowledgeably regulated by the ICU team based on arterial blood gas results. Severe hypoxemia is known to result in irreversible tissue damage within minutes, but hyperoxia can also produce harmful effects within hours. By maximizing alveolar ventilation, gas exchange, and ventilation and perfusion matching, supplemental oxygen can be optimally used and the effects of acidemia minimized.

Treatment for respiratory acidosis is aimed at increasing alveolar ventilation to improve the exchange of carbon dioxide and oxygen. Because the respiratory center is depressed by increased amounts of carbon dioxide (carbon dioxide narcosis), the lowered oxygen tension of the blood becomes the stimulus for respiration. If the patient inhales high concentrations of oxygen, the stimulation for respiration may be removed. For this reason, oxygen is never given to patients with carbon dioxide narcosis.

Low flow oxygen (1 to 3 L/min) is given to a patient with chronic pulmonary disease who maintains a chronically elevated arterial Pco_2 in the presence of arterial hypoxemia. If intermittent positive pressure breathing is indicated, compressed or room air is used instead of oxygen in this situation.

Severe hypoxemia usually suppresses cardiac output to some degree. Cardiac output may be further compromised immediately after a patient is placed on a mechanical ventilator because of impaired venous return by the elevated transpulmonary pressure (Jardin et al., 1981). An attempt is made to carefully balance ventilation with an optimal or adequate cardiac output by shortening inspiratory time and by minimizing transpulmonary pressures by using lower tidal volumes.

Bagging

A common practice in some ICUs is bagging. A self-inflating breathing bag is temporarily connected to the airway. The lungs are manually inflated for a few breaths. The purpose of bagging the patient is to provide some extra-large breaths during treatment, to maintain some degree of positive end-expiratory pressure, to assess lung compliance, and to facilitate the effect of instillation of a small volume of saline solution into the tracheobronchial tree to loosen secretions. Bagging must be performed cautiously. Aggressive bagging can produce bronchospasm. The use of bagging in conjunction with suctioning is controversial. Some clinicians prefer to bag the patient after suctioning to avoid the possibility of the positive pressure pushing the mucus distally. Others maintain that because of the adherent quality of the mucus to the walls of the airway and the dilatation of the airways in response to positive pressure, bagging does not propel the mucus distally. Rather, it is believed that bagging before suctioning promotes air entry distal to the mucous plugs and movement of plugs centrally on expiration.

Certain body positions present a particular problem when a pressure-cycled ventilator is being used. The efficiency of the ventilator is greatly reduced when the patient's head is positioned below the hips because of an increase in total pulmonary resistance caused by the pressure of the abdominal contents. Therefore the use of a self-inflating breathing bag may be required to maintain pressure when changing from one position to another and during some postural drainage positions. Adequate tidal volume can be maintained by an assistant while the physical therapist aids the patient with bronchial drainage. With the use of the self-inflating bag, the physical therapist needs to ensure the patient is adequately ventilated and takes a larger than tidal breath every minute or so. As soon as possible, spontaneous breathing is encouraged in conjunction with postural drainage. The small airways dilate slightly on inspiration and cause mucus to peel away from the walls; thus, during expiration, mucous plugs are moved toward the trachea. The degree to which chest wall percussion, shaking, and vibration facilitate this movement is equivocal in the literature (Kirilloff, Ownes, Rogers, and Mazzocco, 1985; Dean and Ross, 1992a). Thus these less substantiated, less physiological conventional procedures (i.e., manual techniques) should be considered carefully and only after other more supported and physiological treatments have been exploited. Furthermore, because of their documented adverse effects, it is essential that the patient be continuously monitored for safety reasons and to establish a favorable treatment outcome. For the unconscious or paralyzed patient, the ventilator or self-inflating bag can be used to increase inflation volumes. Research is needed to examine the role of bagging and the effect of this technique on mucous removal.

Instillation

Instillation is another procedure that should be used selectively in patients. A mucolytic effect of saline has not been well established. Beneficial effects, however, may be more apparent in neonates.

Mucociliary transport and secretion clearance

The patient in respiratory failure needs special attention to fluid balance to carefully regulate hydration and fluid volume. Inhaled humidified air is a significant additional source of body fluid. Normally the alveolar gas is saturated with water vapor. The lining of the tracheobronchial tree is therefore protected from erosion and potential infection. This is particularly important in the patient requiring frequent suctioning. The effect of humidification can be assessed by the consistency of the patient's secretions. Thick secretions suggest humidification may be inadequate, and the patient may be systemically dehydrated.

If the effects of mobilization on mucociliary transport and secretion accumulation have been exploited and further secretion clearance is warranted, postural drainage may be indicated. Postural drainage may be contraindicated in patients with unstable vital signs and is usually contraindicated immediately after feedings and meals. In some institutions, however, patients on continuous 24-hour tube feedings are tipped after feeding has been discontinued for 15 minutes. The cuff in the artificial airway is inflated to avoid aspiration. A sequence including percussion, shaking, and vibration may be indicated in conjunction with postural drainage. Manual techniques have been associated with desaturation, atelectasis, musculoskeletal trauma, discomfort, cardiac dysrhythmias, and arrest (Kirilloff, et al., 1985); therefore these techniques must be applied rationally and with attention to all monitoring systems and changes in signs and symptoms. The precise sequence, the duration, intensity, and frequency of treatment is based on treatment outcome rather than time. The application of manual techniques in the head-down position is contraindicated in patients with acute myocardial infarction and increased intracranial pressure. Relative contraindications include hemorrhage, bronchopulmonary fistula, acute chest trauma, lung abscess, and gastric reflux (Boggs and Wooldridge-King, 1993).

The specific postural drainage positions to be used are determined based on the pathology, x-ray, and clinical examination. The recommended positions for the bronchopulmonary segments involved should be approximated as closely as possible (Chapter 19) and only modified if there are clear indications to do so. Frequently, specific positioning in the ICU is compromised as a result of the patient's status, intolerance to lying flat or being tipped, or limitations imposed by the monitoring apparatus or ventilator.

Breathing and coughing maneuvers

If the patient is nonventilated or recently extubated, body positioning and breathing and coughing maneuvers are emphasized to promote mucociliary transport and secretion clearance (Bennett, Foster, and Chapman, 1990), decrease minute ventilation and respiratory rate, increase tidal volume, and improve arterial blood gases (Barach, 1974; Casciari, Fairshter, Harrison, Morrison, Blackburn, and Wilson, 1981). Breathing exercises are believed to be most effective if pursed-lips breathing is performed in conjunction with mechanical pressure applied over the abdomen (Irwin and Tecklin, 1985; Mueller, Petty, and Filley, 1970). To derive the maximal benefits, breathing and coughing maneuvers should be performed in body positions that are most mechanically and physiologically optimal. In addition, they are performed in the postural drainage positions to augment mucociliary

clearance. Patients should not breathe below the end of normal tidal ventilation to avoid airway closure.

Weaning from the mechanical ventilator

The physical therapist and the respiratory therapist are primarily responsible for weaning the patient off mechanical ventilation. Thus coordinating their goals and working together to ensure the weaning process is carried out expediently and with the least risk of weaning complications (e.g., postextubation atelectasis, aspiration and hypoxemia) is a priority (Marini, 1984; Shoemaker et al., 1984). Blood gas analysis and pulmonary function provide the indications for weaning. Ideally, the patient's spontaneous tidal volume should approximate that delivered by the ventilator. Forced vital capacity should be two to three times the patient's required tidal volume (Figure 32-2). Weaning is not usually indicated if the patient requires PEEP greater than 5 cm H_2O or FIo_2 greater than 0.4. In addition, patients who are unable to generate a negative inspiratory pressure of –20 mm Hg or greater are unlikely to be able to generate sufficient intrathoracic pressures for deep breathing and airway clearance and thus are poor candidates for weaning. Minute ventilation and maximum voluntary ventilation can be measured at bedside and contribute to the decision whether to wean. Although weaning protocols differ depending on the patient and the ven-

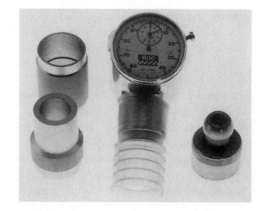

FIGURE 32-2

Spirometer for bedside measurement of TV, VC, and minute volume.

tilatory mode used, general guidelines for this common ICU procedure are outlined in the box below.

PATIENT WITH STATUS ASTHMATICUS
Pathophysiology and medical management

Status asthmaticus is a potentially life-threatening situation (Petty, 1982; Gaskell and Webber, 1988). The pathophysiological features include marked airway resistance secondary to bronchospasm, edema, and mucous secretion and retention. The work of breathing is markedly increased, resulting in respiratory distress. A cycle results in which the patient becomes more hypoxemic and hypercapnic secondary to alveolar hypoventilation, bronchospasm increases, and reactive pulmonary hypertension may ensue along with a further increase in the work of breathing and anxiety.

The classical signs and symptoms of a severe asthmatic attack that may progress to status asthmaticus include tachypnea, dyspnea, labored breathing, audible wheezing, tachycardia, cyanosis, anxiety, and panic. If the patient is able to cooperate with spirometric testing, the degree of reduced vital capacity, peak flow, and forced expiratory volume provide indices of the severity of airway obstruction (Brunner and Wolff, 1988).

Medical management is aimed at administering drugs and fluids to reduce hypoxemia with oxygen, decrease airway inflammation and resistance, and hence reduce the work of breathing and anxiety. Intravenous sodium bicarbonate helps to reverse respiratory acidosis and possibly metabolic acidosis (Civetta, et al., 1988).

Principles of physical therapy management

The prime objective of physical therapy is to optimize oxygen transport and possibly avoid or delay the need for mechanical ventilation. If ventilation becomes

---

General Steps in Weaning a Patient From the Mechanical Ventilator

1. An individualized weaning schedule is designed for each patient in which periods of time are spent off the ventilator and on a T tube that delivers appropriate oxygen and humidity

2. The initial time period off the ventilator is carefully selected; mornings are often good times

3. (a) Physical activity should be at a minimum during this period (e.g., not during or after physical therapy, not after meals, tests, or procedures, and not during family visits) (b) Supplemental oxygen and humidity are given

4. The physical therapist offers support and reassurance

5. Vital signs, and signs and symptoms of respiratory distress are monitored continuously during weaning

6. The patient is not left unattended in the initial weaning sessions until periods off the ventilator are reliably tolerated well for several successive minutes

7. (a) Deterioration of vital signs, blood gases, and evidence of distress indicate that the patient will have to return to ventilatory assistance imminently (b) Rest periods of at least an hour are strategically interspersed in the weaning schedule

8. Blood gases are performed at regular intervals (e.g., 15, 30, 60, 90, and 120 minutes or more or less frequently as indicated)

9. If blood gases stabilize within acceptable limits during the weaning period and the patient is generally tolerating the procedure well, the time off the ventilator is increased

10. Patients with underlying cardiopulmonary disease who are older, malnourished, obese, or smoke can be expected to take longer to be completely weaned from the ventilator

11. Weaning is generally faster in patients who have required a shorter period of mechanical ventilation

12. To hasten the weaning process, intermittent mandatory ventilation (IMV) has been reported to be useful in some patients. Others, however, have observed that the use of IMV tends to fatigue the patient and delay the patient's progress in weaning. Thus IMV must be used cautiously, and individual variability must be considered in terms of its effectiveness.

necessary, prognosis for recovery is poorer (Petty, 1982). Physical therapy can augment the medical management of the patient with status asthmaticus. In an attempt to avert intubation and mechanical ventilation the physical therapist coordinates treatment with the patient's medications (i.e., bronchodilators, muscle relaxants, steroids, and supplemental oxygen). The physical therapist promotes breathing control, enhances ventilation and perfusion matching, promotes mucociliary transport and secretion clearance, reduces hypoxemia, and teaches the patient to coordinate relaxed breathing with general body movement. Caution needs to be observed to avoid stimuli that potentiate bronchospasm and deterioration of the patient's condition (e.g., body positions that increase respiratory distress rather than relieve it, chest wall percussion, forced expiration maneuvers, aggressive bagging and possibly instillation). Attention to relaxation and reduction of excessive oxygen demands is a priority as was described for the patient with chronic airflow limitation. Certain body positions may have to be avoided, for example, because of the patient's intolerance and exacerbation of symptoms in those positions. Because of the relationship of altered pulmonary function in different positions, positioning (especially in patients in respiratory distress) must be applied cautiously within the patient's tolerance. Those body positions that reduce respiratory distress and the work of breathing and maximize alveolar ventilation, oxygen saturation and blood gases, are the positions of choice.

Major problems in status asthmaticus are alveolar hypoventilation, airway obstruction secondary to bronchospasm, mucosal edema, and secretions. Thus maximizing alveolar ventilation and facilitating mucociliary transport are priorities (Bates, 1989). Other problems include significantly increased work of breathing because of an inefficient breathing pattern and an ineffective cough. The physical therapist coordinates treatment with the patient's medications to facilitate relaxation, mucociliary transport, and clearance of secretions with breathing control and modified chest wall percussion, vibration, and huffing or gentle coughing. Obtaining a productive cough without augmenting bronchospasm is a challenge. Deep breathing with pursed-lips expiration helps to prolong expiration and to maintain the patency of the small airways. Deep, slow, and relaxed breathing is emphasized along with periodic effective, controlled huffing and avoidance of forced expiratory maneuvers (Hietpas, Roth, and Jensen, 1979; Nunn, Coleman, Sachithanandan, Bergman, and Laws, 1965).

Despite aggressive noninvasive management, blood gases may deteriorate and mechanical ventilation may be inevitable. Relaxation, maximizing alveolar ventilation, and reducing airway collapse and obstruction continue to be the primary goals; however, means of achieving these goals differ when the patient is mechanically ventilated. Optimal prescriptive body positioning is the intervention of choice. Secretion clearance is achieved by judicious suctioning. Suctioning is performed as required because it can contribute to reduced oxygenation, airway collapse, and atelectasis, increased arousal, increased work of breathing, and generally increased respiratory distress.

PATIENT WITH RESTRICTIVE LUNG DISEASE
Pathophysiology and medical management

Acute respiratory failure can be associated with primary restrictive lung disease (i.e., interstitial pulmonary fibrosis). This is distinct from restrictive defects secondary to neuromuscular and musculoskeletal diseases (e.g., Guillain-Barré syndrome, myasthenia gravis, and neuromuscular poisonings are common neuromuscular disorders that can precipitate respiratory failure in the absence of underlying primary lung disease) (Chapter 33). If paralyzed, the patient will likely be dependent on ventilatory assistance.

Restrictive lung dysfunction may complicate the management of patients admitted to the ICU for reasons other than cardiopulmonary disease. The lung parenchyma, the chest wall, or both may be involved. The underlying cause of respiratory failure may therefore reflect ventilatory pump failure, gas exchange failure, or both. The specific restrictions to cardiopulmonary function need to be identified and treated individually to optimize treatment. Obstructive and restrictive patterns of cardiopulmonary frequently coexist; thus the contribution of both types of defects to a patient's oxygen transport should be determined. Typically, in restrictive lung disease, all lung volumes and capacities are reduced, although tidal volume can be relatively normal (see Figure 8-5, p. 150). Patients with severe interstitial pulmonary fibrosis have increased pulmonary artery pressures with an associated increase in right ventricular work (Chung and Dean, 1989). These patients desaturate very readily.

Principles of physical therapy management

Restrictive ventilatory dysfunction is commonly associated with both medical and surgical conditions. The principles of management of acute respiratory failure associated with these differ in that medical conditions are associated with underlying irreversible lung damage, whereas in the surgical patient the pulmonary restriction is reversible. The natural course of disease in the medical patient will be determined in part by the patient's premorbid status. The majority of surgical patients, however, will have had normal lung function before surgery and the development of cardiopulmonary complications (see Chapter 34). Regardless of whether mechanical ventilation is indicated, tissue oxygenation, carbon dioxide removal, regulation of blood pH, and an effective cardiac output are priorities. Supplemental oxygen is often effective in improving tissue oxygenation in conditions associated with restrictive lung disease in the absence of a right to left shunt. In the presence of shunt, supplemental oxygen does not reverse hypoxemia.

A judicious turning regimen can also be designed to optimize cardiopulmonary function, (even if the patient is mechanically ventilated), reduce risks of cardiopulmonary complications, reduce musculoskeletal deformities and skin breakdown, and promote comfort. It is essential with body positioning for any purpose that the patient is not confined unnecessarily and does not assume any position for too long. Although lines, leads, monitoring devices, and catheters may be required, these are anchored as securely as possible with sufficient length to allow the patient to move spontaneously, be mobilized as much as possible, undergo as many positioning changes as possible, and facilitate routine patient care.

Mobilization and general body movement, particularly in upright positions, is always a priority in the ICU, as much and as often as possible, given the patient's condition and safety considerations. Movements may be totally assisted but more often are likely to be active-assisted and active. No matter how weak the patient may be, active-assisted and active movements are the mainstay of the movement interventions performed by the physical therapist, particularly if these can be performed in near-upright positions. Assisted or passive movements should not be performed unless specifically indicated (i.e., the patient is unable to execute these movements completely alone). Even modest attempts at active-assisted movements, with perhaps only a minimal number of repetitions, benefit the patient considerably more both in terms of treatment goals related to cardiopulmonary and musculoskeletal function than assisted movements that do not contribute to muscle strength, endurance, and coordination. Injudicious application of totally assisted movements will contribute to the patient's deconditioning and physical deterioration. Regardless of the type of mobilization, the patient is observed closely for arterial desaturation, discomfort, respiratory distress, cyanosis, fatigue, and extent of cooperation if assisted-active and active movements are being performed.

Assisted movements are indicated to promote oxygen transport via their effects on ventilatory and circulatory patterns (West, 1995). Additionally, the goal is to maintain joint range of motion and prevent adaptive shortening of periarticular soft tissue in particular. Care must therefore be taken to perform these movements through the complete range of movement for each joint, with special attention to rotatory components of joint movement. Lax joints can maintain range with one complete range of motion daily. Lax joints are unprotected and vulnerable to excessive strain. Protection may best be effected in these joints by moving the joint more slowly through the extremes of joint range and just short of complete range. In the presence of spasticity or limb splinting because of discomfort the involved joints will benefit from two or more excursions through full range daily.

One approach that may be particularly beneficial in altering the distribution of ventilation and blood flow is general body and range of motion exercises, particularly of the upper limbs. If the patient is able to assist, however, greater cardiopulmonary stress occurs with upper limb exercise; thus heart rate, ECG, and blood pressure need monitoring. Lower-extremity movements, such as hip and knee flexion, may help to position the diaphragm for improved excursion. Lower-extremity movements will also increase venous return, which may or may not be desirable, depending on the patient. The goals of upper- or lower-extremity work must therefore be clearly defined. Possible benefits and untoward effects must be identified to ensure the patient benefits optimally from the prescribed exercise.

The treatment of choice in all patients is to stimulate those conditions that maintain optimal oxygen transport in health or approximate those conditions as closely as possible. That is, the most physiological interventions are exploited first and the least physiological interventions are exploited last or when more physiological interventions are not possible. Physiological interventions such as mobilization may be contraindicated in patients whose oxygen delivery is too low. Without some reserve capacity in oxygen transport, the patient cannot sustain the additional metabolic load that mobilization imposes. Patients who are this critical are often put on neuromuscular blocking agents to reduce muscle tone and thereby reduce oxygen demand. Because these patients are in induced paralytic states, mobilization is not possible.

Optimizing oxygen transport using body positioning and then nonphysiological interventions may then need to be considered. Furthermore, extreme caution needs to be observed in positioning these patients and moving their limbs because they are at risk of subluxations, pressure sores, bruising, and strains.

Interventions to promote mucociliary transport and secretion clearance are applicable to all situations in which secretions, mucosal edema, bronchospasm, or a combination of these factors occur. If postural drainage is indicated to further facilitate mucociliary transport and secretion clearance, caution needs to be exercised to avoid inducing bronchospasm and hypoxemia; thus the use of percussion should be considered carefully.

PATIENT WITH RESTRICTIVE LUNG DISEASE
Pathophysiology and medical management

The initial priority of management in the acute phase of myocardial infarction (MI) is the correction of the immediate problems including dysrhythmias, myocardial insufficiency, reduced cardiac output, hypoxemia, chest pain, and anxiety followed by implementation of a progressive rehabilitation program ranging from the acute medically stable phase to post discharge rehabilitation phase (Andreoli, Fowkes, Zipes, and Wallace, 1991; Froelicher, 1987; Irwin

---

Means of Reducing Myocardial Work Load in Patients With Cardiopulmonary Disease

1. A quiet environment without excessive noise and stimulation.

2. Low-intensity activity until medical stability has been maintained and patient shows signs of physical improvement.

3. Progressive mobilization begun in conjunction with patient's medical status, ECG stability, and unchanging or resolving enzyme levels.

4. Reduce patient's anxiety about his or her condition, self-care activities, and family and work responsibilities.

5. Gentle mobilization exercises, deep breathing, and coughing are usually begun immediately as a prophylactic measure, although crepitations are frequently audible in the bases of the lungs of coronary patients; treatments need to minimize pulmonary congestion and cardiac stress.

6. Relaxation is often promoted with low-intensity activity. All levels of activity, including breathing exercises, are performed in a coordinated, rhythmic manner. Breath holding, Valsalva maneuvers, and isometric muscle contractions, (i.e., isometric exercise and exercise involving significant muscle or postural stabilization) are absolutely contraindicated during all activities in patients with coronary artery disease and should not be performed in any stage of a rehabilitation program.

and Tecklin, 1985). Before admission to the coronary care unit, continuous monitoring of the heart rate and rhythm is established. An intravenous line is routinely started for the administration of medications and fluids. An arterial line may be started for serial blood sampling for blood gases and enzyme measures. Initially, pain medications, coronary vasodilators, and diuretics are frequently used to minimize the work of the heart, anginal pain, and discomfort. Drugs such as morphine serve to depress the respiratory drive; thus the physical therapist must be aware of corresponding changes in vital signs. Less potent sedatives and tranquilizers are more routinely prescribed. Increased pain and anxiety potentially worsen the patient's cardiac status by increasing myocardial oxygen demand and altering normal breathing pattern and gas exchange.

The primary purpose of oxygen administration to the cardiac patient is to reduce hypoxemia, myocardial work, and angina. Dyspnea, however, is commonly observed in the initial phases of myocardial infarction and can be effectively controlled by supplemental oxygen administered by nasal cannulae or mask. Oxygen may also correct potential ventilation-perfusion mismatching and hypoxemia. Oxygen is always administered with humidity to avoid drying the airways.

Blood gas analysis is performed within an hour of initiating oxygen therapy to establish a baseline of arterial saturation. In this way, oxygen dose can be altered to regulate blood gases and acid base balance.

MEDICAL CARDIAC PATIENT
Principles of physical therapy management

A primary principle of the management of the patient after myocardial infarction is to reduce myocardial oxygen demand and workload. The myocardium needs rest to promote optimal healing. Judicious rest of the myocardium is a priority that can often be balanced with gentle rhythmic, nonstatic movements. The box on p. 592 illustrates several ways of reducing myocardial workload in patients with cardiopulmonary disease.

The physical therapist should be watchful at all times for signs of impending or silent infarction, including generalized or localized pain anywhere over the thorax, upper limbs, and neck, palpitations, dyspnea, lightheadedness, syncope, sensation of indigestion, hiccups, and nausea.

Depending on the degree of myocardial infarction and damage, varying lengths of modified mobility may be recommended (Andreoli, Fowkes, Zipes, and Wallace, 1991). During this period, the physical therapist concentrates on rhythmic breathing exercises, gentle coughing exercises or huffing, modified positioning with the bedhead elevated at least 15 degrees to facilitate the gravity-dependent mechanical action of the heart and thereby reduce myocardial oxygen demand. The patient is encouraged to perform deep breathing and coughing every hour during the day. Bed exercises including rhythmic, unresisted, hip and knee and foot and ankle exercises are usually performed every 4 hours or so, or when the patient turns in bed. The patient is cautioned to exercise one leg at a time, sliding one heel up and down the bed, guarding against lifting the leg off the bed. These exercises; when performed correctly and coordinated with inspiration and expiration require relatively little effort or additional physical stress to the MI patient. Comparable with the management of the postoperative patient, these exercises are performed prophylactically to reduce the risk of venous stasis and formation of thromboemboli. In addition, they may help to regulate more coordinated breathing, encourage deep breaths and mucociliary transport, and reduce atelectasis. The patient is cautioned against performing the Valsalva maneuver and straining because these activities increase intrathoracic pressure and reduce cardiac output.

Electrocardiographic (ECG) monitoring of the cardiac patient is the responsibility of all members of the health-care team involved in the patient's care. The physical therapist has a special responsibility to be proficient in ECG interpretation in the coronary care unit because physical therapy is one of the most metabolically demanding interventions for patients (Dean et al., 1995; Weissman et al., 1984). The physical therapist often has the responsibility of initiating new activities with the cardiac patient, which might include sitting over the edge of the bed, engaging in self-care (particularly involving the arms being maintained in a raised position), getting in and out of bed, sitting in a chair, going to the bathroom, walking around the room or in the hallways, and eventually exercising on the treadmill or ergometer. Changes in the ECG must be watched for, particularly when introducing new activities and increasing the intensity of workload in activities. Careful attention to ECG changes and serum enzyme levels will contribute to enhanced physical therapy care of the acute MI patient by optimizing the treatments prescribed and the margin of safety with which activities are performed.

Congestive heart failure may be unavoidable in cases of severe infarction or even milder infarction coupled with lung disease. Fluid intake and output and daily weight measurements promote early detection of congestive heart failure. Routine fluid intake by an intravenous line should not exceed 20 to 30 ml per hour. Signs of imminent and established congestive heart failure appear in the box below. The work of the heart can be significantly reduced in the upright position (Levine and Lown, 1952).

All cardiac patients are prone to anxiety about their conditions and prognoses. The patient is given realistic guidelines at each stage of recovery with respect to the level of activity that can be safely performed, which can potentially avert deterioration and promote recovery. Involving the patient in rehabilitation planning from the onset facilitates the patient's planning realistically for the future and may help to reduce the depression often experienced by the acute MI patient.

The initial rehabilitation program is planned with the long-range rehabilitation goals in mind. The program designed for the cardiac patient is progressive in terms of types of activities, usually beginning with activities of daily living and with respect to the intensity,

duration, and frequency of these activities (Bjore, 1972; Froelicher, 1987). The patient's tolerance and changes in ECG and vital signs are used as indicators for establishing and modifying the treatment program. These physiological parameters must be observed carefully as the patient progresses to optimize the potential benefits of the therapeutic regimens as early as possible without endangering the patient.

Patient education and prevention of infarction are particularly important for the cardiac patient. As soon as the patient is alert and able to cooperate, information about his or her condition with guidelines about activity, diet, and stress management is reinforced. The more involved and informed the patient

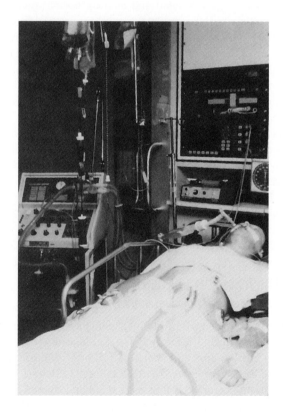

FIGURE 32-3
Patient following open heart surgery (4 hours postoperative). NOTE: patient on mechanical ventilator, mediastinal drains, receiving blood, IV's, on EKG, CVP, Swan Ganz, Arterial Blood Gas lines.

Signs of Imminent Congestive Heart Failure

Development of tachydysrhythmias

Development of a ventricular gallop

Pulmonary crackles and other persistent adventitiae

Development of dyspnea

Development of increased jugular venous pressure and distention

Guidelines to Stages of Physical Therapy in the Open Heart Surgical Patient

Stage 1

Patient may be seen in the postanesthesia and recovery room for a physical therapy assessment; the patient is usually extubated within 24 hours after surgery. Although the patient must be permitted to rest as much as possible in the initial 24-hour period, judicious body positioning is instituted to stimulate physiologic "stir-up." Usually once extubated, the patient is positioned side to side for deep breathing and coughing at least four times in the first 24 hours and low-intensity mobilization is initiated. Medications are administered before treatment to ensure optimal effect during treatment. Depending on the findings of x-ray, physical examination, and arterial blood gases, the patient may require vibrations and possibly percussion. Postural drainage positions are modified to avoid tipping the patient head-down and causing increased myocardial strain. A sputum sample for culture and sensitivity testing may be taken at this time. The patient can usually tolerate being dangled over the edge of the bed for a few minutes. Special care is taken for all heart patients to avoid the Valsalva maneuver, forced coughing, and huffing, and to maintain a semirecumbent or upright position for treatment. Blood pressure is checked before, during, and after treatment. Mobilization is progressed.

Stage 2

Deep breathing and coughing maneuvers coupled with mobilization are continued. Positioning for enhanced alveolar ventilation and ventilation and perfusion matching may be indicated. If secretion accumulation is a problem and the patient too unstable to be optimally mobilized or positioned, postural drainage and possibly percussion and/or vibration may be indicated. Upper limb and neck exercises are introduced. Neck exercises are withheld if central venous pressure lines are still in place in the neck veins. The patient can sit in a chair at bedside as tolerated. The patient is encouraged to stand erect for a minute or so on transferring back and forth to the chair.

Stage 3

The patient can take short walks as tolerated. Ambulation is not begun until arterial lines and the Swan-Ganz catheter have been capped or removed. Vital signs are monitored before and after standing and walking. Deep breathing and coughing maneuvers are continued even if the chest is clear, until the patient is up and about within reasonable limits as tolerated. The patient is encouraged in grooming and self-care.

Stage 4

Deep breathing and coughing should be done by the patient without supervision. The presence of atelectasis on x-ray or from assessment findings, however, would indicate the need for continuation of mobilization and body positioning with breathing exercises. Ambulation is increased as tolerated.

Stage 5

Patient can participate in individual or class activities, concentrating on trunk mobility, upper-extremity range of motion, coordinated breathing activities, posture, biomechanics, and increasing the patient's endurance gradually.

Stage 6

The patient can attempt six to eight stairs if progress has been satisfactory and as indicated. Aortic repairs in the first week or so are prone to rupture. Elevation of the blood pressure is therefore avoided to reduce the risk of breakdown of the aortic suture line.

Stage 7

The patient depends primarily on ambulation for maintaining optimal alveolar ventilation and mucociliary transport rather than breathing and coughing exercises. The patient is cautioned to balance a period of exertion with a period of rest. The patient may be discharged. The physical therapist ensures the patient fully understands the specific details of the home-exercise program. The emphasis of exercise for cardiac patients continues to be on rhythmic, coordinated dynamic movements on discharge, avoiding isometric, static exercise. If possible, the patient is invited to participate in a reconditioning and health promotion program as an outpatient in a physical therapy department.

NOTE: The physical therapist must guard against excessively intense treatment of open heart surgical patients or other patients who are on a prophylactic course of anticoagulants.

is in self-management, the greater the likelihood of receptivity and adherence to a rehabilitation regimen after discharge.

PATIENT AFTER OPEN HEART SURGERY
Principles of physical therapy management

Patients scheduled for open heart surgery are treated as high-risk surgical candidates because of the nature and invasiveness of this type of surgery (Figure 32-3), regardless of their general level of health before surgery (Trekova, Dementyeva, Dzemeshkevich, and Asmangulyan, 1994). Whenever possible, patients prepare for surgery in advance by decreasing or stopping smoking, by avoiding exposure to respiratory tract infections, by avoiding stress, by eating a balanced diet, and by getting adequate sleep. In addition, patients can benefit from a modified, prescriptive exercise program before surgery to maximize their aerobic capacity and thereby improve their perioperative course.

In the preoperative period the physical therapist may spend additional time with patients scheduled for open heart surgery to provide teaching of the basic anatomy and physiology related to surgery to be performed, the effect of anesthesia, the role of intubation and mechanical ventilation, the incision lines to be expected over the chest and the legs if veins are to be removed for bypass surgery, the lines, leads, chest tubes, and catheters that will be in place after surgery, and the course of recovery the patient might expect barring complications (Chapter 26). The emphasis on patient education in most open heart surgery units may contribute to the generally low incidence of complications and mortality.

Some guidelines for physical therapy management of the open heart surgical patient appear in the box on p. 595. These guidelines are to be applied thoughtfully and cautiously with regard to each specific patient's condition and observed recovery. These guidelines suggest the upper limit of intensity of physical therapy if all is progressing well initially and should be reduced if warranted by the patient's condition. Progression from one stage to the next is based on an optimal and reliable treatment response at each level before proceeding. Different institutions may advocate different practices, depending on their facilities, experience of the surgical and ICU team, and the incidence of postoperative complications and survival for that institution.

The physical therapist must guard against excessively intense treatment of open heart surgical patients or other patients for whom periods of relatively restricted mobility (4 to 5 days) are anticipated. In addition to the fact these patients may be hemodynamically unstable initially, these patients may be susceptible to soft tissue bruising from being on a prophylactic course of anticoagulants.

Physical therapy follow-up should continue several months beyond discharge at which point the patient should be well integrated into a cardiac rehabilitation program. Continuity and continuation of physical therapy throughout the entire rehabilitation period, from acute- to long-term, cannot be overemphasized given that achieving a maximal recovery from surgery is the priority.

SUMMARY

This chapter describes the principles of cardiopulmonary physical therapy in the management of critically ill patients with primary cardiopulmonary dysfunction. Cardiopulmonary failure secondary to chronic lung disease and heart disease are described. Cardiopulmonary physical therapy management is based on the specific underlying pathophysiological mechanisms of these various disorders. These principles, however, cannot be interpreted to be guidelines for specific treatment in that each patient is an individual whose condition reflects multiple factors contributing to impaired cardiopulmonary function or threatening it (i.e., the effects of restricted mobility, recumbency, extrinsic factors related to the patient's care, and intrinsic factors related to the patient in addition to the underlying pathophysiology).

REVIEW QUESTIONS

1. With respect to critically ill patients with the following conditions, describe the pathophysiology of *primary* cardiopulmonary dysfunction, cardiopulmonary failure, obstructive lung disease,

status asthmaticus, restrictive lung disease, and coronary artery disease.

2. Relate cardiopulmonary physical therapy treatment interventions to the underlying pathophysiology of *each* of the above conditions in the critically ill patient and provide the *rationale* for your choice.

References

Andreoli, K.G., Fowkes, V.K., Zipes, D.P., & Wallace, A.G. (1991). *Cardiac care* (7th ed.). St. Louis: Mosby.

Austin, G.L., & Greenfield L.J. (1980). Respiratory care in cardiac failure and pulmonary edema. *Surgical Clinics in North America, 60,* 1565-1575.

Barach, A.L. (1974). Chronic obstructive lung disease: Postural relief of dyspnea. *Archives of Physical Medicine & Rehabilitation, 55,* 494-504.

Barach, A.L., & Beck, G.J. (1954). Ventilatory effects of head-down position in pulmonary emphysema. *American Journal of Medicine, 16,* 55-60.

Bates, D.V. (1989). *Respiratory function in disease* (3rd ed.). Philadelphia: WB Saunders.

Bennett, W.D., Foster, W.M., & Chapman, W.F. (1990). Cough-enhanced mucus clearance in the normal lung. *Journal of Applied Physiology, 69,* 1670-1675.

Bjore, D. (1972). Postmyocardial infarction: A program of graduated exercises. *Journal of the Canadian Physiotherapy Association, 24,* 22-25.

Boggs, R.L., & Wooldridge-King, M. (1993). *AACN procedure manual for critical care* (3rd ed.). Philadelphia: WB Saunders.

Brunner, J.X., Wolff, G. (1988). *Pulmonary function indices in critical care patients.* New York: Springer-Verlag.

Burns, J.R., & Jones, F.L. (1975). Early ambulation of patients requiring ventilatory assistance. *Chest, 68,* 608.

Casciari, R.J., Fairshter, R.D., Harrison, A., Morrison, J.T., Blackburn, C., & Wilson, A.F. (1981). Effects of breathing retraining in patients with chronic obstructive pulmonary disease. *Chest, 79,* 393-398.

Chung, F., & Dean, E. (1989). Pathophysiology and cardiorespiratory consequences of interstitial lung disease-review and clinical implications. *Physical Therapy, 69,* 956-966.

Civetta, J.M., Taylor, R.W., & Kirby, R.R. (1988). *Critical care.* Philadelphia: J.B. Lippincott.

Clauss, R.H., Scalabrini, B.Y., Ray, J.F., III, & Reed, G.E. (1968). Effects of changing body position upon improved ventilation-perfusion relationships. *Circulation, 37*(Suppl. 4), 214-217.

Dantzker, D.R. (1991). *Cardiopulmonary critical care.* Philadelphia: W.B. Saunders.

Dean, E. (1985). Effect of body position on pulmonary function. *Physical Therapy, 65,* 613-618.

Dean, E. (1994). Physiotherapy skills: Positioning and mobilization of the patient. In B.A. Webber & J.A. Pryor. (Eds.). *Physiotherapy for respiratory and cardiac problems.* Edinburgh: Churchill Livingstone.

Dean, E., Murphy, S., Parrent, L., & Rousseau, M. (1995). Metabolic consequences of physical therapy in critically-ill patients. *Proceedings of the world confederation of physical therapy congress,* Washington, DC.

Dean, E., & Ross, J. (1992a). Discordance between cardiopulmonary physiology and physical therapy. *Chest, 101,* 1694-1698.

Dean, E., & Ross, J. (1992b). Mobilization and Body Conditioning. In C. Zadai, (Ed.), *Pulmonary management in physical therapy.* New York: Churchill Livingstone.

Douglas, W.W., Rehder, K., Beynen, F.M., Sessler, A.D., & Marsh, H.M. (1977). Improved oxygenation in patients with acute respiratory failure: The prone position. *American Review of Respiratory Disease, 115,* 559-566.

Fell, T., & Cheney, F.W. (1971). Prevention of hypoxia during endotracheal suction. *Annals of Surgery, 174,* 24-28.

Froelicher, V.F. (1987). *Exercise and the heart. Clinical concepts* (2nd ed.). St. Louis: Mosby.

Gallagher, T.J., & Civetta, J.M. (1980). Goal-directed therapy of acute respiratory failure. *Anesthesia & Analgesia, 59*(11), 831-834.

Gaskell, D.V., & Webber, B.A. (1988). *The Brompton hospital guide to chest physiotherapy.* (5th ed.). Oxford: Blackwell Scientific Publications.

Gibson, G.J., Pride, N.B., Davis, J.N., & Loh, L.C. (1977). Pulmonary mechanics in patients with respiratory muscle weakness. *American Review of Respiratory Disease, 115*(3), 389-395.

Hanson, P. & Nagle, F. (1987). Isometric exercise: Cardiovascular responses in normal and cardiac populations. In P. Hansen, (Ed.), *Exercise and the heart.* Philadelphia: W.B. Saunders.

Hietpas, B.G., Roth, R.D., & Jensen, W.M. (1979). Huff coughing and airway patency. *Respiratory care, 24,* 710.

Holten, K. (1972). Training effect in patients with severe ventilatory failure. *Scandinavian Journal of Respiratory Diseases, 53,* 65-76.

Irwin, S., & Tecklin, J.S. (Eds.). (1985). *Cardiopulmonary physical therapy.* St. Louis: Mosby.

Jardin, F., Farcot, J.C., Boisante, L., Curien, N., Margairaz, A., & Bourdarias, J.P. (1981). Influence of positive end-expiratory pressure on left ventricular performance. *New England Journal of Medicine, 304,* 387-392.

Kirilloff, L.H., Owens, G.R., Rogers, R.M., & Mazzocco, M.C. (1985). Does chest physical therapy work? *Chest, 88,* 436-444.

Kumar, A., Pontoppiaan, H., Falke, K.J., Wilson, R.S. & Laver, M.B. (1973). Pulmonary barotrauma during mechanical ventilation. *Critical Care Medicine, 1* 181-186.

Leblanc, P., Ruff, F., & Milic-Emili, J. (1970). Effects of age and body position on "airway closure" in man. *Journal of Applied Physiology, 28,* 448-451.

Levine, S.A., & Lown, B. (1952). "Armchair" treatment of acute coronary thrombosis. *Journal of American Medical Association, 148,* 1365-1368.

Mackenzie, C.F., Imle, P.C., & Ciesla, N. (1989). *Chest physiotherapy in the intensive care unit* (2nd ed.). Baltimore: Williams & Wilkins.

Macklem, P.T., & Roussos, C.S. (1977). Respiratory muscle fatigue: A cause of respiratory failure? *Clinical Science & Molecular Medicine, 53* 419-422.

Marini, J.J. (1984). Postoperative atelectasis: Pathophysiology, clinical importance, and principles of management. *Respiratory Care, 29,* 516-528.

Matthay, M.A. (Ed.). (1985). Pathophysiology of pulmonary edema. *Clinics in Chest Medicine, 6,* 301-314.

Mueller, R.E., Petty, T.L., & Filley, G.F. (1970). Ventilation and arterial blood gas changes induced by pursed lips breathing. *Journal of Applied Physiology, 28,* 784-789.

Nunn, J.F., Coleman, A.J., Sachithanandan, T., Bergman, N.A., & Laws, J.W. (1965). Hypoxemia and atelectasis produced by forced expiration. *British Journal of Anesthesia, 37,* 3-12.

Petty, T.L. (1982). *Intensive and rehabilitative respiratory care* (3rd ed.). Philadelphia: Lea & Febiger.

Petty, T.L. (1985). *Chronic obstructive pulmonary disease* (2nd ed.). New York: Marcel Dekker.

Piehl, M.A., & Brown, R.S. (1976). Use of extreme position changes in acute respiratory failure. *Critical Care Medicine, 4* 13-14.

Ray, J.F., III, Yost, L., Moallem, S., Sanoudos, G.M., Villamena, P., Paredes, R.M., & Clauss, R.H. (1974). Immobility, hypoxemia, and pulmonary arteriovenous shunting. *Archives of Surgery, 109,* 537-541.

Rochester, D.F., & Arora, N.S. (1983). Respiratory muscle failure. *Medical Clinics of North America, 67,* 573-597.

Rochester, D.F., & Esau, S.A. (1984). Malnutrition and the respiratory system. *Chest, 85,* 411-415.

Shoemaker, W.C., Thompson, W.L., & Holbrook, P.R. (Eds.) (1984). *Textbook of critical care.* Philadelphia: W.B. Saunders.

Trekova, N.A., Dementyeva, II, Dzemeshkevich, S.L., & Asmangulyan, Y.T. (1994). Blood oxygen transport function in cardiopulmonary bypass surgery for acquired valvular diseases. *Intensive Surgery, 79,* 60-64.

Underhill, S.L., Woods, S.L., Froelicher, E.S.S., & Halpenny, C.J. (1989). *Cardiac nursing* (2nd ed.). Philadelphia: J.B. Lippincott.

Vincent, J.L., & Suter, P.M. (1987). *Cardiopulmonary interactions in acute respiratory failure.* New York: Springer-Verlag.

Walsh, J.M., Vanderwarf, C., Hoscheit, D., & Fahey, P.J. (1989). Unsuspected hemodynamic alterations during endotracheal suctioning. *Chest, 95,* 162-165.

Webber, B.A., & Pryor, J.A. (Eds.). (1994). *Physiotherapy for respiratory and cardiac problems.* Edinburgh: Churchill Livingstone.

Weber, K.T., Janicki, J.S., Shroff, S.C., & Likoff, M.J. (1983). The cardiopulmonary unit: The body's gas exchange system. *Clinics in Chest Medicine, 4,* 101-110.

Weinstein, M.E., & Skillman, J.J. (1980). Management of severe respiratory failure. *Surgical Clinics of North America, 60,* 1403-1412.

Weissman, C., & Kemper, M. (1993). Stressing the critically ill patient: The cardiopulmonary and metabolic responses to an acute increase in oxygen consumption. *Journal of Critical Care, 8,* 100-108.

Weissman, C., Kemper, M., Damask, M.C., Askanazi, J., Hyman, A.I., & Kinney, J.M. (1984). Effect of routine intensive care interactions on metabolic rate. *Chest, 86,* 815-818.

Weissman, C., Kemper, M., Elwyn, D.H., Askanazi, J., Hyman, A.I., & Kinney, J.M. (1989). The energy expenditure of the mechanically ventilated critically ill patient. *Chest, 2,* 254-259.

West, J.B. (1995). *Respiratory physiology—the essentials* (5th ed.). Baltimore: Williams & Wilkins.

Wilson, R.F. (1992). *Critical care manual* (2nd ed.). Philadelphia: F.A. Davis.

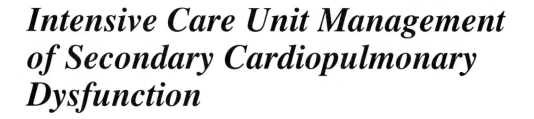

CHAPTER 33

Intensive Care Unit Management of Secondary Cardiopulmonary Dysfunction

Elizabeth Dean

KEY TERMS
Burns
Head injury
Morbid obesity

Musculoskeletal trauma
Neuromuscular dysfunction
Spinal cord injury

INTRODUCTION

This chapter describes the principles and practice of cardiopulmonary physical therapy in the management of secondary cardiopulmonary dysfunction that can lead to cardiopulmonary failure. Some common categories of conditions described include neuromuscular disease, morbid obesity, musculoskeletal trauma, head injury, spinal cord injury, and burns. Each category of condition is presented in two parts. First, the related pathophysiology and pertinent aspects of the medical management of the condition are presented. Second, the principles of physical therapy management are discussed. Guidelines to

management are not mutually exclusive for each category. Rather, considerable overlap may exist when conditions coexist. The principles presented are not treatment prescriptions. Each patient must be assessed and treated individually taking into consideration the contribution of immobility, recumbency, extrinsic factors related to the patient's care, and intrinsic factors related to the individual patient (see Chapter 16), in addition to the underlying pathophysiology. For examples of specific treatment prescriptions refer to the companion volume to this book entitled *Clinical case studies in cardiopulmonary physical therapy.*

PATIENT WITH NEUROMUSCULAR DISEASE
Pathophysiology and medical management

Guillain-Barré syndrome, myasthenia gravis, muscular dystrophy, multiple sclerosis, stroke, poliomyelitis, and neuromuscular poisonings are common neuromuscular disorders that can precipitate respiratory failure in the absence of underlying primary lung disease (Cooper, Trend, and Wiles, 1985; Curran and Colbert, 1989; Dean, Ross, Road, Courtenay, and Madill, 1991; Fugl-Meyer and Grimby, 1984; Griggs and Donohoe, 1982; Lane, Hazleman, and Nichols, 1974). If paralyzed, the patient will likely be dependent on ventilatory assistance. Cardiopulmonary physical therapy has a central role in minimizing the need for mechanical ventilation in these patients because their prognosis for weaning is poor. Progressive respiratory insufficiency is best addressed early with the institution of nighttime ventilation at home (Curran, 1981) before the development of failure and necessity for hospitalization. Patients with progressive neuromuscular diseases (e.g., muscular dystrophy) are living longer; thus cardiopulmonary insufficiency will be compounded by age-related changes of the cardiopulmonary system (Dean, 1994a; Leblanc, Ruff, and Milic-Emili, 1970).

Neuromuscular conditions contribute to cardiopulmonary dysfunction in numerous ways (Chapters 21 and 22). With progressive deterioration of inspiratory and expiratory muscle strength and endurance, respiratory insufficiency and failure can ensue (Black and Hyatt, 1971). Depending on the specific pathology, such deficits include reduced lung volumes and flow rates, reduced alveolar ventilation, increased airway resistance, ventilation and perfusion mismatch, impaired mucociliary transport, mucous accumulation, reduced cough and gag reflexes, relatively unprotected airway secondary to impaired glottic closure and weakness of the pharyngeal and laryngeal structures, and increased work of breathing.

Principles of physical therapy management

A patient with restrictive pulmonary disease secondary to neuromuscular conditions is at considerable risk of succumbing to the negative cardiopulmonary and cardiovascular sequelae of reduced mobility and recumbency, in addition to the pathophysiological consequences of respiratory failure. Provided the patient has some residual muscle power, the balance between oxygen demand and supply will determine the degree to which mobilization can be exploited to maximize oxygen transport. The treatment goals for these patients are to maximize oxygen delivery, enhance the efficiency of oxygen uptake and utilization, and thereby reduce the work of breathing. In these patients, minimizing oxygen demand overall (i.e., during mobilization as well as at rest) is a priority. Mobilization needs to be prescribed in body positions that enhance oxygen transport and its efficiency so that the benefits of mobilization can be exploited more fully without worsening arterial oxygenation (Dean, 1985). The patient requires continuous monitoring of oxygen transport and hemodynamic monitoring to ensure the exercise stimulus is optimally therapeutic and not excessive.

Although the mechanisms are different, patients with neuromuscular dysfunction can benefit from body positioning to reduce respiratory distress much like a patient with chronic airflow limitation (Barach, 1974). Upright and lean-forward positions will reduce distress to the greatest extent.

The patient's body position and length of time in any one position must be carefully monitored and recorded to minimize the risks of positions that are deleterious to oxygenation and to ensure that a beneficial position is not assumed for too long because of the diminishing benefits over time. This is particularly important for the patient who is incapable of positioning him or herself, who is incapable of communicating a need to turn, and in whom muscle wasting, bony prominences, and thinning of the skin may predispose the patient to skin breakdown.

Patients who are hypotonic and generally weak and debilitated fail to adapt normally to position-dependent fluid shifts and thus are more prone to orthostatic intolerance (Marini and Wheeler, 1989). Gravitational stimulation is essential to maintain the volume regulating mechanisms. Tilt tables should be used judiciously given the potential risks in these patients, which is compounded by the loss of the lower-extremity muscle pump mechanism. Because of potential adverse reactions to fluid shifts and the potential for desaturation, falling Pao_2 levels and dysrhythmias, the patient's hemodynamic status must be monitored closely during gravitational challenges.

The importance of chest wall mobility to optimize three-dimensional chest wall excursion in chronic neurological patients is emphasized in Chapters 21 and 22. This goal is particularly challenging in the neurological patient with acute respiratory insufficiency. The goal is to promote alveolar ventilation, reduce areas of atelectasis, and optimize ventilation and perfusion matching and breathing efficiency to augment and minimize reliance on respiratory support (i.e., supplemental oxygen and mechanical ventilation) while minimizing respiratory distress. This is especially important because patients with neuromuscular conditions are poor candidates for being weaned off mechanical ventilation (Petty, 1982). In addition these patient are prone to microaspirations. Promotion of mucociliary transport is therefore essential to facilitate clearing of aspirate and minimize bacterial colonization and risk of infection.

Another major problem for patients with restrictive lung disease secondary to generalized weakness and neuromuscular disease is an ineffective cough. Cough facilitation techniques (e.g., body positioning, abdominal counter pressure, and tracheal tickle can be used to increase intraabdominal and intrathoracic pressures and cough effectiveness. A natural cough, even when facilitated, is preferable and more effective in dislodging mucus from the sixth or seventh generation of bronchi than repeated suctioning. Even a weak, facilitated cough may be effective in dislodging secretions to the central airways for removal by suctioning or for redistributing peripheral secretions (Hasani, Pavia, Agnew, and Clarke, 1991). Huffing, a modified cough performed with the glottis open and with abdominal support, may help to mobilize secretions in patients with generalized weakness (Hietpas, Roth, and Jensen, 1979). In some cases, suctioning may be the only means of eliciting a cough and clearing secretions simultaneously. Coughing attempts are usually exhausting for these patients. Thus ample rest periods must be interspersed during treatment, particularly for the ventilated patient. Coughing maneuvers need to be strategically planned. Even though the patient may be only to effect a series of a few weak coughs, it is es-

sential that these attempts are maximized (i.e., the patient optimally rested and medicated [e.g., bronchodilators, analgesia, reduced sedation and narcotics] is physically positioned to optimize length-tension relationship of the diaphragm and abdominal muscles, positioned vertically to optimize inspiratory lung volumes, and expiratory flows and avoid of aspiration, and is provided thoracic and abdominal support during expiration to maximize intrathoracic and intraabdominal pressures) (see Chapter 21). These supportive measures will ensure that the benefits of the normal physiological cough mechanism, which is the single best secretion clearance technique, is maximized (i.e., the most productive cough with the least energy expenditure) (Bennett, Foster, and Chapman, 1990; Hasani et al., 1991; Kirilloff, Owens, Rogers, and Mazzocco, 1985; Zinman, 1984). Forced chest wall compression or forced expiratory maneuvers are contraindicated (Nunn, Coleman, Sachithanandan, Bergman, and Laws, 1965).

Impaired mobility, inability to cough effectively, decreased airway diameter, and bronchospasm contribute to impaired mucociliary transport and secretion accumulation. In addition, impaired glottic closure and increased risk of reflux in this patient population exposes the airway to risk of aspiration. Prophylactically, multiple body positions and frequent position changes will minimize the risk of secretion accumulation and stasis. If mechanically ventilated, these patients are suctioned as indicated. If pulmonary secretions become a significant problem despite these preventative measures, postural drainage positions are selected to achieve the optimal effect (i.e., secretion mobilization and optimal gas exchange). Given the treatment response, manual techniques of which manual vibration would have the greatest physiological justification, may yield some benefit.

Patients with chronic neuromuscular dysfunction and residual musculoskeletal deformity pose an additional challenge to the cardiopulmonary physical therapist in that cardiopulmonary function is less predictable because of altered lung mechanics (Bake, Dempsey, and Grimby, 1976) and possibly cardiac dynamics. Thus clinical decision making is more experiential in these patients who require close monitoring.

OBESITY
Pathophysiology and medical management

Restriction of cardiopulmonary function secondary to morbid obesity is called the *alveolar hypoventilation syndrome* or *Pickwickian syndrome.* In this syndrome the weight of excess adipose tissue over the thoracic cage and abdominal cavity restricts chest wall movement and movement of the diaphragm and abdominal contents, respectively, during respiration. In very heavy individuals, cardiopulmonary function can be significantly impaired, resulting in hypoxemia and cardiopulmonary failure. The major pathophysiological mechanisms include significant alveolar hypoventilation, reactive hypoxic pulmonary vasoconstriction, increased pulmonary vascular resistance, myocardial hypertrophy, increased right ventricular work, altered position of the thoracic structures, abnormal compression of the heart, lungs, and mediastinal structures, abnormal position of the heart, cardiomegaly, increased intraabdominal pressure, elevated hemidiaphragms with resulting pressure on the underside of the diaphragm, impaired cough effectiveness, impaired mucociliary transport, mucous obstruction of airways, airway narrowing, bronchospasm, impaired mechanical efficiency of diaphragmatic excursion, and impaired respiratory mechanics and breathing efficiency (Bates, 1989). In addition, such patients are likely to have poor cardiopulmonary reserve capacity secondary to increased metabolical rate and minute ventilation at submaximal work rates, increased metabolic cost of breathing, and increased work of breathing. Moderately heavy patients whose pulmonary function is normally not compromised may exhibit cardiopulmonary dysfunction when their oxygen transport systems are stressed because of illness.

Mechanical ventilation can be a challenge in that the system pressure required to inflate the lungs may predispose the patient to barotrauma. Furthermore, high system pressures contribute to reduced stroke volume and cardiac output. Adequate circulation is essential to fulfill the goals of medical management (i.e., to optimize tissue oxygenation and carbon dioxide removal). Thus a delicate balance between adequate alveolar ventilation, cardiac output, and peripheral circulation is maintained.

Principles of physical therapy management

The obese patient can be treated aggressively provided there are no contraindications and he or she is being fully monitored. Treatments need to be intense, to the limits of the patient's tolerance, provided this is not contraindicated. An aggressive approach is essential given that the obese patient is at greater risk of deteriorating between treatments than a nonobese counterpart. Recumbency is tolerated poorly by an obese patient. Positional decrements in PaO_2 and Sao_2 can induce dysrhythmias. The weight of the abdominal viscera limit diaphragmatic descent and elevate the resting position of the diaphragm, impeding its mechanical efficiency.

These patients need to be aggressively mobilized; both whole body exercise stress and range of motion exercises between mobilization sessions. Active and active assisted upper-extremity range-of-motion exercises are associated with increased hemodynamic stress; thus the patient must be monitored closely. Lower-extremity exercise, such as pedaling and hip and knee flexion and extension exercises, may help position and improve the excursion of the diaphragm. Lower-extremity movement will augment venous return. Depending on the patient and the work of the heart, the effect of lower-extremity movement will need monitoring to ensure that myocardial work is not increased excessively.

The erect upright position is optimal to augment ventilation and reduce the work of the mechanical ventilator and the risk of barotrauma. The upright position, coupled with leaning forward, displaces the abdominal contents forward, thereby reducing intraabdominal pressure and facilitating diaphragmatic descent. The posterior lung fields, particularly of the bases, are at risk for dynamic airway closure and atelectasis. Numerous positions and position changes ensure that the dependent alveoli remain open. The time spent in the supine position should be minimized. In fact, greater emphasis should be placed on nursing these patients in the upright position (i.e., the position of least risk and its variants). In addition to its pulmonary benefits, the upright position can reduce compression of the heart and mediastinal structures and there is a potential decrease in stroke volume and cardiac output. The weight of the chest wall, in addition to the weight of internal fat deposits in and around the cardiopulmonary unit, can compromise cardiac output and contribute to dysrhythmias. Thus during all body position changes the patient should be monitored hemodynamically to ensure the position is being tolerated well. Obese patients often slump after being positioned in the upright position. It is crucial that the position of these patients is checked frequently and corrected. The slumped position can be counterproductive in that the benefits of the upright position are significantly reduced and can lead to deterioration.

Although obese patients do not tolerate the prone position well, the semi-prone position can be beneficial by simulating the benefits of the upright lean-forward position on the displacement of the abdominal viscera (Ross and Dean, 1992). This position also simulates the prone abdomen-free position, which is associated with even greater benefit than the prone abdomen-restricted position (Dean, 1985). The benefits of the prone position for the obese individual include increased lung compliance and enhanced gas exchange and oxygenation. The full prone abdomen restricted position is contraindicated in the obese individual with cardiopulmonary failure, however, because this position can compromise diaphragmatic descent and contribute to further cardiopulmonary distress and failure and possibly cardiac arrest.

Mucociliary transport is slowed and ineffective in obese patients with cardiopulmonary failure. Frequent body positioning will facilitate mucociliary transport and lymphatic drainage. The postural drainage positions can be effective in mobilizing secretions should accumulation become a problem. Manual techniques are not likely to add much benefit particularly in the morbidly obese patient. Suctioning is essential to clear pulmonary secretions from the central airways.

The obese individual is at risk for postextubation atelectasis. Thus aggressive mobilization and numerous positions and frequent position changes need to be continued.

The spontaneously breathing obese patient has a weak ineffective cough, which will be even less effective after a period of intubation and mechanical ventilation. Deep breathing and coughing maneuvers are taught comparable with those described for the patient with neuromuscular disease. Body positioning to facilitate coughing and supported coughing need to be instituted to maximize cough effectiveness. These maneuvers should be carried out in conjunction with hourly extreme position shifts.

Morbidly obese patients have a high incidence of upper airway obstruction and sleep apnea secondary to floppy compliant pharyngeal tissue. Thus the quality of their sleep and rest is suboptimal, and they are apt to desaturate significantly while sleeping. These patients are also at high risk for esophageal reflux and aspiration. The optimal resting position is with the head of bed up.

PATIENT WITH MUSCULOSKELETAL TRAUMA
Pathophysiology and medical management

Crush and penetrating injuries of the chest are commonly seen in the ICU (Moylan, 1988). Damage to the chest wall, lung parenchyma, and heart contribute to the risk of cardiopulmonary failure (see box on p. 604). Associated injuries of the head, spinal cord, and abdomen may also contribute. Fractures of long bones and pelvis are associated with fat emboli, which pose the threat of pulmonary embolism. In addition, fluid loss in multiple trauma contributes to loss of blood volume, hypovolemia, and hemodynamic instability. The more extensive the injuries, the greater the pain and need for analgesia. Pain contributes significantly to reduced alveolar ventilation, airway closure, and inefficient breathing patterns.

Paradoxical motion of the chest wall associated with flail chest and rib fractures results from instability of portions of the rib cage after trauma to the chest. If severe, patients may require surgical stabilization of the ribs or stabilization by continuous ventilatory management. Chest wall injuries and rib fractures are particularly painful.

The presence of blood or air in the chest cavity and in the potential spaces of the pericardial sac and intrapleural cavity impairs cardiac distension and contraction, impairs ventilation, promotes retention of secretions, interferes with effective clearance, and impairs lymphatic drainage (Marini and Wheeler, 1989). Resolution of effusions can be facilitated with

---

Factors Contributing to Cardiopulmonary Failure After Trauma and Their Diagnostic Signs

Airway Obstruction

Respiratory insufficiency

Respiratory distress

Impaired blood gases

Inadequate Ventilation

Reduced thoracic movement

Paradoxical thoracoabdominal movement

Tension Pneumothorax

Cyanosis

Unilaterally absent breath sounds

Distended neck veins

Subcutaneous emphysema

Cardiac Tamponade

Distended neck veins

Muffled heart sounds

Narrowed pulse pressure

Paradoxical pulse

Open Pneumothorax

Decreased breath sounds

Penetration of thoracic wall

Myocardial Contusion

Dysrhythmia

Flail Chest

Loose segment

Multiple palpable fractured ribs

Decreased or moist breath sounds

Modified from Moylan, J. A. (Ed.). (1988). *Trauma surgery.* Philadelphia: JB Lippincott.

mobilization and body positioning. These interventions reexpand underlying atelectasis and help restore fluid balance by their effects on lymphatic drainage. Furthermore, by shifting the effusion fluid, atelectatic areas can reexpand. The presence of a pneumothorax or hemothorax can severely compromise lung expansion. A tension pneumothorax results when air collects under tension in the pleural cavity. The tension pneumothorax promotes lung collapse on both the ipsilateral and contralateral sides, which further threatens respiratory failure. Phrenic nerve injuries inhibit diaphragmatic function (Dureuil, Viires, and Cantineau, 1986). The position of the affected hemidiaphragm rests higher in the thoracic cavity, which may restrict ventilation to the lung base and contribute to airway closure and basal atelectasis. Diaphragmatic injuries directly affect ventilation in two ways. First, the bellows action of the lungs is compromised. Second, the lung is displaced by herniation of the abdominal contents into the thoracic cavity.

Analysis of blood gases in the patient with posttraumatic injuries of the chest often shows severe hypoxemia and moderate elevations of arterial PCO_2. The presence of acidemia is common, which may have both respiratory and metabolical components.

Principles of physical therapy management

Severe restlessness and dyspnea in a patient with chest injury are classic indications of respiratory failure. Auscultation and percussion can usually reveal an underlying pneumothorax or hemothorax. Tension pneumothorax is confirmed by chest x-ray or aspiration of the chest with a needle and syringe.

Flail chest refers to fractures involving the chest cage where there are two or more fractured ribs at two or more sites. This results in instability of the chest wall. The so-called flail segment is usually apparent on physical examination. Paradoxical movement of the flail segment can often be observed. The chest is depressed rather than elevated over the site during inspiration. Rib fractures are indicated by tenderness and crepitations on physical examination and from x-ray findings. Nonventilatory management of chest injuries in the absence of severe hypoxemia is preferred in these patients.

Rib Fractures

Simple uncomplicated rib fractures often receive no specific treatment. Pain from complicated fractures may be treated with intercostal nerve blocks and transcutaneous electrical nerve stimulation and analgesia. Optimizing alveolar ventilation and mucociliary transport and avoiding pulmonary complications are primary goals. Strapping the chest is avoided because this further restricts and compromises chest wall expansion.

The current method of therapy for flail chest is internal stabilization of the chest and use of a mechanical ventilator. Slight hyperventilation will usually reduce the respiratory drive of most patients to allow the ventilator to take over the full work of breathing. The flail segment is then stabilized by internal expansion of the lungs. The treatment ensures adequate ventilation with the least pain possible. After 2 weeks, the flail segment is usually stable.

When the patient can maintain a reasonable tidal volume and normal blood gases, weaning is begun. As soon as tidal volume and forced vital capacity are within acceptable limits, oxygen can be administered through an endotracheal tube with a T tube assembly. Arterial blood gases are monitored closely after the ventilator has been discontinued. Once the blood gases are in acceptable ranges over a reasonable period of time (i.e., 12 to 24 hours) the endotracheal tube is removed.

Pneumothorax and Hemothorax

Air or blood in the pleural cavity after chest trauma must be removed through a chest tube. For a pneumothorax the chest tube is positioned in the second or third intercostal space in the midclavicular line. For a hemothorax the chest tube is positioned in the sixth intercostal space in the posterior axillary line. Usually the chest tubes are sutured and taped into position and therefore are not easily dislodged. If the tubes are pulled out, subcutaneous emphysema or a pneumothorax results. A pneumothorax will also result if the tube is disconnected from the underwater seal. This is the reason for securing the collecting reservoirs of a chest tube drainage system with tape to the floor. Mobilizing and frequency repositioning the patient facilitates chest tube drainage and reexpansion of collapsed alveoli. Care is taken to avoid kinking or straining chest tubes during patient treatment.

A bronchopulmonary fistula can be responsible for a major loss of the tidal volume delivered by the ventilator. Small leaks can be tolerated and are usually compensated for by an increase in tidal or minute ventilation.

Multiple Trauma

The management of multiple trauma is a major challenge for the ICU team. Multisystem involvement and complications often present a precarious situation in which priorities have to be defined for each individual situation. Multiple trauma can include head injury, chest wall injuries, fractures, lung contusions, diaphragm injury, pleural space disorders, internal injuries, thromboemboli, fat emboli, and cardiac contusions. Shock and adult respiratory distress syndrome may ensue (see Chapter 34). The clinical picture of the patient with multiple trauma is compounded by the mobilization and positioning restrictions imposed (Ray et al., 1974). Positive end-expiratory pressure (PEEP) is frequently used to reduce the effects of lung congestion secondary to shock or adult respiratory distress syndrome (ARDS) (McAslan and Cowley, 1979). Arterial blood gases are assessed to evaluate the effectiveness of PEEP in effecting improved oxygen transfer.

Multiple Fractures

Multiple trauma patients are assumed to have spinal involvement, particularly of the cervical spine, until ruled out with appropriate scans and x-rays. Meanwhile the physical therapist performs repeated assessments to establish a baseline and recommend positions for the patient that will maximize oxygen transport. Treatment to enhance oxygen transport and mucociliary transport is primarily restricted to body positioning using log rolling maneuvers and a selected range of motion exercises (i.e., not of the head and neck, and possibly shoulders).

Fixation, traction, and casting of fractures and dislocations of the limbs complicate the management of the trauma patient. Restrictions to mobilization and body positioning are primary concerns of the physical therapist (Mackenzie, 1989). Mobilization in the upright position provides both a gravitational stimulus and an exercise stimulus, both of which are essential to optimize oxygen transport. This is preferable to mobilization exercises in the recumbent position. In some cases, traction can be transferred from over the end of the bed to over a chair. A strict routine of body positioning is maintained, although severe limitations often exist with respect to the specific positions and the degree of turning permitted. Lower limb traction can be maintained when the patient is positioned in a modified sidelying position. Coordinating treatments with analgesia schedules reduces the patient's pain and fatigue, thereby improving tolerance to and prolonging the treatment. These patients usually tolerate the head-down position well provided head injury does not complicate the clinical picture.

The acute effects of mobilization that will benefit the patient with musculoskeletal trauma include augmentation of ventilation, perfusion, ventilation and perfusion matching, and promotion of mucociliary transport and cough effectiveness. General mobilization exercises and proprioceptive neuromuscular facilitation (PNF) can be used to promote a mobilization stimulus. Cycle pedals can be attached to a chair or the end of the bed to provide a low-intensity exercise challenge for some patients. Maximal work output can be achieved within the patient's capacity using an interval training type schedule (i.e., schedule of work to rest periods). A mobilization program that promotes the long-term effects of exercise can be prescribed that involves as many large muscle groups as possible in rhythmic, dynamic exercise.

Frequent deep breathing and coughing is continued during and between treatments, depending on whether the patient requires mechanical ventilation. Body positioning is carried out within the limits of the patient's traction and casts. Impaired mucociliary transport is treated with body positioning and frequent position changes. Secretion accumulation may require postural drainage. Modified positions may be indicated because of the positioning restrictions imposed by the fractures, traction, and fixation devices. If indicated manual techniques may be coupled with postural drainage (Mackenzie, Shin, Hadi, and Imle, 1980). Care must be taken to ensure the addition of manual techniques is beneficial and is tolerated by the patient.

Relaxation interventions, both active and passive, should be integrated into the treatment regimen for the trauma patient to reduce excessive oxygen consumption and promote comfort (Malamed, 1989). Active relaxation refers to relaxing the patient through participation of the patient in relaxation procedures. Passive relaxation refers to relaxing the patient using passive procedures (e.g., body positioning, physical supports, talking slowly and calmly, and taking adequate time for conducting treatments). Taking time to implement mobilization is essential. First, mechanically moving and having patients who have multiple injuries move requires a prolonged period of time. In addition, however, the cardiovascular and cardiopulmonary systems of critically ill need time to adapt to new positions physiologically and to control concommitant discomfort. Prolonged periods of time may be required to turn a patient, dangle him or her over the bed, or transfer him or her to chair with continuous monitoring. Every effort is made to maintain the patient's spirits, reduce stress, and encourage a positive attitude toward active participation early in the rehabilitation program that begins in the ICU.

Care must be taken to avoid undertreating or overtreating trauma patients. A clear chest can rapidly regress because of general immobility and limitations to body positioning imposed by traction and pain. Treatments should always be coordinated with the patient's analgesics to optimize treatment response and for the patient's comfort. Whenever possible, the patient should be equipped with slings and pulleys and weights at bedside and a monkey bar overhead for bed mobility and upper-extremity exercise. In addition to their cardiopulmonary benefits, PNF patterns are useful in preparation for slings and pulleys. The use of PNF patterns for trauma and postoperative patients can be well tolerated by these patients. All activities are taught in conjunction with breathing control exercises and coordination with the respiratory cycle.

PATIENT WITH HEAD INJURY
Pathophysiology and medical management

Hypoxemia is observed in many patients with injury to the central nervous system (Demling, 1980). This may reflect primary damage to the cardiopulmonary centers of the brain or secondary effects of associated trauma. Arterial blood gases are therefore closely monitored in these patients.

Acute cerebral edema with sudden increase in intracranial pressure (ICP) and reduction in cerebral perfusion pressure, rapidly affects central control of respiration (Borozny, 1987). Advancing cerebral edema is evidenced by deterioration in level of consciousness, pupillary reflexes, ocular reflexes, pattern of respiration, and exaggerated muscle tone and posture. The sequence of these clinical signs corresponds to progressively increasing ICP from the cortex toward the medullopontine region. With involvement of the brain stem, respiration becomes variable and incoordinate. With loss of central control and imminent cessation of breathing, respiration is shallow and ataxic. The appearance of the jaw and laryngeal jerk with each inspiratory effort suggests a poor prognosis.

Physical therapy and the patient's normal routine may have a dramatic effect on the ICP. ICP can be elevated indirectly by an increase in intrathoracic pressure as a result of physical therapy or suctioning. Turning and positioning may produce obstruction to cerebral venous outflow. Noxious stimuli, such as arterial and venous punctures or cleansing wounds, can elevate ICP and relatively innocuous stimuli, such as noise or pupil checks. Whether these factors elevate

ICP depend on cerebral blood volume and intracranial compliance. On cerebral stimulation, a chain reaction is initiated. Cerebral activity is increased, which in turn elevates metabolic rate, blood flow, and hence volume and ICP. Alternatively, increased cerebral blood volume secondary to gravitational effects, increased ICP, and reduced cerebral perfusion pressure.

The head of the bed is usually maintained between 30 and 40 degrees to promote venous drainage and thereby reduce ICP. The patient's head and neck can be fixed in a neutral position by halo traction or by sand bags positioned on either side (Figure 33-1). Mechanical hyperventilation is used to maintain Pco_2 below normal limits but above 20 mm Hg. Arterial blood gases are checked during or immediately after hyperventilation. Prolonged hyperventilation is avoided.

Barbiturate coma may be induced to decrease the cerebral metabolical rate for oxygen and hence cerebral blood flow. The reduction in cerebral metabolical rate exceeds the reduction in blood flow and thus oxygen supply exceeds demand, which is a desirable treatment outcome. Invasive hemodynamic monitoring is instituted in conjunction with barbiturate coma because barbiturates contribute to hemodynamic instability.

A complication of head injuries is acute lung in-

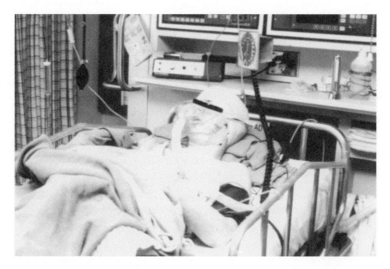

FIGURE 33-1
Patient following neurosurgical procedure; head of bed elevated 20 degrees to help reduce ICP.

jury, specifically, neurogenic pulmonary edema (see Chapter 34). Antonomical nervous system dysfunction contributes to hypertension and neurogenic pulmonary edema. The endothelial tight junctions in the pulmonary capillaries leak protein into the interstitium along with fluid. Constriction of the lymphatic vessels may also contribute to fluid accumulation by impeding the removal of lung water. Increased fluid accumulation in the interstitium may progress to the alveoli contributing further to impaired gas exchange and reduced lung compliance.

Principles of physical therapy management

Physical therapy priorities in the management of the patient with cardiopulmonary dysfunction secondary to head injury appear in the box below.

In cases of abnormally elevated ICP, mechanical hyperventilation and maintenance of Pco_2 around 25 mm Hg are effective measures to reduce cerebral edema by reducing blood flow. Intracranial pressure may increase with treatment and in particular with turning or suctioning. An ICP of up to 30 mm Hg

may be acceptable provided the pressure returns to normal immediately after the removal of the pressure-potentiating stimulus. Prolonged elevation of ICP suggests low cerebral compliance and the possibility of potential brain damage unless pressure is reduced. Thus all interventions must be performed guardedly with due consideration being given to corresponding changes in ICP. Typically, management of patients with central nervous system trauma includes judicious tracheal suctioning, a stringent turning regimen, lung hyperinflation with the manual breathing bag in the nonventilated patient, or deep breathing with occasionally increased tidal volumes or sighs in the ventilated patients.

If the ICP is unstable and a risk of brain damage exists, physical therapy should follow sedation. Ideally, treatments should be performed when the ICP is low and intracranial compliance is satisfactory. The head-down position is contraindicated. Noise and noxious stimulation that increases ICP should be kept to a minimum.

If the ICP is elevated, all noxious stimuli should be removed. In severe conditions a decision may

---

Physical Therapy Priorities in the Management of the Patient with
Cardiopulmonary Dysfunction Secondary to Head Injury

1. Prevention of cerebral hypoxia by maintaining a patent airway
2. Reduction of intracranial pressure and optimal cerebral perfusion pressure
3. Position the patient within the limits of fracture stabilization and elevated intracranial pressure to promote alveolar ventilation and ventilation and perfusion matching
4. Position the patient to reduce pathological patterns of muscle synergy and thereby promote ventilation and reduce oxygen consumption
5. Position the patient to reduce myocardial stress
6. Avoid activities and stimuli that increase ICP
7. Reduce atelectasis
8. Shift lung fluid accumulations and areas of atelectasis
9. Promote lymphatic drainage
10. Promote mucociliary transport and reduce pooling of secretions, and risk of chest infection
11. Reduce the work of breathing and improve the efficiency of the muscles of respiration, particularly if long-term disability is a risk
12. Perform active, active-assisted, or passive movements as soon as possible to enhance cardiopulmonary function and secondarily to preserve musculoskeletal and neuromuscular function and reduce the risk of thromboemboli

have to be made by the team to limit or withdraw interventions that lead to an excessive ICP increase that does not remit instantly (e.g., physical therapy, positioning, suctioning, or neurologic assessment).

Movement of the limbs is performed gently and in a relaxed manner. Patients in a comatose state may experience passive limb movement noxiously. Intracranial pressure may be elevated as a result. Passive movements, however, may have the added benefit of promoting improved tidal ventilation in the nonventilated patient by providing afferent stimulation to the respiratory center via peripheral muscle and joint receptors.

Severe head injury may produce flexor or extensor posturing. These synergies may be inhibited by appropriately positioning the patient. Judicious body positioning, in turn, reduces oxygen consumption and the patient's overall energy requirements.

Neurophysiological facilitation of respiration has been proposed as a treatment intervention to improve ventilation, coughing, and breathing pattern in the unconscious patient (Bethune, 1975). Neurophysiological facilitation techniques include cocontraction of the abdominal muscles, vertebral pressure, intercostal stretch, lifting the posterior basal areas of the lungs, and perioral stimulation. Although these techniques are believed to stimulate reflex involuntary respiratory movements, there is no evidence to support their efficacy in the management of the unconscious patient. Comparable with conventional chest physical therapy procedures, reported benefits associated with neurofacilitation cannot be discriminated from the potent and direct physiological effects of increased arousal, body positioning, and mobilization on oxygen transport (Dean, 1994b). These latter effects have been well documented.

Although arousing the patient and increasing oxygen consumption occurs with cardiopulmonary physical therapy, arousal and oxygen consumption are generally minimized to reduce hemodynamic and metabolical demands in head-injured patients.

PATIENT WITH SPINAL CORD INJURY
Pathophysiology and medical management

The principal cause of death in the early stages of acute spinal cord injury, particularly for the high le-

sions, is cardiopulmonary complications. Lung volumes are reduced with the exception of residual volume that increases. Interestingly, vital capacity increases in the supine compared with the sitting position in quadriplegic patients. However, this does not counter the negative effects of reduced functional residual capacity (FRC) and increased airway closure in this position and reduced flow rates.

Spinal cord injuries above C3 result in loss of phrenic nerve innervation, necessitating a tracheostomy and mechanical ventilation. The lower the level of the spinal cord lesion, the lower the cardiopulmonary risk. All patients with spinal cord injuries are at risk for developing atelectasis and pneumonia. The coughing mechanics of quadriplegic patients are abnormal and contribute to ineffective airway clearance (Estenne and Gorino, 1992). In addition the quadriplegic patient is at risk for developing pulmonary emboli. Prophylactic low-dose heparin is used routinely unless the presence of pulmonary emboli is suspected and higher dosages are indicated.

Patients with suspected spinal cord injuries usually undergo immediate spinal fixation on admission. Depending on the level of injury determined by clinical signs and x-rays, traction, and fixation may be localized to the head and neck or spinal support and casting may be required in the thoracic or lumbar regions.

Principles of physical therapy management

Because of the need to maintain relative immobility in the acute stabilization period of suspected spinal cord injury, therapeutic body positioning rather than mobilization is a primary intervention for optimizing oxygen transport. Although modified body positioning can be achieved, the provision of optimal care under these restricted conditions is a singularly important challenge to the physical therapist, particularly with respect to the management of adequate oxygen transport while the patient is in the ICU. Patients with high spinal cord lesions can be positioned in all positions within the limits of the cervical traction device being used, barring head injury. Both head and foot-tipped positions, however, are introduced cautiously and with hemodynamic monitoring because both positions can have significant cardiopulmonary and hemodynamic consequences secondary to spinal nerve loss and hence sympathetic nerve loss to the peripheral blood vessels. Turning frames such as the Stryker frame facilitate turning and tipping these hemodynamically labile patients in the supine and prone positions (Douglas, Rehder, Beynen, Sessler, and Marsh, 1977).

Effective body positioning, despite the need in some cases for extensive modification, may be sufficient to optimize oxygen transport secondary to improved regional ventilation and perfusion to all lung fields. In the spontaneously breathing patient, deep breathing and coughing maneuvers need to be coupled with position changes to optimize mucociliary transport (Alverez, Peterson, and Lunsford, 1981; Braun, Giovannoni, and O'Connor, 1984). Some patients may not tolerate numerous positions and position changes and thus have impaired mucociliary transport. If secretion accumulation and stasis develop, postural drainage can be instituted; however, tipping must be attempted very cautiously. Patients should be monitored closely during and after treatment. Because of their well-documented side effects (Kirilloff et al., 1985) and the hemodynamic lability of acute quadriplegic patients, percussion and vibration are applied cautiously, should they be indicated, depending on the severity of any complicating fracture-dislocation(s), the stability of fixation, the condition of the lungs, the presence of chest wall injuries, and hemodynamic lability.

The high-frequency oscillating ventilator may have some benefit in the management of multiple trauma patients with spinal injuries who require ventilation. The advantages of the high-frequency oscillating ventilator include improved spontaneous mucociliary clearance and reduced incidence of atelectasis (Gross and King, 1984). Weaning quadriplegic patients off the ventilator requires special skill because of the lost function of the respiratory muscles. For these patients, weaning can be particularly fatiguing, frightening, and frustrating. Patients are weaned lying supine when they are alert and able to cooperate. Short periods off the ventilator on the T piece are used initially. Use of the accessory muscles of respiration and any other muscular reserves are encouraged to compensate for the loss of function of the

respiratory muscles. In some centers, patients are started in the weaning period on respiratory muscle training. The physical therapist must be well versed and practiced in this procedure before using it in conjunction with weaning the quadriplegic patient off the ventilator. Because of the potential risk of inappropriate application and of danger to the patient, respiratory muscle training must be effected knowledgeably to optimize its benefits for each individual patient.

Respiratory Muscle Training

Respiratory muscle weakness and fatigue, two physiologically distinct entities, are probably much more common in the ICU than appreciated. These states need to be recognized and detected early because both can cause respiratory muscle failure (Macklem and Roussos, 1977). The distinction between the two conditions is that weakened muscles respond to resistive muscle training, whereas fatigued muscles do not. Exposing fatigued respiratory muscles to resistive loads can accentuate respiratory failure. The indication for respiratory muscle training, therefore, is weak rather than fatigued respiratory muscles. Rest is indicated for fatigued respiratory muscles. Whether the respiratory muscles are weak or fatigued must be established before prescribing respiratory muscle training.

The combination of immobilization and cardiopulmonary involvement secondary to multiple trauma may result in similar disuse atrophy and weakness of the diaphragm as observed in other skeletal muscles. Respiratory muscle weakness and fatigue can be a component of both obstructive and restrictive patterns of lung disease. Patients with spinal cord injuries do not have the same advantage of performing coordinated general body activity and relaxation maneuvers to help reduce the work of breathing. This contributes to a marked decrease in respiratory muscle strength and endurance resulting in reduced vital capacity, rib cage mobility, and the ability to cough. For these reasons, patients with paralysis and demonstrated respiratory muscle weakness are particularly well suited for respiratory muscle training. The quadriplegic patient has lost the function of the intercostal muscles which are important muscles of inspiration and are responsible for thoracic cage expansion. In addition, the absence of the abdominal muscles, which are the primary expiratory muscles, drastically reduces the ability to cough effectively and to perform a forced expiration. The diaphragm and the accessory muscles of inspiration, namely the scaleni and sternocleidomastoid muscles, then become the quadriplegic patient's respiratory muscles.

These factors as well as the effects of heat, humidity, and the vertical position, all predispose the quadriplegic individual to the development of respiratory muscle weakness and failure. The physical therapist can help avert the effects of respiratory muscle weakness with respiratory muscle training.

Respiratory muscle training with a regimen of progressive resistive breathing has been demonstrated to improve the strength and endurance of respiratory muscles (Gross and King, 1980; Loveridge and Dubo, 1990; Pardy and Leith, 1984) and improve functional capacity in some patients (Reid and Warren, 1984). Resistive breathing exercise is aimed at the prevention of respiratory failure by increasing the strength and particularly endurance of the key muscle of inspiration, the diaphragm. Because the diaphragm is skeletal muscle, it can be reconditioned using a series of inspiratory resistance maneuvers. A stronger, endurance-trained diaphragm will not fatigue as quickly as an untrained diaphragm when exposed to such potentially fatiguing factors as eating a meal, talking, exposure to heat and humidity, sitting upright, overcoming a respiratory tract infection, and so on.

A candidate for respiratory muscle training is equipped with an individual resistive breathing package containing the valve, mouthpiece, noseclip, flow regulator, and a series of resistors that attach to the inspiratory side of the valve (Figure 33-2). It is essential that flow rate is controlled in that patients can negate the training effect of a set resistor by changing flow rate.

An initial pretraining assessment is performed to determine the appropriate resistor with which to commence training. The progression to the next level of resistance is based on specific criteria of endurance on the current resistor. Once the resistor has been chosen, a typical training session includes the steps shown in the box on p. 612.

Maximum inspiratory mouth pressure and vital capacity can be measured routinely to monitor change in diaphragmatic function. The level of inspiratory resistance and the duration for which the patient can use each resistor are indications of the endurance of the inspiratory muscles. Measurement of vital capacity and maximum inspiratory and expiratory mouth pressures provide an index of the strength of the inspiratory muscles.

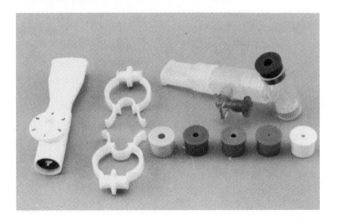

FIGURE 33-2
Handheld resistive breathing training devices. **Left,** P-Flex; resistance level is altered by changing settings on dial. **Right,** DHD device; resistance level is altered by inserting stopper with different size orifice into inspiratory port.

General Steps Involved in Respiratory Muscle Training and Its Prescription

1. The patient is usually in the sitting or upright position for training initially unless sitting is not yet indicated
2. The noseclip is attached snugly
3. The mouthpiece is placed securely in the individual's mouth and allows him or her to select an individual rate and pattern of breathing
4. The patient adjusts flow rate to that designated and maintains it with feedback from the flow regulator
5. Breathing is performed comfortably without force
6. The patient is instructed to stop the exercise by letting go of the valve if the resistance becomes too difficult or if lightheadedness or dizziness occur
7. When the individual has adjusted to the resistance in the initial training position, an attempt can then be made to train at the same load in other positions
8. The parameters of the respiratory muscle training is determined by the patient's baseline; specific parameters of the prescription include initial resistance, the flow rate, the number of repetitions, the number of sets, the frequency of sessions, and progression

---

Modified from Hornstein S: *Ventilatory muscle training. A clinical guide for physiotherapists,* Unpublished manual of the Spinal Cord Injury Unit, Shaughnessy Hospital, 1984, Vancouver, BC.

Certain precautions must be observed with respiratory muscle training. Each time a new resistance is tried, the physical therapist should be with the patient. The patient selects his or her own rate and pattern of breathing. The inspiratory rate is usually constant. Too shallow breathing is inefficient, and too slow, deep breathing may result in accumulation of carbon dioxide. The patient is cautioned about avoiding hyperventilation. The physical therapist, or the patient when he or she is capable, should check the valving system on the respiratory muscle trainer before each training session to ensure it is functioning properly.

PATIENT WITH BURNS
Pathophysiology and medical management

Cardiopulmonary complications are common in patients with smoke inhalation with or without severe burns and are a major cause of death (Marini and Wheeler, 1989). Smoke and chemical inhalation produce edema, bronchospasm, cough, mucosal sloughing, hemorrhage, hoarseness, stridor, and profuse carbonaceous secretions. Irritation of the alveoli and acute pulmonary edema can result in a condition resembling adult respiratory distress syndrome (see Chapter 34). Carbon monoxide poisoning may complicate the clinical picture further and seriously threaten tissue oxygenation (Cahalane and Deming, 1984; Cane, Shapiro, and Davison, 1990). Hemoglobin has a higher affinity for binding with carbon monoxide than oxygen. A carboxyhemoglobin level greater than 20% denotes carbon monoxide poisoning. Levels in excess of 50% may produce irreversible neurological damage. The principal danger of carbon monoxide poisoning is that arterial Pao_2 can be adequate and tissue oxygen tension inadequate. Administration of high levels of oxygen is an initial priority to reduce the half-life of carbon monoxide to 1 hour from several hours.

Depending on the severity and extent of the burns, treatment ranges from conservative medical interventions to multiple surgeries related to progressive debridement and skin grafting. Both second and third degree burns can result in severe disfigurement and disability. Second-degree burns are partial thickness burns and tend to be painful. Third-degree burns are full thickness burns; these tend to be anesthetic in that the nerves themselves have been destroyed. Body positioning to optimize oxygen transport is life-preserving; however, positioning and limb splinting must also be considered from the outset to minimize deformity and restore optimal neuromuscular and musculoskeletal status. Positioning priorities in the burn patients must address both these aspects of management.

Treatment is directed at improving arterial saturation, maintaining fluid balance, and preventing infection. Hypoxemia is effectively treated with the administration of oxygen and maintaining clear airways. If the patient is breathing spontaneously, oxygen is given via nasal cannulae or mask at flows of 1 to 5 L/min, depending on the arterial oxygen saturation. Moisture can be administered through a face tent with a heated nebulizer. Fluid balance is particularly challenging in the burn patient because of the loss of skin, which is essential to the retention and compartmentalization of body fluids and in the regulation of fluid and electrolyte loss from the body. In addition, these patients may lose blood because of injury at the time of the accident. There is also a period without fluid replacement from before the injury to the time medical attention is available and IV fluid resuscitation commenced. Because of the nature of burns, even when fluid resuscitation has begun, fluid and electrolyte balance remains a challenge until considerable healing and repair has occurred. Fluid and electrolyte imbalances have considerable implications for hemodynamics and cardiopulmonary function (see Chapter 15) and contribute to hemodynamic instability, which necessitates modification of the physical therapy management.

An airway may be inserted initially with burns to the face, airway, and lungs in anticipation of progressive edema, which would make the insertion of airway considerably more difficult hours or days later. Ventilatory assistance is indicated with evidence of respiratory insufficiency secondary to smoke inhalation, and burns of the nose, face, throat, airway, lungs, and chest wall. A nasotracheal tube is preferred to a tracheostomy tube because complications with a tracheostomy tube are greater in burn patients.

Cardiopulmonary complications are generally related to sepsis or fluid overload in the initial stage. Acute pulmonary edema and congestion are largely preventable with careful fluid therapy. Central venous pressure can be misleading in the burn patient because of severe fluid loss and may remain at low values despite pulmonary edema. Pulmonary artery pressure more accurately reflects the status of the pulmonary circulation in these patients. Treatment of pulmonary edema consists typically of digitalis, diuretics, and mechanical ventilation. Positive end expiratory pressure is usually indicated in the ventilated burn patient. Mist or aerosol inhalation is also used to reduce the thickness of pulmonary secretions.

On admission of the burn patient to hospital, the patency of the airway is assessed immediately. Inhalation injuries are common in burn patients, resulting from smoke inhalation, heat trauma, and chemical and gas inhalation. Oxygen and humidification are usually administered immediately. Heat may cause laryngeal and bronchial edema. If airway occlusion from impending edema threatens, intubation is performed. If indicated early, intubation may avoid respiratory distress within the critical 24-hour period after admission. Particular care is given to children and older adults with inhalation injury because these patients have a higher risk of developing secondary cardiopulmonary complications.

Complications must be anticipated in the burn patient and prevented (Deming, 1985). These include impaired thermoregulation, hypermetabolism and increased energy expenditure, ileus and gastric distension, pain, and infection. Eschar formation associated with circumferential burns of the chest wall mechanically restricts chest wall movement and can lead to respiratory failure. Tissue edema that can continue for a few days after the burn contributes to increased tissue pressure and impaired tissue perfusion potentiating tissue ischemia and necrosis. Late complications include gastrointestinal bleeding secondary to stress ulceration and the continued high risk of infection.

Principles of physical therapy management

Cardiopulmonary physical therapy is often required immediately for the patient with inhalation damage to maintain the patency of the airways, prevent atelectasis and retention of secretions, and improve or maintain gas exchange. Pulmonary function may be severely impaired as the net result of inhalation damage, burns and trauma to the chest wall, pain and fluid imbalance.

Cardiopulmonary physical therapy often has to be modified in the burn patient (Wright, 1984). Mobilization to enhance oxygen transport is exploited as much as possible, however, because of blood volume and hemodynamic problems, orthostatic intolerance may limit mobilization and positioning alternatives. With more severe burns and more extensive burn distribution, body positioning is the primary intervention. Positioning to effect an optimal therapeutic effect on oxygen transport is challenging because of the significant physical limitations that may exist. Given that body positioning profoundly influences ventilation and perfusion matching (Clauss, Scalabrini, Ray, and Reed, 1968), the reduced number of positioning alternatives will contribute to shunt, ventilation and perfusion mismatch, and hypoxemia. This effect will be accentuated if the patient is mechanically ventilated (see Chapter 32).

Patients who have skin grafts require particular care when moving or positioning because of the danger of sheering forces of the graft, which can disrupt the circulation, nutrition, and healing of the new skin. Sterile procedures must be observed at all times. The physical therapist is usually required to cap, gown, mask, and glove before treating the patient with extensive exposed areas and to cover the chest with a sterile drape. Facilitating mucociliary transport is a priority if the patient has significant mobility and positioning restrictions because of the burn severity. Wherever possible, mobilization in conjunction with multiple body positions and position changes is attempted to maximize mucociliary clearance (Wolff, Dolovich, Obminski, and Newhouse, 1977). If secretions have accumulated, positioning for postural drainage requires the same consideration as positioning for improved alveolar ventilation and ventilation and perfusion matching. In the spontaneously breathing patient, postural drainage positions can be used selectively to increase alveolar volume in the superior lung fields and alveolar ventilation to inferior lung fields, in addition to purposes of drainage of the superior bronchopulmonary segments. However, if the patient is mechanically ventilated, the superior lung fields are preferentially ventilated (see Chapter 32). Should the addition of manual techniques be indicated, percussion may not be comfortably tolerated in the presence of first and second degree burns. Manual vibration may substitute. Manual techniques are con-

traindicated over freshly grafted skin; however, manual vibration may be transmitted from a more distal site to a lung field that cannot be vibrated directly.

Risk of aspiration is increased if tube feedings are not discontinued for at least 1 hour before treatment. A nasogastric tube is often used and should be correctly positioned particularly during treatment.

Stimulating exercise and gravitational stress may initially consist of being in the upright position preferably with the legs dependent, performing selected limb movements and dangling over the edge of the bed for a few minutes if this can be tolerated. however, in patients with severe burns and significant fluid imbalance, active and active-assisted movements in an upright position that can be tolerated, may substitute. As the patient's tolerance increases, free unsupported sitting can progress to standing and walking. Ambulation during ventilator-assisted breathing should always be considered for any patient for whom this activity is not contraindicated. The upright position and physical activity in the upright position are likely to enhance markedly the patient's cardiopulmonary and neuromuscular function, and improve the patient's strength and endurance in preparation for long-term rehabilitation. If sitting up and ambulation are not imminent, appropriate limb movements, preferably active, can help provide an exercise stimulus that can enhance oxygen transport. Passive full range of motion exercises, in addition, are required to maximize joint range (a distinct goal from that to enhance oxygen transport), wherever possible.

Positioning to minimize deformity is a priority given the potential consequences for cardiopulmonary function and oxygen transport, as well as musculoskeletal and biomechanical reasons. Positioning a burn patient regardless of the goal should consider alignment, pressure points, muscle balance, and effect on healing and grafted skin.

Certain precautions have to be observed in the management of the burn patient. First, skin loss contributes to substantial fluid loss, often resulting in labile fluid and electrolyte imbalance. This situation enhances myocardial irritability and the risk of dysrhythmia. Hemodynamic and ECG monitoring is performed routinely during physical therapy treatment. Second, large areas of skin loss increase the risk of infection; therefore the physical therapist must be familiar with sterile technique.

SUMMARY

This chapter describes the principles and practice of physical therapy in the management of cardiopulmonary dysfunction secondary to neuromuscular and musculoskeletal conditions that can lead to cardiopulmonary failure. Categories of conditions included are neuromuscular conditions, musculoskeletal conditions, morbid obesity, head injury, spinal cord injury, and burns. A detailed understanding of the underlying pathophysiology of these conditions and their medical management provides a basis for defining the physical therapy goals and prescribing treatment. The principles described in this chapter cannot be interpreted as treatment prescriptions in that each patient is an individual whose condition reflects multiple factors contributing to impaired oxygen transport or threat to it (i.e., the effects of restricted mobility, recumbency, extrinsic factors related to the patient's care, and intrinsic factors related to the patient in addition to the underlying pathophysiology).

REVIEW QUESTIONS

1. With respect to critically ill patients with the following conditions, describe the pathophysiology of cardiopulmonary dysfunction *secondary to* neuromuscular dysfunction, morbid obesity, musculoskeletal trauma, head injury, spinal cord injury, and burns.
2. Relate cardiopulmonary physical therapy treatment interventions to the underlying pathophysiology of *each* of the above conditions in the critically ill patient and provide the *rationale* for your choice.

References

Alvarez, S.E., Peterson, M., & Lunsford, B.R. (1981). Respiratory treatment of the adult patient with spinal cord injury. *Physical Therapy, 61,* 1737-1745.

Bake, B., Dempsey, J., & Grimby, G. (1976). Effects of shape changes of the chest wall on distribution of inspired gas. *American Review of Respiratory Disease, 114* 1113-1120.

Barach, A.L. (1974). Chronic obstructive lung disease: Postural relief of dyspnea. *Archives of Physical Medicine & Rehabilitation, 55,* 495-504.

Bates, D.V. (1989). *Respiratory function in disease* (3rd ed.). Philadelphia: W.B. Saunders.

Bennett, W.D., Foster, W.M., & Chapman, W.F. (1990). Cough-enhanced mucus clearance in the normal lung. *Journal of Applied Physiology, 69,* 1670-1675.

Bethune, D.D. (1975). Neurophysiological facilitation of respiration in the unconscious adult patient. *Physiotherapy Canada, 27*(5), 241-245.

Black, L.F., & Hyatt, R.E. (1971). Maximal static respiratory pressures in generalized neuromuscular disease. *American Review of Respiratory Diseases, 103,* 641-650.

Borozny, M.L. (1987). Intracranial hypertension: Implications for the physiotherapist. *Physiotherapy Canada, 39,* 360-366.

Braun, S.R., Giovannoni, R., & O'Connor, M. (1984). Improving the cough in patients with spinal cord injury. *American Journal of Physical Medicine, 63,* 1-10.

Cahalane, M., & Deming, R.H. (1984). Early respiratory abnormalities from smoke inhalation. *Journal of the American Medical Association, 25,* 771-773.

Cane, R.D., Shapiro, B.A., & Davison, R. (1990). *Case studies in critical care medicine* (2nd ed.). St. Louis: Mosby.

Clauss, R.H., Scalabrini, B.Y., Ray, J.F., III, & Reed, G.E. (1968). Effects of changing body position upon improved ventilation-perfusion relationships. *Circulation, 37*(Suppl. 4), 214-217.

Cooper, C.B., Trend, P.S., & Wiles, C.M. (1985). Severe diaphragm weakness in multiple sclerosis. *Thorax, 40,* 631-632.

Curran, F.J. (1981). Night ventilation to body respirators for patients in chronic respiratory failure due to late stage muscular dystrophy. *Archives of Physical Medicine and Rehabilitation, 62,* 270-274.

Curran, F.J., & Colbert, A.P. (1989). Ventilator management in Duchenne muscular dystrophy and postpoliomyelitis syndrome: twelve years' experience. *Archives of Physical Medicine and Rehabilitation, 70,* 180-185.

Dean, E. (1985). Effect of body position on pulmonary function. *Physical Therapy, 65,* 613-618.

Dean, E. (1994a). Cardiopulmonary development. In B.R. Bonder & M.B. Wagner. (Eds.). Philadelphia: F.A. Davis.

Dean, E. (1994b). Invited commentary on "Are incentive spirometry, intermittent positive pressure breathing, and deep breathing exercises effective in the prevention of postoperative pulmonary complications after upper abdominal surgery?" A systematic overview and meta-analysis. *Physical Therapy, 74,* 10-15.

Dean, E., Ross, J., Road, J.D., Courtenay, L., & Madill, K. (1991). Pulmonary function in individuals with a history of poliomyelitis. *Chest, 100,* 118-123.

Demling, R.H. (1985). Burns. *New England Journal of Medicine, 31,* 1389-1398.

Demling, R.H. (1980). The pathogenesis of respiratory failure after trauma and sepsis. *Surgical Clinics of North America, 60,* 1373-1390.

Douglas, W.W., Rehder, K., Beynen, F.M., Sessler, A.D., & Marsh, H.M. (1977). Improved oxygenation in patients with acute respiratory failure: The prone position. *American Review of Respiratory Disease, 115*(4), 559-566.

Dureuil, B., Viires, N., & Cantineau, J.P. (1986). Diaphragmatic contractility after upper abdominal surgery. *Journal of Applied Physiology, 61,* 1775-1780.

Estenne, M., & Gorino, M. (1992). Action of the diaphragm during cough in tetrapelgic subjects. *Journal of Applied Physiology, 72,* 1074-1080.

Fugl-Meyer, A.R., & Grimby, G. (1984). Respiration in tetraplegia and in hemiplegia: A review. *International Rehabilitation Medicine, 6,* 186-190.

Griggs, R.C., & Donohoe, K.M. (1982). Recognition and management of respiratory insufficiency in neuromuscular disease. *Journal of Chronic Diseases, 35,* 497-500.

Gross, D. (1980). The effect of training on strength and endurance on the diaphragm in quadriplegia. *American Journal of Medicine, 68,* 27-35.

Gross, D., & King, M. (1984). High frequency chest wall compression: A new non-invasive method of chest physiotherapy for mucociliary clearance. *Physiotherapy Canada, 36,* 137-139.

Hasani, A., Pavia, D., Agnew, J.E., & Clarke, S.W. (1991). The effect of unproductive coughing/FET on regional mucus movement in the human lungs. *Respiratory Medicine, 85,* (Suppl A), 23-26.

Hietpas, B.G., Roth, R.D., & Jensen, W.M. (1979). Huff coughing and airway patency. *Respiratory Care, 24,* 710.

Hornstein, S. (1984). *Ventilatory muscle training. A clinical guide for physiotherapists.* Unpublished manual of the Spinal Cord Injury Unit, Shaughnessy Hospital, Vancouver, B.C.

Kirilloff, L.H., Owens, G.R., Rogers, R.M., & Mazzacco, M. (1985). *Chest, 88,* 436-444.

Lane, D.J., Hazleman, B., & Nichols, P.J.R. (1974). Late onset respiratory failure in patients with previous poliomyelitis. *Quarterly Journal of Medicine, 43,* 551-568.

Leblanc, P., Ruff, F., & Milic-Emili, J. (1970). Effects of age and body position on "airway closure" in man. *Journal of Applied Physiology, 28,* 448-451.

Loveridge, B., & Dubo, H. (1990). Respiratory muscle training in quadriplegic patients. *Archives of Physical Medicine and Rehabilitation.*

Mackenzie, D.F. (Ed.). (1989). *Chest physiotherapy in the intensive care unit* (2nd ed.). Baltimore: Williams & Wilkins.

Mackenzie, C.F., Shin, B., Hadi, F., & Imle, P.C. (1980). Changes in total lung/thorax compliance following chest physiotherapy. *Anesthesia & Analgesia, 59,* 207-210.

Macklem, P.T., & Roussos, C.S. (1977). Respiratory muscle fatigue: A cause of respiratory failure? *Clinical Science & Molecular Medicine, 53,* 419-422.

Malamed, S.F. (1989). *Sedation: A guide to patient management* (2nd ed.). St. Louis: Mosby.

Marini, J.J., & Wheeler, A.P. (1989). *Critical care medicine—The essentials.* Balitmore: Williams & Wilkins.

McAslan, T.C., & Cowley, R.A. (1979). The preventive use of PEEP in major trauma. *American Surgeon, 45,* 159-167.

Moylan, J.A. (Ed.). (1988). *Trauma surgery.* Philadelphia: J.B. Lippincott.

Nunn, J.F., Coleman, A.J., Sachithanandan, T., Bergman, N.A., & Laws, J.W. (1965). Hypoxaemia and atelectasis produced by forced expiration. *British Journal of Anesthesia, 37,* 3-12.

Pardy, R.L., & Leith, D.E. (1984). Ventilatory muscle training. *Respiratory Care, 29,* 278-284.

Petty, T.L. (1982). *Intensive and rehabilitative respiratory care* (3rd ed.). Philadelphia: Lea & Febiger.

Ray, J.F., III, Yost, L., Moallem, S., Sanoudos, G.M., Villamena, P., Paredes, R.M., & Clauss, R.H. (1974). Immobility, hypoxemia, and pulmonary arteriovenous shunting. *Archives of Surgery, 109,* 537-541.

Reid, W.D., & Warren, C.P.W. (1984). Ventilatory muscle strength and endurance training in elderly subjects and patients with chronic airflow limitation: A pilot study. *Physiotherapy Canada, 36,* 305-311.

Ross, J., & Dean, E. (1992). Body positioning. In C. Zadai, (Ed.). *Clinics in physical therapy, pulmonary management in physical therapy.* New York: Churchill Livingstone.

Wolff, R.K., Dolovich, M.B., Obminski, G., & Newhouse, M.T. (1977). Effects of exercise and eucapnic hyperventilation on bronchial clearance in man. *Journal of Applied Physiology, 43,* 46-50.

Wright, P.C. (1984). Fundamentals of acute burn care and physical therapy management. *Physical Therapy, 64,* 1217-1231.

Zinman, R. (1984). Cough versus chest physiotherapy. *American Review of Respiratory Diseases, 129,* 182-184.

CHAPTER 34

Complications, Adult Respiratory Distress Syndrome, Shock, Sepsis, and Multiorgan System Failure

Elizabeth Dean

KEY TERMS
Acute lung injury
Adult respiratory distress syndrome
Multiorgan system failure
Perioperative complications

Respiratory failure
Sepsis
Shock

INTRODUCTION

The purpose of this chapter is to describe some common complications seen in critically ill patients. Complications arising from the following conditions are included: respiratory failure, surgery, acute lung injury and adult respiratory distress syndrome, shock, sepsis, and multiorgan system failure. Second, the implications for cardiopulmonary physical therapy are presented. Complications add further complexity to the diagnosis of the multiple factors contributing to impaired oxygen transport and to the challenge of prescribing effective treatment. Understanding the patho-

physiological deficits in these complex conditions is the basis for efficacious management in addition to reducing the risk of an untoward treatment response and preventing worsening the patient's condition.

RESPIRATORY FAILURE

Metabolical Dysfunction

The range of complications associated with respiratory failure that can further impair tissue oxygenation are described in the box on p. 619. The metabolical consequences of these complications and impairment of oxygen transport are life threatening for the patient. Thus prevention of their development is a priority. Should complications develop, however, early detection and definitive management becomes the priority if the patient is to survive.

A hallmark of these complications is the impairment of multiple steps in the oxygen transport pathway, which adds to the complexity of management (Dantzker, 1991). The three major components of oxygen transport can be affected individually or in combination (i.e., oxygen delivery, consumption, and extraction) (Pallares and Evans, 1992; Wysocki, Besbes, Roupie, and Brun-Buisson, 1992).

In health the ratio of oxygen consumption to delivery is low (i.e., 23%, which ensures an over supply of oxygen as a safety margin) (see Chapter 1). This safety margin also ensures that most patients are able to recover from insults to the oxygen transport system. However, if the insult is extreme, such as that resulting from complications of respiratory failure, surgery, acute lung injury and adult respiratory distress syndrome, shock, sepsis, and multiorgan system failure, significant metabolical dysfunction secondary to tissue hypoxia can result (Guiterrez, 1991).

The relationship between oxygen consumption and delivery has elucidated our understanding of hemodynamic and metabolical changes observed in critical illness (Vincent, 1991). The phenomenon of oxygen-delivery dependence of oxygen consumption occurs when a patient's oxygen transport system is unable to supply sufficient oxygen to meet basal oxygen demand (Phang and Russell, 1993). Oxygen delivery below 300 ml O_2/min/M^2 limits the oxygen diffusion gradient and reduces oxygen extraction and utilization at the cellular level. This is termed the *critical level of oxygen delivery*. When oxygen delivery exceeds 300 ml/min/M^2, oxygen consumption does not depend on delivery. Thus the greater the delivery in relation to consumption the greater the safety margin. When oxygen transport is so severely compromised that oxygen delivery falls below the critical level, anaerobic metabolism is triggered. However, anaerobic metabolism may also be triggered at levels of oxygen delivery that exceed the normal critical threshold for anaerobic metabolism

(Fenwick, Dodek, Ronco, Phang, Wiggs, and Russell, 1990). This so-called pathological dependence of oxygen consumption on oxygen delivery occurs when the cells are inadequately extracting and using oxygen even in the presence of supranormal oxygen delivery levels. This phenomenon is observed in patient with adult respiratory distress syndrome and shock (discussed later this chapter).

Given physical therapy is one of the most metabolically demanding ICU interventions (Dean, Murphy, Parrent, and Rousseau, 1995; Weissman and Kemper, 1993), the physical therapist needs to be able to calculate this safety margin to prescribe the type of treatment and its parameters (i.e., intensity, duration and frequency) such that treatment is maximally beneficial and associated with the least risk to the patient.

The ultimate treatment outcome measures are markers of oxygen tissue metabolism (Dantzker, 1993; Nightingale, 1993; Pallares and Evans, 1992). In addition, hourly assessment of oxygen delivery, consumption, and extraction provide the basis for directing management of oxygen transport deficits.

Pulmonary Dysfunction

Complications of the cardiopulmonary system can lead to respiratory failure (see box on p. 619) (Boggs and Wooldridge-King, 1993; Civetta, Taylor, and Kirby, 1988). Some of these relate to being mechanically ventilated. Certain technical problems related to the cuffs used in conjunction with artificial airways may occur (e.g., overinflation, distortion, and herniation of the orifice of the tube). Mucous plugs can occlude the endotracheal tube or tracheostomy and impede ventilation. The common complications can be reduced if the tube is changed frequently and if minimal amounts of air are used for cuff inflation.

Prolonged endotracheal intubation can result in laryngeal edema, ulceration, and fibrosis. Mechanical ventilation may also rupture a bleb on the surface of the lung and produce a pneumothorax with rapid tension development. Chest tubes are inserted immediately to relieve the tension. Blebs occur when alveoli rupture, causing air to track to subpleural sites.

Mechanical ventilators can be a source of infection.

Complications of Respiratory Failure
Life-threatening impairment of oxygen transport and tissue oxygenation
Fluid and electrolyte imbalances
Cardiac dysrhythmias and hemodynamic instability
Myocardial dysfunction
Metabolical dysfunction
Thromboembolism
Neurological dysfunction
Gastrointestinal dysfunction
Renal dysfunction
Metabolical and blood sugar irregularities
Infection
Nutritional deficits
Complications of intubation and mechanical ventilation, including increased risk of infection
Complications of oxygen therapy

The physical therapist can help minimize this risk by not directly handling the ventilator attachments that communicate with the air flow channels. Condensation from the hose should not be drained toward the ventilator or toward the patient. The physical therapist should be masked and gloved when connecting and disconnecting the patient to and from the ventilator.

Oxygen toxicity is a significant clinical complication of mechanical ventilation. Mechanical ventilators have precise oxygen controls to deliver the lowest possible inspired oxygen concentration needed to maintain arterial oxygen tensions. Because of the iatrogenic complications of high FIo_2 levels (i.e., denitrogen atelectasis and oxygen toxicity) excess oxygen above the patient's needs is never indicated other than short periods of hyperoxygenation before suctioning or in preparation for, during, and immediately after mobilization (Fell and Cheney, 1971; Shoemaker, 1984).

Flow-directed pulmonary artery catheters (i.e., Swan-Ganz catheters), commonly used in the intensive care unit (ICU) for monitoring patients who develop hemodynamic complications, are also associated with some complications (see Chapter 15). Infection may lead to bacteremia and septicemia. Judicious selection and application of any invasive procedure is warranted to minimize undue hazard. The presence of these catheters limits head and neck positions and requires mobilization be carried out cautiously within the patient's hemodynamic tolerance.

Acid-Base Abnormalities

Any combination of acid-base imbalance may occur either acutely or chronically during respiratory failure. Severe alkalemia associated with potassium and chloride losses may occur after mechanical ventilation and can precipitate serious cardiovascular and neurological complications (see Chapter 15) (Petty, 1982). Significantly impaired oxygen delivery to peripheral tissue may contribute to increased anaerobic metabolism and metabolic acidosis (Fenwick, Dodek, Ronco, Phang, Wiggs, and Russell, 1990).

Fluid and Electrolyte Abnormalities

Fluid retention can occur with prolonged mechanical ventilation in a patient with no evidence of cardiac failure. Pulmonary edema, weight gain, decreased pulmonary compliance, and reduced oxygen transport are common signs. Fluid overload is a common cause of this fluid retention. Mechanically ventilated patients are therefore usually maintained underhydrated. Because of a tendency for sodium retention and hence fluid retention, intravenous saline solution is kept to a minimum. Humidifiers attached to mechanical ventilators are responsible for adding a considerable amount of water by absorption through the lungs.

Cardiac Dysrhythmias

Cardiac dysrhythmias are a common complication of respiratory failure. In addition, patients in respiratory failure tend to be older adults who as a group have a greater incidnce of dysrhythmias secondary to cardiac disease. Electrocardiographic monitoring is therefore essential for all patients requiring ventilatory assistance in addition to patients with overt or suspected heart disease. Both atrial and ventricular tachydysrhythmias are seen in acute respiratory failure. Sinus tachycardia and premature ventricular contractions, however, are particularly common. With rapid lowering of arterial P_{CO_2}, ventricular fibrillation, or even death may occur.

In the presence of respiratory failure and in the absence of cardiac disease the management of cardiac dysrhythmias lies predominantly in the correction of blood-gas abnormalities. Effective supportive management can usually be achieved with pharmaceutical agents. Intravenous injection of lidocaine followed by continuous infusion is useful in managing premature ventricular contractions, which may be the precursor of potentially fatal tachydysrhythmias and cardiac arrest. Electrolyte replacement may also be required.

A thorough understanding of the clinical presentation, electrocardiographic diagnosis, and correct management of cardiac dysrhythmias is fundamental to the optimization of physical therapy treatments in the ICU and minimizing any risk to the patient. Cardiac dysrhythmias resulting from any cause necessarily require ongoing evaluation and therapy.

The physical therapist must be able to treat the patient optimally and safely within the restrictions of any dysrhythmia in addition to other medical or surgical conditions. The implications of the dysrhythmia on the patient's clinical presentation and for treatment selection and response must be recognized by the physical therapist and considered in designing the treatment plan.

Thromboembolism

A high incidence of pulmonary thrombosis or embolism exists in patients in acute respiratory failure. Early diagnosis and management of pulmonary thromboembolism have been greatly facilitated by the use of serial ultrasound procedures and scans. Physical therapy has a key role in preventing the development of thromboemboli by promoting frequent changes in position, specific bed exercises, particularly of the lower limbs, and passive range of motion exercises if indicated. It is essential that movement and repositioning are performed regularly to maximize their cardiopulmonary protective benefits. Pneumatic extremity cuffs apply pressure intermittently over the lower legs to minimize venous pooling and assist venous return (see Chapter 32). JOBST® and TED® stockings also may be applied over the feet and legs to increase circulatory transit time in the dependent areas and reduce circulatory stasis.

Myocardial Dysfunction

As in any clinical situation, acute myocardial infarction can occur during the management of acute respiratory failure. The risks are increased because patients in respiratory failure tend to be older and more susceptible to positional hypoxemia. The probability of heart failure and associated dysrhythmias is increased and significantly compounds the problems of the patient in respiratory failure.

Gastrointestinal Dysfunction

Peptic ulcer is commonly associated with chronic airway obstruction. The stress of respiratory failure predisposes the patient to peptic ulceration. Profound hemorrhage may occur and blood replacement is necessitated.

Gastric dilation may occur in patients who are receiving mechanical ventilation. Gastric dilation is best managed by means of a nasogastric tube and intermittent suction. Care must be exercised to avoid hypokalemia and hypochloremia caused by excessive gastric suctioning. Special care is also taken to avoid fecal impaction, particularly in the paralyzed patient. This risk can be reduced with suitable fluid balance, mobilization, frequent turning in conjunction with appropriate trunk and lower limb movements.

Neurological Dysfunction

A close correlation exists between the state of consciousness and the arterial P_{O_2} and P_{CO_2}. In addition, changes occur in alertness, personality, memory, and orientation with altered blood gases. Motor changes also occur, including generalized or localized weakness, tremors, twitching, myoclonic jerks, gross clonic movements, convulsions, and flaccidity. Neurological complications of respiratory failure must be differentiated from those of nonpulmonary origin.

The physical therapist must be aware of the spectrum of neurological complications that can result from respiratory failure and recognize that apparent improvement of neurological signs may reflect improved cardiopulmonary status.

Renal Dysfunction

The development of renal failure greatly compromises the chances of the patient's survival. Renal failure can result from gastrointestinal bleeding, sepsis associated with shock, drug-induced nephrotoxicity, and hypotension. Urinary outputs are maintained with adequate fluid and diuretics, with care not to induce pulmonary edema. Dialysis may need to be instituted if more conservative management fails (Phipps, Long, and Woods, 1991). If dialysis is anticipated, the physical therapist should review existing treatment goals to modify treatment accordingly.

POSTOPERATIVE COMPLICATIONS

Pathophysiology and medical management

Respiratory failure in the postoperative patient is usually associated with a low Pao_2 and a high $Paco_2$. This situation is likely to be more common than generally appreciated. If the patient is in good general health and is free from underlying cardiopulmonary disease, recovery is usually rapid. Otherwise, more severe complications and cardiopulmonary failure may result and progress to a life-threatening situation. The effects of surgery on oxygen transport and on the various organ systems are described in Chapter 28. Common postoperative complications and their causes appear in the box at right and the box on p. 622.

Hypoxemia

The most common postoperative complication is hypoxemia secondary to alveolar hypoventilation, reduced functional residual capacity (FRC), airway closure, and postsurgical atelectasis (Leblanc, Ruff, and Milic-Emili, 1970; Marini, 1984; Ray et al., 1974). Adequate oxygenation, however, can be present despite hypoventilation when oxygen is being administered. The presence or absence of cyanosis may be an unreliable sign because peripheral cyanosis can occur despite adequate arterial Po_2. Morbidity and mortality has been reported to be reduced in patients with severe respiratory failure and system involvement when supranormal levels of oxygen delivery was achieved (Hayes, Yau, Timmins, Hinds, and Watson, 1993; Waxman and Shoemaker, 1980; Yu, Levy, Smith, Takiguchi, Miyasaki, and Myers, 1993).

Common Postoperative Complications
Hypoxemia
Hypercapnia
Increased work of breathing
Increased work of the heart
Fluid shifts and third spacing
Fluid and electrolyte imbalances
Metabolic and blood sugar abnormalities
Reduced blood volume
Cardiac dysrhythmias
Reduced cardiac output
Reduced tissue perfusion and oxygenation
Anemia
Pain
Alveolar hypoventilation
Airway collapse
Atelectasis
Physiological shunting
Ventilation and perfusion mismatching
Impaired mucociliary transport
Mucus accumulation and stasis
Pneumonia
Thromboemboli
Pulmonary embolus
Coagulopathies
Sepsis
Shock
Multiorgan system failure

Factors Contributing to Postoperative Complications That Affect Oxygen Transport

Premorbid cardiopulmonary status

Premorbid oxygen transport (aerobic) capacity

Premorbid systemic disease

Premorbid general health and immune status

Smoking history

Age and gender

Lifestyle factors—nutritional status, stress, work situation, family situation, psychosocial support system, and substance abuse

Obesity

Pregnancy

Perioperative pain and anxiety

Perioperative reduced arousal

Perioperative reduced mobility

Perioperative recumbency

Perioperative medications (e.g., narcotics)

Perioperative nutritional deprivation

Perioperative reduction in normal sleep quality and quantity

Type of surgery

Extent of physical manipulation and compression of lung parenchyma, phrenic nerves, diaphragm, and the heart

Perioperative fever and increased oxygen consumptions

Duration of surgery

Position assumed during surgery

Duration of static positioning during surgery

Type, depth, and duration of anesthesia and sedation

Use of an airway

Use of mechanical ventilation

Oxygen therapy

Neuromuscular blockade

Fluid loss and chest tube drainage

Fluid accumulation and third spacing

Infusion of blood products

Site, number, and extent of incisions

Dressings and binders

Traction and splinting devices

Placement of lines, leads, catheters, and monitoring devices

Invasive monitoring equipment (e.g., Swan-Ganz catheter, Foley catheter, intracranial pressure monitor, central venous line, arterial lines, intravenous lines, and intraaortic balloon counter pulsation pump)

Need for cardiopulmonary bypass machine

Duration on cardiopulmonary bypass machine

Infection

Pain

Pain, in addition to the effects of anesthesia, frequently contributes to alveolar hypoventilation and atelectasis after abdominal or thoracic surgery. Rapid, shallow, and monotonous breathing may be spontaneously adopted by the patient to avoid pain and coughing. Although minute ventilation is favored, alveolar ventilation is compromised by the increased ratio of dead space to tidal volume. Furthermore, in the absence of deep breaths, coughs, and sighs, atelectasis may develop in the underventilated portions of the lungs. The ventilation-perfusion ratio is disturbed because blood flow to underventilated lung segments is ineffective, physiological shunting occurs, and arterial Po_2 tends to drop although Pco_2 may be unchanged. An abnormally high transpulmonary pressure is then needed to reinflate these atelectatic alveoli.

Pulmonary Embolism and Deep Vein Thrombosis

Pulmonary embolism is a potentially life-threatening complication. Pulmonary embolism usually results from a thrombus forming in the veins of the lower limbs, pelvis, in the right atrium, or in the right ventricle. Patients may be at risk if they have varicose veins, chronic heart failure or if they are obese, pregnant, or taking oral contraceptives.

The patient with a pulmonary thromboembolism usually has a sudden onset of tachypnea, radiating chest pain, and apparent anxiety. Occasionally, right heart failure follows. Enzymes are often elevated. Right heart strain may be evidenced on ECG. Right bundle branch block, peaked P waves, and inverted T waves may be seen. No abnormality may be noted on chest x-ray.

Treatment consists of primary ventilatory and circulatory support, with adequate oxygenation of peripheral tissues. Anticoagulants, such as heparin, are infused intravenously to minimize further formation of thromboembolic substrates.

Principles of physical therapy management

Significant impairment of lung volume, mechanics, and gas exchange uniformly occur after anesthesia and tissue dissection. The extent and duration of these changes increase with the magnitude of the operative procedure and degree of anesthesia required and the patient's premorbid risk factors. These abnormalities observed in the postoperative period are characterized by gradual and progressive alveolar collapse. Total lung capacity, FRC, and residual volume are significantly decreased in patients who develop complications. Because of the significant decrease in FRC (30% or more), compliance is decreased, and therefore the work of breathing is increased. Hypoxemia secondary to transpulmonary shunting usually becomes maximal within 72 hours after surgery, and often is completely resolved with conservative management within seven days. The Fio_2 will depend on the mode of 100% oxygen administration. Low oxygen flows and low amounts of Fio_2 tend to be delivered via nasal cannulae. Higher flows can deliver higher amounts of Fio_2 via oxygen masks and masks with reservoir bags. The Fio_2 must always be taken into account when interpreting arterial blood gases. The Fio_2 is selected to provide adequate oxygenation with the lowest oxygen concentration possible.

Based on the patients' assessment, arterial blood gases, fluid and electrolyte balance, hemodynamic status, and x-ray, a decision is made as to which treatments on the physiological hierarchy will optimize oxygen transport and what parameters will be used for each treatment. Positioning these patients upright and mobilizing them wherever possible will maximize FRC and reduce closing volumes and hence enhance gas exchange and oxygenation. What precludes mobilizing these patients even minimally is their lack of alertness which must be explained. If the patient is unable to respond to treatment because of narcotics, for example, this can be discussed at rounds and other medications should be considered so that the patient is able to cooperate more. Thus even extreme body positioning will achieve more favorable results (Barlett, Gazzaniga, and Geraghty (1973; Clauss, Scalabrini, Ray, and Reed, 1968; Douglas, Rehder, Beynen, Sessler, and Marsh, 1977; Piehl and Brown, 1976).

Endotracheal intubation and mechanical ventilation may be indicated if blood gases fail to improve with conservative management. The treatment priorities for the ventilated patient before and during weaning are presented in Chapter 32. Special attention in the postoperative patient is given to the pulmonary complications associated with diminished ability to move spontaneously, surgical pain, restrictions imposed by dressings and binders, diminished ability to cooperate, and to periodically hyperventilate the lungs.

Facilitating mucociliary transport is a primary goal in these patients. Impaired mucociliary transport can be precipitated by alveolar hypoventilation, perhaps the most common cause of postoperative complications. Sufficient impairment can lead to mucous stasis, airway obstruction, atelectasis, and infection. Multiple positions, including upright positions and 360-degree axial turns, and multiple position changes facilitates mucociliary transport. In the event of mucous accumulation and difficulty in removing pulmonary secretions, specific body positions are selected to optimize postural drainage of the affected bronchopulmonary segments and to maximize alveolar volume and ventilation. The addition of manual techniques can be detrimental in severely ill patients (Mackenzie, 1989; Poelaert, Lannoy, Vogelaers, Everaert, Decruyenaere, Capiau, and Colardyn, 1991), thus their use needs to be considered carefully.

Suctioning may be most effective immediately before and after position changes. The appropriate oxygen transport variables are monitored to assess treatment outcome and minimally to ensure the patient who may be unstable is not deteriorating. If the patient begins to deteriorate, treatment is discontinued until the patient stabilizes. Why the patient deteriorated is determined so that a decision can be made as to whether treatment can be reintroduced, and if so, what modifications are indicated.

Pain management is integral to the management of the surgical patient. Noninvasive and nonpharmacological pain control strategies need to be exploited for all surgical patients to augment or reduce the need for potent analgesics especially narcotics. Chapter 28 described some physical therapy pain control strategies for surgical patients that can be applied with modification to the patient with surgical complications. Of these, use of electrotherapy modalities, such as transcutaneous electrical nerve stimulation, may be limited in the ICU because of electrical interference with monitoring devices.

Rest is prescribed as judiciously as treatment interventions to enable the patient to physiologically restore between and within treatments. This is particularly important for ICU patients who are hypermetabolical and have increased oxygen demands. Particular care must be observed in prescribing treatment threshold parameters for these patients. Suprathreshold states can be associated with an inappropriate balance between oxygen delivery and oxygen consumption such that the patient becomes compromised (e.g., hemodynamically unstable, cardiopulmonary distress is precipitated, or both). A greater volume of a mobilization stimulus, however, may be delivered to these patients with an intermittent mobilization regimen than with a single prolonged course of mobilization. Thus the benefits that would be accrued would be correspondingly increased.

Prevention of thromboemboli is a major treatment objective and is best achieved with mobilization, body positioning, passive movements, and physical devices, such as pneumatic cuff devices and stockings, to augment low-dose anticoagulants in patients at risk. Patients who develop pulmonary emboli are treated medically and physical therapy needs to be correspondingly modified to minimize oxygen consumption until the embolus resolves and the patient is in no imminent danger.

ACUTE LUNG INJURY AND ADULT RESPIRATORY DISTRESS SYNDROME

Acute lung injury results from damage to the alveolar epithelium (Gattinoni et al., 1994). The extent of the damage reflects damage to the type I and type II alveolar cells. Damage to the type I cells results in alveolar edema, atelectasis, and loss of lung compliance secondary to loss of structural integrity of the alveoli provided by the type I alveolar cells. Damage to the type II cells also contributes to atelectasis and loss of lung compliance, but the mechanism relates to impairment of the production of surfactant and pulmonary fluid that covers the alveolar epithelium.

Pulmonary edema refers to the accumulation of vascular fluid in the interstitial spaces and alveoli. In acute lung injury the mechanism of pulmonary edema involves increased water movement across the pulmonary endothelial cells and increased permeability of the endothelium to protein. This type of pulmonary edema is referred to as *noncardiogenic pulmonary edema.* Pulmonary edema that is cardiogenic in origin results from left ventricular failure. An increase in hydrostatic pressure damages the interstitial tight spaces, which normally provide an effective barrier between the pulmonary circulation and alveoli. The critical distinction between the two types of pulmonary edema is that cardiogenic pulmonary edema primarily involves the movement of water across the alveolar capillary membrane, whereas noncardiogenic pulmonary edema involves the movement of protein and water into the interstitial and alveolar spaces. The clinical consequences reflect the location of the edema (i.e., interstitial, alveolar or both) and the amount of fluid accumulation.

Acute lung injury is characterized as a clinical spectrum of parenchymal cell dysfunction. Mild injury reflects predominantly endothelial cell dysfunction and noncardiogenic edema. Severe injury reflects a progression to both endothelial and epithelial cell dysfunction and adult respiratory distress syndrome (ARDS). The clinical spectrum of acute lung injury and the clinical manifestations of mild and severe injury are shown in Figure 34-1. The clinical presentation of moderate injury falls between these two extremes.

ARDS results from major insult to the lung and injury to the alveolar-capillary membrane. Some of the causes of ARDS include shock, severe trauma or infection, overwhelming pneumonia, and inhaled toxins. Increased vascular permeability resembling that of the inflammatory response is a common feature.

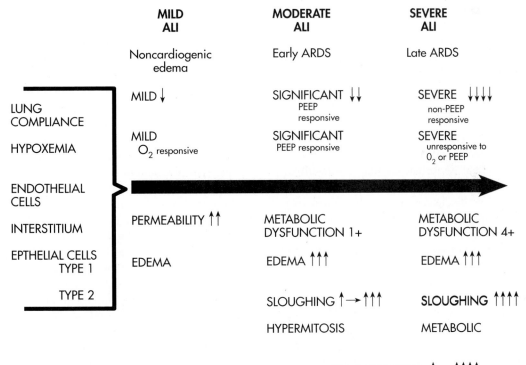

FIGURE 34-1
Major pathophysiologic manifestations comprising the spectrum of acute lung injury from mild to severe disease. (From Shapiro BA, Peruzzi WT: Changing practices inventilatator management: a review of the literature and suggest clinical correlates, *Surgery* 117:121–133, 1991.)

Fluid seeps into the interstitial spaces and overwhelms the alveoli, leading to pulmonary edema. Lung compliance and gas exchange are severely compromised. Thus the patient presents with severe dyspnea and hypoxemia. Diffuse pulmonary infiltrates appear on x-ray. Arterial hypoxemia results primarily from underventilated but perfused lung units and right to left shunt. In this situation, hypoxemia is relatively refractory to increases in FIo_2.

Fibrinogen in the fluids leaking into the alveoli contributes to fibrosis and reduction of lung compliance associated with ARDS. Increased lung surface tension and alveolar collapse tend to result from an inactivation of surfactant with the accumulation of fluid in the alveolar spaces. Thus reduced lung compliance produces a significant decrease in FRC in the patient with ARDS.

The signs and symptoms of ARDS may take up to 48 hours to be fully manifested. The prognosis for survival of patients is 40% to 60%. Hypoxemia is a principal feature of the syndrome, and results from a right to left shunt, whereby fluid-filled alveoli are ineffectively ventilated. Hyperventilation and labored respiration can be expected in conjunction with hypoxemia. Oxygen therapy has little effect in the presence of shunting. Hypercapnia is not usually a major problem in the ARDS patient.

The metabolical perturbations that can result include problems with oxygen delivery, consumption, and extraction as discussed previously. When oxygen delivery falls below the critical level, anaerobic metabolism is triggered resulting in increased lactate production. Elevated serum lactates are associated with a poor prognosis.

Principles of physical therapy management

Intubation and ventilatory support are implemented if arterial blood gases are severely affected and rerspiratory distress worsened. An endotracheal tube can be placed through the nose or mouth or a tracheostomy can be performed. The tidal volume is set at about 10 ml/kg of the patient's body weight. The patient usually establishes the respiratory rate, although it may be rapid. A positive end expiratory pressure (PEEP) of around 12 cm H_2O maintains the alveoli open and thereby optimizes gas transfer at end-expiration. Arterial oxygenation is usually improved with PEEP because the effect of shunting is reduced and a given FIo_2 tends to be more effective. Although the FIo_2 may be reduced, which reduces the possibility of oxygen toxicity, supranormal oxygen delivery can be beneficial in these patients (Bishop et al., 1993). Survival may be improved and frequency of multiorgan system failure reduced.

Further monitoring of respiratory status in conjunction with arterial blood gases is essential for following the progress of the syndrome. In addition to the oxygen transport variables the principal parameters monitored in ARDS are reduced lung compliance, tachypnea, and the concentration of inspired oxygen needed to maintain acceptable levels of the arterial blood gases.

ARDS is characterized by a major pathophysiological restrictive component. Hence the principles of management of restrictive lung disease can be effectively applied. Changes in lung compliance and FIo_2 requirements provide guidelines to treatment required, treatment response, and course of the syndrome. Patients with ARDS require close monitoring and often frequent treatments aimed at promoting optimal gas exchange because of the severity of the syndrome and high incidence of mortality associated with it. Special attention is given to body positioning to promote ventilation and perfusion matching and mucociliary transport and to minimize the effect of restriction of diaphragmatic and chest wall excursion. Some patients, for example, benefit from side lying in which excursion of the inferior hemidiaphragm is favored. Other patients, however, seem to deteriorate from apparent restriction of the inferior lung in side lying. Each patient's condition and specific areas of lung involvement must be taken into consideration when prescribing a turning regimen. The effect of the patient's body position on blood gases helps to establish a suitable regimen on a rational basis.

The sitting position optimizes lung capacity. The use of a reclining chair at the bedside perhaps should be considered more often in the management of patients with acute lung injury. Theoretically, the potential function of all lung fields will be benefited with the lungs in a more upright position. Patients who are too unstable to tolerate upright positions may respond favorably to extreme body positions and the prone position (Albert, Leasa, Sanderson, Robertson, and Hlastala, 1987; Langer, Mascheroni, Marcolin, and Gattinoni, 1988).

Severely affected patients may require neuromuscular blockade to reduce their oxygen demand and enable them to respond to ventilatory assistance more effectively. Handling and positioning patients on neuromuscular blockade requires particular care because these patients lack muscle tone to protect their muscles and joints. Rotating beds can be extremely beneficial for these patients who are either too hemodynamically unstable or difficult to turn manually. These mechanical beds slowly rotate side to side through an arc, thus changing the patient's body position continuously (Gentilello et al., 1988; Pape, Regel, Borgman, Sturm, and Tacherne, 1994).

SHOCK

Common causes of shock include hypovolemia, septicemia, heart failure, and direct insult to the central nervous system. Some of the classical features of shock are hypotension, reduced cardiac output, tachycardia, hyperventilation, diaphoresis, pallor, confusion, nausea, and incontinence. Inadequate tissue perfusion results in extracellular acidemia and loss of potassium ions from the cells. The pulmonary blood vessels constrict in response to hypoxemia, which tends to increase pulmonary artery pressures.

Failure of cellular function secondary to shock can result from a deficiency of substrate for energy production, a reduced ability to use the nutrients for energy production, or both. The pathophysiological mechanisms responsible include hypoperfusion of the tissues, hormonal and metabolical cellular changes, and the toxic effects of the metabolical changes. Collectively, these produce cellular damage. With hypoperfusion and decreased oxygen delivery and other nutrients, the production of adenosine triphosphate is reduced. The maintenance and repair of cell membranes is disrupted, resulting in swelling of the endoplasmic reticular and eventually the mitochondria. Persisting cellular hypoxia contributes to rupture of the lysosomes, which releases enzymes that con-

tribute to intracellular digestion and calcium deposition. Once the lysosomes have ruptured and intracellular digestion is triggered, irreversible cell damage ensues, impairing oxygen extraction and uptake (Wysocki, Besbes, Roupie, and Brun-Buisson, 1992).

The pathology of shock and the effect on the respiratory membranes of the mitochondria follow a similar course regardless of cause. Swelling of the interstitial tissue disrupts the perfusion of the pulmonary capillaries. Congestive atelectasis and pulmonary edema ensue. In the advanced stages, hyaline membrane changes and pneumonitis may occur.

Principles of physical therapy management

Foremost, the physical therapist must be knowledgeable about the relationship of oxygen delivery and consumption in these patients, as well as the implications of the pathophysiological processes on oxygen extraction. The type of treatments and their parameters are based on a careful analysis of oxygen transport variables. Treatments are prescribed within the patient's safety margin. Physical therapists in the ICU must also be knowledgeable about the signs and symptoms associated with impending and frank shock. By recognizing and understanding the components of the different types of shock and the effect on the cardiopulmonary system, the physical therapist can better prescribe a rational treatment plan for the short- and long-term management of the patient.

Although physical therapy may be limited in reversing the signs and symptoms of shock, physical therapy can help to restore and maintain optimal cardiopulmonary function, reduce the risk of complications associated with immobility and with recumbency, and maintain physical status at the best possible optimal level during the episode and in anticipation of the patient's recovery. The primary objective, however, is to minimize oxygen demand. A minimal objective is not to worsen the patient's condition by imposing excessive metabolical demand. This is the case in patients whose oxygen delivery is approaching the critical level with respect to oxygen consumption dependence. Excessive demands in these patients can be life threatening.

Patients in shock are usually unresponsive. The

course of the shock episode is often complicated with the sequelae of immobility and recumbency. The specific goals related to optimization of cardiopulmonary and musculoskeletal function and prevention of further complications associated with cardiopulmonary function in particular are priorities.

Specific concerns for the patient in shock include the need for short, efficacious treatments and avoidance of unnecessary fatiguing of the patient. Treatment goals are therefore critically appraised and prioritized throughout each day to target physical therapy treatment only to the very immediate and essential needs of the patients. Prudent patient positioning is a priority because of the relative immobility and reduced spontaneous movement observed in these patients and recumbency. Approximations to the upright position (i.e., head of bed up and foot of bed down) can augment sympathetic stimulation and improve hemodynamic status and reduce sympathomimetic medications. In addition, this position simulates the upright sitting position (although not perfectly) with respect to its beneficial effects on pulmonary and cardiac function.

Late stages of refractory shock leading to renal failure may necessitate dialysis. In peritoneal dialysis a liter of fluid with a high osmotic fluid content is injected into the patient's abdomen to draw fluid out. The fluid is drained after about 30 minutes. Cardiopulmonary physical therapy is most effective if performed after the fluid has been completely drained from the peritoneum. After drainage of the fluid the diaphragm is at a more optimal functional length for respiration, which potentially can improve treatment response. If hemodialysis is indicated, the patient is connected to a unit that dialyzes the blood externally. This process takes several hours and is usually repeated every few days.

In the end stages of shock, as for other severely ill medically unstable patients, physical therapy may constitute primarily supportive care and comprehensive monitoring.

SEPSIS AND MULTIORGAN SYSTEM FAILURE

Sepsis is the response to bacteremia or other by products of bacteria in the blood. The clinical features of sepsis include fever, tachycardia, tachypnea, and respiratory alkalemia. Metabolical abnormalities are also a common feature of sepsis. Sepsis is the most common predisposing factor contributing to multiorgan system failure (MOSF), which typically involves failure of more than two organ systems (Carrico, Meakins, and Marshall, 1993; Vincent, 1993). Table 34-1 shows the major organs affected and their clini-

TABLE 34-1		
Presentation of Multiorgan System Failure		
ORGAN	**CLINICAL PRESENTATION**	**SYNDROME**
Lungs	Hypoxemia, lung compliance, diffuse infiltrates	Acute lung injury/ARDS
Kidneys	Creatine > 2 mg/dl	
	Urine output < 500 ml/24 hr	Oliguric ARF
	Urine output > 500 ml/24 hr	Nonoliguric ARF
Liver	Bilirubin 2 mg/dl, SGOT and LDH	Jaundice
	Intractible hyperglycemia or hypoglycemia	Hepatocyte failure
	Cholecystitis	Acalculous cholecystitis
Gut	Upper gastrointestinal bleed	Stress ulceration
Coagulation	Thrombocytopenia, prolonged PT and PTT	Hypofibrinogenemia DIC
Heart	Hypotension, CI	Heart failure
CNS	Response only to painful stimuli	Obtundation

Modified from Civetta, J.M., Taylor, R.W., & Kirby, R.R. (1988). Critical care. Philadelphia: JB Lippincott.

ARF, acute renal failure; *SGOT,* serum glutamic oxaloacetic transaminase; *LDH,* lactate, dehydrogenase; *DIC,* disseminating intravascular coagulation; *PT,* prothrombin time; *PTT,* partial prothrombin time; *CI,* cardiac index

cal manifestations (i.e., pulmonary, gastrointestinal, hepatic, renal, cardiovascular, hematological, and central nervous systems). The cascade of pathophysiological features of this MOSF is believed to be precipitated by multiple mediator systems. The release of these mediators impairs oxygen delivery and utilization of oxygen by the cells. Thus the supply of the major energy source to the cell, adenosine triphosphate, is reduced which leads to structural and functional damage of the various organ systems. The mortality rate ranges from 60% to 80%.

Conditions that predispose a patient to MOSF include sepsis, overwhelming infection, multiple trauma and tissue injury, inflammation, and tissue perfusion deficits. Patients who are older, have chronic diseases, are immunosuppressed or have a severe initial presentation have an increased risk of failure and mortality.

Principles of physical therapy management

The patient with sepsis and MOSF, like the patient in shock, is gravely ill and unlikely to be able to cooperate with treatment. The principles for management are comparable with those for managing the patient in shock, however, oxygen delivery is likely to be consistently compromised in these patients. If oxygen delivery is critically low, oxygen consumption depends on oxygen delivery and the patient is in a state of metabolical acidosis (see Chapter 1). In this situation, where oxygen delivery is compromised to the point of not meeting tissue oxygen demands, the goal of treatment is to maximize oxygen delivery (Bishop et al., 1993; Yu, Levy, Smith, Takiguchi, Miyasaki, and Myers, 1993) and minimize oxygen demand so that oxygenation of vital organs is threatened to the least extent. Thus the physical therapist must estimate the oxygen reserve capacity (i.e., the balance between oxygen demand and oxygen) in every assessment to select optimal treatment, which is associated with the least risk. Treatments are selected to improve the efficiency of oxygen transport and utilization and thereby reduce the work of the heart and of breathing. Above all, treatment should not worsen the patient's oxygen transport status. Selective body positioning can augment oxygen transport and maximize the ef-

fective FIo_2. Even though the patient will likely benefit more from some positions than others, frequent body position changes, preferably 360-degree turning regimen, are still necessary to avoid the sequelae of static body positioning. Semi-prone positions can substitute well for full prone positions if the patient is too hemodynamically unstable. Semi-prone positions may be tolerated better by the patient and may be safer. Even though hourly position changes may not be feasible in these severely ill patients, prolonged periods in a static position (more than 2 hours) is deleterious to the patient. Thus a balance between these two concerns must be achieved.

Promoting optimal mucociliary transport remains a priority even in the absence of secretion accumulation. Frequent position changes and numerous positions ensure pulmonary secretions are continually being redistributed to prevent accumulation and enhance removal. Should postural drainage be indicated, these positions may need to be modified. Head-down positions in particular may not be tolerated well. Based on a careful assessment, the relative benefits of superimposing manual techniques must be established in that these procedures are associated with increased metabolical demand to which the patient is not readily able to adapt. Increasing the oxygen demand of these patients may worsen their condition.

SUMMARY

This chapter presents several major complications that occur secondary to various conditions in the intensive care unit. Complications add significantly to the complexity of the physical therapy diagnoses of the patient's underlying problems with respect to oxygen transport and cardiopulmonary management. The complications highlighted in the chapter include those that impair multiple steps in the oxygen transport pathway and hence jeopardize metabolism at the cellular level. This sequence of events is most frequently associated with the complications of respiratory failure, surgery, adult respiratory distress syndrome, shock, sepsis, and multiorgan system failure.

Physical therapy treatments in critical care areas are typically short, frequent, and should always be efficacious. Patients with the complications, however, are usually severely compromised and often unable to cooperate with treatment necessitating particularly short and frequent sessions. Because of the severity of illness, patients with the complications described often require treatments that are more passive (i.e., stress the oxygen transport system minimally, thus are lower on the physiological treatment hierarchy). These patients require frequent and comprehensive monitoring (often several times daily) of their oxygen transport capacity (i.e., the relationship between oxygen delivery and consumption, and oxygen extraction, to establish if and when treatment is indicated, and the specific parameters of treatment. If a patient is thought to be too unstable for treatment at a given time, continued monitoring of her or his status is essential so that small windows of opportunity can be exploited during stable periods. During periods of monitoring rather than active treatment intervention, the physical therapist continues to have an important role in recommending body positions and frequency of body position changes so that these can yield the greatest benefit to oxygen transport.

REVIEW QUESTIONS

1. Describe the complications associated with respiratory failure.
2. Describe the implications for cardiopulmonary physical therapy of respiratory failure, surgical complications, acute lung injury, adult respiratory distress syndrome, shock, sepsis, and multiorgan system failure.

References

Albert, R.K., Leasa, D., Sanderson, M., Robertson, H.T., & Hlastala, M.P. (1987). The prone position improves arterial oxygenation and reduces shunt in oleic-acid-induced acute lung injury. *American Review of Respiratory Diseases, 135,* 626-633.

Bartlett, R.H., Gazzaniga, A.B., & Geraghty, T.R. (1973). Respiratory maneuvers to prevent postoperative pulmonary complications. A critical review. *JAMA, 224,* 1017-1021.

Bishop, M.H., Shoemaker, W.C., Appel, P.L., Wo, C.-J., Zwick, C., Kram, H.B., Meade, P., Kennedy, F., & Fleming, A.W. (1993). Relationship between supranormal circulatory values, time delays, and outcome in severely traumatized patients. *Critical Care Medicine, 21,* 56-63.

Boggs, R.L., & Wooldridge-King, M. (1993). *AACN procedure manual for critical care* (3rd ed.). Philadelphia: WB Saunders.

Cane, R.D., Shapiro, B.A., & Davison, R. (1990). *Case studies in critical care medicine* (2nd ed.). St. Louis: Mosby.

Carrico, C.J., Meakins, J.L., & Marshall, J.C. (1993). Multiple organ failure syndrome. The gastrointestinal tract: the motor of MOF. *Archives of Surgery, 121,* 197-208.

Civetta, J.M., Taylor, R.W., & Kirby, R.R. (1988). *Critical care.* Philadelphia: JB Lippincott.

Clauss, R.H., Scalabrini, B.Y., Ray, J.F., III, & Reed, G.E. (1968). Effects of changing body position upon improved ventilation-perfusion relationships. *Circulation, 37*(Suppl. 4), 214-217.

Dean, E., Murphy, S., Parrent, L., & Rousseau, M. (1995). Metabolic consequences of physical therapy in critically-ill patients. *Proceedings of the World Confederation of Physical Therapy Cogress.* Washington, DC.

Dantzker, D.R. (1991). *Cardiopulmonary critical care* (2nd ed.). Philadelphia: WB Saunders.

Dantzker, D.R. (1993). Adequacy of tissue oxygenation. *Critical Care Medicine, 21,* S40-S43.

Douglas, W.W., Rehder, K., Beynen, F.M., Sessler, A.D., & Marsh, H.M. (1977). Improved oxygenation in patients with acute respiratory failure: the prone position. *American Review of Respiratory Disease, 115,* 559-566.

Fell, T., & Cheney, F.W. (1971). Prevention of hypoxia during endotracheal suction. *Annals of Surgery, 174,* 24-28.

Fenwick, J.C., Dodek, P.M., Ronco, J.J., Phang, P.T., Wiggs, B., & Russell, J.A. (1990). Increased concentrations of plasma lactate predict pathologic dependence of oxygen consumption on oxygen delivery in patients with adult respiratory distress syndrome. *Journal of Critical Care, 5,* 81-86.

Gattinoni, L., Bombino, M., Pelosi, P., Lissoni, A., Pensenti, A., Fumagalli, R., & Tagliabue, M. Lung structure and function in different stages of severe adult respiratory distress syndrome. *Journal of the American Medical Association, 271,* 1772-1779.

Gentilello, L., Thompson, D.A., Tonnesen, A.S., Hernandez, D., Kapadia, A.S., Allen, S.J., Houtchens, B.A., & Miner, M.E. (1988). Effect of a rotating bed on the incidence of pulmonary complications in critically ill patients. *Critical Care Medicine, 16,* 783-786.

Gutierrez, G. (1991). Cellular energy metabolism during hypoxia. *Critical Care Medicine, 19,* 619-626.

Hayes, M.A., Yau, E.H.S., Timmins, A.C., Hinds, C.J., & Watson, D. (1993). Response of critically-ill patients to treatment aimed at achieving supranormal oxygen delivery and consumption. *Chest, 103,* 886-895.

Kariman, K., & Burns, S.R. (1985). Regulation of tissue oxygen extraction is disturbed in adult respiratory distress syndrome. *American Review of Respiratory Diseases, 132,* 109-114.

Langer, M., Mascheroni, D., Marcolin, R., & Cattinoni, L. (1988). The prone position in ARDS patients. A clinical study. *Chest, 94,* 103-107.

Leblanc, P., Ruff, F., & Milic-Emili, J. (1970). Effects of age and body position on "airway closure" in man. *Journal of Applied Physiology, 28,* 448-451.

Mackenzie, C.F. (Ed.). (1989). *Chest physiotherapy in the intensive care unit* (2nd ed.). Baltimore: Williams & Wilkins.

Marini, J.J. (1984). Postoperative atelectasis: pathophysiology, clinical importance, and principles of management. *Respiratory Care, 29,* 516-528.

Nightingale, P. (1993). Optimization of oxygen transport to the tissues. *Acta Anaesthesiologica Scandinavica, 98,* 32-36.

Pallares, L.C.M., & Evans, T.W. (1992). Oxygen transport in the critically ill. *Respiratory Medicine, 86,* 289-295.

Pape, H.C., Regel, G., Borgman, W., Sturm, J.A., & Tacherne, H. (1994). The effect of kinetic positioning on lung function and pulmonary haemodynamics in posttraumatic ARDS: a clinical study. *International Journal of the Care of the Injured, 25,* 51-57.

Petty, T.L. (1982). *Intensive and rehabilitative respiratory care* (3rd ed.). Philadelphia: Lea & Febiger.

Phang, P.T., & Russell, J.A. (1993). When does VO_2 depend on DO_2? *Respiratory Care, 38,* 618-630.

Phipps, W.J., Long, B.C., & Woods, N.F. (Eds.). (1991). *Medical-surgical nursing: concepts and clinical practice* (4th ed.). St. Louis: Mosby.

Piehl, M.A., & Brown, R.S. (1976). Use of extreme position changes in acute respiratory failure. *Critical Care Medicine, 4*(1), 13-14.

Poelaert, J., Lannoy, B., Vogelaers, D., Everaert, J., Decruyenaere, J., Capiau, P., & Colardyn, F. (1991). Influence of chest physiotherapy on arterial oxygen saturation. *Acta Anaesthesiologica Belgica, 42,* 165-170.

Ray, J.F., III, Yost, L., Moallem, S., Sanoudos, G.M., Villamena, P., Paredes, R.M., & Clauss, R.H. (1974). Immobility, hypoxemia, and pulmonary arteriovenous shunting. *Archives of Surgery, 109,* 537-541.

Roukonen, E., Takala, J., & Kari, A. (1991). Septic shock and multiple organ failure. *Critical Care Medicine, 19,* 1146-1151.

Shapiro, B.A., & Peruzzi, W.T. (1995). Changing practices in ventilator management: A review of the literature and suggested clinical correlates. *Surgery, 117,* 121–133.

Shoemaker, W.C. (Ed.). (1984). *Critical care: state of the art.* Fullerton, CA: Society of Critical Care Medicine.

Vincent, J.L. (1991). Advances in the concepts of intensive care. *American Heart Journal, 121,* 1859-1865.

Vincent, J.L. (1993). Oxygen transport in severe sepsis. *Acta Anaesthesiology Scandinavica, 37* (Suppl 98), 29-31.

Waxman, K., & Shoemaker, W.C. (1980). Management of postoperative and posttraumatic respiratory failure in the intensive care unit. *Surgical Clinics of North America, 60,* 1413-1428.

Weissman, C., & Kemper, M. (1993). Stressing the critically ill patient: the cardiopulmonary and metabolic resposnes to an acute increase in oxygen consumption. *Journal of Critical Care, 8,* 100-108.

Wolff, R.K., Dolovich, M.B., Obminski, G., & Newhouse, M.T. (1977). Effects of exercise and eucapnic hyperventilation on bronchial clearance in man. *Journal of Applied Physiology, 43,* 46-50.

Wysocki, M., Besbes, M., Roupie, E., & Brun-Buisson, C. (1992). Modification of oxygen extraction ratio by change in oxygen transport in septic shock. *Chest, 102,* 221-226.

Yu, M., Levy, M.M., Smith, P., Takiguchi, S.A., Miyasaki, A., & Myers, S.A. (1993). Effect of maximizing oxygen delivery on morbidity and mortality rates in critically ill patients: A prospective, randomized, controlled study. *Critical Care Medicine, 21,* 830-838.

PART VII

Guidelines for the Delivery of Cardiopulmonary Physical Therapy: Special Cases

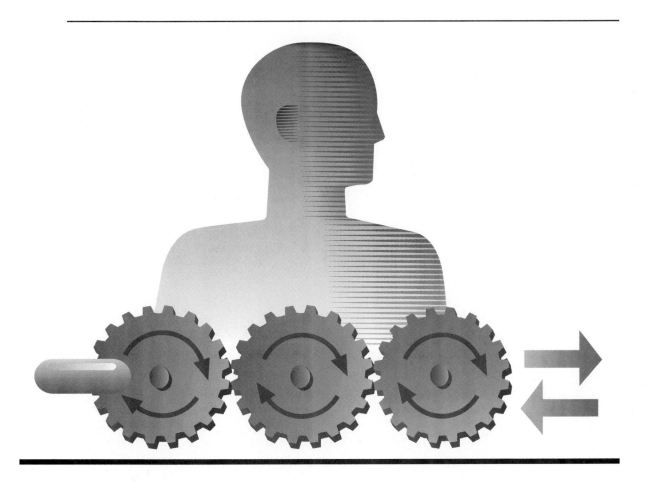

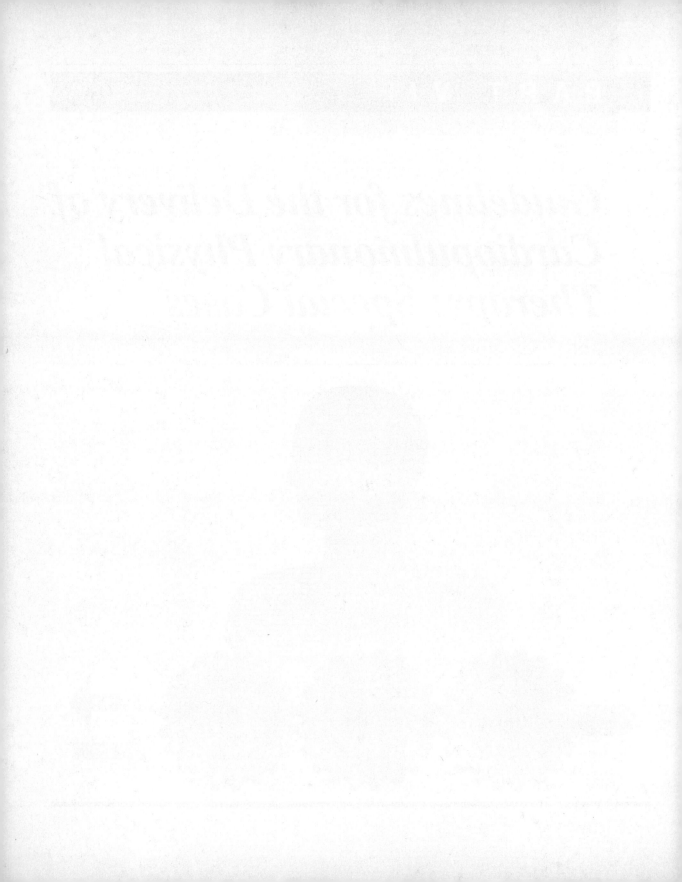

CHAPTER 35

The Neonatal and Pediatric Patient

Victoria A. Moerchen
Linda D. Crane

KEY TERMS

Bronchopulmonary dysplasia

Chest physical therapy with
    infants/children

Childhood asthma

Cystic fibrosis

Endocardial cushion defect

Handling for ventilation

Hyaline membrane disease

Patent ductus arteriosus

Pediatric cardiac rehabilitation

Pediatric pulmonary rehabilitation

Pulmonary development

Transitional circulation

Trunk-ventilation interaction

INTRODUCTION

Pediatrics entails a "special" application of cardiopul-monary physical therapy. This chapter stresses that cardiopulmonary development and its related vulner-abilities form the basis for cardiopulmonary practice with neonatal and pediatric patients.

The objectives of this chapter include to: (1) re-view cardiopulmonary development and related vul-nerabilities; (2) relate developmental pathologies to issues of adequate ventilation and oxygen transport;

(3) present principles and precautions of direct respi-ratory care; and (4) incorporate these principles into suggestions for practice.

This chapter begins with a brief description of crit-ical events and important characteristics of cardiac and pulmonary development. Relevant diagnoses are then presented to build onto this developmental per-spective and to stress that cardiopulmonary pathology and ventilatory compromise are often related to de-velopmental vulnerabilities. Finally, treatment approaches are described, including pediatric cardiac rehabilitation, pulmonary care for neonatal and pediatric patients, pediatric pulmonary rehabilitation, and developmental motor approaches for trunk and ventilatory muscle function.

A knowledge of cardiopulmonary development, congenital and developmental cardiopulmonary pathology, and pediatric cardiopulmonary treatment is essential for any therapist serving children. Most pediatric patients require ongoing attention to respiratory function, whether as a primary focus of physical therapy or as an inherent aspect of motor development. This chapter is relevant to therapists who perform direct cardiopulmonary care and to therapists who incorporate a cardiopulmonary awareness into developmental motor therapy.

CARDIOPULMONARY DEVELOPMENT

The application of cardiopulmonary physical therapy to infants and children requires a special understanding of developmental cardiopulmonary anatomy and physiology. Knowledge of normal development and its inherent points of vulnerability will help the reader understand some of what is known about cardiopulmonary pathology in pediatric patients.

Cardiac Development

Differences in fetal and neonatal gas exchange account for differences in the anatomy and physiology of fetal and neonatal circulation. A basic review of developmental circulation is essential for discussion of congenital heart defects and the role of pediatric cardiopulmonary physical therapy.

Fetal circulation

Placental oxygenation is a major characteristic of fetal circulation. Additionally, in fetal circulation blood flow through the right and left sides of the heart occurs in parallel, such that cardiac output is actually combined ventricular output (CVO) (Heyman and Hanley, 1994). This is possible as a result of shunts in fetal circulation (Parks, 1988).

Two points of shunting during fetal circulation are at the foramen ovale and the ductus arteriosus. The fora-

men ovale allows right-to-left blood flow through the atria, bypassing the lungs (Yao, 1983). Left ventricular output (LVO) is well-oxygenated blood that then enters the ascending aorta and flows to the brain and upper body. The ductus arteriosus similarly allows the lungs to be bypassed, as most of the right ventricular output (less well-oxygenated than the LVO) flows to the descending aorta and from there to the lower body.

Fetal blood flow to the lungs is minimal, secondary to high pulmonary vascular resistance during fetal circulation. Only 10% to 12% of CVO goes to the lungs (Koff, 1993; Phelan, Olinsky, and Robertson, 1994), with the function of nourishing the developing lung tissue rather than providing gas exchange.

Neonatal circulation

Adult-like circulation occurs at or shortly after birth, with separation from the placenta and ventilation of the lungs resulting in closure of the ductus venosus, foramen ovale, and ductus arteriosus. This process, referred to as transitional circulation, occurs early in neonatal life and increases the efficiency of oxygen uptake and transport (Heyman and Hanley, 1994; Rudolph, 1970).

The initiation of breathing and the removal of lung fluid increases pulmonary blood flow. Whereas fetal circulation was characterized by high pulmonary vascular resistance and low systemic resistance, separation from the placenta causes a rise in systemic resistance and a decrease in pulmonary vascular resistance. As this shift in relative pulmonary and systemic resistances occurs, sites of intercommunication (shunts) close, and the ventricles shift from working in parallel to working in series (Heyman and Hanley, 1994).

Closure of Foramen Ovale. The increased left atrial pressure that occurs during transitional circulation results in apposition of the valve of foramen ovale against the interatrial septum, functionally closing this site of fetal circulatory shunting (Rudolph, 1970). In most infants, anatomical closure occurs 2 to 3 months later (Emmanouilides and Baylen, 1988; Yao, 1983).

Closure of Ductus Arteriosus. Functional closure or constriction of the ductus arteriosus occurs postnatally within the first 15 to 72 hours in response to increased arterial oxygen saturation (Daniels, Hopman, Stoelinger, Busch, and Peer, 1982). Anatomical closure of ductus arteriosus occurs by 2 to 3 weeks in most term neonates (Rudolph, 1970). It is important to note that the responsiveness of the ductal smooth muscle to arterial oxygen tension and to endogenous prostaglandins is impacted by gestational age (Pack, 1988; Yao, 1983).

Pulmonary Development

Structural and functional characteristics of pulmonary development in infants and children are significant because they may contribute to aspects of respiratory vulnerability (Muller and Bryan, 1979).

Newborn respiration

The pulmonary anatomy of the term infant is markedly different from the adult but also different from the child. An infant's airways are narrower from the nares to the terminal bronchioles. This presents a point of pulmonary vulnerability because a smaller diameter airway is more easily obstructed by mucus, edema, foreign objects, and enlarged lymphatic tissue. The infant also has a high larynx (Laitman and Crelin, 1980). Although this position of the larynx enables the newborn to breathe and swallow simultaneously, it may also contribute to predominant patterns of infant nasal breathing, which can result in increased work to breathe during any compromise of the nasal airway.

Even without airway compromise, the work of breathing is increased during the neonatal period. The initial low compliance of the newborn's lungs requires increased effort for ventilation, which results in a high rate of respiration and increased oxygen consumption.

Although the process of transitional circulation allows more efficient O_2 transport in the neonate than in the fetus, gas exchange in the newborn is still somewhat inefficient because of immature alveolar structure and function. The surface area for gas exchange is 1/20 that of an adult (Johnson, Moore, and Jefferies, 1980), and the diffusion distance across the alveoli-capillary membrane is increased as a result of thick alveolar walls (Blackburn, 1992).

Functional characteristics of infant pulmonary development are also significant to understanding possible contributions to pulmonary distress in infants. The diaphragm of a newborn has fewer type I (high oxidative) muscle fibers (25% compared with 50% in adult) (Muller and Bryan, 1979). This difference predisposes an infant to earlier diaphragmatic fatigue when stressed.

A biomechanical difference between the infant and child is the circular and horizontal alignment of the ribs and the concomitant horizontal angle at which the diaphragm inserts on the ribs during newborn and early infant chest development (Massery, 1991; Muller and Bryan, 1979). This, along with the more cartilaginous nature of the rib cage, results in less efficient chest wall mechanics. The result, again, is increased work to breathe. (See Chapter 37 for a more complete discussion of chest development).

Respiration in the child

Two residual structural differences exist beyond the newborn period and have potential implications for pulmonary vulnerability in the child. First, the somewhat horizontal angulation of the ribs persists until approximately 7 years of age and results in less efficient chest wall mechanics (Muller and Bryan, 1979). Secondly, lymphatic tissue (especially adenoids) grows rapidly until about 6 years of age (Sinclair, 1978) and can continue to be a potential source of upper airway obstruction.

As infants and children grow and develop, however, most structural and functional disadvantages disappear. An aspect of growth and development that can be protective for infants and younger children is alveolar multiplication. This begins in the first year of life and continues until approximately 8 years of age (Blackburn, 1992; Thurlbeck, 1975).

Cardiopulmonary Considerations in the Preterm Infant

All of the cardiopulmonary structural and functional characteristics of neonates that have been previously discussed apply to the premature infant. Additionally, there are significant gestational characteristics and aspects of cardiopulmonary vulnerability that are more pronounced and create more problems in premature infants (Table 35-1).

Recall that the transitional circulation of a term newborn includes a decrease in pulmonary vascular

TABLE 35-1

Factors Contributing to Cardiopulmonary Dysfunction in the Premature Infant*

ANATOMICAL	PHYSIOLOGICAL
Capillary beds not well developed before 26 weeks' gestation	Increased pulmonary vascular resistance leading to right-to-left shunting
Type II alveolar cells and surfactant production not mature until 35 weeks' gestation; elastic properties of lung not well developed; lung space decreased by relative size of the heart and abdominal distention	Decreased lung compliance
Decreased responsiveness of the ductus arteriosus to oxygen tensions; delayed ductal closure	Left-to-right shunting
Type I, high-oxidative fibers compose only 10% to 20% of diaphragm muscle	Diaphragmatic fatigue: respiratory failure
Highly vascular subependymal germinal matrix not resorbed until 35 weeks' gestation, increasing the vulnerability of the infant to hemorrhage	Decreased or absent cough and gag reflexes; apnea
Lack of fatty insulation and high surface area to body-weight ratio	Hypothermia and increased oxygen consumption

*Modified from Crane, L.D. (1995). Physical Therapy for the Neonate with Respiratory Disease. In S. Irwin & J.S. Tecklin (Eds.). *Cardiopulmonary physical therapy.* St. Louis, Mosby.

resistance over the first day. In preterm infants, however, lung immaturity and abnormal surfactant function (Jobe, 1988) may result in retained high pulmonary resistance (poor lung compliance), hypoperfusion, and respiratory distress syndrome (Walther, Benders, and Leighton, 1992). Persistent pulmonary hypertension will reinforce persistent right-to-left shunting through the ductus arteriosus (Nudel and Gootman, 1983; Rudolph, 1980). In fact, respiratory distress syndrome (RDS) has been identified as the best predictor of prolonged patency of ductus arteriosus (Milne, Sung, Fok, and Crozier, 1989).

As the respiratory distress of the premature infant improves with neonatal intensive care, cardiopulmonary vulnerabilities can then occur in the opposite circulatory direction. Given the gestationally related responsiveness of ductus arteriosus to oxygen, some preterm infants retain patency of the ductus even when pulmonary vascular resistance falls (Archer, 1993). The result is left-to-right shunting that may lead to congestive heart failure (Nudel and Grootman, 1983; Parks, 1988).

Most significantly, the immature status of cardiopulmonary anatomy in preterm infants predisposes them to hypoxia under any conditions that require increased oxygen (Blackburn, 1992). Cardiopulmonary pathophysiology and/or the stressors inherent to medical care often present challenges beyond the adaptive capacities of these fragile little systems.

COMMON PEDIATRIC DIAGNOSES

The sections that follow present and discuss specific cardiac and pulmonary diagnoses. Common neuromuscular or developmental diagnoses that have inherent to them the risk of compromised respiration or associated cardiopulmonary disease are also discussed. The diagnoses presented are not all inclusive but merely represent an attempt to give the reader a preliminary knowledge of underlying pathologies and medical management of diagnoses commonly encountered in the practice of pediatric cardiopulmonary physical therapy.

TABLE 35-2	
Common Pediatric Diagnoses and Associated Heart Defects	
DIAGNOSIS	**HEART DEFECTS**
Duchenne's muscular dystrophy	Cardiomyopathy (adolescence)
Fetal alcohol syndrome	Ventricular septal defect Tetralogy of Fallot Pulmonary value stenosis Patent ductus arteriosus
Friedreich's ataxia	Ventricular hypertrophy Congestive heart failure
HIV-1 infection	Myocarditis Ventricular dysfunction
Juvenile rheumatoid arthritis	Pericarditis
Marfan syndrome	Aortic aneurysm Aortic/Mitral insufficiency
Noonan's syndrome	Dystrophic pulmonary valve (Pulmonary stenosis)
Prematurity	Patent ductus arteriosus
Trisomy 13 (Patau's syndrome)	Ventricular septal defect Atrial septal defect Patent ductus arteriosus
Trisomy 18 (Edwards' syndrome)	Ventricular septal defect Patent ductus arteriosus (large)
Trisomy 21 (Down syndrome)	Endocardial cushion defect Ventricular septal defect Atrial septal defect Tetralogy of Fallot
Turner's syndrome	Coarctation of the aorta
Williams syndrome	Supravalvular aortic stenosis Supravalvular pulmonary stenosis

Cardiac Diagnoses

Patent ductus arteriosus, endocardial cushion defects, and tetralogy of Fallot are the cardiac defects discussed within the limits of this chapter. Additionally, Table 35-2 provides a summary of common developmental diagnoses and their associated cardiac defects.

Patent ductus arteriosus

Patent ductus arteriosus (PDA), already introduced as a cardiopulmonary complication in preterm infants, is the most common heart defect during the neonatal period (Musewe and Olley, 1992). In term newborns, however, PDA accounts for 10% of congenital heart disease (Mitchell, Korones, and Berendes, 1971).

Gestational age, the presence of lung disease, the size of the ductus, and the direction of the shunt mediate the clinical features of PDA (Greene, Mavroudis, and Backer, 1994; Musewe and Olley, 1992). The preterm infant with very low birth-weight will have the most extreme clinical picture. An infant or child with a large ductus will also have an obvious clinical presentation. Tachycardia, an ejection systolic murmur, bounding peripheral pulses, increased respiratory distress, and poor feeding or poor weight gain are the classical signs of PDA (Archer, 1993; Greene et al., 1994; Musewe and Olley, 1992). In the term infant, PDA may be more clinically silent, especially when the ductus is small (Parks, 1988).

Medical management of PDA includes nonsurgical use of indomethacin or direct surgical closure of the PDA (Musewe and Olley, 1992).

Endocardial cushion defects and artrioventricular defects

Endocardial cushion defects (ECD) represent a spectrum of defects characterized by malformation of the atrial septum, the mitral and tricuspid valves, and/or the ventricular septum (Emmanouilides and Baylen, 1988). Combinations of these defects are categorized as complete, transitional/intermediate, and partial, depending on degree of ventricular septal deficiency (Merrill, Hoff, and Bender, 1994; Spicer, 1984). In the complete form of ECD, all of the structures are deficient. In the partial form, only an atrial septal defect with a cleft mitral valve is present (Emmanouilides and Baylen, 1988; Merrill et al., 1994; Parks, 1988).

There is marked variation in the underlying anatomy of this class of cardiac defects, such that clinical features are equally varied and difficult to inclusively summarize. In neonates with a complete defect, heart failure may manifest in infancy. However, neonates with milder forms of this defect may not be symptomatic until much later in development (Parks, 1988). Additionally, endocardial cushion defects are frequently associated with other cardiac defects (Emmanouilides and Baylen, 1988).

Although the total incidence of endocardial cushion defects in infancy is 1% to 4%, the incidence in infants and children with Down syndrome is 40% (Freedom and Smallhorn, 1992). In fact, in these children a complete ECD is the most common cardiac malformation (Spicer, 1984).

Operative management of infants and children with ECD depends on the morphology of the defect, the degree of pulmonary hypertension, and the extent of mitral valve regurgitation (Merrill et al., 1994). For infants with complete ECD, early surgical repairs are indicated (Bender, Hammon, Hubbard, Muirhead, and Graham, 1982; Graham and Bender, 1980).

Tetralogy of Fallot

Tetralogy of Fallot (TOF) is named for its "tetrad" of defects: ventricular septal defects, right ventricular outflow obstruction, right ventricular hypertrophy, and aortic override (Bove and Lupinetti, 1994; Pinsky and Arciniegas, 1990). A neonate with TOF will have symptoms dependent on the extent of right ventricular tract obstruction, which results in decreased pulmonary blood flow and the presence of right-to-left shunting (Bove and Luppinetti, 1994). The classic picture is one of cyanosis, especially with crying (Emmanouilides and Baylen, 1988; Pinsky and Arciniegas, 1990).

In neonates, initial medical management may include treatment of hypoxemia by pharmacologically maintaining patency or reopening the ductus arteriosus for additional pulmonary blood flow (Driscoll, 1990; Freedom and Benson, 1992). The elimination of conditions that produce hypoxemia may also include pharmacological agents to increase systemic vascular resistance and decrease myocardial contractility (Bove and Lupinetti, 1994). Surgical repairs are generally performed within the first year (Bove and Lupinetti, 1994; Starnes, Luciani, Latter, and Griffin, 1994).

Pulmonary Diagnoses

The section that follows provides a brief discussion of common pulmonary disorders for which chest physical therapy is indicated. Additional physical therapy treatment is described later in this chapter.

Hyaline membrane disease

The most common respiratory disorder in premature infants is hyaline membrane disease (HMD) or infant respiratory distress syndrome (IRDS or RDS). Occurring almost exclusively in preterm infants younger than 37 weeks' gestation, HMD results from lung immaturity and an inadequate amount and regeneration of surfactant (Phelan et al., 1994). Surfactant functions to decrease alveolar surface tension and thus enables the neonate to stabilize terminal air spaces (Wallis and Harvey, 1979). Surfactant deficiency results in alveolar collapse and increased effort to breathe.

Clinical signs of respiratory distress resulting from HMD occur early (usually within 1 to 2 hours) and persist for at least 48 to 72 hours (Farrell and Avery, 1975). Respiratory failure is common in these infants, necessitating oxygen therapy and assisted ventilation.

Chest physical therapy (CPT) is commonly indicated in the management of infants with HMD. There is usually a marked increase in airway secretions in the "recovery" state of the syndrome (after approximately 2 to 3 days), which is exacerbated by oxygen therapy and endotracheal intubation (Crane, 1981; Finer and Boyd, 1978).

Bronchopulmonary dysplasia

As more preterm newborns survive neonatal respiratory distress, the prevalence of chronic lung disease or bronchopulmonary dysplasia (BPD) has increased (Parker, Lindstrom, and Cotton, 1992). Although controversial, the etiology of BPD is usually linked with positive pressure ventilation and oxygen therapy in the treatment of respiratory distress during the neonatal period. The risk of BPD is highest in younger, low–birth-weight premature infants (Abman and Groothius, 1994).

Northway, Rosan, and Porter's (1967) classic description of BPD includes four pathological stages. The first stage involves symptoms similar to HMD/RDS, but by the fourth stage, BPD has progressed to include characteristics of chronic lung disease (Voyles, 1981).

Clinically, infants with BPD often present with rales, wheezing, cyanosis, hypoxemia, increased incidence of lower respiratory tract infections, and abnormal chest radiographs by 1 month postnatally (Abman and Groothius, 1994). Medical management of BPD is primarily supportive. Long-term oxygen therapy is often necessary for infants who exhibit persistent severe hypoxemia.

The cardiopulmonary outcome of BPD is variable, ranging from near normal pulmonary function by age 3 to 5 in children who had milder forms of BPD, to continued poor cardiopulmonary function, chronic distress, and ongoing oxygen dependence in children

with severe BPD (Berman, Katz, Yabek, Dillon, Fripp, and Papile, 1986; Gerhardt, Hehre, Feller, Reinfenberg, and Bancalari, 1987). Right-sided heart failure (cor pulmonale) is a common sequelae of this disease, especially in the first few years. Additionally, BPD survivors demonstrate an increased incidence of neurodevelopmental sequelae, including cerebral palsy and general development delay (Northway, 1979; Vohr, Bell, and Oh, 1982).

Chest physical therapy is an important component of the management of an infant with BPD. Airway clearance problems are common due to submucosal and peribronchial smooth muscle hyperplasia, increased mucous secretions, oxygen therapy, and frequent lower respiratory tract infections. Infants with BPD also frequently have poor growth, which may be a consequence of a higher resting VO_2, such that caloric needs are greater (Weinstein and Oh, 1981).

Transient tachypnea of the newborn

Transient tachypnea (TTNB) is another neonatal problem considered in the differential diagnosis of HMD/RDS. It is associated with delayed clearance of amniotic fluid from the lungs, results in early presentation of respiratory distress, and is most common in full-term and postterm neonates (especially if delivered by cesarean) (Avery, Garewood, and Brumley, 1966; Emmanouilides and Baylen, 1988). Chest physical therapy is occasionally indicated for infants with this problem, but TTNB is usually self-limited.

Meconium aspiration syndrome

Meconium is the content of fetal and newborn bowels. Although the cause of meconium passage is highly debated (Bacsik, 1977), once meconium is present in the uterine environment the risk for aspiration is significant. It is generally accepted that meconium aspiration most frequently occurs with the first postnatal breaths of term or postterm infants (Gregory, 1977), but it may also occur with gasping in utero just before delivery (Katz and Bowes, 1992; Wiswell and Bent, 1993). Research has supported the contention that meconium aspiration syndrome (MAS) is often preventable if the upper and lower airways are suctioned immediately after birth (Wiswell, Tuggle, and Turner, 1990). The lower airways especially should be suctioned in infants delivered through thick, particulate ("pea soup") meconium in amniotic material (Gregory, 1977).

Aspiration of meconium can result in serious and devastating pathophysiology. Most commonly, the meconium will partially or completely block the peripheral airways (Wiswell and Bent, 1993). Atelectasis is the classic finding, but with partial obstruction, hyperexpanded areas will also be observed as a result of air that was inspired but then trapped in distal, small airways. Common complications of MAS include tension pneumothorax, persistent pulmonary hypertension, and bronchiolitis and pneumonitis secondary to chemical irritation from the components of the meconium (Wiswell and Bent, 1993). Additionally, long-term pulmonary sequelae have been reported (MacFarlane and Heaf, 1988; Swaminathan, Quinn, Stabile, Bader, Platzker, and Keens, 1989).

Medical management of MAS is supportive, with supplemental oxygen and, if necessary, mechanical ventilation. Chest physical therapy is especially advocated during the first 8 hours of life, although it may be necessary for a longer period of time if the infant requires assisted ventilation.

Pneumonia

Neonatal Pneumonia. The most common organisms producing neonatal septicemia associated with pneumonia in neonates are *group B streptococcus* and *Hemophilis influenzae* (Emmanouilides and Baylen, 1988). Neonatal pneumonia mimics HMD/RDS in clinical presentation and chest radiographs.
Aspiration Pneumonia. Aspiration is an unfortunate result of small children's "indiscreet curiosity" (Waring, 1975) in exploring their environment and relying on their mouths for sensory learning. Aspiration can also result from gastroesophageal reflux and decreased upper airway neuromuscular control (Orenstein and Orenstein, 1988).

Bronchial drainage techniques are often indicated as part of the medical management of infants and children after aspiration to aid with airway clearance and reduce the possibility of bacterial superinfection.
Pneumocystis Carnii Pneumonia/HIV-Infected Children. Pulmonary involvement is often the lead-ing cause of symptoms in children with HIV (Marolda, Pace, Bonforte, Kotin, Rabinowitz, and Katlan, 1991). In infants with perinatally acquired HIV, *pneumocyctis carnii pneumonia* (PCP) frequently occurs within the first 15 months of life (Connor et al., 1991). The risk of mortality during the infant's first episode of PCP is high (Bagarazzi, Connor, McSherry, and Oleske, 1990; Bernstein, Bye, and Rubinstein, 1989; Scott et al., 1989).

The clinical presentation of PCP includes failure to thrive, cough, dyspnea, tachypnea, fever, hypoxemia, and chest radiograph evidence of prominent air bronchograms and multiple cysts or bullae (Bagarazzi et al., 1990; Berdon, Mellins, Abramson, and Ruzal-Shapiro, 1993; Bernstein et al., 1989). PCP is most often diagnosed after bronchoalveolar lavage studies (Phelan et al., 1994).

Treatment is supportive and includes antibiotic therapy, antiretroviral therapy, nutritional support, and mechanical ventilation as needed (Bagarazzi et al., 1990; Phelen et al., 1994).

Asthma

Although asthma is discussed in detail in Chapter 4, a discussion of pediatric pulmonary problems would not be complete without some discussion of this common cause of childhood lung disease. An estimated 8% to 10% of children in the United States have asthma, with asthma accounting for the most lost time from school and 33% of pediatrician visits per year (Magee, 1991).

Childhood asthma can begin at any age, and its clinical etiology and clinical course are variable. Children with early medical histories including very low birth weight, bronchopulmonary dysplasia, and respiratory syncytial virus infection may be at increased risk for developing asthma (Pullen and Hey, 1982; Rickards, Ford, Kitchen, Doyle, Lisseden, and Keith, 1987; Smyth, Tabachnik, Duncan, Reilly, and Levison, 1981).

Medical management usually includes avoidance of known precipitants, adrenergic drugs, and corticosteroids (in chronic, severe cases). Chest physical therapy for this disease includes patient and family education in breathing control, relaxation, effective coughing, and exercise. Older children, in particular, may benefit from CPT especially when they are responding slowly to pharmacological treatment alone (Asher, Douglas, Airy, Andrews, and Trenholme, 1990). Exercise, also highly effective in the treatment and management of asthma, is discussed in a later section on pulmonary rehabilitation.

Cystic fibrosis

Cystic fibrosis (CF) is a complex autosomal-recessive disorder that affects the exocrine glands. Definitive diagnosis of CF includes positive family history, obstructive pulmonary disease, recurrent pulmonary infection, intestinal malabsorption and poor growth, the presence of *Staphylococcus aureus* or *Pseudomonas aeruginosa* in the respiratory tract, and, most importantly, a positive sweat chloride test (Cystic Fibrosis Foundation, 1990).

The chronic pulmonary disease in CF is related to increased secretion of abnormally viscous mucus, impaired mucociliary transport, airway obstruction, bronchiectasis, overinflation, and infection. Radiographic changes are most pronounced in the upper lobes, especially the right (Wood, Boat, and Doershuk, 1976).

The early institution of prophylactic pulmonary physical therapy, including postural drainage and the judicious use of antibiotics, provides effective measures for controlling or slowing the effects of bronchiolar and bronchial obstruction. Involvement of the child and family in pulmonary care is particularly important. Family understanding of the nature of the disease and the purpose of each therapeutic measure promotes successful management of the child. A home program of CPT should be established for each child, taking into consideration the child's ongoing pulmonary needs and the family's unique contributions and constraints.

Bronchial drainage is an aspect of conventional treatment for CF that in recent years has gained several options that allow both efficacy and patient independence (Davis, 1994). Airway clearance techniques are described in detail in Chapter 20, but alternatives to traditional percussion and postural drainage warrant mention within the context of CPT for children with CF. Specifically, the forced-expiration technique (FET) as part of the active cycle of

breathing (ACB) technique, use of a positive expiratory pressure (PEP) mask, autogenic drainage (AD), and use of the flutter device, have been shown to be effective in assisting sputum expectoration, often in greater amounts and in less time per treatment (Konstan, Stern, and Doershuk, 1994; Mahlmeister, Fink, Hoffman, and Fifer, 1991; Pryor, 1991; Pryor and Webber, 1979; Schoni, 1989).

Although postural drainage, percussion, and vibration remain the treatment of choice for infants and children who are unable to be instructed in techniques that use patterns of voluntary breathing, other techniques are available for children who can follow specific breathing instructions and who can perform a reliable pulmonary function test. Children as young as 2 to 3 years can be taught to "huff" as part of FET (Pryor, 1991), the PEP mask has been used with children as young as 3½ years (Mahlmeister et al., 1991), and AD can reportedly be taught to children as early as 4 to 6 years of age (DeCesare and Graybill, 1990; Schoni, 1989). The benefits of each technique should be carefully considered relative to each child's cognitive, respiratory, and motor planning abilities when choosing or modifying the child's program for airway clearance.

Ventilatory muscle training is an important aspect of pulmonary treatment in older children with CF. Studies have demonstrated that training to improve the endurance of ventilatory muscles decreases dyspnea and increases general exercise tolerance in patients with CF (Keens, Krastins, Wannamaker, Levison, Crozier, and Bryan, 1977; Reid and Loveridge, 1983).

The role of general exercise in the cardiopulmonary management of children with CF is specifically discussed within the context of pulmonary rehabilitation. However, it is important to realize that some debate exists as to whether exercise can replace more traditional airway clearance techniques. Pryor (1991) has suggested that exercise should be an additional component rather than a substitute for breathing techniques. Cerney (1989) in contrast, reported that some children with mild disease may be able to use regular exercise in place of bronchial drainage treatments. The severity of the disease process and the child's condition at any one point in time, will clearly mediate the appropriateness and effectiveness of exercise as either a component or as a primary means of airway clearance.

Special respiratory problems associated with intubation and tracheostomy

Once an infant or child develops respiratory failure, intubation and mechanical ventilation are usually required. The goals of medical management are then to treat the cause of the respiratory failure as aggressively as possible and to wean the child from mechanical ventilation as quickly as possible.

If a child's condition necessitates long-term mechanical ventilation, or if an artificial airway is needed to bypass an upper airway obstruction, a tracheostomy is usually performed (Scott and Koff, 1993).

Infants and children who have a tracheostomy and are intubated for long periods of time require vigorous prophylactic airway management, such as bronchial drainage and airway suctioning. Chest PT, including postural drainage and vibration emphasizing right upper lobe segments, has been shown to significantly decrease the incidence of postextubation atelectasis in infants intubated for more than 24 hours (Finer, Moriartey, Boyd, Phillips, Stewart, and Ulan, 1979).

Pulmonary Considerations in Neuromuscular and Motor Diagnoses

Although cardiopulmonary symptoms may not be the primary reason for referral to physical therapy in children with neuromuscular and general motor developmental diagnoses, these children do have motor involvement that can result in respiratory and postural muscle weakness, immobile chests, and hypoventilation. Furthermore, many of these children have had medical histories remarkable for cardiopulmonary complications or have diagnoses that entail progressive processes that will result in cardiopulmonary compromise.

Table 35-3 provides an extensive summary of the interactions between trunk musculature and ventilation in children with atypical development. Although the biomechanical deviations noted are frequently seen in children with atypical tonal presentations, they are also common in children with scoliosis, sternal deformity, or general immobility of the thorax.

These deviations and other aspects of ventilatory compromise are discussed with regard to motor diagnoses common to pediatric practice.

Cerebral palsy

Children with cerebral palsy generally have weak trunk and postural muscles, which, when combined with atypical neural mechanisms, produce atypical movement patterns and functional alignment deviations. The trunk and respiration relationships described in Table 35-3 are consistent with the clinical picture of external pulmonary development in children with cerebral palsy.

Although the extent of mobility impairment is variable between children, hypoventilation, increased work to breathe, inefficient cough, increased risk for aspiration, and poor breath support for vocalization can occur (Alexander, 1993). Limited active mobility and the use of habitual patterns with little deviation

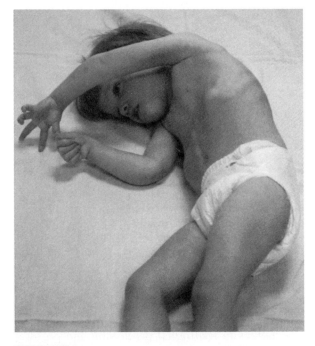

FIGURE 35-1
Flattened anterior chest with marked rib flaring in a child with cerebral palsy.

TABLE 35-3

Functional Relationships of Trunk Control and Respiration

BIOMECHANICAL COMPONENT	POSTURAL/TRUNK CONTROL CONSEQUENCES	RESPIRATORY CONSEQUENCES
Weak abdominal obliques	Passive lumbar lordosis Protruding tummy Lower rib flaring Decreased trunk rotation Unable to weight shift Dependence on rectus abdominis	Ineffective cough High chest Retained horizontal rib alignment Tight rectus abdominis may lead to pectus excavatum Child may use diaphragm for trunk control, limiting its function as a primary muscle of respiration Decreased support of abdominal contents under diaphragm
Tight pectoralis minor	Forward shoulders Scapula pulled laterally and anteriorly, away from the thoracic wall Upper thoracic flexion	Anterior upper chest cannot adequately expand
Weak serratus anterior	Weak upper fibers—medial edge of scapula leaves the thoracic wall	Decreased structural reinforcement of the posterior chest wall Interdigitation of the lower fibers of serratus anterior with the external abdominal oblique will interact to affect the dynamic stability of the rib cage
Decreased active upper thoracic extension	Kyphotic upper trunk Passive overlengthening of the scapular retractors	Approximation of upper ribs → decreased upper chest mobility → decreased oxygenation of the upper lobe → abdominal breathing
Decreased rib cage stability	Serratus anterior will elevate the ribs rather than stabilize the scapula against the thoracic wall	Decreased structural support for the respiratory muscles to work from

Modified from Moerchen VA: Respiration and motor development: a systems perspective, *Neurol Rep 18* (3): 8-10, 1994. Reprinted from the *Neurology Report* with the permission of the Neurology Section, APTA.

of the center of gravity beyond the base of support contribute to thoracic stiffness. A high chest, flattened anteriorly, with excessive rib flaring, is common in these children (Figure 35-1).

Therapeutic attention to respiration should first identify possible aspiration and suggest modifications for positioning during feeding. Additionally, certain postures for sleep and play may be less restrictive for chest excursion and should be incorporated into a home program. Mobilization of the ribs and thoracic spine are important precursors to improving chest excursion during ventilation.

Chest PT may be indicated if the child develops a primary pulmonary complication. Prophylactic postural drainage can also be integrated into many sensory stimulation programs for more severely involved children. Additional "handling" to address ventilatory function will be discussed in a subsequent section on motor approaches to respiratory treatment.

Myelomeningocele

Myelomeningocele or spina bifida are diagnoses that physical therapists generally equate with issues of ambulation and mobility. However, central ventilatory dysfunction is prevalent in infants, children, and adolescents who also have an associated Arnold-Chiari type II malformation (Hays, Jordan, McLaughlin, Nickel, and Fisher, 1989; Swaminathan et al., 1989; Ward, Jacobs, Gates, Hart, and Keens, 1986).

The Arnold-Chiari type II malformation, which occurs in 90% of infants with myelomeningocele, is a hindbrain malformation consisting of a caudal herniation of the cerebellum and brain stem into the cervical canal (Charney, Rorke, Sutton, and Schut, 1987). Ventilatory problems associated with a symptomatic Arnold-Chiari type II malformation include inspiratory stridor (vocal cord paralysis), central apnea, and respiratory distress (Hays et al., 1989; Hesz and Wolraich, 1985; Oren, Kelly, Todres, and Shannon, 1986). However, abnormal ventilatory patterns have also been observed in asymptomatic infants (Ward et al., 1987) and adolescents (Swaminathan et al., 1989).

Ventriculoperitoneal shunting (management of hydrocephalus) and, if necessary, cervical decompression are the surgical approaches to treatment of life-threatening ventilatory complications in this population.

Other pulmonary issues in children with myelomeningocele warrant discussion. Trunk weakness and hypotonia are observed early in the motor development of infants and toddlers who have shunted hydrocephalus. Additionally, in children with thoracic and high lumbar level lesions, abdominal muscle support for diaphragm function may be insufficient. The use of abdominal binders, and spinal othoses/body jackets with (anterior) diaphragm cut-outs and an elastic insert are indicated to aid in diaphragm function (Figure 35-2). Although progressive scoliosis is not the natural history of children with spina bifida, it is a symptom of unstable neurology (tethered cord), and attention to ventilatory ability is necessary both for general monitoring and for possible preoperative evaluation.

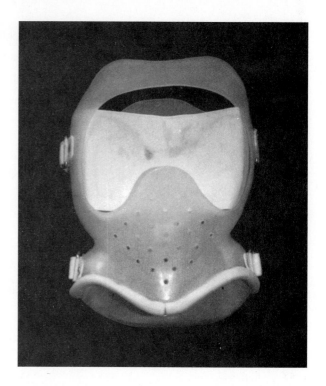

FIGURE 35-2
An anterior cut-out and elastic support in a body jacket/spinal orthosis aids diaphragm function.

Down syndrome

Impaired pulmonary function in children with Down syndrome is clearly related to generalized weakness of trunk musculature (Dichter, Darbee, Effgen, and Palisano, 1993). The postural deviations common in these children reflect (Figure 35-3) inefficient muscle function for both ventilation and movement (Moerchen, 1994). Again the trunk-ventilation relationships delineated in Table 35-3 summarize the subtle but significant clinical presentation of external pulmonary development in these children. Too often only motor development is addressed by physical therapists who are treating children with Down syndrome. Respiration needs to be considered if therapy goals include increased vocalizations or improved tolerance for exercise.

Pulmonary hypoplasia may also challenge the res-

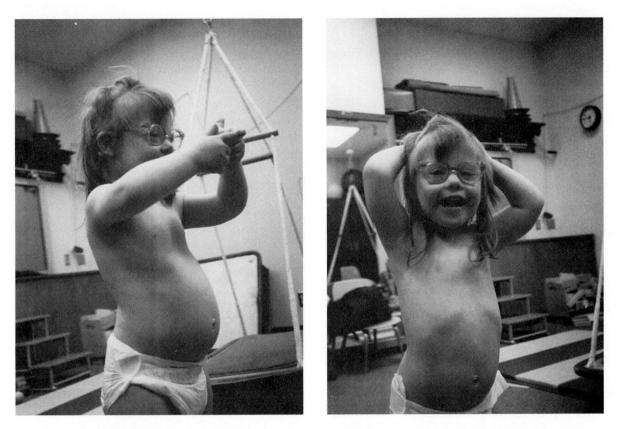

FIGURE 35-3
A, Characteristic posture of a child with Down syndrome/hypotonia. Note the abdominal protrusion and sternal retraction. **B,** Rib flaring with upper extremity movement; the abdominal obliques are not stabilizing the lower ribs.
Photos from Moerchen, V.A. (1994). Respiration and Motor Development: a Systems Perspective. Neurology Report, 18(3), 8–10. Reprinted with the permission of the Neurology Section, APTA.

piratory function of these children. Cooney and Thurl-beck (1982) observed a consistent combination of de-creased numbers of alveoli and larger alveolar ducts in individuals with Down syndrome, not related to age or incidence of heart disease. Although these re-searchers had a small sample size, their results do sug-gest that trisomy 21 may result in lung vulnerability.

Muscular dystrophy

Duchenne's muscular dystrophy involves end-stage respiratory failure that results from progressive respi-ratory muscle weakness, thoracic deformity, reduced lung compliance, retained secretions, ventilation-perfusion imbalance, and hypoxemia (Bach, O'Brien, Krotenberg, and Alba, 1987; Smith, Calverley,

Edwards, Evans, and Campbell, 1987). In 70% to 90% of these patients, death is directly related to restrictive respiratory complications (Bach et al., 1987; Smith et al., 1987).

Physical therapists are typically involved in treatment of these patients for preservation of motor function. Early attention to ventilation, however, is warranted. Prophylactic spinal fusion to prevent scoliosis-related compromise of ventilation in these patients considers both the progression of the spinal curvature and vital capacity (VC) (Rideau, Glorion, Delauber, Tarle, and Bach, 1984).

Chest physical therapy should be a component of the overall physical therapy management of children with muscular dystrophy. Deep breathing, coughing, and activities to address endurance are recommended but will require ongoing modification as the disease progresses. Inspiratory muscle training in these children remains controversial. Although some researchers have demonstrated improved endurance of ventilatory muscles (DiMarco, Kelling, DiMarco, Jacobs, Shields, and Altose, 1985; Martin, Stern, Yeates, Lepp, and Little, 1986; Stern, Martin, Jones, Garrett, and Yeates, 1991), other researchers have suggested that inspiratory resistance may over-tax respiratory muscles that are already near fatigue due to working against incompliant structures (lungs, thorax) (Smith, Coakley, and Edwards, 1988).

Respiratory dependence does occur as the disease progresses. Protocols for point of initiation and type of mechanical ventilation are being studied. There is, however, agreement that close monitoring of VC and of nocturnal hypoventilation can allow respiratory support to be implemented before the onset of acute respiratory failure (Bach, Alba, Pilkington, and Lee, 1981; Bach et al., 1987; Curran, 1981).

Miscellaneous conditions

Multiple other pediatric diagnoses and musculoskeletal conditions include clinical presentations (strength, alignment, and limited mobility) that should cue the therapist's attention to pulmonary function. Syndromes that involve sternal deformity such as Marfan syndrome or Poland's syndrome will clearly entail possible ventilatory compromise. Children with juve-

nile rheumatoid arthritis (JRA) may have inflammation of thoracic joints or may splint through their trunks when they try to move painful extremities. With these children, breathing exercises will have a role both in pulmonary care and in pain management.

Put simply, children who make compensations in their movement patterns to accommodate pain, weakness, or deformity, may limit the mechanics of their thoraces. Conversely, children who cannot adequately oxygenate may make compensations in their movement patterns to support ventilation. Clearly, attention to ventilation should be an inherent aspect of observing motor development and quality of movement in all children.

PHYSICAL THERAPY TREATMENT APPROACHES

Postoperative Pediatric Cardiac Rehabilitation

Postoperative physical therapy consists largely of techniques to increase respiration, mobilize secretions, and progress physical mobility. Positional rotation for pulmonary care is possible if the child has a stabilized sternum. Breathing exercises and coughing will need to be modified based on the child's age and cognitive level. Huckabay and Daderian (1990) reported improved postoperative cooperation in children 3 to 10 years of age when choice making was incorporated into a breathing program.

Immobilization after cardiac surgery is to be avoided as much as medically possible. Passive range of motion may be initiated immediately, with care to avoid compromising arterial lines. Ambulation is generally initiated once the child is extubated and has had atrial and groin lines removed (Johnson, 1991).

Child and family education as part of pediatric cardiac rehabilitation has been observed to reduce parent and child anxiety related to safe levels of physical activity (Balfour, Drimmer, Nouri, Pennington, Hemkens, and Harvey, 1991; Calzolar et al, 1990; Mathews et al, 1983). Although studies of pediatric cardiac rehabilitation have been focused on children older than 6 years, monitored exercise has been shown to safely produce an increase in peak oxygen consumption and a decrease in resting heart rate (Balfour, Drimmer, Nouri, Pennington, Hemkins, and Harvey, 1991; Calzolari et al., 1990; Mathews et al., 1983).

Exercise prescription for cardiopulmonary rehabilitation of older children who have undergone cardiac repairs at an early age will require careful monitoring. Lower exercise VO_2 values, lower cardiac output, and lower values of diffusion capacity of the lung for carbon monoxide have been observed in response to exercise in children who have undergone cardiac surgery as compared with the responses of age-matched controls (Gildein, Mocellin, and Kaufmehl, 1994; Tomassoni, Galioto, and Vaccaro, 1991). Exercise recommendations include submaximal performance (Tommassoni et al., 1991) and technique training to increase the biomechanical efficiency of movement while decreasing the associated metabolical costs (Gildein et al., 1994).

Chest Physical Therapy for Neonates and Infants

The primary goal of chest physical therapy for neonates and infants is to improve airway clearance. If techniques of bronchial drainage can increase the diameter of the airways through secretion mobilization, then ventilation may also be improved and the work of breathing reduced. These techniques should be judiciously applied for prophylaxis and treatment in infants who have or are at risk for developing airway clearance problems. Applying bronchial drainage techniques to infants requires a thorough understanding of each infant's condition and the precautions and considerations inherent to any technique or combination of techniques.

Positional rotation

Frequent changing of position will prevent prolonged dependency of any one portion of the lung, so that pooling of secretions can be limited/avoided and improved ventilation can be achieved (Menkes and Britt, 1980; Ross and Dean, 1989). Whereas positional rotation programs for adults emphasize the lower lobes, positional programs for infants must emphasize all lung areas (Figures 35-4 to 35-6). The upper lobes and right middle lobe are common sites of airway collapse and atelectasis in infants, and the right middle lobe bronchus is surrounded by a collar

of lymph nodes, making it vulnerable to extrinsic compression. Important considerations and essentials of a positional rotation program for infants are outlined in the box below.

It is important to note that premature infants do tolerate and benefit from prone positioning. Studies have demonstrated improved oxygenation, tidal volume, dynamic lung compliance, and synchrony of chest wall movement when preterm infants are put in prone positions (Hutchinson, Ross, and Russell, 1979; Lioy and Manginello, 1988; Martin, Harrell, Rubin, and Fanaroff, 1979).

Positional rotation is generally performed manually every 2 hours, and, although this provides pul-

---

Essentials of a Positional Rotation Program

1. Care should be taken to coordinate any change in the infant's position with other nursing procedures to avoid unnecessary stimulation.

2. Infants should never be left unattended when in a head-down position.

3. Vital signs should be monitored closely by respiration and heart rate monitors. The alarms should be turned on.

4. The infant's chest should be auscultated for adventitious breath sounds after positioning.

5. While the infant is in a drainage position, secretions will be more easily mobilized. The infant's trachea or endotracheal tube should be suctioned as needed.

6. Avoid placing the infant in a head-down position for approximately 1 hour after eating to avoid aspiration of regurgitated food.

7. Any change in the infant's position should be done slowly to minimize stress on the cardiovascular system.

8. Infants with umbilical arterial lines can be placed on their abdomens. However, one should always check that the line has not been kinked.

9. Some infants might require modified drainage positions. Infants with severe cardiovascular instability or suspected intracranial bleeding should not be placed in a head-down position.

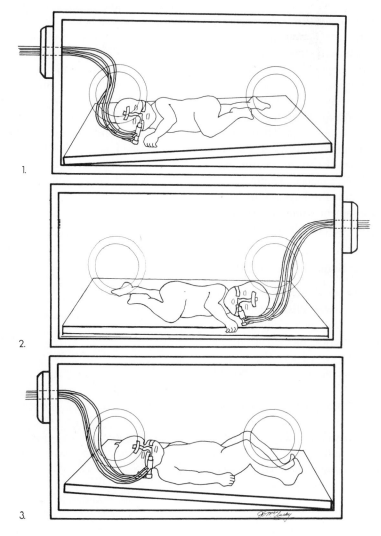

FIGURE 35-4

Sequence for positional rotation.

Position 1.—Segments that come off the left lower bronchus posteriorly are drained by positioning the infant on his right side, three-fourths prone with a head-down angle. ***Position 2.***—The posterior segment of the right upper lobe is drained by positioning on the left side, three-fourths prone with the bed flat. ***Position 3.***—The anterior segments of the upper lobes are drained by positioning supine with the head of the bed elevated or flat. ***Position 4.***—Segments that come off the right lower lobe bronchus posteriorly are drained by positioning on the left side, three-fourths prone with a head down angle.

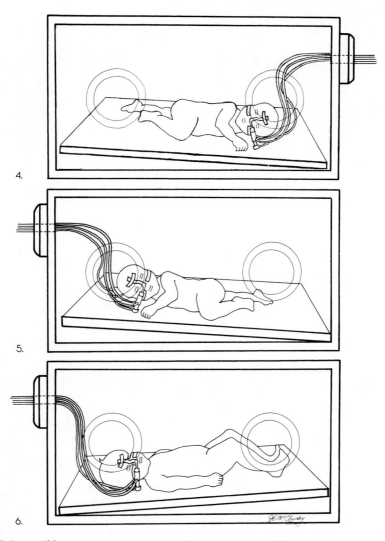

4.

5.

6.

FIGURE 35-4—cont'd

Position 5.—The posterior segment of the left upper lobe is drained by positioning on the right side, three-fourths prone with the head of the bed elevated. *Position 6.*—Segments that come off the tracheobronchial tree anteriorly are drained by positioning supine with a head-down angle. *Positions 7 and 8.*—Segments such as the right middle lobe or lingula that come off the tracheobronchial tree anterolaterally will be drained in a three-fourths spine position, slightly head dow (see Figure 35-5, p. 652).

NOTE: Babies on ventilators may also be positioned prone. This is usually done by the therapist rather than in a *routine* positional rotation (see Figure 35-6, p. 652).

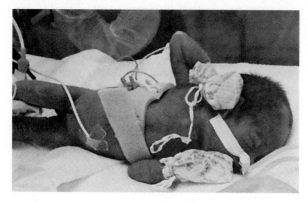

FIGURE 35-5
Three-fourths supine position for right middle lobe. Lingula is the same three-fourths supine position with the patient lying on his right side.

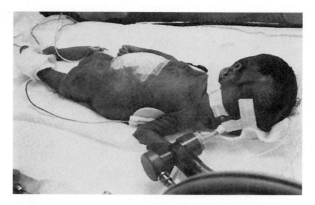

FIGURE 35-6
Premies (even those on ventilators with numerous catheters) may be placed prone when care is taken.

monary benefit, it may also contribute to the disruption of homeostasis that has been documented to occur in the course of neonatal intensive care (Long, Philip, and Lucey, 1980; Yeh, Lilien, Leu, and Pildes, 1984). Use of nursery beds that provide continuous positional oscillation (from right side to supine to left side, and so forth) might provide an option that allows the benefits of position change while also minimizing the homeostatic disruption. Murai and Grant (1994) demonstrated that continuous positional oscillation as part of a total chest physical therapy program decreased the duration of oxygen supplementation without adversely effecting the cardiopulmonary status of the neonates.

Postural drainage

Postural drainage (PD) positions to promote gravity-assisted drainage of specific segmental airways can be safely applied to infants and children. In the acute care setting, however, many of the head-down positions are modified according to tolerance and precautions or contraindications (Table 35-4). The rule for modification of any position for PD is that the position used should be as close to the classical (anatomically correct) position for that segment as safely possible. Examples of the classical PD positions for each bronchopulmonary segment are pictured in Figure 35-7.

Tiny infants (especially premature infants weigh-

ing less than 800 grams) usually require and benefit from modification of the head-down position. Horizontal to slightly elevated positioning of the head may be best (Thoresan, Cowan, and Whitelaw, 1988). This modification primarily is due to the high incidence of intraventricular hemorrhage in premature infants (Crane, Zombek, Krauss, and Auld, 1978; Emery and Peabody, 1983). Other precautions for Trendelenburg positioning of infants include but are not limited to abdominal distention, congestive heart failure, dysrhythmias, hydrocephalus, frequent episodes of apnea and bradycardia, and acute respiratory distress.

Chest percussion and vibration

Percussion and vibration are used in conjunction with postural drainage to augment the effect of gravity in the removal of secretions. There are several ways to perform percussion on infants. For a larger infant, it is possible to use a cupped hand, similarly to percussing an adult's chest. For a smaller infant, some modification of this technique is needed. Chest percussion for a smaller infant is accomplished by the use of tenting three fingers, four fingers, or using any of the commercially available percussion devices made for neonates (Figure 35-8). A small anesthesia mask or "palm cup" can also be used effectively.

Precautions for chest percussion in the infant include but are not limited to unstable cardiovascular or

TABLE 35-4

Precautions and Contraindications for Postural Drainage in a Neonate*

POSITION	PRECAUTION	CONTRAINDICATION
Prone	Umbilical arterial catheter Continuous positive airway pressure in nose Excessive abdominal distention Abdominal incision Anterior chest tube	Untreated tension pneumothorax
Tendelenburg position (head down)	Distended abdomen SEH/IVH* (grades I and II) Chronic congestive heart failure or cor pulmonale Persistent fetal circulation Cardiac dysrhythmias Apnea and bradycardia Infant exhibiting signs of acute respiratory distress Hydrocephalus Less than 28 weeks' gestational age	Untreated tension pneumothorax Recent tracheoesophageal fistula repair Recent eye or intracranial surgery Intraventricular hemorrhage (grades III and IV) Acute congestive heart failure or cor pulmonale

*Subependymal hemorrhage/intraventricular hemorrhage.
From Crane LD: Physical therapy for the neonate with respiratory disease. In Irwin S, Tecklin JS, editors: *Cardiopulmonary physical therapy,* St. Louis, 1995, Mosby.

oxygenation status (although percussion may be provided safely if continuous transcutaneous monitoring is available), coagulopathy, subcutaneous emphysema, or intraventricular hemorrhage. Additionally, percussion is generally contraindicated over a healing thoracotomy incision or if the child displays irritability and signs of respiratory distress with the treatment.

Vibration is accomplished either through manual vibratory motion of the therapist's fingers on the infant's chest wall (Figure 35-9) or through the use of a mechanical vibrator. An electric toothbrush can be adapted by padding the bristle portion with foam (Curran and Kachoyeanos, 1979). Vibration has been observed to occasionally increase irritability and may be less well tolerated than percussion. The most common precaution for vibration is increased irritability with the development of bradycardia and respiratory distress.

The decision to use chest percussion and vibration will depend on the reviewed principles and precautions, the medical condition of the infant, and the infant's tolerance to handling. Continuation of percussion and vi-

bration will depend on the day-to-day medical status of the infant and the infant's response to treatment.

Airway suctioning

Sterile airway suctioning is discussed in detail in Chapter 42. However, some special considerations for suctioning the airway of an infant need to be highlighted (Durand, Sangha, Cabal, Hoppenbrowers, and Hodgman, 1989; McFadden, 1981; Perlman and Volpe, 1983).

1. If possible, suction with a transcutaneous oxygen monitor in place. These monitors give continuous feedback regarding the infant's oxygenation status.
2. Bagging should be done only with a bag attached to a pressure manometer to ensure that sufficient pressures are being used without exceeding the maximum safe levels (these limits should be similar to the ventilator settings).
3. Suction for no more than 5 seconds with each catheter withdrawal.

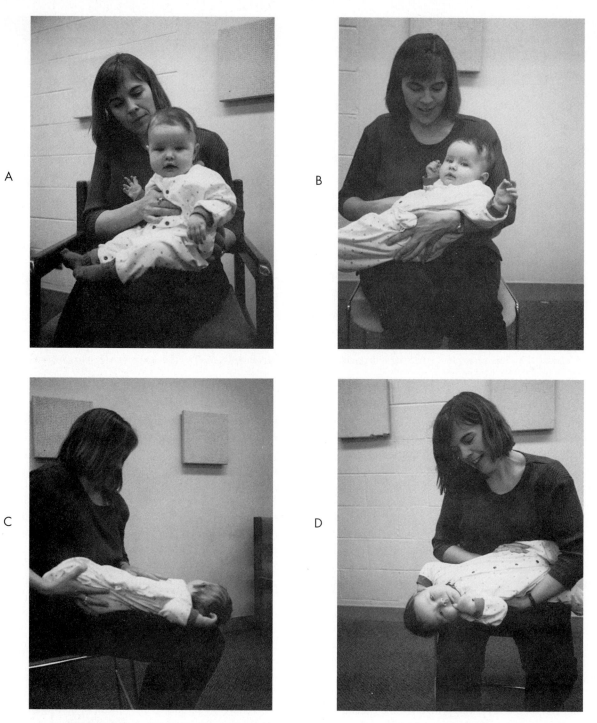

FIGURE 35-7

Postural drainage with an infant. **A,** Both upper lobes—apical segments. **B,** Left upper lobe—anterior segment. **C,** Right upper lobe—anterior segment. **D,** Lingula.

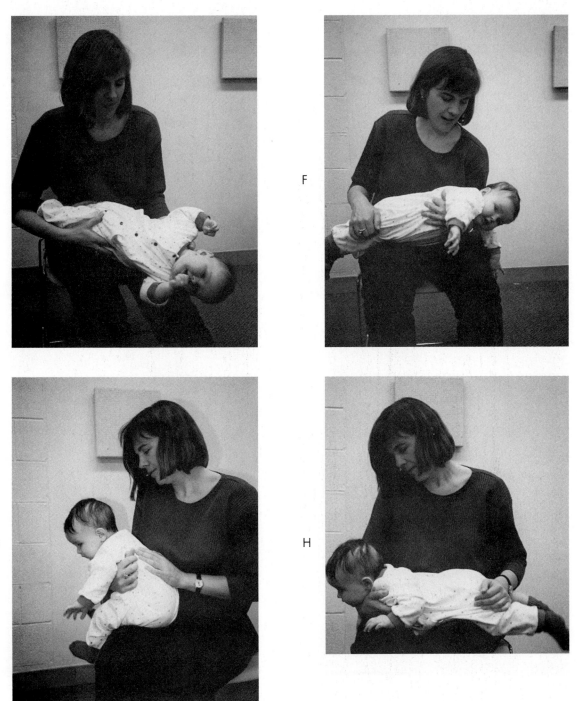

FIGURE 35-7—cont'd

E, Right middle lobe. **F,** Right upper lobe—posterior segment. **G,** Left upper lobe—posterior segment. **H,** Both lower lobes—apical (superior) segments.

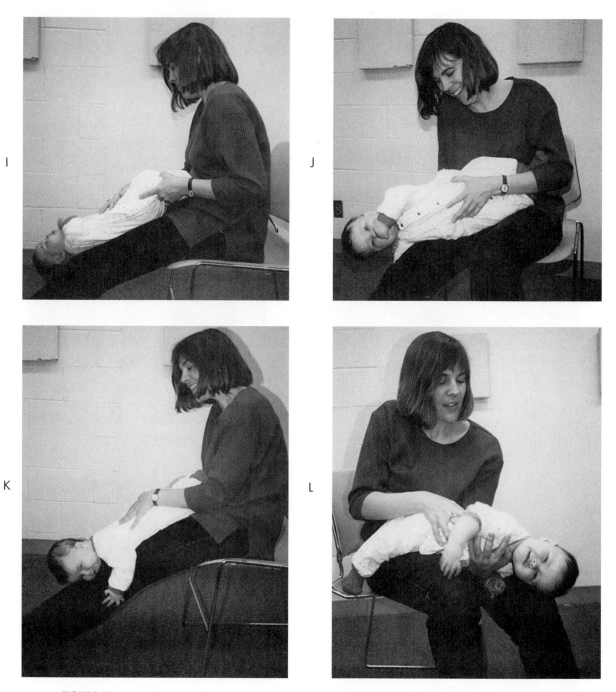

FIGURE 35-7—cont'd
I, Both lower lobes—anterior basal segments. **J,** Left lower lobe—lateral basal segment; Right lower lobe—carduac (medial) segment. **K,** Both lower lobes—posterior basal segments. **L,** Right lower lobe—lateral basal segment.

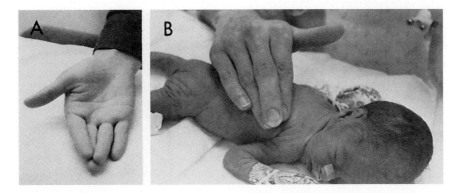

FIGURE 36-8
"Tenting" of the finger for percussion of premies or small children.

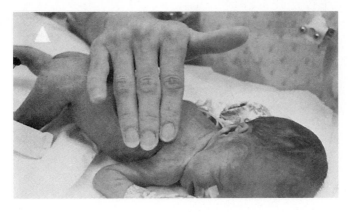

FIGURE 36-9
Manual chest wall vibration of a premie.

4. Infants should be carefully hyperoxygenated when hyperventilated so as to minimize hyperoxia and hypoxia. Bagging usually does not need to continue for more than 5 to 10 seconds to maintain adequate oxygen levels.

5. Monitor the blood pressure of preterm infants before, during, and after suctioning. Change in blood pressure may indicate increased intracranial pressure and risk for intracranial hemorrhage.

Chest Physical Therapy for Children

The goals for chest physical therapy with children (2 years and older) include more than improving airway clearance. Children are capable of following directions and imitating a therapist's demonstration of deep breathing, coughing, and active exercise. Chest physical therapy in children is focused on improving ventilation, improving the efficiency of breathing, increasing general strength and endurance with an emphasis on muscles of respiration, improving posture, and addressing relaxation, breathing control, and pacing.

The application of chest PT with children often requires patience and creative adaptation (Figure 35-10). The challenge is to make it seem less like a treatment and more like a game. It is important, however, to be honest in your explanations and to speak to the child with respect and at a level appropriate to the child's age and development.

Involving the family in PT treatment of a child can

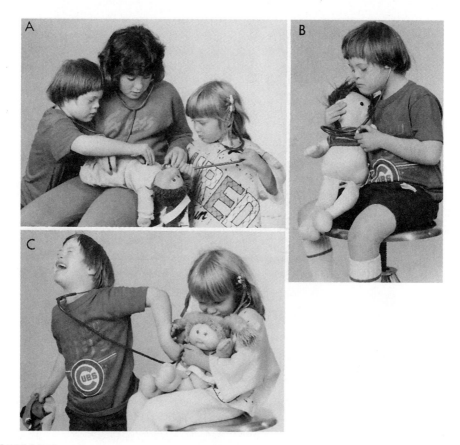

FIGURE 36-10
A, B, C, Few areas of health care delivery require creative adaptation and problem solving to the extent that pediatrics does.

be invaluable. In some cases the parent may do most of the "hands-on" and repeat instructions to the child under the direct guidance of the therapist. This arrangement will also help reinforce parent and family education for carry-over of home therapy.

Positional rotation

The goal of positional rotation and postural drainage is to prevent the accumulation of secretions and to aid in their removal. Any child who is immobile, receiving artificial ventilation, or not expanding his chest adequately should have his position changed at least every 2 hours. Recall that positional changes will enhance oxygen transport and promote pulmonary drainage (Ross and Dean, 1989). If the child is reluc-

tant to have his position changed, changing the location of the television may be helpful. Be creative!
Young Children. In younger children (18 months to 3 years) deep breathing is usually encouraged by blowing bubbles, tissue paper, mobiles, or simple horns. To achieve maximal chest expansion, the child should be positioned on each side while playing blowing games or singing. The theory behind the side lying position is that the downside lung ventilates more effectively (see Chapter 18). Additionally, if the poorly ventilated lung is uppermost, stretch techniques can facilitate deeper breathing (see Chapter 22).

Spontaneous coughing in younger children often occurs with a change in position or with crying. For the child who does not cough spontaneously or whose

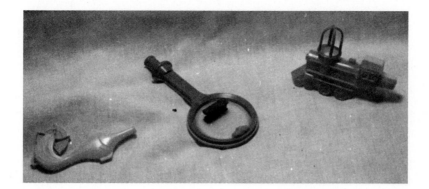

FIGURE 35-11
Whistles such as these encourage increased inspiration and controlled, sustained expiration to make the whistle components move (**left:** a fish with a wheel that moves at its back fin; **middle:** a race car that drives around a track making whirling sounds; **right:** a ball that moves up and down in a train).

cough is inadequate to clear secretions, nasopharyngeal suctioning may be necessary.

Older Children. School-age children can be more specifically instructed in various breathing exercises, such as diaphragmatic breathing, pursed-lip breathing, and segmental lateral costal breathing. They may also be candidates for using relaxed deep breathing for control and pacing of activity. Cooperation with this age group, however, still remains higher if some aspect of therapy is fun. Elaborate whistles are available that encourage deep breathing as a fun means to an end of making the whistle components move (Figure 35-11). Additionally, pediatric incentive spirometers are available with cheerful/"cool" pictures to make respiration exercises more like a game (Figure 35-12).

Older children (not infants) can be stimulated to cough by applying a firm pressure over the trachea in the suprasternal notch. Beware that coughing, whether spontaneous or stimulated, may elicit gagging and vomiting, especially if airway clearance is scheduled too soon after a child has eaten.

Preoperative and postoperative care

The efficacy of postoperative chest PT is highly related to preoperative care. The appropriate application of preoperative assessment, instruction, and treatment by therapists helps to decrease the incidence of postoperative complications.

Preoperative teaching is extremely important for both the child and the family. Parents can often be more anxious than the child, so patient and family education is important. The level of preoperative training with the child will depend on the child's age.

If the child is very young (under 2 years), the therapist will meet with the parents and explain the purpose of bronchial drainage treatments, potential airway clearance problems, and possible complications. The preventative nature of these treatments should be stressed, and procedures that might be done with the child after surgery should be demonstrated and discussed. These might include: (1) positioning, (2) chest percussion, (3) vibration, and (4) airway suctioning. In addition, always allow time for the parents to ask questions.

If the child is able to understand simple concepts, the therapist can, in addition to parent orientation, instruct the child in various breathing games, use of an incentive spirometer, coughing, and general upper and lower extremity exercises.

In older children (8 years or older), postoperative procedures can be explained and demonstrated. The importance of bronchial hygiene should be stressed during demonstration of deep breathing and cough-

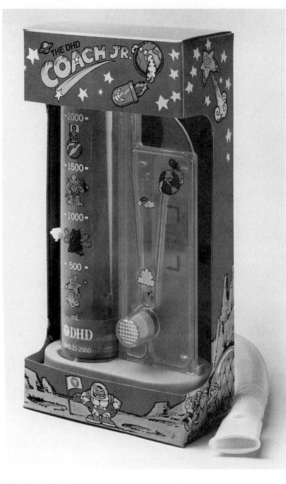

FIGURE 35-12

A pediatric incentive spirometer. (Photo provided courtesy of DHD Medical Products. Used by permission.)

ing. The child can be shown how to splint the incision using a pillow or stuffed animal to assist with comfort while coughing. Do not tell the child that coughing will not hurt; be honest but reinforce that splinting will help. Teach the child diaphragmatic and pursed-lip breathing with an inspiratory-hold maneuver, and, if appropriate, teach the child how to use an incentive spirometer.

Postoperative pulmonary complications may not be as prevalent in the pediatric age group as in adults, but they still occur. The most common complications are atelectasis, infection secondary to pooling of secretions, and airway obstruction. Infants and children with the following characteristics will be at risk for developing postoperative pulmonary complications: (1) preexisting lung disease, (2) thoracic or upper abdominal location of the incision, (3) prolonged postoperative bedrest or restricted mobility, and (4) neuromuscular involvement that affects the ability to be mobile and to cough and deep breathe.

Postoperative treatments generally focus on increasing ventilation, coughing, and active mobility. Specific bronchial drainage is used only if the child is unable to clear his or her airways or is at risk due to chronic lung disease.

After high abdominal or thoracic surgery, there may be a tendency for the child to splint on the side of his or her incision. Arm, shoulder, and trunk movement should be encouraged to prevent any postoperative complications. For the younger child, chest mobility can be encouraged by clapping the hands overhead or by dramatizing songs such as *The Itsy Bitsy Spider.* More conventional exercises may be taught to the older child.

Children tend to mobilize very quickly (unless their movement is limited secondary to motor involvement or to a specific surgical procedure). Once the child is out of bed and moving about, with clear lungs and an effective cough, postoperative CPT treatments can generally be discontinued.

Pediatric Pulmonary Rehabilitation

Rehabilitation programs for pediatric patients with chronic lung disease include the same components and have essentially the same goals as adult pulmonary rehabilitation. The major difference is related to different diagnoses being most prevalent in the children versus adult age groups. Asthma and CF are the most common diagnoses of children who are candidates for pulmonary rehabilitation.

Exercise and asthma

Exercise and conditioning are very important components of the treatment of the child with asthma. Improved chest and trunk mobility, control of breathing, strength, posture, and an increased tolerance to exercise are all goals that can be addressed in the design of exercise programs for these children (Magee, 1991; Seligman, Randel, and Stevens, 1970).

Part of a pulmonary rehabilitation program may involve providing recommendations for the child's participation in physical education (PE). Certain aspects of exercise relative to pulmonary function in children with asthma need to be communicated to the PE teacher. Running is the form of exercise most likely to aggravate exercise-induced asthma, especially if performed in a cool, dry environment. Swimming, by contrast, is an excellent activity. Continuous or high burst exercise might induce bronchospasm, whereas short periods of exercise (less than 6 continuous minutes) may be beneficial for conditioning without bronchial aggravation (Magee, 1991). PE teachers should also be aware that the child may need to use a preexercise aerosol to participate in PE without pulmonary consequence (Magee, 1991).

Exercise and cystic fibrosis

Physical activity designed to improve exercise tolerance helps children with CF to mobilize secretions and to improve body image. The development of an exercise program for children with CF should be done on a individualized basis and a preexercise assessment should include but not be limited to the following:

1. Assessment of range of motion, strength, and posture.
2. Complete chest evaluation.
3. Evaluation of ADL tolerance and limitations.
4. Inspiratory muscle strength (maximal inspiratory negative pressure at the mouth) and endurance testing. This inspiratory endurance testing can be done with an inspiratory muscle training device by having the child breathe for a predetermined length of time at progressively increased resistances until tolerance is reached.
5. Exercise tolerance testing, performed with ECG, blood pressure, and oxygen monitoring.

A basic exercise program for children with CF should include activities to strengthen the back and shoulder extensors, to elongate the trunk flexors, and to address overall endurance. The role of more vigorous exercise and fitness training in these children is a issue of debate, based on inconsistent incidence of oxygen desaturation during exercise in children with CF (Coates, 1992). Loutzenhiser and Clark (1993), however, suggested that severity of CF is not the primary limiting factor in the exercise capacity of these children. Clearly, any aerobic exercise program designed for older children with CF will require careful monitoring of pulmonary support during exercise.

Motor Approaches to Maximize Trunk and Ventilatory Function

Attention to pulmonary function is easily accomplished within any "handling" approach to motor therapy for children with trunk weakness, tightness, alterations in tone, or general immobility. Most "handling" consistent with a neurodevelopmental technique (NDT) approach lends itself readily to a dual focus on movement quality and ventilation. Extrinsic pulmonary development is clearly interrelated with musculoskeletal and motor development of the trunk.

Treatment should begin with assessment and initial handling for functional range of motion through the trunk. This will typically require elongation of the pectoral, sternocleidomastoid, upper trapezius, and rectus abdominis muscles. Manual lowering of the rib cage will also be necessary to work toward maximizing chest mobility (Figure 35-13).

Passive elongation of muscles must always be followed by active elongation. Controlled prone extension off the ball is both fun for the child and effective for the therapist (Figure 35-14). Manual guidance for upper extremity abduction and external rotation will facilitate active elongation of the pectoral muscles via active firing of the scapular retractors. The ball can be used to impart movement and support the lower rib cage. This elongates the anterior trunk (rectus abdominis), lengthens intercostal muscles, and facilitates increased upper chest expansion.

Handling to achieve proprioceptive input of the scapulae on the posterior thorax, will help reinforce active thoracic extension and anterior chest expansion. The therapist's hands can stabilize the rib cage to reinforce abdominal oblique function during movement (Figure 35-15).

Activities requiring alternating extension-rotation

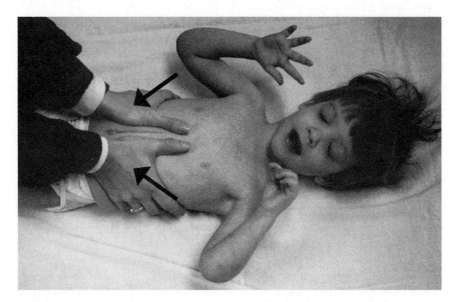

FIGURE 35-13
Manual lowering of the rib cage.
NOTE: Arrows indicate direction of therapist's hand movement (caudal and medial).

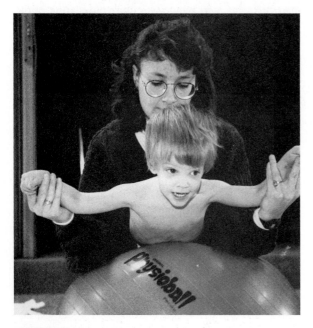

FIGURE 35-14
Handling to facilitate active upper thoracic extension, as a means of actively opening the anterior chest and lengthening rectus abdominis while supporting the lower rib cage on the ball.

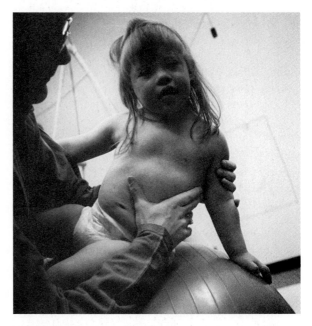

FIGURE 35-15
Handling to reinforce upper chest expansion and abdominal oblique stabilization of the lower ribs.

and flexion-rotation will recruit control of the abdominal obliques and maintain active upper trunk extension. Bubble blowing, whistle toys, and singing are excellent means of monitoring the ventilatory changes that occur with active use of increased upper chest expansion. As tidal volume increases, vocalizations should increase in frequency, sound higher, and become louder.

The concept of functional carry-over is central to the treatment approach presented here. Addressing ventilation and trunk control simultaneously has intuitive appeal based not only on shared musculoskeletal relationships but also on the necessity of pulmonary tolerance for motor activity.

SUMMARY

Cardiopulmonary physical therapy with infants and children is presented starting with issues related to development and developmental vulnerabilities. Specific cardiopulmonary diagnoses in pediatrics are described and treatment recommendations are provided. Cardiopulmonary development and function are presented as the basis for indications and precautions for treatment of neonatal and pediatric patients.

The link between pulmonary and motor function has also been stressed. Many children with motor involvement are at risk for or have had medical histories remarkable for cardiopulmonary dysfunction. Motor approaches to maximize ventilatory function have been included in this chapter to reinforce that efficient oxygenation is a priority not only for children with primary cardiopulmonary diagnoses but also for children with motor compromise.

REVIEW QUESTIONS

1. Discuss the importance of changes in pulmonary blood flow during transitional circulation, and relate these changes to closure of foramen ovale and ductus arteriosus.
2. Describe six characteristics of an infant's pulmonary anatomy that contribute to the increased work of breathing and to the potential for pulmonary distress in this age group.
3. Identify and discuss two aspects of cardiopulmonary vulnerability in the preterm infant.

4. Compare the goals of chest physical therapy for infants and older children. What are the similarities and differences?
5. When treating infants to improve airway clearance, what are the precautions/considerations of:
   • positional rotation?
   • postural drainage?
   • percussion?
   • vibration?
   • airway suctioning?
6. How might neuromotor (neuromuscular) dysfunction affect pulmonary development and contribute to possible postoperative complications?
7. Describe goals, precautions, and suggested monitoring for exercise in children who have the following:
   • a history of cardiac surgery
   • asthma
   • cystic fibrosis?

References

Abel, E.L. (1984). *Fetal alcohol syndrome and fetal alcohol effects.* New York: Plenum Press.

Abman, S.H., & Groothius, J.R. (1994). Pathophysiology and treatment of bronchopulmonary dysplasia. *Pediatric Clinics of North America, 41,* 277-315.

Alexander, R. (1993). Respiratory and oral-motor functioning. In B.H. Connolly & P.C. Montgomery (Eds.). *Therapeutic exercise in developmental disabilities* (2nd ed.). Hixson, TN: Chattanooga Group.

Archer, N. (1993). Patent ductus arteriosus in the newborn. *Archives of Disease in Childhood, 69,* 529-532.

Asher, M.I., Douglas, C., Airy, M., Andrews, D., & Trenholme, A. (1990). Effects of chest physical therapy on lung function in children recovering from acute severe asthma. *Pediatric Pulmonology, 9,* 146-151.

Avery, M.E., Gatewood, O.B., & Brumley, G. (1966). Transient tachypnea of newborn. *American Journal of Disease in Children, 111,* 380-385.

Bach, J., Alba, A., Pilkington, L.A., & Lee, M. (1981). Long-term rehabilitation in advanced stage of childhood onset, rapidly progressive muscular dystrophy. *Archives of Physical Medicine and Rehabilitation, 62,* 328-331.

Bach, J.R., O'Brien, J., Krptenberg, R., & Alba, A.S. (1987). Management of end stage respiratory failure in Duchene muscular dystrophy. *Muscle & Nerve, 10,* 177-182.

Bacsik, R.D. (1977). Meconium aspiration syndrome. *Pediatric Clinics of North America, 24,* 463-479.

Bagarazzi, M.L., Connor, E.M., McSherry, G.D., & Oleske, J.M. (1990). Pneumocystis carnii pneumonia (PCP) among human immunodeficiency virus (HIV) infected children: ten years experience. *Pediatric Research, 27,* 166 (Abstract No. 980).

Balfour, I.C., Drimmer, A.M., Nouri, S., Pennington, D.G., Hemkins, C.L., & Harvey, L.L. (1991). Pediatric cardiac rehabilitation. *American Journal of Disease in Childhood, 145,* 627-630.

Bender, H.W., Hammon, J.W., Hubbard, S.G., Muirhead, J., & Graham, T.P. (1982). Repair of atrioventricular canal malformation in the first year of life. *Journal of Thoracic and Cardiovascular Surgery, 84,* 515-522.

Berdon, W.E., Mellins, R.B., Abramson, S.J., & Ruzal-Shapiro, C. (1993). Pediatric HIV infection in its second decade—the changing pattern of lung involvement. *Radiologic Clinics of North America, 31,* 453-463.

Berman, W., Katz, R., Yabek, S.M., Dillon, T., Fripp, R.R., & Papile, L. (1986). Long-term follow-up of bronchopulmonary dysplasia. *Journal of Pediatrics, 109,* 45-50.

Bernstein, L.J., Bye, M.R., & Rubinstein, A. (1989). Prognostic factors and life expectancy in children with acquired immunodeficiency syndrome and *pneuomocystitis carnii pneumonia. AJDC, 143,* 775-778.

Blackburn, S. (1992). Alterations of the respiratory system in the neonate: Implications for clinical practice. *Journal of Perinatal Nursing, 6,* 46-58.

Boehme, R. (1991). How do I get scapular stability in my patients? *Team Talk, 1,* 1-3.

Boehme, R. (1992). Assessment and treatment of the respiratory system for breathing, sound production, and trunk control. *Team Talk, 2,* 2-8.

Bove, E.L. & Lupinetti, F.M. (1994). Tetralogy of Fallot. In C. Mavroudis & C.L. Backer (Eds.). *Pediatric cardiac surgery* (2nd ed.). St. Louis: Mosby.

Bozynski, M.A., Naglie, R.A., Nicks, J.J., Burpee, B., & Johnson, R.V. (1988). Lateral positioning of the stable ventilated very-low-birth-weight infant: effect on transcutaneous oxygen and carbon dioxide. *AJDC, 142,* 200-202.

Calzolari, A., Turchetta, A., Biondi, G., Drago, F., De Ranieri, C., Gagliardi, G., Giambini, I., Giannico, S., Kofler, A.M., Perrotta, F., Santilli, A., Vezzoli, P., Ragonese, P., & Maecelletti, C. (199). Rehabilitation of children after total correction of tetralogy of Fallot. *International Journal of Cardiology, 28,* 151-158.

Cerney, F.J. (1989). Relative effects of bronchial drainage and exercise for hospital care of patients with cystic fibrosis. *Physical Therapy, 69,* 633-639.

Charney, E.B., Rorke, L.B., Sutton, L.N., & Schut, L. (1987). Management of Chiari II complications in infants with myelomeningocele. *Journal of Pediatrics, 11,* 364-71.

Coates, A.L. (1992). Oxygen therapy, exercise, and cystic fibrosis. *Chest, 101,* 2-4.

Connor, E., Bagarazzi, M., McSherry, G., Holland, B., Boland, M., Denny, T., & Oleske, J. (1991). Clinical and laboratory correlates of Pneumocystis carnii pneumonia in children infected with HIV. *JAMA, 265,* 1693-1697.

Cooney, T.P., & Thurlbeck, W.M. (1982). Pulmonary hypoplasia in Down's syndrome. *New England Journal of Medicine, 307,* 1170-1173.

Crane, L. (1981). Physical therapy for neonates with respiratory dysfunction. *Physical Therapy, 61,* 1764-1773.

Crane, L.D., Zombek, M., Krauss, A.N., & Auld, P.A.M. (1978). Comparison of chest physiotherapy in infants with HMD. *Pediatric Research, 12,* 559 (Abstract No. 1173).

Curran, F.J. (1981). Night ventilation by body respirators for patients in chronic respiratory failure due to late stage Duchenne muscular dystrophy. *Archives of Physical Medicine and Rehabilitation, 62,* 270-273.

Cystic Fibrosis Foundation Center Committee and Guidelines Subcommittee (1990). Cystic fibrosis foundation guidelines for patient services, evaluation, and monitoring in cystic fibrosis centers. *AJDC, 144,* 1311-1312.

Daniels, O., Hopman, J.C.W., Stoelinga, G.B.A., Busch, H.J., & Peer, P.G.M. (1982). Doppler flow characteristics in the main pulmonary artery and the Lratio before and after ductal closure in healthy newborns. *Pediatric Cardiology, 3,* 99-104.

Davis, P.B. (1994). Evolution of therapy for cystic fibrosis. *New England Journal of Medicine, 331,* 672-673.

Dichter, C.G., Darbee, J.C., Effgen, S.K., & Palisano, R.J. (1993). Assessment of pulmonary function and physical fitness in children with Down syndrome. *Pediatric Physical Therapy, 5,* 3-8.

DiMarco, A.F., Kelling, J.S., DiMarco, M.S., Jacobs, I., Shields, R., & Altose, M.D. (1985). The effects of inspiratory resistive training on respiratory function in patients with muscular dystrophy. *Muscle & Nerve, 8,* 284-290.

Driscoll, D.J. (1990). The cyanotic newborn. *Pediatric Clinics of North America, 37,* 1-23.

Durand, M., Sangha, B., Cabal, L.A., Hoppenbrowers, T., & Hodgman, J.E. (1989). Cardiopulmonary and intracranial pressure changes related to endotracheal suctioning in preterm infants. *Critical Care Medicine, 17,* 506-510.

Emery, J.R., & Peabody, J.L. (1983). Head position affects intracranial pressure in newborn infants. *Journal of Pediatrics, 103,* 950-953.

Emmanouilides, G.C. & Baylen, B.G. (1988). *Neonatal cardiopulmonary distress.* St. Louis: Mosby.

Farrel, P.M., & Avery, M.E. (1975). Hyaline Membrane Disease. *American Review of Respiratory Disease, 111,* 657-688.

Finer, N.N., & Boyd, J. (1978). Chest physiotherapy in the neonate: a controlled study. *Pediatrics, 61,* 282-285.

Finer, N.N., Moriartey, R.R., Boyd, J., Phillips, H.J., Stewart, A.R., & Ulan, O. (1979). Postextubation atelectasis: a retrospective review and a prospective controlled study. *Journal of Pediatrics, 94,* 110-113.

Freedom, R.M., & Benson, L.N. (1992). Tetralogy of Fallot. In R.M. Freedom, L.N. Benson, & J.F. Smallhorn. (Eds.). *Neonatal heart disease.* London: Springer-Verlag.

Freedom, R.M., & Smallhorn, J.F. (1992). Atrioventricular septal defect. In R.M. Freedom, L.N. Benson, & J.F. Smallhorn. (Eds.). *Neonatal heart disease.* London: Springer-Verlag.

Gerhardt, T., Hehre, D., Feller, R., Reifenberg, L., & Bancalari, E. (1987). Serial determination of pulmonary function in infants with chronic lung disease. *Journal of Pediatrics, 110,* 448-456.

Gildein, P., Mocellin, R., & Kaufmehl, K. (1994). Oxygen uptake transient kinetics during constant-load exercise in children after operations of ventricular septal defect, tetralogy of Fallot, transposition of the great arteries, or tricuspid valve atresia. *American Journal Cardiology, 74,* 166-169.

Graham, T.P., & Bender, H.W. (1980). Preoperative diagnosis and management of infants with critical congenital heart disease. *Annals of Thoracic Surgery, 29,* 272-288.

Greene, M.A., Mavroudis, C., & Backer, C.L. (1994) Patent ductus arteriosus. In C. Mavroudis & C.L. Backer. (Eds.). *Pediatric cardiac surgery.* St Louis: Mosby.

Gregory, G.A., Gooding, C.A., Phibbs, R.H., & Tooley, W.H. (1974). Meconium aspiration in infants—a prospective study. *Journal of Pediatrics, 85,* 848-852.

Hays, R.M., Jordan, R.A., McLaughlin, J.F., Nickel, R.E., & Fisher, L.D. (1989). Central ventilatory dysfunction in myelodysplasia: an independent determinant of survival. *Developmental Medicine and Child Neurology, 31,* 366-370.

Heymann, M.A. & Hanley, F.L. (1994). Physiology of circulation. In C. Mavroudis & C.L. Backer. (Eds.). *Pediatric cardiac surgery.* St Louis: Mosby.

Hesz, N., & Wolraich, M. (1985). Vocal-cord paralysis and brainstem dysfunction in children with spina bifida. *Developmental Medicine and Child Neurology, 27,* 522-531.

Huckabay, L., & Daderian, A.D. (1990). Effect of choices on breathing exercises post-open heart surgery. *Dimensions of Critical Care Nursing, 9,* 190-201.

Hutchinson, A.A., Ross, K.R., & Russell, G. (1979). The effects of posture on ventilation and lung mechanics in preterm and light-for-date infants. *Pediatrics, 64,* 429-432.

Jobe, A. (1988). The role of surfactant in neonatal adaptation. *Seminars in Perinatology, 12,* 113-123.

Johnson, B. (1991). Postoperative physical therapy in the pediatric cardiac surgery patient. *Pediatric Physical Therapy, 3,* 14-22.

Johnson, T.R., Moore, W.M., & Jeffries, J.E. (1978). *Children are different: developmental physiology* (2nd ed.). Columbus, OH: Ross Laboratories.

Kapandji, I.A. (1982). *The physiology of the joints* (Vol. 1). New York: Churchill Livingstone.

Katz, V.L., & Bowes, W.A. (1992). Meconium aspiration syndrome: reflections on a murky subject. *American Journal of Obstetrics and Gynecology, 166,* 171-183.

Keens, T.G., Krastins, I.R.S., Wannamaker, E.M., Levison, H., Crozier, D.N., & Bryan, A.C. (1977). Ventilatory muscle training in normal subjects and patients with cystic fibrosis. *American Review of Respiratory Disease, 116,* 853-860.

Koff, P.B. (1993). Development of the cardiopulmonary system. In P.B. Koff, D. Eitzman, & J. Neu. (Eds.). *Neonatal and pediatric respiratory care.* St Louis: Mosby.

Konstan, M.W., Stern, R.C., & Doershuk, C.F. (1994). Efficacy of the Flutter device for airway mucus clearance in patients with cystic fibrosis. *Journal of Pediatrics, 124,* 689-693.

Laitman, J.T., & Crelin, E.S. (1980). Developmental change in the upper respiratory system of human infants. *Perinatology and Neonatalogy, 4,* 15-21.

Lioy, J., & Manginello, F.P. (1988). A comparison of prone and supine positioning in the immediate postextubation period of neonates. *Journal of Pediatrics, 112,* 982-984.

Long, J.G., Phillip. A.G.S., & Lucey, J.F. (1980). Excessive handling as a cause of hypoxemia. *Pediatrics, 65,* 203-207.

Loutzenhiser, J.K., & Clark, R. (1993). Physical activity and exercise in children with cystic fibrosis. *Journal of Pediatric Nursing, 8,* 112-119.

MacFarlane, P.I., & Heaf, D.P. (1988). Pulmonary function in children after neonatal meconium aspiration syndrome. *Archives of Disease in Childhood, 63,* 368-372.

Magee, C.L. (1991). Physical therapy for the child with asthma. *Pediatric Physical Therapy, 3,* 23-28.

Mahlmeister, M.J., Fink, J.B., Hoffman, G.L., & Fifer, L.F. (1991). Positive-expiratory-pressure mask therapy: theoretical and practical considerations and a review of the literature. *Respiratory Care, 36,* 1218-1229.

Marolda, J., Pace, B., Bonforte, R.J., Kotin, N.M., Rabinowitz, J., & Kattan, M. (1991). Pulmonary manifestations of HIV infection in children. *Pediatric Pulmonology, 10,* 231-235.

Martin, A.J., Stern, L., Yeates, J., Lepp, D., & Little, J. (1986). Respiratory muscle training in muscular dystrophy. *Developmental Medicine and Child Neurology, 28,* 314-318.

Martin, R.J., Herrell, N., Rubin, D., & Fanaroff, A. (1979). Effects of supine and prone positions on arterial oxygen tension in the preterm infant. *Pediatrics, 63,* 528-531.

Massery, M. (1991). Chest development as a component of motor development: implications for pediatric physical therapists. *Pediatric Physical Therapy,3,* 3-8.

Mathews, R.A., Nixon, P.A., Stephenson, R.J., Robertson, R.J., Donovan, E.F., Dean, F., Fricker, F.J., Beerman, L.B., & Fischer, D.R. (1983). An exercise program for pediatric patients with congenital heart disease: Organizational and physiologic aspects. *Journal of Cardiac Rehabilitation, 3,* 467-475.

McFadden, R. (1981). Decreasing respiratory compromise during infant suctioning. *American Journal of Nursing, 81,* 2158-2161.

Mellins, R.B., & Berdon, W.E. (1994). The lung in human immunodeficiency virus infection. In P.D. Phelan, A. Olinsky, C.F. Robertson. *Respiratory illness in children* (4th ed.). Boston: Blackwell-Scientific Publications.

Merrill, W.H., Hoff, S.J., & Bender, H.W. (1994). Surgical treatment of atrioventricular septal defects. In C. Mavroudis & C.L. Backer. (Eds.). *Pediatric cardiac surgery.* St. Louis: Mosby.

Milne, M.J., Sung, R.Y.T., Fok, T.F., & Crozier, I.G. (1989). Doppler echocardiographic assessment of shunting via the ductus arteriosus in newborn infants. *American Journal of Cardiology, 64,* 102-105.

Mitchell, S.C., Korones, S.B., & Berendes, H.W. (1971). Congenital heart disease in 56,109 births: incidence and natural history. *Circulation, 43,* 323-331.

Moerchen, V.A. (1994) Respiration and motor development: a systems perspective. *Neurology Report, 18,* 8-10.

Muller, N.L., & Bryan, A.C. (1979). Chest wall mechanics and respiratory muscle in infants. *Pediatric Clinics of North America, 26,* 503-516.

Murai, D.T., & Grant, J.W. (1994). Continuous oscillation therapy improves pulmonary outcome of intubated newborns: results of a prospective, randomized, controlled trial. *Critical Care Medicine, 22,* 1147-1154.

Musewe, N.N., & Olley, P.M. (1994). Patent ductus arteriosus. In R.M. Freedom, L.N. Benson, & J.F. Smallhorn. (Eds.). *Neonatal heart disease*. London: Springer-Verlag.

Northway, W.H., Rosan, R.C., & Porter, D.Y. (1967). Pulmonary disease following respirator therapy of hyaline membrane disease: bronchopulmonary dysplasia. *New England Journal of Medicine, 276*, 357-368.

Northway, W.H. (1979). Observations on bronchopulmonary dysplasia. *Journal of Pediatrics, 95*, 815-818.

Nudel, D.B., & Gootman, N. (1983). Clinical aspects of neonatal circulation. In N. Gootman & P.M. Gootman. (Eds.) *Perinatal cardiovascular function*. New York: Marcel Dekker.

Oren, J., Kelly, D.H., Todres, D., & Shannon, D.C. (1986). Respiratory complications in patients with myelodysplasia and Arnold-Chiari malformation. *AJDC, 140*, 221-224.

Orenstein, S.R., & Orenstein, D.M. (1988). Gastroesophageal reflux and respiratory disease in children. *Journal of Pediatrics, 112*, 847-858.

Parker, R.A., Lindstrom, D.P., & Cotton, R.B. (1992). Improved survival accounts for most, but not all, of the increase in bronchopulmonary dysplasia. *Pediatrics, 90*, 663-668.

Park, M.K. (1988). *Pediatric cardiology for practitioners*. St. Louis: Mosby.

Perlman, J.M., & Volpe, J.J. (1983). Suctioning in the preterm infant: Effects on cerebral blood flow velocity, intracranial pressure, and arterial blood pressure. *Pediatrics, 72*, 329-334.

Phelan, P.D., Olinsky, A., & Robertson, C.F. (Eds.). (1994). *Respiratory illness in children*. Boston: Blackwell-Scientific Publications.

Pinsky, W.W., & Arciniegas, E. (1990). Tetralogy of Fallot. *Pediatric Clinics of North America, 37*, 179-192.

Pullan, C.R., & Hey, E.N. (1982). Wheezing, asthma, and pulmonary dysfunction 10 years after infection with respiratory syncytial virus in infancy. *British Medical Journal, 284*, 1665-1669.

Pryor, J.A. (1991). The forced expiration technique. In J.A. Pryor. *Respiratory care* (pp. 79-100). London: Churchill-Livingstone.

Pryor, J.A., & Webber, B.A. (1979). An evaluation of the forced expiration technique as an adjunct to postural drainage. *Physiotherapy, 65*, 304-307.

Reid, W.D., & Loveridge, B.M. (1983). Ventilatory muscle endurance training in patients with chronic obstructive airway disease. *Physiotherapy Canada, 35*, 197-205.

Rickards, A.L., Ford, G.W., Kitchen, W.H., Doyle, L.W., Lissenden, J.V., & Keith, C.G. (1987). Extremely-low-birthweight infants: neurological, psychological, growth and health status beyond five years of age. *Medical Journal of Australia, 147*, 476-481.

Rideau, Y., Glorion, B., Delaubier, A., Tarle, O., & Bach, J. (1984). The treatment of scoliosis in Duchene muscular dystrophy. *Muscle & Nerve, 7*, 281-286.

Ross, J., & Dean, E. (1989). Integrating physiological principles into the comprehensive management of cardiopulmonary dysfunction. *Physical Therapy, 69*, 255-259.

Rudolph, A.M. (1970). The changes in the circulation after birth: Their importance in congenital heart disease. *Circulation, 41*, 343-359.

Rudolph, A.M. (1980). High pulmonary vascular resistance after birth: Physiologic considerations and etiologic classification. *Clinical Pediatrics, 19*, 585-590.

Scott, G.B., Hutto, C., Makuch, R.H., Mastrucci, M.T., O'Connor, T., Mitchell, C.D., Trapido, E.J., & Parks, W.P. (1989). Survival in children with perinatally acquired human immunodeficiency virus type 1 infection. *New England Journal of Medicine, 321*, 1791-1796.

Scott, A.A., & Koff, P.B. (1993). Airway care and chest physiotherapy. In P.B. Koff, D. Eitzman, & J. Neu. (Eds.) *Neonatal and pediatric respiratory care*. St. Louis: Mosby.

Seligman, T., Randel, H.O., & Stevens, J.J. (1970). Conditioning program for children with asthma. *Physical Therapy, 50*, 641-647.

Shoni, M.H. (1989). Autogenic drainage: A modern approach to physiotherapy in cystic fibrosis. *Journal of the Royal Society of Medicine, 82*, Supl 16, 32-37.

Sinclair, D. (1978). *Human growth after birth*. London: Oxford University Press.

Smith, P.E.M, Calverley, P.M.A, Edwards, R.H.T., Evans, G.A., & Campbell, E.J.M. (1987). Practical problems in the respiratory care of patients with muscular dystrophy *New England Journal of Medicine, 316*, 1197-1205.

Smith, P.E.M., Coakley, J.H., & Edwards, R.H.T. (1988). Respiratory muscle training in Duchene muscular dystrophy. *Muscle & Nerve*, 784-785.

Smyth, J.A., Tabachnik, E., Duncan, W.J., Reilly, B.J., & Levison, H. (1981). Pulmonary function and bronchial hyperreactivity in long-term survivors of bronchopulmonary dysplasia. *Pediatrics, 68*, 336-340.

Spicer, R.L. (1984). Cardiovascular disease in Down syndrome. *Pediatric Clinics of North America, 31*, 1331-1343.

Starnes, V.A., Luciani, G.B., Latter, D.A., & Griffin, M.L. (1994). Current surgical management of tetralogy of Fallot. *Annals of Thoracic Surgery, 58*, 211-215.

Stern, L.M., Martin, A.J., Jones, N., Garrett, R., & Yeates, J. (1991). Respiratory training in Duchene dystrophy. *Developmental Medicine and Child Neurology, 33*, 649.

Swaminathan, S., Paton, J.Y., Ward, S.L.D., Jacobs, R.A., Sargent, C.W., & Keens, T.G. (1989). Abnormal control of ventilation in adolescents with myelodysplasia. *Journal of Pediatrics, 115*, 898-903.

Swaminathan, S., Quinn, J., Stabile, M.W., Bader, D., Platzker, A.C.G., & Keens, T.G. (1989). Long-term pulmonary sequelae of meconium aspiration syndrome. *Journal of Pediatrics, 114*, 356-361.

Thoresen, M., Cowan, F., & Whitelaw, A. (1988). Effect of tilting on oxygenation in newborn infants. *Archives of Disease in Childhood, 63*, 315-317.

Thurlbeck, W.M. (1975). Postnatal growth and development of the lung. *American Review of Respiratory Disease, 111*, 803-844.

Tomassoni, T.L., Galioto, F.M., & Vaccaro, P. (1991). Cardiopulmonary exercise testing in children following surgery for tetralogy of Fallot. *AJDC, 145*, 1290-1293.

Vohr, B.R., Bell, E.F., & Oh, W. (1982). Infants with bronchopulmonary dysplasia: Growth pattern and neurologic and developmental outcome. *American Journal of Disease in Childhood, 136*, 443-447.

Voyles, J.B. (1981). Bronchopulmonary dysplasia. *American Journal of Nursing, 81*, 510-514.

Wallis, S., & Harvey, D. (1979). Respiratory distress: its cause and management. *Nursing Times, 75,* 1264-1272.

Walther, F.J., Benders, M.J., & Leighton, J.O. (1992). Persistent pulmonary hypertension in premature neonates with severe respiratory distress syndrome. *Pediatrics, 90,* 899-903.

Ward, S.L.D., Jacobs, R.A., Gates, E.P., Hart, L.D., & Keens, T.G. (1986). Abnormal ventilatory patterns during sleep in infants with myelomeningocele. *Journal of Pediatrics, 4,* 631-634.

Waring, W.W. (1975). Respiratory diseases in children—An overview. *Respiratory Care, 20,* 1138-1145.

Weinstein, M.R., & Oh, W. (1981). Oxygen consumption in infants with bronchopulmonary dysplasia. *Journal of Pediatrics, 99,* 958-961.

Wiswell, T.E., & Bent, R.C. (1993). Meconium staining and the meconium aspiration syndrome. *Pediatric Clinics of North America, 40,* 955-981.

Wiswell, T.E., Tuggle, J.M., & Turner, B.S. (1990). Meconium aspiration syndrome: have we made a difference? *Pediatrics, 85,* 715-721.

Wood, R.E., Boat, T.F., & Doershuk, C.F. (1976). Cystic Fibrosis. *American Review of Respiratory Disease, 113,* 833-878.

Yao, A.C. (1983). Cardiovascular changes during the transition from fetal to neonatal life. In N. Gootman & P.M. Gootman. (Eds.). *Perinatal cardiovascular function.* New York: Marcel Dekker.

Yeh, T.F., Lilien, L.D., Leu, S.T. & Pildes, R.S. (1984). Increased O_2 consumption and energy loss in premature infants following medical care procedures. *Biology of the Neonate, 46,* 157-162.

CHAPTER 36

The Aging Patient

Elizabeth J. Protas

KEY TERMS   Aging   Exercise changes
                     Autonomic   Pulmonary changes
                     Cardiovascular changes

INTRODUCTION

Cardiopulmonary and autonomic nervous system functions are dynamic and undergo changes as people age. It is important for physical therapists to be aware of changes that are to be expected with normal aging to better understand the impact of disease and impairment on these functions. In addition, a clear understanding of how these systems respond to exercise training will assist the clinician in prescribing and evaluating exercise interventions in elders.

Unfortunately, aging is a bit more complicated to understand than just the issue of chronological age. As people age, greater variability occurs between individuals, making predications about any one individual more difficult. The trends of some changes are probably not

linear but curvilinear, with changes accelerating after age 65. Thus many of the physiological studies that have been done with 60 year olds may not apply to individuals who are 80, 90, or 100 years old. Most of the studies that are available on exercise in older individuals have been conducted with subjects who are under age 65. A vast majority of these studies only used men as subjects or had a small number of women in the sample. Gender may be an important variable in relation to exercise and aging, but there is limited data available on this issue. Another consideration is the composition of study populations. With increasing age, there is a greater incidence of disease. Latent cardiovascular disease and histories of chronic illnesses are common in older populations. Comorbidities are frequently encountered in elders. It may be more uncommon to have a person over age 75 without any problems than to have a healthy older individual. As a physical therapist, I may be more interested in the responses of a frail 85- or 90-year-old woman who has a history of hypertension, coronary artery disease, and diabetes than someone who is healthy at this age because this reflects the population who is referred to physical therapy. The occurrence of disease states in study populations may impact the cardiopulmonary responses to exercise. Finally, the study of the physiological aspects of exercise and aging is still evolving. The literature can be confusing and contradictory, making conclusions and generalizations difficult. An attempt is made to provide some direction in this confusing maze of information.

An additional issue is a model of aging that might sort out some of the determinants of aging. (Figure 36-1) The model identifies biological factors, disuse, disease, and psychosocial concerns as determinants of aging. Biological factors address genetics, gender, cellular mechanisms, and metabolical, and physiological responses that influence aging. Disuse is implicated in more sedentary life styles led by many elders, which results in loss of exercise capacity (Bortz, 1993). Capacities that decline as a result of disuse should be reversible or attenuated with exercise training. The emphasis in this chapter is on the biological and disuse characteristics of aging. The impact of various diseases is discussed in other chapters. Psychosocial issues related to exercise and aging are not discussed.

CARDIAC CHANGES WITH AGING

Aerobic Capacity

The aerobic capacity is the maximum ability to perform exercise with large muscle groups. This ability is produced by the interaction of the lungs, heart, and peripheral tissues. The most common indirect measure of the aerobic capacity is the maximum oxygen consumption (Vo_{2max}), or the maximum oxygen used during exercise. The Vo_{2max} is directly related to the cardiac output (the amount of blood pumped by the heart) and the arteriovenous oxygen difference (the amount of oxygen extracted in the periphery). The cardiac output is the product of the heart rate times the stroke volume. The aerobic capacity reflects the central cardiac function and the efficiency of the peripheral tissues to extract and use oxygen.

The Vo_{2max} declines with age between 0.40 to 0.50 ml/kg/min per year in men and between 0.20 to 0.35 ml/kg/min per year in women (Figure 36-2) (Buskirk and Hodgson, 1987). The reduction is approximately 10% per decade. The decline is larger in

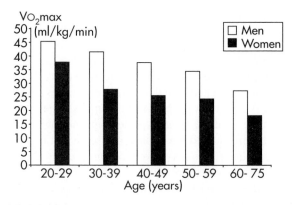

FIGURE 36-2
Decline in maximum oxygen consumption (Vo_{2max}) from age 20 to 75 in both men and women. (Redrawn with permission Hossack KF, Bruce RA: Maximal cardiac function in sedentary normal men and women: comparison of age-related changes, *J Appl Physiol* 53:799-804, 1982.)

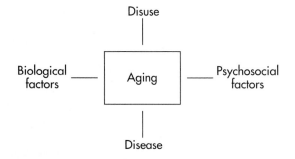

FIGURE 36-1
A model of aging which identifies the major determinants underlying the aging process.

men than women; however, the capacity of the males is larger than the females (Hossack and Bruce, 1982). Vo_{2max} is related to body size, which tends to be smaller in women than men. Increases in body weight as people age results in reduced Vo_{2max} even if the aerobic capacity remains the same, since relative oxygen consumption is related to body weight. Reduced physical activity with aging also contributes to a loss of Vo_{2max}.

Considerable disagreement exists about the mechanisms that contribute to the decline in Vo_{2max} with age. Both cardiac and peripheral changes contribute to the loss. A reduction in maximum cardiac output accounts for 50% to 100% of the total reduction in Vo_{2max} (Dempsey and Seals; Ogawa et al., 1992; Saltin, 1986). Decreased maximum arteriovenous oxygen consumption accounts for whatever is not due to decreased maximal cardiac output. A major component to the decline in maximal cardiac output is a decreased maximal heart rate (Ogawa et al., 1992; Hagberg, 1987). The decline in heart rate is linearly related to age and occurs in both sedentary and active elders (Sidney and Shephard, 1977). Reduced maximal stroke volume has also been observed as people age (Ogawa et al., 1992) Recent studies suggest decreased stroke volume is associated with a decrease in total blood volume in healthy older men and women (Dempsey and Seals, 1995; Davy and Seals, 1994; Stevenson, Davy, Reiling, and Seals, 1995). Most evidence suggests that decreased Vo_{2max} with aging is related to decreased maximal heart rate, stroke volume, and arteriovenous oxygen difference, although each component's contribution varies (Dempsey and Seals, 1995; Lakatta, 1993).

Cardiac Mechanics

The most consistent cardiac structural change is a modest increase in left ventricular wall thickness in 80 year olds compared with 20 year olds (Lakatta, 1993), attributed to an increase in size of cardiac myocytes and is exaggerated by hypertension and/or coronary artery disease (Lakatta, 1993). After age 80, the left ventricular wall thickness again decreases.

The cardiac filling or diastolic properties of the heart are altered with age. Diastole requires a relax-

ation of the myocardial fibers, sufficient venous return to rapidly fill the heart, and the timing of the atrial contraction to contribute to the end diastolic volume. Relaxation is hampered possibly by an increase in ventricular stiffness, although there is limited evidence of this in humans (Lakatta, 1993). The period of the isovolumic myocardial relaxation (between aortic valve closing and mitral valve opening) is prolonged. Likewise the peak rate of left ventricular filling during early diastole is reduced in older, healthy men and women compared with younger individuals. Despite the changes in early diastole, the resting left ventricular end-diastolic volume remains the same because of an enhanced left atrial contribution to ventricular filling. This is accompanied by an enlarged left atrium and an audible fourth heart sound in most older adults (Lakatta, 1993; Fleg, Gerstenblech and Lakatta, 1988).

Considerable disagreement exists about what happens to diastolic function during exercise. Some recent studies suggest that end-diastolic volume during exhaustive exercise increases in older men but not it women (Lakatta, 1993). Filling pressures during exercise in men increase with age (Ehrsam, Perruchoud, Oberholzer, Burkhart, and Herzog, 1983). In addition, peak left ventricular diastolic filling rate during submaximal and maximal exercise decreases with aging (Levy, Cerqueria, Abrass, Schwartz, and Stratton, 1993; Schulman, Lakatta, Fleg et al. 1992) Decreased filling rate is associated with increased ventricular stiffness and prolonged relaxation times (Ehsani, 1987).

Resting measures of systolic and cardiac pump function do not change with aging. The resting end-systolic volume and stroke volume do not change with age. Likewise, the ejection fraction at rest (end-diastolic volume – end-systolic volume/end-diastolic volume) is similar in healthy older and younger individuals (Lakatta, 1993).

Unlike resting systolic function, the pumping function of the heart changes considerably in response to exercise. Myocardial contractility as measured by the ratio of end-systolic volume to systolic arterial pressure declines during exercise as people age (Lakatta, 1993). The end-systolic volume increases, whereas the ejection fraction decreases during exercise. These changes reduce stroke volume during exercise. Reduced contractile performance is related to a decrease in the response to beta-adrenergic stimulation, changes in the myocardium, increased systolic blood pressure, and ventricular wall abnormalities (Dempsey and Seals, 1995).

Impact of Exercise Training on Aerobic Capacity and Cardiac Mechanics

Older persons who continue to be active reduce the rate of decline in Vo_2max to 5% per decade compare with an anticipated decline of 10% per decade in sedentary adults (Haberg, 1987). A recent metaanalysis of 29 studies including 1030 men and 466 women between the ages of 61 and 78 and endurance training, concluded that endurance training significantly increases functional capacity in young elders (Green and Crouse, 1995). Less improvement was seen with increasing age, a shorter length of training, low Vo_{2max} before training, and short duration of exercise sessions. The analysis suggests that a healthy 68-year-old individual who exercises for 30 minutes three times per week for 4 to 6 months can improve Vo_{2max} by 14% (Green and Crouse, 1995). Similar improvements occur in both men and women (Kohrt, Malley, Coggan et al., 1991; Warren et al., 1993).

The mechanisms underlying improvements in Vo_{2max} in the elderly with endurance training are not clear. One consistent finding is greater extraction of oxygen in the exercising skeletal muscle, which produces a wider arteriovenous oxygen difference in both older men and women (Ogawa et al., 1992; Ehsani, 1989). This implies that adaptations in the peripheral skeletal muscles account for some of the increase in Vo_{2max} in elders. The impact of exercise training on maximal cardiac output is uncertain (Ehsani, 1989). Maximum cardiac output can either remain the same or increase after exercise training, depending on the effect of training on maximal stroke volume and maximal heart rate. Maximal heart rate remains the same in older men regardless of activity level, suggesting that the decline in maximal heart rate depends on factors other than exercise and physical fitness (Seals, Hagberg, Hurley, Ehsani, and Holloszy, 1985). A decrease in response to circulating

catecholamines is most often cited as the reason for changes in maximal heart rate with aging (Rodeheffer, Gerstenblith, Becker, Fleg, Weisfeld, and Lakatta, 1984). Relatively intense endurance training for a year or more can increase peak stroke volume in men (Ehsani, Ogawa, Miller, Spina, and Jilka, 1991; Seals, Hagberg, Spina, Rogers, Schectman, and Ehsani, 1994). Adaptations to exercise training in older women have been attributed predominantly to peripheral changes in arteriovenous oxygen difference rather than central changes in cardiac function (Spina, Ogawa, Kohrt, Martin, Holloszy, and Ehsani, 1993). This apparently occurs despite intensive endurance training over a year-long period.

The diastolic changes that occur with aging can be reversed by exercise training (Levy et al., 1993). Levy et al. intensively endurance trained 13 rigorously screened older men aged 60 to 82 (mean age 68) and 11 younger men in their twenties for 6 months. The training increased resting, submaximal, and peak filling rates for the older group comparable with the changes seen in the younger group (Levy et al., 1993). End-diastolic peak volume at rest and exercise also increase after lengthy endurance training (Ehsani et al., 1991). Thus training reduces the age-associated diastolic changes. The mechanisms of this response are uncertain in humans. Studies in rats have shown that exercise training increases calcium uptake in cardiac sarcoplasmic reticulum, decreases relaxation time, reduces the decline of left ventricular pressure, enhances fatty acid oxidation, and increases cytochrome c oxidase levels (Levy, Cerqueira, Abrass, Schwartz, and Stratton, 1993; Tate, Taffet, Hudson, Blaylock, McBride, and Michael, 1990; Starnes, Beyer, and Edington, 1983). All of these changes have been associated with reduced diastolic function with aging.

Exercise training can also improve systolic performance in older men as reflected by the increase in the exercise stroke volume. Increased peak stroke volume occurs with an increased exercise ejection fraction, a decrease in end-systolic volume, and greater left ventricular wall mass (Ehsani et al., Seals et al., 1994). These changes apparently do not occur in older, estrogen-deficient women (Spina et al., 1993). Table 36-1 contains a summary of these changes.

TABLE 36-1		
Cardiac Changes With Aging*		
	BECAUSE OF AGING	AFTER EXERCISE TRAINING
Maximum Exercise		
Oxygen consumption	↓	↑
Heart rate	↓	↔
Stroke volume	↓	↑, ↔
Arteriovenous oxygen difference	↓	↑
Cardiac output	↓	↑, ↔
Cardiac function		
Diastolic		
Left ventricular wall thickness	↑, ↓ after 80	↑
Left ventricular filling rate	↓	↑
End-diastolic volume	↔	↑
Systolic		
Myocardial contractility	↓	↑, ↔[†]
End-systolic volume	↑	↓, ↔[†]
Ejection fraction	↓	↑,↔[†]

*↑ = increase; ↓ = decrease; ↔ = no change;
[†]in women

Vascular and Autonomic Changes with Aging

Aging results in an increase in arterial stiffness because of a loss of elastin and an increase in collagen (Lakatta, 1993; Roach and Burton, 1959). Arterial wall thickness and diameter and resting systolic pressure also increase (Figure 36-3) (Lakatta, 1993). It is unclear whether peripheral vascular resistance increases in normotensive older adults. Changes in the structure, size, and reactivity of the arteries increase the work of the left ventricle and have been directly implicated in the increase in cardiac myocyte size.

Complaints of dizziness when an older patient moves from supine to standing are frequently encountered by the physical therapist. Postural hypotension, or orthostatic intolerance, generally does not occur in healthy community dwelling elders but is common in debilitated, institutionalized individuals

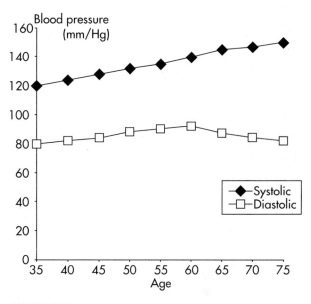

FIGURE 36-3

Changes in systolic and diastolic blood pressures as people age. (Redrawn with permission from Timiras PS: Cardiovascular alterations with age: atherosclerosis, coronary heart disease and hypertension. In Timiras, PS: *Physiological basis of aging and geriatrics,* Boca Raton, Fla., 1988, CRC.)

over the age of 70 (Lipsitz, 1989). Orthostatic intolerance is associated with decreased resting diastolic function, decreased stroke volume, extreme inactivity, and, in individuals with hypertension, high levels of systolic blood pressure (Harris, Lipsitz, Kleinman, and Cornoni-Huntley, 1991).

There are decreases in baroreceptor and cardiopulmonary reflexes with aging (Lakatta, 1993; Cleroux, et al., 1989) Arterial and venous dilation are reduced, but vasoconstriction is relatively spared. The heart demonstrates an overall decrease in responsiveness to autonomic stimulation. Older individuals experience higher central venous and mean arterial pressures, but lower forearm blood flow and forearm vascular resistance in response to passive leg raising (Cleroux et al., 1989). During submaximal and maximal exercise, arterial blood pressure is either unchanged or increased when comparing younger and older subjects (Seals, 1993). There also appears to be impaired peripheral vasodilation in skeletal muscle in response to exercise (Ogawa et al., 1992). Redistribution of blood flow during exercise normally involves the shunting of blood from inactive limbs and viscera. There seems to be an enhanced vasoconstriction in inactive muscles during dynamic exercise in healthy older men (Taylor, Hand, Johnson, and Seals, 1992).

Effect of Exercise Training on Vascular and Autonomic Function in Aging

Exercise training improves peripheral bloodflow in skeletal muscle in 60-year-old men and women (Martin, Ogawa, Kohrt, Malley, Korte, and Stoltz, 1991). Systolic and mean arterial blood pressure responses to submaximal exercise are lower in physically active adults compared with sedentary individuals (Martin et al., 1991). Endurance training also increases muscle sympathetic nerve activity and plasma norepinephrine concentrations at rest and during a moderate isometric handgrip, indicating elevated sympathetic nerve activity in response to exercise (Table 36-2) (Ng, Callister, Johnson, and Seals, 1994).

PULMONARY FUNCTION

Structural and Functional Changes With Aging

Two major changes with aging of the pulmonary system are decreased elastic recoil and stiffening of the

---

TABLE 36-2

Vascular and Autonomic Changes With Aging*

	BECAUSE OF AGING	AFTER EXERCISE TRAINING
Arterial wall thickness	↑	?
Systolic blood pressure	↑	↓
Diastolic blood pressure	↑ and ↔	↓
Orthostatic tolerance	↔	?
Arterial and venous dilation	↓	?
Vasoconstriction	↔	↔
Central venous pressure	↑	?

*↑ = increases; ↓ = decreases; ↔ = unchanged;
? = insufficient data on older adult subjects

---

chest wall (Dempsey and Seals, 1995). The lung's elastic recoil depends on the composition of the connective tissue, the structure of the connective tissue, and alveolar surface tension produced by surfactant (Dempsey and Seals, 1995). Very limited evidence suggests that the structure of the connective tissue may be the primary mechanism for age-associated change in elastic recoil. Chest wall stiffness is accompanied by an increase in chest anterioposterior diameter, coastal cartilage calcification, narrowing of the intervertebral disks, and changes in the rib to vertebrae articulations (Crapo, 1993).

Decreases occur with the alveolar-capillary surface area, the alveolar septal surface area, and the total surface area of lung parenchyma (Brody and Thurlbeck, 1985). This reduces the surface area available for gas exchange.

Loss of elastic recoil with aging is directly associated with reduced forced expiratory flow. Limitations in exhalation are caused by airway narrowing and closure at all lung volumes; thus reducing forced expiratory volume in 1 second (FEV_1) (Dempsey and Seals, 1995) Early airway closure also produces an early closing volume and a relative increase in the total residual volume. The combination of reduced elastic recoil and increased chest wall stiffness leads to a decrease in the forced vital capacity in older individuals. Flow rates are also significantly lower in women and African-Americans than in Caucasian men at any age (Dempsey and Seals, 1995).

Respiratory muscle strength, as reflected by the ability to create pressure over a range of lung volumes and flow rates, is similar when comparing healthy 30 and 70 year olds (Johnson and Dempsey, 1991) This suggests that respiratory muscle strength does not change with aging; however, maximal inspiratory and expiratory pressures have been reported to decrease 15% between the sixth and eighth decades (Figure 36-4) (Enright, Kronmal, Manolio, Shanker, and Hyatt, 1994). Perhaps these observed differences are similar to the differences observed with submaximal and maximal cardiac responses with the dynamic pressure measures over different volumes and flows considered submaximal.

Changes in the surface area result in a decrease in the diffusion capacity of the lung (Murray, 1986). Both the loss of surface area and a decrease in pulmonary capillary blood volume contribute to reduced and uneven ventilation to perfusion matching in elders. The resting partial arterial pressure of oxygen declines 5 to 10 mm Hg between ages 25 and 75 (Dempsey and Seals, 1995). These changes do not affect the arterial oxymyoglobin saturation or oxygen content. Paralleling changes in the peripheral vasculature, pulmonary vascular resistance and pulmonary arterial pressure at rest increase (Table 36-3).

Changes in Pulmonary Responses to Exercise With Aging

In addition to the structural and functional changes at rest, a number of significant changes occur in breathing during acute exercise. Expiratory flow limitations occur at lower exercise intensities as people age. A normal, healthy 69 year old will begin to experience flow limitations even in response to moderate exercise (Dempsey and Seals, 1995). Practically, this may be experienced by the individual as having greater difficulty "catching his or her breath" during exercise.

Normally as people exercise, the tidal volume increases directly with increasing exercise intensity up to about 50% to 60% of the vital capacity. This re-

mains unchanged as people age, although the vital capacity for elders is reduced. Likewise, as exercise and the tidal volume increase there is a slight drop in the ratio of dead space to tidal volume. This drop is not effected by aging, although the older person will breathe more (have a higher minute ventilation) in response to submaximal exercise.

The work of breathing is increased during exercise as people age as a result of a number of factors. Higher ventilation during exercise requires the development of higher pleural pressures; thus increasing the work required. In addition, an increase in the end-expiratory lung volume with increasing exercise results in breathing that occurs at a stiffer point in the lung-volume relationship. The increased stiffness im-

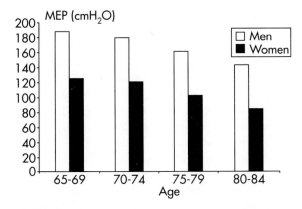

FIGURE 36-4
Decrease in maximum expiratory pressures between ages 65 to 84 for both men and women. This is a measure of respiratory muscle strength. (Redrawn with permission from Enright PL, Kronmal RA, Monlio TA, Schenker MB, Hyatt RE: Respiratory muscle strength in the elderly, *Am J Respir Crit Care Med* 149:430-438, 1994.)

TABLE 36-3

Pulmonary Function Changes With Aging*

	BECAUSE OF AGING	AFTER EXERCISE TRAINING
Structure and Function		
Elastic recoil	↓	
Chest wall stiffness	↑	
Alveolar-capillary surface area	↓	
Forced expiratory flow	↓	↔
Total residual volume	↑	↔
Forced vital capacity	↓	↔
Maximum inspiratory and expiratory pressure	↓	
Ventilation-perfusion matching	↓	
Partial arterial pressure oxygen	↓	↔
Oxygen saturation	↔	↔
Pulmonary vascular resistance	↑	
Exercise response		
Expiratory flow limitation	↑	↔
Minute ventilation	↑	↓[†], ↑[‡]
Work of breathing	↑	↓
Respiratory muscle oxygen consumption	↑	↓
Arterial hypoxemia	↔, ↑	↑
Pulmonary artery pressure	↑	↔
Pulmonary wedge pressure	↑	↔

*↑ = increases; ↓ = decreases; ↔ = unchanged
[†]submaximal
[‡] maximal

poses a higher elastic recoil on the ventilatory muscles, requiring greater pressure development by the inspiratory muscles. The increase in expiratory flow resistance likewise requires greater pressure development by the expiratory muscles. Both the inspiratory and expiratory changes increase the work of breathing. The increase in the work of breathing increases the respiratory muscle oxygen consumption so that the respiratory muscles alone can require 10% to 12% of the total body oxygen consumption during maximal exercise in a sedentary 70-year-old man (Dempsey and Seals, 1995).

What is also apparent is that the reserves used to respond to exercise represent a greater percent of the available capacity. An older individual can exceed 50% of inspiratory muscle capacity even during moderate exercise. This is in contrast to the younger individual who rarely exceeds 50% of the capacity with exercise (Dempsey and Seals, 1995) Thus the reserve capacity to generate pleural pressure is reduced in elders by virtue of the fact that greater capacity is needed even for moderate exercise.

The variability characteristic of exercise responses in older individuals is particularly evident when considering gas exchange and pulmonary-vascular hemodynamics. In general, most individuals demonstrate only slight changes in arterial blood-gas homeostasis, but a small number of individuals demonstrate arterial hypoxemia with exercise (Dempsey and Seals, 1995). Some studies suggest that this response may be a factor of fitness level. More fit older individuals showed progressive arterial hypoxemia and carbon dioxide retention during mild-to-moderate exercise (Prefaut, Anselme, Caillaud, and Masse-Biron, 1994; Anselme, et al., 1994).

The pulmonary artery pressure is increased with aging at any oxygen consumption or cardiac output during exercise (Reeves, Dempsey, and Grover, 1989). In addition, the maximal pulmonary artery pressure at maximal exercise is reached at substantially lower oxygen consumption and cardiac outputs in older individuals compared with younger persons. The pulmonary wedge pressure also increases with age and can exceed 25 mm Hg during peak supine exercise (Dempsey and Seals, 1995). Limited data suggest that these high pressures may in turn induce pulmonary edema during intense exercise in elders. Pulmonary edema would limit

diffusion and may contribute to ventilation perfusion maldistribution (Dempsey and Seals, 1995)

Effects of Exercise Training on Pulmonary Function

Aerobic training in elders can reduce some of the changes that have been described. There are limited or no studies that address some of the changes, such as chest wall compliance or pulmonary artery pressure. The studies that are available deal with relatively young subjects who are 60 to 70 years old, which does not provide insights into what exercise might do for the those in their seventies, eighties, or beyond.

Aerobic training can significantly decrease submaximal minute ventilation (Makrides, Heigenhauser, Jones, 1986; Warren et al., 1993). One study used a walking program with 70-year-old women over a 12-week period and demonstrated a 7.7% drop in the submaximal minute ventilation (Figure 36-5) (Warren et al., 1993). Decreased minute ventilation is accompanied by a decrease in carbon dioxide production, the respiratory exchange ratio (carbon dioxide production/oxygen consumption), and the blood lactate level for any given level of submaximal exercise (Makrides et al., 1986; Warren et al., 1993). Thus the improved ventilatory efficiency after training may have more to do with improved efficiency in the periphery rather than an impact on the pulmonary system directly. Improved peripheral metabolical efficiency results in the production of less carbon dioxide; therefore the lungs do not have to work as hard to eliminate the carbon dioxide. The important functional results of these changes are that the older adults will experience less breathlessness, experience a lower perceived exertion, and use a lower percentage of their maximal ventilatory capacity during exercise (Jones, 1986).

Exercise training also increases maximal ventilatory responses during maximal exercise (Warren et al., 1993; Jones, 1986). The 12-week walking program referred to above increased maximum minute ventilation by 14% in 70-year-old women (see Figure 36-5) (Jones, 1986). These women walked 5 days/week at an intensity of 78% of the maximal treadmill heart rate or 118 beats/minute on average, so the program was not very strenuous but produced substantial changes in maximum ventilation. Exercise training can improve submaximal ventilatory effi-

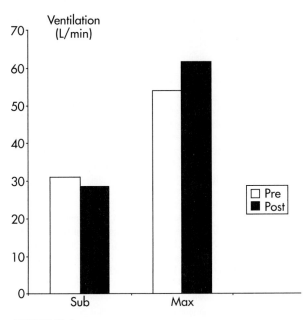

FIGURE 36-5

Submaximal and maximal minute ventilation pre- and post-exercise training with a 12-week walking program in women whose mean age was 72.5 years. (Redrawn with permission from Warren BJ, Nieman DC, Dotson RG, Adkins CH, O'Donnell KA, Haddock BL, Butterworth DE: Cardiorespiratory responses to exercise training in septuagenarian wormen, *Int J Sports Med* 14:60-65, 1993).

ciency and increase maximum ventilation in elders. Table 36-3 on p. 675 summarizes the pulmonary changes with aging and exercise.

Summary

Profound changes occur at rest and in response to submaximal and maximal exercise as people age. Many of these changes are reduced or reversed as a result of exercise training. The implication is that many of these changes may have more to do with disuse than aging per se. Sedentary individuals tend to show these changes to a greater extent than more active seniors. Prevailing evidence suggests that elders at any age can derive benefits from exercise training. Even very modest, short-term interventions have proved efficacious. Older individuals should be encouraged to engage in regular physical activity to improve their exercise capacity.

REVIEW QUESTIONS

1. What are the major changes which occur with aging in the cardiovascular system?
2. What outcomes will exercise training produce in an older adult's cardiovascular system?
3. What are the major changes that occur with aging in the autonomic nervous system in response to exercise, and which of these changes can be influenced by execise training?
4. What are the major changes that occur in the pulmonary system with aging and in responding to exercise?
5. Describe the possible impact of exercise training on the aging pulmnary system.

References

Anselme, F., Caillaud, C., Couret, I., et al. (1994). Histamine and exercise-induced hypoxemia in highly trained athletes. *Journal of Applied Physiology 76*, 127-132.

Bortz, W.M. (1993). The physics of frailty. *Journal American Geriatric Society, 41*, 1004-1008.

Brody, J.S., & Thurlbeck, W.M. (1985). Development, growth, and aging of the lung. In Fishman, A.P. (Ed.). *Handbook of physiology.* (Vol 3).

Buskirk, E.R., & Hodgson, J.L. (1987). Age and aerobic power: the rate of changes in men and women. *Federation Proceedings, 46*, 1824-1829.

Cleroux, J. et al. (1989). Decreased cardiorespiratory reflexes with aging. *American Journal of Physiology 257*, H961-H968.

Crapo, R.O. (1993). The aging lung. In Mahler, D.A. (Ed.). *Pulmonary disease in the elderly.* New York: Marcel Dekker.

Davy, K.P., & Seals, D.R. (1994). Total blood volume in healthy young and older men. *Journal of Applied Physiology, 76*, 2059-2062.

Dempsey, J.A., & Seals, D.R. (1995). Aging, exercise, and cardiopulmonary function. In Holloszy, J. (Ed.). *Perspectives in exercise science.* New York: Williams & Wilkins.

Ehrsam, R.E., Perruchoud, A., Oberholzer, M., Burkhart, F.& Herzog, H. (1983). Influence of age on pulmonary hemodynamics at rest and during supine exercise. *Clinical Science, 65*, 653-660.

Ehsani, A.A. (1989). Cardiovascular adaptations to exercise training in the elderly. *Federation Proceedings, 46*, 1840-1843.

Ehsani, A.A., Ogawa, T., Miller, T.R., Spira, R.J., & Jilka, S.M. (1991). Exercise training improves left ventricular systolic function in older men. *Circulation, 83*, 96-103.

Enright, P.L., Kronmal, R.A., Manolio, T.A., Shenker, M.B., & Hyatt, R.E. (1994). Respiratory muscle strength in the elderly. *American Journal Respiratory Critical Care Medicine, 149*, 430-438.

Fleg, J.L., Gerstenbleth, G., & Lakatta, E.G. (1988). Pathophysiology of the aging heart and circulation. In Messerli, F.H. (Ed.). *Cardiovascular disease in the elderly* (2nd ed.). Boston: Martinus Nihoff.

Green, J.S., & Crouse, S.F. (1995). The effects of endurance training on functional capacity in the elderly: a meta-analysis. *Med Science Sport Exercise, 27,* 920-926.

Hagberg, J.M. (1987). Effect of training on the decline of VO_2max with aging. *Federation Proceedings, 46,* 1830-1833.

Harris, T., Lipsitz, L.A., Kleinman, J.C., & Cornoni-Huntley, J. (1991). Postural change in blood pressure associated with age and systolic blood pressure. *Journal Gerontology Medicine Science 46,* M159-M163.

Hossack K.F., & Bruce, R.A. (1982). Maximal cardiac function in sedentary normal men and women: comparison of age-related changes. *Journal of Applied Physiology, 53,* 799-804.

Johnson, B.D., & Dempsey, J.A. (1991). Demand vs capacity in the aging pulmonary system. In Holloszy, J. (Ed.). *Exercise and sport sciences review.* (Vol 19). Baltimore: Williams & Wilkins.

Jones, N.L. (1986). The lung of the Master's athlete. In Sutton, J.R., & Beck, R.M. (Eds.). *Sports medicine for the mature athlete.* Indianapolis Benchmark Press.

Kohrt, W.M., et al. (1991). Effects of gender, age, and fitness level on response of VO_2max to training in 60-71 yr olds. *Journal of Applied Physiology, 71,* 2004-2011.

Lakatta, E.G. (1993). Cardiovascular regulatory mechanisms in advanced age. *Physiology Review, 73,* 413-467.

Levy, W.C., et al. (1993). Endurance exercise training augments diastolic filling at rest and during exercise in healthy young and older men. *Circulation 88,* 116-126.

Lipsitz, L.A. (1989). Orthostatic hypotension in the elderly. *New England Journal Medicine 321,* 952-957.

Makrides, L., Heigenhauser, G.J., Jones, N.L. (1986). Physical training in young and older healthy subjects. In Sutton, J.R., Brock, R.M. (Eds.). *Sports medicine for the mature athlete.* Indianapolis: Benchmark Press.

Martin, III, W.H., Ogawa, T., Kohrt, W.M., Malley, M.T., Korte, E., & Stolz, S. (1991). Effects of aging, gender, and physical training on peripheral vascular function. *Circulation, 84,* 654-664.

Murray, J.F. (1986) *Aging in the normal lung.* (2nd ed.). Philadelphia: WB Saunders.

Ng, A.V., Callister, R., Johnson, D.G., & Seals, D.R. (1994) Endurance exercise training is associated with elevated basal sympathetic nerve activity in healthy older humans. *Journal of Applied Physiology, 77,* 1366-1374.

Ogawa, T., et al. (1992). Effects of aging, sex, and physical training on cardiovascular responses to exercise. *Circulation, 86,* 494-503.

Prefaut, C., Anselme, F., Caillaud, C., & Masse-Biron, J. (1994). Exercise-induced hypoxemia in older athletes. *Journal of Applied Physiology 76,* 120-126.

Reeves, J.T., Dempsey, J.A., & Grover, R.F. (1989). Pulmonary circulation during exercise. In Weir, E.K., & Reeves, J.T. (Eds.). *Pulmonary vascular physiology and pathophysiology.* New York: Marcel Dekker.

Roach, M.R., & Burton, A.C. (1959). The effect of aging on the elasticity of human iliac arteries. *Canadian Journal Biochemistry Physiology, 37,* 557-570.

Rodeheffer, R.J., Gerstenblith, G., Becker, J.L., Fleg, J.L., Weisfield, M.L., & Lakatta, E.G. (1984). Exercise cardiac output is maintained with advancing ages in healthy human subjects: cardiac dilatation and increased stroke volume compensate for diminished heart rate. *Circulation, 69,* 203-213.

Saltin, B. (1986). The aging endurance athlete. In Sutton, J.R., & Brock, R.M. (Eds.). *Sports medicine for the mature athlete.* Indianapolis: Benchmark Press.

Schulman, D.D. Lakatta, E.G., & Fleg, J.L., Lakatta, L., Beder, L.C., & Gerslenblith, G. (1992). Age-related decline in left ventricular filling at rest and exercise. *American Journal of Physiology, 263,* H1932-H1938.

Seals, D.R. (1993). Influence of aging on autonomic-circulatory control in humans at rest and during exercise. In Gisolfi, C.V., Lamb, D.R., & Nadel, E.R. (Eds.). *Perspectives in exercise science and sports medicine.* (Vol 6) *Exercise, heat, and thermoregulation.* Dubuque: Brown & Benchmark.

Seals, D.R., Hagberg, J.M., Hurley, B.F., Ehsani, A.A., Holloszy, J.O. (1985) Endurance training in older men and women. I. Cardiovascular response to exercise. *Journal of Applied Physiology, 57,* 1024-1029.

Seals, D.R., Hagberg, J.M., Spina, R.J., Rogers, M.A., Schechtman, K.B., & Ehsani, A.A. (1994). Enhanced left ventricular performance in endurance trained older men. *Circulation, 89,* 198-205.

Sidney, K.H., & Shephard, R.J. (1977). Maximum and submaximum exercise tests and men and women in the seventh, eighth, and ninth decades of life. *Journal of Applied Physiology 43,* 280-287.

Spina, R.J., Ogawa, T., Kohrt, W.M., Martin III, W.H., Holloszy, J.O., & Ehsani, A.A. (1993). Differences in cardiovascular adaptations to endurance exercise training between older men and women. *Journal of Applied Physiology, 75:849-855.*

Starnes, J.W., Beyer, R.E., & Edington, D.W. (1983). Myocardial adaptations to endurance exercise in aged rats. *American Journal of Physiology, 245,* H560-H566.

Stevenson, E.T., Davy, K.P., Reiling, M.J., & Seals, D.R. (1995). Maximal aerobic capacity and total blood volume in highly trained middle-aged and older female endurance athletes. *Journal of Applied Physiology, 77,* 1691-1696.

Tate, C.A., Taffet, G.E., Hudson, E.K., et al. (1990). Enhanced calcium uptake of cardiac sarcoplasmic reticulum in exercise-trained old rats. *American Journal of Physiology, 27,* H431-H435.

Taylor, J.A., Hand, G.A., Johnson, D.G., & Seals, D.R. (1992). Augmented forearm vasoconstriction during dynamic exercise in healthy older men. *Circulation, 86,* 1789-1799.

Timiras, P.S. (1988). Cardiovascular alterations with age: atherosclerosis, coronary heart disease and hypertension. In Timiras, P.S. (1988). *Physiological basis of aging and geriatrics.* Boca Raton, FL: CRC.

Warren, B.J., et al. (1993). Cardiorespiratory responses to exercise training in septuagenarian women. *International Journal of Sports Medicine, 14,* 60-65.

CHAPTER 37

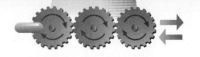

The Patient with Neuromuscular or Musculoskeletal Dysfunction

Mary Massery

KEY TERMS

Adverse musculoskeletal changes

Chest development

Effects of gravity

Gravity

Impaired phonation support

Musculoskeletal deficits

Neuromuscular deficits

Nighttime hypoxemia

Paradoxical breathing

Planes of ventilation

Pulmonary function tests

Respiratory impairments

Respiratory muscles

Sleep disorders

Triad of ventilation

INTRODUCTION

It is often observed in a rehabilitation setting that patients with neurological deficits continue to acquire respiratory problems long after their acute phases have subsided. Research has repeatedly documented a decrease in pulmonary function for the chronic neurologically impaired patient, yet many therapists do not appear to fully comprehend why this occurs. This section tries to elaborate the causes of respiratory complications secondary to neuro-muscular and/or musculoskeletal deficits and what clinicians can do to minimize or eliminate these complications. The focus of this treatment approach is primarily aimed at the physical therapist (PT). Every effort is made to explain specific physical therapy concepts so that all clinicians, occupational therapists (OTs), speech language pathologists (SLPs), respiratory therapists (RTs), and nurses (RNs), family members, and others can benefit from the ideas presented in this chapter.

DIAGNOSES ADDRESSED

The following treatment ideas are applicable for all neurological and orthopedic diagnoses including the following: spinal cord injuries (SCI), head traumas, cerebral vascular accidents (CVA), multiple sclerosis (MS), amyotrophic lateral sclerosis (ALS), Parkinson's disease, cerebral palsy (CP), muscular dystrophy (MD), polio myelitis (polio), spina bifida, and neuropathies as well as back, neck, and shoulder injuries or dysfunction. However, it is by no means an exhaustive list. The primary consideration for application of these treatment techniques is the residual physical deficits left by a neurological or musculoskeletal insult. Therefore a patient presenting with hemiplegia will be treated with techniques geared toward promoting increased function on the involved side, regardless of how the original deficit was acquired (e.g., from a CVA, head trauma, or CP). Likewise, tetraplegia or paraplegia not only refers to patients that have suffered from SCIs but any patient that presents with tetraplegic or paraplegic deficits.

However, three aspects of neurological/musculoskeletal disorders must be clarified here to assist the therapist in discerning which techniques, described later, are appropriate for his or her particular patient. The three aspects follows: (1) progressive vs. nonprogressive injuries, (2) cerebral vs. noncerebral injuries, and (3) rehabilitation vs. habilitation. Single-insult injuries, such as SCIs, traumatic brain injuries, CVAs, CPs, or cervical whiplash, are nonprogressive. The damage was only inflicted once and does not repeat itself. Progressive diseases, on the other hand, such as MS, ALS, Parkinson's disease, MD, or scoliosis, show increasing physical deficits over time. Goals for these groups will be different, with maximal respiratory functioning stressed for the single-insult diagnoses and comfort and ease of ventilation stressed for progressive diagnoses. Similar treatment consideration is given for patients with detrimentally affected cerebral functioning, such as with traumatic brain injuries, CVAs, and Parkinson's disease, versus those whose deficits are at the spinal level, such as with SCIs, neuropathies, myopathies, and polio. Patients with only spinal involvement may respond favorably to complex techniques and demonstrate better conscious carryover, whereas those with impaired cerebral function-

ing may respond better to techniques that act primarily on the subconscious and require little cognitive participation. Finally, the difference between rehabilitation and habilitation must be understood. Rehabilitation involves restoring function, and habilitation teaches functioning for the first time. Children with acquired deficits in utero or shortly after birth have never experienced normal movement patterns. Therefore they cannot depend on the memory of past motor experiences to help correct abnormal motor patterns the way adults going through rehabilitation can. This important difference must be accounted for when developing their treatment programs.

PLANES OF VENTILATION

This neuromuscular/musculoskeletal treatment approach is based on the premise that ventilation does not take place in a one-dimensional plane but rather as a three-dimensional activity. The chest expands in an anterior-posterior plane, an inferior-superior plane, and a lateral plane (Figure 37-1). Too often, therapists treat patients with neuromuscular and/or musculoskeletal dysfunctions with apparent disregard for this extremely important fact. This one-dimensional fallacy has been perpetuated by techniques taught to new therapists that describe the patient's breathing program in only one or two postures, most often supine and sitting. To be effective, we must acknowledge this three-dimensional movement of the thorax and use this concept when determining treatment protocol.

EFFECTS OF GRAVITY

If chest expansion takes place in three planes, the effect of gravity on these planes must be considered. Physical therapists would not exercise a weak muscle without taking into account the effect of gravitational pull on that muscle, thereby making the positioning of the limb in space an important consideration in treatment planning. This same consideration must be given for the weakened ventilatory muscles. Gravity can assist, resist, or have no effect on the movement of the chest wall, according to the chest's position in space. Consider weakened intercostal muscles. Plac-

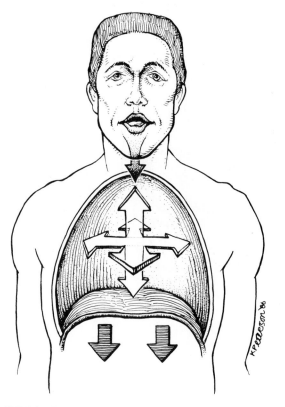

FIGURE 37-1

Planes of respiration (anterior-posterior, inferior-superior, and lateral).

ing a patient with this deficit in a supine position for initial treatment in his or her rehabilitation program and then asking the patient to "breathe up into your hands" is asking the patient to attempt the most difficult gravitational posture first (breathing into the anterior plane with gravity resisting the movement). It would seem more appropriate to start retraining techniques in a gravity-eliminated posture for anterior chest expansion, such as side lying, or a gravity-assisted posture, such as hands-knees, and then progress to gravity-resisted postures, such as supine.

Gravity also affects the positioning of the intestines under the diaphragm. In the normal, neurologically intact person, this seems to have a minor effect on respiratory functioning. However, for many neurologically impaired persons with a marked loss

in abdominal tone (many SCIs, Guillian-Barré syndrome, or spina bifida), intestinal positioning becomes an important factor in respiratory functioning.

The abdominal wall acts as the anterior support for the intestines, causing the intestines to sit high in the abdominal cavity (see Chapter 2). This forces the diaphragm to rest high, at approximately the level of the fifth rib in an erect posture (Figure 37-2). The diaphragm contracts, drawing its origins toward its insertion (concentric contraction). These muscle fibers, which originate down as low as the tenth rib, must rise up superiorly and then medially toward the central tendon (see Chapter 2). This movement pattern causes primarily superior and lateral expansion of the lower chest. Without abdominal wall support, the intestines shift inferiorly and anteriorly, the "beer-belly" effect, allowing gravity to position the diaphragm lower in the abdominal cavity (Figure 37-3). This puts the diaphragm at an extreme mechanical disadvantage. Instead of having to rise up and over the intestines, the lateral fibers of the diaphragm can now move more horizontally to reach the central tendon, thereby significantly reducing excursion in all three planes of expansion. This adverse positioning may be so significant as to cause a negative lower chest expansion on inspiration for patients with tetraplegia. Quantitatively, this may be seen as much as $\frac{1}{2}$- to 1-inch decrease rather than increase in overall lower chest expansion, measured at the xiphoid process, when the patient proceeds from maximal expiration to maximal inspiration.

Since gravity causes the intestines to shift, the effect on the diaphragm will be most dramatic in a gravity-dependent position, such as sitting or standing, rather than in a gravity-eliminated position, such as supine. Thus the importance of providing the patient with an external abdominal wall support in these upright postures should be undeniably clear. Although not as effective as the abdominal muscles themselves, abdominal supports help restore the natural mechanical advantage of the diaphragm (see Chapter 22).

In addition to changing muscle effectiveness, gravity also affects bony structures. Obviously, this affects a growing child more so than a fully devel-

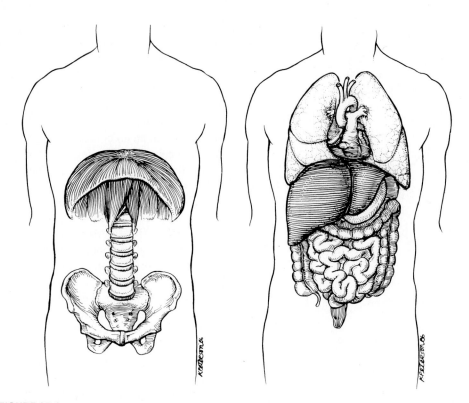

FIGURE 37-2
Proper mechanical positioning of the diaphragm relative to the abdominal viscera. Note the high dome shape of the diaphragm.

oped adult, but both will be affected. Bones grow according to stress laid on them, thus abnormal stresses produce abnormal bony developments. For persons with severe neurological deficits, gravity becomes the main force acting on the bones and joints, unopposed by normal muscle action. This can result in many skeletal deformities, such as flattening or flaring of the lower anterior rib cage, narrowing of the upper chest, loss of normal spinal curves, and chest cavus deformities. Prevention of these deformities, rather than their cure, must be the aim of a good long-term ventilatory program for the neurologically impaired.

GRAVITY: EFFECTS ON CHEST DEVELOPMENT

Thus far the effects of gravity on the planes of ventilation, muscle function, and bony changes in the adult have been discussed. This same force, gravity,

plays an extremely crucial role in the skeletal development of the chest in the newborn. Normal, neurologically intact infants move freely in and out of postures, such as prone, hands-knees, and standing, as they progress developmentally, allowing gravity to alternately assist or resist the movements. Through this, the infant begins to strengthen and develop muscle groups and learn to interact with the gravitational force in his or her environment.

This combination of normal movement patterns in a gravitational field, along with genetic predisposition, accounts for the normal development of the bones, muscles, and joints that comprise the chest wall. Conversely, infants with severe neurological impairments do not have that same freedom of movement within their environments. This applies to children with congenital deficits, such as CP or spina bifida, or for children who acquire deficits at an early

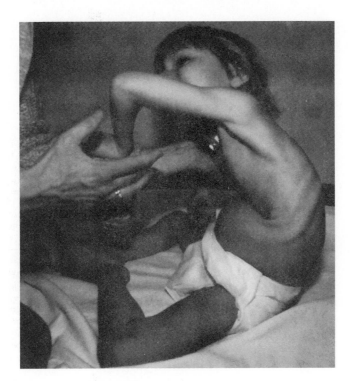

FIGURE 37-3
Independent upright posturing in a patient with congenital quadriplegia. Note relationship of rib cage and abdominal viscera.

developmental age, such as some CVAs, head traumas, or SCIs. These children become subjugated to the effects of gravity on their growing and developing bodies because they are unable to independently counteract its constant presence. A variety of reasons may account for their inability to change their own positions in space: (1) muscle weakness, (2) tonal problems (e.g., spasticity or flaccidity), (3) reflex dominance, (4) incoordination, or (5) a combination of the above. Typically, these children spend significantly more time in supine than in any other posture, which can lead to undesirable changes in the thorax.

Understanding the basic steps and principles in normal chest development is essential for accurately assessing abnormal chest deformities often seen in this physically challenged population. Initially, the newborn's chest is triangular in shape, narrow and flat in the upper portion, and wider and more rounded in the lower portion (Figure 37-4). The infant's short

neck renders the upper accessory muscles nonfunctional as a ventilatory muscle. The infant's arms are held in flexion and adduction across the chest, significantly hampering lateral or anterior movement of the chest wall. This all points to underdevelopment of the upper chest region in the newborn. The infant, forced to be a diaphragmatic breather, shows greater development of the lower chest and hence leads to the triangular shaping of the rib cage.

From 3 to 6 months of age, the infant begins to develop more trunk extension tone, they spend more time in a prone on elbows position, and they begin to reach out into the environment with the upper extremities. This facilitates development of the anterior upper chest. Constant stretching helps to expand the anterior upper chest both anteriorly and laterally. An increase in intercostal and pectoralis muscle strength improves the infant's ability to counteract the force of gravity on the anterior upper chest in supine, leading

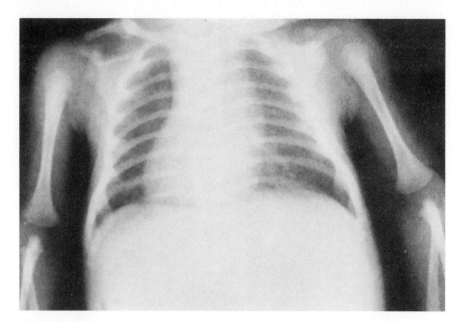

FIGURE 37-4
Newborn chest configuration. Note triangular shape.

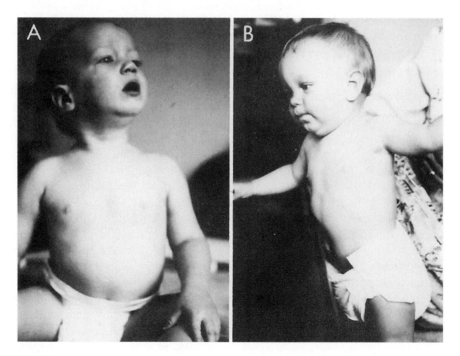

FIGURE 37-5
A and **B,** 10-month old infant chest configuration. Note shape of chest changes and angle of ribs.

to the development of a slight convex configuration of the area and a more rectangular shaping of the thorax from a frontal plane.

The next significant development occurs when the child begins to independently assume erect postures (e.g., sitting, kneeling, or standing). Until this time, the ribs are aligned fairly horizontally, with narrow intercostal spacing (see Figure 37-4). In fact the newborn's chest only comprises approximately one third of the total trunk cavity. As the child begins to move up against the pull of gravity, the ribs rotate downward (more so in the lower ribs), creating the sharper angle of the ribs as seen in the adult (Figures 37-5 and 37-6). This markedly elongates the rib cage until it eventually occupies more than half of the trunk cavity. A comparison of chest x-rays of newborns and adults, as well as pictures of infants, clearly shows these developmental trends (see Figure 37-4 to 37-6). Development trends are summarized in Table 37-1.

Children with severe neurological deficits often show a very different picture of chest development. Frequently, they do not develop adequate upper-extremity and neck muscle control (e.g., weak muscles, tone problems, reflex dominance, or incoordination), causing their upper chests to retain the more primitive triangular, flattened shape. Inadequate muscle control or chronically shortened neck muscles also renders the accessory muscles less able to assist if needed in ventilation. In some cases the child's diaphragm remains so strong and unbalanced by the abdominal and intercostal muscles that it creates a cavus deformity (pectus excuvatum) at the sternum (Figure 37-7). This occurs when the intercostal muscles are incapable of maintaining the anterior chest wall's position against gravity and the abdominal muscles are weak or flaccid, thus not stabilizing the lower borders of the thorax. This may also eventually cause an anterior flaring of the lower ribs.

Most of these children with severe neuromuscular

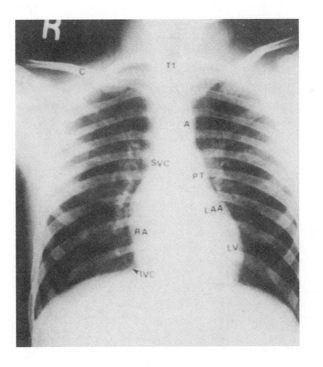

FIGURE 37-6
Normal adult chest x-ray. Chest shape is rectangular, ribs angled downward, upper and lower chest equally developed.

impairments require significant assistance to maintain an upright posture, therefore they spend more time in a recumbent position. Thus the rib cage tends to show less downward rotation and elongation than that of the normally developing child. In some cases of prolonged supine posturing combined with hyperactivity of the rectus abdominus, as seen in many children with spastic tetraplegia CP, the chest will become flattened anteriorly, yet flared laterally in the lower ribs (Figure 37-8). These children are unable to stabilize the lower lateral borders of their rib cage and are unable to counteract gravity's influence on the anterior chest wall move-

TABLE 37–1		
Chest Development Table		
Chest	**Infant**	**Adult**
Size	Occupies one third of the trunk cavity	Occupies greater than one half trunk cavity
Shape	Triangular frontal plane	Rectangular frontal plane
	Circular anterior-posterior plane	Elliptical anterior-posterior plane
Upper chest	Narrow	Wide
	Flat apex	Convex apex
Lower chest	Circular	Elliptical
	Flared lower ribs	Integrated with abdominals
Ribs	Evenly horizontal	Rotated downward; especially inferiorly
Intercostal spacing	Narrow	Wide
	Limits movement of ribs	Allows for individual movement of ribs
Diaphragm	Adequate	Adequate
	Minimal dome shape	Large dome shape, greater excursion
Accessory muscles	Nonfunctional	Functional

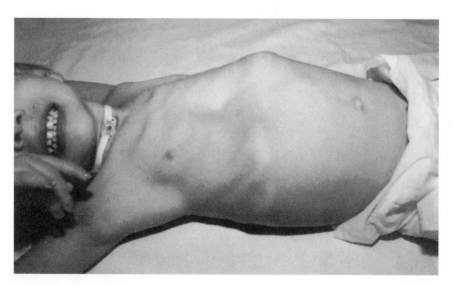

FIGURE 37-7
Pectus excavation deformity (secondary to spinal cord injury and resultant muscle imbalance).

ments. Thus we see these adverse musculoskeletal changes, which limits the breathing patterns options.

As long as the neurological deficits are present, these children will never develop normally. However, frequent position changes, inhibition of undesired tone, facilitation of weakened chest muscles, promotion of preferred breathing patterns, and incorporation of ventilatory strategies with movement will stimulate normal chest development. Optimum respiratory function cannot be expected from a severely underdeveloped chest.

MUSCULAR AND TONAL INFLUENCES ON CHEST DEVELOPMENT

Adverse effects of gravity are counteracted by functioning musculature. Recall that inspiration/expiration

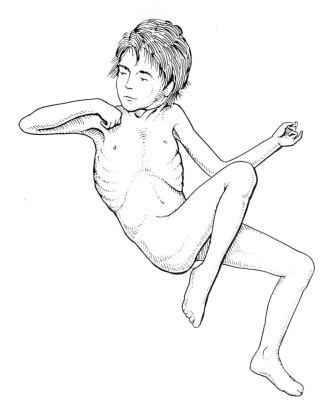

FIGURE 37-8
Musculoskeletal changes secondary to static positioning and neurological deficit.

occurs because of pressure gradients between the air outside the lungs and the air inside. These gradients are achieved through movements in the chest wall. Muscle contractions provide the power to move the chest wall. If these muscles do not overcome the effect of gravity because of weakness, paralysis, abnormal tone, or inadequate muscle control, the chest will be unable to expand in all three planes of ventilation, thus limiting pulmonary function. Because of this important fact, all muscles originating or inserting into the chest wall become "ventilatory muscles." The box on p. 688 lists these muscles and how they affect chest expansion and other specific respiratory function. They are listed in the following two distinct groups: the primary muscles needed for normal ventilation (the triad of normal ventilation) and all other accessory muscles of ventilation. Impairment to any of these muscles may result in respiratory deficits.

Another factor that determines a muscle's effectiveness as a chest wall mover is neurological tone in the muscle. Rigidity of movement, as seen in some patients with head traumas and Parkinson's disease will render the chest immobile, severely limiting its ability to expand in any plane. Spasticity, more often to a lesser degree than rigidity, can render the chest immobile. Spasticity (i.e., SCI, CP, some head trauma), is frequently activated by quick movement of the affected muscle either actively or passively. A quick activity like coughing may activate this abnormal tone and work against the patient as he or she tries to produce an effective cough. The other extreme of abnormal muscle tone is flaccidity or lack of any muscular tone, as seen with some SCIs, CVAs, and MD. In this case the muscle is entirely unable to move the chest wall or to counteract the effects of gravity. Of the three types of abnormal tone, flaccidity is the most adversely influenced by the effects of gravity.

At the same time, postural reflexes and their effect on muscle tone must be considered. For instance, the tonic labrinthyne reflex (TLR) increases extensor tone when the person is supine and increases flexor tone when that person is prone. For patients with CP, for example, this reflex may stay a dominant force in their motor control, interfering with their ability to move freely in supine and prone positions. Because of this, a child with CP with increased extensor tone

Trunk Muscles and Their Function in Ventilation

Muscles of Ventilation—Three-Dimensional Movements

Triad of normal ventilation

Diaphragm

- Major muscle of passive ventilation
- Innervation—phrenic nerve—C3 to C5
- Primary movement—all three planes
- Dependency on intercostal and abdominal muscles
- Concentric contractions—quiet and forceful inhalation
- Eccentric contractions—controlled exhalation and speech

Intercostals

- Primary function—stabilizes rib cage
- Innervation—T1 to T2
- Primary movement—concentric contractions
  - Lateral and superior expansion in lower chest during both quiet and forceful inhalation. Anterior expansion occurs to a lesser degree.
  - Anterior and superior expansion in upper chest, lateral expansion occurs to a lesser degree.
  - Forceful exhalation—primarily medial and inferior compression in lower chest, posterior and inferior compression in upper chest
- Eccentric contractions—needed for controlled exhalation and speech

Abdominals

- Stabilizes inferior border of rib cage—provides mid trunk control
- Innervation T6 to L1
- Provides visceral support
- Provides positive pressure support for the diaphragm
- Provides necessary intrathoracic pressure for an effective cough

Accessory muscles

Erector spinae

- Stabilizes thorax posteriorly to allow for normal anterior chest wall movement to occur
- Innervated at T1 to S3

Pectoralis muscles

- Provides upper chest anterior and lateral expansion
- Innervated C5 to T1
- Can be a substitute rib cage stabilizer after paralysis of the intercostal muscles

Serratus anterior

- Provides posterior expansion of rib cage when upper extremities are fixated
- Innervated C5 to C7
- Only inspiratory muscle that is paired with trunk flexion movements rather than trunk extension movements

---

> *Trunk Muscles and Their Function in Ventilation—cont'd*
>
> Scalenes
> - Provides superior and anterior expansion of the upper chest
> - Innervated C3 to C8
>
> Sternocleidomastoid
> - Provides superior and anterior expansion of upper chest
> - Innervated C2 to C3 and accessory cranial nerve
>
> Trapezius
> - Provides superior expansion of the upper chest
> - Innervated C2 to C4 and accessory cranial nerve

---

will see an even greater increase in that abnormal tone if placed supine. That will make it more difficult for the child to attempt any flexion phase of a breathing pattern in supine (coughing or exhalation). Children should not be left supine as the therapist teaches them altered breathing patterns. If the goal of that treatment session is to promote controlled exhalation maneuvers, the child would have been positioned for failure rather than success. Therefore positioning of the patient and tonal inhibitory or facilatory techniques become of vital importance when developing a treatment plan for maximizing respiratory function.

SPECIFIC RESPIRATORY IMPAIRMENTS

The first half of this chapter discusses the forces that influence the functioning of the neurologically impaired chest. Understanding these forces allows one to discern the impairments that will appear as a direct or indirect result of those neurological deficits. Decreased chest expansion, abnormal or inefficient breathing patterns, abnormal bony changes, decreased cough effectiveness, decreased coordination of breathing with functional activities, decreased ability to phonate, and decreased ability to self-maintain bronchial hygiene can all be direct results of severe neurological deficits. These specific impairments are addressed now in detail.

DECREASED CHEST EXPANSION

Muscle weakness or abnormal tone, combined with the effects of gravity that were previously discussed, serve to decrease the ability of the chest to expand in one or all three planes of ventilation. Quantitatively, chest expansion can be measured via lung volumes by taking vital capacity readings and comparing them with the norms, and it can be measured by taking chest excursion measurements during inhalation with a tape measure in three places: under the axilla, just beneath the nipple line, and on the lowest most ribs (8, 9, and 10). Although both methods give an objective measurement, neither technique can assess which planes of ventilation are being compromised. Subjective assessment skills are needed to determine limiting factors. The box on p. 690 gives detailed summaries of such assessments for persons with all levels of SCIs. These characteristics can be extrapolated to subjective chest assessments of other neurological and/or musculoskeletal disorders, especially where weakness is present.

COMPENSATORY BREATHING PATTERNS

Limitations in chest expansion inevitably lead to changes in breathing patterns. Severely involved CVAs or head trauma patients may show severe abnormalities in their breathing patterns in response to

Neuromuscular Effects on Respiratory Function in Spinal Cord Injuries

Paraplegia: Primarily T1 to T5

1. Weakened and/or absent
   - Abdominal
   - Intercostal
   - Erector spinae
2. Planes of ventilation limited
   - Slight decrease in anterior and lateral expansion
3. Resulting in
   - Slight to moderate decrease in chest expansion and vital capacity (VC)
   - Decreased ability to build up intrathoracic and intraabdominal pressures
   - Decreased cough effectiveness
   - Possible paradoxical breathing

Tetraplegia: C5 to C8

1. Missing aforementioned muscles and weakened
   - Pectoralis
   - Serratus anterior
   - Scalenes
2. Planes of ventilation limited
   - Marked decrease in anterior and lateral expansion
   - Slight decrease in posterior expansion
3. Resulting in
   - Significant decrease in chest expansion and VC
   - Significant decrease in forced expiratory volume (FEV)
   - Significant decrease in cough effectiveness
   - Paradoxical breathing in acute phase and perhaps longer

Tetraplegia: C4

1. Missing aforementioned muscles and weakened
   - Scalenes
   - Diaphragm
2. Planes of ventilation limited
   - Marked decrease in anterior and lateral expansion
   - Slight decrease in inferior and superior expansion
3. Resulting in
   - More pronounced limitations in all three planes of ventilation
   - Possible decrease in tidal volume (TV)
   - Possible need for mechanical ventilation

Neuromuscular Effects on Respiratory Function in Spinal Cord Injuries—cont'd

Tetraplegia: C1 to C3

1. Missing aforementioned muscles and weakened and/or absent, the last of the remaining accessory muscles
   - Sternocleidomastoid (SCM)
   - Trapezius
2. Planes of ventilation limited
   - All severely limited including superior expansion
3. Resulting in
   - Significant decrease in TV
   - The need for full-time mechanical ventilation (at least in acute phase)

---

impairments to their respiratory centers in the brain stem. This chapter focuses on compensatory breathing patterns that develop as a result of muscular weakness or paralysis, high tone, or pain. Details of breathing pattern changes secondary to brain stem lesions can be found in Chapter 22. The compensatory patterns discussed here are itemized in the box at right.

There are two types of paradoxical, or "see-saw," breathing. The first is caused by a strong diaphragm in the absence of the two other triad muscles, intercostal muscles and abdominal muscles (e.g., polio, tetraplegia, or paraplegia). Normal diaphragmatic excursion requires the muscular support and function of the intercostal and abdominal muscles to optimize the diaphragm's contractions. In this type of paradoxical breathing the diaphragm contracts, the abdomen rises excessively because of flaccid abdominal muscle tone, and the upper chest collapses because of a lack of the stabilizing contraction of the intercostal muscles (Figure 37-9). This is the more common form of paradoxical breathing.

The second type of paradoxical breathing occurs when there is diaphragm paralysis while the upper accessory muscles are still intact. The abdominal muscles may or may not be functional. The see-saw action here is the opposite motion of that described previously (Figure 37-10). With this type of paradoxical breathing, the abdomen draws inward during inspiration and the upper chest rises. The upper accessory muscles contract, expanding the rib cage

Possible Compensatory Breathing Patterns after a Neurological Injury/Disease

- Paradoxical breathing (see-saw breathing)
  - Paralyzed intercostals and/or abdominals
    - upper chest collapses
    - abdomen rises excessively
  - Paralyzed diaphragm
    - lower chest collapses
    - upper chest rises excessively
- Diaphragm and upper accessory muscles only (paralyzed intercostals)
- Upper accessory muscles only (all three "triad" muscles paralyzed)
- Asymmetrical breathers (hemiplegia, unilateral disorders)
- Lateral or "gravity eliminated" breathers (weakness not paralysis)
- Shallow breathers (typically associated with high-tone)

primarily in a superior plane. Anterior and lateral expansion may also occur if the intercostal and pectoralis muscles are functioning. Generally, this compensatory breathing pattern requires some kind of assisted ventilation, at least part time, because the diaphragm normally supplies most of the expansion

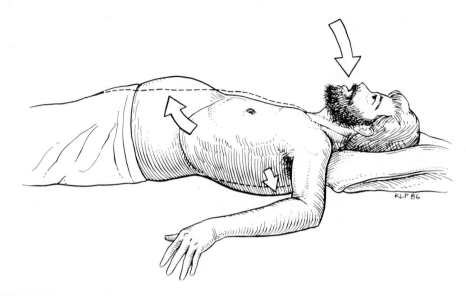

FIGURE 37-9
Paradoxical breathing, strong diaphragm, absent accessory muscles and abdominal muscles.

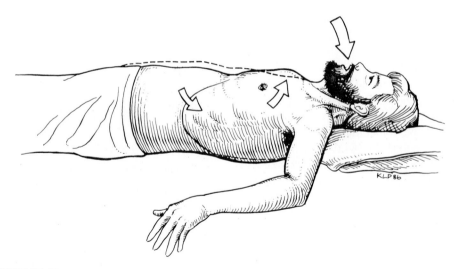

FIGURE 37-10
Paradoxical breathing, diaphragm paralysis.

necessary to maintain adequate oxygenation levels. Total accessory muscle breathing is generally incapable of providing adequate independent long-term ventilation because of the likelihood of respiratory muscle fatigue.

Another type of compensatory breathing pattern occurs when the intercostal and abdominal muscles are paralyzed but the diaphragm and upper accessory muscles still function (i.e., tetraplegia, C_5 to C_8; and paraplegia, T_1 to T_5). These patients learn to counterbal-

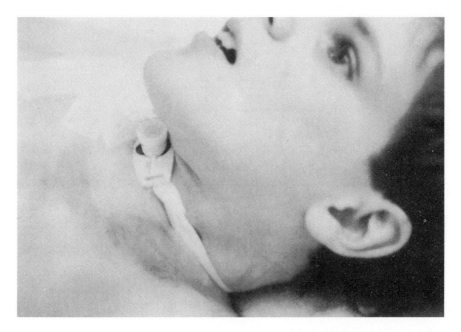

FIGURE 37-11
Shortened neck musculature secondary to accessory muscle breathing pattern.

ance the strength of the diaphragmatic pull by using their sternocleidomastoid muscles and possibly their scalene, trapezius, and pectoralis muscles. Allowing for superior and possibly some anterior and lateral expansion of the chest, this compensatory breathing pattern prevents the collapse of the upper chest seen in paradoxical breathing. This must be cognitively coordinated with the inspiratory phase and is generally a more effective breathing pattern. On subjective breathing assessment, these patients often present with shortened neck muscles (Figure 37-11). Intercostal retractions, or the collapsing of the intercostal spaces on inspiration, may be seen here. The paralyzed intercostal muscle tissue will be sucked in toward the lungs during the creation of negative pressure within the chest, thus the observance of the retractions (Figure 37-12). This may be the most accurate way of assessing intercostal paralysis without an EMG test.

If the patient lacks all "triad ventilatory muscles," they may be able to breathe using their upper accessory muscles only. Generally they will need mechanical ventilation to augment their independent effort.

Neurological insults that affect the chest asymmetrically, such as with CVAs and some head traumas, show another type of compensatory breathing pattern. These patients can still actively expand their unaffected side in all three planes of ventilation. Often, they accentuate this asymmetry to achieve more expansion on their unaffected sides. This may be seen as increased sidebending toward their involved side (Figure 37-13). This leads to inadequate ventilation on the affected side, which puts these patients at a higher risk of developing respiratory complications secondary to inadequate ventilation. In addition, the adverse effects on their posture can lead to undesired musculoskeletal changes over a prolonged period of time especially for the pediatric patient. Prevention of these secondary changes is of utmost importance.

Patients with generalized weakness, such as with Guillain-Barré syndrome, some myopathies, neuropathies, or incomplete SCIs, may show a tendency toward lateral breathing, or breathing that takes place primarily in gravity-eliminated planes. For example, in supine, patients with weakened chest muscles could not

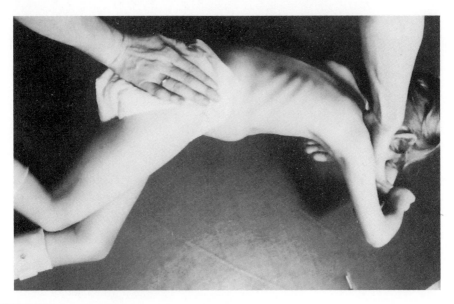

FIGURE 37-12
Intercostal retractions noted during inspiration.

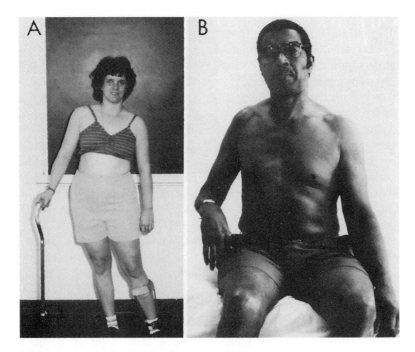

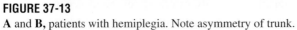

FIGURE 37-13
A and **B,** patients with hemiplegia. Note asymmetry of trunk.

effectively oppose the force of gravity in the anterior plane, thus they alter their breathing pattern to cause expansion in the lateral plane where gravity is eliminated. In sitting, these same patients would tend to breathe inferiorly where gravity would assist the movement. Likewise, in side lying, they would tend to breathe in an anterior plane. Overall, these patients have the best prognosis for effective breathing retraining methods because they have weakness, not complete paralysis.

The last breathing pattern to be discussed involves patients with central nervous system deficits resulting in high tone, such as MS, Parkinson's disease, and some head traumas. Their breathing patterns are altered not so much by muscle weakness as by the following: (1) chest immobility because of abnormally high neuromuscular tone (spasticity, rigidity, tremors), which severely limits chest expansion in any plane, (2) cerebellar incoordination, or (3) improper sequencing because of lesions in the brain, most commonly seen with medullary lesions. Breathing is usually symmetrical, shallow, sometimes asynchronous, and frequently tachypneic (respiratory rates over 25 breaths/minute). Initiation and follow-through of a volitional maximal inspiration is difficult or impossible for these patients. This will markedly curtail the ability to produce an effective cough and to maintain bronchial hygiene.

SLEEP DISORDERS

The patients described in this chapter frequently need to use their accessory muscles cognitively, to arrive at a work-efficient, ventilation-efficient, breathing pattern. Because of this, they should be evaluated for nighttime ventilatory assistance. Muscle weakness or breathing inefficiency may cause a state of chronic hypoventilation and/or sleep apnea episodes during sleep. Drowsiness, lack of concentration, disturbed sleep, and/or irritability are common complaints of this state. In the clinical setting, we see many tetraplegic patients and other severely involved neurological patients who are lethargic after awakening. Hospital staff may incorrectly label these patients as lazy or uncooperative. It should be assessed whether this behavior is volitional or whether it is due to a state of chronic nighttime hypoxemia. Assessments can be made by screening high-risk patients for this

disorder with oximetry during sleep. Patients showing deficiencies may need repositioning of their sleep postures, nighttime ventilation, oxygen support, or a combination of these. Rigorous exercising or activities of daily living (ADL) training may be more appropriately scheduled later in the day for these patients until their sleep problems have been rectified.

CHANGES IN PULMONARY FUNCTIONS

The abnormal breathing patterns discussed previously develop secondary to the patient's neurological deficits. However, those new patterns then change the patient's pulmonary function, which in turn affects functional respiratory status. Specifically, changes in respiratory rates (RR), tidal volume (TV), and vital capacity (VC) are addressed here.

Alveolar minute ventilation is the product of TV times RR. The optimal relationship between these two parameters is those values that result in minimizing the mechanical work that the lungs must perform with a particular breathing pattern. In other words, it is the combination of RR and TV that requires the body to put out the least muscular effort per breath. Because most of the compensatory breathing patterns that have been discussed thus far reduce the patient's TV, the only recourse this patient has is to increase RR. Normal RR is between 12 to 20 breaths/minute; however, for this neurological population, it is not uncommon to see RRs at least twice that figure.

Although adjusting RR does bring the patient's respiratory system back to a state of equilibrium, it may not produce the most efficient pattern in the long run. The idea of the oxygen cost of breathing in that pattern must be considered in its long-term functional use. Ideally, TV at rest should be about 10% of one's actual VC. At this level, the able-bodied person needs less than 5% of the total oxygen available to the body to operate the respiratory mechanisms. When performing a normal physical task or low-level exercise, this oxygen consumption rate increases slowly, never quite reaching a point where the oxygen cost of operating the respiratory system outweighs the cost of performing the activity. However, for patients with impaired chest functions, such as in this population, the total oxygen consumption level of the respiratory muscles at rest can be as much as 4 to 10 times that amount. These patients may have TV/VC ratios that are already in the 33% to 67% range at rest, indicating inefficient breathing patterns, reduced VCs, inadequate respiratory reserves, or both. When they attempt a mild exercise, they become quickly short of breath. They do not have adequate oxygen reserves to supply the respiratory and the nonrespiratory muscles simultaneously, thus severely limiting exercise tolerance. Therefore although these patients may show adequate maintenance of alveolar minute ventilation at rest, a mild increase in activity level may magnify respiratory insufficiencies.

An adequate VC is imperative in restoring a patient's functional status. Without the ability to expand the chest maximally under his or her own muscle power, VC will decrease after a neurological insult. For example, studies show that tetraplegia resulting from SCIs may reduce the patient's VC to 33% of the predicted value, increasing the TV/VC ratio to 30%. For SCIs, an adequate VC is generally considered to be 66% of the expected value. This would restore the TV/VC ratio to approximately 15%, thus decreasing

the work of breathing. If VC remains less than 60% of the predicted value, most research indicates that these patients will demonstrate inadequate coughs. Similarly, a FEV_1 less than 60% indicates lack of sufficient power behind the cough. When VC remains or decreases to only 25% to 30% of the predicted norm, then ventilation assistance usually becomes necessary.

ADVERSE MUSCULOSKELETAL CHANGES

Neuromuscular weakness and the compensatory breathing patterns may cause adverse musculoskeletal changes over a prolonged period of time. Previous discussion in this chapter revolved around the adverse effects that gravity can play on the skeleton if the body is unable to counteract its force. Pronounced deformities are more prevalent in children, of course; however, both children and adults are effected. Several examples of specific changes are presented.

A common musculoskeletal deformity secondary to muscle weakness is seen as a flattened anterior chest wall, as seen with many paraplegic and tetraplegic patients. (Figure 37-14) For the patient

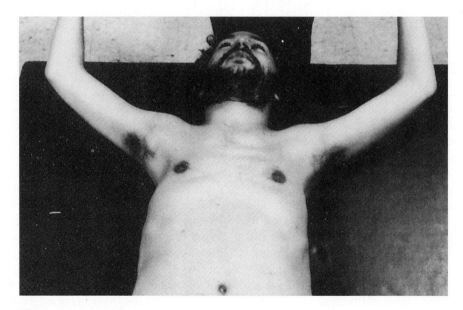

FIGURE 37-14
Musculoskeletal changes in adult chest secondary to spinal cord injury (SCI). Note flattening of the anterior chest wall and narrowing of the upper chest.

with weak or paralyzed intercostal muscles, this flattening often occurs because of prolonged supine positioning along with the significant resistance that anterior chest expansion meets from gravity.

Another common deformity is a pectus excuvatum at the base of the xiphoid process. Patients who have a strong diaphragm but no muscular support from the intercostals and abdominal muscles may develop this type of musculoskeletal deformity (see Figure 37-7, p. 686). It can result from the diaphragm pulling inward so hard that the sternum, without intercostal muscle support, cannot maintain its neutral position. Over time, it caves in, resulting in a permanent deformity.

Anterior or lateral flaring of the lower rib cage may also be noted. This is usually a result of insufficient abdominal strength, thus the lower ribs are not stabilized and integrated into the abdominal area (see Figure 37-8, p. 687). In upright, this is seen as a marked delineation between the rib cage and abdominal area in the mid-trunk region (see Figures 37-3, p. 683 and 37-15).

Upper chest adverse musculoskeletal changes occur when the intercostal and/or other upper accessory muscles are impaired. The diaphragm is not positioned to assist in expansion of this area. Therefore, without those accessory muscles, the anterior wall of the upper chest will become flattened and appear

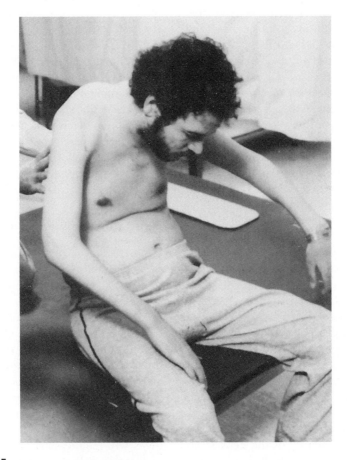

FIGURE 37-15
Independent upright posturing. Adult with tetraplegia. Kyphosis restricts chest movement for respiration. Note folding at mid-trunk line.

more narrow than that of the normal upper chest (see Figure 37-14, p. 696), resembling the more primitive triangular shaping of the chest seen in the newborn (see Figure 37-4, p. 684).

Spinal curves are not spared deformities. In a weakened, low-tone patient, scoliosis is common because the patient cannot adequately maintain himself or herself upright against gravity. Slowly, the spine collapses on itself, seeking stability; therefore scoliosis is developed. All types of patients with the neurological diagnoses discussed in this chapter are at risk for developing scoliosis. The second possible spinal change, a lumbar and thoracic kyphosis, can occur as well because of the force of gravity on a mobile spine and lack of paraspinal muscle support. Secondary to these kyphoses, many patients develop an excessive cervical lordosis to maintain eye contact. In sitting the patient hunches over his or her trunk, making eye contact and head righting difficult (see Figures 37-3, p. 683 and 37-15, p. 697).

These spinal changes affect the functioning of the respiratory system adversely. With a kyphotic thorax in an upright posture, expansion of the chest in all three planes of ventilation will be impaired. The ribs require a stable base from which to become properly mobilized. A kyphotic, weak posterior support does not provide the necessary stability for optimal rib mobility and function. Therefore proper elevation and angulation of the ribs becomes impossible. This limits overall chest expansion and vital capacity.

Musculoskeletal changes in children must be addressed. They are in a state of habilitation rather than rehabilitation. Because of this, the neurological deficit affects their developing chests more severely. Their rib cages remain more triangular in shape, since the muscles of the upper chest never develop fully or normally. The ribs also remain more horizontal than in the normal adult, probably because of less upright posturing and lack of intercostal and abdominal muscle contractions on the rib frames. Their necks and shoulders do not mature developmentally, often because of overuse of the neck accessory muscles. This leads to a permanent shortening of the neck strap muscles, making the child appear to lack a cervical area (see Figures 37-7, p. 686, and 37-8, p. 687).

Proper elongation of the cervical spine cannot occur, resulting in skeletal changes to that area. Scoliosis, along with thoracic kyphosis, tends to be more pronounced than in the adult.

DECREASED COUGH EFFECTIVENESS

With decreased chest expansion, the presence of compensatory breathing patterns, and the adverse musculoskeletal changes, the patient's ability to cough will be drastically reduced. Vital capacity will be impaired as will the ability to build up sufficient intraabdominal pressure, especially for patients with weakened, flaccid, or uncoordinated abdominal musculature. For many patients with traumatic brain injuries, Parkinson's disease, CP, and CVA, the inability to coordinate an effective cough will be significantly impaired. This inability may be due to cerebellar damage or to high neuromuscular tone (spasticity, rigidity, tremors). Frequently, the quick action required to produce an effective cough will be the same action that will trigger a sudden increase in the abnormal neuromuscular tone. Objectively, when the patient can not expel at least 60% of his or her actual vital capacity in 1 second (FEV_1), he or she will often be incapable of producing an effective cough without some assistance or retraining.

MAINTAINING BRONCHIAL HYGIENE

All these changes in respiratory functioning lead to a decreased ability of the neurologically impaired patient to independently maintain bronchial hygiene. Complete expansion of the chest in all three planes of ventilation and in all postures is impaired, so the ability to properly aerate all lung segments is impaired. Thus the ability to perform independent bronchial drainage will likewise be impaired. Inefficient breathing patterns may cause them to remain in a state of chronic hypoventilation. Inability to produce an effective cough impairs the ability to clear the lungs of secretions. Therefore most of these patients will require some assistance, either physically or through verbal instruction, to achieve adequate bronchial hygiene.

IMPAIRED PHONATION

Aphasia, as a secondary impairment to neurological deficits, is generally recognized by all members of the medical team as a problem that necessitates speech therapy. However, many persons with neurological impairments display serious deficits in communication that remain untreated and the deficits remain unacknowledged. Primarily, that deficit is inadequate breath support for phonation; in other words the patient's inability to control the force and duration of exhalation for the purpose of phonation. Duration of phonation and voice intensity are regulated by a delicate balance between airway resistance, provided by the laryngeal muscles, and the force of exhalation, provided by the muscles of ventilation (Figure 37-16). When the respiratory muscles are malfunctioning, as in the neurological diseases discussed, the patient's ability to regulate the flow of air out of the lungs may be impaired. Good eccentric control of the inspiratory muscles (the ability to slowly release these muscle during exhalation) is needed to produce normal lengths of phonation. Otherwise, the air may be expelled from the lungs too quickly because of the natural elastic recoil of the diaphragm, rendering that volume of air useless for phonation. Therefore both a decrease in tidal volume and a decrease in eccentric control of the respiratory muscles will lead to impairments in functional speech.

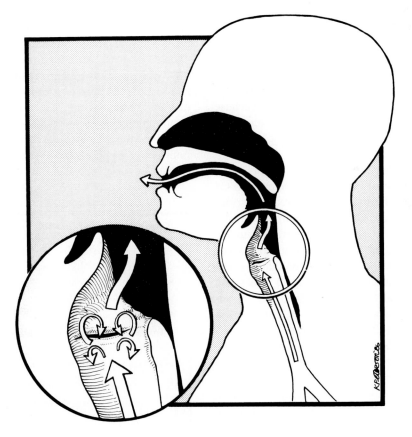

FIGURE 37-16
Relationship of air flow and vocal folds.

The average adult breathes at a ratio of 1:1 or 1:2 (inhalation time: exhalation time) during quiet breathing. The average ratio during phonation becomes 1:5, with 8 to 10 syllables per breath being a comfortable speaking length. Clinically, many patients are seen to struggle with two- to thee-syllable phrases because of inadequate breath support. Often these same patients are not referred to speech therapy for training because they are not diagnosed as having a "speech" problem (e.g., many patients with SCIs, MDs, polio, or spina bifida). Optimally, these patients should be able to phonate (an "ah" or "oh" sound) for at least 10 to 12 seconds during a controlled expired vital capacity. Many of their voices fade away after 3 to 4 seconds. Without the ability to communicate with normal speaking lengths and normal voice intensities, these patients' successful reentry into society's mainstream becomes significantly more difficult.

Another misconception about these patients is that they are mentally slow or retarded because they do not use all the proper figures of speech. In reality, these patients may exclude figures of speech because of the extended time it takes them to communicate something. For them, it is more expedient to forego their inclusion.

A marked example of this was seen in our clinic. A 3-year-old girl who sustained a complete C4 to C5 spinal cord lesion at birth and had not received prior rehabilitation was seen. On initial examination, her speech was choppy, brief, and grammatically incorrect. She rarely initiated conversation and her voice intensity was very low. It was suspected that she perhaps suffered some anoxic brain damage to account for her developmentally delayed speech. After an intense breathing retraining program in conjunction with a physical rehabilitation program, her speech changed drastically. She spoke fluently, with 8 to 10 syllables/breath, correct inclusion of grammar, and louder and more varied voice intensities. Instead of being quiet and more reserved as she had been before treatment, the mother reported that the child was a regular chatterbox. Her new communication skills appeared to improve her self-esteem. At that point, it became understood that her cognitive skills were well underestimated on initial screening.

Air flow out of the lungs should be as important to clinicians as airflow into the lungs. An evaluation of expiratory eccentric control is necessary for all neurological patients regardless of diagnoses. All disciplines should incorporate a phonation facilitation program into their rehabilitation program, especially for those patients who would otherwise not receive any speech training.

GOALS OF A NEUROMUSCULAR OR MUSCULOSKELETAL RESPIRATORY PROGRAM

In conclusion, the combination of secondary effects that follow a neurological and/or musculoskeletal insult are responsible for leaving the person with residual musculoskeletal or neuromuscular deficits at greater risk for developing respiratory complications long after their acute phases have subsided. The long-term goal of any respiratory rehabilitation program for these patients is obvious; reduce their risk for developing these complications. First and foremost is the need to increase or maintain chest expansion in all three planes of ventilation. Second, educating the patient and/or family in methods to maintain good bronchial hygiene must be emphasized to prevent infections. Logically, improving cough effectiveness will improve airway clearance. Next, increasing the patient's vital capacity

---

Respiratory Rehabilitation Goals

- Increase or maintain chest expansion in all three planes of ventilation
- Educate the patient and/or family in methods for maintaining good bronchial hygiene
- Improve cough effectiveness
- Increase the patient's vital capacity and tidal volume
- Reduce high respiratory rates
- Modify inadequate breathing patterns
- Improve eccentric control of the diaphragm and other ventilatory muscles for improved phonation skills
- Incorporate effective ventilatory strategies with all motor tasks

and tidal volume, where indicated, will help to improve aeration of the lungs. If necessary, reducing high respiratory rates to improve pulmonary functions will be a goal. Other goals include modifying inadequate breathing patterns, which could mean increasing or decreasing the use of accessory muscles to achieve maximal breathing efficiency, and improving eccentric control of the diaphragm and other ventilatory muscles for improved phonation skills. These concepts lead us to realize the need for incorporating effective ventilatory strategies with all motor tasks. These goals are summarized in the box on p. 700. When implementing this program, it is necessary to recall that the patient's respiratory needs do not exist in a vacuum. They must be able to apply what they learn from this program into all phases of their lives. Thus incorporation of these goals into ADL or multipurpose activities will yield the most successful results.

REVIEW QUESTIONS

1. What differences are noted in patients suffering deficits acquired as adults versus a child with acquired deficits in utero or shortly after birth?
2. Which orthopedic and neurologic diagnoses can be associated with cardiopulmonary dysfunction?
3. How should the effect of gravity on ventilation be considered during exercise and positioning?
4. What factors contribute to normal chest development?
5. What symptoms would be noted in patients that have sleep disorders?
6. Why should a therapist be concerned about phonation in patients with neurological dysfunction?
7. What are the goals of a neuromuscular/musculoskeletal cardiopulmonary program?

Bibliography

Alexander, H., et al. (1982). Breathing alterations in head injured patients. *Journal of Neurological Sciences 51:*209-218.

Annoni, J.M., Ackermann, D., & Kresslring, J. (1990). Respiratory function in chronic hemiplegia. *Int Disabil Studies.* May:78-80.

Aronson, A. (1985). *Clinical voice disorders: An interdisciplinary approach.* (2nd ed.). New York, Thieme Inc.

Ashworth, B. & Hunter, A.R. (1971). Respiratory failure in myasthenia gravis. *Proc R Soc London* (Biol) 64:489-90.

Bach, J.R. (1991). New approaches in the rehabilitation of the traumatic high level quadriplegic. *Americal Journal of Physical Medicine and Rehabilitation 70(1):*13-9.

Bach, J.R. (1995). Respiratory muscle aids for the prevention of pulmonary morbidity and mortality. *Seminars in Neurology 15(1):*72-82.

Boehme, R. (1992). Assessment and treatment of the respiratory system for breathing, sound production and trunk control. *Teamtalk 2(4):*2-8.

Borden, G., Harris, K. Speech Science Primer: Physiology, Acoustics, and Perception of Speech, 2nd ed. Baltimore, Williams & Wilkens, 1984.

Boughton, A., Ciesla, N. (1986). Physical therapy management of the head injured patient in the intensive care unit. *Topics in Acute Care Trauma Rehabilitation 1(1):*1-18.

Boyden, E. (1977). Development of the newborn lung. In hudson, W.A. (Ed) *Development and growth of the airways.* New York: Marcel Dekker.

Braun, N.T. (1982). Force-length relationship of the normal human diaphragm. *Journal of Applied Physiology 53:*405-412.

Brown, J.C., Swank, S.M., Matta, J., & Farras, D.M. (1984). Late spinal deformity in quadriplegic children and adolescents. *Journal of Pediatric Orthopedics 4(4):*456-61.

Byran, A.C. Mansell, A.I., & Levison, H. (1977). Regulation of pulmonary alveolar development in late gestation and the perinatal period. In Hudson, W.A. (Ed). *Development and growth of the airways.* New York: Marcel Dekker. 399-418.

Cartwright, R.D. (1984) Effect of sleep position on sleep apnea severity. *Sleep 7(2):*110-14.

Cherniak, R.M. Cherniak, L., Naimark, A. (1972). *Respiration in health and disease.* (Second Edition). Philadelphia: PA Saunders.

Cherniak, N.S. *Abnormal breathing patterns: Their mechanisms and clinical significance. JAMA 230:*57-58.

Clough, P., Lindenauer, D., Hayes, M., & Zekany, B. (1986). Guidelines for routine respiratory care of patients with spinal cord injury. *Physical Therapy 66(9):*1395-402.

Cooper, C.B., Trend, P.S. & Wiles, C.M. (1985). Severe diaphragm weakness in multiple sclerosis. *Thorax 40:*631-32.

Corrado, A., Gorini, M., & De Paola, E. (1995). Alternative techniques for managing acute neuromuscular respiratory failure. *Seminars in Neurology 15(1):*84-88.

Dean, E., Ross, J. Road, J.D., et al. Pulmonary function in individuals with a history of poliomyelitis. Chest 1991; 100:118-123.

DeGroodt, W., et al. (1988). Growth of the lung and thorax dimensions during the pubertal growth spurt. *Eur Prespir J 1:*102-108.

DeReuck, A.V., & Porter, R. (1967). *Ciba foundation symposium: Development of the lung.* Boston: Little, Brown.

DeTroyer, A. (1983). Mechanical action of the abdominal muscles. *Bulletin of European Physiopathology and Respiration 19:*575.

DeTroyer, A., et al. (1985). Mechanics of intercostal space and actions of external internal intercostal muscles. *Journal of Clinical Investigation 75:*85-87.

DeVivo, M.J., Kartus, P.L., Stover, S.L., Fine, P.R. (1990). Benefits of early admission to an organised spinal cord injury care system. *Para 28:*545-555.

DeVivo, M.J., Black, K.J., & Stover, S.L. (1993). Causes of death during the first 12 years after spinal cord injury. *Archives of Physical Medicine and Rehabilitation 74:*248-254.

Donovon, W.H., et al. (1984). Incidence of medical complications in spinal cord injury: patients in specialised, compared with non-specialized centres. *Para 22:*282-290.

Edwards, P.R., Howard, P. (1993). Methods and prognosis of non-invasive ventilation in neuromuscular disease. Monaldi *Archives for Chest Disorders 48(2):*176-182.

Fishburn, M.J., Marino, R.J., Ditunno, J.F. (1990). Atelectasis and pneumonia in acute spinal cord injury. *Archives of Physical Medicine and Rehabilitation 71:*197-200.

Fulford, F.E., & Brown, J.K. (1976). Position as a cuase of deformity in children with cerebral palsy. *Dev Med Child Neuro 18:*305-14.

George, C.F., Millar, T.W., & Kryger, M.H. (1988). Sleep apnea and body position during sleep. *Sleep 11(1):*90-99.

Griggs, R.C., & Donohoe, K.M. (1981). Recognition and management of respiratory insufficiency in neuromuscular disease. *Archives of Neurology 38:*9-12.

Hixon, T.J. (1991). *Respiratory function in speech and song.* San Diego: Singular Publishing Group.

Hoffman, L.A. (1987). Ineffective airway clearance related to neuromuscular dysfunction. *Nursing Clinics of North America 22(1):*151-66.

Jaeger, R.J., Turba, R.M., Yarkony, G.M., & Roth E.J. (1993). Cough in spinal cord injured patients: comparison of three methods to produce cough. *Archives of Physical Medicine and Rehabilitation 74:* 1358-61.

Jasper, N., Kruger, M., Ectors, P., & Sergysels, R. (1986). Unilateral chest wall paradoxical motion mimicking a flail chest in a patient with hemilateral C7 spinal injury. *Intensive Care Medicine 12(6):*396-98.

Kelling, J.S., DiMarco, A.F., Gottfried, S.E., & Altose, M.D. (1985). Respiratory responses to ventilatory loading following low cervical spinal cord injury. *Journal of Applied Physiology 59(6):*1752-56.

Kerby, G.R., Mayer, L.S., & Pingleton, S.K. (1987). Nocturnal positive pressure ventilation via a nasal mask. *American Review of Respiratory Diseases 135:*738-40.

Levitt, S., & Miller, C. (1973). The interrelationship of speech therapy and physiotherapy in children with neurodevelopmental disorders. *Dev Med Child Neurol 15:*188-93.

Maloney, F.P. (1979). Pulmonary function in quadriplegia: effects of a corset. *Archives of Physical Medicine and Rehabilitation 60:*261-65.

Mellin, G., & Harjula, R. (1987). Lung function in relation to thoracic spinal mobility and kyphosis, *Scandinavian Journal of Rehabilitation Medicine 19(2):*89-92.

Mosconi, P., Langer M., Cigada, M., & Mandelli, M. (1991). Epidemiology and risk factors of pneumonia in critically ill patients. *European Journal of Epidemiology 7(4):* 320-327.

Netscher, D.T., & Peterson R. (1990). Normal and abnormal development of the extremities and trunk. *Ped Plastic Surg 17:*13-21.

Nolan, S. (1994). Current trends in the management of acute spinal cord injury. *Critical Care Nursing Quarterly 17(1):*64-78.

Rochester, D. (1986). Respiratory effects of respiratory muscle weakness and atrophy. *American Review of Respiratory Diseases 134:*1083-86.

Ross, J., & Dean, E. (1989). Integrating physiological principles into the comprehensive management of cardiopulmonary dysfunction. *Physical Therapy. 69(4):*255-259.

Saumarez, R.C. (1986). An analysis of possible movements of human upper rib cage. *Journal of Applied Physiology 60(2):*678-689.

Sharp, J.T., Goldberg, N.B., & Druz, W.S. (1975). Relative contributions of rib cage and abdomen to breathing in normal subjects. *Journal of Applied Physiology 60(2):* 608-618.

Sharp, J.T., Beard, G.A., & Sunga, M. et al. (1986). The rib cage in normal and emphysematous subjects: a roentgenographic approach. *Journal of Applied Physiology 61:*2050-59.

Tator, C.H. Duncan, E.G., & Edmonds, V.E., et al. (1993). Complications and costs of management of acute spinal cord injury. *Para 31:*700-714.

Whiteneck, G.G., Charlifue, S.W., & Frankel, H.L., et. al. (1992). Mortality, morbidity and psychosocial outcomes of persons spinal cord injured more than 20 years ago. *Para 30:*617-630.

CHAPTER 38

The Transplant Patient

Susan Scherer

KEY TERMS

Cardiac rehabilitation
Denervation of the heart
Immunosuppression
Organ donation

Organ rejection
Psychosocial
Pulmonary rehabilitation
Secretion management

HISTORY

The ability to transplant an organ from one individual to another is a relatively new phenomenon. Early attempts at transplant were barely successful. New advances in surgical techniques and immunosuppressive drugs, however, have made transplantation of solid organs a viable treatment option. The increased life expectancy of transplant patients means that physical therapists have many opportunities to treat patients after transplant in various settings. Trends in patient demographics indicate that a physical therapist may see a transplant patient not only in a regional medical center setting but also in outpatient and rural clinics. This chapter contains guidelines for treating patients with heart or lung transplants.

BACKGROUND

Early transplant experiments were carried out on animals in the early 1900s, with success at maintaining life for 90 minutes to 8 days (Hosenpud, Cobanoglo Norman, Starr, 1991). Medical advances in cardiopulmonary bypass and immunosuppressive medications provided the opportunity for successful transplants. After many trials and failures, the first successful orthotopic heart transplant was performed in 1967 by Barnard; the first successful lung transplant was performed in 1963 by Hardy and Webb.

Improvements in surgical technique, detection of rejection, and immunosuppressive drugs means transplants are increasing in number. Virtually every solid organ can be transplanted from one individual to another of the same species if there are similarities in immune system markers. Kidney transplants are the simplest and most common, whereas heart-lung block transplants are uncommon.

Purpose of Transplants

Although transplants are considered an acceptable treatment option, a solid organ transplant is usually considered a last-resort therapeutic intervention. Medical intervention for diseases, such as cardiomyopathy and interstitial pulmonary fibrosis, is limited. When conventional medical therapy has failed, a transplant may be considered. Although a transplant offers a patient a second chance at life, the medical management of a transplant causes a patient to require medical intervention on a long-term basis.

Availability of Transplants

The number of medical centers who perform transplants has grown to approximately 175 worldwide in 1989 (Hosenpud et al., 1990). Because of the success rates, many types of transplants are no longer considered experimental but are considered appropriate treatment for organ failure. In 1994 approximately 10,000 kidney transplants were performed and 2500 heart transplants were completed (Colorado Organ Recovery Systems [CORS], Denver, Colorado 1994).

Rejection Issues

Although transplants are successful, some health professionals believe that patients are merely exchanging one set of problems for another. For a transplant to be successful, a patient must remain on powerful immunosuppressive drugs for the remainder of his or her life. Some of these medications have crippling side effects. The effects of long-term prednisone are well known: osteoporosis, muscle weakness, and glucose intolerance, whereas the long-term effects of cyclosporine and azathioprine impact on the patient's ability to fight infection. Patients also need to manage medication side effects on a day to day basis. It is these medications, however, that make for impressive survival rates.

National 1-year survival rates are as follows:*

Kidney	93.8%
Liver	76.7%
Heart	82.6%
Heart-lung	57%
Lung	68%

Organ Donation

The major limitation of organ transplantation is a supply and demand issue. The number of patients who could benefit from transplant significantly exceeds the number of organs available. Media coverage assists with identifying the issues and may play a role in increasing the number of donors. To become an organ donor, check with your state about specific requirements; often a driver's license has a space to identify you as an organ donor. Make sure that you discuss your wishes with your family. If you are hospitalized, family members or close personal friends will often be approached about donating your organs. If your family is confident that you wished your organs to be donated, they will more likely say "yes" to organ donation.

CURRENT TRANSPLANT ISSUES

Transplant trends include early detection of rejection, development of new immunosuppressive medications, and donor management. For donor organs to be viable, the donor must be managed in a way that preserves organs. In the past, fluids were pushed to preserve kidney function for transplant. This extra fluid, however, made the lungs unusable. New donor management techniques are increasing the viability of multiple organs from the same donor.

Ethical Considerations

Should a person who has developed end-stage chronic obstructive pulmonary disease (COPD) from smoking be allowed to receive a lung transplant? Should a heart transplant be given to someone who developed alcoholic cardiomyopathy? Should a pa-

*Source: CORS, Denver, 1994.

tient with cystic fibrosis receive a double-lung transplant even though the donor lungs could go to two different individuals with pulmonary fibrosis? These are some of the ethical issues with which transplant teams struggle. There are no easy answers nor is there unanimous agreement on each case. Despite the difficulty of making wise choices, each team carefully considers each candidate for transplant. Criteria are used so that individual preferences of team members are not given priority. When and if health-care resources become more limited, the decisions may become more difficult. If transplant success improves and donor organs increase in number, transplants could become a mainstream of treatment.

Criteria for Being Listed on a Transplant Waiting List

Virtually every medical center with a transplant program has developed criteria for patient selection. Although each center may set its own criteria, there are similarities among the medical centers (see box below).

Waiting Time

The time spent waiting for a transplant can vary considerably. Some patients wait less than a week; others wait up to 18 months. During the waiting period, patients struggle with the need to carry on their lives, all the while knowing that at any moment they may be called to the hospital for transplant.

The number of transplant centers in the United States is limited. State of the art hospital facilities and surgeons are necessary components of a successful

---

Criteria for Transplant Waiting List

Age: under 65 (60 in some centers)

Terminal illness (expected life span less than 1 year

Nonsmoker

Adequate social support system

Disease free in other systems

---

transplant program. Because of these needs, most transplants are performed at large, regional medical centers, often those associated with a medical school. Because donor organs are viable for only hours after removal from the donor, patients waiting for transplant are required to live within a several-hour radius of the transplant center. Some patients may arrange air transportation to the medical center, others may relocate themselves and family to temporary housing within the metropolitan area. Most patients are given a beeper to maintain contact in a timely manner.

Psychosocial Implications

A strong support system is considered an essential component of a successful transplant. Demands of waiting and relocation to the transplant city put considerable stresses on the patient and significant others. The patient is torn between wanting to remain hopeful that a transplant will provide new life and the reality of knowing that death may come before the transplant. Patients feel these oppositional forces continuously and struggle to keep a balance between hope and reality. Therapists can assist patients by listening to feelings, being supportive, and encouraging participation in support groups. Because most patients experience these feelings, support groups offer invaluable intervention. Groups which include patients both before and after transplant probably have the most to offer in terms of psychosocial support. Those patients who relocate to transplant centers may have the most difficult time psychologically, especially as they leave family and significant others behind. Feelings of being useless are common because patients waiting in a foreign city must find something to do.

Spouses and significant others also benefit from group support. The psychological stresses are somewhat different on spouses. Spouses speak of the struggle to remain hopeful, yet plan for a future that may not include their loved one. If the patient and spouse move to a new city to wait for transplant, they may find themselves with more time together than they have ever spent before. In this forced retirement, new stresses are added to relationships. Transplant teams usually include a psychologist or social worker to whom patients may be referred for individual or family counseling if the stresses limit function or participation in pretransplant programs.

After transplant, patients struggle with conflicting feelings. Patients are often emotionally overwhelmed with a feeling of gratefulness that they are alive and feel guilty that someone else's grief has given them a chance to rejoice. Psychological or spiritual support may be requested or suggested after transplant (Craven, Bright, and Dear, 1990).

Patient Education

The waiting period time provides an ideal opportunity for patient education. Nursing generally provides much of the education regarding preoperative procedures, postoperative course, and medication. Rehabilitation teaching includes breathing training, airway clearance techniques, and activity progression.

TRENDS IN TRANSPLANT CARE

Transplants are being made available to a broader group of patients. Although transplants are only performed in certain centers, patients from rural areas are being evaluated at regional centers. Because transplant criteria differ slightly from center to center, some patients may be evaluated at several centers. The increased availability of transplants and the reliability of air transportation means that even patients from outlying geographical areas may be considered for transplant. After transplant, improved medical care has led to shorter hospital stays. For the patient who has relocated to the transplant city this means that he may be discharged to an apartment and return to the hospital several times a week for physician follow-up and rehabilitation. Once medically stable, patients may be allowed to return to their homes as early as 2 to 3 months after transplant, if medical support and rehabilitation needs can be met.

SURGICAL PROCEDURES

The surgical approach for transplant is chosen to provide the surgeon the optimal working area and visual field. The choice of incision may affect patient comfort and function after surgery. The physical therapist should be familiar with the surgical incisions and impact on rehabilitation.

Heart transplants are usually performed through a median sternotomy incision and cardiopulmonary bypass is used. A midline incision from sternal notch distally allows the sternum to be accessed and split. Although the native heart is excised, a portion of the right atrium and the SA node is preserved. The donor heart is sutured to the atrial cuff and the major vessels reattached. After surgery, the two halves of the sternum are wired together, the new heart defibrillated, bypass reversed, and the patient awakened.

Lung transplantation surgical incisions depend on whether a single or double-lung transplant is to be performed. Single lung transplants are performed through a posterolateral thoracotomy incision, with the patient side lying on the opposite side. To allow visual access for the surgeon, the latissimus dorsi and lower trapezius muscles are cut. The incision through the fourth or fifth intercostal space also means the intercostal muscles at this level may be incised. If the rib at the surgical level fractures, it is resected so that the bone ends do not rub or puncture the lung. The serratus anterior muscle is preserved if at all possible, but the lateral portion of the rhomboid may be cut to allow more access for the surgeon. Postoperative pain and impaired upper quarter movement patterns may present significant problems for patients.

Double-lung transplants are performed through an anterior incision sometimes described as a clamshell approach. A horizontal incision above the level of the diaphragm is performed, but the distance needed for adequate visualization means that the pectoralis major and minor may be incised bilaterally.

PHYSICAL THERAPY CONSIDERATIONS

As important members of the transplant team, physical therapists need an understanding of the physiological components of both the pretransplant disease and posttransplant state, the influence of surgery or physiology on musculoskeletal structure and function, and how medical management may necessitate modification of therapeutic interventions.

Physiology

The cardiovascular and respiratory systems are critical elements of functional ability, in areas of endurance and movement. Adequate oxygenation and circulation are needed to provide fuel to perform daily activities. In the patient awaiting heart transplant, cardiac output is significantly compromised, and hemodynamics may be unstable. Because of these limitations, pretransplant exercise is inappropriate. Posttransplant, however, the main interventions will be to restore normal cardiac output. Knowledge of physiology allows the therapist to choose appropriate interventions.

In patients with terminal lung disease, the primary limitation is ventilation. Pulmonary rehabilitation has been beneficial in improving daily function (Toronto Lung Transplant Group, 1988; Petty, 1980; Moser, Bokinsky, Savage, Archibald, Hansen, 1980) and may be used in the pretransplant period. Supplemental oxygen can be used during exercise to maintain adequate oxygenation. The waiting period before transplant is an ideal time to optimize muscle function and flexibility.

Musculoskeletal Considerations

The musculoskeletal problems of patients with pulmonary disease are well documented (see Chapter 4). Patients undergoing lung transplants are unique in that after transplant the musculoskeletal system returns to normal structure. The chest wall adapts in size to the new lung. The need to use accessory muscles of respiration is reduced. The physical therapist needs to optimize breathing in the preoperative period, yet prepare the chest and shoulder musculoskeletal system for normal function.

Medical Management

Knowledge of medical management including medications, ventilatory support, and hemodynamic monitoring assists the therapist in determining whether modifications are needed during rehabilitation. Table 38-1 lists suggested areas to monitor during both before and after transplant rehabilitation. For example, patients often complain of tremors during rest and activities. Therapists should be knowledgeable enough to question other health professionals as to whether the tremors are a result of medications, such as cyclosporine, a metabolic abnormality, a seizure disorder, or muscle weakness.

PHYSICAL THERAPY ASSESSMENT

The purpose of physical therapy before transplant is to identify baseline function and to screen for impairments that may limit rehabilitation goals. In some instances, physical therapists will provide treatment in the pretransplant period; in other cases, the information gained from early assessment allows the therapist to identify areas needing attention or modification after transplant. Physical therapy assessment in the postoperative period addresses specific impairments and functional limitations of the individual.

TABLE 38-1

Recommended Monitoring
√ = heart   x = lung

	BLOOD PRESSURE	HEART RATE	Sao₂	RATING OF PERCEIVED EXERTION
Before exercise	x √	x √	x	
During exercise	√	x √	x	x √
After exercise	√	x √	x	

Cardiac Patients

Pretransplant assessment of the cardiac patient includes functional ambulation (6-minute walk) and screening for deficits in muscle strength or range of motion. Exercise training is not generally recommended pretransplant. Range of motion may be increased or specific muscle strengthening may be accomplished, however, if the need is determined to be significant. All patients will be limited in functional endurance, therefore the results of the 6-minute walk is compared with posttransplant functional status.

Pulmonary Patients

Because rehabilitation in the pretransplant period is often indicated in patients waiting for lung transplant, the physical therapy assessment information may be used to design a more effective rehabilitation program. Upper and lower extremity muscle strength and range of motion is assessed, as well as posture, shoulder and trunk mobility, breathing pattern, breath sounds, and functional mobility.

Posttransplant Assessment (Heart and Lung)

After transplant, physical therapy assessment addresses all areas of functional limitations and the corresponding impairments. Patients should be evaluated in the immediate postoperative phase, and reevaluated on admission to the outpatient treatment phase. Because of the surgical intervention, bed mobility, ventilation, secretion management, range of motion, and pain control are important areas to address.

REHABILITATION OF THE TRANSPLANT PATIENT

To assist in treatment planning, rehabilitation is categorized into the following four phases: pretransplant, postoperative acute phase, postoperative outpatient phase, and community- or home-based phase. Although the ultimate goal of transplant rehabilitation is to improve the patient's function and quality of life, each phase of rehabilitation has its own emphasis.

PRETRANSPLANT REHABILITATION

Heart Transplant

Because the patient awaiting heart transplant has significantly compromised cardiac output and may be hemodynamically unstable, preoperative rehabilitation is generally not recommended. Some patients with moderate congestive heart failure may be able to tolerate a mild level of exercise (Roubin, Anderson, et al., 1990; Hillegass and Sadowsky, 1994). Most patients, however, are unable to tolerate endurance training.

Some patients may need musculoskeletal intervention for decreased range of motion, muscle weakness, or general discomfort. If physical intervention is needed, heart rate, blood pressure, and ECG monitoring is used to guide treatment. If heart rate or blood pressure decreases during exercise, exercise should be stopped.

The main goal in the preoperative period is to prevent losses of function. Maintenance of range of motion, soft tissue extensibility, and muscle strength are suggested goals.

Lung Transplant

Although each patient is treated individually, there are similarities among patients, resulting in a standard program for pretransplant rehabilitation (Figure 38-1). Pretransplant rehabilitation resembles pulmonary rehabilitation programs in existence for patients with COPD, CF, and restrictive diseases (Toronto Lung Transplant Group, 1988; Conners and Hilling, 1993; Malen and Boychuck, 1989).

General Considerations for Rehabilitation

Since the primary limitation in pulmonary disease is ventilatory, oxygen needs are essential to monitor. A pulse oximeter with finger or ear probe is mandatory in a pretransplant pulmonary rehabilitation program. Oxygen saturation should be maintained above 88% at all times. A source of supplemental oxygen is necessary, whether the patients bring their own oxygen or it is supplied by the center. In patients with severe disease, oxygen-conserving devices may need to be

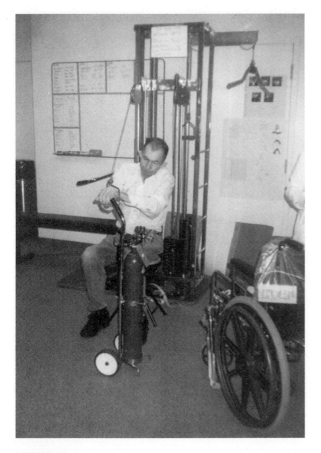

FIGURE 38-1
Pre-lung transplant rehabilitation.

used. Patients with COPD should have blood gases monitored for carbon dioxide retention, since increasing exercise often requires an increase in supplemental oxygen. Several of our patients has carbon dioxide levels in the 88 to 100 range. Although heart rate is not a good measure of exercise intensity, patients with lung disease may demonstrate signs of right heart failure and should have heart rate and blood pressure monitoring on a regular basis.

Goals

The overall goal of pretransplant pulmonary rehabilitation is to maximize function and reduce all muscu-

loskeletal impairments to function. Using the waiting time to maximize muscle strength and range of motion means that less time is needed posttransplant to return to functional activities. Pretransplant rehabilitation programs have been shown to decrease posttransplant hospital stay (Scherer, 1995). It is reasonable to set goals to achieve normal muscle strength in lower extremity musculature, increase upper extremity muscle strength, increase shoulder and chest wall range of motion to normal or within functional limits, demonstrate coordinated diaphragmatic breathing with exercise and activities, and improve cardiovascular endurance. An example of a preoperative pulmonary rehabilitation program is in the box on p. 710.

Interventions

Deficits which are found in any of the above areas may be addressed in the pulmonary rehabilitation program, except in patients with primary pulmonary hypertension or Eisenmenger's syndrome. In those patients, exercise which increases cardiac workload is contraindicated. However, if cardiac output is monitored and the physician agrees, range of motion exercises may be taught and light strengthening exercises may be performed. For example, a 22-year-old female with primary pulmonary hypertension was found to have injured her shoulder 4 weeks previously, resulting in decreased range of motion in a capsular pattern. She has been on the lung transplant waiting list for 3 months. The physician wants her only to walk as necessary for her daily activities. With consultation with the physician, joint mobilization, range of motion activities, and modalities may be used with few precautions. Strengthening exercises may be used cautiously, avoiding breath-holding and Valsalva maneuvers.

Other Transplants

Patients awaiting other organ transplants may also be referred to physical therapy for treatment of musculoskeletal problems. Because of the level of metabolic abnormality in patients awaiting liver and kidney transplants, endurance training is difficult to perform. Other physical therapy interventions, how-

---

Preoperative Pulmonary Rehabilitation

Warm-up (group)		**10 minute**
Active range of motion		
Upper body		
Lower body		
Trunk		
Light resistance (5 to 10 reps)		
Individualized Endurance Program		
Bike (Airdyne)	25 to 30 watts	10 to 20-minute intervals
Treadmill	0.8 to 1.5 mph	
	0% to 5% grade	10 to 30 minutes
Arm ergometer	0 to 25 watts	10 to 15 minutes forward and backward
Individualized Strength Program		**15 to 20 minutes**
Pulleys	Theraband	
Latissimus pull-downs	Rhomboids	
Diagonal arms	Shoulder extension rotation	
Pectoral	Shoulder flexion	
Latissimus		
Triceps		
Subscapularis		
Lower Extremity		
Quadriceps		
Hip extensors		
Hip abductors		
Cool-down (group)		**10 minutes**
Stretching (full-body)		
Breathing		
Relaxation		

---

ever, may be used as appropriate (i.e., muscle strengthening, range of motion).

ACUTE PHASE REHABILITATION

The acute phase of rehabilitation begins in the intensive care unit and continues throughout the patient's hospital stay. Interventions are focused on facilitating normal cardiovascular and pulmonary function and increasing functional abilities in self-care and ambulation.

Heart Transplant (Acute)

Considerations

In the immediate postoperative period after heart transplant, cardiac output is compromised and hemodynamic responses slowed. A transplanted heart is

University Hospital Cardiovascular Rehabilitation Supervised Exercise/Activity Plan/Surgical Patients

Physician _____ DX _____ MEDS _____

Step/Date	Exercise	Activity
1 ICU 1/5 METS __/__/__ __/__/__	—Active/Passive ROM, in bed × 5 reps —Teach hourly ROM exercise	—Partial self care —Feed self —Use of bedside commode —UP in chair for meals as —Turn, cough, deep breathe & use incentive spriometer, q2-4° —Sitting bed bath
2 ICU 1.5-2.0 METS	—Active ROM, sit on edge of bed × 5 reps —Teach Rating Perceived Exertion	—Sit in chair as tol —Partial/complete self care —Up in chair for meals —Turn, cough, deep breathe and use incentive spriometer, q2-4° —Sitting bed bath
3 FLOOR 2.0 METS	—Active ROM/warmups, standing × 10 reps —Walk 100 ft. slow pace	—Sit in chair 2-3×/day (20 min) —Complete self care —Sitting bed bath —Incentive spriometer indep, TID
4 FLOOR 2.5 METS	—Warmups, standing × 10 reps —Walk 150 ft, average pace —Teach pulse counting	—Complete self care —Use of bathroom w/assist —Walk around room —May take warm shower after pacer wire removed —Incentive spriometer indep, TID
5 FLOOR 3 METS	—Warmups, standing × 10 reps —Walk 300 ft, average pace	—Dressing indep —May stand at sink for ADLs
6 FLOOR 3.5 METS	—Warmups, standing × 10 reps —Walk 500 ft, average pace —Walk down flight of stairs —Instruct in home exercise	—As above —Introduce to phase II
7 FLOOR 4 METS	—Warmups, standing × 10 reps —Walk up flight stairs —Walk 500 ft average pace —Schedule submax ETT —Enroll in Phase II	—All self care indep —As above

Guidelines for Exercise

—Pt HR to be 50-120 bpm

—Exercise HR not more than 20 beats above rest

—No worsening ST changes

—RPE of 10 or less

—no significant arrhythmias

—SBP < 200, DBP < 120 during exercise

—< 10-15 DBP drop during exercise

—no angina or other symptoms

stiff for several days, and the sympathetic nervous system input to the heart is destroyed in the transplant process. To maintain cardiac output (HR x SV) in a heart with decreased stroke volume a fixed rate pacemaker is used at a rate of approximately 120 beats/minute for several days. ECG readings may be normal because the donor heart has an intact conduction system, although the atrial cuff left from the native heart may cause the ECG to have two P waves. The therapist working with heart transplant patients in the ICU should be aware that heart rate cannot increase significantly, therefore blood pressure and patient response should be monitored. Surgical cardiac rehabilitation guidelines can be used to guide treatment, with increases of 0.5 to 1 metabolic equivalent (MET) per day (see box on p. 711). Complications of heart transplant include sternum instability, infection or pain, and potential nerve or circulatory damage to the femoral area because of intraaortic balloon pump (IABP) cardiac assist. Acute rejection episodes are characterized by flu-like symptoms including low-grade fever and muscle achiness and is often accompanied by dysrhythmias. Rejection episodes can only be confirmed by tissue biopsy.

Goals

Goals of the acute phase of rehabilitation include the following: (1) regain normal postural cardiovascular responses (no postural hypotension) and (2) increase functional activities. The former is primarily focused on the patient being able to tolerate changes in position, increase time in upright sitting, and transfer independently. Upper and lower extremity range of motion and strength need to be adequate to perform activities of daily living.

Exercise Guidelines

Deconditioning and lack of sympathetic input to increase heart rate response contribute to the possibility of hypotension. Because of the high incidence of postural hypotension, patients need to change positions slowly and be given time to adapt to the new position. Exercise may be continued during mild-to-moderate rejection episodes but is not performed during periods of severe rejection. The main consideration for exercise in patients with heart transplants is that

the heart is denervated. Because of the lack of sympathetic input, heart rate cannot increase quickly and contractility is not under sympathetic control. The only mechanism by which heart rate can be increased is by circulating catecholamines, which take 10 to 15 minutes to influence a response. Therapists working with heart transplant patients should allow time for patients to adapt to changes in position and may want to use light active bed exercises as a warm-up activity (Irwin and Tecklin, 1995).

Lung Transplant

Considerations

After lung transplantation, patients are generally mechanically ventilated for 24 to 72 hours. Often, paralytic agents are used in this period so that ventilation can be optimized. Patients who received double-lung transplants may be more hemodynamically compromised if they were on bypass during surgery. Chest tubes are likely in place, and patients are medicated for pain. Infection control is imperative; isolation rooms with negative-pressure ventilation are used and medical personnel at minimum are required to wash their hands and wear masks when in the patient's room. Isolation or reverse-isolation procedures are followed (the patient wears the mask when leaving the room). The primary monitoring is oxygen saturation, followed by heart rate and blood pressure. A common complication in the immediate postoperative period is pneumothorax.

Goals

In the immediate postoperative period the major goals are to increase time out of bed, optimize ventilation-perfusion ratio, and increase active range of motion on the surgical side (Malen and Boychuck, 1989). Major problems and goals are listed in Table 38-2.

Interventions

The range of therapeutic interventions are many. In general an intervention may continue until an abnormal exercise response is reached. Abnormal responses include a decrease in heart rate or blood pressure with an increase in exercise, a decrease in oxygen saturation below recommended levels (88%

TABLE 38–2

Problems and Goals for Acute Posttransplant Rehabilitation: Lung Transplant

PROBLEM	GOAL
Decreased secretion clearance Because the lungs are denervated, there is decreased sensation of secretions.	Independent secretion management
Incisional pain Postoperative pain is related to the surgical incision and decreased movement of muscles	Pain management Pain medication
Abnormal postural hemodynamic responses (i.e., postural hypotension and fatigue)	Normalize hemodynamic response (i.e., no postural hypotension, normal heart rate, respiratory rate, and blood pressure response to exercise)
Increased oxygen/ventilatory requirements	Adequate oxygenation without supplemental (SaO_2 94% to 96% on room air) Diaphragmatic breathing Normal vital capacity
Decreased functional mobility Decreased shoulder range of motion	Independent activities of daily living (dressing, hygiene, shower, toilet) Need adequate shoulder range of motion to perform these activities
Decreased exercise tolerance	Independent transfers Out of bed most of day Independent ambulation 500 ft Bicycle 10 minutes, no resistance
Compromised nutrition	No supplemental feedings (IV)

to 90%), or symptoms of dizziness and diaphoresis. Suggested treatments are shown in Table 38-3.

POSTOPERATIVE OUTPATIENT REHABILITATION

Heart Transplant

Once the patient leaves the hospital, rehabilitation looks much like phase II cardiac rehabilitation. The overall objective is to increase functional activity to within normal limits.

Duration of this phase of rehabilitation generally continues for 8 to 12 weeks, at which time the patient is encouraged to continue exercise on his or her own or at a fitness facility. Many heart transplant patients return to predisease levels at this stage.

Considerations

As mentioned before, transplanted hearts lack autonomic innervation. Implications for exercise response are that heart rate increases can only be accomplished, using circulating catecholamines. For the phase II cardiac rehabilitation patient, this means that the warm-up and cool-down portions of exercise should be increased to 10 to 15 minutes and progressed slowly. Resting heart rates are close to the intrinsic heart rate of 100, and heart rate should not be used as an indication of fitness nor to establish exercise intensity. Rating of perceived exertion is a more appropriate indication of exercise intensity. Recommended guidelines are 11 to 13 on the 20-point Borg scale (Irwin and Tecklin, 1995; Hosenpud et al., 1990). Both endurance and strength exercise can be

TABLE 38–3

Acute Rehabilitation Interventions

GOALS	INTERVENTIONS
Independent secretion management	Incentive spirometer Secretion removal (positioning, percussion, and vibration) Assisted cough or instruction
Pain management Pain medication	Active range of motion shoulder girdle Positioning Mild heat Massage/soft tissue techniques
Normalize hemodynamic response (i.e., no postural hypotension, normal heart rate, respiratory rate, or blood pressure response to exercise)	Sitting on edge of bed Out of bed to chair day 1 or 2 Ambulation to bathroom day 2 or 3
Adequate oxygenation without supplemental oxygen Diaphragmatic breathing with activity Normal vital capacity	Instruction of diaphragmatic breathing Facilitation of diaphragmatic breathing Lateral costal expansion techniques (surgery side) Incentive spirometry
Independent activities of daily living (dressing, hygiene, shower, toilet) Need adequate shoulder range of motion to perform these activities	Encourage and assist with activities of daily living Active and active-assisted range of motion All motions shoulder girdle Wand exercises Side lying shoulder abduction
Independent transfers Out of bed most of day Independent ambulation 500 ft Bicycle 10 minutes, no resistance	Daily schedule Assisted ambulation in room initially, to hallway within 2 to 3 days Bicycle in room, 2 minutes initially, progress to 10 minutes
No supplemental feedings (IV)	Schedule rehabilitation around meals Medical management of nausea

performed in this rehabilitation stage, although upper extremity strengthening should only be started after the sternum has healed. To protect the sternum, lifting should be limited to less than 10 lbs for 6 to 8 weeks. Treadmill, bike, arm ergometry, and indoor cross-country ski equipment are all appropriate choices.

Signs of Rejection

The primary signs and symptoms of rejection include flu-like symptoms including low-grade fever and muscle aches. Dysrhythmias and bradycardia below 60 or relative bradycardia (decreased compared with patient's normal resting heart rate) are significant and

should be reported to the physician immediately. Rejection episodes are monitored by biopsy. Exercise can continue if the rejection episode is mild or moderate as determined by biopsy. Summary guidelines for postoperative rehabilitation for heart transplant are outlined in the box below.

Lung Transplant

Because patients are discharged from the hospital as early as 8 days after transplant, much of their medical management and rehabilitation occurs on an outpatient basis. In the early stages of this postoperative outpatient phase, patients are medically labile and need

> **Summary Cardiac Guidelines**
>
> Cardiac phase II protocols
>
> Heart rate is not intensity regulator
>
> Increase warm-up and cool-down to 10 to 15 minutes
>
> RPE 11 to 13 (20-point Borg scale)
>
> No exercise in severe rejection (biopsy)
>
> Continue exercise in mild rejection

once- or twice-a-week monitoring of medical status. Rehabilitation should progress in this phase, but close communication with medical personnel is recommended because of the many medication changes. Blood levels of immunosuppressive drugs are monitored and metabolic function (fluid and electrolyte levels, kidney and liver function) are followed.

General Considerations

Patients in the outpatient phase of rehabilitation begin at low levels of function and progress to having few functional limitations. Therapists need to adapt and progress the rehabilitation program appropriately. If rehabilitation is not aggressive, patients may succumb to the effects of prednisone and cyclosporine. Because of the debilitating side effects of immunosuppressive medications, rehabilitation needs to be aggressive and preventive in nature. Rehabilitation can occur in a group setting and/or on an individual basis.

Monitoring

The areas of emphasis in the lung transplant patient follow from the physiology and surgery performed. The primary limitation pretransplant is ventilatory, with the surgery intended to improve ventilation. Monitoring of ventilatory status should be the primary consideration of the therapist. Respiratory rate and oxygen saturation should be followed closely during exercise sessions.

Rejection

The primary symptoms of acute rejection are shortness of breath, exercise intolerance, and desaturation at rest or with exercise. Patients generally have a portable oximeter at home and may report episodes of desaturation. Rejection should be suspected and reported if a decrease in Sao_2 of 4% to 5% for the same amount of activity is seen (Malen and Boychuck, 1989).

Goals

Patients are generally excited about the improvement in shortness of breath and surprised at the level of muscle weakness seen especially in the lower extremities. Once ventilation is no longer a limiting factor in function, other deficits emerge. In the initial stages of outpatient rehabilitation, patients may have multiple complaints about the side effects of medications and often generally do not feel well. Rehabilitation should continue through these periods of malaise. The overall objective of outpatient rehabilitation is to improve function to levels appropriate for the patient's age and interests. Generally, patients are closely followed by the medical staff for 2 to 3 months after transplant, and rehabilitation 2 to 3 times per week continues throughout this period.

The most common impairments that limit function are decreased cardiopulmonary endurance, decreased muscle strength and endurance, range of motion limitations, and abnormal movement patterns of the shoulder or trunk. Impairments may be caused by the surgical procedure itself or as a result of years of abnormal muscle mechanics, posture, and decreased activity. Cardiopulmonary endurance training is emphasized at this stage of rehabilitation, as is posture reeducation, range of motion, and upper extremity movement patterns. Lower extremity strengthening can begin early, but upper extremity resistive training should be delayed until wound and tissue healing is complete, generally about 6 weeks because of the delays in wound healing caused by prednisone. Goals which specifically address impairments may include normal shoulder range of motion, normal muscle strength in all major muscle groups of upper and lower extremities, and normal thoracic mobility (Figure 38-2).

Interventions

To achieve the goals of rehabilitation and address impairments, a pulmonary rehabilitation protocol may be

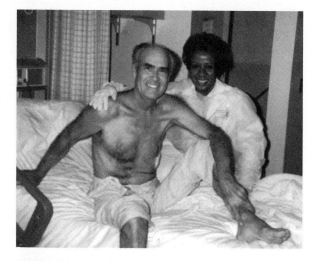

FIGURE 38-2
Post-single lung transplant inpatient.

Lung Transplant Guidelines
Keep Sao_2 above 90%
Add supplemental oxygen if necessary during treated acute rejection episodes
Patient should wear mask when with people
Increase strength program during prednisone bursts

used, or the therapist may creatively design a rehabilitation program. Except for delaying upper extremity strengthening for 6 weeks after surgery, no therapeutic interventions are contraindicated. For endurance training, stationary bicycles, treadmills, arm ergometers, indoor nordic ski machines, rowers, and stair climbers may be used. Pulleys, weight equipment, free weights, resistive elastic bands, or gymnastic balls all may be appropriate for strengthening and facilitation of normal movement patterns. Because of the effects of prednisone, proximal muscle function must be addressed, and strengthening programs should be aggressive, keeping the repetitions to 10 or less. Once a patient has achieved a satisfactory level of function (determined by the therapist and patient), formal rehabilitation may be discontinued.

The general considerations for lung transplant patients are to monitor oxygen saturation and prevent the patient from contracting respiratory infections. A summary of lung transplant treatment guidelines are listed in the box below.

COMMUNITY OR HOME-BASED REHABILITATION

Patients are generally followed at the transplant center until the medical staff is satisfied with patient progress.

Return to home can occur at this point in time, whether or not rehabilitation goals have been met. The major goal of community-based rehabilitation is return to normal function with minimal limitations. Many patients feel so good after transplant that return to prior level of function, including employment, is a natural phenomenon. Formal rehabilitation may only be necessary in complicated cases or after rejection episodes or illness. Patients may also seek physical therapy advice for musculoskeletal problems unrelated to the transplant. Therapists should be comfortable treating patients in many settings, addressing the common complications, and watching for signs of rejection.

Heart Transplant

Ironically, the medications used to prevent rejection in transplant patients may increase the incidence of coronary artery disease. It is recommended that patients participate in a regular exercise program to manage the effects of the medications and to prevent coronary artery disease complications. Hospital-based phase III cardiac rehabilitation programs are appropriate, or patients may elect to independently exercise in a fitness facility. Some follow-up by the center is important to encourage compliance in exercise programs.

Lung Transplant

For patients who have left their home community to wait for lung transplant, the transition to home frequently occurs at 3 months after transplant. Ideally, rehabilitation goals from the outpatient phase will have been accomplished, and the patient will be able

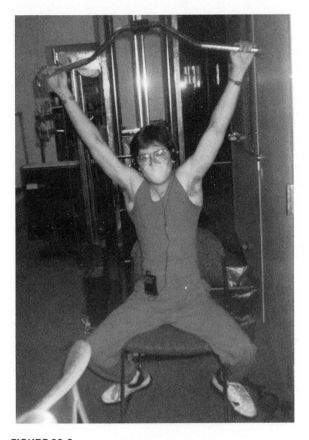

FIGURE 38-3
Post-double lung transplant outpatient at approximately 3 months post-surgery.

to return home to pursue his or her own interests. Success stories are many. One patient returned home and progressed to walking 5 miles a day, fishing 4 to 5 times/week, and bow hunting with a 50-lb bow. One gentleman reported at a 6-month follow-up visit that he was pleased to be riding around his ranch and checking up on things. The therapist asked if he was riding in the truck, and he replied, "no, on my horse." A 21-year-old male (130 lb) with cystic fibrosis resumed weight lifting and bench pressed 110 lbs, 8 months after a double-lung transplant (Figure 38-3).

Other patients have more rehabilitation needs. For example, a 40-year-old single-lung transplant patient sustained a brachial plexus injury from the surgery

and needed long-term therapy. A 55-year-old male had a bowel obstruction after surgery, which lengthened his recovery time. If the patient is medically stable but has rehabilitation needs, the patient may be referred for physical therapy in his or her home town, possibly away from the transplant center. Other patients may have multiple episodes of rejection, which are treated with high-dose steroids, and develop steroid myopathy, requiring intensive and progressive strength training.

Goals

Physical therapy assessment is critical to identify problem areas and evaluate progress toward goals. Goals at this stage should be primarily guided by specific patient quality of life issues. Common long-term impairments are chest wall soreness, abnormal upper quarter movement patterns, and low back and knee pain from overuse.

Influence of Medications on Treatment

Patients are on a multitude of medications after transplant, and additional medications may be added to decrease the side effects of the primary immunosuppressive drugs (Miller, 1995). Prednisone, cyclosporine, and azathioprine (Imuran) are the mainstay of immunosuppression, with OKT 3 and FK 506 being additional options.

Prednisone

Because organ rejection is primarily an inflammatory response, corticosteroids are usually used in transplant patients. Steroid therapy may be delayed until primary wound closure is certain (1 to 2 weeks) at which time the patient is begun on low-dose oral steroids. Acute rejection episodes are treated with oral or intravenous steroid pulses. Corticosteroids work by immobilizing macrophages and decreasing B and T lymphocytes.

Cyclosporine

Cyclosporine is a very powerful immunosuppressive agent that works by inhibiting T lymphocyte growth factor and T helper cells. Side effects are common and annoying to patients. It is considered a peripheral

Side Effects of Immunosuppressive Medications	
Prednisone	**Cyclosporine**
Hypertension	Tremors
Glucose intolerance	Hypertension
Osteoporosis	Increased cholesterol
Muscle weakness	Nephrotoxicity
Delayed wound healing	

nerve irritant. Therapists should watch for muscle tremors and peripheral neuropathy.

Azathioprine

Azathioprine (Imuran) is a powerful drug that inhibits RNA and DNA synthesis of most immune system cells. Bone marrow suppression (leukopenia, anemia) is common as are gastrointestinal symptoms of nausea, vomiting, and anorexia.

New Drugs

Research has added drugs such as OKT 3 and FK 506 to the immunosuppression regimen. OKT 3 is a monoclonal antibody that is used for management of acute rejection and is not used on a daily basis. OKT 3 blocks all T lymphocyte functions for a short time after administration and can help remove T cell byproducts from the graft site. Because of its dramatic and potentially dangerous side effects, this medication is given in a controlled setting where the patient can be carefully monitored at 15- or 30-minute intervals. Pulmonary edema, bronchospasm, fever, chills, and hypokalemia are common reactions.

Rehabilitation should not be given during administration of these medications. The box above summarizes the effects of common immunosuppressive medications.

SUMMARY

Physical therapy has an important role in maintaining and improving functional levels of patients both before and after organ transplant. Knowledge of cardiovascular and pulmonary physiology along with the ability to analyze movement and function allow rehabilitation professionals to maximize a patient's quality of life. The field of organ transplant is exciting and growing. New advances in long-term management of transplant recipients means that rehabilitation professionals need to continue to develop and evaluate approaches to care.

REVIEW QUESTIONS

1. What feelings do patients and family commonly experience before and after an organ transplant?
2. What is the role of pretransplant pulmonary rehabilitation?
3. How does the surgical incision affect the musculoskeletal function of a posttransplant patient?
4. What are the signs of organ rejection in the cardiac transplant patient? the lung transplant patient?
5. How is the rehabilitation of the heart transplant patient similar and different than traditional cardiac rehabilitation?
6. How is the rehabilitation of the lung transplant patient different than other forms of pulmonary rehabilitation?
7. How do immunosuppressive drugs affect a patient's neuromuscular function? Muscle strength? Cardiopulmonary endurance?

References

Conners, G., & Hilling, L. (1993). *AACVPR guidelines for pulmonary rehabilitation programs.* Champaign, Ill.: Human Kinetics Publishers.

Craven, J.L., Bright, J., & Dear, C.L. (1991). Psychiatric, psychosocial, and rehabilitative aspects of lung transplantation. *Clinics Chest Medicine, 11*(2), 247-57.

Hillegass, E., & Sadowsky, S.A. (1994). *Essentials of cardiopulmonary rehabilitation.* Philadelphia: WB Saunders.

Hosenpud, J.D., Cobanoglu, A., et al. (1991). *Cardiac transplantation.* New York: Springer-Verlag.

Irwin, S., & Tecklin, J.S. (1995). *Cardiopulmonary physical therapy.* St. Louis: Mosby.

Malen, J.F., & Boychuck, J.E. (1989). Nursing perspectives on lung transplantation. *Critical Care Nursing Clinics of North America, 1*(4), 707-722.

Moser, K.M., Bokinsky, G.E., et al. (1990). Results of a comprehensive rehabilitation program: physiologic and functional effects on patients with chronic obstructive pulmonary disease. *Archives of Internal Medicine 140(12):*1596-1601.

Scherer, S.A. (1995). *Preoperative pulmonary rehabilitation reduces pot-operative length of hospital stay after lung transplant.* Denver: International Conference on Pulmonary Rehabilitation and Home Ventilation, abstract.

Toronto Lung Transplant Group. (1988). Experience with Single-lung transplantation for pulmonary fibrosis. *JAMA, 259*(15), 2258-2262.

University Hospital surgical cardiac rehabilitation protocol. (1994). Denver.

CHAPTER 39

The Patient in the Community

Donna Frownfelter

KEY TERMS

Assisted living
Continuity of care
Home care
Managed care

Outpatient
Skilled nursing and rehabiliatation facilities
Subacute hospitals
Transitional care units

INTRODUCTION

Physical therapy in the community may take on a wide variety of forms. The practice has certainly changed dramatically over the last few years. Diagnostic related groupings (DRGs) began the trend of patients leaving the hospital earlier and often in a more acute stage of recovery. Subacute hospitals, Medicare skilled nursing, and rehabilitation facilities with transitional care units provide therapy and facilitate patient progression so that he or she will be back home within a short (perhaps a month) period of time. Managed care has had a significant impact on diagnoses and treatment authorization, which affects the type of diagnosis given to patients and the number of therapy sessions authorized for given diagnoses or symptoms.

This chapter focuses on patients in the skilled nursing home, home care, and alternative long-term care settings. These concepts and ideas could easily be used in an adult day care or outpatient setting, senior housing, or a transitional or an assisted living facility. The settings described in this chapter will be used only as examples on which to focus the discussion.

Continuity of care is an essential component of quality health care in light of the trend toward earlier hospital discharge either to a skilled nursing/rehabilitation facility or to home with nursing and therapy support. A colleague in hospital practice recently commented that she feels more like a triage therapist than a physical therapist. At times the absolute basics of therapy (i.e., transfers and gait with an assistive device) are all that a patient is able to receive before leaving the hospital setting. An exercise sheet may accompany the patient home but, in general, after discharge from the hospital, most patients do not know their exercise programs. In addition, they have poor endurance because they are generally still healing from the insults or injuries for which they were hospitalized. In the geriatric population the caregiver is often an elderly spouse who also has medical problems and is limited in the ability to assist the patient.

The types and diagnoses of patients seen in the community may vary; often they are the very young and the very old. With the medical community's ability to save premature, low-birth-weight infants we have had an influx of ventilator-assisted, oxygen-dependent infants with bronchopulmonary dysplasia (BPD). They may be slow to develop and need intervention to prevent pulmonary infections and to improve in the natural developmental sequence. Often they may have difficulty swallowing, and nutritional issues may delay their physical gains, as well as their speech and language, secondary to poor breath support.

Specialty hospitals have been developed to care for the medically fragile, ventilator-assisted (dependent) patient who is not stable enough to be at home or lacks the resources to be at home. Many patients, especially children on ventilators whose parents can provide some care and are assisted by nursing staff, are coming home successfully on ventilators. They integrate into the community in school and recreation, function well, and perceive a high quality of life.

Elderly patients will often try valiantly to remain at home and independent, amazing the most seasoned clinician with their inventiveness and family/friend supports. Others will recognize that they no longer are able to care for themselves and that the caregiver, who is often also elderly (often a frail spouse), cannot continue in that role.

Nursing homes, long thought of as a place "to go to die," have become centers of skilled nursing and rehabilitation. The trend is moving toward "transitional care units" where a patient will go for approximately 1 month to gain strength and practice activities of daily living, transfers, and gait and develop endurance that will allow them to return home.

The focus of long-term care is to help residents live fuller and more satisfying lives even if they are unable to return home after rehabilitation. Many nursing home chains have developed beautiful, hotel-like atmospheres with a range of services. The residents may live in independent apartments and, if a disease or trauma occurs, may return to the skilled nursing area to receive rehabilitation services. When they are able, they transfer to an assisted living area and continue to live there or will transfer back to their apartments when they are sufficiently recovered.

Even after an acute incident (e.g., a cerebrovascular accident [CVA]), a patient may not be able to return home in a month but may continue to make gains up to a year or more as strength, balance, and endurance improve. Therapists can screen residents and continue to try to improve their physical status and to enable them to live to their fullest capacity.

MANAGED CARE

Managed care groups are having a significant impact on placement and case management of individuals who are able to return home. We are seeing many patients in home care 5 days a week with caregivers present around the clock. Significant cost savings may be noted compared with an extended hospitalization or stay in a skilled nursing facility. Most managed care companies are willing to listen to suggestions that save money and improve customer satisfaction.

When we think of these practice settings, it becomes obvious that cardiopulmonary concerns are highlighted. From the very young to the very old, primary and secondary cardiopulmonary issues are often the limiting factor in a patient's rehabilitation progress.

Before considering some specific differences in community settings, we will look at the commonalities in the principles of exercise training and prescription.

GENERAL PRINCIPLES OF EXERCISE TRAINING AND PRESCRIPTION

Specificity of Training

Exercise programs are individually developed to meet specific goals. To develop muscle strength, a high-resistance, low-repetition program (i.e., weight lifting) is prescribed. To develop muscle endurance, a low-resistance, high-repetition program (i.e., walking, treadmill) is prescribed. The benefits of exercise depend on the targeted exercise. Strength training increases muscle fibers (white) and endurance training increases the number of capillaries and mitochondrial content (Celli, 1994).

It is noted that a weight lifter is usually not a long-term runner, and few runners are able to lift heavy arm weights. In developing exercise programs, we must keep in mind the goals for the individual. Generally, some form of both strength and endurance is desired. However, programs often focus on one or the other, not both.

Intensity and Duration of Training

Both intensity and duration have significant consequences on the amount of training effect. Olympians often train at maximal or near maximal levels to achieve their "superstar" level of fitness. However, it has been noted that middle-aged, nonathletic individuals benefit from lesser levels of exercise. Siegel et al. (1970) demonstrated that training sessions of 30 minutes about three times a week significantly improved Vo_{2max} when the heart rate was raised over 80% of predicted maximal heart rate.

Casaburi et al. (1991) studied 19 COPD patients who could achieve either 50% or 80% of maximal exercise (anaerobic threshold). They found that patients who participated in the higher intensity training program benefited more than the lower intensity training patients. However, significant training did occur in the lower intensity group (Casaburi, 1991).

The number and length of treatments have a significant effect on endurance training. An intense period of care followed by a maintenance or managed-care period prevents the effects of stopping exercise training. Carry-over and maintenance is extremely important (Make, 1991).

Deconditioning Effect

Training effect can be lost after the exercise has stopped. Bed rest in normal individuals was shown to result in a significant decrease in Vo_{2max} with 21 days

of resting. Even more troublesome were the results that it took 10 to 50 days for the values to return to the level before resting (Saltin et al., 1968).

In normal individuals who received ventilatory muscle training followed by a month without training, the subjects lost the achieved training effect (Keens et al., 1977).

SPECIFIC CARDIOPULMONARY CONCERNS IN THE COMMUNITY

Patients in nursing homes, alternative long-term care and independent living facilities, and the home after disease or trauma often have several problems in common. They may have decreased independence, mobility level, strength, and endurance, as well as poor posture, and are at risk for falls secondary to poor balance and weakness. Often they are poorly nourished, either from lack of appetite or dysphagia or as a result of depression brought on by their physical limitations and feelings of being overwhelmed with their situations. At times there is a sense of hopelessness and a feeling that things will not be the same again. This depression is especially common when patients are placed in nursing homes when they wanted to go home but realized they could not take care of themselves or their families insisted on the placement.

Many patients have a preexisting cardiopulmonary disease, such as asthma, emphysema, bronchitis, coronary artery disease, prior myocardial infarction, hypertension, dysrhythmias, or congestive heart failure. In addition to those diagnoses, they often have fractured hips, knee replacements, or CVA. The cardiopulmonary factors may in fact be the limiting consideration to the progress with therapy. These concerns need to be dealt with so that the patient reaches his or her full rehabilitation potential.

IF YOU CANNOT BREATHE YOU CANNOT FUNCTION

Functioning depends on the ability to breathe. An example of this was seen in a patient that fell in the parking lot of a hospital while going to a pulmonary rehabilitation program. She was in a long leg cast at home and became very short of breath with sit-to-stand transfers. Limited by severe shortness of breath, she could barely ambulate across the room with her pick-up walker. When observed using her bronchodilator metered-dose inhaler (MDI), she was found to be using it improperly. After she was instructed on how to use it properly, she used the bronchodilator before transfer and gait and was like a different patient. She was able to coordinate her breathing pattern with control to match her activity and her endurance was remarkably improved.

With these principles in mind, we can look at some of the considerations in nursing home and home health settings.

LONG-TERM CARE FACILITIES AND NURSING HOMES

As mentioned previously, with the changes in health care, much rehabilitation is now taking place in transitional care units, Medicare skilled nursing homes, and assisted living facilities.

The following are special considerations when working in a long-term care setting.

- There are several layers of care from geriatric specialist nurse consultants to head nurses to general floor nurses to aides.
- Most patient care is given by aides.
- Communication and cooperation are the keys to achieving patient goals and success.
- Input and involvement of the patient and family or significant others is essential in developing goals.
- Clear and achievable goals need to be developed and revisited as the patient progresses or regresses in therapy. Is the goal to transition to home, to assisted living, or to living at the nursing home?
- Quality of life issues need to be taken into consideration. How mobile is the patient? Is he or she independent? Is he or she a morning person? When is therapy going to be most efficient timewise? Will it conflict with his or her other interests and activities, which may give him or her moral support or act as a distractor and provide real recreation?
- Nutritional concerns need to be taken seriously. Is the patient losing or gaining weight? Do his or her

dentures fit or is he or she not eating or chewing food because of poor dentition or denture fit? Is he or she aspirating? Does he or she have dysphagia?

- Is the patient sleeping? Many patients after surgery, trauma, or a CVA are left supine or in a side-lying position to sleep. They may not have ever slept in that position before. However, they do not recognize that may be the reason they are not sleeping. If the patient states he or she cannot sleep ask him or her about previous sleep positions and try to work with the nursing aide staff on positioning for sleep.
- Follow-through of methods of working with the patient should be consistent so as not to confuse the patient. For example, breathing exercises in conjunction with activities should be consistent. If the patient is taught in therapy to inspire when extending the trunk, that should be communicated to other caregivers and consistently encouraged. If the goal is for the patient to walk to meals, a coordinated effort should be made to try to have the patient accomplish this as a transition plan. For example, when the therapist talks with the aide and a care plan is established, the patient can start walking to one meal or as far as he or she can toward the dining room. When that is accomplished, the goal will be to walk to two meals, and so on. Then additional goals can be added to walk to activities, social settings, out to the car to meet the family, and other functional, appropriate goals.
- In-services to reinforce the therapy techniques and goals should be done individually and in formal classes. Classes are helpful, on a one-time basis, to discuss and instruct on a particular topic. However, an ongoing one-on-one therapist/aide patient-specific mini-in-service is essential. The classes need to be repeated on a regular basis for new staff and as a refresher for some aides who have not used or practiced the techniques. The aides may at first feel they are "too busy and unable to do the job," but you can convince them that it will be of benefit to the aide, as well as the patients. The patient will be able to do more and in the long run, the aide will have less work. In ad-

dition, the family members will be pleased and regard the work of the aide more highly. This will also benefit the nursing home because it will be known for its individualized, excellent patient care, which will make the director of nursing and the administrator pleased. Most aides would like to do the best for their patients and provide the best care they can render.

- Try to get other programs and nursing home activity groups to follow-through with therapeutic goals. Talk with the activity department if patients need extra encouragement or help with oxygen to participate. If patients need to drink more water for increased hydration, ask them to remind the patient and provide water.
- As a therapist, be willing to pitch in and help whenever you are able, even if it "isn't in your job description." Your willingness to be a team player will be noticed. If an aide is off sick and you are available at lunch and see there is a problem passing out trays, offer to help. The next time you ask an aide for help there will probably be more willingness. If there is a patient that is difficult to transfer, offer to help in getting the patient up for physical therapy. This will serve as both a teaching opportunity and as a help to the aide. Look for ways of blending your therapy with the needs of the nursing staff.
- Give recognition to aides who have been re-markable in their patient care follow-through for therapy goals. Be on the look out for ways to praise and thank them in a sincere manner. They will be more willing to help in the future.
- Sponsor open house times in the therapy department so that the staff come in and can see the therapists. You can provide educational material for the staff (and food). Welcome their input and suggestions for patients who may benefit from therapy but are not on the physical therapy caseload.
- Prepare a bulletin board to show the accomplishments of patients in pictures and description. We all love success stories and being part of the success. Show pictures of aides, as well as therapists, helping the patients.
- In addition to chart reviews and talking about patients with the nurses, screen patients in the dining rooms and activity sessions and walking in the hall. The aides will be a terrific source of patient referrals; they are with the patients more than anyone else.

MONITORING CARDIOPULMONARY STATUS IN THE LONG-TERM CARE FACILITY

With the increase in patient acuity, it is more important than ever to monitor the patient's response to mobilization and exercise. Many long-term care and subacute facilities are purchasing pulse oximeters and portable ECG monitors because they have more

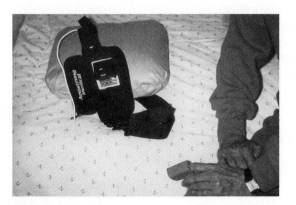

FIGURE 39-1
Pulse oximeter.

unstable patients (Figure 39-1). In addition, all therapists should be competent in blood pressure monitoring and taking pulse rates; auscultation training is highly recommended (see Chapter 14).

During the initial evaluation the vital signs and oximetry should be taken. The readings should be taken at rest in a supine or semi-Fowler's position for a baseline. Readings should then be taken in sitting and standing positions. It is helpful to take the blood pressure on both arms to see if there is a difference in the readings.

When the patient begins treatment, vital signs and oximetry should be performed before and after the mobilization or gait activity. A normal exercise response would be that the blood pressure and pulse would increase in relation to the activity. An increase of 20% to 30% might be expected and would be within normal limits. The time the vital signs take to return to normal (recovery time) should be within 5 to 10 minutes.

Many patients who are not considered cardiopulmonary patients have an abnormal response to exercise. If we are not observing and measuring objectively, we will not know the cardiopulmonary response is abnormal, and deleterious effects may occur.

An example of this was seen in a patient one month after a CVA. The patient was very fatigued and complained that his knees felt like they were going to buckle. This patient had been doing quite well and was not being monitored. However, after the patient expressed the feeling of weakness the therapist took the vital signs after the patient rested and walked again. The blood pressure and heart rate dropped during the exercise. The doctor was informed and ordered a blood test that revealed the patient did not have an appropriate blood level of digitalis. The medication was increased and the patient improved. Had the therapist not checked the vital signs and continued to push the patient, there could have been serious consequences.

SPECIAL MONITORING CONSIDERATIONS FOR PATIENTS ON OXYGEN

Patients receiving oxygen therapy have usually been placed on oxygen because of hypoxemia (low levels of oxygen in the arterial blood) or to relieve the myocardial work, such as in a patient with a severe myocardial infarction or other cardiac dysfunction (see Chapters 4 and 27).

It is important to note that the arterial blood gas is drawn at rest with no patient activity unless specifically noted otherwise (such as an exercise test blood gas). Generally the Medicare guidelines require that the patient has a Po_2 of 55 mm Hg (Torr) to be placed on oxygen. This is on the steep part of the oxyhemoglobin dissociation curve (see Chapter 3).

When the patient exercises he or she consumes more oxygen than at rest. Consequently if a patient is on oxygen at rest and the Po_2 is 55 or 60 mm Hg he or she may desaturate during exercise. This means that the red blood cell Hg will give up more oxygen to supply the exercising muscle. However, it is enough oxygen for exercise and the patient will experience increased shortness of breath, the oximeter will note a drop below 90%, and the blood pressure and heart rate may initially increase because of the stress and later drop as the heart cannot compensate for the decrease in oxygen level.

The pulse oximetry reading of normals is 97.5% oxygen saturation. It is clinically acceptable to maintain oxygen saturation at 90% or above. This saturation corresponds with keeping the Po_2 generally at above 55 mm Hg. When the Po_2 drops below 55 mm Hg, a dramatic drop in oxygen saturation will occur for a small drop in Po_2.

If the nursing home does not have an oximeter, the durable medical equipment company that supplies the oxygen may be called and will bring an oximeter when they check the oxygen. However, any patient on oxygen at rest should be tested for desaturation. Another option is to call the patient's doctor to request an increase in oxygen during exercise. For example, a patient on 1 L/min at rest can have a prescription written for 1 L/min at rest and 2 or 3 l/min during exercise. The increase in oxygen is no problem as long as the oxygen is decreased back to the resting amount as soon as the patient recovers back to baseline. This is even true for carbon dioxide retainers whose oxygen is carefully titrated to prevent taking away the hypoxic drive to breathe.

DOCUMENTATION

Functional outcomes are key to documentation. As we evaluate patients and write care plans, we set goals that are both short and long term. Each goal should be linked to functional outcomes that enable the patient to be more mobile, safe, as independent as possible, and functional in the care setting in which he or she lives.

Documentation needs to show progress toward the functional outcomes the therapist has developed with the patient. Goals should be attainable and realistic. If there is poor or slow progress to a goal, there needs to be documentation and explanation in the notes of what has occurred and how the treatment program will be modified or how the goals need to be changed.

When the functional outcomes have been met, the patient is reassessed to see if they can accomplish more or if the patient should be discharged from therapy with a maintenance program. A screening date should be set to check back and monitor the patient to ensure maintenance, improvement, or decline in condition. At times patients who have "plateaued" will improve and may be picked up on a screening to request a doctor's order to have additional therapy with specific increased goals defined. If a patient's condition has declined, the patient can be reevaluated to see if the patient's former status can be resumed or maintained.

It should be remembered that third party payors are reading the notes to understand what the evaluation and treatment plan for the patient is and how the patient has progressed in meeting functional outcomes. Because the patient is receiving long-term therapy, the more therapy the patient needs, the more documentation is necessary to tell the story to the third party payor or the managed care group. A good quote to remember is, "If it wasn't written, it wasn't done!"

In summary, every patient in a long-term facility is a patient with cardiopulmonary concerns. The cardiopulmonary system needs to be optimized for full rehabilitation to occur. Cooperation with the nurses and aides, as well as special activities staff, is essential for follow-through of treatment programs and patient success. Teamwork is the key, and communication and documentation are vital.

CARDIOPULMONARY CONCERNS IN HOME CARE

Home care takes the practice setting one step further from the hospital. Managed care is having major impacts on changes in this area of therapy and nursing care. Cost effective yet excellent therapy is the goal of managed care. There is a great deal of creativity; deals can be made if a provider group can demonstrate that the patient will benefit and a cost savings to the managed care group will occur. We are seeing coalitions form between contract service therapy agencies, durable medical equipment companies, nursing agencies, and enteral feeding companies to provide "one-stop shopping" groups. The managed care companies prefer to make one call that will provide them with nursing service, therapists, and home medical equipment, such as walkers, canes, tub seats, raised toilet seats, oxygen, IVs, and enteral feeding.

Home care involves not only seeing more acutely ill patients but also seeing some interesting cardiopulmonary situations. For example, in working with major medical centers who perform transplant surgery the therapist works with patients before and after heart and lung and other transplant surgeries. It has been demonstrated that patients, even as seriously ill as pretransplant patients, can improve their functional abilities, strength, and endurance to be better candidates for surgery. Postoperative care is also improved when the patient is in better physical condition before surgery. Other diagnoses are also being treated effectively before and after surgery. It makes sense to begin preoperative orthopedic consults to evaluate patients and teach them the exercises they will be doing after surgery. In addition, any patient facing abdominal or thoracic surgery could benefit from a preoperative visit if coming to the hospital presents difficulty. Consequently, therapists who never thought they would be required to work with cardiopulmonary patients are needing to increase their knowledge bases to treat these patients appropriately.

In the home-care setting the therapist is alone with supports through the nursing and home-care agencies. However, in the home they usually must be prepared to evaluate patients and their progress with very little supervision or consultation. In addition, they must be able to handle emergencies and crisis situations. All home-care therapists must have a basic CPR certification renewed annually. Policies and procedures dealing with how to handle emergencies, infection control, and safety are essential for any therapist in the home.

Therapists need to know how to obtain necessary information and equipment for the patient. They need to be creative in adapting equipment and be innovative if the patient cannot afford to purchase medical equipment. This is not the setting for new graduates, but rather for the experienced therapists.

HOME SETTING

In the hospital or outpatient center the patient comes to your place of business. They come where you work. With long-term care and home care, you go to work where they live. A certain etiquette is required when going into a patient's residence. Permission needs to be requested to enter the residence, alter their living space, put in grab bars, remove scatter rugs and telephone cords that are seen as a safety hazard, or rearrange rooms that you may consider too cluttered and unsafe. The therapist must remember that this is the patient's home and must be tactful in the way recommendations are made. The cluttered room may hold treasures that have been accumulated over a lifetime. They may surround themselves with items that are all they have left to remember. It may be true that a path needs to be made for safe walker ambulation, but how this is communicated may make all the difference in developing good rapport between a home-care therapist and the patient.

Initially, an evaluation of the patient's home needs to be made. What equipment do they have, is it in working order, do they know how to use it? Often a patient borrows "grandpa's cane" and does not realize that he or she is eight inches shorter than grandpa. Modifications may need to be made so that existing equipment fits properly and is functional.

Safety is a primary consideration. Are there cords across the floor? Are scatter rugs loose or tacked down with carpet tape? Can the patient pick up his or her foot sufficiently to walk over the scatter rug without tripping? Are there pieces of kitchen linoleum that have come up and might trip the patient? Are the kitchen chairs on rollers and the patient's balance poor?

Is the patient on oxygen and you discover that he or she has a gas stove? Are the close relatives,

friends, or a caretakers smokers? Signs need to be posted to warn of danger of smoking and flames around oxygen. Patients who are smokers need to have this reinforced very clearly.

Does the patient have stairs? Is the bedroom upstairs? Is there a first floor bathroom? If the bathroom is on the second floor can the patient get up the stairs safely and in a timely manner, or does a commode on the lower level seem more appropriate?

Is the bed the proper height? Are there handrails? Is it difficult for the patient to transfer into bed? Is a device needed to help the patient transfer independently?

The question of the bed arose with one home-care patients who had a fractured pelvis. When I first visited her, I asked how she had broken her pelvis and she replied, "Hopping into bed." I questioned what she meant and she said, "I'll show you." I followed her to her bedroom watching her gait with her walker. When we got to her bedroom, it was quickly noted that this very short patient had a very tall bed. The mattress was between her iliac crest and waist when she backed up to the bed. She stated, "I used to have a stool that I climbed into bed on, but my son thought it wasn't safe and took it away. Now I have to hop up into bed!" She had returned home to do the same activity that had put her in the hospital with a fractured pelvis. Looking at the bed, I noted that there were 3-inch rolling casters and a caster pad under the bed. The son was called and the casters and pads removed. The patient was quite pleased that the bed was 4 inches lower and she could transfer in quite easily.

Is there family support or a caretaker if the patient is not independent? If the spouse needs to work or go out, how long can the patient be safely left alone? Does the patient know how to obtain a caretaker? Are they able to financially afford the support?

Most home-care agencies have social worker support to help patients discover resources available to them. A physician's referral is needed and the service is generally covered under Medicare.

COMMUNICATION AND CROSS REFERRALS TO OTHER DISCIPLINES

It is essential that communication take place between the members of the home-care team. Communication is difficult because everyone is on the road and traveling to patients' homes. Generally, pager numbers of therapists and nurses are exchanged and compliance with answering pages is good. However, consideration needs to be given to the realization that we do not like to be interrupted frequently when seeing patients. Generally a system of timing the calls or pages is welcomed. A 911 can be placed after the page number to identify an urgent call if the call is very important or information needs to be given immediately.

Physical therapy is the most common therapy. However, at times another therapy will be indicated but not made when the patient is discharged. When a patient expresses a problem that could be handled better or could provide increased service to a patient, a cross referral should be made by calling the home-care agency or the patient's nurse case manager. Identify the problem and why you feel the additional therapy is indicated. The physician will be called and the order generally obtained. It would then be helpful for the referring therapist to call the new therapist and update him or her on the patient and reason for the referral. This communication should be documented to show the necessary communication between the therapists and nurses.

An example of this was seen in a patient that I received a referral on for home care that had been on a ventilator for a month in the hospital. She had been intubated, was very hoarse, and complained that she was having trouble swallowing and eating. Liquids especially were going down the wrong way. The home-care referral said that the patient had a swallowing study in the hospital that demonstrated she was aspirating. A speech language pathologist had been working with her on swallowing in the hospital. However, speech therapy had not been ordered at home. Nothing had changed on the day the patient had been discharged. Since the patient was still aspirating, a speech consult was requested.

At times it is helpful to do a joint treatment session with another discipline. This can be done to coordinate therapy and provide focus and continuity of goals. It will also lead to success for the patient. For example, a physical therapist and a speech language therapist may meet to focus on a patient with poor posture who lacks breath support for phonation. Another patient who is having difficulty feeding because of trunk weakness and is sitting in flexion with a forward head and neck and is having difficulty swallowing may benefit from speech and occupational therapists working on seating systems and feeding. The interaction and communication between therapists facilitates ideas for both therapists, provides continuity and follow-through, and helps to optimize patient care.

MONITORING CARDIOPULMONARY STATUS AT HOME

Cardiopulmonary status at home is similar to that in a long-term care facility. However, at home there is not usually an oximeter available. This is unfortunate, since many more patients are coming home on oxygen and ventilators. This trend should change and home-care therapists should have oximeters available for evaluation of patient status and exercise desaturation. The durable medical equipment company has oximeters and the therapist may request an oximetry study done with a physician referral. It is helpful to make an appointment and meet the therapist to see the results and to try to reenact the therapy to see if the patient desaturates with exercise.

The same blood pressure and pulse monitoring should be done at rest on both arms and in sitting, standing, and before and after exercise as mentioned previously in this chapter.

HOME OXYGEN

Home oxygen may be supplied by an oxygen concentrator, by tanks or as a liquid oxygen system (Figure 39-2) (Chapter 41). One consistent problem that must be dealt with in exercise with patients at home on oxygen is the incredibly long oxygen tubing needed to allow patients to go to the bathroom, out to the kitchen, and to the living room (Figure 39-3). Often 60 to 90 feet of tubing must be used. The question often arises, "Does the patient get the right amount of oxygen with such long tubing?" The answer is yes because the flow meter is a compensated one, which means it reads what really is occurring. If more tubing is added and a lesser flow was occurring, the flow meter would drop to indicate that had happened. Then it would be readjusted to the proper liter flow as ordered.

It has been found that the portable oxygen systems, in particular the demand oxygen system, do not always

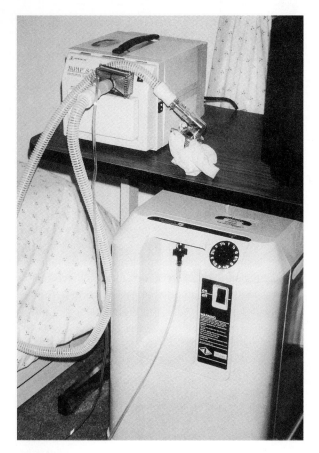

FIGURE 39-2
Oxygen concentrator.

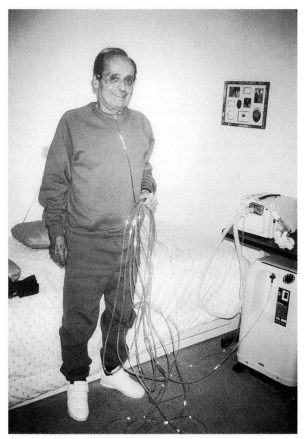

FIGURE 39-3
Oxygen tubing presents a significant safety hazard.

deliver the exact amount expected (Figure 39-4). It is necessary to use oximetry to determine whether the patient has an appropriate oxygen saturation reading.

Patients need to be taught either to coil the tubing or to develop a means to make sure that they do not trip over the tubing because it creates a safety hazard. Some patients have more than one tank or concentrator in the home to prevent having long lengths of tubing.

THERAPEUTIC GOALS FOR HOME-CARE PATIENTS WITH CARDIOPULMONARY DYSFUNCTION

To be independent at home, patients with cardiopulmonary dysfunction need to:
- Understand the dysfunction or disease.

- Be compliant with medications and health precautions.
- Learn preventative care (i.e., prevent pulmonary infections and not increase salt/water intake if on cardiac precautions or taking steroids).
- Learn ventilatory strategies to increase comfort and function (see Chapter 00).
- Learn to monitor themselves for signs of impending trouble (i.e., increased shortness of breath, swelling in ankles, productive cough, change in mucus, decreased urine output, or rapid weight gain) (Figure 39-5).
- Train to pace activity and use energy conservation techniques and rest periods to accomplish more with less stress.

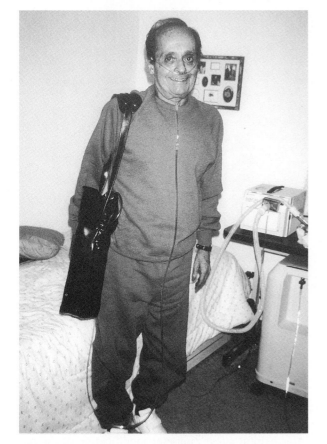

FIGURE 39-4
Portable demand oxygen system.

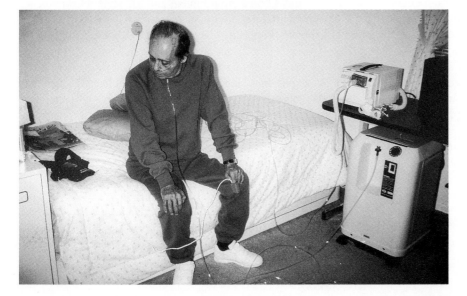

FIGURE 39-5
Patient monitoring oximeter with exercise.

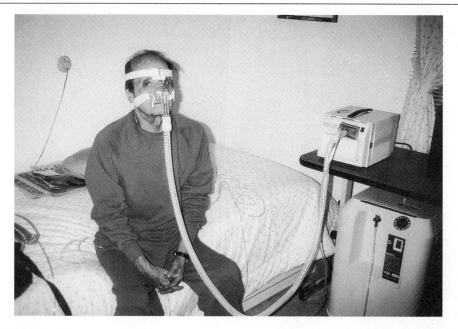

FIGURE 39-6
Nasal CPAP unit.

- Maintain proper nutrition and hydration.
- Develop a support network to help when needed and to check on the patient occasionally.
- Maintain walking program and general exercise to continue functional gains.

Some patients may need noctural nasal continuous positive airway pressure (CPAP) (Fig. 39-6). This may be ordered to treat sleep apnea or to rest the patient and assist with ventilation. A Bt-PAP unit allows the patient to rest and let the machine assist ventilation by providing pressure support on inspiration and exhalation. Often at first, the patient may have difficulty adjusting to the nasal CPAP, but in time, the patient will adapt to the assistance and feel it is beneficial.

SUMMARY

Education, self-monitoring, compliance to medication, reduction of risk factors, nutrition, and hydra-

tion are essential in the progress and maintenance of patients at home. As health-care practitioners, we offer helpful suggestions for modification of the patient's home environment and life style. However, we cannot force a patient to comply or accept what we have proposed. The patient in the home setting is independent in his or her judgments and activities. We need to respect that and at the same time provide our experience and therapeutic judgment and expertise. This setting is often the most rewarding a therapist can have, although at times it also may be the most frustrating. One thing is certain, if you ask a patient where they want to be, the answer sounds like, "There's no place like home!"

REVIEW QUESTIONS

1. What are some common problems patients in the community have in common?
2. What role does a preexisting cardiopulmonary

condition play in a new diagnosis or trauma (e.g., CVA, hip fracture)?

3. What are some uniques situations or concerns about patient care being delivered in a nursing home, assisted living center, home care?

4. What role can a physical therapist play in optimizing the patient's care in the above settings?

5. How can cardiopulmonary function be monitored outside the hospital?

6. What special considerations should be taken with a patient on oxygen?

References

Emlet, C., Cragtree, J., Condon, V., & Tremel, L. (1995). *In-home assessment of older adults, an interdisciplinary approach.* Gaithersburg, Md.: Aspen Publishers.

Harrington, J. (1983). The case for home health specialization. *Clinical Management in Physical Therapy, 3:*17.

Jackson, B.N. (1984). Home health care and the elderly in the 1980's. *American Journal of Occupational Therapy. 38:*717.

Jackson, D.E., & Wilhoire, M.J. (1985). Home health physical therapy, considerations for the provision of care. *Clinical Management in Physical Therapy, 5:*10.

May, B.J., (1993). Home health and rehabilitation, *Concepts of Care,* Philadelphia. F.A. Davis.

May, B.J. (1990). Principles of exercise for the elderly, In Basmajian, J.V. & Wolf, S.L. (Eds.). (1990). *Therapeutic exercise,* (5th ed.). Baltimore: Williams & Wilkins. 1990.

Pfau, J. (1989). *Adult exercise instruction sheets: Home exercise for rehabilitation therapy skill builders.* Tucson.

Polich, C. (1990). The provision of home health care services through health maintenance organizations: Conflicting roles for HMOs. *Home Health Care Quarterly, 11:*17.

Sallade, J. & Adam, L. (1986). Geriatric exercise booklet, *Clinical Management in Physical Therapy, 6:*32, 1986.

Schaefer, K. & Lewis, C. Marketing geriatric programs—A home care example, *Clinical Management in Physical Therapy,* 6:11–17, 1986.

Vassif, J.A. (1985). The Home Health Care Solution, New York: Harper & Row.

Zola, I.K. (1990). Aging, disability and the home care revolution, *Archives of Physical Medicine and Rehabilitation, 71:*93.

PART VIII

Related Aspects of Cardiopulmonary Physical Therapy

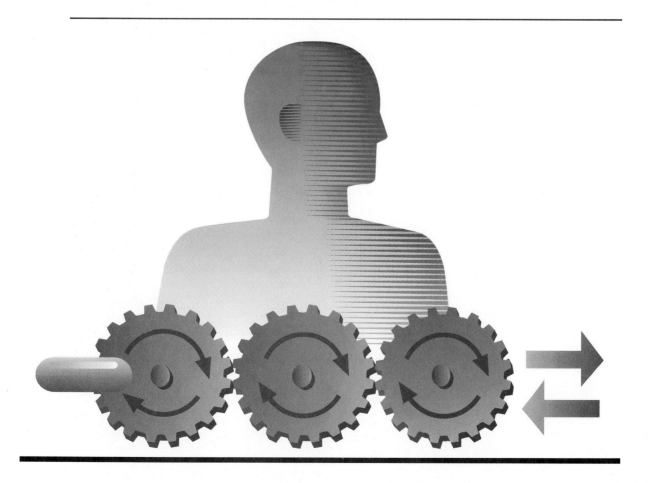

CHAPTER 40

Body Mechanics—The Art of Positioning and Moving Patients

Mary Massery
Donna Frownfelter

KEY TERMS	Body mechanics	Ventilation related to:
	Dependent patients	Supine
	Lifting and moving	Sidelying
		Upright
		Upright
		Neutral alignment of trunk, head and shoulders

INTRODUCTION

Body mechanics may be defined as the efficient use of one's body as a machine and a locomotive entity. In working with critically ill or chronically dependent patients, it is essential that optimal body positioning is accomplished to facilitate maximal ventilatory potential. Therapists and nurses attempting to position or move dependent patients must understand and use proper body mechanics (Neil, 1959; Fuerst and Wolff, 1969). This is necessary to reduce stress and trauma and to promote success for both the patient and the nurse or therapist. Positioning and moving dependent patients is an art that is quite different than working with a patient who can move independently and assume any given position with ease. In this chapter, the principles of body positioning and moving dependent patients are discussed.

POSITIONING FOR OPTIMAL VENTILATION

Because of the three-dimensional nature of breathing, the therapist's goal is to facilitate chest excursion in all three planes of ventilation—anterior-posterior, superior-inferior, and lateral (Massery, 1994). This can be accomplished by improving the length-tension relationships of the muscles used in inspiration (Crosbie and Myles; 1985; Kendall, 1993). Massery reasons that the success of proper positioning to enhance inspiratory muscles will do the following:

1. Improve the length-tension relationship of the accessory ventilatory muscles involved in that posture
2. Incorporate a passive stretch of the chest wall
3. Use the natural coordination of the trunk-chest wall movement with inspiration and exhalation patterns to maximize movement

The following are some common improvements that can be incorporated into normal positioning.

Supine Position

As mentioned in Chapter 37, all activity is performed in the field of gravity. Patients in a supine position may find breathing difficult because they must overcome gravity to move the chest wall with each breath. Using towel rolls or pillows to facilitate a better position may significantly improve the patient's opportunity for improved respiration.

Upper chest expansion can be increased by removing pillows under the patient's head to increase thoracic extension. This will increase the length-tension relationship of the neck accessory muscles (scalene and sternocleidomastoid muscles). Increased movement will be noted in the upper chest in a superior and anterior plane. Further anterior expansion can be achieved by using a towel roll placed longitudinally at the vertebral spine to open the anterior chest of a patient who tends toward excessive flexion of the trunk (Figure 40-1).

If the patient needs some support under his or her head to achieve a neutral chin tuck to protect his or her swallowing ability, then a thin pillow or horizontal towel roll under the occiput, may be used (Figure 40-2).

External rotation of the shoulders with the scapula in a neutral or retracted position will place the pectoralis and intercostal muscles on stretch. This will improve lateral and anterior chest wall movement (Kendall 1993). If a patient has full range of motion (ROM) and is comfortable with the arms placed overhead or in full flexion/abduction/external rotation for

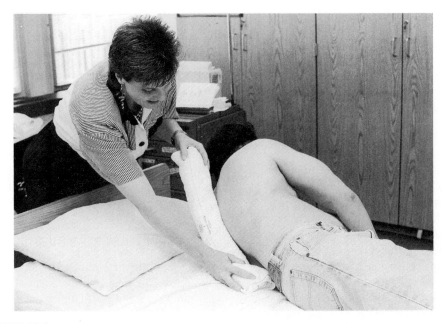

FIGURE 40-1
Placement of vertical towel roll.

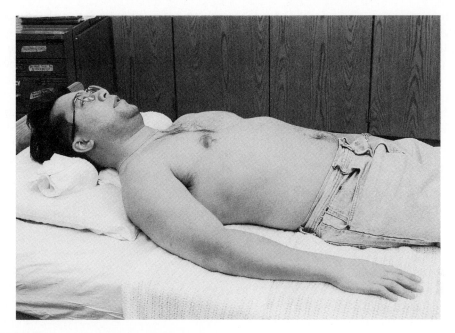

FIGURE 40-2
Increased openness of anterior chest wall with the vertical thoracic towel roll and the occipital towel roll combined.

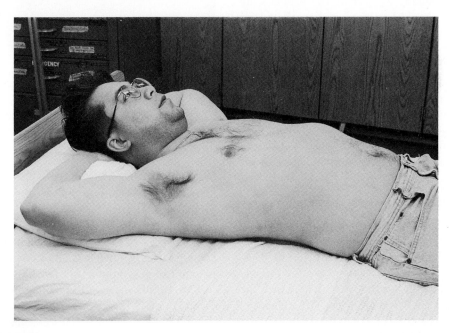

FIGURE 40-3
Butterfly position with thoracic towel roll to open anterior chest.

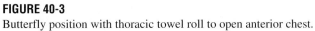

maximal stretch, this is the optimal position for full excursion of the anterior chest wall (Figure 40-3). If there are significant shoulder limitations, moderate shoulder abduction with forearm supination may be the best position available to facilitate chest excursion. Whenever significant limitations are found, the therapist should try to modify the position to accommodate the patient and achieve optimal ventilation.

Sidelying Position

Sidelying is an optimal position for improving breathing patterns. Gravity is eliminated for anterior expansion and the diaphragm moves freely. In addition sidelying is a reflex-inhibiting posture, and some high-tone patients will be able to relax and breathe more freely. It is important to consider the shunt effects if a patient has lung pathology. For example, if a patient has right lower lobe pneumonia or atelectasis, sidelying on the good side will improve oxygenation. Conversely, sidelying with the affected side down will cause a decrease in oxygenation (differential shunt) because a poorly ventilated patient receives more perfusion to the down lung and more shunting will occur. The patient's hip and knee joints should be flexed and supported for comfort. The upper extremities can be moved up and away from the body to allow for free movement of the upper chest wall. A pillow can be used to support the upper arm anteriorly, or the patient can be placed in a three-quarter supine position and a pillow behind the back to support the uppermost arm. If the patient has full range of motion and is comfortable, a butterfly position of the arms can be used. This will automatically open up the rib cage and facilitate inspiration.

Upright Postures

Upright postures create new challenges to breathing by adding the component of balance and an unsupported spinal column. Pelvic alignment is a key component. An anteriorly tilted pelvis in healthy flexible adults will tend to do the following: (1) reduce the kyphotic curve in the thoracic spine, (2) adduct the scapula toward a neutral position, (3) produce a more neutral or externally rotated upper-extremity position, and (4) pull the head back into a neutral chin tuck

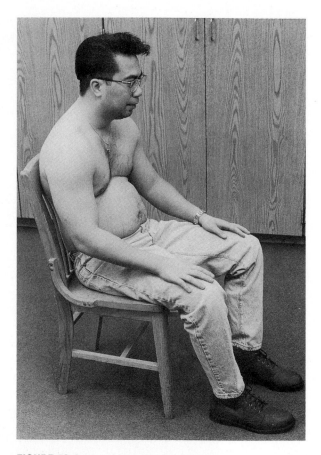

FIGURE 40-4
Unsupported upright position of patient with T1 paraplegia. NOTE: Posterior plevic tilt and excessive thoracic khyphosis with resulting collapse of anterior chest wall.

(Woodhall-McNeal, 1992; Borello-France, Burdett, and Gee, 1988). The anterior tilt of the pelvis will improve upper-extremity ROM and ventilation potential. Attending to this one consideration may be all that is necessary to improve the breathing capacity in some patients, allowing them to continue to advance in their exercise programs or rehabilitation courses.

One simple means of attaining an anterior pelvic tilt in sitting is to have the patient lean forward over his or her legs, then slide a towel roll horizontally just behind the ischial tuberosities, which will prevent the pelvis from rolling back into a posterior tilt (Johnson,

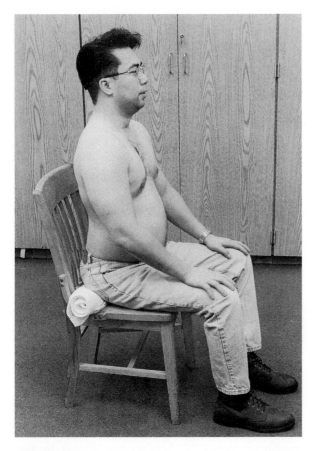

FIGURE 40-5
Ischial towel roll to support pelvis in anterior tilt in patient with T1 paraplegia. Note: chenges in the thoracic spine and open anterior chest wall as well as improved head and neck alignment.

1989) (Figures 40-4 and 40-5). This is well tolerated for many patients with intact sensation and a pelvis that is at least minimally mobile. For neurological patients with impaired sensation or less pelvic mobility, a wedge may be substituted; however, caution must be used because some sliding may occur.

Neutral Alignment of the Head and Shoulders

A vertical or horizontal towel roll may also be used with wheelchair positioning to bring the shoulders and head back into a more neutral alignment. The anterior chest wall will also be more open with this technique.

A neutral head and neck position is important for patients with impaired speech volume or endurance and for patients with swallowing or aspiration dysfunction. A neutral chin tuck will optimize the length-tension relationship of the vocal folds, minimize vocal strain, and improve protective airway reflexes (Massery, 1994).

It is also vital to evaluate the patient's shoulder positioning. Internal rotation of the shoulders and scapular protraction tends to block the upper chest from reaching its full expansion potential. Alternately, external rotation of the shoulders will markedly increase upper chest wall movements and thoracic extension. Clinically, improved lung volumes will be noted when these positioning considerations are taken into consideration. Often these small, seemingly insignificant changes will position the patient for success with other therapeutic activities. If unattended, these small factors can impede patient progress. Positioning has everything to do with increasing ventilation and functional skills.

LIFTING AND MOVING DEPENDENT PATIENTS

There has been a change from earlier concepts and principles of lifting. As discussed, the body has been thought of as a machine. It was believed that improper mechanics of lifting would result in tremendous loads on the disks. The key components of lifting were to "keep it close," "bend knees," "lift with the legs." Later the spinal posture was the center of attention during lifting (*Physical Therapy Forum,* 1985).

During observation, lifting seemed to occur "naturally" from slightly bent knees and then, during the raise lift butt-end first, with the patient rearing backward at the start as the therapist started to extend the knees before lifting. The predominance of injuries seems to occur with the back in flexion. There is a rationale for strengthening abdominal muscles to promote safer lifting. Abdominal strength is necessary to support a pelvic tilt during lifting. Many commercially available lumbar and abdominal elastic velcro supports are now available and widely accepted. They provide additional abdominal wall support.

Another current school of thought advocates lifting with the lordotic lumbar curve intact. This is the technique used by weight lifters. When these individuals are questioned about backaches, they usually deny any problems.

The lifting technique may be modified by other factors, such as limited space (i.e., small hospital rooms), clothing, or degenerative knee joints.

The first consideration in body mechanics is the need for maintenance of proper posture and balance (body stability). Consideration should be paid to the relationship between gravity, posture, and body stability (Figure 40-6). It is commonly known that gravitational force is always exerted in a vertical direction toward the center of the earth. In addition, that point in a patient or object at which all of its mass is centered is called the *center of gravity* (the point at which the patient's maximum weight is concentrated). In the standing position the human body's center of gravity is approximately 55% of the body's total height and in the pelvic cavity, slightly anterior to the upper part of the sacrum. The lower the center of gravity, the greater the body stability. Consequently, when the human body is used as a machine to lift an object, muscular effort great enough to maintain stability and to lift against the force of gravity is necessary, especially when the patient's center of gravity is further removed from your own. Therefore one way to conserve energy and maintain stability is to carry the weight of the patient (or object) as close to one's own center of gravity as possible. This allows maximal concentration of one's own energy toward movement of the patient, with minimal stress or injury to oneself. To help accomplish this, the bed should be adjusted so the therapist or nurse can reach the patient comfortably. Usually adjusting the bed to one's hip level is adequate. This makes the patient close to the therapist's center of gravity.

The majority of lifting should be done with the legs (knees) and not by straining to lift with the arms and back (Figure 40-7). Whenever there is a question about one's ability to lift a patient alone, generally it should not be done, and assistance should be obtained (Rantz & Courtial, 1977).

Another point to consider is the base of support while lifting. The base of support is defined as the area between the feet that provides the body's stability. It is easily appreciated that the wider the base of support, the greater the body's stability. To enlarge on this concept, one also needs to define the line of gravity and its relationship to body stability. The line of gravity is an imaginary line passing through the center

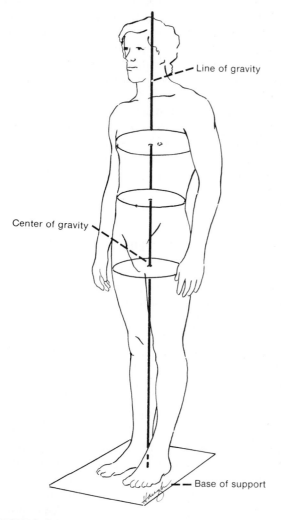

FIGURE 40-6
The line of gravity passes through the center of gravity and the base of support to maintain body stability.

of gravity of an object and perpendicular to the surface on which the object (body) rests (see Figure 40-6). The closer the line of gravity passes to the center of the base of support, the greater the body's (object's) stability. Increased muscular effort needs to be exerted in proportion to the distance the line of gravity shifts away from the base of support (Rauch, 1971).

To summarize and apply these concepts, one can list the following guidelines:

1. The lower the center of gravity, the wider the base of support, and the nearer the line of gravity falls to the center of the base of support, the greater the body's (object's) stability. When lifting, stand with feet well apart, knees slightly flexed, and one foot forward. Keep head and trunk in proper alignment.

2. When our bodies are used as machines, the external weight on which we are working displaces the center of gravity in the direction of the weight being lifted. To conserve energy and maintain stability, carry the weight as close to your own center of gravity as possible. Lower your hips to the level of the surface supporting the weight you plan to lift by flexing your hips and knees. Adjust the bed up as high or down as low as you need for comfortable and efficient work.

3. The effort to perform a given activity depends on the weight of the object to be lifted. Know your limits. Do not attempt to lift alone if you have any doubts about your ability to do so. Don't be a hero in a back brace. Obtain assistance for the sake of both the patient and yourself.

4. Other general tips for lifting are as follows (Figure 40-7):
   - Lift with your legs. Keep legs in a position that permits them to supply most of the force for shifting your trunk.
   - Do not attempt to lift with your arms and back.
   - When lifting, avoid rotation of the spine. Shift feet into position for weight shift when moving or lifting patient.
   - Stabilize your body against a stationary object whenever possible.
   - For best efficiency, coordinate the move by a synchronized verbal expression understood by therapists and patient, such as "1–2–3 lift."

One additional consideration must be noted—moving against the resistance of friction. *Friction* is defined as a force that opposes the movement of one object over the surface of another. Friction is reduced as the amount of surface area contact between two objects is reduced.

When moving a patient side to side or up and down in bed, the therapist or nurse attempts to reduce the contact of the patient's body surface with the bed. This can be accomplished by several maneuvers—use a turning sheet (placed just above the patient's shoulders to just below the patient's hips), cross the patient's arms over the chest or abdomen, flex the patient's knees and hips, and ask the patient to flex his or her neck and raise the head as he or she is lifted (if the patient is unable to do this, the therapist or nurse will assist) (Figure 40-8).

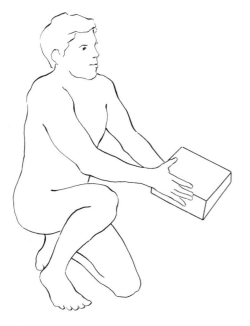

FIGURE 40-7
Reach work level by bending the knees and hips rather than the back. Lift with the legs! This can also be done with a full double knee squat similar to techniques by weightlifters.

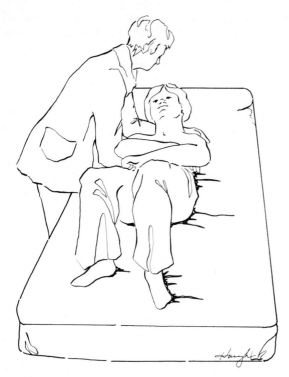

FIGURE 40-8

The patient should be prepared for a position chenge: knees bent, arms crossed over chest and head lefted up to reduce friction between the patient's body and the bed.

MOVING DEPENDENT PATIENTS

I. Moving the patient up or down (Roper, 1973; Lewis, 1976; Neil, 1976).

A. Using a turning sheet (Figures 40-9 to 40-11).
1. Sheet should cover from shoulders to hips.
2. Gather material as close to the patient's body as possible.
3. Hold at shoulders and hips, with a flexion pattern (see Figure 40-10).
4. Cross patient's arms over chest, flex knees and hips.
5. Ask patient to raise head if possible.
6. Synchronize action by counting "1–2–3 lift."
7. Shift weight from one leg to the other rather than lifting up and pulling on back.

B. Without turning sheet (up or down), two people.
1. Follow basic procedure—cross arms, lift head, flex knees and hips.
2. The therapist places his or her hands and forearms under the patient's shoulders and hips.
3. If patient is extremely heavy or tall, another person can bend knees and assist.

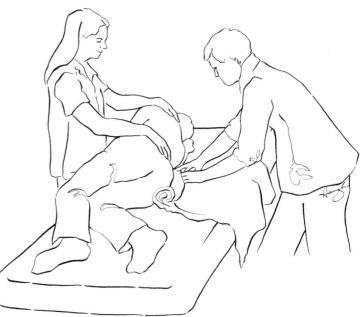

FIGURE 40-9

To insert the drawsheet, the patient is turned to his side and the half-rolled drawsheet is tucked under him (from just above the shoulders to just below the hips). He rolls over the drawsheet and it is pulled out behind him.

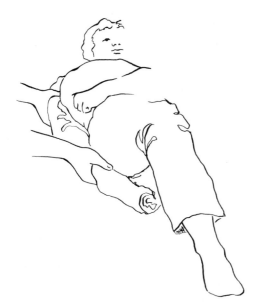

FIGURE 40-10
The drawsheet should be rolled close to the patient's body. A flexion hand grip at the patient's shoulders and hip is most efficient.

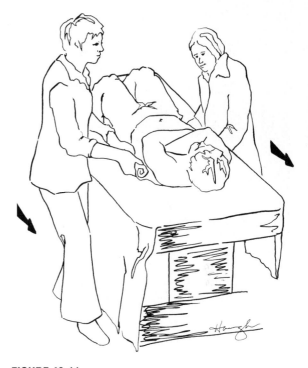

FIGURE 40-11
Moving the patient toward the head of the bed. The patient is prepared. The therapist is positioned to move toward the head of the bed in order to shift his body weight to move the patient.

II. Moving the patient to the side of the bed.
  A. With turning sheet.
    1. Cross arms, and other body parts, toward the side to which the patient is to be moved.
    2. Therapist's hands at patient's hips and shoulder on material close to patient's body.
    3. One therapist pushes, the other pulls.
  B. Without turning sheet.
    1. Both persons stand on the desired side.
    2. One therapist's forearms under patient's shoulder, the others under patient's hips.
    3. Synchronize action by counting "1–2–3 pull."
III. Turning the patient to his side.
  A. With turning sheet (to right side) (Figures 40-12 and 40-13).
    1. Move patient supine to opposite side of turn (e.g., if turning to right side, move patient to left side of bed).

    2. Bring right arm to the side at a 90-degree angle up and away from body.
    3. Place left arm across chest.
    4. Place left leg over right leg.
    5. Pull sheet at patient's back to turn.
  B. Without turning sheet (to right side).
    1. Move to opposite side (therapist's hands and forearms under patient's shoulders and hips).
    2. Same steps as 2, 3, and 4 above.
    3. Roll to right side using left shoulder and left hip to push or pull.
IV. Turning the patient prone (e.g., roll to right side) (Figure 40-14).

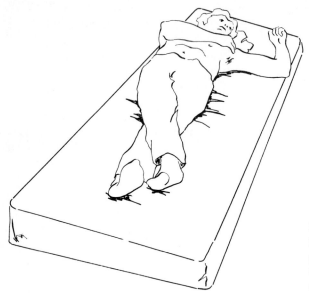

FIGURE 40-12

Preparation for the patient to turn to his left side: move patient to the right side of the bed, position his left arm up to the side at a 90-degree angle, cross the right leg and arm over his body and turn the patient's head to the left.

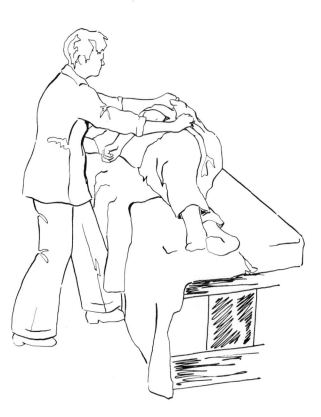

FIGURE 40-13

A one-person turn to the right side using a drawsheet. The patient's body position is the same as for the turn to the side. The therapist is positioned with one foot forward, the other back. He pulls the sheet with his hands positioned at the hips and shoulders of the patient.

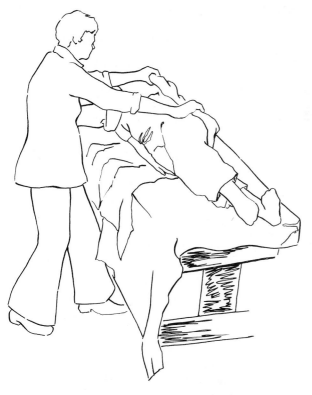

FIGURE 40-14
Positioning patient prone (EXAMPLE: Rolling to the right side). The patient's right arm is tucked in at his side with the left arm and leg crossed over.

A. With or without turning sheet.
   1. Move patient to opposite side of bed from side toward which he or she is turning.
   2. Cross left arm and left leg over body.
   3. Right hand and arm at body side tucked in as close as possible.
   4. Use hips and shoulders to turn.
   5. Free both arms, do not allow patient to lie on arm or hand.
   6. May want pillow under hips and lower legs to bend knee and relieve back strain at lumbar spine.

To summarize, we find patient positioning and movement is a necessary and integral function of physical therapy. It is so often taken for granted and performed with little thought or planning. Therapists and nurses need to analyze beforehand their physical activities in relation to the principles of efficient movement and the proper application of body mechanics. A "tube index", counting and identifying each technical attachment, (e.g., IV, Foley cather, arterial blood gas stint, or chest tubes) should be done before moving a patient. Extra care needs to be taken to prevent dislodging important medical equipment. This could prove life threatening if ventilator tubing was pulled and a patient was extubated. The practical application of body mechanics will not only conserve energy and preserve muscles and joints but will also allow the patient to be moved with a minimum amount of pain and discomfort, with greater safety.

REVIEW QUESTIONS

1. Why is it important to utilize efficient body mechanics when positioning and moving dependent patients?
2. How can changing a patient's position affect ventilation?
3. How can therapist use towel rolls and easily accessible equipment to improve a patient's position and potential for improved ventilation?
4. What ventilation/perfusion changes occur when a patient is turned from the "bad" side down to the "good" side down?
5. Can positioning alone be considered therapeutic when it accomplishes the plan of treatment goal?

References

Borello-France, D.P., Burdett, R.G., & Gee, Z.L., (1988). Modification of sitting posture of patients with hemiplegia using seat boards and backboards, *Physical Therapy, 68*(1), 68-71.

Crosbie, W.J., & Myles, S. (1985). An investigation into the effect of postural modification on some aspects of normal pulmonary function. *Physiotherapy, 7*,(7), 311-314.

Fuerst, E., & Wolff, L. (1959). *Fundamentals of nursing* (4th ed) Philadelphia: JB Lippincott.

Is there a right way to lift? (1985). *Physical Therapy Forum, 4,* 23.

Johnson, G. (1989). Functional *Orthopedics I.* San Ansellmo, Calif: Institute of Physical Art. Chicago: Course presentation June 8-11, 1989.

Kendall, F.P., McCreary, E.K., & Provance, P.G. (1993). *Muscles testing and function.* Baltimore: Williams & Wilkins.

Lewis, L. (1976). *Fundamental skills in patient care.* Philadelphia: JB Lippincott.

Massery, M. (1994). What's positioning got to do with it? *Neurology Report, 18* (3), 11-14.

Neil, C. (1959). Body management in nursing. *Nursing Times, 55,* 163.

Rantz, M. & Courtial, D. (1977). *Lifting, moving and transferring patients: a manual.* St. Louis, Mosby.

Rauch, B. (1971). *Kinesiology and applied anatomy,* Philadelphia: Lea & Febiger.

Roper, N. (1973). *Principles of nursing,* (2nd ed). New York: Churchill Livingstone.

Woodhall-McNeal, A. P. (1992). Changes in posture and balance with age, *Aging, 4* (3), 219-225.

CHAPTER 41

Respiratory Care Practice Review

Michael Wade Baskin

KEY TERMS
Aerosol
Humidity
Intermittent positive pressure
  breathing (IPPB)

Mechanical ventilation
Oxygen
Oxygen delivery

INTRODUCTION

Proper care of the pulmonary patient involves a multi-disciplinary approach, and all professionals involved should have a working knowledge of each individual profession's scope of care. As respiratory therapists, physical therapists, occupational therapists, and nurses apply their expertise in providing care for pulmonary patients, it becomes evident that coordinated team work is essential to ensure effective treatment programming. The purpose of this chapter is to provide nonrespiratory therapist health-care professionals with an overview of respiratory care principles and modalities frequently encountered in the various settings. It is also the intention of this chapter to eliminate the anxiety experienced by professionals because of the plethora of attachments to the cardiopulmonary patient. Interaction with the various modalities and pieces of equipment is also discussed.

OXYGEN THERAPY

The atmosphere around us contains 20.95% oxygen, one of the most essential elements needed to sustain human life. Oxygen exerts a partial pressure of 159.6 mm Hg at sea level (dry air) and approximately 97 mm Hg in arterial blood. The normal range as measured by arterial blood gas analysis is 80 to 100 mm Hg. Under normal circumstances, this molecule travels from the atmosphere to the mitochondria at the cellular level where it is used to produce ATP in a process called *aerobic metabolism*. The pathway involves the lungs, blood, circulation, and the muscle tissue where the mitochondria reside. Any process that inhibits the transport of oxygen from the atmosphere to the cellular level can cause tissue hypoxia and ultimately death.

One of the most common drugs that a respiratory therapist uses is oxygen. Patients with cardiopulmonary problems frequently need oxygen supplementation. Respiratory therapists and the nursing staff are generally responsible for administration of this drug under a physician's order. There are several different methods a therapist may choose to deliver oxygen in the most effective way.

The purpose of oxygen therapy is to treat and to prevent hypoxemia, excessive work of breathing, and excessive myocardial work (Kacmarek, Mack, and Dimas, 1990). Although individual oxygen appliances offer suggested guidelines regarding oxygen administration, the only way to ensure effective delivery from a given device is blood gas monitoring of Pao_2, partial pressure of oxygen in the arterial blood or by monitoring hemoglobin saturation by oximetry. Oxygen therapy can be administered by one of two methods—low-flow and high-flow systems.

Low-Flow Systems

A low-flow oxygen system is that which does not intend to meet the total inspiratory requirements of the patient. This method of oxygen delivery is not used when a specific concentration of oxygen is needed (Burton, Hodgkin, and Ward, 1991).

The nasal cannula, also called *nasal bi-prongs,* is one of the most common low flow devices encountered because of its low expense and high patient compliance (Figure 41-1). This device supplies between 24% and 40% oxygen with flow rates from 1 L/min to 6 L/min. Flow rates above 6 L/min can cause nasal mucosa irritation and drying. The approximate liter flow and resultant FIo_2 values are shown in Table 41-1.

Nasal canulas deliver 100% oxygen, however, this percentage significantly lessens as the oxygen mixes with inspired air from the room. The amount of oxygen delivered depends on the flow rate and the ventilatory pattern of the patient. A larger minute volume (TV × RR) would dilute the oxygen at any given flow rate causing a greater decrease in the percentage delivered to the lungs. In other words, the faster and deeper a patient breathes, the more diluted the oxygen will become. On the other hand, if a patient has a low minute volume, the oxygen percentage delivered will increase (Kacmarek et al., 1990). If precise control of FIo_2 is needed, the nasal cannula should not be used (Bazuaye, Stone, Corris, and Gibson, 1992).

Mouth breathing by patients on a nasal cannula typically causes the attending health-care provider to switch the patient to a mask; however, this may be unnecessary. If the nasal passages are unobstructed, then oxygen is able to collect in the oral and nasal cavity (anatomical reservoir). On inspiration, the oxygen collected in this area is drawn into the airway system. If a patient with a nasal cannula is mouth breathing, the practitioner should ensure the nasal passages are unobstructed. If there is concern that the patient is not

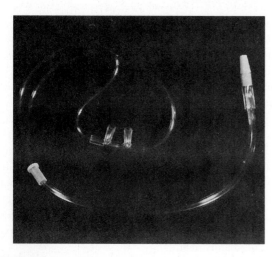

FIGURE 41-1
Oxygen cannula.

TABLE 41-1	
Approximate liter flow and resultant FIo_2 values.	
FLOW (L/min)	**FIo_2(%)**
1	24
2	28
3	32
4	36
5	40
6	44

receiving adequate oxygen, an oxygen saturation measurement should be obtained. If this is not feasible, or if the patient is unable to breathe through the nose, it would be appropriate to switch the patient to a mask.

Breathing through the nose should be encouraged to receive maximum benefit from the nasal cannula; however, mouth breathing does not mean the patient is not receiving oxygen (Dunlevy & Tyl, 1992).

The simple mask, or open-face mask, is another low-flow oxygen delivery device commonly used. It can deliver from 40% to 60% oxygen, depending on the flow rate and the patient's ventilatory pattern. This device requires a flow rate of 5 to 6 L/min to prevent rebreathing and excessive respiratory work (Jensen, Johnson, and Sandstedt, 1991). As with the nasal cannula, this type of oxygen delivery method should not be used if precise control of oxygen concentration (FIo_2) is required.

The partial rebreathing mask is basically a mask with a reservoir bag attached. The oxygen source supplies the bag with 100% oxygen where it mixes with exhaled anatomical dead-space–air that has not taken place in gas exchange. This exhaled air is rich in oxygen. The exhaled air that has taken place in gas exchange and contains CO_2 is vented through the open ports on each side of the mask. This mask can deliver oxygen concentrations from 70% to more than 80%, and it requires flows between 7 and 10 L/min to keep the bag from fully collapsing during inspiration (Kacmarek et al., 1990).

The nonrebreathing mask is another low-flow delivery device that also contains a bag reservoir, but it can deliver up to 100% oxygen. This mask contains valves at the reservoir bag and the side vents to prevent ambient air mixing on inspiration and exhaled air mixing on expiration. In order for this mask to operate effectively, a good seal between the patient's face and the mask should be achieved. The bag should partially deflate during inspiration (Figure 41-2).

Another interesting form of low-flow oxygen delivery is the transtracheal oxygen catheter. This method has gradually gained wider acceptance as a long-term oxygen delivery device. It is surgically placed into the trachea via a small incision between the second and third tracheal rings. Generally, these devices are seen in home-oxygen patients. Transtra-

cheal oxygen catheters are more efficient than nasal cannulas, and they have a high patient acceptance rate with low complications (Kent, et al., 1987). Because the oxygen is administered directly into the trachea, 50% less oxygen is needed (Kacmarek et al., 1990). For people who use portable oxygen systems, and for those who require high oxygen flow rates, tracheal oxygen catheters may be beneficial (Jackson, King, Wells, and Shneerson, 1992). The catheter can be covered by the patient's clothing, therefore, it is cosmetically appealing.

HIGH-FLOW SYSTEMS

A high-flow oxygen delivery system is that which delivers a specific oxygen concentration despite the patient's ventilatory pattern. If it is found that a patient requires oxygen delivered at an FIo_2 of 50% to keep the oxygen saturation at a safe level, then a high-flow system would be the method of choice.

This type of system is also used when there is fear of administering too much oxygen to a hypercapneic patient. The respiratory drive to breath could be reduced and possibly result in apnea. Precise control of low-concentration oxygen is warranted in such cases.

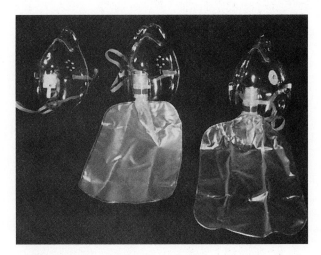

FIGURE 41-2
Left to right, mask without bag, partial rebreathing bag, nonbreathing bag. NOTE: the valves on the mask and at the junction between the mask and bag.

The Venturi mask is a common method of delivering high-flow oxygen concentrations from 24% to 50%. This mask operates via the Venturi principle, which provides for a mixing of 100% oxygen and entrained ambient air. The oxygen flows though a narrow orifice at a high velocity causing a subatmospheric pressure. This drop in pressure is what causes the ambient air to be entrained through a port. The size of the port determines the amount of air to be entrained and thus the percentage of oxygen delivered. The Venturi mask has a rotating air entrainment port that allows the health-care provider to "dial in" the desired FIo_2 (Figure 41-3).

Mechanical aerosol systems also operate via air entrainment, but the mask is connected to the aerosol unit by large-bore tubing to allow a specific FI_{O2} to be delivered with high humidity (Figure 41-4). Although drainage bags are usually attached to the tubing to collect condensation, the tubing must be monitored for possible pooling of water causing flow obstruction to the patient. If partial obstruction occurs, a mild back pressure results in the tubing, causing less air entrainment. This means that a higher concentration of oxygen will result and possibly deliver a higher dosage of oxygen to the patient than desired.

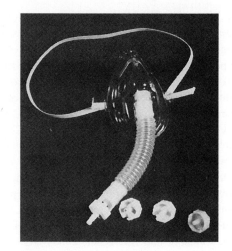

FIGURE 41-3
Venturi mask.

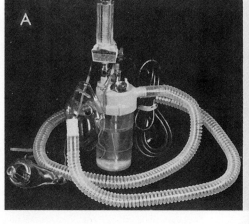
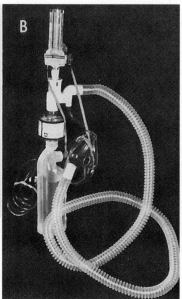

FIGURE 41-4
A, Heated aerosol. **B,** Nebulizers.

HOME AND PORTABLE OXYGEN

As health care continues to move out of the hospital setting and into the home, more health-care practitioners will be providing care to oxygen patients in their homes. Oxygen is most commonly delivered in the home for those needing long-term oxygen, usually chronic obstructive pulmonary disease (COPD) patients. Generally 1 to 2 L/min is prescribed via nasal cannula, but the flow rate will depend on the patient's need.

Home oxygen-delivery systems can be divided into three categories: high-pressure oxygen cylinders, low-pressure liquid oxygen, and oxygen concentrators (Burton et al., 1991).

High-pressure oxygen tanks come in various sizes. The larger ones such as the H and K sizes are used as a base unit or reservoir. Long oxygen tubing connected to these tanks allows for patient mobility.

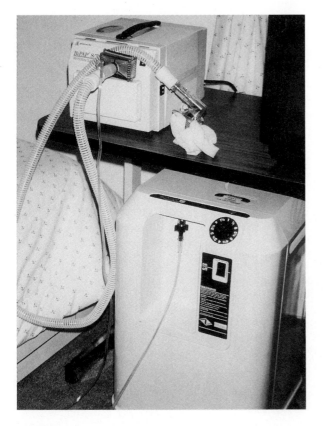

FIGURE 41-5
Oxygen concentrator.

Smaller tanks are used for portability and can provide up to 3 hours of use. They can be refilled by transferring gas from the larger reservoir tank.

Liquid oxygen is a low-pressure oxygen delivery method, and it tends to be more convenient than using the high-pressure tanks, especially for the active oxygen patient. The canisters are lightweight and allow patients to be away from the home reservoir for up to 8 hours. The down side is that liquid oxygen costs more, and the reservoirs need to be filled up to twice a week with continuous use. If high flows are needed, these units are not recommended.

Oxygen concentrators are commonly seen in the home health setting, especially since Medicare offers coverage for these devices (Figure 41-5). Generally, they tend to be expensive initially but are actually less expensive for long-term use. They are electrically powered and create oxygen by drawing ambient air across a semipermeable membrane, separating oxygen from nitrogen. They generally operate at 2 L/min and provide 90% oxygen. Long oxygen tubing, up to 50 ft, allows patients extra mobility. Patients using concentrators should have a back-up device, such as a portable tank, in case of a power outage.

RESPIRATORY MODALITIES
Intermittent Positive Pressure Breathing

Intermittent positive pressure breathing (IPPB) is mentioned here not to educate the reader about its use but to inform the reader about its declining use. Although this particular modality continues to be used in some hospital settings, there is little evidence to supports its efficacy.

This particular technology was developed during World War II to assist pilots breathing in unpressurized cabins at high altitudes. IPPB subsequently became a very popular respiratory therapy device in the 1960s and 1970s (Figure 41-6). However, its use began to decline in the 1980s. In 1983 the National Heart, Lung, and Blood Institute reported that IPPB has limited therapeutic benefit. This clinical trial is only one of several studies that show IPPB is an outmoded medical technology. In fact, research dating back to the 1950s questions the efficacy of this device (Duffy and Farley, 1992).

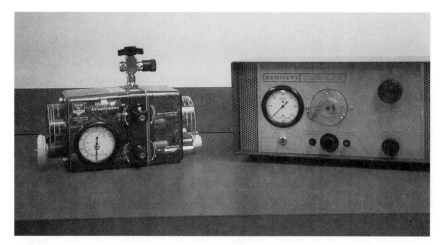

FIGURE 41-6
Left, Bird Mark and *right,* Bennett AP-5 IPPB machines.

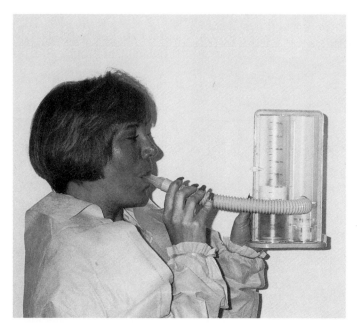

FIGURE 41-7
Incentive spirometry device in use.

The purpose of the IPPB machine is to increase alveolar ventilation, to improve the ventilation-perfusion ratio, to mobilize and facilitate expectoration of thick secretions, to decrease the work of breathing, and to deliver aerosolized medications. It is a pressure-cycled ventilator that, when triggered by a patient's inhalation, delivers ambient air or oxygen to the patient until a preset pressure is reached. It is basically a lung expansion device that helps deliver an increased tidal volume. IPPB is used for a variety of pulmonary conditions, and treatment sessions usually last 10 to 15 minutes.

This modality comes into question in the clinical setting because it has not shown to provide benefits over that of other simpler respiratory treatment methods. It also introduces potential complications and hazards that the other treatments do not. Typically, IPPB has been used to treat asthma, COPD, and postoperative atelectasis; however, other therapies, such as incentive spirometry (IS), postural drainage, and aerosol therapy, tend to prevail as the treatment of choice over IPPB.

Although IPPB is questionable regarding its clinical efficacy, it may be a beneficial form of treatment in acute asthma or COPD that is refractory to standard therapy, atelectasis that has not responded to simpler therapy, and the prevention of respiratory failure in patients with kyphoscoliosis and neuromuscular disorders (Handelsman, 1991).

INCENTIVE SPIROMETRY

Incentive spirometry (IS), also called *sustained maximum inspiration* (SMI), is simply a visual and/or audio feedback device that encourages slow, deep inspiration (Figure 41-7). Generally, this treatment is performed frequently, up to every hour, and its purpose is to treat and prevent atelectasis, especially in postoperative thoracic and abdominal patients.

HUMIDITY AND AEROSOL THERAPY
Humidity Therapy

Under normal circumstances, when inhalation takes place, air becomes 100% saturated with water vapor before entering the lower airway tracts below the ca-

rina. This humidification process is important to mucous production, ciliary activity, and a healthy respiratory tract. When this normal humidification process is interferred with, other methods of adding moisture to the respiratory system must be employed.

Humidification is the addition of water vapor in its molecular form to a gas. When a dry gas is being administered to a patient (e.g., via a nasal cannula), some type of humidification appliance would be used to prevent unnecessary complications. Flows of 2 L/min or less may not require humidification when using a nasal cannula. Humidification therapy is also indicated in the presence of thick tenacious secretions and when an artificial airway is in place. Artificial airways, such as endotracheal and tracheostomy tubes, bypass the normal humidification system (the upper airway); therefore, supplementation is essential (Frownfelter, 1987).

There are basically two types of humidifiers. Bubble-through humidifiers are those which are generally used with simple oxygen appliances. The pass-over type of humidifier is usually found in conjuction with a mechanical ventilator. Both bubble-through and pass-over humidifiers are available for ventilators, and they are usually heated to warm the humidified air to body temperature before entering the airway (Kacmarek et al., 1991).

Aerosol Therapy

An aerosol is created when a suspension of liquid or solid particles exists in a gas. Today, the two most common forms of medication aerosol delivery in the clinical setting are the small volume nebulizer (SVN) and the metered dose inhaler (MDI). A bland aerosol is administration of water or saline solution to the patient's lungs.

In general the goals of aerosol therapy are to hydrate dried retained secretions, to improve cough efficiency, to restore and maintain function of the mucociliary elevator, to deliver medications, and to humidify gases delivered through artificial airways. The MDI is strictly used for medication delivery.

Other forms of aerosol delivery are the spinning disk, such as in a room humidifier or mist tent, and the ultrasonic nebulizer. Both of these are electri-

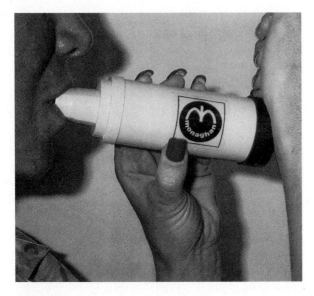

FIGURE 41-8
Commonly used spacer device.

cally powered as opposed to the SVN, which is pneumatically powered (Figure 41-8) (Branson and Seger, 1988).

A key element in aerosol delivery is particle size. The size of the aerosol particle will determine its ability to penetrate into the airway before depositing or raining out. The therapeutic range is considered 1 μ with the smaller range of particles having the greatest penetrating ability. The larger particles deposit sooner. If they are greater than 5 μ then the chances of entry into the airway are less. The particles may deposit in the nose and proximal airway. The greatest amount of alveolar deposition (95% to 100%) occurs in the 1 to 2 μ range. On the other hand, aerosol particles smaller than 1 μ are so stable that they may not deposit at all (Kacmarek et al., 1991).

Although particle size is important in determining appropriate deposition, a patient's ventilatory pattern is probably more important in that it is the more variable and controllable of the two. Gravity also plays a factor, and it too can be used to benefit particle deposition. Patients should be sitting up as much as possi-

ble while taking slow, deep breaths with a short 3- to 4-second inspiratory hold. Mouth breathing is encouraged if aerosol therapy is delivered by mask. Nasal breathing may filter out particles of optimal size. Of course, not all patients will be able to achieve this position and ventilatory pattern, and the therapist must modify accordingly.

In comparing SVN with MDI's ability to deliver medications, it is found that the MDI is either equal in efficacy or outperforms nebulizers. Significant cost savings are also realized by those institutions who recognize MDI usage as an effective means of aerosol medication delivery over SVN (Orens, Kester, Fergus, and Stoller, 1991).

To further enhance the efficacy of the MDI treatment, a spacer or holding chamber may be attached to trap the aerosol particles before inhalation. This device allows greater drug particle deposition to the airways and reduces oropharyngeal deposition (Ashworth, Wilson, Sims, Wotton, and Hardy, 1991). Ventilator patients that are receiving drug aerosol therapy also receive greater benefit from an in-line MDI with a holding chamber as compared with a jet nebulizer (Fuller, Dolvich, Posmituck, Pack, and Newhouse, 1990).

Aerosol-Therapy Precautions

It should be mentioned that there are hazards associated with aerosol therapy. Bronchospasm may occur as the smooth muscle of the bronchial passages react to foreign particles entering the lung. Shortness of breath and respiratory distress may also occur as a result of dried retained secretions swelling and occluding portions of the lung. Cross contamination is a concern in that aerosol devices may harbor organisms that can be transmitted to patients. Frequent equipment changes and proper sterilization and cleaning techniques are key in preventing this occurrence.

MECHANICAL VENTILATION

The subject of mechanical ventilation is vast and highly technical. The purpose of this section is to give the reader a concise overview of mechanical ventila-

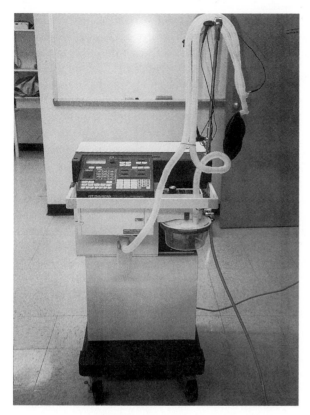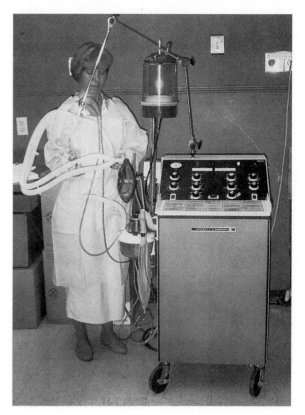

FIGURE 41-9

A, Puritan Bennett 7200a microprocessor driven ventilator. **B,** Bennett MA-1 ventilator-bellows system driven by an electric compressor.

tion and provide a foundation from which to make appropriate decisions when working in this environment.

Many disease states that lead to cardiac and/or respiratory failure will require mechanical ventilation to support the patient's effort to ventilate and oxygenate (Figure 41-9). Today, patients receiving mechanical ventilator support can be found in both the hospital and the home. Acute exacerbations of disorders such as emphysema, COPD, and chronic bronchitis commonly require mechanical ventilation and are generally seen in hospital ICUs. Disorders requiring long-term ventilation, such as spinal cord injury, brain injury, and certain neuromusculoskeletal diseases, may be found receiving mechanical ventilation in the home or long-term care facility.

Today, mechanical ventilator assistance is provided primarily by machines that deliver preset posi-

tive pressure breaths to a patient. Positive pressure ventilation is opposite of normal physiological ventilation in that normal ventilation occurs when negative pressure, created by contraction of the diaphragm, causes air to enter the lungs. Whereas normal inspiration occurs by "pulling" air into the lungs, ventilators "push" air into the lungs. This is important in that the thoracic cavity becomes an area of higher pressure, which may create adverse cardiovascular and hemodynamic events.

Modes of Mechanical Ventilation

The physician and respiratory therapist have a never-ending sea of choices in which to choose the most appropriate method of ventilation. This area sometimes presents confusing terminology and a lack of consistency. In fact, choosing the appropriate mode of ventilation may be considered more of an art than a science. Before describing the modes of ventilation, the following terms should be defined:

1. **Trigger**—Variable that causes a breath to be delivered by the ventilator. A patient may inhale causing the ventilator circuit pressure to drop to a preset number (i.e., less than 1 or 2 cm H_2O). This is called a *pressure trigger.* Some ventilators are volume and flow triggered.

2. **Flowrate**—The speed at which the ventilator breath is delivered. This parameter is usually measured in liters per minute.

3. **Frequency**—Refers to the number of breaths delivered over time (e.g., 10 breaths per minute).

4. **Spontaneous breath**—Breathing through the ventilator circuit without assistance.

The following is a description of common current ventilator modes:

- **Controlled mechanical ventilation (CMV).** The control mode is a lesser used method of ventilation and generally requires the patient be sedated and paralyzed. The ventilator delivers all breaths at a preset frequency, volume or pressure, and flowrate. The patient cannot take spontaneous breaths or trigger the machine.

- **Assist control (AC).** The patient receives a preset pressure or volume, frequency or number of breaths, and flowrate. In between machine-cycled breaths, the patient can trigger the machine to deliver another breath at the preset parameters. All breaths are machine delivered. No spontaneous breathing can occur.

- **Assisted mechanical ventilation.** This mode is similar to AC, however, there is no set frequency. The patient triggers the machine at will to deliver a set pressure or volume at a set flowrate.

- **Intermittent mandatory ventilation (IMV).** As the ventilator delivers a set mandatory frequency and volume or pressure, the patient is allowed to take spontaneous breaths between cycles. This is a former popular mode.

- **Synchronized intermittent mandatory ventilation (SIMV).** This mode improves on that of IMV in that it synchronizes the machine delivered

breaths with the patient's spontaneous breaths. In IMV the machine may cycle a breath before the patient can completely exhale a spontaneous breath. If no inspiratory effort is present, the machine delivers the mandatory breaths.

- **Continuous positive airway pressure (CPAP).** The patient spontaneously breathes and a preset level of pressure is constantly maintained. This method of ventilation can also be achieved through use of commercially available pneumatically powered units that hook directly into the oxygen wall outlet. A tight fitting mask is secured around the patient's mouth and nose, and a preset pressure and oxygen percentage is delivered.

- **Airway pressure release ventilation (APRV).** The patient is allowed to spontaneously breathe with a set amount of CPAP. If additional ventilation is required, the CPAP will be dropped periodically, releasing the pressure, causing the patient to exhale. When the exhalation is complete, CPAP is restored. Proponents of this mode claim that by allowing the patient control, patient comfort and compliance are high.

- **Pressure support ventilation (PSV).** In using pressure support the patient is allowed to breathe spontaneously and receives a preset amount of inspiratory support until the flowrate reaches a minimal level. The patient controls the frequency, tidal volume, inspiratory time. This mode is often used in conjunction with SIMV. This mode is also popular due to high patient compliance.

- **Mandatory minute ventilation (MMV).** The patient is allowed to breathe spontaneously; however, a minimal level of minute ventilation will be achieved through ventilator-assisted breaths. This is usually accomplished by using PSV.

- **Volume-assured pressure support (VAPS).** This is one of the newest modes of ventilation. It allows the patient to breathe spontaneously in the PSV mode and monitors each breath's tidal volume. If the breath is not going to reach the set volume, the ventilator will hold the flowrate constant and increase the pressure until the desired volume is reached (Branson and Chatburn, 1992).

Alarm Management and Precautions

When working around ventilators, it is inevitable that alarms will sound. Alarms are important indicators of a patient's condition or machine malfunction. All alarms should be recognized and valued as excellent sources of information. If alarms are silenced or ignored without interpretation, patient fatalities may result.

The most common alarms are those which monitor high and low pressure, FI_{O2}, apnea, disconnection, and volume. Generally, if the high-pressure alarm continues to sound, the patient should be checked for secretion buildup. Suctioning can remedy this problem. The ventilator tubing should also be checked for possible occlusion from compression or excessive water buildup (Figure 41-10). Low pressure may signify a leak in the ventilator circuitry or a bad patient connection.

If you are unfamiliar with a particular ventilator and an alarm sounds that you are unable to identify and/or remedy, first ensure the patient is not in any extra distress. Assess the overall appearance and, most of all, rise and fall of the chest as the ventilator cycles. If the patient does not appear to be receiving breaths, immediate action should be taken to remove the ventilator from the patient and to begin manual ventilation with a self-inflating bag. The respiratory care practioner should be called to rectify the situation. When the problem is resolved, the patient should be returned to the mechanical ventilator.

One primary precaution to keep in mind when working with a ventilator patient is to watch for condensation in the tubing that could accidentally be poured directly into the patients lungs. When moving a ventilator patient, plan ahead by securing all lines, wires, and tubing. Follow the appropriate procedure for emptying any water from the ventilator tubing before moving the patient. Aspiration of water from ventilator tubing can be fatal.

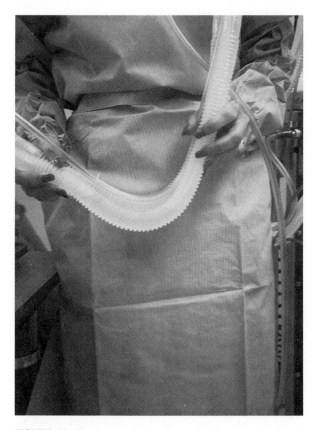

FIGURE 41-10
Condensation build-up in ventilator tubing—a potential hazard.

SUMMARY

Physical therapists need to understand the basic equipment and principles of respiratory care in order to optimize functional outcomes of their patients.

REVIEW QUESTIONS

1. If precise control of oxygen percentage to a patient is warranted, what type of delivery system is indicated?
2. Does mouth breathing by a patient on a nasal cannula indicate that he is receiving no oxygen?
3. Why do low-flow oxygen masks require a certain minimum liter flow, that is, 5 to 6 L/min for a simple mask?
4. Why is IPPB come into question as an effective modality?
5. What are two concerns regarding condensation collecting in mechanical ventilator tubing?

References

Ashworth, H.L., Wilson, C.G., Sims, E.E., Wotton, P.K., & Hardy, J.G. (1991). Delivery of propellant soluble drug from a metered dose inhaler. *Thorax, 46*(4), 245-247.

Barbarash, R.A., Smith, L.A., Godwin, J.E., & Sahn, S.A. (1990). Mechanical ventilation. *DICP, The Annals of Pharmacotherapy, 24,* 959-970.

Bazuaye, E.A., Stone, T.N., Corris, P.A., & Gibson, G.J. (1992). Variability of inspired oxygen concentration with nasal cannulas. *Thorax, 47*(8), 609-611.

Branson, R.D., & Seger, S.M. (1988). Bronchial hygiene techniques. In R.M. Kacmarek, & J.K. Stoller. *Current respiratory care* (pp. 24-28). Philadelphia: B.C. Decker.

Branson, R.D., & Chatburn, R.L. (1992). Technical description and classification of modes of ventilator operation. *Respiratory Care, 37*(9), 1026-1044.

Burns, S.M. (1990). Advances in ventilatory therapy: high-frequency, pressure support, and nocturnal nasal positive pressure ventilation. *Focus on Critical Care, 17*(3), 227-237.

Burton, G.G., Hodgkin, J.E., & Ward, J.J. (1991). *Respiratory care a guide to clinical practice* (3rd ed.) (pp. 524-525). Philadelphia: J.B. Lippincott.

Duffy S.Q., & Farley, D.E. (1992). The protracted demise of medical technology: the case of intermittent positive pressure breathing. *Medical Care, 30*(8), 718-734.

Dunlevy, C.L., & Tyl, S.E. (1992). The effect of oral versus nasal breathing on oxygen concentrations received from nasal cannulas. *Respiratory Care, 37*(4), 357-60.

Frownfelter, D.L. (1987). *Chest physical therapy and pulmonary rehabilitation an interdisciplinary approach* (2nd ed.). St Louis: Mosby.

Fuller, H.D., Dolovich, M.B., Posmituck, G., Pack, W.W., & Newhouse, M.T. (1990). Pressurized aerosol versus jet aerosol delivery to mechanically ventilated patients. Comparison of dose to the lungs. *American Review of Respiratory Disease, 141*(2), 440-444.

Handelsman, H. (1991). Intermittent positive pressure breathing (IPPB) therapy. *Health Technology Assessment Reports, 1,* 1-9.

Hodgkin, J.E., Connors, G.L., & Bell, C.W. (1993). *Pulmonary rehabilitation guidlines to success* (2nd ed.). Philadelphia: JB Lippincott.

Jackson, M., King, M.A., Wells, F.C., & Shneerson, J.M. (1992). Clnical experience and physiologic results with an implantable intratracheal oxygen catheter. *Chest, 102*(5), 1413-8.

Jensen, A.G., Johnson, A., & Sandstedt, S. (1991). Rebreathing during oxygen treatment with face mask. The effect of oxygen flow rates on ventilation. *Acta Anaesthesiologica Scandinavica, 35*(4), 289-292.

Kacmarek, R.M., Mack, C.W., & Dimas, S. (1990). *The essentials of respiratory care* (3rd ed.). St. Louis: Mosby.

Kent, C., et al. (1987). A program for transtracheal oxygen delivery: Assessment of safety and efficacy. *Annals of Internal Medicine, 107,* 802-808.

Orens, K.D., Kester, L., Fergus L.C., & Stoller, J.K. (1991). Cost impact of metered dose inhalers vs small volume nebulizers in hospitalized patients: the cleveland clinic experience. *Respiratory Care, 36*(10), 1099-1104.

Pilbeam, S.P. (1992). *Mechanical ventilation physiological and clinical applications.* St. Louis: Mosby.

Zadai, C.C. (1992). *Pulmonary management in physical therapy.* New York: Churchill Livingstone.

CHAPTER 42

Care of the Patient With an Artificial Airway

Lisa Sigg Mendelson

KEY TERMS

Airway clearance
Artificial airway
Suctioning

Tracheostomy
Tracheostomy tube/cuff

HISTORICAL PERSPECTIVE

An artificial airway is a tube inserted in the trachea either through the mouth or nose or by a surgical incision. Artificial airways have been known to medical science for 3000 years. George Washington ultimately died of upper airway obstruction because his physicians could not agree on the use of tracheostomy. It was not until 1909, when Chevalier Jackson published his classical paper on tracheotomy, that this procedure gained some acceptance. The procedure did not become a highly specialized technique in patient care until the invention of modern tracheostomy tubes and the development of intermittent positive-pressure ventilators. In today's clinical practice, artificial airways have the following four basic

purposes: (1) to bypass upper airway obstruction, (2) to assist or control respirations over prolonged periods, (3) to facilitate the care of chronic respiratory tract infections, and (4) to prevent aspiration of oral and gastric secretions. Multiple disease processes and traumatic problems can require an artificial airway, but each situation, simple or complex, can fit into one or several of these categories (see box on p. 762).

INDICATIONS OF NEED—OBSERVATION

The respiratory care team can play a vital role in recognizing patient need for a tracheostomy from physiological changes that indicate respiratory distress. Cardinal signs of dangerous airway obstruction are

---

Disease Processes that Could Require an Artificial Airway because of Respiratory Insufficiency

1. Primary lung disease (e.g., emphysema, chronic bronchitis, pulmonary fibrosis, cystic fibrosis, severe pneumonia, burned lung, and toxic inhalation).

2. Systemic disease with secondary lung involvement (e.g., cardiac failure, renal failure (fluid overload), and multi-organ system failure).

3. Neuromuscular disease (e.g., polio, Guillain-Barré syndrome, myasthenia gravis, use of muscle relaxants, and tetanus).

4. Central nervous system depression (e.g., drugs, postanesthesia, metabolical coma, cerebrovascular accident, meningitis, and central nervous system tumors).

5. Trauma (e.g., head/neck/chest surgery or injuries).

6. Diseases complicated by extremes of age (e.g., premature infant or elderly).

7. Mechanical obstruction (e.g., upper airway infection, laryngeal paralysis, tumor, edema, bleeding, foreign body, and thyroid malignancy).

8. Recurrent aspiration (e.g., glottic incompetence, occlusive diseases of the esophagus, and swallowing disorders of various causes).

From Selecky PA: Tracheostomy—a review of present day indications, complications and care, *Heart Lung* 3: 272-283, 1974.

---

stridor and chest wall retractions. Early clinical signs may include restlessness, agitation, tachycardia, confusion, motor dysfunction, and decreased oxygen saturation on pulse oximetry. These signs may be accompanied by headache, flapping tremor, and diaphoresis. Cyanosis from impaired oxygenation of the blood is a late, ominous sign.

In children, restlessness must be due to lack of oxygen unless another factor (e.g., thirst) is clearly evident. Extreme fatigue and an inability to sleep indicate impending danger. Apprehension, restlessness, and mental confusion at any age may be taken as early signs of hypoxia.

Complications of Tracheostomy

The selection of the appropriate airway is made by the following factors: (1) What is the best means of accomplishing the goal? (2) Is it an emergency or a controlled, determined situation? (3) Will the airway be needed for long-term care? In general, oral endotracheal tubes are inserted in emergencies. They are the quickest and easiest tubes to insert even for relatively untrained personnel. A nasotracheal tube will generally replace the oral endotracheal tube for a long-term intubation. The nasal tube is more efficient in that it is better secured, the patient may eat, it is easier to suction, and it is generally more comfortable for the patient.

There are certain complications with nasotracheal tubes. Among these are sinus blockage and pain, vocal cord damage, or pressure necrosis to the cartilaginous structure of the nose. To reduce these complications, the airway should be evaluated daily. The tube should be removed as quickly as possible when the indication for intubation is reversed. However, if there appears to be a need for a more long-term airway, a tracheostomy should be considered. The procedure should not be taken lightly because many additional complications may occur.

Complications of tracheostomy can be surgical, postoperative, or physiological. Complications that occur at the time of the operation are more frequently direct results of the surgical procedure itself. Delayed complications may result directly or indirectly from surgery, from postoperative care, or from the abrupt physiological changes resulting from tracheostomy. Nursing objectives in caring for the patient after a tracheostomy are to maintain patency of the tube, cleanliness of the wound site, and good aeration and to observe any changes in the patient's vital signs and oxygenation by pulse oximetry.

In patients with artificial airways the normal physiological mechanism for adding moisture to the air via the nasal mucosa obviously is bypassed. Therefore supplemental humidification is extremely important to protect the mucosa from drying and crusting, which results in obstruction.

The dressing under the tracheostomy tube and tracheostomy ties should be changed when they become soiled because dried blood and other secretions near the incision can encourage bacterial growth. The incision should be checked frequently for bleeding. The skin may be cleaned with half-strength hydrogen peroxide and sterile saline when a new dressing is applied. The dressing should be folded into place—never cut. This eliminates the possibility of lint or frayed threads being aspirated. Commercially prepared dressings best meet these criteria.

When changing the tapes that hold the tube in place, it is best to have one nurse hold the tube in place while another replaces the old tapes. An angle is cut at the end of the tape to facilitate its placement through the flange of one side of the tube. The tape is then threaded through the back of the tracheostomy tube and through the other flanged opening and tied securely with a square knot placed on one side of the patient's neck. One finger should be placed under the twill tape while tying to prevent the tape from being tied too tight.

Pneumothorax can occur immediately after tracheostomy because of laceration of the mediastinal pleura at the time of surgery or within 24 hours (arises often in children and patients with chronic obstructive lung disease). Other problems include air embolism, aspiration, and subcutaneous and mediastinal emphysema. Recurrent laryngeal nerve damage or posterior tracheal penetration may occur but is uncommon.

Postoperative Physiological Complications

Attentive nursing care is the single most essential factor in postoperative management. A ratio of one nurse for each patient is the ideal; however, since this is not often possible, increased vigilance by the entire respiratory care team is of vital importance.

A patient with an artificial airway is understandably apprehensive and has special communication needs. He or she should also be reminded that the inability to phonate is only temporary. The patient must be reassured that he or she will be attended to constantly and will be able to trust and depend fully on the nursing staff to attend to his or her needs. If alert, the patient must be equipped with a signal light or bell, paper and pencil, magic slate, or picture board for communication.

Airway obstruction is the foremost complication that exists for the postoperative tracheostomy patient. Tracheal secretions are the major source of obstruction, particularly if they are excessive or viscous. When using cuffed tube, acute obstruction might occur from overinflating the cuff, which would allow it to balloon over the end of the tube. Other causes of obstruction are dislodgement of the tube into a false tract anterior to the tube tracheal opening, occlusion by an overinflated cuff, and kinking of softened plastic cannula.

Tracheobronchitis, inflammation of the trachea and bronchus, is a complication resulting primarily from irritation resulting from incorrect suctioning technique.

Crusting is a common and complex problem that may result from inadequate humidification of inspired air or may result from dehydration. In many instances, ulceration of the tracheal mucosa results from irritation by the airway or incorrect suctioning. This ulcerated area becomes infected with various organisms and is virtually covered by crust. Further suctioning removes the crust, causing discharge of serum and bleeding. The discharge produces a wet eschar that is covered with mucus. Because of the drying effect of air passing over this mass, a hard crust can form. This process can compound the difficulty because the development of this crust in the trachea might eventually produce a mass large enough to completely plug the tracheal cannula and almost completely obstruct the trachea. Cases have been cited where an entire cast of the tracheobronchial tree has been removed.

Other physiological complications may be related to the following: (1) hypoxia developing before or during the procedure and resulting in an uncontrollable patient, cardiac arrest, and increased myocardial sensitivity to adrenalin; (2) alkalosis developing from rapid carbon dioxide wash-out after establishment of the airway, resulting in myocardial fibrillation and apnea; (3) cardiac failure, resulting in profuse bronchorrhea caused by pulmonary edema and shock.

Other chronic complications cited by Dailey, Simon, Young, and Stewart (1992) include the following: (1) infection at the surgical site, (2) aspiration, (3) aerophagia, (4) persistent stoma, and (5) tracheal stenosis.

Postoperative Mechanical Complications

Dislocation of the tube may result from unsatisfactory nursing care, poor attention to the airway during positioning, or ventilator tubing pulling on the airway. If the tracheostomy tube tapes are not kept tight and tied with a square knot or if they become loose as a result of cervical emphysema or edema, the tube may be coughed out of the trachea and become lodged in the tissues of the neck and obstruct the airway.

Stay sutures are useful in tracheostomy patients when there is the possibility of tube displacement. These sutures are valuable during recannulization of the tube if it comes dislodged before a tract has been well established. Stay sutures will prevent entry into a false tract. Advantages of this technique include the following: (1) blockage or displaced tubes can be rapidly replaced, (2) exposure of the trachea at surgical intervention is improved, (3) firm anchoring of the trachea at the moment of incision, (4) decreased trauma associated with extubation, and (5) uniform tracheostomy technique for all ages.

Dislodgement of the outer cannula or required removal before a tract has been well established (usually 5 to 10 days) again requires diligence and quick action by the nurse. No attempt at reinsertion should be made without adequate light, satisfactory tissue retraction, tracheal hook, and a Trousseau's dilator. A Trousseau's dilator and tracheal hook should be readily available. A spare tracheostomy tube of the correct size should be kept at the patient's bedside at all times. Then, should the tube be coughed out, the nurse uses the Trousseau's dilator to hold the wound apart while summoning the physician. Tragedies have occurred from inserting the tube into the soft tissues of the neck or mediastinum because of a dislodged cannula and the frantic efforts to replace it. Once the tracheostomy tract has been firmly established, the tube can be replaced by the nurse on written order of the physician.

TRACHEOSTOMY TUBES

Metal Tubes

Tracheostomy tubes are of two basic types—metal and polyvinyl chloride (hard and soft). Metal tubes can be made of either stainless steel or sterling silver and composed of the following three parts: (1) an outer cannula that fits into the tracheal incision, (2) an inner cannula that fits into the outer cannula, and (3) an obturator. Before the outer cannula is inserted into the tracheal incision, the obturator is placed inside. The lower end of the obturator protrudes from the end of the outer cannula and facilitates its insertion into the trachea. This is the only purpose of the obturator. The protruding end of the obturator obstructs the lumen of the outer cannula. When the obturator is removed, immediately replace it with the inner cannula. When dealing with metal tubes, the parts of each set are not interchangeable and fit only one particular set. If one part is lost or damaged, the entire set is useless. Therefore each part, including obturator, is accounted for carefully. Plastic tubes generally have interchangeable parts. Care should be exercised in handling sterling silver tubes, since silver is easily dented.

Mucus that has dried inside the inner cannula cannot be cleaned by merely rinsing in water. The cannula should be soaked in hydrogen peroxide and scrubbed with a tracheostomy brush and rinsed with saline to be sure all secretions have been removed. If a silver inner cannula becomes discolored, it may be cleaned with silver polish.

The inner cannula should always be inspected to be sure it is clean and clear of secretions before it is reinserted. Be sure to lock the inner cannula in position after reinsertion.

Polyvinyl Chloride (Plastic) Disposable Tubes and Cuff Inflation

The development of plastic tracheostomy tubes came about for the following three important reasons:

(1) application of silicone to the inner surface of the plastic tube minimizes crusting and adherence of secretions; (2) there is greater ease in attaching a safe, dependable, permanent inflatable cuff to the plastic tube that cannot slip off and occlude the tracheal opening; and (3) lower costs allow the tube to be disposable. Plastic tubes come with and without cuffs.

The cuffed tracheostomy tube is primarily used in conjunction with a positive-pressure ventilator to form a closed system (Figure 42-1). It is also used to reduce the possibility of aspiration because of absent, protective laryngeal, and pharyngeal reflexes. The inflatable cuff is located around the lower portion of the tube and, when inflated, seals the trachea from most airflow except through the tube itself (see Figure 42-1). The cuff, usually made of pliable plastic, is inflated by injecting air into the fine-bore tubing. A small pilot balloon is located proximally in the tubing and indicates that the cuff is inflated. The nurse must check the inflation end of the cuff and the balloon be-

fore insertion of the tube into the trachea to be certain that there are no leaks. The Luer valve inflation port to the pilot balloon is self-sealing. Some Luer valves have a relief valve when pressure exceeds 25 mm Hg.

Cuff Inflation

There are two commonly used methods of cuff inflation. These are the minimal air leak, in which a small amount of air escapes on inspiration, and minimal occlusive volume, in which just enough air is placed in the cuff to stop air from escaping on inspiration. According to Crabtree Goodnough (1988), the minimal leak cuff technique may produce less injury than the minimal occlusive volume inflation technique. Regardless of which technique is used, the pressure of the cuff should be checked every 4 to 8 hours and the pressures documented. With continued research and monitoring of tracheal cuff pressures, potential tracheal injury can be prevented.

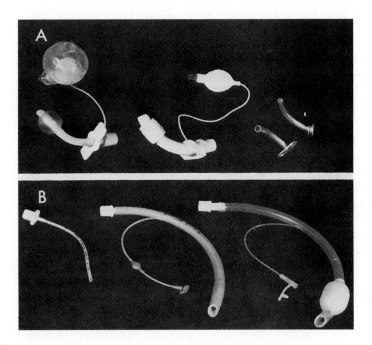

FIGURE 42-1
A, Cuffed adult tracheostomy tubes, uncuffed pediatric tracheostomy tube (far left). **B,** Cuffed adult endotracheal tubes, uncuffed pediatric endotracheal tube (far left).

Once the cuff is inflated, the only route for air exchange is through the patient's tracheostomy tube; therefore careful observation of the patient by the nurse is essential. If the patient is on mechanical ventilation, observation is essential if there is ventilator failure because asphyxiation may occur. Alarms are always in the "on" position when a patient is being mechanically ventilated. Some means of resuscitation, such as a manual resuscitating bag with mask, must be available at the bedside to ventilate the patient in case the tracheostomy tube comes out or is dislodged.

Considerable emphasis has been given to the incidence of tracheal ischemia and resulting stenosis from the use of a cuffed tube. This ischemia results from the pressure of the cuffed tube against the tracheal wall, which heals with scar formation, resulting in subsequent stenosis. This complication can be reduced or eliminated by minimal air leak or minimal occlusive volume. For the minimal occlusive volume, the cuff must be inflated to eliminate any air leak on inspiration. Cuff pressures should be monitored and documented every 4 to 8 hours to prevent tracheal injury. The recommended cuff pressure is 15 to 25 mm Hg. Inflate the cuff until there is no air leak between the wall of the trachea and the cuff, and then release a small amount of air to allow only a slight air leak between the walls of the trachea and the cuff. This reduces the pressure of the cuff, still allows the ventilator to function properly, and reduces the likelihood of tracheal ischemia. Any difficulty in properly inflating the cuffed tracheostomy tube should be immediately reported to the physician.

If the tracheotomized patient is conscious, he or she may attempt to speak. If the cuff is properly inflated, he or she will be aphonic, since no air can pass over the vocal cords. If he or she needs to speak, the cuff can be deflated, and the patient may be given a sterile dressing to hold over the tube. This will allow him or her to speak and also simulate a cough by rapid exhalation to clear secretions.

Inspired air must be continuously and adequately humidified by means of nebulizing equipment to prevent the formation of crusts. The equipment used for this purpose can be a possible source of infection. Therefore the nebulizer and tubing should be changed ideally every 8 hours but at least once every 24 hours.

The Communitrache I is a tracheostomy tube that permits the removal of secretions above the inflation cuff without nasotracheal suctioning. The other plus factor to this tracheostomy tube is the patient's ability to communicate, especially while on a ventilator. When the patient is weaned from the ventilator, a fenestrated tube may be used. Fenestrated comes from the French word *fenestre,* meaning window. There is a window (fenestration) in the outer cannula. When the tube is used for speaking the cuff is down, the inner cannula removed, and an external plug is inserted to cap the tracheostomy tube to allow the patient to speak. The cuff must be deflated when the cap is in place. If the cuff was inflated, the patient would be unable to breathe air into the lungs. The patient exhibits immediate distress if this mistake is made. If a patient with fenestrated tube needs to be suctioned, the inner cannula must be placed so that the suction catheter does not enter the fenestration and cause injury to the tracheal wall mucosa.

Other Airway Devices

The Olympic tracheostomy button is used as an interim airway after tracheostomy tube removal (Figure 42-2). This method is another example of weaning a patient from tracheostomy tube but still maintaining the stoma should a tracheostomy be again needed. The patient that benefited most from the procedure was the COPD patient. This was one method used to facilitate secretion removal after hospitalization when it became necessary because of the disease process. The Olympic tracheostomy button allowed the tracheostomy patient the opportunity to reestablish an unobstructed airway and at the same time allowed the patient to speak.

The Passy-Muir valve is used for patients with upper airway obstruction and with difficult decannulation (Figure 42-3). The Passy-Muir is a one-way valve, allowing inspiration only and forcing exhalation through the upper airway. By using the valve the upper airway muscles gradually recover, allowing for transition to a fenestrated tube or a smaller size tracheostomy tube and preparing the patient for eventual decannulation (Pierson and Kacmarek, 1992).

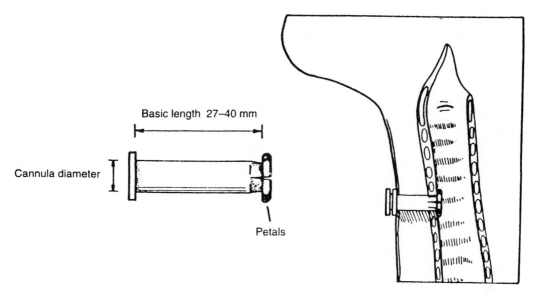

FIGURE 42-2

Dimensions and actual positioning of an Olympic tracheostomy button. (From Pierson DJ and Kacmarek RM: *Foundations of respiratory care,* Churchill Livingstone, 1992, Edinburgh © David J. Pierson.)

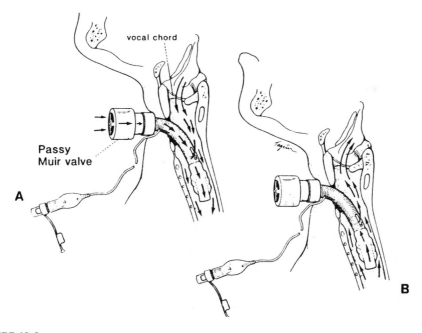

FIGURE 42-3

The Passy Muir Valve. This valve attaches to a standard 15-mm tracheostomy adapter. It allows inspriation **A,** via the valve, but exhilation **B,** must occur via the upper airway. (From Pierson DJ and Kacmarek RM: *Foundations of respiratory care,* Churchill Livingstone, 1992, Edinburgh © David J. Pierson.)

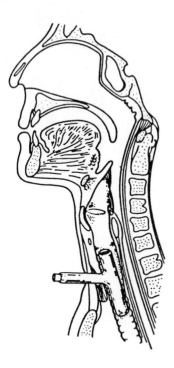

FIGURE 42-4
The Montgomery T-tube. (Reprinted with permission from Montgomery WW: Manual care of the Montgovery silicone tracheal T-tube. *The annals of otology rhinology & laryngology (supplement 73)* 89(4): 3, 1980.)

The management of major airway obstruction by tracheal tumor, external compression, or tracheal disease below the thoracic inlet still present difficult problems. The Montgomery T tube is a bifurcated silicone rubber stent designed to preserve patency of the airways in a patient with injury to the trachea or main bronchi (Figure 42-4). When the T tube is in place, the patient breathes normally through nose and mouth and can speak. The T tube is a method in which secretions can be removed if necessary and is helpful in long-term therapy to alleviate obstruction or during reconstructive surgery. This device does not cause any adverse tissue reaction on a long-term basis, according to Montgomery.

Airway Care

Normally, the mucociliary escalator and the cough reflex provide airway clearance. When these mechanisms fail, suctioning of the airways is indicated. Suctioning does have potential hazards, but it should be a safe procedure with proper guidance and care.

Suctioning

Proper explanation of the suctioning technique to the patient helps allay apprehension and enhance cooperation. Medicate your postoperative patient before suctioning to decrease the pain of coughing. Always maintain a calm and reassuring manner.

Maintain aseptic technique throughout the entire procedure. Use sterile gloves and a sterile disposable catheter for each suctioning.

Position the patient properly unless contraindicated. Nasotracheal and/or pharyngeal suctioning should be done with the patient in Fowler, 60 to 70 degrees, or semi-Fowler position, approximately 45 degrees, with the neck hyperextended (Figure 42-5). The supine position is best for the patient with tracheostomy or endotracheal tubes (Figure 42-6).

Pharyngeal suctioning may be necessary before deflating the cuffed tracheostomy tube. The nurse should not suction the pharynx and then the trachea with the same catheter, but the trachea may be suctioned first and then the pharynx with the same catheter.

Duration of suctioning is of extreme importance. Each suctioning procedure should last no longer than 5 to 10 seconds to avoid hypoxia.

Prolonged suctioning may result in precipitating a dysrhythmia or cardiac arrest. A good way to judge the elapsed time is to hold one's own breath and be guided by the development of discomfort. This is most important for the patient who depends on ventilatory assistance.

The lowest possible vacuum settings are to be used (below 120 mm Hg) that will still support suctioning the tracheostomy tube. The higher the setting is raised, the greater the risk of trauma to the tracheal mucosa. Caution should be exercised to avoid kinking the suction tubing or catheter. When negative pressure is excessive and released suddenly, inadvertent removal of portions of tracheal mucosa may occur.

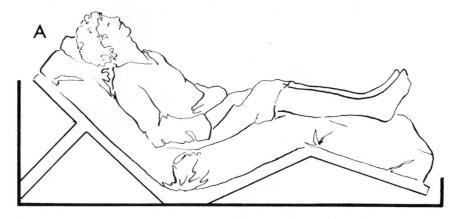

Fowler 60-70 degrees

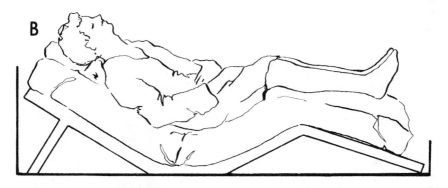

Semi-Fowler 10-12″

FIGURE 42-5
A, Fowler's and **B,** Semi-Fowler's positions.

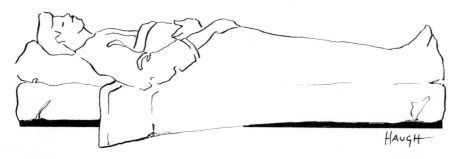

FIGURE 42-6
Supine position.

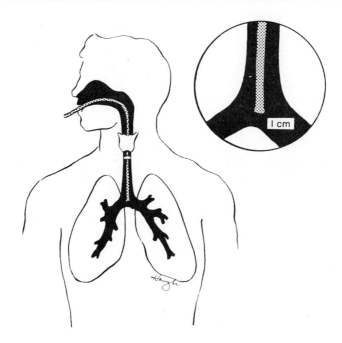

FIGURE 42-7
The catheter will simulate coughing when it contacts the carina (in a patient with cough reflex).

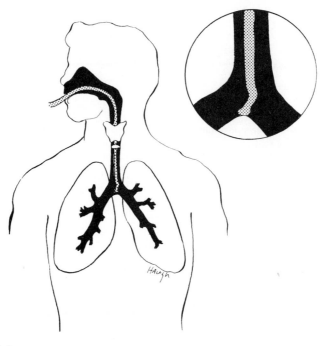

FIGURE 42-8
The catheter is withdrawn 1 cm after it reaches the carina, before applying suction.

Insertion of the suction catheter should be done gently, using aseptic technique and sterile gloves. Goggles are used as part of universal precautions if there is any danger of coughed-out secretions. The catheter should first be moistened in sterile saline or with a water-soluble gel. Suction is not applied while the catheter is passed down into the trachea. Proper insertion of the catheter will stimulate coughing when it contacts the carina (Figure 42-7). It is then immediately withdrawn 1 cm before suction is applied (Figure 42-8). Do not force the catheter up and down while suctioning. Suction is applied only while the catheter is being withdrawn. Rotating the catheter during withdrawal results in suctioning a larger area and increases the surface contact of the trachea and tracheostomy tube (Figure 42-9).

Left main-stem bronchus aspiration is more difficult because of the anatomical arrangement of the bronchus. It was formerly thought that left bronchial aspiration was facilitated by turning the patient's head to the right. Studies by Kirimli et al. (1970) and Panacek et al. (1989) indicate that left bronchial aspiration is best accomplished by using a Coudé tip catheter. After its insertion into the trachea, the curved tip should be positioned to point toward the left main-stem bronchus. Even so, insertion is difficult, and auscultation by stethoscope is necessary to thoroughly access the suctioning.

Right main-stem bronchus aspiration is the usual case because of the more direct alignment of this bronchus with the trachea. This can be carried out almost always with a straight tracheal catheter.

Excessive suctioning can be harmful. Use judgment to determine just how often a patient requires suctioning. Auscultation by stethoscope should be used to determine the thoroughness of suctioning. Suction only when it is needed (Carroll, 1994). Allow the patient to rest and breathe between each insertion of the suction catheter and, if necessary, ventilate him or her for few minutes before further suctioning. Remember each suctioning attempt removes air as well as secretions. Hyperoxygenation and hyperinflation with 100% oxygen has been suggested with better results and fewer complications. Complications from tracheal suctioning include the following: (1) hypoxemia, (2) cardiac dysrhythmia, (3) bronchospasm, and (4) infection. Suctioning can lead to hypoxemia because oxygen is removed from the airways, and this could lead to tissue hypoxia. To minimize this problem, preoxygenation is recommended. This can be done by hyperinflating the patient with $1\frac{1}{2}$ times their normal tidal volume on a ventilator and hyperox-genating with 100% oxygen for 3 to 5 breaths. Cardiac dysrhythmias, such as premature ventricular contractures, bradycardia, and tachycardia, can be diminished by hyperinflating and hyperoxygenating the

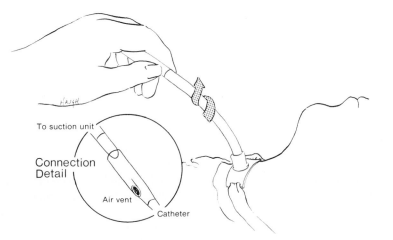

To suction unit

Connection
Detail

Air vent

Catheter

FIGURE 42-9

The catheter is rotated during withdrawal in order to suction a larger surface area.

patient with 100% oxygen. If any dysrhythmias occur on the monitor, the suctioning procedure should be discontinued. Bronchospasm may be effectively prevented by a few puffs of a bronchodilator, such as albuterol, to the tracheostomy tube before suctioning. Infection can be decreased by maintaining sterile technique with sterile gloves and sterile catheters when suctioning.

Suctioning Artificial Airway

Nasotracheal, Endotracheal, and Tracheostomy

1. Check equipment, be sure you have all necessary equipment and maintain sterile field.
2. Check monitors.
3. Wash your hands.
4. Inform patient of the procedure.
5. Hyperoxygenate with 100% oxygen for three to five breaths with manual resuscitation bag.
6. Place patient's neck in extension.
7. Put on sterile gloves.
8. Lubricate catheter with sterile saline or water soluble gel.
9. Place catheter (without suction) upward and backward in short increments. Continue until an obstruction (the carina) is reached.
10. When the carina is stimulated, the patient will generally cough unless his or her reflexes are obtunded.
11. The catheter should be pulled back slightly, from the carina, then suction applied with no more than 120 mm Hg pressure as catheter is withdrawn in a rotating motion.
12. The aspiration time should be within 10 to 15 seconds total. (A good guideline is for the therapist to hold his or her breath during suctioning as the patient is also not breathing. This gives the therapist a better sensitivity for what the patient experiences.)
13. The patient should be allowed to rest for several seconds and again be preoxygenated.
14. Check the patient's breath sounds and repeat the procedure if necessary to remove more secretions.
15. Suction pharynx.
16. The monitor is to be watched for any dysrhythmias.
17. Pulse oximetry is to be used for indications of desaturation.
18. Discard used equipment and remove gloves.
19. Wash your hands.

Nasopharyngeal Airways

When frequent, aggressive nasopharyngeal suctioning is indicated in a semicomatose patient, a nasopharyngeal airway (NPA) will lessen the trauma of frequent passage of the catheter. The NPA is a soft latex material that provides easy access to the trachea for nasopharyngeal suctioning. The nasal and pharyngeal mucosa are protected and the procedure thus becomes more comfortable to the patient. In addition, a fiberoptic bronchoscope may be passed through the airway if the procedure is indicated.

Endotracheal or Tracheostomy Suctioning

The procedures are the same except sterile technique is followed and no lubrication is usually necessary, although it may be used if there is difficulty passing the catheter.

Sterile Suctioning

The technique for correct sterile suctioning of artificial airways is perhaps the most important and vital segment of care for the patient because it removes secretions that would otherwise obstruct the airway. If suctioning is not performed properly, it can cause physiological or psychological trauma to the patient.

The equipment necessary for proper sterile suctioning includes proper mechanical apparatus, connecting tubing, sterile gloves, sterile saline, suction catheters, dressings, and goggles as indicated with universal precautions. While suctioning the patient, it should be remembered that the patient's only air passage is being partially occluded. Thus the suction catheter should never be larger than one half the diameter of the tube opening; if it is larger, it may completely occlude the patient's air passage.

One method of determining the size of the catheter used for suctioning is to double the size of the tracheostomy tube in place and add two. For example, if the patient has a #6 tube, the calculation would be as follows: 6 + 6 = 12 + 2 = 14. Therefore a 14-fr catheter

TABLE 42–1

The Pediatric Trach Card

TRACHEOSTOMY SIZE	RECOMMENDED CATHETER SIZE
Pediatric Tubes	
00 PT	6.5 FR
0 PT	6.5 FR
1 PT	8 FR
2 PT	8 FR
3 PT	10 FR
4 PT	10 FR
Neonatal Tubes	
00 NT	6.5 FR
0 NT	6.5 FR
1 NT	6.5 FR
SCT—Single Cannula Tracheostomy Tubes	
5 SCT	10 FR
6 SCT	12 FR
7 SCT	14 FR
8 SCT	14 FR

Reprinted with permission of Janetti Publications, Inc., publisher *Pediatric Nursing,* Volume 20, Number 2, (March-April, 1994).

would be the largest catheter that could be used to suction the #6 tracheostomy. See Table 42-1 for a correlation of tracheostomy sizes to catheter sizes.

The catheter used for pharyngeal suctioning should never be used for subsequent suctioning of the artificial airway, but using an artificial airway suction catheter for pharyngeal suction is acceptable. Aseptic technique is absolutely necessary to minimize the risk of infection and, ideally, only disposable catheters should be used.

Suctioning may be necessary every few minutes when the patient initially returns from surgery because there is an increase in secretions, which usually results from irritation of the endotracheal tube plus a reflex mechanism initiated by the surgical trauma. Usually by paying attention to the patient's color, respiratory rate, lung sounds, and oxygen saturation on pulse oximetry, the nurse or therapist can determine the amount of secretions present. Excessive mucus in

the trachea or large bronchi is usually indicated by coarse rattling sounds. Fine bubbling sounds usually suggest fluid located more peripherally (i.e., in the alveolar spaces). If accumulated secretions are not cleared, they can cause respiratory and cardiac rates to increase; effective oxygen and carbon dioxide transfer is impaired causing cyanosis to appear and low-grade fever to develop.

Extubation/Decannulation

Extubation or decannulation is the removal of the artificial airway. The patient is helped to gradually relearn normal breathing through his or her upper respiratory tract before the tube is removed. This can be a time of considerable fear and anxiety for patients because they have learned they can breathe safely through their tracheostomy, and they may become apprehensive when asked to breathe in a normal manner. The relearning process can be accomplished under the physician's direction by reducing the lumen of the tube for a day or two or by partially obstructing the tube's outer opening for increasing lengths of time. Eventually, the patient is able to tolerate the complete occlusion of the tracheostomy opening. This is sometimes difficult and similar to breathing through a straw.

When occluding the tracheostomy opening with a cuffed tube, the cuff must be deflated first. Failure to do this will result in total obstruction of the patient's airway as the tube opening is occluded.

Fenestrated tubes have also been excellent for weaning the patient from the tracheostomy tube. Actually, they do not increase the airway resistance as in the above method and are probably more effective. They also allow the patient to talk and attempt to cough to mobilize secretions. Other methods used in decannulation include the Olympic tracheostomy button and the Passy-Muir valve. The Olympic tracheostomy button allows the airway to remain patent for suctioning and reinsertion of a tracheostomy tube should it become necessary. The Passy-Muir valve allows for normal recovery of the upper airway muscle, making it possible to reduce the size of tracheostomy tube leading to eventually plugging and decannulating. Careful observation and documentation of the patient's ability to ventilate must be done when either of these devices are used in the decannulating process.

Close supervision should continue after extubation. After a tracheostomy tube is removed, the skin edges are usually taped together with butterfly strips for a few days until the wound heals. While healing, air will escape through the wound and reduce the effectiveness of the patient's cough. The patient should be instructed that the noise from the partially closed trachea is normal and small secretions should be removed from this area. The patient should be taught to hold a sterile dressing firmly over the incision when coughing until the opening healed.

REVIEW QUESTIONS

1. What physiological changes occur with surgical placement of tracheostomy tube?
2. Discuss possible psycosocial concerns of patients with a tracheostomy.
3. List information that you would include in a teaching plan for the tracheostomized patient.
4. How does the patient care team prepare the tracheostomized patient for self care?
5. Compare emergency care, acute care, and long term care for a patient with upper airway obstruction and tracheostomy placement.

References

Carroll, P. (1994). Safe suctioning PRN. *RN, May,* 32-37.

Class, P. (1992). Nursing considerations for airway management in the PACU. *Current Reviews for Post Anesthesia Care Nurses, 14*(1), 1-8.

Crabtree Goodnough, S.K. (1988). Reducing tracheal injury and aspiration. *Dimension of Critical Care Nursing, 7*(6), 324-331.

Dailey, R.H., Simon, B., Young, G.P., & Stewart, R.D. (1992). Airway maneuvers. In *The airway emergency management.* St. Louis: Mosby.

Frost, E.A. (1976). Tracing the tracheostomy. *Annals of Otolaryngology, 85,* 618-624.

Furtan, N.D, Dutcher, P.O., & Roberts, J.K. (1993). The safety and efficacy of bedside tracheostomy. *Otolaryngology-Head and Neck Surgery,* (109), 707-711.

Goodwell, E.W. (1934). The story of tracheostomy. *British Journal of Children's Diseases, 31*(367-369), 167-176.

Goodwell, E.W. (1934). The story of tracheostomy. *British Journal of Children's Diseases, 31*(370-372), 253-271.

Jackson, C. (1909). Tracheostomy. *Laryngoscope, 18,* 285-290.

Jackson, C. (1921). High tracheostomy and other errors. The chief causes of chronic laryngeal atenosis. *Surgery, Gynecology, Obstetrics, 32,* 392-395.

Jackson, D., & Albamonte, S. (1994). Enhancing communication with the Passy-Muir valve. *Pediatric Nursing, 20,*(2), 149-153.

Kirchner, J.A. (1980). Tracheostomy and its problems. *Surgical Clinics of North America, 60,*(5), 1093-1104.

Kirimli, B., King, J.E., & Pfaeffle, H.H. (1970). Evaluation of tracheobronchial suction technique. *Journal of Thoracic and Cardiovascular Surgery, 59,* 340-344.

Lull, J.M., Pierson, D.J., & Tyler, M.L. (1993). Methods of Airway Maintenance. In *Intensive respiratory care.* Philadelphia: WB Saunders.

Mocaluso, S., & Roman, M. (1994). Managing post-intubation injuries. *Medsurg Nursing, 3*(3), 192-202.

Montgomery, W.W. (1989). Manual of care of the Montgomery silicone tracheal T-tube. *Annals of Otology, Rhinology and Laryngology (Supp. 73), 89(4),* 3.

Montanari, J., & Spearing, C. (1986). Of measuring tracheal cuff pressure. *Nursing, 86*(7), 46-49.

Noll, M.L., Hix, C.D., & Scott, G. (1990). Closed tracheal suction systems: effectiveness and nursing implications. In *AACN clinical issues in critical care nursing.* Philadelphia: JB Lippincott.

Panacek, E.A., Albertson, T.E., Rutherford, W.F., Fisher, C.J., & Foulke, G.E. (1989). Selections left endobronchial suctioning of the intubated patient. *Chest, 95,* 885-87.

Patton, C. (1991). The critical airway classic problems. *Current Reviews for the Post Anesthesia Care Nurses, 13*(5), 33-40.

Pierson, D.J., & Kacmarek, R.M. (1992). In *Foundations of respiratory care.* New York: Churchill Livingstone.

Roberts, J.T. (1994). In Clinical Management of the Airway, Philadelphia: WB Saunders.

Selecky, P. (1974). Tracheostomy—a review of present day indication, complications and care. *Heart Lung, 3,* 272.

Tracheostomy tube adult homecare guide. (1993). Irvine: Mallinckrodt Medical TPT.

Traver, J.A., Mitchell, J.T., & Flodquist-Priestly, G. (1991). Artificial airway care. In *Respiratory care: a clinical approach.* Gaithersberg, Md.: Aspen Publishers.

Traver, J.A., Mitchell, J.T., & Flodquist-Priestly, G. (1991). Suctioning. In *Respiratory care: a clinical approach.* Gaithersberg, Md.: Aspen Publishers.

Warnoch, C., & Porpora, K. (1994). A pediatric trache card: transforming research into practice. *Pediatric Nursing, 20*(2), 186-188.

Weilitz, P.B., & Dettenmeier, P.A. (1994). Back to basics test your knowledge of tracheostomy tubes. *American Journal of Nursing, 94*(2), 46-50.

CHAPTER 43

Respiratory and Cardiovascular Drug Actions

Arthur V. Prancan

INTRODUCTION

The respiratory and cardiovascular systems have many built-in mechanisms for controlling their functions during health and disease. In healthy individuals, both systems act quickly and positively to maintain proper functioning under the most complicated conditions. Even during trauma or disease, these systems often overcome distress and regain normal function. The physiology of respiration or circulation is sometimes altered by a disease so that the homeostatic mechanisms are no longer effective. In such a case, a drug with the appropriate action becomes necessary to restore normal physiological function.

Before a drug can be used effectively, the system it is to modify must be understood. How the mechanism of the drug action relates to the biological system must be clear before an effect can be predicted.

This chapter describes much of the basic respiratory and cardiovascular physiology that underlies the action of the drugs presented. Hopefully, the relationship between basic physiology and the drug mechanism of action is also evident.

All pharmacological interventions for the respiratory and cardiovascular systems are not covered. Certainly no attempt has been made to describe the pharmacology of other systems or disease states.

For further study, one of the books listed in the reference section at the end of the chapter is highly recommended.

AUTONOMIC PHARMACOLOGY

This section introduces the basic aspects of drug action related to both components of the autonomic nervous system—the sympathetic and parasympathetic nervous systems. For both systems, synthesis, storage, and release of the chemical neurotransmitter are described to emphasize the places in the metabolical scheme where drugs can intervene. The sites of action for the adrenergic (sympathetic) and cholinergic (parasympathetic) transmitters and blockers is also described.

The autonomic nervous system controls all of the bodily functions over which you have no voluntary control, and perhaps which you might not control as well if you had the opportunity. The functions include regulation of respiratory airway diameter, respiratory secretions, blood vessel diameter, heart rate, intestinal motility, pupil size, and many others. It is easy to see that it might take more than the talents of a well-trained expert to keep an active person functioning day and night.

The sympathetic nervous system is the half of the autonomic system that takes a dominant role in the cardiovascular and respiratory systems when some sort of bodily activity is necessary. This includes actions such as increasing ventilation capacity, elevating blood pressure, and shunting blood flow to the skeletal muscles. Classically, the sympathetic component of the autonomic nervous system has been called the fight-or-flight system. The other half of the autonomic system is called the parasympathetic nervous system. It is most important in maintaining the less exciting functions of the body like digestion, salivation, and urination. In some organs the two systems work against each other to provide very fast and very fine control. For example, the size of the pupil responds quickly to a change in light intensity. The parasympathetic system actively functions to decrease the size of the opening while the sympathetic system relaxes, thereby causing a quick decrease in pupil size. If the light is turned down, the opposite occurs just as fast. This is a good example of the antagonistic action of the two components of the autonomic nervous system.

Some organs, however, have only one innervation. Much of the arterial blood vessel network is controlled only by sympathetic nerves. Also, gastric secretion and gastric motility are primarily regulated by one system—the parasympathetic.

SYMPATHETIC NEUROTRANSMISSION

Sympathetic nerves transport impulses from the vasomotor center in the medulla of the brain through the spinal cord and out to the smooth muscle, heart muscle, and secretory cells. These tissues have receptor sites that will accept the norepinephrine released from the nerve ending. Norepinephrine, also called *noradrenalin,* is synthesized in the nerve ending only in the sympathetic neurons. It is stored in the terminal until an electric impulse reaches the terminal, then it is released into the synapse.

The norepinephrine molecule attaches to a receptor molecule on a cell surface in the immediate vicinity of its release. This drug-receptor combination causes a biological change, such as stimulation of the pacemaker cells in the heart to fire more frequently (increased heart rate). The effect is terminated when the norepinephrine is reabsorbed into the nerve terminal. About 90% of the released norepinephrine is taken back into the neuron. There, it is either restored into granules for future release or it is destroyed by the enzyme monoamine oxidase (MAO).

There are two types of sympathetic receptors—alpha and beta. The alpha-receptor is found in the arterioles, and the beta-receptor is found in the arterioles, heart, and bronchioles. Stimulation of the alpha-receptor in the arteriole causes vasoconstriction that results in increased blood pressure. The beta-receptor in the arterioles causes vasodilation and a lowered blood pressure. Some drugs stimulate both receptors, and in those cases the effect will be determined by the degree of alpha or beta activity of the drug. An example is norepinephrine. It has 90% alpha activity and 10% beta activity, and it always causes vasoconstriction. Epinephrine is 50% alpha and 50% beta and may cause a rise or drop in blood pressure.

Stimulation of the beta-receptor in the heart results in increased heart rate (beats per minute) and increased stroke volume (number of milliliters of blood the left ventricle pumps out into the aorta every time it contracts). Incidentally, the combination of these two changes (heart rate [HR] × stroke volume [SV]) is another way of saying cardiac output (CO) (milliliters of blood pumped per minute):

$$\text{beats/min(HR)} \times \text{ml/beat(SV)} = \text{ml/min(CO)}$$

This expression, cardiac output, is a common one and it constitutes half of the blood pressure regulation equation: CO × TPR = BP, where CO is cardiac output, TPR is total peripheral resistance, and BP is blood pressure. Total peripheral resistance is determined by vasoconstriction or vasodilation in the arterioles. Vasoconstriction increases resistance so TPR and BP goes up.

Stimulation of smooth muscle beta-receptors will relax these tissues wherever they are found. Respiratory airway smooth muscle will decrease tension when the beta-receptor is activated by beta-acting drugs like epinephrine or isoproterenol. The functional result will be an increase in air flow because of a larger airway diameter. Likewise, blood vessels respond to beta-acting drugs by increasing in diameter, allowing a greater rate of flow. In this case, TPR has decreased and blood pressure will drop.

Adrenergic Drugs

Norepinephrine (Levarterenol, Levophed)

As mentioned previously, norepinephrine (Levarterenol, Levophed) is a mixed-activity drug (90% alpha, 10% beta). It stimulates beta-receptors in the heart, which results in an increase of heart rate and stroke volume (increased cardiac output). In the arterioles, norepinephrine causes vasoconstriction via the alpha-receptor, resulting in increased total peripheral resistance. The total effect, of course, is an increase in blood pressure. Norepinephrine has little effect on the bronchioles. This drug is given only intravenously, and it can be used clinically to raise blood pressure. The natural sympathetic compounds are known as catecholamines.

Epinephrine (Adrenalin)

Epinephrine (Adrenalin) is also a mixed activity drug (50% alpha, 50% beta). It is naturally produced in the adrenal medulla and can be released during sympathetic nervous system activation. When this occurs, it acts as a circulating hormone, stimulating both alpha- and beta-receptors. This drug will increase heart rate and stroke volume and may slightly increase or decrease total peripheral resistance at the arterioles. In any case, cardiac output always goes up; blood pressure may go up or down slightly.

In the bronchioles, epinephrine exerts a dramatic dilating effect that is mediated by the beta-receptor. Epinephrine can be administered by inhalant aerosol to reverse a bronchoconstrictive episode. It is also administered intramuscularly and subcutaneously to treat asthma, anaphylactic reactions to an allergic response, cardiac arrest, heart block, and as a mild vasoconstriction to keep local anesthetics at the injection site.

Isoproterenol (Isuprel)

Isoproterenol (Isuprel) is a synthetic compound that has 100% beta activity. This means that it can increase heart rate and stroke volume to produce a great rise in cardiac output, and it stimulates the beta-receptor on the arterioles to effect a profound vasodilation. The final result can be a high cardiac output with low blood pressure. This drug improves blood circulation in shock patients by increasing local blood flow (vasodilation) and elevating cardiac output. Isoproterenol is considered very useful for treating acute asthmatic conditions because of its bronchodilating action.

Phenylephrine (Isophrin, Neo-Synephrine) and Metaraminol

Both phenylephrine (Isophrin, Neo-Synephrine) and metaraminol are powerful and prolonged stimulators of alpha-receptors. The action is directly on the receptor site itself. The response to the administration of either of these drugs is a rise in blood pressure because of vasoconstriction accompanied by a reflex bradycardia, which causes a decrease in cardiac output. Reflex alterations of cardiovascular function are explained later in this chapter. The primary usefulness of these drugs is in various hypotensive states.

Phenylephrine is used as a nasal decongestant and mydriatic and for the relief of paroxysmal atrial tachycardia. Phenylephrine affords relief from the tachycardia because it increases blood pressure and evokes the cardiovascular reflex that is marked by high vagal tone and bradycardia.

Ephedrine

Ephedrine has both alpha and beta activity as direct effects and it also causes release of epinephrine and norepinephrine. Its pharmacological actions are similar to epinephrine, with the main exception that duration of action of ephedrine is longer. Ephedrine increases cardiac output and vascular resistance, resulting in increased blood pressure. Ephedrine also causes bronchial muscle relaxation, which is less potent than that of epinephrine but has a longer duration. This drug is useful in controlling milder cases of bronchoconstriction that require long-term drug therapy.

Amphetamine (Dextroamphetamine, Dexedrine)

Amphetamine (Dextroamphetamine, Dexedrine) drug has pharmacological properties related to the catecholamines because it causes release of norepinephrine from the nerve terminal. Amphetamine has both alpha- and beta-receptor activity, although indirectly, through its release of norepinephrine. The usual cardiovascular response is an increase in blood pressure often accompanied by a reflex bradycardia. Amphetamine also has potent central nervous system (CNS) activity. It is a stimulant of the medullary respiratory center, and it can antagonize drug-related central nervous system depression. Respiratory depression often accompanies overdoses of CNS depressant drugs and this effect may be overcome by amphetamine. This drug is usually used for its central nervous system effects and not for peripheral cardiovascular or respiratory effects.

Beta$_2$-Receptors Stimulants

There are several drugs that act primarily at the beta$_2$ smooth muscle receptor site, causing selective actions in the bronchioles and arterioles but not in the heart. These drugs will produce a bronchodilation without increasing cardiac output. This particular lack of cardiovascular effect makes them safer than isoproterenol or epinephrine in treatment of bronchial

asthma. The drugs are metaproterenol (Alupent, Metaprel), terbutaline (Brethine, Bricanyl), albuterol (Proventil, Ventolin), isoetharine (Bronkosol, Bronkometer), and salmeterol (Servant).

Alpha-Adrenergic Blocking Drugs

Phentolamine (Regitine)

Phentolamine (Regitine) is a competitive alpha-receptor blocker. Its action is reversible. This drug prevents the hypertensive effect of norepinephrine, and it reverses the blood pressure elevating effect of epinephrine (epinephrine reversal). Epinephrine reversal looks like an isoproterenol effect with high cardiac output and low blood pressure. Phentolamine may be used clinically as a vasodilator. It is also useful as a clinical diagnostic agent in evaluating hypertensive patients who may have pheochromocytoma, which is a tumor that grows in the gastrointestinal chromaffin tissue. The tumor produces epinephrine and norepinephrine and may be responsible for one aspect of a clinical hypertension.

Phenoxybenzamine (Dibenzyline)

Phenoxybenzamine (Dibenzyline) is also an alpha-adrenergic blocking agent. It has effects similar to phentolamine in the cardiovascular system but it is less reversible. This drug is gaining some usefulness in the treatment of shock syndromes characterized by high vascular tone.

Prazosin (Minipress), Doxazosin (Cardura), and Terazosin (Hytrin)

Prazosin (Minipress), doxazosin (Cardura), and terazosin (Hytrin) are selective for arterioles and venules and are the most useful against hypertension of the drugs in this class. Although they act by vasodilation, these drugs exert minimal reflex tachycardia because they do not potentiate the vasomotor center and the increased venous capacitance reduces venous return and cardiac output.

Beta-Adrenergic Blocking Drugs

Propranolol (Inderal)

Propranolol (Inderal) is a beta-adrenergic blocker. This drug occupies the beta-receptor sites of the heart, the blood vessels, and the bronchioles. It prevents the beta-adrenergic effect usually seen with drugs like epinephrine, norepinephrine, and isoproterenol. In the arterioles, when epinephrine is given after propranolol, the usual mixed alpha and beta effect is eliminated, leaving only an alpha-adrenergic action. This causes profound vasoconstriction, allowing greater increase in blood pressure than is normally seen with epinephrine alone. In the heart the beta-receptors are blocked and, since there are no alpha-adrenergic receptors in this organ, all effects of catecholamine drugs on the heart are effectively eliminated, allowing the vagal influence on the heart to predominate. Propranolol decreases the heart's requirement for oxygen because it blocks the cardiac stimulant action of norepinephrine. In the respiratory system the administration of propranolol results in bronchoconstriction. This effect is increased dramatically in patients who are susceptible to asthma. The main use for propranolol is in conditions related to hypertension and tachycardia, where a decrease in cardiac output is beneficial.

Metoprolol (Lopressor) and Atenolol (Tenormin)

Metopolol (Lopressor) and atenolol (Tenormin) are beta-adrenergic antagonists that have been designed to be cardioselective. This offers an advantage in safety when a beta-blocker must be used in asthmatic patients, in whom this disease would be aggravated if respiratory beta-receptors were blocked. The natural beta-adrenergic agonist, epinephrine, is bronchodilating, and an important class of bronchodilating drugs acts at bronchiolar beta-adrenergic receptors.

Sympatholytic Drugs

Reserpine

Reserpine is an alkaloid of *Rauwolfia serpentina,* also known as the Indian snake root plant. There are many commercial preparations of this compound, but it is widely sold as the simple plant extract. This compound depletes norepinephrine from the nerve endings in the various tissues of the body that produce and store norepinephrine, including the brain. The depletion takes several days to accomplish, and it may take several weeks to restore catecholamine levels to normal after therapy is discontinued. During this time, there is a de-

crease in catecholamine response to sympathetic stimulation. Blood pressure in humans does not drop dramatically with therapeutic doses of reserpine, but when reserpine is used in combination with diuretics or other antihypertensive agents, a significant antihypertensive effect is obtained. Reserpine is used in this way to treat essential hypertension. One serious side effect related to reserpine use is the behavioral modification that can result in severe depression and suicide.

Guanethidine (Ismelin)

Guanethidine (Ismelin) is an adrenergic neuron-blocking agent that works by replacing norepinephrine in the nerve terminal. Norepinephrine is usually taken up by the nerve terminal after its discharge and is reused to maintain granule concentrations. Guanethidine takes the place of norepinephrine in the granules and prevents the reuptake of norepinephrine, thereby causing its metabolism outside of the neuron and its eventual depletion. The result on the cardiovascular system of this action is postural hypotension. The patient is unable to control blood pressure by sympathetic activity. This drug is used in treatment of severe hypertension, usually after diuretics and reserpine are shown to be ineffective.

Methyldopa (Aldomet) and Clonidine (Catapress)

Methyldopa (Aldomet) and clonidine (Catapress) decrease the activity of the sympathetic nervous system at its control center in the brain. The consequence is a total decrease in sympathetic activity in the heart and blood vessels leading to a reduction in blood pressure.

PARASYMPATHETIC NEUROTRANSMISSION

The center for parasympathetic control is the vagal nucleus in the medulla. The vagus nerves pass through the spinal cord and out to the heart, the smooth muscle, and exocrine glands (salivary glands and pancreas). In all of these tissues, acetylcholine is released from the nerve terminals and combines with receptor sites to cause an effect such as bradycardia (slowing of the heart) or an increasing gastric motility. Acetylcholine is found in many parts of the central and peripheral nervous system. Acetylcholine is the only transmitter used in the parasympathetic system. It is used to transmit impulses from the nerve that comes out of the spinal cord to the nerve that finally reaches the cells in the organ being affected. This connection is called a ganglion and exists in both sympathetic and parasympathetic systems. Acetylcholine is also the neurotransmitter that makes the connection between the voluntary (somatic) nerves and the skeletal muscle.

There are two types of receptors in these systems. Acetylcholine affects both, but some drugs affect only one and not the other. The two types of receptors are called nicotinic and muscarinic. They are named after the drugs that selectively stimulate them. Nicotine stimulates only those receptors in the ganglia and at the neuromuscular junction. The muscarinic receptor site is found everywhere a parasympathetic nerve terminal synapses at a tissue. The biological effects usually attributed to the parasympathetic nervous system, such as bradycardia, salivation, and bronchoconstriction, for example, are produced when the muscarinic receptors are stimulated. Of course, it is also possible to stimulate muscarinic receptors indirectly with a nicotinic drug by activating the parasympathetic ganglia. In fact, in a similar way, it is possible to stimulate the entire sympathetic nervous system. The neurotransmitter at the sympathetic ganglia is acetylcholine and it affects nicotinic receptor sites there. One of the toxic effects of acetylcholine and drugs that act like it is hypertension with tachycardia because of stimulation of the sympathetic postganglionic fibers.

To better understand the action of acetylcholine and related drugs, let us consider the synthesis, release, and inactivation of this transmitter. Acetylcholine is synthesized inside the nerve terminal from acetyl-CoA and choline. The acetylcholine is then stored in granules and is released out into the synapse when an action potential reaches the terminal. The acetylcholine molecule attaches to a receptor site, muscarinic or nicotinic, or to the enzyme that breaks it apart. Combination with the receptor site results in biological action, and coupling with the enzyme ends in destruction. The enzyme, acetylcholinesterase, is found at all cholinergic synaptic sites. A nonspecific variety of the enzyme is also prevalent in many other tissues. It too will break down acetylcholine. The final action of either enzyme is the production of acetic acid and choline. The acetic acid is washed away for further metabolism, and the choline is reabsorbed into the nerve terminal for resynthesis to acetylcholine.

Cholinergic Drugs

Acetylcholine

Acetylcholine is the endogenous cholinergic transmitter that accounts for nicotinic and muscarinic actions within the autonomic nervous system. It is rapidly hydrolyzed by acetylcholinesterase and the nonspecific cholinesterase and therefore has a short duration of action if administered parenterally. This makes acetylcholine (ACh) a poor drug. Nicotinic effects of acetylcholine are (1) stimulation of parasympathetic ganglia, causing occurrence of all muscarinic effects, (2) stimulation of sympathetic ganglia, causing increase in vascular resistance and cardiac output to produce hypertension, and (3) stimulation of the neuromuscular junction (NMJ) at the skeletal muscle (muscle contraction and movement). Muscarinic effects of acetylcholine are bradycardia, salivation, pinpoint pupils, bronchial constriction, gastric and intestinal hypermotility, increased gastric acid and mucous secretion, and facilitated urination. Toxic effects of cholinergic stimulation include diarrhea, urinary incontinence, bradycardia, bronchoconstriction, excessive salivation, CNS excitement, and respiratory collapse. In all of these toxic effects, atropine, a competitive muscarinic blocker, is the antidote of choice.

Bethanecol (Urecholine)

Bethanecol (Urecholine) is a synthetic choline ester that is not destroyed as easily as acetylcholine by cholinesterase enzymes. It is useful in treating patients with urinary retention and paralytic ileus, and it is administered orally or subcutaneously. The side effects and toxicities for this drug are exactly those for ACh. However, since the drug is not given intravenously, cardiac and respiratory effects are minimized.

Carbachol (Carcholin)

Carbachol (Carcholin) is a mixed nicotinic and muscarinic drug because it releases acetylcholine from the nerve ending, producing the expected cholinergic effects at all receptor sites. The drug is useful for treatment of glaucoma (applied topically), paralytic ileus, and urinary retention (orally and subcutaneously).

Pilocarpine

Pilocarpine is a cholinomimetic that is useful in ophthalmology as an antiglaucoma agent. Cholinergic compounds decrease intraocular pressure by relieving the obstruction to the canal of Schlemm, a drainage circuit for the eye. Miosis (pinpoint pupils) is one feature of cholinergic therapy and may be beneficial to glaucoma treatment because the muscular base of the relaxed iris may contribute to the drainage block. Another use of pilocarpine is to promote salivary flow in patients with a ganglionic blockade.

Anticholinesterases

Before proceeding to specific anticholinesterase drugs, it is important to understand the basic mechanism of action for these compounds. Acetylcholinesterase is the enzyme responsible for destroying acetylcholine at the various nerve junctions where it is released. The class of drugs that interfere with this function is called anticholinesterases. These drugs attach to the enzyme and thereby block the enzymatic hydrolysis of ACh, causing ACh to accumulate outside of the nerve ending. This results in a greater response than normal to any cholinergic nerve stimulation. Some of these anticholinesterases are relatively short-acting compounds and are therapeutically important, whereas others are extremely long-lasting and potent compounds that are important only as poisons. The long-acting compounds have been used as insecticides and as nerve gases in chemical warfare. The therapeutically useful anticholinesterases are beneficial in problems related to the eye, intestine, and the skeletal neuromuscular junction (NMJ). In these applications, these drugs increase the amount of ACh available for activity, an effect that is especially important in cases where the synthesis or release of acetylcholine is lower than normal, as in myasthenia gravis.

There is also great medical interest in the toxicology of the anticholinesterases, especially the extremely potent irreversible anticholinesterases. Toxicity because of these compounds is not uncommon and is often severe. When a toxic irreversible anti-

cholinesterase, such as diisopropylfluorophosphate (DFP) or sarin, is ingested, inhaled, or absorbed across the skin, a great variety of toxic cholinergic effects are seen. The first effects seen after exposure to an anticholinesterase are often ocular and respiratory effects. In the eyes, marked miosis is produced quickly. In the respiratory system, bronchoconstriction and bronchial secretions combine to produce tightness in the chest and wheezing. Gastrointestinal symptoms include nausea, vomiting, cramps, and diarrhea. Other muscarinic effects are severe salivation, involuntary defecation and urination, sweating, lacrimation, bradycardia, and hypotension.

Further effects are related to nicotinic functions of acetylcholine. These include skeletal muscle twitching, weakness, and paralysis. CNS effects include depression of the respiratory and cardiovascular control centers, leading to respiratory collapse. At the time of death, respiratory paralysis is evident and it is because of a combination of bronchoconstriction, bronchosecretions, respiratory muscle paralysis from overstimulation, and CNS and control depression. The treatment of this toxicity is closely related to preserving respiratory function. Administration of atropine, a muscarinic blocker, will effectively decrease bronchoconstriction and secretion. Another drug, pralidoxime (Protopam), is used to reactivate the acetylcholinesterase. It is most effective shortly after exposure to the toxic agent because it breaks down the anticholinesterase so it can be removed from the enzyme site. Additional measures are related to physiological support of the patient. Maintenance of an airway, artificial respiration, and oxygen administration are important therapeutic applications for these patients.

Physostigmine (Eserine)

Physostigmine (Eserine) is useful in glaucoma and in selected therapeutic measures where a cholinergic effect is beneficial. It functions as an indirect cholinomimetic by blocking the acetylcholinesterase.

Neostigmine (Prostigmine)

Neostigmine (Prostigmine) is useful in patients with nonobstructive paralytic ileus to increase tone and motility of the small and large intestines. It is also useful for stimulating skeletal NMJ. Neostigmine is used for treating myasthenia gravis because it indirectly increases acetylcholine at the NMJ and it acts directly at the nicotinic receptor site itself. The disease is marked by subnormal response to acetylcholine, resulting in skeletal muscle weakness. Neostigmine temporarily restores muscle strength.

Edrophonium (Tensilson)

This a very short-acting anticholinesterase. It is primarily useful as a diagnostic agent in myasthenia gravis to reveal, for a few minutes, if the dose of neostigmine is appropriate. A longer-acting drug would risk a serious cholinergic toxicity if the neostigmine dose was already at the therapeutic limit.

Cholinergic Blocking Drugs

Cholinergic antagonists block the various receptor sites where acetylcholine is a transmitter. There are specific blocking drugs for each type of acetylcholine receptor. Atropine blocks all cholinergic action right at the muscarinic receptor site on smooth muscle, exocrine glands, and myocardium. Another cholinergic antagonist, curare, works only at the neuromuscular junction to block the nicotinic effect of acetylcholine, resulting in paralysis of skeletal muscle. Still another type of nicotinic blocker is the ganglionic blocker, hexamethonium, which blocks both sympathetic and parasympathetic ganglia by occupying the acetylcholine receptor there. These drugs are useful wherever sympathetic or parasympathetic tone needs to be decreased. It is possible to selectively inhibit cholinergic effects in the body to produce a desired effect or to eliminate an undesirable effect. Because of this selectiveness, cholinergic antagonists have widespread use in many areas of medicine.

Atropine

Atropine is an extract from the plant *Atropa belladonna,* also known as the deadly nightshade. Another plant extract, scopolamine, has action similar to atropine. Atropine works by establishing a competitive blockage at the muscarinic receptor site, which is the effector at all tissues innervated by the parasympathetic nervous system. This blockade is selective for the tissue effect of the parasympathetic system

and does not counteract the nicotinic ganglionic effects or the nicotinic effects at the NMJ.

Because heart rate is controlled by both sympathetic and parasympathetic tone, atropine will eliminate the parasympathetic effect on the heart, allowing the sympathetic system to increase heart rate and stroke volume to cause an increase in cardiac output. In fact, tachycardia may occur after atropine administration. In cases where bradycardia exists because of high vagal tone, atropine can be used to reverse this depression.

In the respiratory tract, atropine is a bronchodilator. It is also possible to delay respiratory depression associated with anesthetic, tranquilizing, and anticholinesterase drugs by using atropine, either as a pretreatment agent or as an antidote during overdose.

Atropine is used widely as preanesthetic medication to prevent bronchiolar secretions and laryngeal spasm, as well as bradycardia. A more general medical use for atropine exists as an emergency tool. It is the antidote of choice for all cholinergic toxicities.

One of the most important clinical uses for atropine is in the gastrointestinal (GI) tract as an antiulcer and antispasmodic agent. This drug acts to decrease motility in the GI tract so that other antiulcer agents can remain in contact with the GI mucosa longer, and it is possible that it also decreases acid secretion. Other problems related to hypermotility of the GI tract are treated with atropine, mainly to decrease gastric muscle activity during treatment of conditions such as cramping and diarrhea.

In ophthalmology, atropine is useful for producing mydriasis, which is pupillary dilation. It is contraindicated in glaucoma patients because it may precipitate an acute attack.

Atropine itself is also capable of producing toxic effects. These are mydriasis, tachycardia, dry mouth, constipation, and urinary retention. Effects related to the central nervous system are also apparent, and these include sedation initially, followed by delirium and hallucinations, which lead to a coma. In severe toxicities the patient convulses and experiences severe respiratory depression, which may be the final course. Anticholinesterase drugs, such as physostigmine and neostigmine, are effective antidotes for atropine because they increase the amount of acetylcholine that will compete with atropine for the receptor site.

Homatropine (Novatrin) and Cyclopentolate (Cyclogyl)

Homatropine (Novatrin) and cyclopentolate (Cyclogyl) are anticholinergic drugs related in action to atropine. They are useful in ophthalmology to produce mydriasis.

Dicyclomine (Bentyl)

Dicyclomine (Bentyl) is considered very useful in the gastrointestinal tract to decrease secretions and motility. It is sometimes called a chemical vagotomy.

Trihexyphenidyl HCL (Artane) and Benztropine Mesylate (Cogentin)

Trihexyphenidyl HCL (Artane) and benztropine mesylate (Cogentin) are antiparkinson drugs that enter the CNS to reverse the imbalance between the cholinergic and dopaminergic systems in this disease. They have some of the same side effects as atropine.

Pentolinium (Ansolysen) and Hexamethonium (Methium)

Pentolinium (Ansolysen) and hexamethonium (Methium) are nicotinic antagonists. They block the acetylcholine receptor site in the ganglia in both the sympathetic and parasympathetic nervous systems. They are used to control hypertension, which is due to a high sympathetic tone. Because of their blocking action at the sympathetic ganglion, these drugs produce a postural hypotension. They will also decrease cholinergic effects at the parasympathetic effector sites because they block the ganglia for the entire parasympathetic nervous system as well. This means that a patient may experience blurred vision, dryness of mouth, and tachycardia, as well as other atropine-like peripheral effects.

THE CARDIOVASCULAR REFLEX

The cardiovascular reflex involves many of the components of the autonomic nervous system to maintain a normal blood pressure. This mechanism is important for maintaining blood pressure within certain limits during all phases of physical activity. Even the simple act of standing from a sitting position requires prompt compensation by this reflex system. If in some way this reflex is interrupted, a condition known as orthostatic hypotension will exist. A common manifestation of this condition is fainting on standing because of inadequate blood flow to the brain. This section is devoted to the functional aspects of the reflex after a change in blood pressure.

The Carotid Baroreceptors

Neuronal elements, known as baroreceptors, exist in the sinus of the carotid arteries supplying the brain. These are stretch receptors that fire electrical impulses at a rate directly related to the blood pressure. As the pressure in the artery increases, the vessel wall (and baroreceptor) stretches, causing an increase in the receptor firing rate. Conversely, a decrease in blood pressure results in a decrease in stretch receptor firing rate. This firing rate signal is sent directly to the brain, where the vasomotor center and vagal nucleus respond to it.

The Functional Reflex

To create an example for demonstrating this reflex, let us assume we have just experienced a loss of blood pressure. The carotid baroreceptors shorten and slow their firing. This message is then delivered to the brain, and the vasomotor center responds by increasing sympathetic nerve activity. This control always responds to information regarding blood pressure in the carotid artery by doing the opposite of the baroreceptors. If the pressure had risen, the baroreceptors would have increased their firing rate and the vasomotor center would have responded by slowing the sympathetic nerve firing rate. Since the blood pressure in this example is low, the vasomotor center increases sympathetic nerve firing, resulting in increased release of norepinephrine from the nerves that reach the heart and arterioles. Norepinephrine increases the heart rate and stroke volume, thereby producing an increase in cardiac output. In the arterioles, norepinephrine stimulates the alpha-receptors, producing vasoconstriction, which results in increased resistance result in raised blood pressure. A third component of the sympathetic nervous system can be involved during sympathetic activation. Epinephrine released from the adrenal medulla also increases cardiac output.

Meanwhile, the vagal nucleus is responding to the decreased baroreceptor firing by decreasing its own activity. The vagus nerve to the heart will release less acetylcholine, allowing the sympathetic effect to predominate. The total effect becomes an increase in blood pressure, which is the response required to return the systemic pressure to normal. If the original pressure alteration had been an increase above normal, the opposite reflexive actions would have occurred to return pressure to a normal range. In this case the predominant effect would have been an increase in vagal nerve tone, releasing high amounts of acetylcholine at the heart, causing a dramatic slowing of heart rate, accompanied by a decrease in stroke volume. This combination produces a decrease in cardiac output. The sympathetic system would have responded to the increased baroreceptor firing by decreasing firing in all sympathetic nerves, thereby decreasing norepinephrine and epinephrine release. All of these factors combine to decrease blood pressure to normal.

DRUGS USED IN AIRWAY OBSTRUCTIVE DISEASE

Patients suffering from asthma, emphysema, and chronic bronchitis may have an obstructed airway for several reasons. Acute asthmatic obstruction and some chronic airway obstruction are due to bronchial smooth muscle contraction, resulting in a smaller diameter airway. Inflamed passageways, which are swollen because of edema, may also constitute an airway obstruction. A further complication seen in many respiratory diseases is the thickening and collection of secretions that cannot be eliminated from the respiratory tree and subsequently block the airway. In this section the various drugs that can reverse smooth muscle contraction, inflammatory edema, and collection of secretions are presented.

A variety of therapeutic mechanisms are useful against this collection of obstructive conditions. The single most effective mechanism for relief of smooth muscle spasm is the beta$_2$ activity that is available in some of the adrenergic agents. Other useful mechanisms aim at potentiating the beta activity of adrenergic agents, decongesting the inflamed airway, de-

creasing release of histamine, and in a broader approach, the general stabilization of cells that can release mediators of the disease, thereby lowering the severity of the disease.

Sympathomimetic Drugs

Isoproterenol (Isuprel) and Epinephrine (Adrenalin)

The muscle relaxant bronchodilator effect attributed to the beta-adrenergic sympathomimetic compounds is most commonly required for asthmatic or allergic emergencies. Isoproterenol (Isuprel) is often self-administered by inhalation to reverse mild-to-moderate obstructive episodes. However, during a severe acute obstruction, the airway is unable to pass the drug to the alveoli, and the intramuscular or subcutaneous routes for epinephrine (adrenaline) and isoproterenol are used. Isoproterenol is a purely beta compound. Epinephrine has 50% beta-adrenergic activity and also exerts a great bronchodilating effect. Both of these agents are useful when given parenterally or by inhalation. The most common side effects of isoproterenol are flushing of the skin, headache, palpitation, and tachycardia. Epinephrine may cause an anxiety reaction in a patient along with headache, palpitations, and respiratory difficulty. Both drugs can cause serious cardiac reactions (dysrhythmias), which have resulted in death.

Metaproterenol (Alupent), Isoetharine (with Phenylephrine, Bronkosol-2), and Salmeterol (Servant)

Metaproterenol (Alupent), isoetharine (with Phenylephrine, Bronkosol-2), and salmeterol (Servant) are isoproterenol analogs that exert most of their action on respiratory or vascular smooth muscle but have little effect on the heart. They are useful compounds for selectively relaxing bronchial smooth muscles without directly affecting the heart. The major advantage of these drugs is that their action on the heart is minimal or absent, and their potential for inducing cardiac toxicities is correspondingly reduced. However, because vascular smooth muscle responds much like respiratory smooth muscle to these drugs, arterial resistance can be decreased, leading to a drop in blood pressure and a reflexive tachycardia. The beta agonists are often given by inhalation, which minimizes their systemic absorption and potential for side effects.

Ephedrine

Ephedrine is a sympathomimetic that acts by liberating norepinephrine and epinephrine from storage sites in addition to having a possible direct effect on adrenergic receptors. Its usefulness and side effects are similar to those of epinephrine. One beneficial factor in ephedrine use is that it can be administered orally for convenient long-term therapy.

Xanthines

Xanthines have effects similar to the catecholamines in the respiratory and cardiovascular systems. This similarity in effect may be due to the elevation of cyclic AMP. Both the catecholamines and xanthines are known to produce elevated cyclic AMP levels in the tissues they stimulate. The catecholamines activate adenylate cyclase, the enzyme that converts ATP to cyclic AMP. The newly formed cyclic AMP exerts its effects on the local tissue (e.g., bronchial muscle relaxation) and is inactivated by the enzyme phosphodiesterase. The xanthines inhibit phosphodiesterase, conserving cyclic AMP and thereby promoting its effects. Additional actions of xanthines may be direct smooth muscle relaxation that could increase airway diameter, and antagonism of adenosine, which is bronchoconstricting.

Theophylline and Aminophylline

Theophylline and aminophylline are structurally very similar to caffeine. They are used to control asthma when given orally or intravenously. Theophylline is often used orally for long-term maintenance of mild-to-moderate disease. One of the most common uses for aminophylline is the treatment of acute asthmatic airway obstruction, especially in cases that do not respond to epinephrine alone. Intravenous administration of this drug increases the opportunity for serious side effects, which are hypotension and cardiac dysrhythmias.

Corticosteroids

The antiinflammatory steroids are related to the naturally occurring glucocorticoid, cortisol (Prednisone,

Methylprednisolone, and Beclomethasone). Many compounds have been synthetically derived to produce a variety of antiinflammatory potencies. The usefulness of corticosteroids in treating respiratory diseases depends on the ability of these drugs to depress the symptoms of inflamed tissue. The mechanism of action for the drugs, however, has not clearly been defined. Some specific effects of corticosteroids that relate to the antiinflammatory action are decreased capillary dilation and permeability, and stabilization of lysosomal membranes in white blood cells. In addition, these compounds decrease the synthesis of compounds that can promote broncho-obstructive disease—prostaglandins and leukotrienes. The long-term use of the corticosteroids is recommended only after other measures fail. The reason for this caution is that they produce serious side effects and permanent changes if used for 2 weeks or longer. After 1 week of corticosteroid therapy, behavioral changes and acute peptic ulcers may be observed. However, when longer therapy is instituted and adrenal suppression occurs, the patient requires supplemental corticosteroid therapy until normal adrenal cortex function is restored. This state of insufficiency may last for as long as several months after suppression. Most patients who receive corticosteroids for long-term therapy develop a condition called Cushing's syndrome. It is characterized by wasting of muscles because of the breakdown of protein and by redistribution of fat from the extremities to the face and the trunk. Eventually these patients develop osteoporosis and diabetes. Other serious complications are peptic ulcers, psychosis, glaucoma, intercranial hypertension, and growth retardation. The time to onset of side effects can be prolonged and the severity of effects can be minimized by applying dosing strategies that provide antiinflammatory benefit in the lung at low systemic doses. Corticosteroids can be given at low doses in alternate day administration or they can be given by inhalation in a form that is not systemically absorbed.

Antihistamine

Cromolyn Sodium (Intal) and Nedocromil Sodium (Tilade)

Cromolyn sodium (Intal) and nedocromil sodium (Tilade) have limited usefulness compared with the other drugs presented here—they can only prevent an asthmatic episode. The mechanism of action is probably the stabilization of the mast cell that synthesizes, stores, and releases histamine. Since histamine can precipitate broncho-obstructive reactions, these drugs are useful by preventing its release. They are administered by inhalation.

Mucolytics and Expectorants

Acetylcysteine (Mucomyst) and Pancreatic Dornase (Dornavac)

Acetylcysteine (Mucomyst) and pancreatic dornase (Dornavac) act by breaking the chemical bonds that hold together the large protein structure that contributes to the viscosity of mucus. Mucolytics are inhaled to liquify mucus so that it can be moved out of the bronchial tract to prevent airway obstruction. Side effects associated with these drugs are bronchospasm, nausea, and vomiting. Acetylcysteine also inactivates the penicillin antibiotics and is contraindicated in their presence.

Trypsin (Tryptar)

Trypsin (Tryptar) is a proteolytic enzyme that may also be useful for liquefying respiratory secretions. It can be administered by inhalation, although it can cause irritation to the eyes, nose, and throat. An additional problem with this drug is a possible anaphylactic reaction in sensitized patients. There is a variety of other enzymes with specific actions on protein that may be useful in liquefying secretions.

Sodium Iodide and Potassium Iodide

Sodium iodide and potassium iodide are expectorants that act by increasing the amount of respiratory secretion so that is relatively less viscous and can be more easily removed. The iodide salts are often used in late bronchitis, bronchiectasis, and asthma, and they break up especially tough bronchial secretions by attracting fluid to the respiratory tract. Characteristic side effects with these compounds are gastric irritation, nausea, and vomiting. More serious complications occasionally involve the respiratory tract. These patients wheeze and experience bronchial spasm. Other expec-

torants that are usually used in mixtures or administered as cough syrups are ammonium chloride, syrup of ipecac, and glyceryl guaiacolate. These are useful for patients who cannot tolerate the iodide salts.

DRUG INHALATION DEVICES

Most drugs given by inhalation in respiratory disease are delivered by pressurized metered-dose inhalers (MDI). These devices rely on pressurized chlorofluorocarbon propellants to deliver very small drug particles (less than 5 micron diameter) into the airway. Each activation of the metered valve allows an accurately determined volume (dose) of propellant and drug mixture to be released at a high velocity.

The delivery of drugs to the site of action in the airway by any type of inhalation is inefficient, and therefore, correct technique in use of the MDI is an important concern. The MDI will allow delivery of 20% of the metered drug to the airway if the patient correctly coordinates the proper rate of inhalation with activation of the device and then adequately holds the breath before exhalation. It is estimated that 50% or fewer patients manage the drug delivery correctly. In response, patient education on correct MDI technique is an important part of therapy, and additional devices, called spacers, have been developed to allow success with variations in technique. The spacers come in various configurations, but they all provide a chamber between the patient and the MDI, which can be charged with the drug-propellant mixture that is then inhaled without concern for critical timing. Patients with poor MDI technique should benefit from the addition of a spacer.

An alternative to the MDI, in patients who have difficulty with inhalation technique, is the single-dose or multi-dose powder inhaler. This device offers a drug compounded into a fine powder, which is delivered from a container on simple inhalation by the patient. Coordination of drug delivery is simple and not a problem, because only inspiration by the patient drives powder delivery to the airway. The method offers the same or lower efficacy of drug delivery (6% to 20%), compared with MDI.

REVIEW QUESTIONS

1. Why is it important to have an understanding of the system a drug is to modify?
2. What are the primary and secondary effects of the commonly used bronchodilators, Ventolin and Alupent?
3. What is the cardiovascular reflex and why is it important to physical therapists?
4. What is the pharmacologic rationale for treatment of patients with chronic obstructive airways disease. (COPD)?
5. Why is patient compliance with their medications a concern of the physical therapist?

References

Clark, T.J.H., Godfrey, S., & Lee, T.H., (Eds.). (1992). *Asthma*, London: Chapman and Hall.

Hardman, J., Gilman, A.G., Limbird, L., & Rall, T.W., (Eds.). (1995). *The pharmacological basis of therapeutics.* New York: McGraw-Hill.

Kaliner, M.A. (1993). How the current understanding of the pathophysiology of asthma influences our approach to therapy. *Journal of Allergy and Clinical Immunology, 92*(1 pt. 2), 144-147.

Katzung, B.G., (Ed.). (1995). *Basic and clinical pharmacology.* East Norwalk, CT: Appleton & Lange.

O'Brien-Ladner, A. (1994). Asthma: new insights in the management of older patients. *Geriatrics, 49*(11), 20-25, 30-32.

Powell, C.V. (1993). Management of acute asthma in childhood.*British Journal of Hospital Medicine, 50*(5), 272-275.

Whelan, A.M., & Hahn, N.W. (1991). Optimizing drug delivery from metered-dose inhalers. *Drug Intelligence and Clinical Pharmacology, 25,* 638-645.

Acid-base balance: a condition existing when the net rate at which the body produces acids or bases equals the net rate at which acids or bases are excreted. The result of acid-base balance is a stable concentration of hydrogen ions in body fluids. The amount of acid or base in the arterial blood is measured by pH.

Acidosis: a process causing acidemia, which is a blood pH of less than 7.38.

Acute exacerbation of chronic airflow limitation: an increase in the severity of the signs and symptoms of chronic airflow limitation usually triggered by infection, inflammation, or increased sputum production.

Acute lung injury: injury to the lung characterized by a clinical spectrum of parenchymal lung dysfunction resulting from multiple etiologies and leading to alveolar capillary membrane leaking (high protein content). Mild-to-moderate lung injury results in noncardiogenic edema and severe injury results in adult respiratory distress syndrome. The hallmarks of worsening lung injury include refractory hypoxemia, right-to-left shunt, and reduced lung compliance.

Adult respiratory distress syndrome (ARDS): a respiratory syndrome characterized by respiratory insufficiency and hypoxemia. Triggers include aspiration of a foreign body, cardiopulmonary bypass surgery, gram-negative sepsis, multiple blood transfusions, oxygen toxicity, trauma, pneumonia, or other respiratory infection.

Aerosol: nebulized particles suspended in a gas or air.

Airway clearance: the removal of mucus and foreign material from the airways.

Airway-clearance deficits: deficits in the ability to remove mucus and foreign material from the airways.

Alveolar proteinosis: a disorder marked by the accumulation of plasma proteins, lipoproteins, and other blood components in the alveoli of the lungs. The cause is unknown and clinical symptoms vary, although only the lungs are affected. Some patients are asymptomatic, whereas others show dyspnea and an unproductive cough.

Alveolar ventilation: the volume of inspired air that reaches the alveolar level and participates in gas exchange, measured by P_{CO_2}.

Alveolitis: an allergic pulmonary reaction to the inhalation of antigenic substances characterized by acute episodes of dyspnea, cough, sweating, fever, weakness, and pain in the joints and muscles lasting from 12 to 18 hours. Recurrent episodes may lead to chronic obstructive lung disease with weight loss, increasing exertional dyspnea, and interstitial fibrosis.

Anesthesia: the absence of normal sensation, especially sensitivity to pain, as induced by an anesthetic substance or by hypnosis or as occurs with traumatic or pathophysiological damage to nerve tissue.

Angina: angina pectoris, the paroxysmal chest pain caused by anoxia of the myocardium.

Angina pectoris: a paroxysmal thoracic pain caused most often by myocardial anoxia as a result of atherosclerosis of the coronary arteries. The pain usually radiates down the inner aspect of the left arm and is frequently accompanied by a feeling of suffocation and impending death. Attacks of angina pectoris are often related to exertion, emotional stress, and exposure to intense cold.

Ankylosing spondylitis: a chronic inflammatory disease of unknown origin, first affecting the spine and adjacent structures and commonly progressing to eventual fusion (ankylosis) of the involved joints. In addition to the spine the joints of the hip, shoulder, neck, ribs, and jaw are often involved. Physical therapy aids in keeping the spine as erect as possible to prevent flexion contractures. In advanced cases, surgery may be performed to straighten a badly deformed spine.

Arrhythmia: an abnormal heart rhythm represented by an irregularity of the timing or the appearance of the ECG tracing. This term is often used synonymously with dysrhythmia.

Arterial blood gas: a test to evaluate the acid-base balance and partial pressures of oxygen and carbon dioxide in the arterial blood.

Arteriovenous-oxygen difference (a-vo₂ difference):   the difference between the oxygen content of arterial blood and the amount in venous blood.

Artifact: extraneous deflection of the ECG waveform caused by movement or electrical interference. Artifact may be mistaken for a dysrhythmia.

Artificial airway: a plastic or rubber device that can be inserted into the upper or lower respiratory tract to facilitate ventilation or the removal of secretions.

Assessment: an evaluation or appraisal of a condition.

Assisted cough: the physical assistance of a cough, either by the patient or an assistant.

Asthma: a respiratory disorder characterized by recurring episodes of paroxysmal dyspnea, wheezing on expiration/inspiration because of constriction of the bronchi, coughing, and viscous mucoid bronchial secretions. Treatment may include elimination of the causative agent, hyposensitization, aerosol or oral

bronchodilators, beta-adrenergic drugs, methylxanthines, and short-term use of corticosteroids.

Atelectasis: an abnormal condition characterized by the collapse of lung tissue, preventing the respiratory exchange of carbon dioxide and oxygen. Symptoms may include diminished breath sounds, a mediastinal shift toward the side of the collapse, fever, and increasing dyspnea.

Atherosclerosis: a common arterial disorder characterized by yellowish plaques of cholesterol, lipids, and cellular debris in the inner layers of the walls of large and medium-sized arteries. The vessel walls become thick, fibrotic, and calcified, and the lumen narrows, resulting in reduced blood flow to organs normally supplied by the artery. Antilipidemic agents do not reverse atherosclerosis, but a diet low in cholesterol, calories, and saturated fats, adequate exercise, and the avoidance of smoking and stress may help prevent the disorder.

Blood: the liquid pumped by the heart through all the arteries, veins, and capillaries. The blood is composed of a clear yellow fluid, called plasma, and the formed elements, and a series of cell types with different functions. The major function of the blood is to transport oxygen and nutrients to the cells and to remove from the cells carbon dioxide and other waste products for detoxification and elimination.

Body mechanics: using one's body effectively to prevent injury.

Bradycardia: an abnormally slow heart rate.

Bradypnea: a decreased respiratory rate under 10 breaths per minute.

Bronchiectasis: an abnormal condition of the bronchial tree, characterized by irreversible dilatation and destruction of the bronchial walls. Symptoms of bronchiectasis include a constant cough productive of copious purulent sputum, hemoptysis, chronic sinusitis, clubbing of fingers, and persistent moist, coarse rales. Treatment includes mobilization, frequent postural drainage, antibiotics, and, rarely, surgical resection of the affected part of the lungs.

Bronchiolitis: an acute viral infection of the lower respiratory tract that occurs primarily in infants under 18 months of age, characterized by expiratory wheezing, respiratory distress, inflammation, and obstruction at the level of the bronchioles.

Bronchitis: an acute or chronic inflammation of the mucous membranes of the tracheobronchial tree. Acute bronchitis is characterized by a productive cough, fever, hypertrophy of mucous-secreting structures, and back pain. Most common in adults, it is often a complication of cystic fibrosis in children. Treatment includes the cessation of cigarette smoking, avoidance of airway irritants, the use of expectorants, and postural drainage. Currently, prophylactic antibiotics, steroids, and desensitization therapy are not recommended.

Bronchopulmonary dysplasia: an iatrogenic condition observed in neonates that resembles chronic airflow limitation and is associated with positive pressure mechanical ventilation and oxygen therapy.

Burns: an injury to tissues of the body caused by heat, electricity, chemicals, radiation, or gases in which the extent of the injury is determined by the amount of exposure of the cell to the agent and to the nature of the agent. The treatment of burns includes pain relief, careful asepsis, prevention of infection, maintenance of the balance in the body of fluids and electrolytes, and good nutrition. Severe burns of any origin may cause shock, which is treated before the wound.

Cardiac output (Q): the amount of blood ejected from the heart into the aorta each minute.

Cardiac rehabilitation: a supervised program of progressive exercise, psychological support, and education or training to enable a myocardial infarction patient to resume the activities of daily living on an independent basis. Special training may be needed to adapt the patient to a new occupation and lifestyle.

Cardiopulmonary failure: progressive insufficiency of cardiopulmonary function resulting in significant impairment of cardiac output and/or ventilation that cannot be adequately compensated without ventilatory support.

Cardiopulmonary function: the integrated function of the heart and lungs.

Cardiopulmonary physical therapy: *see* p. ix.

Cardiopulmonary unit: the heart and lungs, which function interdependently as a unit.

Catabolic: relating to catabolism, which is the breaking down in the body of complex chemical compounds into simpler ones, often accompanied by the liberation of energy.

Cellular respiration: the processes involved with cellular metabolism, including energy transfer, oxygen utilization, and carbon dioxide production.

Cerebral palsy: a motor function disorder caused by a permanent, nonprogressive brain defect or lesion present at birth or shortly thereafter. Early identification of the disorder facilitates the handling of infants with cerebral palsy and the initiation of an exercise and training program. Treatment is individualized and may include the use of braces, surgical correction of deformities, speech therapy, and various indicated drugs, such as muscle relaxants and anticonvulsants.

Childhood asthma: reversible airway hyperreactivity and edema affecting children that is often triggered by dust or animals; hallmarked by narrowing of the airways, wheezing, shortness of breath, accessory muscle use, and impaired oxygenation.

Chronic bronchitis: a lung condition characterized by the presence of a chronic productive cough for at least 3 months in each of 2 successive years.

Chronic renal insufficiency: impaired function of the kidneys manifested by impaired blood urea nitrogen, creatinine clearance, and reduced urinary output. Renal insufficiency may precipitate renal failure.

Chronic airflow limitation: a more precise term for chronic obstructive pulmonary disease (e.g., chronic bronchitis and emphysema).

Clinical decision making: the process of making decisions based on a thorough history, assessment, integration of the results of laboratory tests and investigations, and the patient's needs and wants.

Complications with coughing: Complications associated with an impaired cough (e.g., impaired mucociliary transport, mucous accumulation, pulmonary aspiration, and increased risk of infection).

Congestive heart failure (CHF): an abnormal condition that reflects impaired cardiac pumping, caused by myocardial infarction, ischemic heart disease, or cardiomyopathy. Failure of the ventricle to eject blood efficiently results in volume overload, chamber dilatation, and elevated intracardiac pressure. Retrograde transmission of increased hydrostatic pressure from the left heart causes pulmonary congestion; elevated right heart pressure causes systemic venous congestion and peripheral edema.

Connective tissue dysfunction: impaired function of connective tissue observed in connective tissue and vascular collagen conditions.

Continuity of care: the provision of continuous care from one setting to another (e.g., inpatient to outpatient facilities).

Controlled breathing: teaching a patient ventilatory strategies to exert cognitive control over ineffective breathing patterns.

Control of breathing: the central and peripheral regulation and control mechanisms of breathing.

Control of the heart: the central and peripheral regulation and control mechanisms of the heart.

Coronary artery disease: any one of the abnormal conditions that may affect the arteries of the heart and produce various pathological effects, especially the reduced flow of oxygen and nutrients to the myocardium. Any of the coronary artery diseases, such as coronary atherosclerosis, coronary arteritis, or fibromuscular hyperplasia of the coronary arteries, may produce the common characteristic symptom of angina pectoris. Studies over the last 30 years confirm that coronary atherosclerosis occurs most frequently in populations with regular diets high in calories, total fat, saturated fat, cholesterol, and refined carbohydrates. Other risk factors include cigarette smoking, hypertension, serum cholesterol levels, coffee intake, alcohol intake, deficiencies of vitamins C and E, water hardness, hypoxia, carbon monoxide, social overcrowding, heredity, climate, and viruses.

Cough: a sudden, audible expulsion of air from the lungs. Coughing is preceded by inspiration, the glottis is partially closed, and the accessory muscles of expiration contract to expel the air forcibly from the respiratory passages. Coughing is an essential protective response that serves to clear the lungs, bronchi, or trachea of irritants and secretions or to prevent aspiration of foreign material into the lungs. It is a common symptom of diseases of the chest and larynx. Because the function of coughing is to clear the respiratory tract of secretions, it is important that the cough bring out accumulated debris. Where it does not, because of weakness or inhibition of the force of the cough caused by pain, instruction and assistance in effective coughing and deep-breathing exercises are required.

Cough pump: the integrated thoracic and abdominal mechanisms involved in cough resulting in forced expiration and evacuation and clearance of the airways.

Cough stages: the stages of cough include maximal inspiration, closure of the glottis, increased intraabdominal pressure, opening of the glottis, and forced expiration.

Cystic fibrosis: an inherited disorder of the exocrine glands, causing those glands to produce abnormally thick secretions of mucus, elevation of sweat electrolytes, increased organic and enzymatic constituents of saliva, and overactivity of the autonomic nervous system. The glands most affected are those in the pancreas, the respiratory system, and the sweat glands. Because there is no known cure, treatment is directed at the prevention of respiratory infections, which are the most frequent cause of death. Mucolytic agents and bronchodilators are used to help liquefy the thick, tenacious mucus. Physical therapy measures, such as exercise, postural drainage, and breathing exercises, can also dislodge secretions. Life expectancy in cystic fibrosis has improved markedly over the past several decades, and with early diagnosis and treatment, most patients can be expected to reach adulthood.

Dead space: the amount of lung in contact with ventilating gases but not in contact with pulmonary blood flow. Alveolar dead space refers to alveoli that are ventilated by the pulmonary circulation but are not perfused. The condition may exist when pulmonary circulation is obstructed, as by a thromboembolus. Anatomical dead space is an area in the trachea, bronchi, and air passages containing air that does not reach the alveoli during respiration. As a general rule the volume of air in the anatomical dead space in millimeters is approximately equal to the weight in pounds of the involved individual. Certain lung disorders, such as emphysema, increase the amount of anatomical dead space. Physiological dead space is an area in the respiratory system that includes the anatomical dead space together with the space in the alveoli occupied by air that does not contribute to the oxygen-carbon dioxide exchange.

Denervation of heart: the transplanted heart initially loses its innervation (i.e., it is denervated and relies on exogenous catecholamines for cardiac acceleration and deceleration).

Dependent patients: patients unable to help themselves.

Depolarization: the changes in ionic concentrations across muscle cell membranes leading to contraction of the cell.

Diabetes: a clinical condition characterized by the excessive excretion of urine. The excess may be caused by a deficiency of antidiuretic hormone (ADH), as in diabetes insipidus, or it may be the polyuria resulting from the hyperglycemia occurring in diabetes mellitus.

Diaphragmatic breathing pattern: involves teaching patients with COPD how to relax the accessory muscles and to perform controlled diaphragmatic breathing.

Diffusion: the process in which solid, particulate matter in a fluid moves from an area of higher concentration to an area of lower concentration, resulting in an even distribution of the particles in the fluid. No energy is required.

Documentation: written material associated with the history, the compilation of laboratory reports and investigations, and the results of the clinical assessment.

Dyspnea: the sensation of difficulty in breathing.

ECG monitoring: electrocardiographic monitoring involving electrode placement on the chest wall and on the limbs for a 12-lead ECG; such monitoring provides a tracing of the electrical activity of the heart.

Echocardiography: evaluation of cardiac structure and function by using the properties of sound. Quantitative and qualitative measurements can be derived. The most common types include two-dimensional, Doppler, and transesophageal echoes.

Ejection fraction: a measure of myocardial function, it is the amount of ventricular volume ejected with each heart beat. Expressed as a percent, the ejection fraction = (end-diastolic volume – end-systolic volume) × 100 end-diastolic volume.

Electrocardiogram (ECG):   the tracing produced by the sequential depolarization and repolarization of myocardial cells as detected by surface electrodes placed on the skin.

Electromechanical coupling: the coupling of electrical and mechanical events of the heart to effect cardiac output.

EMG power spectrum: electromyography is the process of recording the electrical activity of muscle on a cathode-ray oscilloscope. The electromyographic (EMG) power spectrum is the full range of electrical activity of the muscle.

Emphysema: a lung condition characterized by an abnormal permanent enlargement of the air spaces distal to the terminal bronchioles, accompanied by destruction of their walls.

Endocardial cushion defect: any cardiac defect resulting from the failure of the endocardial cushions in the embryonic heart to fuse and form the atrial septum.

Endocrine function: the function of the endocrine glands responsible for normal physiological function.

Evidence-based practice: practice based on evidence from the physiologic and scientific literature.

Exercise: (1) The performance of any physical activity for the purpose of conditioning the body, improving health, or maintaining fitness or as a means of therapy for correcting a deformity or restoring the organs and bodily functions to a state of health. (2) Any action, skill, or maneuver that exerts the muscles and is performed repeatedly in order to develop or strengthen the body or any of its parts. (3) To use a muscle or part of the body in a repetitive way to maintain or develop its strength. The physical therapist constantly assesses the patient's needs and provides the proper type and amount of exercise, taking into account the patient's physical or mental limitations. Exercise has a beneficial effect on each of the body systems, although in excess it can lead to the breakdown of tissue and cause injury.

Exercise blood gases: blood gases taken before, during, and after exercise to determine the effect of exercise on oxygen transport.

Exercise stress: the physical stress imposed by movement (i.e., mobilization and exercise.)

Expiratory reserve volume (ERV):   the maximum volume of gas that can be expired from the resting expiratory level.

Extrinsic factors: factors related to the patient's care that contribute to cardiopulmonary dysfunction and impaired gas exchange.

Fluid and electrolyte status: the status of blood volume and distribution, and the status of electrolyte balance in the body; fluid balance often has a direct effect on electrolytes.

Forced expiratory volume in one second (FEV$_1$):   the amount of air expired in 1 second during a forced exhalation after a maximal inhalation.

Forced vital capacity (FVC):   the total amount of air exhaled during a forced exhalation after a maximal inhalation.

Functional residual capacity: the volume of gas in the lungs at the end of a normal expiration. The functional residual capacity is equal to the residual volume plus the expiratory reserve volume.

Function optimization: optimal functioning of the patient as a whole person based on optimal physiological functioning at an organ system level.

Gas exchange: the movement of oxygen and carbon dioxide between the pulmonary capillary blood and the alveolar tissue and between the systemic capillary blood and peripheral tissue cells.

Gastrointestinal dysfunction: abnormal function of the gastrointestinal system.

Gravitational stress: stress imposed on the human body by gravity and its physiological effects.

Gravity: the heaviness or weight of an object resulting from the universal effect of the attraction between any body of matter and any planetary body. The force of the attraction depends on the relative masses of the bodies and on the distance between them.

Head injury: any traumatic damage to the head resulting from blunt or penetrating trauma of the skull. Blood vessels, nerves, and meninges can be torn; bleeding, edema, and ischemia may result.

Health behavior: an action taken by a person to maintain, attain, or regain good health and to prevent illness. Health behavior reflects a person's health beliefs. Some common health behaviors are exercising regularly, eating a balanced diet, and obtaining necessary inoculations.

Heart: the muscular, cone-shaped organ, about the size of a clenched fist, that pumps blood throughout the body and beats normally about 70 times per minute by coordinated nerve impulses and muscular contractions. Enclosed in pericardium, the heart rests on the diaphragm between the lower borders of the lungs, occupying the middle of the mediastinum. The sinoatrial node of the heartbeat sets the rate. Other factors affecting the heartbeat are emotion, exercise, hormones, temperature, pain, and stress.

Heart-lung interdependence: the heart and lung are structurally and functionally interdependent and form a cardiopulmonary unit.

Hemiplegia: paralysis of one side of the body.

Hemodynamic status: status of the heart and its capacity to effect blood movement to perfuse the tissues of the body.

Hibernating myocardium: contractile dysfunction of the myocardium as a result of prolonged ischemia, appearing as a regional wall motion abnormality.

Home care: a health service provided in the patient's place of residence for the purposes of promoting, maintaining, or restoring health or minimizing the effects of illness and disability.

Humidity: pertaining to the level of moisture in the atmosphere, the amount varying with the temperature. The percentage is usually represented in terms of relative humidity, with 100% being the point of air saturation or the level at which the air can absorb no additional water.

Hyaline membrane disease: disease of the newborn, characterized by airless alveoli, inelastic lungs, more than 60 respirations a minute, nasal flaring, intercostal and subcostal retractions, grunting on expiration, and peripheral edema. The condition occurs most often in premature babies. The disease is self-limited; the infant dies in 3 to 5 days or completely recovers with no after-effects. Treatment includes measures to correct shock, acidosis, and hypoxemia and use of positive airway pressure to prevent alveolar collapse. This is also called *respiratory distress syndrome (RDS) of the newborn.*

Hypercapnia: the presence of an abnormally large amount of carbon dioxide in the circulating blood.

Hyperpnea: rapid shallow breathing.

Hypertension: a common, often asymptomatic disorder characterized by elevated blood pressure persistently exceeding 140/90 mm Hg. Patients with high blood pressure are advised to follow a low-sodium, low-saturated-fat diet, to reduce calories to control obesity, to exercise, to avoid stress, and to take adequate rest.

Hypoxemia: a low level of oxygen in the blood, often characterized by a Pao_2 of less than 80 mm Hg.

Immune function: function of the immunological system and its components in effecting optimal immunological protection.

Immunological dysfunction: abnormal function of the immunological system.

Immunosuppression: of or pertaining to a substance or procedure that lessens or prevents an immune response.

Inspiratory capacity (IC):   the maximum volume of gas that can be inhaled from the resting expiratory level. Equal to the sum of the tidal volume and the inspiratory reserve volume, it is measured with a spirometer.

Inspiratory muscle training: resistance ventilatory training designed to increase the strength and endurance of the inspiratory muscles.

Inspiratory resistance breathing: a method of respiratory muscle training that includes normal ventilation with added external threshold loading on inspiration consisting of 15 to 30 minutes of training 5 days per week. External loading is increased from 30% of maximal inspiratory pressure to 60% of maximal inspiratory pressure as patient's tolerance increases.

Inspiratory reserve volume: The maximum volume of gas that can be inspired from the end-tidal inspiratory level.

Intermittent positive pressure breathing (IPPB): a form of assistive or controlled respiration produced by a ventilatory apparatus in which compressed gas is delivered under positive pressure into the person's airways until a preset pressure is reached. Passive exhalation is allowed through a valve, and the cycle begins again as the flow of gas is triggered by inhalation. This is also called *intermittent positive pressure ventilation (IPPV)*.

Interstitial pulmonary fibrosis: a classification of restrictive lung disease including conditions that result in a final common pathway of bouts of chronic lung infection and irreversible fibrosis.

Intraaortic balloon counter pulsation: procedure for assisting left ventricular function and coronary perfusion involving the insertion of a balloon in the femoral artery. The inflation and deflation of the balloon is synchronized with the ECG such that it inflates during diastole and deflates during systole.

Intracardiac pressures: pressures within the chambers of the heart. Optimal movement of blood through the heart depends on pressure gradients throughout the heart. Normal pressures within each heart chamber are within a restricted range.

Intracranial pressure monitoring: invasive monitoring instituted to measure changes in cranial pressure usually resulting from increased volume of the brain because of injury, bleeding, fluid accumulation, or an intracranial mass.

Isocapnic hyperpnea: a method of respiratory muscle training that includes high ventilation with low external loading consisting of sustained periods of hyperpnea lasting 15 to 30 minutes daily for several weeks with the addition of carbon dioxide to maintain a normal level.

Jacobsen's progressive relaxation exercise: a technique involving contraction followed by relaxation to progressively relax muscle groups.

Kidneys: a pair of bean-shaped urinary organs in the dorsal part of the abdomen, one on each side of the vertebral column. The kidneys produce and eliminate urine through a complex filtration network and reabsorption system comprising more than 2 million nephrons. All the blood in the body passes through the kidneys about 20 times every hour but only about one fifth of the plasma is filtered by the nephrons during that period. The kidneys remove water as urine and return water that has been filtered to the blood plasma, thus helping to maintain the water balance of the body. Hormone, especially the antidiuretic hormone (ADH), produced by the pituitary gland, control the function of the kidneys in regulating the water content of the body.

Kyphoscoliosis: an abnormal condition characterized by an anteroposterior curvature and a lateral curvature of the spine. It occurs in children and adults and can be associated with cor pulmonale.

Late sequelae of poliomyelitis: the late effects of poliomyelitis that may occur in poliomyelitis survivors 30 to 35 years after onset. These effects include disproportionate fatigue, weakness, pain, reduced endurance, choking and swallowing problems, altered temperature sensitivity, and psychological problems.

Learning theory: a group of concepts and principles that attempts to explain the learning process. One concept, Guthrie's contiguous conditioning premise, postulates that each response becomes permanently linked with stimuli present at the time so that contiguity rather than reinforcement is a part of the learning process.

Liver: the largest gland of the body and one of its most complex organs. More than 500 of its functions have been identified. It is divided into four lobes, contains as many as 100,000 lobules, and is served by two distinct blood supplies. Some of the major functions performed by the liver are the production of bile by hepatic cells, the secretion of glucose, proteins, vitamins, fats, and most of the other compounds used by the body, the processing of hemoglobin for vital use of its iron content, and the conversion of poisonous ammonia to area.

Lung cancer: a pulmonary malignancy attributable to cigarette smoking in 50% of cases. Lung cancer develops most often in scarred or chronically diseased lungs and is usually far advanced when detected, because metastases may precede the detection of the primary lesion in the lung. Symptoms of lung cancer include persistent cough, dyspnea, purulent or blood-streaked sputum, chest pain, and repeated attacks of bronchitis or pneumonia. Surgery is the most effective treatment, but only one half of cases are operable at the time of diagnosis and of these 50% are not resectable. Thoracotomy is contraindicated if metastases are found in contralateral or scalene lymph nodes. Irradiation is used to treat localized lesions and unresectable intrathoracic tumors and as palliative therapy for metastatic lesions. Radiotherapy may also be administered after surgery to destroy remaining tumor cells and may be combined with chemotherapy.

Lung capacities: lung volumes that consist of two or more of the four primary nonoverlapping volumes. Functional residual capacity is the sum of residual volume and expiratory reserve volume. Inspiratory capacity is the sum of the tidal volume and inspiratory reserve volume. Vital capacity is the sum of the expiratory reserve volume, the tidal volume, and the inspiratory reserve volume. Total lung capacity, at the end of maximal inspiration, is the sum of the functional residual capacity and the inspiratory capacity.

Lung compliance: the volume change per unit of pressure change in the lungs.

Lungs: a pair of light, spongy organs in the thorax, constituting the main component of the respiratory system. The two highly elastic lungs are the main mechanisms in the body for inspiring air from which oxygen is extracted for the arterial blood system and for exhaling carbon dioxide dispersed from the venous system.

Lung volume: the volume of the lungs that may be compartmentalized into component volumes and capacities.

Malnutrition: any disorder of nutrition. It may result from an unbalanced, insufficient, or excessive diet or from the impaired absorption, assimilation, or use of foods.

Managed care: a health care system in which there is administrative control over primary health care services in a medical group practice. Redundant facilities and services are eliminated and costs are reduced. Health education and preventive medicine are emphasized. Patients may pay a flat fee for basic family care but may be charged additional fees for secondary care services of specialists.

Measurement: the determination, expressed numerically, of the extent or quantity of a substance, energy, or time.

Mechanical ventilation: the use of artificial mechanical means to support ventilation.

Metabolic demand: the energy and oxygen demands of the body required to support metabolism.

Metabolical demand fluctuates depending on the activity level of the individual, the presence of illness and increased temperature, and the requirements of healing and repair.

Method: a technique or procedure for producing a desired effect, such as a surgical procedure, a laboratory test, or a diagnostic technique.

Minute ventilation (VE): the amount of air inspired in 1 minute. It is the product of tidal volume and respiratory rate.

Minute ventilation: the total expired volume of air per minute.

Mobilization: the therapeutic and prescriptive application of low-intensity exercise in the management of cardiopulmonary dysfunction usually in acutely ill patients. The primary goal of mobilization is to exploit the acute effects of exercise to optimize oxygen transport.

Morbid obesity: an excess of body fat that threatens normal body functions, such as respiration.

Mucous blanket: the normal layer of mucous lining the bronchopulmonary tree. This blanket provides a medium through which foreign material and bacteria can be wafted centrally by the cilia for eventual removal by coughing or swallowing.

Multiple sclerosis (MS): a progressive disease characterized by disseminated demyelination of nerve fibers of the brain and spinal cord. It begins slowly, usually in young adulthood, and continues throughout life with periods of exacerbation and remission. As the disease progresses, the intervals between exacerbations grow shorter and disability becomes greater. There is no specific treatment for the disease; corticosteroids and other drugs are used to treat the symptoms accompanying acute episodes. Physical therapy may help to postpone or prevent specific disabilities. The patient is encouraged to live as normal and active a life as possible.

Multisystem assessment: the assessment of multiple organ systems based on clinical examination and investigative laboratory reports. Such assessment helps identify all factors that contribute to deficits in oxygen transport.

Muscle endurance: the ability to sustain repetitive contraction against a given load.

Muscle strength: the maximum force that a muscle can develop with maximal stimulation.

Muscular dystrophy (MD): a group of genetically transmitted diseases characterized by progressive atrophy of symmetrical groups of skeletal muscles without evidence of involvement or degeneration of neural tissue. In all forms of muscular dystrophy, there is an insidious loss of strength with increasing disability and deformity, although each type differs in the groups of muscles affected, the age of onset, the rate of progression, and the mode of genetic inheritance. The basic cause is unknown but appears to be an inborn error of metabolism. Treatment of the muscular dystrophies consists primarily of supportive measures, such as physical therapy and orthopedic procedures to minimize deformity.

Myocardial infarction: necrosis of a portion of cardiac muscle caused by obstruction in a coronary artery from either atherosclerosis or an embolus. Also called a heart attack.

Needs assessment: assessment of the patient's specific physical, functional, and psychological needs.

Nocturnal ventilation: the selective use of mechanical ventilation during the night. Patients with cardiopulmonary dysfunction are at greater risk during the night when they are recumbent and the respiratory drive is depressed.

Obesity: an abnormal increase in the proportion of fat cells, mainly in the viscera and subcutaneous tissues of the body. Obesity may be exogenous or endogenous. Hyperplastic obesity is caused by an increase in the number of fat cells in the increased adipose tissue mass. Hypertrophic obesity results from an increase in the size of the fat cells in the increase adipose tissue mass.

Objective: (1) A goal. (2) Of or pertaining to a phenomenon or clinical finding that is observed; not subjective. An objective finding is often described in health care as a sign, as distinguished from a symptom, which is a subjective finding.

Obstructive lung disease: a classification of lung disease referring to airflow limitation secondary to obstruction and increased airway resistance (e.g., chronic bronchitis and emphysema).

Osteoporosis: a disorder characterized by abnormal rarefaction of bone, occurring most frequently in postmenopausal women, in sedentary or immobilized individuals, and in patients on long-term steroid therapy. The disorder may cause pain, especially in the lower back, pathological fractures, loss of stature, and various deformities.

Outpatient: a patient, not hospitalized, who is being treated in an office, clinic, or other ambulatory care facility.

Oxygen (O_2):   a tasteless, odorless, colorless gas essential for human respiration.

Oxygen consumption (Vo_2):   the difference between oxygen that is inspired and the amount of oxygen exhaled. The difference between inspired and expired oxygen is a primary measure of aerobic fitness.

Oxygen delivery (Do_2):   the delivery of oxygen to the tissues of the body, an essential component of oxygen transport.

Oxygen desaturation: the desaturation of oxygen from the hemoglobin molecule in the blood in response to a reduction of tissue oxygen levels.

Oxygen transport: the process by which oxygen is absorbed in the lungs by the hemoglobin in circulating deoxygenated red cells and carried to the peripheral tissues. The process is made possible because hemoglobin has the ability to combine with oxygen present at a high concentration, such as in the lungs, and to release this oxygen when the concentration is low, such as in the peripheral tissues.

Oxygen transport pathway: the pathway for oxygen delivery to the tissues from the ambient air, through the airways and lungs, across the alveolar capillary membrane, into the pulmonary circulation through the chambers of the heart, via the peripheral and regional circulation to the tissues and the mitochondria where oxygen is used in cellular respiration.

Oxygen saturation: a measurement of the amount of oxygen attached to a hemoglobin molecule.

Oxyhemoglobin dissociation: the dissociation of oxygen from the hemoglobin molecule in peripheral tissues when the concentration of oxygen is low.

Parenchyma: the tissue of an organ as distinguished from supporting or connective tissue.

Parkinson's disease: a slowly progressive, degenerative, neurological disorder characterized by resting tremor, pill rolling of the fingers, a masklike expression, shuffling gait, forward flexion of the trunk, loss of postural reflexes, and muscle rigidity and weakness. It is usually an idiopathic disease of people over 60 years of age, although it may occur in younger people, especially after acute encephalitis or carbon monoxide or metallic poisoning, particularly by reserpine or phenothiazine drugs.

Partial pressure of gases: the pressure exerted by an individual gas, a percent of the total pressure of gases.

Patent ductus arteriosus (PDA):   an abnormal opening between the pulmonary artery and the aorta caused by failure of the fetal ductus arteriosus to close after birth. The defect, which is seen primarily in premature infants, allows blood from the aorta to flow into the pulmonary artery and to recirculate through the lungs, where it is reoxygenated and returned to the left atrium and left ventricle, causing an increased workload on the left side of the heart and increased pulmonary vascular congestion and resistance.

Pediatric cardiac rehabilitation: specialized cardiac rehabilitation for children instituted in the chronic stage of heart disease or after cardiovascular surgery when the patient is through the acute phase.

Pediatric pulmonary rehabilitation: specialized pulmonary rehabilitation for children instituted in the subacute or chronic stages of lung disease or after thoracic surgery when the patient is through the acute phase.

Perfusion: the passage of a fluid through a specific organ or an area of the body.

Perioperative complications: complications before, during, and after surgery.

Peripheral circulation: the systemic circulation, which excludes the circulation to the heart and lungs (the central circulation).

Peripheral vascular disease: any abnormal condition that affects the blood vessels outside the heart and the lymphatic vessels.

Pneumonia: an acute inflammation of the lungs, usually caused by inhaled pneumococci of the species *Streptococcus pneumoniae*. The alveoli and bronchioles of the lungs become plugged with a fibrous exudate. Pneumonia may be caused by other bacteria, as well as by viruses, rickettsiae, and fungi.

Positron emission scans: tomographic scans using positron emitting radionuclides. The tracers used are often taken up in the metabolical pathways of the tissues being studied (e.g., oxygen metabolism or glucose metabolism).

Prescription: an order for medication, therapy, or a therapeutic device given by a properly authorized person to a person properly authorized to dispense or perform the order. A prescription is usually in written form and includes the name and address of the patient, the date, the [4]+ symbol (superscription), the medication prescribed (inscription), directions to the pharmacist or other dispenser (subscription), directions to the patient that must appear on the label, the prescriber's signature, and, in some instances, an identifying number.

Prevention: any action directed toward preventing illness and promoting health to avoid the need for secondary or tertiary health care.

Primary cardiopulmonary dysfunction: cardiopulmonary dysfunction resulting from a primary condition of the heart, lungs, or both.

Pulmonary rehabilitation: rehabilitation of cardiopulmonary dysfunction including the acute, subacute, and chronic phases of the disease or after thoracic surgery. The long-term management includes a comprehensive program of exercise, ventilatory support, additional airway clearance interventions as needed, nutrition, stress reduction, smoking cessation, pacing and energy conservation, vocational rehabilitation, sexual rehabilitation, and education.

Pulmonary development: the anatomical and physiological development of the cardiopulmonary system during normal growth and development.

Pulmonary circulation: the blood flow through a network of vessels between the heart and the lungs for the oxygenation of blood and removal of carbon dioxide.

Quality care: the provision of holistic care in which the needs and wants of the patient are considered.

Recumbency: the state of lying down or leaning against something.

Reflex cough: a cough stimulated reflexively.

Reliability: the extent to which a test measurement or a device produces the same results with different investigators, observers, or administration of the test over time. If repeated use of the same measurement tool on the same sample produces the same consistent results, the measurement is considered reliable.

Residual volume: the volume of air remaining in the lung after a maximal expiration.

Resources: services, personnel, and treatment options that can be drawn on to maximize treatment delivery and effectiveness.

Respiratory muscle fatigue: a loss in the capacity of a muscle underload to develop force or velocity that is reversible by rest.

Respiratory muscles: the muscles that produce volume changes of the thorax during breathing. The inspiratory muscles include the hemidiaphragms, external intercostals, scaleni, sternomastoids, trapezius, pectoralis major, pectoralis minor, subclavius, latissimus dorsi, serratus anterior, and muscles that extend the back. The expiratory muscles are the external intercostals, abdominals, and the muscles that flex the back.

Respiratory muscle weakness: a chronic loss in the capacity of a rested muscle to generate force.

Respiratory mechanics: the physical properties of the lung including resistance and compliance characteristics.

Respiratory failure: the inability of the cardiac and pulmonary systems to maintain an adequate exchange of oxygen and carbon dioxide in the lungs. Respiratory failure may be oxygenation or hypercapniac. Treatment of respiratory failure includes maximizing ventilation, clearing the airways by suction, bronchodilators, or tracheostomy, antibiotics for infections usually present, anticoagulants for pulmonary thromboemboli, and electrolyte replacement in fluid imbalance. Oxygen may be administered in some cases; in others it may further decrease the respiratory reflex by removing the stimulus of a decreased elevated level of oxygen.

Restrictive lung disease: a category of lung disease involving restriction of the lung parenchyma and characterized by stiffness (reduced compliance) and reduced lung volume.

Rheumatoid arthritis: a chronic, destructive, sometimes deforming collagen disease that has an autoimmune component. Rheumatoid arthritis is characterized by symmetric inflammation of the synovium and increased synovial exudate, leading to thickening of the synovium and swelling of the joint. Rheumatoid arthritis usually first appears in early middle age, between 36 and 50 years of age, and most commonly in women. The course of the disease is variable but is frequently marked by remissions and exacerbation.

Risk factors: factors that cause a person or a group of people to be particularly vulnerable to an unwanted, unpleasant, or unhealthful event, such as immunosuppression, which increases the incidence and severity of infection, or cigarette smoking, which increases the risk of developing a respiratory or cardiovascular disease.

Routine body positioning: the routine use of body positioning in the management of patients to minimize the negative effects of static positioning and maximize comfort. The purposes of routine body positioning are distinct from the specific goals of prescriptive body positioning, which are related to optimizing particular components of cardiopulmonary function and gas exchange.

Scleroderma: a relatively rare autoimmune disease affecting the blood vessels and connective tissue. The disease is characterized by fibrous degeneration of the connective tissue of the skin, lungs, and internal organs, especially the esophagus, digestive tract, and kidneys. Scleroderma is most common in middle-aged women.

Secretion management: management of airway secretions.

Sedation: an induced state of quiet, calmness, or sleep, as by means of a sedative or hypnotic medication.

Sepsis and multiorgan system failure: overwhelming systemic infection and pathogens leading to failure within multiple organ systems.

Shock: an abnormal condition of inadequate blood flow to the body s peripheral tissues, with life-threatening cellular dysfunction, hypotension, and oliguria. The condition is usually associated with inadequate cardiac output, changes in peripheral blood flow resistance and distribution, and tissue damage. Causal factors include hemorrhage, vomiting, diarrhea, inadequate fluid intake, or excessive renal loss, resulting in hypovolemia.

Skilled nursing and rehabilitation facilities: an institution or part of an institution that meets criteria for accreditation established by the sections of the Social Security Act that determine the basis for Medicaid and Medicare reimbursement for skilled nursing care, including rehabilitation and various medical and nursing procedures.

Spinal cord injury: any one of the traumatic disruptions of the spinal cord, often associated with extensive musculoskeletal involvement. Common spinal cord injuries are vertebral fractures and dislocations, such as those commonly suffered by individuals involved in car accidents, airplane crashes, or other violent impacts. Such trauma may cause varying degrees of paraplegia and quadriplegia. Treatment of spinal cord injuries varies considerably and involves numerous approaches, such as exercise, ambulatory techniques, and special physical and psychological therapy.

Stable angina: anginal pain that is well-controlled, medically stable, and has a predictable activity/exercise threshold.

Status asthmaticus: an acute, severe, and prolonged asthma attack. Hypoxia, cyanosis, and unconsciousness may follow. Treatment includes bronchodilators given intravenously or by aerosol inhalation, corticosteroids, controlled positive pressure ventilation, sedation, frequent therapy, and emotional support. A bronchodilator may be given by aerosol inhalation from a ventilator.

Stroke volume (SV):   the amount of blood ejected from the ventricles during systole.

Stunned myocardium: contractile dysfunction of the myocardium as a result of an acute episode of ischemia that persists even after perfusion has returned to normal.

Subacute hospitals: hospitals that specialize in the management of nonacute conditions.

Subjective: (1) Pertaining to the essential nature of an object as perceived in the mind rather than to a thing in itself. (2) Existing only in the mind. (3) That which arises within or is perceived by the individual, as contrasted with something that is modified by external circumstances or something that may be evaluated by objective standards.

Suctioning: the use of mechanical airway suctioning that uses a catheter and negative pressure to remove oropharyngeal or airway secretions when the patient is unable to spontaneously or voluntarily take deep breaths and cough effectively.

Supraventricular: pertaining to a feature or event occurring superior to the ventricles of the heart.

Surgery: the branch of medicine concerned with diseases and trauma requiring operative procedures.

Syncytium: the arrangement of cells, as in the myocardium, such that stimulation of one cell causes stimulation of adjacent cells, thus causing an action potential to spread from the initial focus.

Systemic disease: dysfunction or condition affecting one or more systems.

Systemic lupus erythematosus (SLE):   a chronic inflammatory disease affecting many systems of the body. The pathophysiology of the disease includes severe vasculitis, renal involvement, and lesions of the skin and nervous system. The primary cause of the disease has not been determined; viral infection or dysfunction of the immune system has been suggested. Adverse reaction to certain drugs also may cause a lupus like syndrome. SLE occurs four times more often in women than in men.

Tachycardia: an abnormally rapid heart rate.

Tachypnea: an increased respiratory rate over 20 breaths per minute.

Thallium-201 scan: a radionuclide scan that evaluates myocardial perfusion. The tracer is taken up in the myocardium based on perfusion of the area. This agent can be used for rest studies, exercise stress studies, and pharmacological stress studies.

Thoracic cavity: the cavity enclosed by the ribs, the thoracic portion of the vertebral column, the sternum, the diaphragm, and associated muscles.

Thoracic surgery: the branch of medicine that deals with disease and injuries of the thoracic area by manipulative and operative methods.

Throat clearing: the spontaneous elicitation of a coughlike maneuver to clear secretions or an obstruction from the oropharynx that may be threatening the upper airway.

Tidal volume (TV):   the amount of air inhaled and exhaled during normal ventilation. Inspiratory reserve volume, expiratory reserve volume, and tidal volume make up vital capacity.

Total lung capacity (TLC):   the volume of gas in the lungs at the end of a maximum inspiration. It equals the vital capacity plus the residual capacity.

Tracheobronchial tree (TBT):   an anatomic complex that includes the trachea, the bronchi, and the bronchial tubes. It conveys air to and from the lungs.

Tracheostomy: an opening through the neck into the trachea through which an indwelling tube may be inserted.

Tracheostomy tube/cuff: a tube/cuff that is positioned directly through the trachea in the neck to provide a functioning airway that bypasses the nares and oropharynx.

Transitional care units: settings that specialize in providing care between the acute, subacute, and long-term stages of a patient's illness.

Transitional circulation: a transition from one type of blood vessel to another on moving peripherally through the circulation.

Treatment selection and prioritization: the process of selecting treatments and then prioritizing the order in which these treatments are administered. This process is based on the relative contribution of the pathogenesis that each treatment addresses with respect to oxygen transport deficiencies.

Trunk-ventilation interaction: the interrelationship of the shape and movement of the trunk or chest wall on alveolar ventilation. Trunk and ventilation interaction depends on body positioning and movement.

Tuberculosis: a chromic granulomatous infection caused by an acid-fast bacillus, mycobacterium tuberculosis, generally transmitted by the inhalation or ingestion of infected droplets and usually affecting the lungs, although infection of multiple organ systems occurs.

Type I fibers: a type of skeletal muscle fiber that is also called slow-twitch and is suitable for sustained tonic activity (e.g., the maintenance of posture or breathing, which require resistance to fatigue).

Type IIA fibers: a type of skeletal muscle fiber that is also called fast-twitch; this type of fiber is used for short-term, fast, powerful activity in which endurance to fatigue is not required.

Validity: the extent to which a test measurement or other kind of device measures what it is intended to measure.

Valvular heart disease: an acquired or congenital disorder of a cardiac valve, characterized by stenosis and obstructed blood flow or by valvular degeneration and regurgitation of blood.

Ventilation: the process by which gases are moved into and out of the lungs.

Ventilatory strategies: teaching patients to control breathing with the utilization of ventilatory patterns (e.g., combining inspiration with trunk extension and exhalation with trunk flexion).

Ventilation-perfusion scan: two scans which are used to assess patients for the presence of pulmonary emboli. Criteria (BIELLO or PIOPED) are used to determine if matched defects present with high, intermediate, or low probability of pulmonary embolus.

Ventilation and perfusion matching: the matching of ventilation and perfusion in the lungs. Optimal ventilation and perfusion matching occurs in the mid zones of the upright lung where the ratio is 0.8 to 1.0.

Vital capacity (VC):   a measurement of the amount of air that can be expelled at the normal rate of exhalation after a maximum inspiration, representing the greatest possible breathing capacity. The vital capacity equals the inspiratory reserve volume plus the tidal volume plus the expiratory reserve volume. The average normal values of 4000 to 5000 ml are affected by age, physical dimensions of the chest cage, posture, and gender. The vital capacity may be reduced by a decrease in functioning lung tissue, resulting from atelectasis, edema, fibrosis, pneumonia, pulmonary resection, or tumors; by limited chest expansion, resulting from ascites, chest deformity neuromuscular disease, pneumothorax, or pregnancy; or by airway obstruction.

Work of breathing: the total amount of effort required to expand and contract the lungs; the physiological "cost" of breathing. Generally, quiet breathing consumes 2% to 3% of the oxygen consumption and requires 10% of the vital capacity. If a greater amount is used, one would say the work of breathing is increased.